Practitioner's Guide to
Evidence-Based Psychotherapy

Practitioner's Guide to Evidence-Based Psychotherapy

Edited By:

Jane E. Fisher
University of Nevada
Reno, NV

and

William T. O'Donohue
Nicholas Cummings Professor of Organized Behavioral
Healthcare Delivery
University of Nevada
Reno, NV

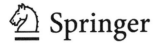 Springer

Jane E. Fisher
Dept. Psychology/298
University of Nevada, Reno, NV, USA
Reno 89557-0062
fisher@unr.edu

William T. O'Donohue
Dept. Psychology/298
University of Nevada, Reno, NV, USA
Reno 89557-0062
wto@unr.edu

Library of Congress Control Number: 2005936798

ISBN-10: 0-387-28369-2   e-ISBN 0-387-28370-6   Printed on acid-free paper.
ISBN-13: 978-0387-28369-2

Printed in the United States of America.   (SPI/SBA)

9 8 7 6 5 4 3 2 1

springer.com

Contents

Introduction: Clinician's Handbook of Evidence-Based Practice Guidelines: The Role of Practice Guidelines in Systematic Quality Improvement

William T. O'Donohue • Jane E. Fisher

In this chapter we will: (1) argue that clinical practice is difficult. Consistently delivering high quality treatments is very demanding; (2) discuss some of the major problems associated with quality clinical practice as well as place these problems in the context of similar problems with general healthcare delivery in the United States; (3) argue that although the exact quality of contemporary behavioral healthcare is unknown—including a detailed understanding of areas of improvement or of excellence—there is evidence to suggest that it is problematic; (4) argue that systematic and thoroughgoing adoption of quality improvement strategies and techniques is the major solution. This solution focuses on systems and common causes of undesirable variation (Walton, 1986) within systems instead of auditing or policing systems to detect and punish "bad apple" individuals. This quality improvement orientation and practice has had tremendous benefits in many industries (consumer electronics, retailing, auto industry) but behavioral healthcare has been very slow, at best, to adopt these practices; and (5) argue that practice guidelines—the focus of this book—are an important component of quality improvement systems but, in themselves, are not meant to be either a panacea for problems of quality or exempt from these quality improvement processes.

In addition, we will argue for the following conclusions which we anticipate will be somewhat controversial:

- That too much discussion that pertains to quality practice has been oriented toward the role of science in clinical practice (see O'Donohue and Lilienfeld, in press). This abstract discussion is interesting and important but it has in all likelihood had all the beneficial effects on participants that it likely to have. Some of the problem may be that this level is too abstract as it raises philosophical questions about what is science, what are the limits of science when applied to human behavior, and what some research literature actually implies for practice. Instead we will argue more focus should be placed on the implementation of sound quality improvement systems which can refine any starting point, including both science-based and non-science-based points, to more common end points (see for example McFall, 1991).
- That much of the controversy over practice guidelines and evidence-based practice has assumed a static model in which, for example, the practice guideline with all its inadequacies constrains clinical practice for some prolonged period. Instead within a quality improvement system, errors and limitation in the practice guideline are continually searched for and improvements, both big and small, are constantly sought. Thus, over time—and the organizations or individuals that are better at quality improvement have a competititive advantage in an increasingly difficult

O'Donohue, W. T. & Fisher, J. E. (2006). Clinician's Hand book of evidence-based practice guidelines: The role of practice guidelines in systematic quality improvement. In J. E. Fisher & W. T. O'Donahue (Eds.), *Practioner's guide to evidence-based psychotherapy*. New York: Springer.

marketplace—these should converge on a practice that more clearly meets specifications and exceeds customers' expectations.

- That a quality improvement system should consist of an overall philosophy (see below for a primer); as well as a practice technology which includes management understanding and buy in; accurately understanding customers' expectations and dissatisfactions; continuing education for quality for all members of the organization; designation of quality indicators; useful information technology; learning loops, transparent report cards; etc. More education is needed for management, academics, managed care personnel, and practitioners on quality improvement.

Currently, some of the key components of best practices in healthcare delivery consist of:

1. basic education in quality improvement philosophy and practices for all members of an organization
2. technologies to understand consumers' expectation, needs, desires, and dissatisfactions
3. understanding the processes in the organization that affect outcome. The focus is in improving processes through "profound knowledge" of these rather than on detecting "bad apple" individuals
4. designations of quality indicators such as patient satisfaction, clinical change, safety, improved functioning, cost impact, among others
5. reliable and affordable, information systems that capture quality indicators
6. evidence-based practice guidelines that are continually improved. Learning trials are used to provide feedback that improves all components of the system
7. incentive systems for meeting or exceeding quality goals as well as for rewarding suggestions that work
8. benchmarking to compare to national averages, ideals, competitors, etc
9. transparent report cards so that purchasers, among others, can be educated on the quality of the services provided

- In addition, we argue that there should be an ethical mandate that all behavioral health practice be delivered in a context of a sound quality improvement system. To be specific: the American Psychological Association should change its Ethical Code. The new principle should state that: "All psychological services should only be offered in the context of a meaningful quality improvement system". "By meaningful quality improvement system", we mean a system which has transparent report cards, benchmarking, continuing education around QI, etc.

QUALITY CLINICAL PRACTICE CAN BE DIFFICULT

Clinical practice is difficult. It can be difficult to accurately understand what the client's problems are. It can be difficult to construct an effective and efficient treatment plan that is evidenced-based. It can be difficult to keep the client motivated to continue in treatment. Ensuring that the client has been provided adequate informed consent also can be challenging. Helping the client not relapse presents additional challenges. In addition, managing all the logistics of therapy: the precertfications, submitting claims, answering questions, keeping notes, updating credentials, and scheduling can present further challenges. Finally, using the diverse amounts of information available that bears on all of these—particularly on evidence-based practice– can be impossible or impractical for individual practitioners as well as even systems of delivery.

Despite these difficulties we, as behavioral health providers, owe our clients excellence. They are in pain, and/or causing pain to others. Their problems may impede their functioning in important roles such as a parent, a spouse, or employee.

In addition, a failure to remedy a problem may cause further and even more serious problems. For example, a failure to successfully treat a substance abuse problem may result in divorce or serious traffic accidents, or physical morbidity resulting from the abuse. As humans we all want to pursue happiness and overcome obstacles to our goals and psychotherapy is, for many, the option they pursue to lessen pain and to increase their chance at happiness. There is often a lot on the line for clients and for this we owe them excellence.

Some practitioners handle the difficulties associated with psychotherapy better than others. Part of this may be due to differences in the quality of training, some to their values, some to their talent, some to the nature of the clients they see, some to their degree of energy v. burnout, and some to the kinds of support that they receive in their practice. However, the degree of variance in what is practiced and what outcome produced is currently enormous and this enormous variability is problematic for several reasons. Our ability to predict what diagnoses clients will receive is poor (Hamann, 1994). In addition, our ability to predict the treatment a client will receive for a given diagnosis is also very poor (Adelman, 1995). Finally, the ability to predict outcomes for a particular client—positive outcomes as well as negative outcomes (iatrogenic) is also poor. These are all serious problems as this lack of predictability means that practice has not been standardized but rather is a function of a variety of unknown variables and variables that do not positively contribute to better outcomes. Generally, consumers find this state of affairs very unsatisfactory; when one orders French fries at a restaurant one is dissatisfied if it takes two hours, if what comes is a baked potato, or if they fries are raw. Consumers want their purchases to be a good value, to be a predictable, and to be a high quality product that brings them high satisfaction. It appears that few consumers experience this now when they purchase psychotherapy.

Psychotherapy has an image problem but it also has a substantive problem underlying this image problem. Our image problem is derived from the fact that many people do not think psychotherapy is effective (Bremer et.al., 2001). Why might people believe this? There may be several reasons:

1. *Problems for which there are no known effective treatments.* For some clinical problems such as antisocial personality disorder (see Lilienfeld this volume) there are in fact currently no effective treatment. Thus, perception is correct for some problems.
2. *Complex comorbidity.* Some clients come with multiple problems and this complexity can make case formulations more difficult and decrease positive outcomes.
3. *Controversies in the evidence-base.* At times the literature is not clear or is controversial concerning the effectiveness or the relative effectiveness of some therapies, e.g., SSRIs for depression (Antonuccio, 1995).
4. *Treatment fidelity and competency.* Some therapists may say they practice a certain evidence-based treatment but actually do so with little competence or adherence to the protocol. Thus therapist competence and treatment fidelity can be a problem (O'Donohue, Fisher, & Hayes, 2003).
5. *Limited effectiveness of treatment.* Our most effective treatments do not work with a sizeable number of people.
6. *Cultural Issues.* Some protocols are not suitable for some clients, e.g., due to cultural influences (Duckworth, in press).
7. *Problematic treatment values and treatment.* Many therapists are not oriented toward evidence-based treatments but rather practice therapies they commit to for reasons other than their demonstrated effectiveness in controlled trials. These therapists may give clients failure experiences or be so off-putting in their presentation (e.g., rebirthing) that potential clients see the therapy as quackery. We unfortunately also see the professional community doing little to stop this malpractice (O'Donohue & Ferguson, 2003).

The problem is not that rebirthing that kills is sometimes practiced, but that rebirthing at all is practiced, given its total lack of evidence for its effectiveness.

8. *Lack of commitment to quality improvement in systems.* Most importantly therapists are not practicing in a system in which quality improvement systems are operating. Thus, they do not receive the support they need to make their practice better. It is our view that too much time has been spent debating very abstract issues such as those found in the philosophy of science and not enough time has been spent in developing and demonstrating practical quality improvement systems to be used in behavioral health services.

We believe that the last two problems are key and are in part this book was designed in part to address. We will discuss each of these in a bit more detail.

PSYCHORELIGIONS OR QUALITY HEALTHCARE?

The penultimate problem described above is of significant concern. There seems to be an acceptance of this "nearly anything goes" orientation within the profession, (sometimes hidden under the honorific "eclecticism"). As most allow a self-labeling of orientation or approach with little evidence asked or offered to ensure that this orientation is being faithfully implemented, it can even be the case that the practitioner who self labels that he or she is offering some particular therapy may not actually be doing this. It is difficult to accurately discern the exact extent of this problem. It may even be the case that a majority of mental health professionals adhere to a view that the therapists are free to choose those that they follow independent of evidence. Mental health professionals seem to believe that it is permissible for them to choose a treatment orientation for other reasons than the evidence for its effectiveness. There seems to be a cult of "psychoreligions" (Cummings, personal communication) rather than an orientation to providing therapies based on their demonstrated effectiveness. This view and tolerance for this view needs to end if we are to truly be a profession committed to quality services for our customers. O'Donohue & Henderson (2001) have argued that we as professionals have "epistemic duties"—roughly duties to have knowledge and practice within this expertise—to our clients and that they should be consistently upheld.

However, there has not been a systematic appraisal of the extent to which behavioral health practice is of high quality and is evidenced based. In general practitioners and systems of behavioral health delivery do not know:

1. how satisfied their various customers are (including areas of dissatisfaction)
2. the extent to which clients are being accurately diagnosed, including their major health risks are accurately identified and appropriately treated
3. the extent to which therapists are practicing interventions for which there is less evidence (particularly much less evidence) for effectiveness than some alternative treatment (see Lilienfeld & Lynn, 2003)
4. the extent to which interventions are harming clients
5. the extent to which therapists are using the "minimally intrusive interventions". A stepped care approach is most conducive to this ethic but rarely used. We have asked authors of the guidelines in this book to discuss several steps that vary in the level of intensity and intrusiveness
6. the extent to which consumers have been given high quality informed consent (including a valid description of all other major options, with the evidence for their effectiveness, probabilities of effects, negative effects, etc.)
7. the extent to which cost-effective therapies are prescribed

8. the extent to which preventative interventions are given appropriately
9. the extent to which a population's health is being adequately addressed. Access problems to typical services may make it difficult or impossible for certain clients to come to therapy. Thus, a question has to be, who am I not seeing that I should be and what can be done about this?

The final problem is that for reasons that are unclear the field has not embraced quality improvement philosophies and practices (Walton, 1986). This is despite the fact that such clear improvements have resulted in many of the industries that mental health professionals have direct experience with, e.g., the auto industry, retail industry, food industry, etc. What can be done about this problem? First, *transportable systems* need to be developed to encourage evidence-based practice. Certainly there are barriers to evidenced based practice. Understanding and remaining current with the literature can be difficult. Clinicians as individual practitioners rarely have the time to analyze and sometimes even lack the access to this literature, particularly if they do not specialize. Moreover it is unnecessary for each clinician to collect, read, critique, and synthesize all the relevant literature for each problem. It seems much for efficient for this to be done once for them *in a system* dedicated to quality improvement and evidence-based practice. Part of the argument in this chapter is that the solo practice model has predominated much therapy and system design in our field, and that this model needs to be replaced by a systems model (even if the clinician has a private office) in which tools are given to the clinician that can result in quality improvement.

PROBLEMS IN THE AMERICAN HEALTHCARE SYSTEM

It is important to understand some of the context of these problems. There has been recent attention to the general problem of quality in healthcare practice although most of the focus has been on physical medicine. In December 1999, the Institute of Medicine (IOM) released a report estimating that 98,000 people die every year in the United States from medical mistakes made by health care professionals. More people die from medical errors than breast cancer, AIDS, or motor vehicle accidents. Leape (2004) showed that healthcare encounters result in higher rates of fatalities than mountain climbing, bungee jumping, and driving.

McGlynn and Shuster (1998) showed that only 50% of American patients received recommended preventative care. With acute illness only 70% received recommended treatment and that 30% received contraindicated treatments. With patients with chronic illnesses, 60% received recommended care while 20% received contraindicated treatments. The report also suggested that cost for these errors could be as high as $29 billion a year, and listed medical mistakes as the fifth leading cause of death in this country. The Institute of Medicine's second report concluded:

"Between the healthcare we have and the healthcare we could have lies not just a gap but a chasm."

Brent James, at Intermountain Health, has been one of the leaders in creatively applying and measuring the results of quality improvement practices to physical health. They have concentrated on analyzing processes, developing information management systems to track outcomes, providing incentives to key players, and administrative and clinical support integrated into the quality improvement efforts. The model involves dividing savings from improvements between the providers, the

TABLE 1.1 Fifty percent reduction in pneumonia costs. At Intermountain Health Care, the use of practice guidelines and protocols has reduced mortality rates, saved considerable amounts of money, shortened lengths of stay, and reduced medical complications.

Community-acquired pneumonia				
Both inpatient and outpatient care				
	1994 without guideline	*1995 with guideline*		
Percent patients admitted	39%	29%		
Average length of stay	6.4 days	4.3 days		
Time to antibiotic	2.1 hours	1.5 hours		
Average cost per case	$2,752	$1,424		
Inpatient care only				
	Without protocol	*With protocol*	*Percent change*	*P*
"Outlier" (complication) DRG at discharge	15.3%	11.6%	↓24.7	<0.001
In-hospital mortality	7.2%	5.3%	↓26.3	0.015
Relative resource units (RRUs) per case	55.9	49.0	↓12.3	<0.001
Cost per case	$5,211	$4,729	↓9.3	0.002

Source: Intermountain Health Care
http://www.managedcaremag.com/archives/0412/0412.james.html

healthcare organization, and the health plan. At Intermountain Health Care Services savings in overall costs from just a few dozen quality improvement projects have run into the tens of millions of dollars. An example is described in Table 1.1.

In 1996 the largest business coalition in the nation, the Pacific Business Group on Health, negotiated a contract with 13 of California's largest health plans that put $8 million in premium income at risk if the plans did not meet specific performance measure targets. Poor performance in the frequency of childhood immunization resulted in a $2 million refund for the employers on whose behalf the coalition had been negotiating.[9]

O'Donohue and Oser (2005) have attempted to address similar questions in mental health services. They have pointed out that there are several difficulties in even understanding the scope of the problem including:

1. no clear definition of what a "mental health error" is. This problem is partly due to a lack of consensus regarding treatment standards
2. little prior orientation to this sort of question in the field
3. a reliance on a "detect and punishment" strategy (i.e., the bad apple theory) which drives errors underground
4. a relativistic ethic in which all perspectives are held to have equal value
5. an idiographic view of case formulation in which few if any general principles are viewed as applying to the uniqueness of each case

WHAT IS EVIDENCED-BASED PRACTICE?

This is a more difficult question than it might seem. There are controversies concerning:

1. What counts as evidence? Do case studies count at all? Single subject experimental designs? "clinical experience?"

2. How should different types of evidence be weighed? How important are randomly controlled trials? What about quasi-experimental designs? How much weight should be given to simple pre–post designs, perhaps in the context in which the intervention has been shown to consistently beat a no treatment or placebo control?

3. What are the appropriate control conditions: no treatment, placebo treatment, treatment as usual, some combination of these, etc.? Is double blindness essential? Are there good measures of whether blinds have been penetrated?

4. How much does it matter if the analysis is done on a basis of intent to treat vs. treatment completers?

5. What are reasonable dependent variables and how should these be weighed? Client satisfaction, diagnostic change, change on a clinical measure, clinical significance, cost-effectiveness, or some combination of these, etc.?

6. What measurement periods ought to be included to assess possible relapse?

7. What is the relative weight of effectiveness (in more natural settings) vs. efficacy trials?

8. What if this patient does not meet the "caseness" assumed in the studies?

9. What are other design characteristics that are important, e.g., manualized therapy with adherence measures?, an explication and statement of process variables so that principles of therapy are elucidated?

10. How are therapy allegiance effects to be investigated? How many independent replications are needed in order to validly infer that the effect is reliable?

11. How much evidence is needed and of what kind in order for some therapy to receive the categorical designation of "evidence-based", empirically supported or something similar? In addition, can evidence be ordered to present a hierarchy of evidence for a set of therapies?

12. How is cost to be weighed in evidence-based practice? Cost should be considered not only in monetary terms but in the use of any resource expended in therapy (e.g., therapist or patient time). If therapy y has slightly more evidence for its effectiveness but costs 10x, and therapy z costs 1x, what ought to be the practice implications?

13. How well do potential negative effects of the therapy need to be measured in order to believe that one has thoroughly assessed these?

14. How important is social validity or consumer acceptability? Who are all the stakeholders and how is their satisfaction with treatment to be weighed?

15. What needs to be shown to demonstrate that the therapy is "culturally sensitive" (Duckworth, in press)?

16. How does one handle comorbidity or any other issue that may threaten the generalization of the evidence to the case at hand?

17. Is implementing an evidenced-based practice also a matter of skill? Can a practitioner be in the right ballpark at least conceptually, but deliver the intervention is such a manner that it falls outside of what is meant by evidenced-based practice?

18. What if anything in a particular case can override the evidence? Can patient preferences? What role do these factors play in treatment formulation?

19. If the clinical problem is a relatively large scale one (e.g., smoking, obesity, depression) how should the scalability and dissemination of the proposed therapy be weighed?

20. Is there service-delivery research showing how the evidenced based practice can be competently and satisfactorily delivered?

These are complex questions but ones that must be addressed if behavioral health is to move from a field with an enormous amount of variability in practice (process) and outcomes to a field in which practice and outcomes are made more predictable because they conform to a relatively restricted set of "best practice" options regarding key choice points.

It is fair to say that randomly controlled trials have had the most weight in developing recommendations in practice guidelines. Following this design nonrandomized controlled trials, cohort studies, single subject designs, uncontrolled descriptive studies and expert opinion have also influenced guideline development.

We argue here that these questions need to be considered and debated but the resolution of these abstract questions does not need to occur prior to practical progress in improving treatment delivery. These questions at times parallel the questions philosophers have proposed in epistemology concerning the exact nature of knowledge. The field of epistemology is still unsettled. However, most of us can proceed with our everyday tasks and affairs despite the fact that the philosophers have not agreed on what the general properties of knowledge are. We believe a similar condition exists in behavioral healthcare for reasons we shall argue below.

A Brief Review of Prior Work in Evidenced-Based Practice

A large question also is concerned with whether evidenced-based practice is the sole consideration in developing a treatment plan. For instance the Institute of Medicine (2001) report Crossing the Quality Chasm: A New Health System for the 21st century it states: "Evidence-based practice is the integration of the best research clinical expertise and patient values (p. 147). However this raises the questions of what exactly are "clinical expertise" and "patient values" and how do these relate to the "best research?" Regarding the former, questions arise such as:

1. How much total experience does a clinician need to have before their claims of "clinical experience" should be taken seriously?
2. How much experience with the particulars of the phenomena clinicians are opining about do they need before they are deemed to have the requisite "clinical experience."
3. What documentation should be presented to support 1 and 2 above?
4. Has a consensus developed from all individuals who meet 1–3 such that the claims are univocal? If not how are these competing claims to be resolved?

Interestingly another definition does not include these factors:

Evidence-based medicine is defined as `The conscientious, explicit and judicious use of current best evidence in making clinical decisions about the care of patients... (thereby) integrating individual clinical care with the best available clinical evidence from systematic review.'* (Eddy, 2001)

There have also been a variety of attempts to answer these questions in clinical psychology. One of the first was the so called "Chambless Report" in which the American Psychological Association Division 12 Task Force on Promotion and Dissemination of Psychological Procedures convened a diverse (on theoretical commitments) committee to both determine both standards for evidence-based treatments (what they initially called "empirically validated") and treatments that actually met these standards.

The Chambless report has been updated (Chambless et al., 1998) and it has been critiqued on several grounds. However, we believe that this is a step in the right direction as it attempts to define evidenced-based treatment as well as practically see these can be disseminated. However, other problems have been that these have not had a wide impact on how therapy is actually practiced. Few (or no) managed care companies have adopted these in their utilization review procedures. These therapies have not dominated or driven out other competing continuing education offerings. And these have not been integrated into systematic quality improvement practices (see below).

In physical medicine the evidenced-based practice movement has had a longer history and more effort has been expended upon it. There have been additional systematic reviews to define evidenced-based practice. The Cochrane Database has been established to review outcome studies and groups of experts in over 40 clinical subspecialties write reviews of the findings. These generally have focused on medical as opposed to psychological problems. These are also meant to be clinician friendly. An interesting website that compares some of the major reviews is http://www.aafp.org/fpm/20030700/ 49prac.html#box_a (see Table 1.2).

TABLE 1.2 A Comparison of Featured Sites Information included is based on descriptions from each resource's web site

	Clinical Evidence	DynaMed	InfoRetriever	PDxMD	UpToDate
Uses systematic searching[1]	X	X			
Uses systematic surveillance[2]	X	X			
Cites best available evidence where rigorous evidence is lacking[3]	X		X		
Provides guidance when there is no evidence	X	X[4]	X	X	
Provides ICD-9 codes	X	X	X		
Includes patient education materials		X	X	X	X
Number of topics[5]	211	1,796	1,036[4]	450+[6]	See note 7 below
Update frequency	Every 6 months in print; monthly online	Daily	Every 4 months; InfoPOEms added monthly online	Monthly	Every 4 months
Annual price[8]	$135[9]	$200[10]	$249	$149[11]	$495[12]
Other formats available	Print; desktop computer; Palm and Pocket PC personal digital assistants (PDAs)	Desktop computer	Desktop computer; PDA (Pocket PC and Palm)	Desktop computer; PDA (Palm and Pocket PC)	Desktop computer; PDA (Pocket PC only)

[1]Web site explicitly specifies which resources are searched for every topic summary.

[2]Web site explicitly describes a systematic process for reviewing and selecting new research reports.

[3]High likelihood of finding research citations when the best available evidence consists of less rigorous studies (e.g., retrospective cohort studies).

[4]Includes "Griffith's 5-Minute Clinical Consult," which is not evidence-based, and summaries of more than 250 treatment guidelines.

[5]Number of clinical topics, where one clinical topic is typically one disease summary, as of July/August 2003.

[6]Also contains more than 550 differential diagnosis lists.

[7]While UpToDate covers more than 6,000 topics, the number is not directly comparable, since one disease is typically listed as many different topics.

[8]Annual price for practicing physicians. For pricing for students, residents and groups, see Web site.

[9]Provided free to US physicians by the United Health Foundation.

[10]25% discount by using "MAFP" group access code (Colorado AFP members use "COAFP" code). Available at no cost to clinicians who participate through peer review, authoring or editing. See Web site for details.

[11]$40/year discount to AAFP members.

[12]Price is for first year; renewals are $395 annually.

Clinical Evidence Clinical Evidence (www.clinicalevidence.com) identifies important clinical questions and answers them by systematically searching for randomized controlled trials and then summarizing the best evidence. The initial literature search includes the Cochrane Library, MEDLINE and Embase.

Studies selected for inclusion are based on validated criteria, and information is summarized using a simple top-down approach, starting with a listing of interventions shown to be beneficial and followed by interventions shown to be harmful and interventions with uncertain effectiveness.

Clinical Evidence is published in print (two issues annually) and online and can also be used on a personal digital assistant (PDA). Several subscription packages are available. For example, an individual subscription to the full print edition including online access costs $135. A free trial subscription and a pay-per-view option are also available.

DynaMed DynaMed (www.dynamicmedical.com) systematically surveys original research reports, journal review services, systematic review sources (such as Clinical Evidence and the Cochrane Library), drug information sources and guideline collections as well as accompanying letters, editorials or review articles that may also be clinically useful, selecting information based on relevance and validity. Article summaries start with the "bottom line," followed by key methods, clinically relevant results and references linked to PubMed abstracts or to the full-text articles, if they are available free of charge online. DynaMed is designed for intuitive browsing; users can jump to a topic of interest (e.g., a disease name) and then click on the appropriate sections (e.g., diagnosis, prognosis or treatment). Individual article summaries are used to update the overall topic summary. DynaMed seeks to involve the health care community by offering users free subscriptions in return for agreeing to serve as peer reviewers and by encouraging users to submit comments online.

A key advantage of DynaMed is that it is updated daily, typically within days of publication of the original research. The annual subscription to DynaMed is $200 for a practicing health care professional, and access is also provided for health care professionals who assist with peer review. DynaMed is primarily used via the Internet, but a desktop version is available. A free 30-day trial is also offered.

InfoRetriever InfoRetriever (www.infopoems.com) is a search engine that allows the search of multiple databases, including InfoPOEms (concise evidence-based summaries selected for clinical relevance and validity from more than 100 journals), Cochrane Database abstracts, selected guidelines, clinical decision rules, diagnostic test calculators and the complete "Griffith's 5-Minute Clinical Consult." Information from these resources is cataloged according to clinical topic. To search InfoRetriever, enter a search term. InfoRetriever organizes multiple hits first by type of information (e.g., diagnosis, therapy or prognosis) and then by source database and levels of evidence.

A key advantage to InfoRetriever is that it includes clinical calculators, allowing interactive look-ups with numerically dependent data, such as calculating risks for specific diseases. A key disadvantage is the need to read multiple hits from different sources to synthesize the available evidence. A one-year subscription costs $249 and includes online access as well as InfoRetriever versions for the desktop computer and either Palm or Pocket PC PDAs. A free 30-day trial is also available.

PDxMD PDxMD (www.pdxmd.com) is designed for intuitive browsing. Topics are created using information from Cochrane Reviews, Clinical Evidence and the National Guideline Clearinghouse. References are hyperlinked to the home pages of these sites, making it easier to search for the relevant report or article. PDxMD also searches for information in reference books, journals, guidelines and position papers. Content is assessed and updated on a rolling basis, and certain updates (e.g., drug approvals or withdrawals) are posted immediately, if necessary.

A key advantage to PDxMD is its differential diagnosis section, which organizes potential conditions by age and prevalence within a signs-and-symptoms matrix. A key disadvantage is that it does not provide direct references for many assertions, except in the treatment section.

PDxMD may be downloaded to a PDA (Palm and Pocket PC) and a desktop version is also available. An annual subscription to PDxMD costs $149 for physicians. A free 30-day trial is also available.

UpToDate UpToDate (www.uptodate.com) is a collection of well-referenced reviews. Beginning as a specialty resource, it has grown considerably by identifying "the most eminent physicians" in multiple specialties. UpToDate is more valid than most textbooks because authors are asked to include evidence where there is any. The UpToDate site does not describe any systematic process for selecting the research included in the reviews, saying only "its guiding principle is whether the material being reviewed is well supported by data and would be useful in a clinical setting." Updates are made three times a year, and new information goes through a multi-level peer-review process. Although UpToDate presents reviews in a dense text format, using the left-hand navigation frame makes it easy to jump to the text section of interest.

A key advantage to UpToDate is that it contains specialty-focused information and includes multiple specialties. A key disadvantage is the lack of an explicit, systematic method for identifying and analyzing the relevant literature.

An individual subscription to UpToDate costs $495 for the first year (plus shipping and handling) and includes three CD releases per year as well as online access. Renewal rates are $395/year. A PDA version (for Pocket PCs only) and a free online demo are also available.

Free resources Although this article has focused on subscription-based clinical information resources, there are several free resources that may also be of interest (see Table 1.3).

It is important to note that there also has been some progress in physical medicine regarding how clinical trials should be reported. There is also some movement for psychology to learn from this as one of the major problems in judging what treatments have empirical support has been the variability and ambiguity in the ways clinical trials have been reported. There have been several attempts to make the reporting of clinical trials more uniform and more clear. CONSORT criteria have been proposed for the reporting on randomized clinical trials (RCTs). These criteria are reported in Table 1.4. Transparent Reporting of Evaluation with

TABLE 1.3 Free Clinical Resources

Web site	URL	Description	Comments
Turning Research Into Practice (TRIP)[1]	www.tripdatabase.com	Search engine covering many high-quality sources	Updated monthly
National Guideline Clearinghouse	www.guideline.gov	Summaries of nearly 1,100 guidelines	Updated weekly
Dr. Alper's links	www.myhq.com/ public/a/l/alper	Internet portal designed by the author with several hundred links organized primarily for patient care	Updated when improvements are identified

[1]TRIP+, an enhanced version with greater coverage and better features, is available by subscription

TABLE 1.4 Chambless Report Criteria

Criteria for empirically validated treatments

Well-Established Treatments

I. At least two good between group design experiments demonstrating efficacy in one or more of the following ways:
A. Superior (statistically significantly so) to pill or psychological placebo or to another treatment.
B. Equivalent to an already established treatment in experiments with adequate sample sizes.

OR

II. A large series of single case design experiments ($n > 9$) demonstrating efficacy. These experiments must have:
A. Used good experimental designs and
B. Compared the intervention to another treatment as in IA.

Further Criteria for Both I and II
III. Experiments must be conducted with treatment manuals.
IV. Characteristics of the client samples must be clearly specified.
V. Effects must have been demonstrated by at least two different investigators or investigating teams.

Probably Efficacious Treatments
I. Two experiments showing the treatment is superior (statistically significantly so) to a waiting-list control group.

OR

II. One or more experiments meeting the Well-Established Treatment Criteria IA or IB, III, and IV, but not V.

OR

III. A small series of single case design experiments ($n > 3$) otherwise meeting Well-Established Treatment

The treatments that met these standards included:

Examples of empirically validated treatments

Well-established treatments citation for efficacy evidence
Anxiety and stress
Cognitive behavior therapy for panic disorder Barlow et al. (1989)
with and without agoraphobia Clark et al. (1994)
Cognitive behavior therapy for Butler et al. (1991)
generalized anxiety disorder Borkovec et al. (1987)
Exposure treatment for agoraphobia Trull et al. (1988)
*Exposure/guided mastery for specific Bandura et al. (1969)
phobia Öst et al. (1991)
Exposure and response prevention for van Balkom et al. (1994)
obsessive-compulsive disorder
Stress Inoculation Training for Coping Saunders et al. (1996)
with Stressors

Depression
*Behavior therapy for depression Jacobson et al. (1996)
McLean & Hakstian (1979)

Volume 51, Number 1, Winter 1998 The Clinical Psychologist
Well-Established Treatments Citation for Efficacy Evidence
Cognitive therapy for depression Dobson (1989)
Interpersonal therapy for depression DiMascio et al. (1979)
Elkin et al. (1989)

Health problems
Behavior therapy for headache Blanchard et al. (1980)
Holroyd & Penzien (1990)
Cognitive-behavior therapy for bulimia Agras et al. (1989)

Thackwray et al. (1993)
*Multi-component cognitive-behavior therapy Keefe et al. (1990a,b) for pain associated with rheumatic disease Parker et al. (1988)
*Multi-component cognitive-behavior therapy Hill et al. (1993) with relapse prevention for smoking cessation Stevens & Hollis (1989)

Problems of Childhood
Behavior modification for enuresis Houts et al. (1994)
Parent training programs for Walter & Gilmore (1973) children with oppositional behavior Wells & Egan (1988)

Marital discord
Behavioral marital therapy Azrin et al. (1980a)
Jacobson & Follette (1985)

The Clinical Psychologist Volume 51, Number 1, Winter 1998
Probably Efficacious Treatments Citation for Efficacy Evidence

Anxiety
Applied relaxation for panic disorder Öst (1988)
Applied relaxation for generalized Barlow et al. (1992) anxiety disorder Borkovec & Costello (1993)
*Cognitive behavior therapy for Heimberg et al. (1990) social phobia Feske & Chambless (1995)
*Cognitive therapy for OCD van Oppen et al. (1995)
*Couples communication training adjunctive Arnow et al. (1985) to exposure for agoraphobia
*EMDR for civilian PTSD Rothbaum (in press)
Wilson et al. (1995)
Exposure treatment for PTSD Foa et al. (1991)
Keane et al. (1989)
*Exposure treatment for social phobia Feske & Chambless (1995)
Stress Inoculation Training for PTSD Foa et al. (1991)
Relapse prevention program for Hiss et al. (1994) obsessive-compulsive disorder
*Systematic desensitization for animal Kirsch et al. (1983) phobia Öst (1978)
*Systematic desensitization for public Paul (1967) speaking anxiety Woy & Efran (1972)
*Systematic desensitization for social anxiety Paul & Shannon (1966)

Chemical Abuse and dependence
Behavior therapy for cocaine abuse Higgins et al. (1993)
Brief dynamic therapy for Woody et al. (1990) opiate dependence

Volume 51, Number 1, Winter 1998 The Clinical Psychologist
Probably Efficacious Treatments Citation for Efficacy Evidence
*Cognitive-behavioral relapse prevention Carroll et al. (1994) therapy for cocaine dependence
Cognitive therapy for opiate dependence Carroll et al. (1994)
Cognitive-behavior therapy for benzodiazepine Otto et al. (1993) withdrawal in panic disorder patients Spiegel et al. (1994)
*Community Reinforcement Approach for Azrin (1976) alcohol dependence Hunt & Azrin (1973)
*Cue exposure adjunctive to inpatient Drummond & Glautier (1994) treatment for alcohol dependence
*Project CALM for mixed alcohol abuse and O'Farrell et al. (1985) dependence (behavioral marital therapy O'Farrell et al. (1992) plus disulfiram)
*Social skills training adjunctive to Eriksen et al. (1986) inpatient treatment for alcohol dependence

Depression
Brief dynamic therapy Gallagher-Thompson & Steffen (1994)
Cognitive therapy for geriatric patients Scogin & McElreath (1994)
Reminiscence therapy for geriatric patients Arean et al. (1993)
Scogin & McElreath (1994)
Self-control therapy Fuchs & Rehm (1977)
Rehm et al. (1979)
*Social problem-solving therapy Nezu (1986) Nezu & Perri (1989)

Health Problems
Behavior therapy for childhood obesity Epstein et al. (1994) Wheeler & Hess (1976)
*Cognitive-behavior therapy for binge eating Telch et al. (1990) disorder Wilfley et al. (1993)
*Cognitive-behavior therapy adjunctive to Nicholas et al. (1991) physical therapy for chronic pain

Continued

TABLE 1.4 (continued)

The Clinical Psychologist Volume 51, Number 1, Winter 1998
Probably Efficacious Treatments Citation for Efficacy Evidence
*Cognitive-behavior therapy for chronic Turner & Clancy (1988) low back pain
*EMG biofeedback for chronic pain Flor & Birbaumer (1993) Newton-John et al. (1995)
*Hypnosis as an adjunct to cognitive-behavior Bolocofsky et al. (1985) therapy for obesity*Interpersonal therapy for Wilfley et al. (1993) binge-eating disorder
*Interpersonal therapy for bulimia Fairburn et al. (1993)

*Multicomponent cognitive therapy for Lynch & Zamble (1989) irritable bowel syndrome Payne & Blanchard (1995)
*Multicomponent cognitive-behavior therapy Gil et al. (1996) for pain of sickle cell disease
*Multicomponent operant-behavioral therapy Turner & Clancy (1988) for chronic pain Turner et al. (1990)
*Scheduled, reduced smoking adjunctive to Cinciripini et al. (1994) multicomponent behavior therapy for smoking Cinciripini et al. (1995) cessation
*Thermal biofeedback for Raynaud's syndrome Freedman et al. (1983)
*Thermal biofeedback plus autogenic Blanchard et al. (1978) relaxation training for migraine Sargent et al. (1986)

Marital discord
*Emotionally focused couples therapy James (1991) for moderately distressed couples Johnson & Greenberg (1985)
Insight-oriented marital therapy Snyder et al. (1989, 1991)

Problems of childhood
Behavior modification of encopresis O'Brien et al. (1986)
*Cognitive-behavior therapy for Kendall (1994) anxious children (overanxious, Kendall et al. (1997) separation anxiety, and avoidant disorders)
*Exposure for simple phobia Menzies & Clarke (1993)
Family anxiety management training Barrett et al. (1996) for anxiety disorders

Volume 51, Number 1, Winter 1998 The Clinical Psychologist
Probably Efficacious Treatments Citation for Efficacy Evidence

Sexual dysfunction
*Hurlbert's combined treatment approach Hurlbert et al. (1993) for female hypoactive sexual desire
*Masters & Johnson's sex therapy for female Everaerd & Dekker (1981) orgasmic dysfunction
*Zimmer's combined sex and marital therapy Zimmer (1987) for female hypoactive sexual desire

Other
Behavior modification for sex offenders Marshall et al. (1991)
Dialectical behavior therapy for Linehan et al. (1991) borderline personality disorder
*Family intervention for schizophrenia Falloon et al. (1985)
Randolph et al. (1994)
Habit reversal and control techniques Azrin et al. (1980b)
Azrin et al. (1980c)
*Social skills training for improving Marder et al. (1996) social adjustment of schizophrenic patients
*Supported employment for severely Drake et al. (1996) mentally ill clients

Note: Studies cited for efficacy evidence are linked to specific treatment manuals or to procedures well described in the study's report. The operational definition of the treatment is to be found in those manuals; the labels used here do not suffice to identify the particular treatment judged to be efficacious.
* Indicates a treatment added or a recommendation altered since the publication of Chambless et al. (1996).
Two treatments have been deleted, not because of negative evidence, but because, unlike the other treatments, we do not have specific target problems identified yet for these approaches: token economy (target problem not specified) and behavior modification for people with developmental disabilities (target unspecified references).

TABLE 1.4 (continued) Checklist of items to include when reporting a randomized trial (56–58)

Paper section And topic	Item	Description	Reported on page #
Title & abstract	1	How participants were allocated to interventions (e.g., "random allocation," "randomized," or "randomly assigned")	
Introduction Background	2	Scientific background and explanation of rationale	
Methods Participants	3	Eligibility criteria for participants and the settings and locations where the data were collected	
Interventions	4	Precise details of the interventions intended for each group and how and when they were actually administered	
Objectives	5	Specific objectives and hypotheses	
Outcomes	6	Clearly defined primary and secondary outcome measures and, when applicable, any methods used to enhance the quality of measurements (e.g., multiple observations, training of assessors)	
Sample size	7	How sample size was determined and, when applicable, explanation of any interim analyses and stopping rules	
Randomization— sequence generation	8	Method used to generate the random allocation sequence, including details of any restriction (e.g., blocking, stratification)	
Randomization— allocation concealment	9	Method used to implement the random allocation sequence (e.g., numbered containers or central telephone), clarifying whether the sequence was concealed until interventions were assigned	
Randomization— Implementation	10	Who generated the allocation sequence, who enrolled participants, and who assigned participants to their groups	
Blinding (masking)	11	Whether or not participants, those administering the interventions, and those assessing the outcomes were blinded to group assignment. When relevant, how the success of blinding was evaluated	
Statistical methods	12	Statistical methods used to compare groups for primary outcome(s); Methods for additional analyses, such as subgroup analyses and adjusted analyses	
Results Participant flow	13	Flow of participants through each stage (a diagram is strongly recommended). Specifically, for each group report the numbers of participants randomly assigned, receiving intended treatment, completing the study protocol, and analyzed for the primary outcome. Describe protocol deviations from study as planned, together with reasons	
Recruitment	14	Dates defining the periods of recruitment and follow-up	
Baseline data	15	Baseline demographic and clinical characteristics of each group	
Numbers analyzed	16	Number of participants (denominator) in each group included in each analysis and whether the analysis was by "intention-to-treat". State the results in absolute numbers when feasible (e.g., 10/20, not 50%)	
Outcomes and estimation	17	For each primary and secondary outcome, a summary of results for each group, and the estimated effect size and its precision (e.g., 95% confidence interval)	
Ancillary analyses	18	Address multiplicity by reporting any other analyses performed, including subgroup analyses and adjusted analyses, indicating those pre-specified and those exploratory	

Continued

TABLE 1.4 (continued)

Paper section And topic	Item	Description	Reported on page #
Adverse events	19	*All important adverse events or side effects in each intervention group*	

Discussion
    Interpretation
	20	*Interpretation of the results*, taking into account study hypotheses,
		    sources of potential bias or imprecision and the dangers
		    associated with multiplicity of analyses and outcomes	

Generalizability	21	*Generalizability (external validity) of the trial findings*	
Overall evidence	22	*General interpretation of the results in the context of current evidence*	

Nonrandomized Designs (TREND) criteria have been developed for non-RCT trials (see Kaplan and Christensen, 2004).

CLINICAL PRACTICE GUIDELINES

Clinical guidelines were developed as an efficient way of providing information on evidence-based practice to clinicians. They have been defined by the Institute of Medicine as "systematically developed statements to assist practitioner and patient decision-making about appropriate health care for specific clinical circumstances" (Edmunds, 1966, p. 127). Their major functions include to:

1. help clinicians in treatment decisions
2. assist organizations in developing clinical risk management protocols
3. guide payers in setting reimbursement policies
4. to assist consumers to choose their care

Clinical practice guidelines have influenced policy makers. In a 1989 report to Congress, the Physician Payment Review Commission recommended increases in federal funding for the development, implementation and evaluation of practice guidelines. In the next year Congress passed legislation to establish the Public Health Service, Agency for Health Care Policy and Research (AHCPR) to carry out these tasks (Edmunds, 1996).

Prior to these efforts there has been a series of efforts to provide and disseminate guidelines: in the 1950s the American Academy of Pediatrics using expert consensus on immunization guidelines. In the mid-1970s the American College of Physicians, the professional organization for internal medicine, along with Blue Cross Blue Shield Organizations developed practice guidelines for laboratory tests. In 1984, the US Preventive Services Task Force developed guidelines for preventive interventions such as screening tests and immunizations. A Seattle-based healthcare consulting firm, Milliman and Robertson, Inc., developed practice guidelines that are used for over 50 million covered lives (Edmunds, 1966). In fact there has been a proliferation of these guidelines for physical health. The American Medical Association has listed 1,600 guidelines from 45 national medical groups. In addition a variety of proprietary guidelines have been developed by managed care companies. (Edmunds, 1966).

There has also been a question of what else should flow from a practice guideline. Suggestions include: paper and pencil tests, work flow diagrams for medical charts, wall charts, and guides for self-monitoring and self-management.

Edmunds (1996) lists two key impediments to guideline implementation: (1) provider autonomy; and (2) disagreements about evidence. More research is needed to more fully understand these issues and to provide means to appropriately handle these.

EVIDENCE-BASED GUIDELINES AND QUALITY IMPROVEMENT

It is the major thesis of this chapter that current mental health services are problematic because they are usually not delivered in a context in which serious, systematic quality improvement procedures are faithfully and continuously implemented. There needs to be a thoroughgoing commitment to this ethos in our field. Quality improvement practices have had tremendous impact on a variety of key industries and are making important headway in physical medicine. However, behavioral health practice has lagged decades behind and as a result our system is often shoddy, inefficient, disreputable, and smaller than it need be. We argue that practice guidelines such as those that are part of this book should be a part of a quality improvement system that constantly recycles corrective feedback to consistently improve practice. We will discuss some of the main components of a such a system below.

OVERVIEW OF QUALITY IMPROVEMENT: THE GENERAL PHILOSOPHY AND STRATEGY

Berwick (1999) has suggested that in contemporary American health care, there are two approaches to quality improvement: (1) the "Theory of Bad Apples" that posits that quality is best achieved by discovering and removing defective practitioners. The "bad apple" approach improves quality by inspection and includes procedures such as licensing and adjudication of complaints, recertification, establishment of thresholds for acceptability, and requires research into better tools for inspection (e.g., increasing sensitivity and specificity). Essential to this approach is the search for outliers, by for example examination of mortality or morbidity data, as well as "vigilant regulation". In this approach outlook, one uses deterrence to improve quality and punishment or the threat of punishment to control health care workers who do not care enough or have problems in doing the right thing. This approach leads to a defensive and fearful workforce who attempt to hide their perceived mistakes or weaknesses. Behavioral health has relied almost exclusively on this approach.

The second approach is the "Theory of Continuous Improvement." This approach holds that problems, and which are viewed as opportunities to improve quality, are built into production processes and that defects in quality are only rarely attributed to particular individual's lack of will, skill, or intention. Even when individuals are at the root of the defect, the problem is generally not one of motivation or effort, but rather of poor job design, failure of leadership or unclear purpose. According to this outlook, real improvement in quality depends on understanding and revising the production processes on the basis of data about the processes themselves. Continuous improvement is sought throughout the organization through constant effort to reduce waste, errors, rework and complexity. The focus is on the average producer, not the outlier, and on learning, not being defensive.

Unfortunately behavioral health services have focused on the bad apple theory with a wide range of therapies tolerated until thresholds of ethicality are breached. Thus, therapists who sleep with their clients or kill their clients (such as the Denver rebirthing case) are detected and punished. However, much of therapy that does not fall outside these ethical boundaries is tolerated and never improved.

What is Quality Improvement?: A Primer

Shewhart. Walter Andrew Shewhart received his Ph.D. in physics in 1917 from the University of California at Berkley. After a brief teaching career, he joined the Western Electric Company, a forerunner to the famous Bell Telephone Laboratories. This work necessitated ensuring reliability of telephone communication devices.

Dr. Shewhart applied what he learned about statistical techniques in graduate school to the task of producing a consistently high-quality telephone. Shewhart proposed that a high quality reliable product need not be "perfect" (the standard expectation of the factory's engineers) but "in control." He proposed that the finished product meet specifications that would and could vary to a certain irreducible extent. He called this normal difference "common cause' variation. Common cause variation can be reduced by understanding the variables in the processes that produce it. On the other hand, he also described "special cause" variation. Special cause variation was a difference in an outcome of a process that required investigation in order to assure quality and maximize productivity. Attempts to eliminate special cause variation were time consuming, costly, wasteful, and made things in the factory worse rather than better. In order to differentiate common cause variation from special cause variation, Shewhart mathematically calculated values that would be displayed on a "control chart". A statistical process control chart indicates whether or not observed variations in a defective apparatus of a given type are significant by plotting individual values, which included statistically generated upper and lower limits.

Malcolm Baldrige The Baldrige program identifies seven key action areas or categories in quality improvement:

Leadership involves efforts by senior leadership and management leading by example to integrate quality improvement into the strategic planning process and throughout the entire organization and to promote quality values and QI techniques in work practices.

Information and Analysis concerns managing and using the data needed for effective QI. Since quality improvement is based on management by fact, information and analyses are critical to QI success.

Strategic Quality Planning involves three major components: (1) developing long- and short-term organizational objectives for structural, performance and outcome quality standards; (2) identifying ways to achieve those objectives, and (3) measuring the effectiveness of the system in achieving quality standards.

Human Resource Development and Management involves working to develop the full potential of the workforce. This effort is guided by the principle that the entire workforce is motivated to achieve new levels of service and value.

Process Management concerns the creation and maintenance of high quality services. Within the context of quality improvement, process management refers to the improvement of work activities and work flow across functional or department boundaries.

System Results entails assessing the quality results achieved and examining the organization's success at achieving quality improvement.

Satisfaction of Patients and Other Stakeholders involves ensuring ongoing satisfaction by those internal and external to the behavioral healthcare system with the services provided.

Health care organizations that follow the Baldrige program have the option of asking for an external review of their progress and are eligible for the Malcolm Baldrige National Quality Award. Baldrige Awards, The Malcolm Baldrige National Quality Award was created by Public Law 100–107 and signed into law on August 20, 1987. The award is named for Malcolm Baldrige, who served as secretary of commerce from 1981 until his untimely death in a rodeo accident in 1987. Baldrige's managerial excellence contributed to long-term improvement in the efficiency and effectiveness of government. The award not only recognizes quality: but, also establishes a framework within which quality initiatives take place. Most organizations that apply for the award, believe that even greater gains accrue through evaluating their system than may result from being awarded one of the coveted awards. Through the Baldrige performance excellence criteria any organization can improve overall performance in seven categories—leadership, strategic planning, customer and market focus, information analysis, human resource focus, process management, and business results.

W. Edwards Deming. Deming made an important contribution to the science of improvement by recognizing that there are certain elements of knowledge that underpin all improvements in the entire spectrum of applications. He gave these elements of knowledge the name "System of Profound Knowledge." According to Deming, to comprehend the workings of a system and thus be able to improve it, one has to have an appreciation of the system as an entity onto itself, have an understanding of its variation, a theory of knowledge of how to bring about change, and psychology of personnel. Understanding variation helps us to understand that all processes in a behavioral healthcare system constantly exhibit variation.

The pursuit of improvement relies on cycles of learning. But it is not enough to show in a test that a change is an improvement. The change must be fully integrated into the system. This takes some planning, and usually some additional learning in matters of dealing with those who the change will affect and who will implement the change and make these changes sustainable.

Deming developed his famous "14 points" to transform management practices:

1. *Create constancy of purpose.* A behavioral health organization's highest priority is to provide the best quality care at the lowest cost possible. A healthcare organization must strive to maximize efficiency and effectiveness through constant improvement.

2. *Adopt the new philosophy.* Everyone working in the organization can find ways to promote quality and efficiency, to improve all aspects of the system, and to promote excellence and personal accountability. Pride of workmanship must be emphasized from recruitment to retirement..

3. *Cease dependence on inspection to achieve quality.* Reliance on routine inspection to improve quality (i.e., a search for errors, problems, or deficiencies) assumes that error is highly likely. Instead, there should be a continuous effort to minimize error. As Deming points out, "Inspection (as the sole means) to improve quality is too late!" Lasting quality comes not from inspection, but from improvements in the system.

4. *Do not purchase on the basis of price tag alone.* Purchasers must account for the quality of the item being purchased, as well as the cost. High quality organizations tend to think of their suppliers as "partners" in their operation. Successful partnerships require clear and specific performance standards and feedback on whether those standards are being met. Supplier performance can also be improved through an understanding of the suppliers' QI efforts; longer-term contracts that include explicit milestones for improvement in key features; joint planning for improvement; and joint improvement activities.

5. *Constantly improve the system of production and service.* Quality can be built into all health delivery activities and services and can be assured by continuous examination to identify potential improvements. This requires close cooperation between those who provide services and those who consume services. Improved efficiency and service can result from focusing not only on achieving present performance targets, but more importantly, by breaking through existing performance levels to new, higher levels.

6. *Institute QI training on the job.* On-the-job QI training ensures that every worker has a thorough understanding of: (1) the needs of those who use and/or pay for behavioral

services; (2) how to meet those needs; and (3) how to improve the system's ability to meet those needs. Incorporating QI into the fabric of each job can speed learning.

7. *Institute effective leadership.* The job of management is leadership. Effective leaders are thoroughly knowledgeable about the work being done and understand the environment and complexities with which their workers must contend. Leaders create the opportunity for workers to suggest improvements and act quickly to make needed changes in production process. Leaders are concerned with success as much as with failure and focus not only on understanding "substandard," but also "super-standard" performance. The effective leader also creates opportunities for below- and above-average performers to interact and identify opportunities for improvement.

8. *Drive out fear.* The Japanese have a saying: "Every defect is a treasure," meaning that errors and failures are opportunities for improvement. Errors or problems can help identify more fundamental or systemic root causes and ways to improve the system. Yet, fear of identifying problems or needed changes can kill QI programs. Also, some may feel that the idea of making improvements is an admission that the current way of doing things is flawed or that those responsible are poor performers. Improved performance cannot occur unless workers feel comfortable that they can speak truthfully and are confident that their suggestions will be taken seriously.

9. *Break down barriers between departments.* Barriers between organizations or between departments within one organization are obstacles to effective QI. Inter-departmental or intra-organizational friction or lack of cooperation result in waste, errors, delay, and unnecessary duplication of effort. A continuous and lasting QI program requires teamwork that crosses traditional organizational lines. QI requires that all workforce members, departments, and units share a unified purpose, direction, and commitment to improve the organization. Intra-organizational pathways are developed and cultivated as mechanisms by which to improve performance.

10. *Eliminate slogans, exhortations, and targets for the workforce for zero defects and new levels of productivity.* The problem with such exhortations is that they put the burden for quality on worker performance instead of poor system design. QI requires that the organization focus on improving its work processes. In so doing, service quality will increase, productivity and efficiency will rise, and waste will diminish.

11. *Eliminate management by numbers and objective. Substitute leadership.* Work production standards and rates, tied to incentive pay, are inappropriate because they burn out the workforce in the long run. Alternatively, a team effort should be marshaled to increase quality, which will lead to increased profits/savings that can then be translated to, for example, higher salaries or better benefits. Improvement efforts should emphasize improving processes; the outcome numbers will change as a consequence.

12. *Remove barriers to pride of workmanship.* The workforce is the most important component of a behavioral health delivery system. The behavioral health delivery system cannot function properly without workers who are proud of their work and who feel respected as individuals and professionals. Managers can help workers be successful by making sure that job responsibilities and performance standards are clearly understood; building strong relationships between management and the workforce; and providing workers with the best tools, instruments, supplies, and information possible.

13. *Institute a vigorous program of education and self-improvement.* Behavioral healthcare workers can improve their lives through education and ever-broadening career and life opportunities. The field needs not just good people; it needs people who are growing through education and life experiences. Management, as well as members of the workforce, must continue to experience new learning and growth.

14. *Put everybody to work to accomplish the transformation.* The essence of QI is an organization-wide focus on meeting the needs of those who use and/or pay for behavioral

health services. Effective quality management programs go beyond emphasizing one or two efforts or areas to improve performance. Every activity, every process and every job in behavioral healthcare can be improved. Everyone within the organization can be given an opportunity to understand the QI program and their individual role within that effort. Improvement teams that include broad representation throughout the organization can help ensure success of initial efforts and create opportunities for cross-disciplinary dialogue and information exchange.

CONCLUSIONS: THE UNMET QUALITY AGENDA IN BEHAVIORAL HEALTH

We view this book as a contribution to the unmet quality improvement agenda in behavioral health. We by no means think that it can stand alone or that it does most of the work that needs to be done. Rather it is an important start. Additional work needs to be done in:

1. *Developing a level of knowledge of quality improvement and commitment to quality improvement in management and other leadership in our field.* Although this has transformed other industries and is making significant inroads in physical medicine, in behavioral health a quality improvement perspective has made few inroads. Leadership is essential in promoting QI in behavioral health. Managers of all organizations need to view that a basic competency for them is a knowledge of quality improvement systems.

2. *Understanding the consumers of our services.* There needs to be an increased focus on our consumers and their expectations and experience of our services. What do they like and dislike about our present services? How can we exceed their expectations? Do they view our services as timely, as a good value proposition, as safe? What do they view as our competition? How are they performing? Where are there gaps in services?

3. *Developing quality indicators.* This is a interesting and complex task. We need to understand what indices denote quality in different domains; in an intake; in the treatment of depression, in billing, etc.

4. *Developing information technologies that efficiently and accurately track quality indicators.* These systems should routinely track outcome and processes so that cycles of learning can occur to improve these. Too much of current behavioral health is based on paper and is done in a pre-information technology revolution manner.

5. *Develop process analysis and cycles of learning.* We need to understand the process that produce outcomes. Who we hire, how we supervise, what guidelines if any we give them, how they follow these, what types of clients are seen, what assessment devices, etc. form the process that produce the outcomes. We need to develop profound knowledge of these, get suggestions for improvements from everyone concerned for all key elements and then conduct cycles of learning in which we see to what extent modifications produce improvements.

6. *Develop and implement continuing education.* The workforce needs to be constantly given new knowledge tools both in quality improvement techniques so that the entire workforce is participating in quality improvement efforsts and more specific information relevant to their tasks (how does one accurately detect an alcoholic?).

7. *Develop benchmarks.* We need to understand how our outcomes compare to national averages, outcomes from efficacy trials, etc. McFall and his colleagues (Stuart, Treat & Wade, 2000; Wade, Treat & Stuart, 1998) have developed an interesting and useful approach to this issues.

8. *Develop transparent report cards.* Our consumers and other interested parties need to see how we are doing. Web-based report cards are current for hospitals (see for example, myhealthfinder.com; hospitalquality.org; or hospitalcompare.hhs.org.)

These sites include comparisons to national averages and top 10% of hospitals, patient volumes, mortality rates, and patient satisfaction data. It would be useful if behavioral health organizations produced similar report cards.

9. *Develop incentive systems.* We also need to develop financial incentive systems for implementing the above. Brent James has developed a useful model. Quality produces medical cost savings (see Cummings, O'Donohue & Ferguson, 2003) and these savings can be split between key parties (employer, insurer, instutitution, provider).

The Organization of The Guidelines

Finally, we wanted to make the guidelines as user friendly as possible. To do this we requested that each expert confine their guideline to approximately 15–20 pages. Most complied but there were a few exceptions in areas that are more complex. We also tried to distill information into subtopics that were most useful. These were:

1. What is x? (this should describe key features and perhaps give diagnostic criteria of the problem).
2. Basic facts about x; Comorbidity, prevalence, age at onset, gender distribution, course and other descriptive information.
3. Assessment :What should be ruled out?
4. What assessments are not helpful?
5. Treatment: What treatments are effective?
6. What are effective self-help treatments? This section was included to address access problems, promote choice and to develop a stepped care approach in which less instrusive and expensive evidence-based treatments are reported, if any.
7. What are effective therapist-based treatments? References of treatment manuals, if any, was required.
8. What is effective medical treatment? Because there is often medical alternatives such as medications and consumers are often faced with a choice; evidence for effective medical treatments was requested.
9. Combination treatments
10. Other issues in management
11. How does one select among treatments?

REFERENCES

Adelman, H. S. (1995). Clinical psychology: Beyond psychopathology and clinical interventions. *Clinical Psychology: Science & Practice 2(1)*, 28–44.

Antonuccio, D. (1995). Psychotherapy for depression: No stronger medicine. *American Psychologist 50*(6), 450–452.

American Psychological Association (2002). Ethical principles of psychologists and code of conduct. *American Psychologist.*

Berwick, D. & Nolan, T. (1998). Physicians as leaders in improving health care: A new series in Annals of Internal Medicine. *Annals of Internal Medicine 128 (4)*, 289–292.

Bremer, B., A. Foxx, R. M., Lee, M., Lykins, D., Mintz, V. R. & Stine, E. (2001). Potential client's beliefs about the relative competency and caring of psychologists: Implications for the profession. *Journal of Clinical Psychology 52(12)*, 1479–1488.

Chambless, D. L., Sanderson, W. C., Shoham, V., Bennett Johnson, S., Pope, K. S., Crits-Christoph, P., Baker, M., Johnson, B., Woody, S. R., Sue, S., Beutler, L., Williams, D. A., & McCurry, S. (1996). An update on empirically validated therapies. *The Clinical Psychologist, 49,* 5–18.

Chambless, D. L., Baker, M. J., Baucom, D. H., Beutler, L., Calhoun, K. S., Crits-Christoph, P., Daiuto, A., DeRubeis, R., Detweiler, J., Haaga, D. A. F., Bennett Johnson, S., McCurry, S., Mueser, K. T., Pope, K. S., Sanderson, W. C., Shoham, V., Stickle, T., Williams, D. A., & Woody, S. A. (1998). Update on empirically validated therapies, II. *The Clinical Psychologist, 51,* 3–16.

Chambless, D. (1996). In defense of dissemination of empirically supported psychological interventions. *Clinical Psychology: Science & Practice 3(3)*, 230–235.

Chambless, D. L., Baker, M. J., Baucom, D. H., Beutler, L., Calhoun, K. S., Crits-Christoph, P., Daiuto, A., DeRubeis, R., Detweiler, J., Haaga, D. A. F., Bennett Johnson, S., McCurry, S., Mueser, K. T., Pope, K. S., Sanderson, W. C., Shoham, V., Stickle, T., Williams, D. A., & Woody, S. A. (1998). Update on empirically validated therapies, II. *The Clinical Psychologist, 51*, 3–16.

X. Chambless D, Hollon S. Defining empirically supported therapies. Journal of Consulting Clinical and Psychology 1998; *66(1)*, 7–18.

Clinton, J. J., McCormick, K., & Besteman, J. (1994). Enhancing clinical practice: The role of practice guidelines. *American Psychologist, 49*, 30–33.

Crits-Christoph, P., Frank, E., Chambless, D. L., Brody, C., & Karp, J. F. (1995). Training in empirically validated treatments: What are clinical psychology students learning? *Professional Psychology: Research and Practice, 26*, 514–522.

Cummings, N. (2005). Personal communication.

Cummings, N. O'Donohue, W., & Ferguson, K (Eds.). (2003). *Behavioral health as primary care: beyond efficacy to effectiveness.* Reno, NV: Context Press.

Cyr, F., King, M. C., & Ritchie, P. L.-J. (1995). Quality management for psychology services in health care facilities. *Canadian Psychology.*

Duckworth (in press). Adjunctive treatments with ethnic and racial minorities. In Cummings & O'Donohue (Eds.), *Evidence Based Adjunctive Treatments.* New York: Elsevier.

Eddy D M. (2001). *Evidence-based clinical improvements.* Presentations at "Directions for success: Evidence-based health care symposium" sponsored by Group Health Cooperative, May 7–9, 2001. Tucson, AZ.

Eddy DM. Evidence-based clinical improvements. Presentations at "Directions for success: Evidence-based health care symposium" sponsored by Group Health Cooperative, May 7-9, 2001. Tucson, AZ.

Edmunds, M. (1996). Clinical practice guidelines: Opportunities and implications. *Annals of Behavioral Medicine, 18*, 126–132.

Hamann, E. E. (1994). Clinicians and diagnosis: Ethical concerns and clinician competence. *Journal of Counseling & Development 50(6)*, 450–452.

Institute of Medicine (2001). *Crossing the quality chasm: A new health system for the 21st century.* Washington, DC: National Academy Press.

Kaplan, R. M. & Christensen, A. J. (2004). Annals of behavior medicine endorses transparent reporting of evaluations with nonrandomized designs (TREND). *Annals of Behavior Medicine 27(3)*, 147–148.

Kenagy, J. W., Berwick, D. M., & Shore, M. F. (1999). Service quality in health care. *Journal of the American Medical Association 281(7)*, 661–665.

Leape, L. L. (2003). Patient safety: the new accountability. Presented at the CDC quality institute in Atlanta, GA April 2003.

Leebov, W. & Scott, G. (1994). *Service quality improvement: the customer satisfaction strategy for healthcare.* New York: American Hospital Publishing.

Lilienfeld, S. O. & Fowler, K. (in press). Antisocial Personality Disorder. In J. E. Fisher & W. T. O'Donohue (Eds.) *Clinician's guide to evidence based psychotherapy.* New York: Springer.

Lilienfeld, S. O. & Lynn, S. J. (2002). *Science and pseudoscience in clinical psychology.* New York: Guilford Press.

McFall, R.M. (1991). Manifesto for a science of clinical psychology. *The Clinical Psychologist 44 (6)*: 75–88.

Nathan, P. E. (1998). Practice guidelines: Not yet ideal. *American Psychologist, 53*, 290–299.

O'Donohue, W., Fisher, J. E., & Hayes, S.C. (Eds.) (2003). *Cognitive Behavior Therapy: A step-by-step guide for clinicians.* NY: John Wiley.

O'Donohue, W. & Ferguson, K. (Eds.). (2003). *Handbook of professional ethics.* San Diego: Academic Press.

O'Donohue, W., & Henderson, D. (1999). Epistemic and ethical duties in clinical decision-making. *Behaviour Change, 16(1)*, 10–19.

O'Donohue, W. T. & Lilienfeld, S. O. (in press). The Epistemological and Ethical Dimension of Clinical Science. In T. Treat (Ed.). *A Festschrift for Richard McFall.* New York: Springer.

O'Donohue, W. & Oser, M. (2005). Psychological errors. Unpublished manuscript.

Strosahl, K. (1996). Three "gold mine-land mine" themes in generation 2 of health care reform. *the Behavior Therapist, 19*, 52–54.

Schuster, M. A., McGlynn, E. A. & Brook, R. H. (1998). How good is the quality of healthcare in the United States? *The Milbank Quarterly 76 (4)*, 517–563.

Shuster, M. A. & Mcglynn, E. A. (1998). How good is the quality of healthcare in the United States? *Merrill Quarterly, 76(4)*, 517–563.

Stuart, G. L., Treat, T. A., & Wade, W. A. (2000). Effectiveness of an empirically based treatment for panic disorder delivered in a service clinic setting: 1-year follow up. *Journal of Consulting & Clinical Psychology 68(3)*, 506–512.

Wade, W. A., Treat, T. A., & Stuart, G. L. (1998). Transporting an empirically based treatment for panic disorder to a service clinic setting: A benchmark strategy. *Journal of Consulting & Clinical Psychology 66(2)*, 231–239.

Walton, M. (1986). *The Deming management method.* New York: Perigee.

Agoraphobia

Holly Hazlett-Stevens

WHAT IS AGORAPHOBIA?

Agoraphobia literally means "fear of the marketplace," based on *agora*, the word for the Greek marketplace (Durand & Barlow, 2003). The term "agoraphobia" was first introduced by Westphal in 1871 to describe the fear and avoidance of public places, although this condition was not widely recognized until the late 1970s (Barlow, 2002). Diagnosis of Agoraphobia first appeared in the *Diagnostic and Statistical Manual of Mental Disorders* in its third edition (DSM-III; American Psychiatric Association [APA], 1980). Agoraphobia was then considered a primary diagnosis, which may or may not be accompanied by recurrent panic attacks (Mennin, Heimberg, & Holt, 2000). However, since publication of the DSM-III-R (APA, 1987), a diagnosis of Panic Disorder is considered primary and is diagnosed either with or without Agoraphobia. Under the current DSM-IV (APA, 1994) diagnostic system, individuals exhibiting symptoms of Agoraphobia but never meeting full diagnostic criteria for Panic Disorder are given a diagnosis of Agoraphobia Without History of Panic Disorder (AWHPD).

The DSM-IV (APA, 1994) describes Agoraphobia as anxiety about several different places or situations from which escape would be either difficult or embarrassing if some sort of unexpected or unwanted bodily symptoms occurred (Criterion A). As a result, such situations are either avoided, require the presence of a trusted person, or are endured with great distress (Criterion B). This anxiety and situational avoidance is not better explained by another anxiety disorder, such as Social Phobia or Specific Phobia (Criterion C). Although panic attacks or "panic-like" bodily sensations are often feared, other feared symptoms include loss of bladder or bowel control, vomiting, or severe headache. Agoraphobia is not recognized by DSM-IV as a diagnosis on its own. An individual meeting criteria for Agoraphobia is then diagnosed with either Panic Disorder With Agoraphobia (PDA) (if diagnostic criteria for Panic Disorder are also met) or AWHPD. Both diagnoses require that the symptoms cannot be fully explained by a general medical condition and do not reflect the direct physiological effects of a substance.

Common agoraphobic situations include shopping malls, public transportation, supermarkets, restaurants, theaters, additional situations involving crowds or waiting in line, travel far from home, and being alone (Barlow & Craske, 2000). Such agoraphobic situations are avoided because of feared bodily sensations or physical symptoms; therefore it is not surprising that other daily activities causing such interoceptive sensations are also avoided. Activities involving physical exertion, such as aerobic exercise, running up flights of stairs, heavy lifting, and dancing, may be avoided because they induce sensations of physiological arousal. Similar interoceptive activities include hot and stuffy spaces, sexual relations, watching suspenseful movies or sporting events, expressing anger or engaging in emotionally arousing discussions, and ingesting caffeine or chocolate (Barlow & Craske, 2000). Individuals with AWHPD who fear sensations other than "panic-like" symptoms might avoid

Hazlett-Stevens, H. (2006). Agoraphobia. In J. E. Fisher & W. T. O'Donohue (Eds.), *Practitioner's guide to evidence-based psychotherapy*. New York: Springer.

additional activities causing other feared sensations. For example, an individual with AWHPD stemming from gastrointestinal distress and fear of losing control of his bowels might avoid eating spicy foods or heavy meals to prevent unwanted gastrointestinal sensations. Nevertheless, the actual agoraphobic situations avoided by individuals with AWHPD do not seem to differ from those avoided by individuals with Panic Disorder With Agoraphobia (Pollard, Tait, Meldrum, Dubinsky, & Gall, 1996).

DSM-IV conceptualizes Agoraphobia as a condition most often secondary to Panic Disorder or sub-clinical panic symptoms. This view rests on the assumption that avoidance of public places and other agoraphobic situations develops as a behavioral reaction to the unexpected physiological arousal of panic (Barlow, 2002). Indeed, re-assessment of 26 AWHPD patients revealed that 57% appeared to suffer from panic attacks containing too few symptoms to meet criteria for Panic Disorder (Goisman et al., 1995). In a longitudinal naturalistic study of 562 participants suffering from panic and agoraphobia symptoms, only 6% were assigned diagnoses of AWHPD (Goisman et al., 1994). These researchers proposed that AWHPD might be best conceptualized as part of a panic syndrome, in which AWHPD lies on a single continuum with PDA and Panic Disorder Without Agoraphobia (PD). Similarly, Andrews and Slade (2002) concluded that these three diagnoses represent three variations of a single disorder after finding strong similarities among AWHPD, PDA, and PD clinical groups.

Although AWHPD is not often seen in mental health treatment settings (Pollard, Bronson, & Kenney, 1989), Agoraphobia can develop in response to somatic conditions other than panic. For example, AWHPD has been associated with Generalized Anxiety Disorder (Hoffart, Thornes, & Hedley, 1995), Irritable Bowel Syndrome (IBS; Mennin et al., 2000), headache (Spierings, Reinders, & Hoogduin, 1989), and fear of vomiting (Pollard et al., 1996). Wittchen, Reed, and Kessler (1998) found that most agoraphobic individuals in their community sample reported no history of uncued panic-related symptoms, challenging the predominant view that panic-like experiences are usually responsible for the development of Agoraphobia. They argued that AWHPD is not often seen in mental health settings because such individuals seldom seek treatment, not because it is a rare condition. Regardless of whether or not panic-related sensations are responsible for the development of an individual's Agoraphobia, the behavioral avoidance is driven by a fear of some sort of internal bodily sensation or event.

BASIC FACTS ABOUT AGORAPHOBIA

The American Psychiatric Association estimates the 1-year prevalence of Panic Disorder between 1% and 2%, with up to one-half of these individuals also suffering from Agoraphobia (APA, 1994). The US National Comorbidity Survey (NCS) lifetime prevalence estimate for PD with or without Agoraphobia is 3.5% (Kessler et al., 1994). Determining the prevalence of AWHPD has proven much more complicated. Initial epidemiological results suggested that AWHPD was more common than PDA. The NCS found the lifetime prevalence for AWHPD to be 5.3% (Kessler et al., 1994). Similarly, the Epidemiological Catchment Area (ECA) survey based on DSM-III criteria reported a 4.2% lifetime prevalence of AWHPD compared to only 0.9% for Panic Disorder (Robins et al., 1984). However, the high rates of AWHPD found in large-scale epidemiological research might reflect overestimates due to methodological difficulties. Both the ECA and NCS relied on structured diagnostic interviews conducted by lay interviewers rather than trained clinicians: the ECA determined DSM-III diagnoses with the Diagnostic Interview Schedule (DIS;

Robins, Helzer, Croughan, & Ratcliff, 1981) and the NCS assigned DSM-III-R diagnoses after administering the Composite International Diagnostic Interview (CIDI; World Health Organization, 1990).

Researchers have since taken a closer look at AWHPD cases from epidemiological studies. Horwath, Lish, Johnson, Hornig, and Weissman (1993) blindly re-interviewed 22 AWHPD participants from the original ECA study. Only two received a diagnosis of AWHPD, one of which had sub-clinical panic attacks. The remaining participants were reclassified with simple (specific) phobias or PDA. In a more recent study using DSM-IV criteria, Andrews and Slade (2002) reported a 1-year prevalence rate of 1.3% for PD, 1.6% for AWHPD, and 0.6% for PDA in their Australian community sample. Although AWHPD and PD groups were mutually exclusive, 18% of those with AWHPD reported recurrent and unexpected panic attacks that did not meet criteria for PD. Thus, the prevalence of AWHPD and its relationship to panic attacks and Panic Disorder remains the subject of much debate.

The prevalence of PDA does not seem to differ among ethnic groups (Eaton, Dryman, & Weissman, 1991; Horwath, Johnson, & Hornig, 1993). However, African Americans are rarely found in treatment outcome research studies (Paradis, Hatch, & Friedman, 1994). Early epidemiological research based on DSM-III criteria consistently revealed that Agoraphobia was more common for women than men (see Pollard & Henderson, 1987). In the later NCS study, women were more than twice as likely as men to meet diagnostic criteria for Agoraphobia (ratio of 2.2:1.0; Magee, Eaton, Wittchen, McGonagle, & Kessler, 1996). According to the DSM-IV-TR (APA, 2000), approximately 75% of those suffering from PDA are women. One explanation for this gender difference is that avoidance behavior is more culturally acceptable for women than for men. Agoraphobic individuals' tendency to avoid situations correlated with "masculinity" scores, such that the lower the score, the greater the avoidance behavior (Chambless & Mason, 1986). Consistent with this view, men are more likely than women to cope with unwanted anxiety and panic symptoms by using alcohol and other psychoactive substances (Kushner, Abrams, & Borchardt, 2000). For a thorough review of gender difference research see Craske (1999, 2003).

Although little is known about the course of AWHPD, the course of PDA is often quite chronic. One longitudinal investigation reported a 1-year remission rate of only 17%, and relapse among these individuals was common (Keller et al., 1994).The onset of Agoraphobia usually occurs in the late-twenties, with a median age of onset of 29 years (Magee et al., 1996). Panic Disorder begins as early as the mid-teens (Burke, Burke, Regier, & Rae, 1990), but PDA is rarely found in younger children (Albano, Chorpita, & Barlow, 1996). More than half the time, individuals with PDA are diagnosed with additional comorbid conditions. This most often involves another anxiety disorder such as Generalized Anxiety Disorder, Specific Phobia, or Social Phobia, or a mood disorder such as Major Depressive Disorder or Dysthymia. Substance use disorders and Axis II personality disorders are also common (see Barlow, 2002; Craske, 1999 for reviews).

Agoraphobia can become quite disabling. Although the NCS study found that only 26.5% of those with Agoraphobia reported that their avoidance interfered "a lot" with their life (Magee et al., 1996), severe functional impairment across many life domains is common among clinical samples (Mennin et al., 2000). Interpersonal problems and marital difficulties have been documented with PDA (Hoffart, 1997; Marcaurelle, Bélanger, & Marchand, 2003), although it is unclear whether these problems were present before the onset of PDA. Other important costs include medical utilization and work disability. PDA often leads to increased use of nonpsychiatric general medical services and emergency room visits (Markowitz, Weissman,

Ouellette, Lish, & Klerman, 1989). Unemployment and other forms of work impairment are also common. Studies of treatment-seeking clinical populations have documented unemployment rates of 50%, and 33% of individuals suffering from PDA may be financially dependent on public assistance programs (Edlund & Swann, 1987; Massion, Warshaw, & Keller, 1993). Although little information about the social costs of AWHPD is available, severe agoraphobic avoidance associated with sub-clinical panic or conditions other than panic can also lead to significant impairment.

WHAT CAUSES AGORAPHOBIA?

Early theories of agoraphobia viewed avoidance behavior as a conditioned fear response. One influential model was the two-factor theory of Mowrer (1960). He proposed that fear is first acquired from a classical conditioning experience, then escape from or avoidance of the conditioned stimulus situation maintains the fear by preventing extinction of this fear response. According to this view, the fear of certain public places would originate when some sort of noxious or aversive event happened to occur in that context and the person became motivated to avoid that particular situation due to their conditioned fear response. In support of this model, Öst and Hugdahl (1983) found that 81% of their agoraphobia sample could identify a specific conditioning experience to account for their fear. Later behavioral theories focused on fears of what might happen in the feared situation rather than fears of the situation itself. For example, Goldstein and Chambless (1978) proposed that agoraphobic avoidance resulted from a fear of impending panic or other feared bodily sensations, a model labeled "fear of fear." From this perspective, innocuous bodily sensations become classically conditioned to the aversive physiological arousal associated with panic attacks. Because these classically conditioned sensations could trigger an unwanted panic attack across situations, individuals avoid various agoraphobic situations out of fear that they would be unable to cope with their panic if it were to occur in that situation.

Modern approaches view the development of Agoraphobia and PDA as a complex interaction between both biological and psychological influences. Agoraphobia is believed to begin with a general predisposition or vulnerability common to all the anxiety disorders (Craske, 1999). This temperament risk factor is often referred to as "negative affectivity" (Watson & Clark, 1984), and is quite similar to constructs such as neuroticism (Eysenck, 1967) and behavioral inhibition (Kagan, 1997). Genetic influences for negative affectivity are well established, but genes only explain half the picture (Craske, 2003). Environmental influences can also make a person vulnerable to experience negative emotional states across situations. Early experiences with stressful situations, particularly those in which the individual perceived the event(s) to be unpredictable and difficult to control, also contribute to the negative affectivity temperament (Craske, 1999). Other developmental experiences that can predispose a person to anxiety disorders include parental modeling of anxious behavior, overprotective treatment, and parental encouragement of anxious behavior and avoidance (Vasey & Dadds, 2001).

More specific physiological and psychological factors could make an individual prone to experience Panic Disorder and Agoraphobia symptoms in particular. Evidence for an overactive hypothalamic–pituitary–adrenal (HPA) axis and autonomic hyperactivity in Panic Disorder exists, although research results are mixed (Craske, 1999). Psychological factors center on a specific fear of unwanted bodily sensations. Cognitive components include attributions and beliefs that certain innocuous sensations are dangerous. For example, accelerated heart rate might be interpreted as a sign of heart attack or stroke, shortness of breath could be taken as a sign of suffocation, and dizziness could be perceived as evidence that the person will faint (Barlow, 2002). Other feared consequences of unwanted bodily sensations include losing control over one's body and going crazy. Clark (1988) described these cognitions as "catastrophic misinterpretations," in which normal anxiety sensations and sometimes other harmless physical sensations are interpreted in a catastrophic way to signal immediate and impending physical and/or mental disaster.

Along similar lines, Reiss et al. (1986) defined "anxiety sensitivity" as the tendency to interpret anxiety sensations as harmful. They suggested that anxiety sensitivity represents a specific vulnerability to Panic Disorder and agoraphobic avoidance, and longitudinal research supports this idea (Ehlers, 1995). Anxiety sensitivity among treatment-seeking agoraphobic clients reflected fears of heart and breathing symptoms, loss of mental control, gastrointestinal difficulties, and other people detecting anxiety symptoms (Wardle, Ahmad, & Hayward, 1990). Individuals with PDA appear more likely to fear physical catastrophes than AWHPD individuals (Hoffart, Friis, Strand, & Olsen, 1994).

Barlow (2002) proposed a comprehensive etiological model of PDA that integrates these various components. He suggested that an individual may be predisposed to experience anxiety through both biological and psychological generalized vulnerability factors. When a stressful event triggers an exaggerated physiological fear response, the individual becomes fearful of the associated interoceptive cues due to a specific tendency to interpret unexplained physical sensations as dangerous. This fear leads to anticipation of future unwanted somatic sensations, or "anxious apprehension." Agoraphobia develops when the individual responds to feared somatic sensations and anticipation of future interoceptive cues with behavioral avoidance of certain situations. This avoidance maintains the fear of unwanted sensations, reinforcing beliefs that such sensations are indeed harmful and need to be avoided in certain situations. This model might also be applied to cases of AWHPD. For individuals fearing panic-like sensations, the same physiological fear response might lead to interoceptive conditioning and the development of avoidance behavior even though full-blown panic attacks are not experienced. Individuals with AWHPD in the absence of subclinical panic may also possess a specific psychological vulnerability to interpret unexplained physical sensations as dangerous. In this case, unwanted bodily sensations other than panic could lead to the same cycle of anxious apprehension and behavioral avoidance seen in PDA.

ASSESSMENT

What Should be Ruled Out?

Before PDA or AWHPD is diagnosed, the clinician should rule out any medical conditions that might account for the client's feared bodily sensations. For example, certain thyroid and vestibular problems can cause panic-like sensations (see Panic Disorder chapter, this volume). Similarly, the clinician should determine that the somatic sensations associated with the client's Agoraphobia are not merely due to the effects of a substance. If the client uses psychoactive substances, careful assessment of when the physiological effects of these substances were experienced is necessary. This allows the clinician to determine whether the direct effects of the substance can account for the avoidance behavior.

Clinicians must also determine that a client's avoidance behavior is not better accounted for by another DSM-IV diagnosis. As reviewed above, epidemiological survey results may have been confounded by misdiagnosed cases of Agoraphobia. Specific Phobia and Social Phobia are easily confused with PDA and AWHPD because all involve behavioral avoidance of in vivo situations. However, the defining feature of Agoraphobia is that fear and avoidance of certain situations stems from a fear that escape would be difficult or embarrassing or that help would be unavailable in the event of a panic attack or other unwanted bodily sensations. If an individual's avoidance is driven by a fear of negative evaluation or fear that he or she might behave in a way that other people would scrutinize, an alternative diagnosis of Social Phobia (Social Anxiety Disorder) should be considered. If the situational avoidance is confined to specific types of situations or objects, a diagnosis of Specific Phobia (formerly Simple Phobia) may be more appropriate. An individual might avoid various public places due to contamination fears or other intrusive obsessive thoughts, but this avoidance behavior would be best conceptualized as a symptom of Obsessive-Compulsive Disorder. Sometimes individuals suffering from Posttraumatic or Acute Stress Disorder will avoid certain places, people, or activities because these stimuli remind them of the traumatic event or because they fear additional harm from the environment. From a diagnostic perspective, this form of behavioral avoidance is usually subsumed under the "avoidance of stimuli" criterion required for both stress disorder diagnoses and does not warrant a separate AWHPD diagnosis.

What is Involved in Effective Assessment?

In clinical settings, Agoraphobia is often detected at the initial diagnostic interview. Structured diagnostic interviews such as the DIS (Robins et al., 1981) and the CIDI (World Health Organization, 1990) have been developed for administration by lay interviewers, but this practice may not always yield a valid diagnosis. Ideally, diagnosis is obtained with a semi-structured clinician administered diagnostic interview so that differential diagnosis issues can be explored fully. Empirically supported semi-structured interviews such as the Anxiety Disorders Interview Schedule for DSM-IV (ADIS-IV; Brown, Di Nardo, & Barlow, 1994) allow the clinician to systematically assess the function of reported anxiety symptoms and avoidance behavior. This information prepares the clinician to conduct a functional analysis of the individual's ideographic cognitions, interoceptive avoidance, situational avoidance, and subtle avoidance and safety behaviors that maintain the disorder (see Barlow, 2002).

Additional information regarding specific cognitive and behavioral features of Agoraphobia can be obtained with self-report questionnaires. Widely used self-report measures include the Anxiety Sensitivity Index (ASI; Reiss et al., 1986), the Anxiety Control Questionnaire (AnxCQ; Rapee, Craske, Brown, & Barlow, 1996), the Body Sensations Questionnaire and the Agoraphobic Cognitions Questionnaire (BSQ and ACQ; Chambless, Caputo, Bright, & Gallagher, 1984), and the Mobility Inventory for Agoraphobia (MI; Chambless, Caputo, Jasin, Gracely, & Williams, 1985). Complete descriptions of these and many other measures, along with reviews of available psychometric data, are available from Antony (2001).

What Assessments are Not Helpful?

Personality inventories such as the Minnesota Multiphasic Personality Inventory (MMPI) and its revision, the MMPI-2, are not particularly useful in the assessment of Agoraphobia. Neither projective psychological tests, including the Rorschach inkblot test and the Thematic Apperception Test (TAT), nor neuropsychological tests such as those found in the Luria-Nebraska and Halstead-Reitan batteries are useful in the diagnosis of Agoraphobia. Medical markers or tests for this condition are not available.

TREATMENT

What Treatments are Effective?

Situational exposure has been central to the psychological treatment of agoraphobic individuals for decades. Although variations in procedures exist, effective exposure involves repeated contact with the avoided situation while the client experiences moderate levels of anxiety (Gelder, 1991). See Hazlett-Stevens and Craske (2003) for a description of in vivo exposure procedures. Teaching clients how to apply progressive relaxation in agoraphobic situations may also prove beneficial, and this Applied Relaxation approach was about as effective as in vivo exposure alone (Öst, Westling, & Hellström, 1993).

When Agoraphobia is present in the context of PDA, treatment typically begins with educational information about the physiology of panic and the harmless nature of the fight or flight response. Cognitive restructuring addresses misappraisals of feared bodily sensations, and the client is encouraged to engage in activities within and between sessions that induce their feared interoceptive cues. Finally, a hierarchy of agoraphobic situations is constructed, and treatment continues with systematic live exposure to each of these feared situations for the remainder of treatment.

What are Effective Self-Help Treatments?

A number of self-help books containing these cognitive-behavioral elements are available to the public. Many of these resources are designed for people suffering from PDA (see Panic Disorder chapter in this volume). However, a few books target Agoraphobia symptoms exclusively:

- Pollard, C.A., & Zuercher-White, E. (2003). *The agoraphobia workbook: A comprehensive program to end your fear of symptom attacks.* Oakland, CA: New Harbinger Publications, Inc.
- Eisenstadt, M. (2003). *Freedom from agoraphobia.* Anchorage, AK: Mark Eisenstadt, M.D.
- Weekes, C. (1990). *Agoraphobia: Simple effective treatment.* New York, NY: HarperCollins Publishers.

One additional self-help resource might be beneficial to friends and family members of people suffering from Agoraphobia:

- Chope, R.C. (2001). *Healing options for you and the agoraphobic in your life.* Oakland, CA: New Harbinger Publications, Inc.

While much empirical research supports the practice of therapist-administered cognitive-behavioral treatment for Agoraphobia, bibliotherapy approaches have been studied much less. Ghosh and Marks (1987) administered a self-help book instruction coupled with only three therapist contacts to treat mild agoraphobic avoidance. Results suggested that this treatment approach was as effective as therapist-guided treatment in less severe cases of Agoraphobia. However, these results do not seem to generalize to more severe agoraphobic individuals, possibly due to difficulties engaging in self-guided exposure exercises (Holden, O'Brien,

Barlow, Stetson, & Infantino, 1983). Self-administered bibliotherapy appears to be an effective treatment approach in some cases of PDA as well (Gould, Clum, & Shaprio, 1993).

Further information about Agoraphobia can be found on the following websites:

- http://www.adaa.org/Anxiety DisorderInfor/PanicDisAgor.cfm
- http://www.nimh.nih.gov/ HealthInformation/panicmenu.cfm
- http://www.anxiety network.com/pdhome.html
- http://pages. infinit.net/drnayman/agorapho.htm

What are Effective Therapist-Based Treatments?

Barlow and colleagues (Craske & Barlow, 2001; Craske, Barlow, & Meadows, 2000) have developed a widely used cognitive-behavioral therapy for PDA known as Panic Control Treatment (PCT). This therapist-based treatment has received much empirical support (see Craske, 1999 and Barlow, 2002 for reviews). However, recent research suggests that situational exposure targeting agoraphobic avoidance might not be necessary for effective treatment of PDA (Craske, DeCola, Sachs, & Pontillo, 2003). See Panic Disorder chapter (this volume) for more information about cognitive-behavioral treatment approaches for PDA. Therapist-guided exposure was moderately effective for severe Agoraphobia when administered over 4–8 weeks (Holden et al., 1983). Öst and colleagues found that their Applied Relaxation (AR) approach coupled with self-exposure instructions was also an effective treatment for PDA agoraphobic avoidance (Öst et al., 1993).

What is Effective Medical Treatment?

Pharmacotherapy for Agoraphobia has been widely studied in the context of PDA. Tricyclic antidepressants such as imipramine have effectively treated agoraphobic avoidance symptoms (Lydiard, Brawman-Mintzer, & Ballenger, 1996). More recently, several selective serotonin reuptake inhibitors (SSRIs) have received empirical support in the treatment of PDA (see White & Barlow, 2002 for a review). Benzodiazepines were the first approved for PDA treatment, but these medications have the potential to undermine effective situational exposure when combined with cognitive-behavioral therapy.

Other Issues in Management

Many theoretical and practical issues remain unresolved. The role of panic attacks and feared anxiety sensations, while clear in cases of PDA, might not always explain the development of AWHPD. Some researchers have suggested that the pathway leading to Panic Disorder differs from the pathway leading to Agoraphobia (Wittchen et al., 1998). Alternatively, comprehensive PDA models (e.g., Barlow, 2002) might be extended to explain how fears of unexplained bodily sensations lead to AWHPD clinical presentations involving sensations other than panic. Nevertheless, careful assessment of any feared sensations associated with agoraphobic avoidance is crucial. The clinical nature and treatment of AWHPD needs to be further explored, particularly in medical settings where individuals experiencing IBS, headaches, and other physical conditions that might lead to Agoraphobia would likely present for treatment.

How Does One Select Among Treatments?

Exposure-based cognitive-behavioral therapy treatments are a good choice for individuals willing to confront their feared situations. This treatment can be quite difficult for severely agoraphobic individuals. Therefore, clinicians must assess whether the individual can endure the distress involved in exposure. Individuals at a heightened risk for suicide may need additional intervention before exposure is attempted. In cases involving domestic violence, avoidance behavior that appears to be Agoraphobia might be serving an adaptive self-protective purpose. Exposure treatment may also be inappropriate for individuals suffering from comorbid psychosis, mania, or dementia. As with all psychological disorders, the potential for side-effects and medical contraindications should be addressed with individuals considering medication treatment.

REFERENCES

Albano, A. M., Chorpita, B. F., & Barlow, D. H. (1996). Childhood anxiety disorders. In E. J. Mash & R. A. Barkley (Eds.), *Child psychopathology*. New York: Guilford Press.

American Psychiatric Association. (1980). *Diagnostic and statistical manual of mental disorders* (3rd ed.). Washington, DC: American Psychiatric Association.

American Psychiatric Association. (1987). *Diagnostic and statistical manual of mental disorders* (3rd ed., rev.). Washington, DC: American Psychiatric Association.

American Psychiatric Association. (1994). *Diagnostic and statistical manual of mental disorders* (4th ed.). Washington, DC: American Psychiatric Association.

American Psychiatric Association. (2000). *Diagnostic and statistical manual of mental disorders* (4th ed., text revision). Washington, DC: American Psychiatric Association.

Andrews, G., & Slade, T. (2002). Agoraphobia without a history of panic disorder may be part of the panic disorder syndrome. *Journal of Nervous and Mental Disease, 190,* 624–630.

Antony, M. M. (2001). Measures for panic disorder and agoraphobia. In M. M. Antony, S. M. Orsillo, & L. Roemer (Eds.), *Practitioner's guide to empirically based measures of anxiety*. New York: Kluwer Academic/Plenum Publishers.

Barlow, D. H. (2002). *Anxiety and its disorders: The nature and treatment of anxiety and panic* (2nd ed.). New York: Guilford Press.

Barlow, D. H., & Craske, M. G. (2000). *Mastery of your anxiety and panic (MAP-3): Client workbook for anxiety and panic* (3rd ed.). San Antonio, TX: Graywind/Psychological Corporation.

Brown, T. A., Di Nardo, P. A., & Barlow, D. H. (1994). *Anxiety Disorders Interview Schedule for DSM-IV (ADIS-IV)*. San Antonio, TX: Graywind/Psychological Corporation.

Burke, K. C., Burke, J. D., Regier, D. A., & Rae, D. S. (1990). Age at onset of selected mental disorders in five community populations. *Archives of General Psychiatry, 47,* 511–518.

Chambless, D. L., Caputo, G. C., Bright, P., & Gallagher, R. (1984). Assessment of 'fear of fear' in agoraphobics: The Body Sensations Questionnaire and the Agoraphobic Cognitions Questionnaire. *Journal of Consulting and Clinical Psychology, 52,* 1090–1097.

Chambless, D. L., Caputo, G. C., Jasin, S. E., Gracely, E. J., & Williams, C. (1985). The Mobility Inventory for Agoraphobia. *Behaviour Research and Therapy, 23,* 35–44.

Chambless, D. L., & Mason, J. (1986). Sex, sex-role stereotyping, and agoraphobia. *Behaviour Research and Therapy, 24,* 231–235.

Clark, D. M. (1988). A cognitive model of panic attacks. In S. Rachman & J. D. Maser (Eds.), *Panic: Psychological perspectives*. Hillsdale, NJ: Erlbaum.

Craske, M. G. (1999). *Anxiety disorders: Psychological approaches to theory and treatment*. Boulder, CO: Westview Press.

Craske, M. G. (2003). *Origins of phobias and anxiety disorders: Why more women than men?* Oxford: Elsevier Ltd.

Craske, M. G., & Barlow, D. H. (2001). Panic disorder and agoraphobia. In D. H. Barlow (Ed.), *Clinical handbook of psychological disorders* (3rd ed.). New York: Guilford.

Craske, M. G., Barlow, D. H., & Meadows, E. A. (2000). Mastery of your anxiety and panic: Therapist guide for anxiety, panic, and agoraphobia (MAP-3). San Antonio, TX: Graywind/Psychological Corporation.

Craske, M. G., DeCola, J. P., Sachs, A. D., & Pontillo, D. C. (2003). Panic control treatment for agoraphobia. *Journal of Anxiety Disorders, 17,* 321–333.

Durand, V. M., & Barlow, D. H. (2003). *Essentials of abnormal psychology* (3rd ed.). Pacific Grove, CA: Wadsworth.

Eaton, W. W., Dryman, A., & Weissman, M. M. (1991). Panic and phobia. In L. N. Robins & D. A. Regier (Eds.), *Psychiatric disorders in America: The Epidemiological Catchment Area study*. New York: Free Press.

Edlund, M. J., & Swann, A. C. (1987). The economic and social costs of panic disorder. *Hospital and Community Psychiatry, 38,* 1277–1279.

Ehlers, A. (1995). A 1-year prospective study of panic attacks: Clinical course and factors associated with maintenance. *Journal of Abnormal Psychology, 104,* 164–172.

Eysenck, H. J. (1967). *The biological basis of personality*. Springfield, IL: Thomas.

Gelder, M. G. (1991). Psychological treatment of agoraphobia. *Psychiatric Annals, 21*, 354–357.

Ghosh, A., & Marks, I. M. (1987). Self-directed exposure for agoraphobia: A controlled trial. *Behavior Therapy, 18*, 3–16.

Goisman, R. M., Warshaw, M. G., Peterson, L. G., Rogers, M. P., Cuneo, P., Hunt, M. F., et al. (1994). Panic, agoraphobia, and panic disorder with agoraphobia: Data from a multicenter anxiety disorders study. *Journal of Nervous and Mental Disease, 182*, 72–79.

Goisman, R. M., Warshaw, M. G., Steketee, G. S., Fierman, E. J., Rogers, M. P., Goldenberg, I., et al. (1995). DSM-IV and the disappearance of agoraphobia without a history of panic disorder: New data on a controversial diagnosis. *American Journal of Psychiatry, 152*, 1438–1443.

Goldstein, A. J., & Chambless, D. L. (1978). A re-analysis of agoraphobia. *Behavior Therapy, 9*, 47–59.

Gould, R. A., Clum, G. A., & Shaprio, D. (1993). The use of bibliotherapy in the treatment of panic: A preliminary investigation. *Behavior Therapy, 24*, 241–252.

Hazlett-Stevens, H., & Craske, M. G. (2003). Live (In vivo) exposure. In W. O'Donohue, J. E. Fisher, & S. C. Hayes (Eds.), *Cognitive behavior therapy: Applying empirically supported techniques in your practice.* Hoboken, NJ: Wiley.

Hoffart, A. (1997). Interpersonal problems among patients suffering from panic disorder with agoraphobia before and after treatment. *British Journal of Medical Psychology, 70*, 149–157.

Hoffart, A., Friis, S., Strand, J. & Olsen, B. (1994). Symptoms and cognitions during situational and hyperventilatory exposure in agoraphobic patients with and without panic. *Journal of Psychopathology and Behavioral Assessment, 16*, 15–32.

Hoffart, A., Thornes, K., & Hedley, L. M. (1995). DSM-III-R Axis I and II disorders in agoraphobic inpatients with and without panic disorder before and after psychosocial treatment. *Psychiatry Research, 56*, 1–9.

Holden, A. E., O'Brien, G. T., Barlow, D. H., Stetson, D., & Infantino, A. (1983). Self-help manual for agoraphobia: A preliminary report of effectiveness. *Behavior Therapy, 14*, 545–556.

Horwath, E., Johnson, J., & Hornig, C. D. (1993). Epidemiology of panic disorder in African-Americans. *American Journal of Psychiatry, 150*, 465–469.

Horwath, E., Lish, J. D., Johnson, J., Hornig, C. D., & Weissman, M. M. (1993). Agoraphobia without panic: Clinical reappraisal of an epidemiologic finding. *American Journal of Psychiatry, 150*, 1496–1501.

Kagan, J. (1997). Temperamental contributions to the development of social behavior. In D. Manusson (Ed.), *The lifespan development of individuals: Behavioral, neurological, and psychosocial perspectives, a synthesis.* New York: Cambridge University Press.

Keller, M. B., Yonkers, K. A., Warshaw, M. G., Pratt, L. A., Golan, J., Mathews, A. O., et al., (1994). Remission and relapse in subjects with panic disorder and agoraphobia: A prospective short interval naturalistic follow-up. *Journal of Nervous and Mental Disease, 182*, 290–296.

Kessler, R. C., McGonagle, K. A., Zhao, S., Nelson, C. B., Hughes, M., Eshleman, S., et al., (1994). Lifetime and 12-month prevalence of DSM-III-R psychiatric disorders in the United States. *Archives of General Psychiatry, 51*, 8–19.

Kushner, M. G., Abrams, K., & Borchardt, C. (2000). The relationship between anxiety disorders and alcohol use disorders: A review of major perspectives and findings. *Clinical Psychology Review, 20*, 149–171.

Lydiard, R. B., Brawman-Mintzer, O., & Ballenger, J. C. (1996). Recent developments in the psychopharmacology of anxiety disorders. *Journal of Consulting and Clinical Psychology, 64*, 660–668.

Magee, W. J., Eaton, W. W., Wittchen, H.-U., McGonagle, K. A., & Kessler, R. C. (1996). Agoraphobia, simple phobia, and social phobia in the National Comorbidity Survey. *Archives of General Psychiatry, 53*, 159–168.

Marcaurelle, R., Bélanger, C., & Marchand, A. (2003). Marital relationship and the treatment of panic disorder with agoraphobia: A critical review. *Clinical Psychology Review, 23*, 247–276.

Markowitz, J. S., Weissman, M. M., Ouellette, R., Lish, J. D., & Klerman, G. L. (1989). Quality of life in panic disorder. *Archives of General Psychiatry, 46*, 984–992.

Massion, A. O., Warshaw, M. G., & Keller, M. B. (1993). Quality of life and psychiatric morbidity in panic disorder and generalized anxiety disorder. *American Journal of Psychiatry, 150*, 600–607.

Mennin, D. S., Heimberg, R. G., & Holt, C. S. (2000). Panic, agoraphobia, phobias, and generalized anxiety disorder. In M. Hersen & A. S. Bellack (Eds.), *Psychopathology in adulthood* (2nd ed.). Needham Heights, MA: Allyn & Bacon.

Mowrer, O. H. (1960). *Learning theory and behavior*. New York: Wiley.

Öst, L.-G., & Hugdahl, K. (1983). Acquisition of agoraphobia, mode of onset, and anxiety response patterns. *Behaviour Research and Therapy, 21*, 623–631.

Öst, L.-G., Westling, B. E., & Hellström, K. (1993). Applied relaxation, exposure in vivo and cognitive methods in the treatment of panic disorder with agoraphobia. *Behaviour Research and Therapy, 31*, 383–394.

Paradis, C. M., Hatch, M., & Friedman, S. (1994). Anxiety disorders in African Americans: An update. *Journal of the National Medical Association, 86*, 609–612.

Pollard, C. A., Bronson, S. S., & Kenney, M. R. (1989). Prevalence of agoraphobia without panic in clinical settings. *American Journal of Psychiatry, 146*, 559.

Pollard, C. A., & Henderson, J. G. (1987). Prevalence of agoraphobia: Some confirmatory data. *Psychological Reports, 60,* 1305.

Pollard, C. A., Tait, R. C., Meldrum, D., Dubinsky, I. H., & Gall, J. S. (1996). Agoraphobia without panic: Case illustrations of an overlooked syndrome. *Journal of Nervous and Mental Disease, 184,* 61–62.

Rapee, R. M., Craske, M. G., Brown, T. A., & Barlow, D. H. (1996). Measurement of perceived control over anxiety-related events. *Behavior Therapy, 27,* 279–293.

Reiss, S., Peterson, R. A., Gursky, D. M., & McNally, R. J. (1986). Anxiety sensitivity, anxiety frequency and the prediction of fearfulness. *Behaviour Research and Therapy, 24,* 1–8.

Robins, L. N., Helzer, J. E., Croughan, J., & Ratcliff, K. S. (1981). National Institute of Mental Health Diagnostic Interview Schedule: Its history, characteristics, and validity. *Archives of General Psychiatry, 38,* 381–389.

Robins, L. N., Helzer, J. E., Weissman, M. M., Orvaschel, H., Gruenberg, E., Burke, J. D., et al. (1984). Lifetime prevalence of specific psychiatric disorders in three sites. *Archives of General Psychiatry, 41,* 949–958.

Spierings, E. L. H., Reinders, M. J., & Hoogduin, C. A. L. (1989). The migraine aura as a cause of avoidance behavior. *Headache, 29,* 254–255.

Vasey, M. W., & Dadds, M. R. (2001). An introduction to the developmental psychopathology of anxiety. In M. W. Vasey & M. R. Dadds (Eds.), *The developmental psychopathology of anxiety.* Oxford: Oxford University Press.

Wardle, J., Ahmad, T., & Hayward, P. (1990). Anxiety sensitivity in agoraphobia. *Journal of Anxiety Disorders, 4,* 325–333.

Watson, D., & Clark, L. A. (1984). Negative affectivity: The disposition to experience aversive emotional states. *Psychological Bulletin, 96,* 465–490.

White, K. S., & Barlow, D. H. (2002). Panic disorder and agoraphobia. In D. H. Barlow (ed.), *Anxiety and its disorders: The nature and treatment of anxiety and panic* (2nd ed). New York: Guilford Press.

Wittchen, H.-U., Reed, V., & Kessler, R. C. (1998). The relationship of agoraphobia and panic in a community sample of adolescents and young adults. *Archives of General Psychiatry, 55,* 1017–1024.

World Health Organization. (1990). *Composite International Diagnostic Interview (CIDI), Version 1.0.* Geneva: World Health Organization.

Amnestic Disorder

Barry A. Edelstein • Angela S. Lowery

WHAT IS AN AMNESTIC DISORDER?

Amnestic Disorder is characterized by memory impairment due to a medical condition or the persisting effects of a substance (e.g., toxin, drug abuse). The memory impairment must cause marked impairment in social or occupational functioning and represent a significant decline from previous functioning (American Psychiatric Association, 2002). There are three diagnostic categories of amnestic disorder that are based upon their etiologies: Amnestic Disorder Due to a General Medical Condition (due to the direct physiological effects of a general medical condition), Substance-Induced Persisting Amnestic Disorder (due to the persisting effects of a substance [i.e., a drug of abuse, a medication, or toxin exposure], and Amnestic Disorder Not Otherwise Specified (American Psychiatric Association, p. 156). For the purposes of this chapter, we will address only the first two categories.

Some of the many causes of amnestic disorder associated with general medical conditions include stroke, closed head trauma, herpes simplex encephalitis, anoxia, and hypoglycemia (American Psychiatric Association, 2002; Cummings & Trimble, 2002). Substances that can cause substance-induced amnestic disorder include, for example, alcohol, sedatives, anxiolytics, and hypnotics (American Psychiatric Association, 2002).

IMPORTANT MEMORY CATEGORIES AND TERMS

Short-term memory. Short-term memory is memory demonstrated immediately after presentation of material to be learned without presentation of an intervening distractor (Cummings & Trimble, 2002; Squire, 1987).

Long-term memory. Long-term memory is memory that is not short term and includes semantic memory (memory for general knowledge), episodic memory (memory for autobiographical events), and procedural memory (memory for skills or cognitive operations (Cummings & Trimble, 2002; Squire, 1987).

Recall. Recall of information is divided into retrieval (activation of long term memory) and recognition (identification of previously learned information).

Retrograde amnesia. Inability to recall or recognize information or events from before the onset of amnesia.

Anterograde amnesia. Inability to recall or recognize new information or events.

Post-traumatic amnesia. Inability to recall memories that are lost after a trauma.

Memory may be classified in terms of the sensory modality through which information is coded and recalled (e.g., visual, auditory, tactile, olfactory).

BASIC FACTS ABOUT AMNESTIC DISORDER

- No prevalence figures are available for Amnestic Disorder, perhaps because it can accompany so many different conditions and disorders, and because of the multitude of possible etiologies.

Edelstein, B. A. & Lowery, A. S. (2006). Amnestic disorder. In J. E. Fishers & W. T. O'Donohue (Eds.), *Practitioner's guide to evidence-based psychotherapy.* New York: Springer.

- The course of amnestic disorders tend to be variable depending upon the etiology, with head trauma or stroke causing acute onsets and prolonged exposure to toxic substances often leading to a lengthy onset.
- The disorder can occur at all ages.
- Individuals with Amnestic Disorder can retain a limited amount of information for a short period of time. Immediate and working memory are usually unimpaired (O'Connor & Verfaellie, 2002).
- Many individuals with severe Amnestic Disorder may deny their memory impairment even when evidence to the contrary is presented.
- Most individuals with Amnestic Disorder lack insight into their memory impairment, although some may acknowledge the impairment but appear unconcerned (American Psychiatric Association, 2002).
- The nature of the memory impairment in amnestic disorders is determined in part by the etiology. One type of memory can be affected without any apparent impairment in other types.
- The greatest impairment is with episodic memory (Tulving, 1983).
- Procedural memory involving previously learned skills, habits, and classically conditioned responses tend to be spared.
- General reasoning abilities are spared (O'Connor & Verfaellie, 2002).

ASSESSMENT

What should be ruled out?

Delirium and dementia, which both can present with memory impairment, must be ruled out. Dementia involves other cognitive deficits such as problems with executive functioning, and delirium involves problems with the ability to focus, shift, or sustain attention. Amnestic disorder must also be distinguished from the amnesia that accompanies dissociative disorders. By definition, amnesia associated with amnestic disorder must result from a medical condition or substance use; however, dissociative amnesias typically do not. Also, dissociative amnesias often involve difficulty recalling events, but no difficulty with learning new information. Amnestic Disorder must be distinguished from memory blackouts that may accompany substance intoxication or substance withdrawal. If the memory loss occurs during intoxication or withdrawal, Amnestic Disorder should not be diagnosed. Amnestic Disorder must be distinguished from malingering or factitious disorder. Finally, amnestic disorder should be distinguished from age-related decline in memory.

What is Involved in Effective Assessment

Memory can be assessed informally through a conversation with the patient that includes some discussion of the patient's history. For example, recent episodic memory can be assessed by noting whether the patient is oriented to person and time. Information about recent personal and public events can be requested. Long-term or remote memory can be informally assessed by asking questions about work history, children, education, and so on.

Memory assessment is one element of a comprehensive cognitive assessment and might include the following (Wilson, 2002, p. 617–618):

- What is the person's general level of intellectual functioning?
- What was the probable level of premorbid functioning
- Does this person have an organic memory deficit?
- Is there a difference in ability between recognition and recall tasks?
- Is there a difference between verbal and visual memory ability?

- To what extent are the memory problems due to language, perceptual or attention deficits?
- How do these scores compare with people of the same age in the general population?

Information is necessary for establishing the context in which the memory assessment results are interpreted and how memory impairment may be affecting the individual's life. Though standardized tests are useful for establishing the nature of the memory impairment and a diagnosis, they are less useful for identifying deficits that affect everyday activities and that might be considered when formulating treatment or rehabilitation (Chaytor & Schmitter-Edgecombe, 2003; Wilson, 2002). More ecologically valid assessment is necessary in such cases, which is often accomplished through functional assessment (e.g., Rivermead Behavioural Memory Test (RBMT: Wilson, Cockburn, & Baddeley, 1985).

When considering treatment or rehabilitation, Wilson (2002, p. 618) recommends addressing the following questions:

- What problems are causing the greatest difficulty for this person and the family?
- What coping strategies are used?
- Are the problems exacerbated by anxiety or depression?
- Can this person return home/to school/to work?
- Should we try to restore lost functioning or teach compensatory strategies?

For a thorough memory assessment, Wilson (2002, p. 624) recommends attention to the following:

- Orientation to time, place, and person.
- Immediate memory, including verbal, visual and spatial short-term/immediate memory.
- Delayed episodic memory, including visual recall, visual recognition, verbal recall and verbal recognition.
- New episodic learning, including verbal, visual, and spatial.
- Implicit memory, including, perhaps, motor, verbal and visual aspects of implicit memory.
- Remote memory, to look at retrograde amnesia—one may want to subdivide this into personal/autobiographical memory and memory for public information.
- Prospective memory, perhaps subdivided into remembering to do things (a) at a given time, (b) within a certain time interval, and (c) when a certain event happens.
- Semantic memory, for both verbal and visual material.

Commonly Used Empirically Supported Instruments

Standardized, empirically supported assessment instruments should be used in determining diagnosis, and may be useful in evaluating the effects of treatment (cf. Hunsley, Crabb, & Mash, 2004).

Anterograde memory (memory for new information) *Wechsler Memory Scale (WMS-III; The Psychological Corporation, 1997).*

- Examines initial learning, learning over trials, short-term memory, working memory, and long-term memory after a short delay.
- Thirty to 35 minutes to administer all primary subtests.
- The normative sample for ages 16–89 years.
- Includes 11 subtests (six primary and five optional) measuring eight indexes.

- Visual immediate and delayed index scores reflect memory of material presented visually.
- Auditory immediate and auditory delayed index scores reflect memory of material presented verbally.
- Working memory index reflects ability to hold information and to give a response based on that information.
- Auditory recognition delayed index reflects recognition of verbal tasks presented previously.
- General memory index consists of the summation of delayed subtest scores, and the immediate memory index consists of the summation of immediate subtest scores.
- New edition is currently under development.

The Rivermead Behavioral Memory Test (RBMT; Wilson et al., 1985)

- Useful for assessing memory for tasks needed in everyday life (de Wall, Wilson, & Baddeley, 1994; van Balen, Westzaan, & Mulder, 1996, Wills, Clare, Sheil, & Wilson, 2000;)
- Consists of 12 tasks such as remembering where an item was hidden, pictures, a route, or names.
- Test requires approximately 25 minutes to administer.
- Four parallel forms available.
- Normative sample for ages 5–96 years (Martin, West, Cull, & Adams, 2000).
- Extended version (Wilson et al., 1999) combines two parallel forms
- Second Extended RBMT created for those with restricted mobility (Clare, Wilson, Emslie, Tate, & Watson, 2000).

The Rey Auditory Verbal Learning Test (RAVLT; Rey, 1964).

- Assesses immediate memory span, short-term memory, and long-term memory.
- Consists of five presentations of 15 words, a single presentation of 15 different words, a recall of the original 15 words, and a delayed recall and recognition of the original 15 words.
- Administration of the initial presentation trials takes about 15 minutes.
- Normative data for ages 7–89 years.
- Requires 10–15 minutes to administer.

Hopkins Verbal Learning Test-Revised (HVLT-R; Benedict, Schretlen, Groninger, & Brandt, 1998; Brandt, 1991)

- Assesses learning, short-term retention, and long-term retention of word lists.
- Includes three trials in which the list of 12 words are read at two second intervals.
- Trials are followed by a 20–25 minutes delay before recall.
- Final recognition memory trial.
- Normative data for ages 16 and older.
- Requires 5–10 minutes to complete plus a 25 minute delay.
- Six forms of HVLT-R (Shapiro, Benedict, Schretlen, & Brandt, 1999).

Rey–Osterrieth Complex Figure Test (ROCFT; Osterrieth, 1944; Rey, 1942).

- Measure of long-term visual and episodic memory (Deckersbach et al., 2000; Lu, Boone, Cozolino, & Mitchell, 2003).
- Involves copying a complex design and then reproducing it from memory after a delay (anywhere from 30 seconds to 30 minutes).
- Normative sample for ages 6–89.
- Requires 45 minutes to administer, including a 30-minute delay.

Retrograde memory (memory for previously acquired information). *Autobiographical Memory Interview (AMI; Kopelman, Wilson, & Baddeley, 1990a,b)*—comprises two subtests: the Personal Semantic Memory Schedule and the Autobiographical Incidents Schedule (Kopelman, 1994; Mayes, 1995)

- Personal Semantic Memory Schedule—examinees answer questions related to past (e.g., schools attended, dates and places of marriages, addresses).
- Autobiographical Incidents Schedule—examinees given prompts to recall.
- Normative data for ages 18 and older.

Public Events Test (Cohen & Squire, 1981)
- Requires answers to questions related to public events from the 1950s and later (Mangels, Gershberg, Shimamura, & Knight 1996)

The Famous Faces Test (Hodges, Salmon, & Butters, 1993)

- Requires naming of person shown in each of 85 black-and-white photographs of famous actors, politicians, etc. (Mangels et al., 1996).

    One of the potential problems of using published standardized tests is that they are not necessarily ecologically valid (see Chaytor & Schmitter-Edgecombe, 2003). Nevertheless, they can offer important information for establishing a diagnosis and the monitoring of treatment progress.

    When training memory for everyday material (e.g., when to take a pill, where one's room is located), clinicians often create their own, perhaps more externally valid, indices of memory.

Treatment Much of the evidence-based literature on the treatment of amnestic disorder has not been critically reviewed in recent years. The last such review (Franzen and Haut, 1991), found little systematic research and well controlled treatment outcome studies. Unfortunately, this continues to characterize the literature, though to a lesser degree.

    Most researchers agree that the direct restoration of memory among individuals with amnestic disorder is not possible (Berg, Koning-Haanstra & Deelman, 1991; Wilson & Moffat, 1992). Thus, most approaches to the psychological treatment of amnestic disorder have involved *environmental adaptations, techniques to improve memory, and external memory aids*, while attempting to optimize preserved cognitive abilities.

    Several approaches to the treatment of amnestic disorder have some empirical support, although many treatment studies involve case studies, small sample sizes, and single-subject designs without replications.

Environmental Adaptations
Many memory-impaired individuals can be helped through adaptations of their environments to provide environmental support (see Craik et al., 1995). The goal is to provide cues that facilitate the retrieval of information or that merely set the occasion for automatic responses.

Examples:

- Labeling of kitchen cabinets with regard to their contents.
- Placing a stop sign at a point beyond which the individual is not to proceed.
- Using cookers that turn themselves off after a period of time.
- Positioning of objects to be remembered in the home so they cannot be missed.
- Placing a chalkboard in a conspicuous with a list of activities and their times for each day.

Techniques for Improving Memory

Most research that has attempted to teach new learning through simple repetitive practice has been unsuccessful (Godfrey & Knight, 1988; Prigatano et al., 1984; Wilson, 2003). Rehearsal strategies can improve memory by repetition when performed using specific mnemonic strategies.

- *Spaced retrieval strategy (Landauer and Bjork (1978).* Involves gradually increasing the interval between rehearsal and testing through distributed practice. The material to be learned is rehearsed repeatedly, with increasingly longer delays between rehearsal and information retrieval (see Wilson & Moffat, 1992; Schacter, Rich, & Stampp, 1985).
- *Errorless discrimination training (Baddeley & Wilson, 1994).* This is perhaps the most well supported approach to memory impairment. The learner is not permitted to make errors. While memory intact individuals can learn from errors, a memory impaired person cannot recall the errors and therefore cannot use this information in the future. Through the repetition of errors, they can be strengthened over time. This approach has been successful with amnestic individuals (see Kessels & de Haan, 2003, for a meta-analysis).

External Memory Aids

External aids can be used to compensate for memory loss. For example, these might take the form of calendars, tape recorders, personal digital assistants (PDAs), notebooks, and diaries. Wilson (2003) has concluded that these aids are perhaps the most beneficial for compensating for memory loss but are often difficult to learn to use. One of the problems is that the appropriate utilization of some of these aids involves the use of memory. Thus, individuals tend to forget to use, enter data, or retrieve it from these devices. Cicerone, et al. (2000) conducted an exhaustive review and analysis of existing research concerning the effectiveness of cognitive rehabilitation for individuals with traumatic brain injury or stroke. The authors of this manuscript comprised the Cognitive Rehabilitation Committee of the Brain-Injury-Interdisciplinary Special Interest Group of the American Congress of Rehabilitation Medicine. Their goal was to establish evidence-based recommendations for clinical practice. Among the topics addressed was the remediation of memory deficits. The Committee found the evidence for the effectiveness of compensatory memory training for subjects with mild memory impairments compelling enough to recommend it as a Practice Standard. The evidence also suggests that memory remediation is most effective when subjects are fairly independent in daily function, are actively involved in identifying the memory problem to be treated, and are capable and motivated to continue active, independent strategy use (Cicerone et al., p. 1605).

Examples *Memory book/journal (see Donaghy & Williams, 1998; Ownsworth and McFarland, 1999; Sohlberg & Mateer, 1989).* These books often contain autobiographical material and other information that the individual would find useful on a daily basis. Implementation of memory books can be challenging due to patient overestimation of cognitive abilities, failure to accept methods that call attention to the memory loss, and unwillingness to admit the need for a memory book (see Fluharty & Priddy, 1993).

Portable timer (e.g., Gouvier, 1982). Timers are used to cue indivduals to perform specific behaviors at specific times.

Computers (e.g., Kirsch, Levin, Simon, Fallon-Krueger, & Jaros, 1987). Computers are used in many ways, for example, to guide amnestic individuals through the steps of a household task.

NeuroPage system (Hersh & Treadgold, 1994). NeuroPage system is a centralized system that permits memory impaired individuals to be electronically paged (i.e., receive a specific message) to cue them to perform a behavior (e.g., take a pill, feed the cat). See the work of Wilson and colleagues (e.g., Evans, Emslie & Wilson, 1998; Wilson, Emslie, Quirk & Evans, 1999). A system similar to the NeuroPage developed by Davis (1999, as cited in Wilson, 2003) permits individuals to program their own page message using the internet. See Wilson, Evans, Emslie & Malinek (1997) for more detail on the NeuroPage system.

CONCLUSIONS

In their review of psychological treatments of memory impairment, Franzen & Haut (1991) concluded that "...it may be possible to positively intervene with memory impairment. However, there are multiple shortcomings in the extant literature that may limit the confidence that we can place in such a conclusion" (p. 54). Almost 15 years later the picture has improved but continues to suffer from a paucity of research addressing the treatment of amnestic disorders. Some approaches are effective but require so much time and effort (e.g, Glisky & Schacter, 1987) that they are impractical in these times of managed care. The compensatory strategies appear to hold the most hope for amnestic individuals, particularly those with severe memory impairment. There are many possible ways of enabling amnestic individuals to compensate for some of their memory loss. However, as Kapur (1995) has observed, the literature is not sufficiently well developed to permit us to state with confidence which memory aids benefit which memory problems in particular amnestic individuals. Kapur concluded that we need to know if the magnitude of any benefit to clients is significant and makes a meaningful difference in their everyday adjustment, if the change is permanent and if it is cost-effective in terms of money and in therapists' time (p. 550).

What are Effective Self-Help Treatments?

Numerous self-help guides for the improvement of memory appear in the literature and bookstores. However, these guides are intended for relatively mild, nonpathological memory loss. There are no empirically supported self-help treatments for amnestic disorders, as the associated memory impairment usually precludes the learning of new information.

Useful websites http://www.biausa.org—Brain Injury Association
http://naric.com—National Rehabilitation Information Center
http://www.ninds.nih.gov—National Institute of Neurological Disorders and Stroke

Other issues in management A significant problem with psychological interventions for memory impairment that involve skill training is the transfer or generalization of training across situations (Edelstein, 1989; Franzen & Haut, 1991). Treatment may need to continue for months to achieve generalization.

How Does One Select Among Treatments?

Selection among treatments is not straightforward because of the difficulty of matching the specific memory deficits to the available treatments, as noted by Franzen & Haut (1991). For the most part the treatment should take into consideration the deficits and spared abilities of the individual. Though memory training may be effective with mild memory impairment, severely impaired individuals will undoubtedly benefit most from compensatory and environmental modification strategies.

KEY READINGS

Butters, N. & Delis, D. C. (1995). Clinical assessment of memory disorders in amnesia and dementia. *Annual Review of Psychology, 46,* 493–523.

Glisky, E. L., & Glisky, M. L. (1999). Cognitive neurorehabilitation. In D. T., Stuss, G. Winocur, & I. H. Robertson (Eds.). *Cognitive rehabilitation.* United Kingdom: Cambridge University Press.

Kapur, N., Glisky, E. L., & Wilson, B. A. (2002). External memory aids and computers in memory rehabilitation. In A. D. Baddeley, M. Kopelman, & B. A. Wilson (Eds). *The Handbook of memory disorders* (2nd ed., pp. 757–783). New York: Wiley.

O'Connor, M., & Verfaellie, M. (2002). The amnestic syndrome: Overview and subtypes. In A. D. Baddeley, M. Kopelman & B. A. Wilson (Eds.) *The handbook of memory disorders* (2nd ed., pp. 145–166). West Sussex, England: Wiley.

Wilson, B. A. (2000). Compensating for cognitive deficits following brain injury. *Neuropsychology Review, 10,* 233–243.

Wilson, B. A. (2002). Assessment of memory disorders. In A. D. Baddeley, M. Kopelman & B. A. Wilson (Eds.) *The handbook of memory disorders* (2nd ed., pp. 617–654). West Sussex, England: Wiley.

REFERENCES

American Psychiatric Association. (2000). *Diagnostic and Statistical Manual of Mental Disorders* (4th ed., text revision). Washington, DC: Author.

Baddeley, A. D., & Wilson, B. A. (1994). When implicit learning fails: Amnesia and the problem of error elimination. *Neuropsychologia, 32,* 53–68.

Benedict, R. H., Schretlen, D., Groninger, L., & Brandt, J. (1998). Hopkins Verbal Learning Test-Revised: Normative data and analysis of inter-form and test-retest reliability. *The Clinical Neuropsychologist, 12,* 43–55.

Berg, I., Konning-Haanstra, M., & Deelman, B. (1991). Long term effects of memory rehabilitation: A controlled study. *Neuropsychological Rehabilitation, 1,* 97–111.

Brandt, J. (1991). The Hopkins Verbal Learning Test: Development of a new memory test with six equivalent forms. *The Clinical Neuropsychologist, 5,* 125–142.

Chaytor, N., & Schmitter-Edgecombe, M. (2003). The ecological validity of neuropsychological tests: A review of the literature on everyday cognitive skills. *Neuropsychology Review, 13,* 181–197.

Cicerone, K. D., Dahlberg, C., Kalmar, D., Langebahy, D. M., Malec, J. M., Berquist, T. F., et al. (2000). Evidence-based cognitive rehabilitation: Recommendations for clinical practice. *Archives of Physical Medicine and Rehabilitation, 81,* 1596–1615.

Clare, L., Wilson, B. A., Emslie, H., Tate, R., & Watson, P. (2000). Adapting the Rivermead Behavioural Memory Test Extended Version (RBMT-E) for people with restricted mobility. *British Journal of Clinical Psychology, 39,* 363–369.

Cohen, N. J., & Squire, L. R. (1981). Retrograde amnesia and remote memory impairment. *Neuropsychologia, 19,* 337–356.

Craik, F. I. M., Anderson, N. D., Kerr, S. QA., & Li, K. Z. H. (1995). Memory changes in normal aging. In A. D. Badeley, B. A. Wilson, & F. N. Watts (Eds.) *Handbook of memory disorders* (pp. 211–241). Chichester: Wiley.

Cummings, J. L., & Trimble, M. R. (2002). *Concise guide to neuropsychiatry and behavioral neurology* (2nd ed.). Washington, DC: American Psychiatric Publishing.

de Wall, C., Wilson, B. A., & Baddeley, A. D. (1994). The Extended Rivermead Behavioural Memory Test: A measure of everyday memory performance in normal adults. *Memory, 2,* 149–166.

Deckersbach, T., Savage, C. R., Henin, A., Mataix-Cols, D., Otto, M. W., Wilhelm, S., et al. (2000). Reliability and validity of a scoring system for measuring organizational approach in the Complex Figure Test. *Journal of Experimental Neuropsychology, 22,* 640–648.

Delaney, R. C., Prevey, M. L., Cramer, J., & Mattson, R. H. (1992). Test–retest comparability and control subject data for the Rey–Auditory Verbal Learning Test and Rey–Osterrieth/Taylor Complex Figures. *Archives of Clinical Neuropsychology, 7,* 523–528.

Donaghy, W., & Williams, W. (1998). A new protocol for training severely impaired patients in the usage of memory journals. *Brain Injury, 12,* 1061–1076.

Edelstein, B. A. (1989). Generalization: Terminological, methodological, and conceptual issues. *Behavior Therapy, 20,* 311–324.

Edelstein, B. A. & Couture, E. T. (Eds.) (1984). *Behavioral assessment and rehabilitation of the traumatically brain-damaged.* New York: Plenum Press.

Evans, J. J., Emslie, H., & Wilson, B. A. (1998). External cueing systems in the rehabilitation of executive impairments of action. *Journal of the International Neuropsychological Society, 4,* 399–408.

Fluharty, G., & Priddy, D. (1993). Methods of increasing client acceptance of a memory book. *Brain Injury, 7,* 85–88.

Franzen, M. D., & Haut, M. W. (1991). The psychological treatment of memory impairment: A review of empirical studies. *Neuropsychology Review, 2,* 29–63.

Glisky, E. L. & Schacter, D. L. (1987). Acquisition of domain-specific knowledge in organic amnesia: Training for computer-related work. *Neuropsychologia, 25,* 893–906.

Godfrey, H. P. D., & Knight, R. G. (1988). Memory training and behavioral rehabilitation of a severely head-injured adult. *Archives of Physical Medicine and Rehabilitation, 69,* 458–460.

Gouvier, W. D. (1982). Using the digital alarm chronograph in memory training. *Behavioral Engineering, 7,* 134.

Hersh, N., & Treadgold, L. (1994). NeuroPage: The rehabilitation of memory dysfunction by prosthetic memory and cueing. *NeuroRehabilitation, 4,* 187–197.

Hodges, J. R., Salmon, D. P., & Butters, N. (1993). Recognition and naming of famous faces in Alzheimer's disease: A cognitive analysis. *Neuropsychologia, 31,* 775–788.

Kapur, N. (1995). Memory aids in the rehabilitation of memory disordered patients. In A. D. Baddeley, B. A. Wilson, & E. N. Watts (Eds.), *The Handbook of memory disorders* (pp. 533–556). New York: Wiley.

Kessels, R., & de Haan, E. H. (2003). Implicit learning in memory rehabilitation: A meta-analysis on errorless learning and vanishing cues methods. *Journal of Clinical and Experimental Neuropsychology, 6,* 805–814.

Kirsch, H., Levine, S.P., Fallon-Krueger, M., & Jaros, L. A. (1987). The microcomputer as an "orthotic device" for patients with cognitive deficits. *Journal of Head Trauma Rehabilitation, 2,* 77–86.

Kitchener, E. G., & Squire, L. R. (2000). Impaired verbal category learning in amnesia. *Behavioral Neurosciences, 114,* 907–911.

Kopelman, M. D. (1994). The Autobiographical Memory Interview (AMI) in organic and psychogenic amnesia. *Memory, 2,* 211–235.

Kopelman, M. D., Wilson, B. A., and Baddeley, A. (1990a). *The Autobiographical Memory Interview* (Manual). Bury Saint Edmunds, UK: Thames Valley Test Company.

Landauer, T. K., & Bjork, R. A. (1978). Optimum rehearsal paterns and name learning. In M. M. Gruneberg, P. E. Morris, & R. N. Sykes (Eds)., *Practical aspects of memory* (pp. 625–632). London: Academic Press.

Lu, P., Boone, K. B., Cozolino, L., & Mitchell, C. (2003). Effectiveness of the Rey-Osterrieth Complex Figure Test and the Meyers and Meyers Recognition Trial in the detection of suspect effort. *The Clinical Neuropsychologist, 17,* 426–440.

Mangels, J. A., Gershberg, F. B., Shimamura, A. P., & Knight, R. T. (1996). Impaired retrieval from remote memory in patients with frontal lobe damage. *Neuropsychology, 10,* 32–41.

Martin, C., West, J., Cull, C., & Adams, M. (2000). A preliminary study investigating how people with mild intellectual disabilities perform on the Rivermead Behavioural Memory Test. *Journal of Applied Research in Intellectual Disabilities, 13,* 186–193.

Mayes, A. R. (1995). The assessment of memory disorders. In A. D. Baddeley, B. A. Wilson, & F. N. Watts (Eds.), *Handbook of memory disorders* (pp. 367–391). New York: Wiley.

Moffat, N. (1992). Strategies of memory therapy. In B. A. Wilson & N. Moffat (Eds.). *Clinical management of memory problems* (pp. 86–119). London: Chapman & Hall.

O'Connor, M., & Verfaellie, M. (2002). The amnestic syndrome: Overview and subtypes. In A. D. Baddeley, M. Kopelman & B. A. Wilson (Eds.) *The handbook of memory disorders* (2nd ed., pp. 145–166). West Sussex, England: Wiley.

Osterrieth, P. A. (1944). Le test du copie d'une figure complex. *Archives of Psychology, 30,* 206–356.

Ownsworth, T. L., & McFarland, K. (1999). Memory remediation in long-term acquired brain injury: Two approaches in diary training. *Brain Injury, 13,* 605–626.

Prigatano, G. P., Fordyce, D. J., Zeiner, H. K., Roueche, J. R., Pepping, M., & Wood, B. C. (1984). Neuropsychological rehabiltation afater closed head injury in young adults. *Journal of Neurology, Neurosurgery, and Psychiatry, 47,* 505–513.

Rey, A. (1942). L'examen psychologique dans les cas d(encephalopathie traumatique. *Archives of Psychology, 28,* 286–340.

Rey, A. (1964). *L'examen clinique en psychologie.* Paris: Presses Universitaires de France.

Schacter, D. L., Rich, S. A., & Stampp, M. S. (1985). Remediation of meory disorders: Experimental evaluatin of the spaced-retrieval technique. *Journal of Clinical and Experimental Neuropsychology, 7,* 79–96.

Shapiro, A. M., Benedict, R. H., Schretlen, D., & Brandt, J. (1999). Construct and concurrent validity of the Hopkins Verbal Learning Test-Revised. *The Clinical Neuropsychologist, 13,* 348–358.

Sohlberg, M. M., & Mateer, C. A. (1989). Training use of compensatory memory books: A three-stage behavioral approach. *Journal of Clinical and Experimental Neuropsychology, 11,* 871–891.

Squire, L. (1987). *Memory and brain.* New York: Oxford University Press.

The Psychological Corporation. (1997). *WMS-III technical manual.* San Antonio, TX: The Psychological Corportation.

Tulving, E. (1983). *Elements of episodic memory.* New York: Oxford.

van Balen, H. G., Westzaan, P. S., & Mulder, T. (1996). Stratified norms for the Rivermead Behavioural Memory Test. *Neuropsychological Rehabilitation, 6,* 203–217.

Wills, P., Clare, L., Shiel, A., & Wilson, B. A. (2000). Assessing subtle memory impairments in the everyday memory performance of brain injured people: exploring the potential of the Extended Rivermead Behavioural Memory Test. *Brain Injury, 14,* 693–704.

Wilson, B. A. (1989). Models of cognitive rehabilitation. In R. L. Wood & P. Eames (Eds.). *Models of brain injury rehabilitation* (pp. 117–141). London: Chapman & Hall.

Wilson, B. A. (1991). Long term prognosis of patients with severe memory disorders. *Neuropsychological Rehabilitation, 1,* 117–134.

Wilson, B. A. (2002). Assessment of memory disorders. In A. D. Baddeley, M. Kopelman & B. A. Wilson (Eds.) *The handbook of memory disorders* (2nd ed., pp. 617–654). West Sussex, England: Wiley.

Wilson, B. A. (2003). Memory rehabilitation. In J. Grafman & I. H. Robertson (Eds.), *Handbook of neuropsychology* (2nd Ed, pp. 37–53). Oxford: Elsevier Science.

Wilson, B. A., Clare, L., Baddeley, A. D., Cockburn, J., Watson, P., & Tate, R. (1999). *The Rivermead Behavioural Memoy Test-Extended Version (RBMT-E).* Bury Saint Edmunds: Thames Valley Test Company.

Wilson, B. A., Cockburn, J., & Baddeley, A. D. (1985). *The Rivermead Behavioural Memory Test.* Titchfield, Fareham, Hants: Thames Valley Test Company.

Wilson, B. A., & Moffat, N. (1992). The development of group memory therapy. In B. A. Wilson & N. Moffat (Eds.), *Clinical management of memory problems* (2nd ed, pp. 243–273). London: Chapman & Hall.

Anorexia Nervosa

Kathleen M. Pike • B. Timothy Walsh • Christina Roberto

WHAT IS ANOREXIA NERVOSA?

The hallmark feature of anorexia nervosa (AN) is a refusal to maintain weight at or above that which is recommended based on age and height. The DSM-IV suggests a guideline of 85% of ideal body weight as the threshold for AN. The International Classification of Mental and Behavioral Disorders, tenth edition (ICD-10, World Health Organization, 1992) utilizes the measure of body mass index (BMI) and specifies a more stringent weight threshold of 17.5 kg/m^2 for AN. Although the principle of low weight as a defining feature of AN is consistent across diagnostic systems, the exact weight threshold necessary to diagnose AN varies and assessment of this criterion requires clinical judgment that takes into consideration an individual's age, stage of physical maturation, pre-morbid weight status, weight history, and (for females) weight at which menses were regularly cyclical.

In addition to the prominent feature of emaciation, AN is also characterized by psychological disturbances related to weight and shape concern, perception of weight and shape, and overvaluation of oneself as a function of weight and shape. These dimensions of disturbance are captured in the second and third diagnostic criteria for AN. The second diagnostic criterion for AN is an intense fear of gaining weight or becoming fat. Similar to the assessment of low weight, this criterion is clear in principle but oftentimes difficult to assess clinically. In particular, younger patients and those not motivated for treatment often deny a fear of weight gain, despite exhibiting behaviors that indicate an intense fear of fatness. In addition, cultural differences have been reported on this dimension (Eating Disorders Commission, 2005). AN is also characterized by an undue influence of shape and weight on self-evaluation and disturbed cognitions regarding body image. Such cognitive distortions may include a lack of concern about the health risks associated with extremely low body weight or a distorted perception that one is fat in spite of his or her visibly emaciated state (Eating Disorders Commission, 2005).

The final symptom included in the DSM-IV is an absence of three or more consecutive menstrual cycles in pre-menopausal females and a lack of sexual potency or drive in males. The absence of menses is an important clinical indicator of potential disturbances in hypothalamic function, osteoporosis, and/or infertility (Herzog & Delinsky, 2001). Yet, recent research finds no difference between individuals who meet full criteria for AN and those who experience all of the symptoms except amenorrhea (Cachelin & Maher, 1998; Garfinkel et al., 1996). Although its nosological importance is currently unclear, amenorrhea unequivocally has clinical significance as a marker of physical health on numerous biological systems, and therefore is important to assess and monitor in clinical practice.

Subtypes. The DSM-IV specifies two subtypes of AN, which are distinguished by the presence or absence of bulimic behaviors. Individuals who rely on dieting, fasting or excessive exercise to lose or maintain a low weight are classified as having

Pike K. M., Walsh, T. & Roberto, C. (2006). Anorexia nervosa. In J. E. Fisher & W. T. O'Dononue (Eds.), *Practitioner's guide to evidence-based psychotherapy.* New York: Springer.

restricting type AN. AN individuals who engage in bulimic behaviors such as binge eating and purging are classified as having AN-Binge/Purge type. People with Binge/Purge type tend to engage in more impulsive self-harming behaviors, such as self-mutilation, stealing, suicide attempts, and alcohol/substance abuse, than those with restricting AN (DaCosta & Halmi., 1991; Halmi et al, 2002; Stock, Goldberg, Corbett, & Katzman, 2002).

Differentiating between Anorexia Nervosa and Bulimia Nervosa. The eating disorder most closely related to AN is bulimia nervosa (BN). Differentiating these disorders is based on the primary distinction of weight status. Whereas individuals with AN have suppressed weight status, individuals with BN typically fall within the normal weight range of the population. If individuals engage in the bulimic behaviors of binge eating and/or purging and meet criteria for low weight status they almost always receive a diagnosis of AN restricting type. If they are normal weight and engage in binge eating and compensatory behaviors at the thresholds specified in the DSM-IV they receive a diagnosis of BN. It is notable that the disturbances of binge eating and compensatory behaviors are more thoroughly defined with clear behavioral guidelines for BN as compared to AN. Behavioral definitions of binge eating and frequency thresholds are not specified for AN, and individuals with AN may meet criteria for AN-Binge/Purge type if they engage in *either* binge eating or purging, i.e, both disturbances are not required.

AN and BN are closely related disorders, particularly for a subgroup of individuals. A significant minority of individuals with AN will go on to develop BN (Bulik, Sullivan, Fear & Pickering,1997; Herzog & Delinsky, 2001) and a significant minority of individuals with BN report past histories of AN (Braun, Sunday, & Halmi 1994; Keel, Mitchell, Miller, Davis & Crow, 2000).

Associated psychopathology. In addition to potential migration within eating disorders, for individuals with AN, lifetime co-morbidity of other psychiatric conditions is approximately 80% (Halmi et al., 1991). Lifetime co-morbidity of major depressive disorder is approximately 50–65% (Herzog, Nussbaum, & Marmor, 1996). Similarly high rates of comorbid anxiety disorders have been reported (Godart, Flament, Perdereau, & Jeammet, 2002; Halmi et al., 1991).

Epidemiology. AN occurs in approximately 1% of the female population and prevalence rates for men are approximately one tenth of rates for women (Hoek, 2002). Some data suggest that prevalence rates among Caucasian populations are greater among higher socioeconomic status groups, though this is not the case in all cultures (Walters & Kendler, 1995). Emerging epidemiological data from around the globe suggest a rise of eating disorders, including AN, among a wide range of non-Caucasian groups (Nasser, Katzman, & Gordon, 2001). Research across cultures suggests that immigration, greater levels of Western acculturation, and industrialization are related to higher rates of eating disorder symptoms (Becker, Burwell, Gilman, Herzog, & Hamburg, 2002; Davis & Katzman, 1999; Gowen, Hayward, Killen, Robinson & Taylor, 1999; Hooper & Garner, 1986; Nasser et al., 2001).

Course of illness. The typical period of onset for the disorder is adolescence and early adulthood (Mitrany, Lubin, Chetrit, & Modan, 1995; Stice, Killen, Hayward, & Taylor, 1998; Walters & Kendler, 1995; Woodside & Garfinkel, 1992). Approximately 40% of individuals with AN recover (Herzog, Deber, & Vandereycken, 1992) Thirty percent improve and 20% are chronically ill, with 10–20% losing their life to the physical complications of starvation or suicide (Steinhausen et al., 1991). Adolescent onset of the disorder is linked to a better prognosis than adult or childhood onset.

What are the Risk Factors for Anorexia Nervosa?

AN is a multi-determined disorder, and a variety of environmental and genetic factors may increase the risk of developing this life threatening illness. The primary risk factors that have been documented for AN are highlighted below. For a comprehensive review of risk factors for eating disorders readers are referred to Jacobi, Hayward, de Zwaan, Kraemer, & Agras (2004).

Gender. One of the most established risk factors for AN is gender, with women comprising more than 90% of AN cases (American Psychiatric Association, 1994).

Dieting. Several studies have found that adolescent fear of weight gain; negative body image, body dissatisfaction, and particularly dieting behavior predict later eating disturbances (Attie & Brooks-Gunn, 1989; Ghaderi & Scott, 2001; Hsu, 1990; Polivy & Herman, 1985; Jacobi et al., 2004).

Sexual abuse and adverse events. Adverse life events and sexual abuse are associated with eating disorders (Wonderlich, Brewerton, Jocic, Dansky, & Abbott, 1997). Within the studies on sexual abuse, some data suggest that childhood sexual abuse is more strongly associated with the binge/purge subtype of AN as compared to restricting AN. Although a risk factor for a significant minority of individuals with eating disorders, the data consistently indicate that childhood sexual abuse is not a specific risk factor for the development of eating disorders. The rate of childhood sexual abuse among individuals with eating disorders is comparable to the rate reported among women with other psychiatric disorders (Webster & Palmer, 2000; Wonderlich et al., 1997).

Family and early eating and digestive problems. Individuals with eating disorders describe more eating conflicts, struggles around meals, and general family dysfunction than do healthy controls (Kotler, Cohen, Davies, Pine, & Walsh, 2001). They also recall severe gastrointestinal problems and picky eating in childhood (Kotler et al., 2001; Marchi & Cohen, 1990; Friedmann, Wilfley, Welch, & Kunche, 1997; Shisslak, Mckeon & Crago, 1990, as cited in Jacobi et al., 2004). Research finds that mothers of individuals with AN are more likely to report complications with the afflicted child's birth, including prematurity and birth trauma, as well as difficult infant sleep patterns (Horesh et al., 1996; Shoebridge & Gowers, 2000; Foley, Thacker, Aggen, Neale, & Kindler, 2001; Cnattingius, Hultman, Dahl, & Apren, 1999, as cited in Jacobi et al., 2004).

Personality characteristics & Axis II personality disorders. Individuals with AN often have negative self-evaluation, low self-esteem, obsessionality, perfectionism, neuroticism, harm avoidance, and low perceived social support (Anderlluh, Tchanturia, Rabe-Hesketh, & Treasure, 2003; Brewerton, Dorn, & Bishop, 1992; Bulik, Sullivan, Weltzin & Kaye, 1995, as cited in Jacobi et al., 2004; Fairburn, Cooper, Doll, Davies, & O'Connor, 1999; Fairburn, Cooper, Doll, & Welch, 1997). In addition, approximately 50% of individuals with AN also meet criteria for Cluster C personality disorders (e.g., avoidant, dependent, obsessive-compulsive, and passive-aggressive personality disorders) (Herpertz-Dahlmann, Wewetzer, Schulz, Remschmidt, 1996; Herzog et al., 1992; Wonderlich & Mitchell, 2001).

Athletic competition. Some evidence suggests that exposure to certain competitive athletic environments may be correlated with the development of eating disorders (Garner, Garfinkel, Rockert & Olmsted, 1987; Fulkerson et al., 1999; Sundgot-Borgen, 1994). In particular, ballet dancers and individuals who engage in large amounts of aerobic activity and maintain a low weight status throughout adolescence may be at a higher risk for development of disturbed eating patterns, and a subset of that group may be at increased risk specifically for AN (O'Connor, Lewis, Kirchener, & Cook, 1996; Davis, Kennedy, Ravelski, & Dionne, 1994).

Genetics. Compared to the general population, female relatives of individuals with AN have a fivefold increased risk of having an eating disorder and a significantly higher risk of EDNOS (Strober, Morrell, Burroughs, Salkin, & Jacobs, 1985). Twin studies have revealed higher concordance of eating disorders among monozygotic versus dizygotic twins (Bulik, Sullivan, Wade, & Kendler, 2000; Kipman, Gorwood, Mouren-Simeoni, & Ades, 1999; Klump, Wonderlich, Lehoux, Lilenfeld & Bulik, 2002, as cited in Jacobi et al., 2004). These studies suggest that genetics may be an important risk factor for developing eating disorders, and research is currently investigating potential genes that may be associated with AN.

In sum, there exist a multitude of risk factors for developing AN. Among the variables studied to date, further research is necessary to more carefully understand the complex relationship among the factors that increase risk of onset, those that are significant in the maintenance of AN, and those that impede recovery.

ASSESSMENT

What is Involved in Effective Assessment of Anorexia Nervosa?

Careful and thorough assessment of AN across a wide range of domains is critical, especially given that the best prognosis for AN accompanies those cases where the disorder is identified early and treatment is pursued without delay. Assessment of AN should include the core behavioral and attitudinal dimensions necessary for diagnosis, assessment of physical and medical status, and assessment of co-morbid conditions. For in-depth discussions of assessment of eating disorders, readers are referred to: Anderson, Lundgren, Shapiro, & Paulosky (2004); Levine (2002); Pomeroy (2004); Pike (in press); Pike, Wolk, Gluck, & Walsh (2000).

Crowther & Sherwood (1997) provide a thoughtful and comprehensive discussion of therapy issues and strategies for maximizing the utility of nonstandardized clinical assessments. In addition, there are multiple advantages to incorporating standardized interviews and self-report instruments into all treatment protocols. Standardized instruments: (1) provide consistent and comprehensive diagnostic assessment; (2) facilitate reliable monitoring of course and outcome for an individual; (3) provide norms for comparison of clinical status and severity; and (4) are often a source of self-learning for the individual.

There are several standardized interviews that may be used in a comprehensive assessment of AN. The Structured Clinical Interview for Diagnosis (SCID: First et al., 1998) provides a categorical diagnosis based on the DSM-IV. The Eating Disorders Examination (EDE; Fairburn & Cooper, 1993) provides both descriptive, continuous data of eating pathology and operationally defined DSM-IV eating disorder diagnoses. In addition, the Interview for Diagnosis of Eating Disorders (IDED; Williamson, Davis, Duchmann, McKenzie, & Watkins 1990) and the Structured Interview for Anorexia and Bulimia (SIAB; Fichter, Elton, Engel, & Meyer, 1991) provide categorical and continuous data for assessment of eating disorders.

Self-report instruments are a useful complement to interview assessment of eating disorders because they can be administered frequently, at low cost and are particularly useful in generating continuous data of eating behaviors (e.g., binge eating, purging, restraint) and attitudinal dimensions (e.g., body shape and weight concerns, drive for thinness). The following self-report instruments assess general eating pathology: Eating Disorder Diagnostic Scale (EDDS; Stice, Telch, & Rizvi, 2000); Eating Disorders Inventory-2 (EDI-2, Garner, Olmsted, & Polivy, 1983; Garner, 1991); and Eating Disorders Inventory-Kids' Eating Disorders Survey (EDI-KEDS; Childress, Brewerton, Hodges et al., 1993). Two instruments provide detailed assessment of dietary restraint: the Dutch Eating Behavior Questionnaire (DEBQ, Van Strien, Frijters, Bergers, & Defares, 1986) and the Three-Factor Eating Questionnaire (TFEQ-R, Stunkard & Messick, 1985). The Body Shape Questionnaire (BSQ, Cooper, Taylor, Cooper & Fairburn, 1987) provides data on body dissatisfaction and the Body Image Avoidance Questionnaire (Rosen, Srebnik, Saltzberg, & Wendt, 1991) assesses body image disturbance. The Binge Eating Scale (Gormally, Black, Daston, & Rardin, 1982) provides In-depth assessment of binge eating. For more detailed review of these instruments the reader is referred to Pike (in press).

What Should be Ruled Out?

Differential diagnosis for AN requires that clinicians rule out the possibility that the weight loss and psychological dimensions associated with AN are not better attributed either to another psychiatric disorder or to a primary medical condition. Other serious psychiatric illnesses, particularly Major Depressive Disorder and Schizophrenia, may occasionally be accompanied by weight loss, but the concerns about shape and weight characteristic of AN are not present. A great variety of serious medical illnesses are associated with weight loss, but a much smaller number typically affect young adults and adolescents. In particular, medical disorders that have been mistaken for AN include gastrointestinal illnesses such as Crohn's disease, brain tumors, and malignancies. The clinician should be especially alert to other diagnostic possibilities when an individual presents with atypical features.

TREATMENT

How Do You Engage Individuals with Anorexia Nervosa in Treatment?

Perhaps the single most distinguishing feature of AN is the ego syntonic nature of the disorder, making it one of the most recalcitrant psychiatric conditions to treat (Vitousek, Watson, & Wilson, 1998). Individuals with AN frequently resist treatment with fierce determination. Especially early in the course of the disorder, it is uncommon for individuals with AN to seek treatment voluntarily. If they do, it will often be for immediate relief of medical symptoms or cognitive preoccupation with food, but not because they desire weight gain and full recovery from the disorder. Given this particular feature of AN, initiation of treatment is often complicated, requiring support and assistance from family or significant others, and an explicit focus on engaging and motivating individuals on the part of therapists.

In recent years a significant amount of work has been devoted to understanding the role of motivation in treatment and articulating approaches for enhancing motivation (Prochaska & DiClemente, 1983; Prochaska, DiClemente & Norcross, 1992; Miller & Rollnick, 1991). Vitousek et al. (1998) have articulated specific applications for eating disorders treatment, stressing the role of Socratic questioning in facilitating discussion about motivation and change. Given the ego syntonic nature of AN, and the frequently protracted course of the disorder, it is important to recognize that investment in recovery will wax and wane and issues of motivation are likely to require attention throughout the course of treatment.

What Treatments are Effective for Anorexia Nervosa?

The empirical data base providing clear directions for clinical care is modest in comparison to the voluminous and longstanding knowledge base we have regarding the clinical symptoms and significance of AN. Recent studies provide empirical support for certain subgroups and certain stages of AN care; however, the gaps in the knowledge base are substantially greater than the empirically supported recommendations.

Outpatient family therapy for new onset adolescent AN. Although multiple models of family therapy for AN exist, the Maudsley family therapy approach has the strongest empirical support for treatment of AN (Dare & Eisler, 2000; Lock, Le Grange, Agras & Dare, 2001). Findings from the original Maudsley study (Russell, Szmukler, Dare, & Eisler, 1987) found family therapy to be more effective than individual supportive therapy for those patients 18 years or younger and whose illness had a duration of less than 3 years. For these cases, treatment gains were largely maintained at five-year follow up (Eisler et al., 2000; Lock et al., 2001; Robin et al., 1999).

Inpatient treatment. While individuals who require hospitalization represent the most severely ill segment of the population, the majority of those hospitalized respond to treatment (Anderson, Bowers, & Evans, 1997; Attia, Haiman, Walsh, & Flater, 1998; Baran, Weltzin & Kaye, 1995). Achieving weight restoration is generally the cornerstone of inpatient treatment given its centrality to recovery. In addition, most inpatient programs employ a multidisciplinary team approach including individual, family and group psychotherapy. However, despite successful progress while in hospital, relapse rates range from 30 to 70% following inpatient care (Pike, 1998; Lay, Jennen-Steinmetz, Reinhard, & Schmidt, 2002). As a result, recent years have witnessed a significant increase in attention focused on post-hospital care and relapse prevention.

Post-hospital CBT for weight restored AN. Although a number of interventions have been evaluated for post-hospital care for AN, CBT has the strongest empirical support for relapse prevention among adults (Pike, Walsh, Vitousek, Wilson, & Bauer, 2003). A survival analysis based on a sample of 33 patients revealed a statistically significant advantage of CBT over a baseline treatment of Supportive Nutritional Counseling. In addition, after employing the Morgan Russell criteria for classifying treatment outcome, 44.4% of the CBT group compared to 6.7% of the nutritional counseling group met criteria for good outcome and 16.7% of the CBT group met even more stringent criteria for full recovery (Pike et al., 2003). CBT is a structured psychotherapy that emphasizes a collaborative therapeutic approach focusing on cognitive, behavioral and affective components that serve to put an individual at risk for and perpetuate the disorder. CBT conceptualizations of eating disorders have also been articulated for BN (Fairburn, 1985; Fairburn, Marcus, & Wilson 1993; Wilson, Fairburn, & Agras, 1997), AN (Garner & Bemis, 1982, 1985; Garner, Vitousek, & Pike, 1997; Pike, Loeb, & Vitousek, 1996; Pike, Devlin, & Loeb, 2004), and BED (Marcus, 1997).

Partial hospitalization. A structural alternative to inpatient treatment is partial hospitalization. Nutritional rehabilitation is a critical component of care, and typically partial hospitalization programs employ multidisciplinary teams similar to inpatient programs (e.g. Toronto Hospital, Kaplan & Olmsted, 1997). Beyond reduced costs, a day program has other advantages over inpatient treatment. It requires that a patient maintain normal psychosocial functioning outside of the hospital, thereby promoting autonomy and reducing regression and dependence.

What are Effective Medication Treatments?

Four placebo controlled trials have examined the possible benefits of antidepressants in alleviating the acute symptoms of AN, but none of the studies yielded successful findings (Attia et al., 1998; Biederman et al., 1985; Halmi, Eckert, LaDu & Cohen, 1986; Lacey & Crisp, 1980). One explanation for this may be that the depletion of neurotransmitters associated with malnourishment may interfere with the body's capacity to benefit from the antidepressant medication effects (Delgado et al., 1990). A limited body of data suggests that fluoxetine may have clinical efficacy in the role of relapse prevention (Kaye et al., 2001), and studies are underway to further examine its potential role in relapse prevention once weight is normalized.

While antidepressant medication for acute AN has not been particularly fruitful, atypical antipsychotics have garnered recent attention. Case reports and open studies report improvement among children, adolescents and adults who have taken olanzapine for AN (Boachie, Goldfield & Spettigue, 2003; Hansen, 1999; Jensen & Mejlhede, 2000; La Via, Gray & Kaye, 2000; Mehler et al., 2001; Powers, Santana & Bannon, 2002). However, the data are not fully consistent (Gaskill, Treat, McCabe, & Marcus, 2001), and double blind clinical trials are necessary to evaluate more thoroughly the clinical utility of such medication interventions for acute AN.

How is Treatment Setting Determined?

As with all psychiatric disorders, the treatment for individuals with AN should be provided in the least restrictive setting appropriate to the severity of their disorder. However, many patients with AN require intensive hospital or partial hospitalization programs at some point in the course of treatment. Determination of level of care depends partially on the severity of the disorder, medical status, the age of onset, stage of recovery and other individual factors.

What are Some Other Important Aspects of Clinical Care for Anorexia Nervosa?

Monitoring medical status and nutritional counseling. A wide range of potential disturbances in physical functioning can accompany AN. The single most important measure of physical state is the patient's weight, which should be obtained at frequent intervals. Vital signs (blood pressure and pulse), ECG, and routine blood tests (e.g., hemoglobin concentration, white blood cell count, serum electrolytes, measures of liver and kidney function) should also be assessed, but all of these parameters may be surprisingly normal and therefore falsely reassuring in individuals who are seriously underweight. A thorough discussion of medical monitoring and medical complications associated with AN is available elsewhere (Walsh, in press). In addition to monitoring medical status, it is often useful to include nutritional counseling in the treatment protocol. If a therapist is sufficiently knowledgeable, this work may be integrated into the psychotherapy. Alternatively, it may be appropriate to establish a treatment team, including a psychotherapist, a physician to monitor medical status and a nutritionist to provide nutritional education and counseling.

What are Effective Self-Help Treatments?

Several self-help books as well as informational websites about AN and other eating disorders are listed below. However, it is important to note that many individuals with AN are unlikely to make use of self-help materials on their own initiative due to the fact that individuals with AN are often quite invested in the disorder and ambivalent about seeking care. At least initially, it is likely that self-help books will be more useful for family and friends of individuals with AN to assist them in understanding the disorder and to provide guidance to them about how to help the individual with AN pursue treatment.

Books:

- Gilbert, S. & Commerford, M. (2000). *The unofficial guide to managing eating disorders.* Foster City: CA: IDG Books Worldwide, Inc.
- Natenshon, A. (1999). *When your child has an eating disorder: A step by step workbook for parents and other caregivers.* San Francisco, CA: Jossey-Bass Inc.

- Schmidt, U. & Treasure, J. (1993). *Getting Better (Bit (e) by Bit (e)—a survival kit for suffers of bulimia nervosa and binge eating disorders*. East Sussex, UK: Psychology Press.
- Siegel, M., Brisman, J., & *Weinshel, M. (1997). Surviving an eating disorder: Strategies for family and friends*. New York, NY: Harper Perrennial.
- Treasure, J. (1997). Anorexia *Nervosa: A survival guide for families, friends & sufferers.* East Sussex, UK: Psychology Press.
- Teachman, B., Schwartz, M. Gordic, B. & Coyle, B. (2003). *Helping your child overcome an eating disorder*. Oakland, CA: New Harbinger Publications, Inc.

Websites:

- Academy for eating Disorders: http://www.aedweb.org/
- American Academy of Pediatrics (AAP): http://www.aap.org/
- The American Psychiatric Association: http://www.psych.org/
- Eating Disorders Coalition: www.eatingdisorderscoalition.org
- Something Fishy: www.something-fishy.org
- The National Institute for Clinical Excellence: http://www.nice.org.uk/
- The National Eating Disorders Association: http://www.nationaleatingdisorders.org
- The Society for Adolescent Medicine: http://www.adolescenthealth.org/
- Eating Disorder Referral and Information Center: edreferral.com

Recommendations for future research on AN

The data base informing clinical decisions regarding AN is quite limited, and the field is in need of developing more comprehensive and empirically supported guidelines for treatment. Given the relatively high rates of comorbid disorders that accompany AN, one strategy for developing new interventions is via adaptation of therapies with proven efficacy for comorbid conditions. Harm reduction models of treatment adapted from the substance abuse field may also offer significant direction in guiding treatment planning for individuals with AN. In addition, new models that promote the development of novel approaches to treatment are of tremendous importance to the field. For example, the application of the principles of fear conditioning to AN (Strober, 2004) may catalyze the development of intervention strategies that have untapped potential in treatment of AN.

We currently have limited support for CBT among weight restored adult AN patients and for Maudsley family therapy among new cases of adolescents with AN. Both these treatment approaches should be further expanded and evaluated for their therapeutic efficacy among additional subgroups of individuals with AN and at different stages of treatment. Although the extant data are quite limited for medication, given the impressive biological disturbances characteristic of AN, it is likely that biological interventions will eventually be found to assist with recovery. Thus, innovative medication trials will continue to be essential to furthering empirically based treatment guidelines for AN. As promising psychotherapy and medication interventions are developed, well-controlled multi-site trials will be required to establish their utility and to analyze the complex interplay of variables that impact prognosis and outcome.

REFERENCES

American Psychiatric Association (1994). *Diagnostic and Statistical Manual of Mental Disorders* (4th ed). Washington DC: Author.

Anderluh, M. B., Tehantaria, K., Rabe-Hasketh, S. & Treasure, J. (2003). Childhood obsessive-compulsive personality traits in adult women with eating disorders: defining a broader eating disorder phenotype *Am. J. Psychiatry*, 160, 242–247.

Andersen, A., Bowers, W., & Evans (1997). Inpatient treatment of anorexia nervosa. In D. Garner, P. & Garfinkel (Eds.) *Handbook of treatment for eating disorders,* (pp. 327–353). New York: Guilford Press.

Anderson, D., Lundgren, J, Shapiro, J., & Paulosky, C. (2004). Assessment of eating disorders: Review and recommendations for clinical use. *Behavior Modification, 28,* 763–82.

Attia, E., Haiman, C., Walsh, B.T., & Flater, S. (1998). Does fluoxetine augment the inpatient treatment of anorexia nervosa? *American Journal of Psychiatry, 155,* 548–551.

Attie, I., & Brooks-Gunn, J. (1989). Development of eating problems in adolescent girls: A longitudinal study. *Developmental Psychology, 25,* 70–79.

Baran, S., Weltzin, T., & Kaye, W. (1995). Low discharge weight and outcome in anorexia nervosa. *American Journal of Psychiatry, 152,* 1070–1072.

Becker, A., Burwell, R., Gilman, S., Herzog, D., & Hamburg, P. (2002). Eating behaviours and attitudes following prolonged exposure to television among ethnic Fijian adolescent girls. *British Journal of Psychiatry, 180,* 509–14.

Biederman, J., Herzog, D., Rivinus, T., Harper, G., Ferber, R., Rosenbaum, J. et al. (1985). Amitriptyline in the treatment of anorexia nervosa: A double-blind placebo-controlled study. *Journal of Clinical Psychopharmacology, 5,* 10–16.

Boachie, A., Goldfield, G., & Spettigue, W. (2003). Olanzapine use as an adjunctive treatment for hospitalized children with anorexia nervosa: Case reports. *International Journal of Eating Disorders, 33,* 98–103.

Braun, D., Sunday, S. & Halmi, K. (1994). Psychiatric comorbidity in patients with eating disorders, *Psychological Medicine, 6,* 859–867.

Brewerton, T., Dorn, L., & Bishop, E. (1992). The tri-dimensional personality questionaire in eating disorders. *Biological Psychiatry 31,* 91a.

Bulik, C., Sullivan, P., Fear, J., & Joyce, P. (1997). Eating disorders and antecedent anxiety disorders: A controlled study. *Acta Psychiatrica Scandanavica, 96,* 101–107.

Bulik, C., Sullivan, P., Fear, J., & Pickering, A. (1997). Predictors of the development of bulimia nervosa in women with anorexia nervosa. *Journal of Nervous and Mental Disease, 135,* 704–707.

Bulik, C. M., Sullivan, P. F., Wade, T. D. & Kendler, K. S. (2000) Twin studies of eating disorders: a review. Int J. Eat Disord, 27, 1–20.

Cachelin, F., & Maher, B. (1998). Is amenorrhea a critical criterion for anorexia nervosa? *Journal of Psychosomatic Research, 44,* 435–40.

Childress, A., Brewerton, T., Hodges, E., & Jarrell, M. (1993). Eating disorders inventory-kids' eating disorders survey (KEDS): A study of middle school students. *Journal of the American Dietetic Association,* 32, 843–850.

Cooper, P., Taylor, M., Cooper, Z., & Fairburn, C. (1987). The development and validation of the Body Shape Questionnaire. *International Journal of Eating Disorders, 6,* 485–494.

Crago, M. Shisslak, C. & Estes, L. (1996). Eating disturbances among American minority groups: A review. *International Journal of Eating Disorders, 19,* 239–248.

Crowther, & Sherwood, N. (1997). Assessment. In D. Garner & P. Garfinkel (Eds.) *Handbook of Treatment for Eating Disorders* (2nd ed., pp. 34–49). New York: Guilford Press.

DaCosta, M., & Halmi, K. (1992). Classification of anorexia nervosa: Question of subtypes. *International Journal of Eating Disorders, 11,* 305–312.

Dare, C., & Eisler, I. (2000). A multi-family group day treatment programme for adolescent eating disorder. *European Eating Disorders Review, 8,* 4–18.

Dare, C., Eisler, I., Russell, G., Treasure, J., & Dodge, L. (2001). Psychological therapies for adults with anorexia nervosa: Randomised controlled trial of out-patient treatments. *The British Journal of Psychiatry, 178,* 216–221.

Davis, C., Kennedy, S., Ravelski, E., & Dionne, M. (1994). The role of physical activity in the development and maintenance of eating disorders. *Psychological Medicine,* 957–967.

Davis, C., & Katzman, M. (1999). Perfection as acculturation: Psychological correlates of eating problems in Chinese male and female students living in the United States. *International Journal of Eating Disorders, 25,* 65–70.

Delgado, P., Charnedy, D., Price, L., Aghajanian, G., Landis, H., & Neninger, G. (1990). Serotonin function and the mechanism of antidepressant action: Reversal of antidepressant-induced remission by rapid depletion of plasma tryptophan. *Archives of General Psychiatry,* 411–418.

Eating Disorders Commission (2005). Part IV: Eating Disorders. In D. Evans, E. Foa, R. Gur, H. Hendin, C. O'Brien, M. Seligman, & BT. Walsh (Eds.) *Treating and preventing adolescent mental health disorders: What we know and what we don't know.* Oxford: Oxford University Press.

Eisler, I., Dare, C., Hodes, M., Russell, G., Dodge, E. & LeGrange, D (2000). Family therapy for adolescent anorexia nervosa: The results of a controlled comparison of two family interventions. *Journal of Child Psychology and Psychiatry, 41,* 727–736.

Fairburn, C. G., (1985). Cognitive behavioral treatment for bulimia Handbook of Psychotherapy for Anorenia Nervosa and Bulima, Edited by Garner, D. M., Garfinkel, P. E, New York, Guilford Press, 160–192.

Fairburn, C., & Cooper, Z. (1993). The Eating Disorder Examination (12th edition). In C. Fairburn, T. Wilson (Eds.). *Binge eating: Nature, assessment, and treatment.* (pp. 317–360). New York: Guilford Press.

Fairburn, C., Marcus, M. & Wilson, G. (1993). Cognitive-behavioral therapy for binge eating and bulimia nervosa: A comprehensive treatment manual. In C. Fairburn & G. Wilson (Eds.), *Binge eating: Nature, assessment and treatment* (pp. 361–404). New York: Guilford Press.

Fairburn, C., & Shafran, C. (1999). A cognitive behavioural theory of anorexia nervosa. *Behavior Research and Therapy, 37,* 1–13.

Fairburn, C., Welch, S., Doll, H., Davies, B., & O'Connor, M. (1997). Risk factors for bulimia nervosa: A community-based case-control study. *Archives of General Psychiatry, 54,* 509–517.

Fichter, M., Elton, M., Engel, K., Meyer, A. (1991). Structured Interview for Anorexia and Bulimia Nervosa (SIAB): Development of a new instrument for the assessment of eating disorders. *International Journal of Eating Disorders, 10,* 571–592.

First, M., Spitzer, R., Gibbon M, & Janet B. (1998). Structured Clinical Interview for DSM-IV Disorders.

Foley, D., Thacker, L., Aggen, S., Neale, M., & Kendler, K. (2001). Pregnancy and perinatal complications associated with risks for common psychiatric disorders in a population-based sample of female twins. *American Journal of Medical Genetics, 105,* 426–431.

Foley, D. L., Thacker, L. R, Aggen, S. H., Neale, M. C. & Kendler, K. S. (2001). Pregnancy and perinatal complications associated with risks for common psychiatric disorders in a population based sample of female twins. *American Journal of Medical Genetice, 105,* 426–431.

Fulkerson, J., Keel, P., Leon, G., & Dorr, T. (1999). Eating-disordered behaviors and personality characteristics of high school athletes and non-athletes. *International Journal of Eating Disorders, 26,* 73–79.

Friedmann, M. A., Wiltey, D. E., Welch, P. R., & Kunce, J. T. (1997). Self-directed hostility and family functioning in normal weight bulimis and overweight binge eateis. *Addictive Behaviors, 22,* 367–375.

Garfinkel, P., Goering, P., Spegg, C., Goldbloom, D., Kennedy, S., Kaplan, A., & Woodside, D. (1996). Should amenorrhea be necessary for the diagnosis of anorexia nervosa? Evidence from a Canadian community sample. *British Journal of Psychiatry, 168,* 500–506.

Garner, D., & Bemis, K. (1982). Anorexia nervosa: A cognitive-behavioral approach to AN. *Cognitive Therapy and Research, 6,* 123–150.

Garner, D., & Bemis, K. (1985). Cognitive therapy for AN. In D. Garner & P. Garfinkel (Eds.), *Handbook of psychotherapy for anorexia nervosa and bulimia* (pp. 107–146. New York: Guilford Press.

Garner, D., Garfinkel, P., Rockert, W., & Olmsted, M. (1987). A prospective study of eating disturbances in the ballet. *Psychotherapy and Psychosomatics, 48,* 170–175.

Garner, D., Olmstead, M., & Polivy, J. (1983). Development and validation of a multidimensional Eating Disorder Inventory for anorexia nervosa and bulimia. *International Journal of Eating Disorders, 2,* 15–34.

Garner, D., Vitousek, K., & Pike, K. (1997). Cognitive behavioral therapy for anorexia nervosa. In D. Garner & P Garfinkel (Eds.), *Handbook of treatment for eating disorders* (pp. 94–144). New York: Guilford Press.

Garner, D. M. (1991). *The Eatings Disorders Inventory-2. Professional Manual.* Odessa, FL: Psychological Assessment Resources.

Gaskill, J., Treat, T., McCabe, E., & Marcus, M. (2001). Does olanzapine effect the rate of weight gain among inpatients with eating disorders? *Paper presented at the International Conference on Eating Disorders.* Vancouver, BC.

Godart, N. T., Flament, M. F., Perdereau, F., & Jeammet, P. (2002). Comorbidity between eating disorders and anxiety disorders: A review. *International Journal of Eating Disorders, 32,* 253–270.

Ghaderi, A. & Scott, B. (2001). Prevalence, incidence and prospective risk factors for eating disorders. *Acta Psychiatric Scandinavica,* 104, 122–130.

Gormally, J., Black, S., Daston, S., & Rardin, D. (1982). The assessment of binge eating severity among obese persons. *Addictive Behaviors, 7,* 47–55.

Gowen, L. Hayward, C., Killen, J., Robinson, T., & Taylor, C. (1999). Acculturation and eating disorder symptoms in adolescent girls. *Journal of Research on Adolescents, 9,* 67–83.

Halmi, K., Eckert, K. LaDu, T., & Cohen, J. (1986). Anorexia Nervosa: Treatment efficacy of cyproheptadine and amitriptyline. *Archives of General Psychiatry, 43,* 177–181.

Halmi, K., Eckert, E., Metchi, P., Sampugnaro, V., Apple, R., & Cohen, J (1991). Comorbidity of psychiatric diagnoses in anorexia nervosa. *Archives of General Psychiatry, 48,* 712–718.

Hansen, L. (1999). Olanzapine in the treatment of anorexia nervosa. *The British Journal of Psychiatry, 175,* 592.

Herpertz-Dahlmann, B., Wewetzer, C., Schulz, E., & Remschmidt, H. (1996). Course and outcome in adolescent anorexia nervosa. *International Journal of Eating Disorders, 19,* 335–45.

Herzog, D., Deber, H., & Vandereeycken, W. (1992). *The course of eating disorders: Long-term follow-up studies of anorexia and bulimia nervosa.* New York: Springer-Verlag.

Herzog, D., & Delinsky, S. (2001). In R. Striegel-Moore, L. Smolak (Eds.), *Eating disorders: innovative directions in research and practice,* APA: Washington, D.C.

Herzog, D., Nussbaum, K., & Marmor, A. (1996). Comorbidity and outcome in eating disorders. *Psychiatric Clinics of North America, 19,* 843–859.

Hoek, H. W. (2002). Distribution of eating disorders. In C. G. Fairburn & K. D. Brownell (Eds.), *Eating disorders and obesity: A comprehensive handbook* (pp. 233–237). New York: The Guilford Press.

Hooper, M., & Garner, D. (1986). Application of the Eating Disorders Inventory to a sample of Black, White and Mixed-race schoolgirls in Zimbabwe. *International Journal of Eating Disorders, 5,* 161–168.

Hsu, L. K. G. (1990). *Eating Disorders.* New York. Guilford Press.

Horesh, N., Apter, A. Ishai, J., Danziger, Y., Miculincer, M., Stelin, D. et al. (1996). Abnormal psychosocial situations and eating disorders in adolescence. Journal of the American Academy of Child & Adolescent Psychiatry, 35, 921–927.

International Classification of Mental and Behavioral Disorders. (1992). *International statistical classification of diseases and related health problems, tenth revision.* Geneva: World Health Organization.

Jacobi, C., Hayward, C., de Zwaan, M., Kraemer, H., & Agras, W. (2004). Coming to terms with risk factors for eating disorders application of risk terminology and suggestions for a general taxonomy. *Psychological Bulletin, 13,* 19–65.

Jensen, V., & Mejlhede, A., (2000). Anorexia nervosa: Treatment with olanzapine. *The British Journal of Psychiatry, 177,* 87.

Kaplan, A., & Olmsted, M. (1997). Partial hospitalization. In D. Garner & P. Garfinkel (Eds.) *Handbook of Treatment for Eating Disorders* (2nd ed). (pp. 354–360). New York: Guilford Press.

Keel, P. Mitchell, J., Miller, K. Devis, T., & Crow, S. (2000). Predictive validity of bulimia nervosa as a diagnostic category. *American Journal of Psychiatry, 157,* 136–138.

Kipman, A., Gorwood, P., Mouren-Simeoni, M. & Ades, J. (1999). Genetic factors in anorexia nervosa. *European Psychiatry, 14,* 189–198.

Kotler, L., Cohen, P., Davies, M., Pine, D., & Walsh, B. T. (2001). Longitudinal relationships between childhood, adolescent, and adult eating disorders. *Journal of the American Academy of Child and Adolescent Psychiatry, 40,* 1434–1440.

Lacey, J., & Crisp, A. (1980). Hunger, food intake and weight: The impact of clomipramine on a refeeding anorexia nervosa population. *Post Graduate Medical Journal,* 79–85.

La Via, M., Gray, N., & Kaye, W. (2000). Case reports of olanzapine treatment of anorexia nervosa. *International Journal of Eating Disorders, 27,* 363–366.

Lay, B., Jennen-Steinmetz, C., Reinhard, I., & Schmitt, M. (2002). Characteristics of inpatient weight gain in adolescent anorexia nervosa: Relation to speed of relapse and readmission. *European Eating Disorders Review, 10,* 22–40.

Levine, R. (2002). Endocrine aspects of eating disorders in adolescents. Adolescent Medicine, 13, 129–143.

Lock, J., Le Grange, D., Agras, W., & Dare, C. (2001). *Treatment manual for anorexia nervosa.* New York: Guilford Press.

Marcus, M. (1997). Adapting treatment for patients with binge-eating disorder. In D. Garner & P. Garfinkel (Eds.), *Handbook of treatment for eating disorders* (2nd ed., pp. 484–493). New York: Guilford Press.

Marchi, M., & Cohen, P., (1990). Early childhood eating behaviors and adolescent eating disorders. *Journal of the American Academy of Child and Adolescent Psychiatry, 29,* 112–117.

Mehler, C., Wewetzer, C., Schulze, U., Warnke, A., Theisen, F., & Dittmann, R. (2001). Olanzapine in children and adolescents with chronic anorexia nervosa: A study of five cases. *European Child and Adolescent Psychiatry, 10,* 151–157.

Miller, W., & Rollnick, S. (1991). *Motivational interviewing.* New York: Guilford Press.

Mitrany, E., Lubin, F., Chetrit, A., & Modan, B. (1995). Eating disorders among Jewish female adolescents in Israel: A five year study. *Journal of Adolescent Health, 16,* 454–457.

Nasser, M., Katzman, M., & Gordon, R. (Eds.) (2001). *Eating disorders and cultures in transition.* New York: Taylor & Francis.

O'Connor, P., Lewis, R., Kirchner, E., & Cook, D., (1996). Eating disorder symptoms in former female college gymnasts: Relations with body composition. *American Journal of Clinical Nutrition, 64,* 840–843.

Pike, K., Loeb, K., & Vitousek, K. (1996). Cognitive behavioral treatment for anorexia nervosa and bulimia nervosa. In K. Thompson (Ed.), *Eating disorders, obesity and body image: A practical guide to assessment and treatment* (pp. 253–302). Washington, DC: American Psychological Association.

Pike, K. (1998). Long-term course of anorexia nervosa. *Clinical Psychology Review, 18,* 447–475.

Pike, K., Wolk, S., Gluck, M., & Walsh, B. T. (2000). In the task force for the handbook of psychiatric measures. *The handbook of psychiatric measures* (pp. 647–672). Washington, DC: American Psychiatric Association.

Pike, K., Devlin, M., & Loeb, K. (2003). Cognitive-behavioral therapy in the treatment of anorexia nervosa, bulimia nervosa, and binge eating disorder. In J. Thompson (Ed.) *Handbook of eating disorders and obesity* (pp. 130–162). New York: Wiley.

Pike, K., & Streigel-Moore, R. (1997). Disordered eating and eating disorders. In S. Gallant, G.,Kerta, R. Royak-Schaler (Eds.), *Health care for women: Psychological, social and behavioral influences,* Washington, DC: APA.

Pike, K., Walsh, B.T., Vitousek, K., Wilson, G.T., & Bauer, J. (2003). Cognitive behavioral treatment in the post-hospital treatment of anorexia nervosa. *American Journal of Psychiatry, 160,* 2046–2049.

Pike, K. (in press). Assessment of anorexia nervosa. In Striegel-Moore, R. & Bulik, C. (Eds.), *Special issue on anorexia nervosa.* New York: Wiley.

Polivy, J., & Herman, C. P. (1985). Dieting and bingeing casual analysis. *American Psychologist, 40,* 193–201.

Pomeroy, C. (2004). Assessment of medical status and physical factors. In J. K. Thompson (Ed.), *Handbook of eating disorders and obesity* (pp. 81–111). Hoboken, NJ: Wiley.

Powers, P., Santana, C., & Bannon, Y. (2002). Olanzapine in the treatment of anorexia nervosa: An open label trial. *International Journal of Eating Disorders, 32,* 146–154.

Prochaska, J. & DiClemente, C. (1983). Stages and processes of self-change in smoking: Toward an integrative model of change. *Journal of Consulting and Clinical Psychology, 5,* 390–395.

Prochaska, J. DiClemente, C., & Norcross, J. (1992). In search of how people change: Applications to addictive behavior. *American Psychologist, 47,* 1102–1114.

Robin, A., Siegel, P., Moye, A., Gilroy, M., Baker-Dennis, A., & Sikand, A. (1999). A controlled comparison of family versus individual therapy for adolescents with anorexia nervosa. *Journal of the American Academy of Child and Adolescent Psychiatry, 38,* 1482–1489.

Rosen, J., Srebnik, D., Saltzberg, E., & Wendt, S. (1991). Development of a body image avoidance questionnaire. *Psychological Assessment, 3,* 32–37.

Russell, G., Szmukler, G., Dare, C., & Eisler, I. (1987). An evaluation of family therapy in anorexia nervosa and bulimia nervosa. *Archives of General Psychiatry, 44,* 1047–1056.

Shisslak, C., McKeon, R., & Crago, (1990). Family dysfunction in normal weight bulimic and bulimic anorexic families. *Journal of Clinical Psychology, 46,* 185–189.

Shoebridge, P., & Gowers, S. G. (2000). Parental high concern and adolescent-onset anorexia nervosa. British *Journal of Psychiatry, 176,* 132–137.

Steinhausen, H.-C., Rauss-Mason, C., & Seidel, R. (1991). Follow-up studies of anorexia nervosa: a review of four decades of outcome research. *Psychological Medicine, 21,* 447–454.

Stice, E., Killen, J., Hayward, C., & Taylor, C. (1998). Age of onset for binge eating and purging during adolescence: A four year survival analysis. *Journal of Abnormal Psychology, 107,* 671–675.

Stice, E., Telch, C., & Rizvi, S. (2000). Development and validation of the Eating Disorder Diagnostic Scale: A brief self-report measure of anorexia, bulimia, and binge-eating disorder. *Psychological Assessment, 12,* 123–131.

Stock, S., Goldberg, E., Corbett, S., & Katzman, D. (2002). Substance use in female adolescents with eating disorders. *Journal of Adolescent Health, 31,* 176–82.

Strober, M. (2004). Pathologic fear conditioning and anorexia nervosa: On the search for novel paradigms. *International Journal of Eating Disorders, 35,* 504–508.

Strober, M., Morrell, W., Burroughs, J., Salkin, B., & Jacobs, C. (1985). A controlled family study of anorexia nervosa. *Journal of Psychiatric Research, 19,* 239–246.

Stunkard, A. & Messick, S. The three-factor eating questionnaire to measure dietary restraint, disinhibition and hunger. *Journal of Psychosomatic Research, 29,* 71–83.

Sundgot-Borgen, J. (1994). Risk and trigger factors for the development of eating disorders in female elite athletes. *Medicine and Science in Sports and Exercise, 26,* 414–419.

Van Strien, T., Frijters, J., Bergers, G., & Defares, P. (1986). The Dutch Eating Behavior Questionnaire (DEBQ) for assessment of restrained, emotional, and external eating behavior. *International Journal of Eating Disorders, 5,* 295–315.

Vitousek, K., Watson, S., & Wilson, G. (1998). Enhancing motivation in eating disorders. *Clinical Psychology Review, 18,* 476–498.

Walsh B. T. (in press). Eating disorders. In D. Kasper, E. Braunwald, A. Fauci, S. Hauser, D. Longo, & J. Jameson (Eds.), *Harrison's principles of internal medicine* (16th ed.). New York: McGraw Hill.

Walters, E., & Kendler, K. S. (1995). Anorexia nervosa and anorexic-like syndromes in a population-based female twin sample. *American Journal of Psychiatry, 152,* 64–71.

Webster, J., & Palmer, R. (2000). The childhood and family background of women with clinical eating disorders: A comparison with women with major depression and women without psychiatric disorder. *Psychological Medicine, 30,* 53–60.

Williamson, D., Davis, C., Duchmann, E., McKenzie, S., & Watkins, P. (1990). *Assessment of eating disorders: Obesity, anorexia, and bulimia nervosa.* New York: Pergamon Press.

Wilson, G. T., Fairburn, C., & Agras, W. (1997). Cognitive-behavioral therapy for bulimia nervosa. In D. Garner & P. Garfinkel (Eds.), *Handbook of treatment for eating disorders* (2nd ed., pp. 67–93). New York: Guilford Press.

Wonderlich, S., Brewerton, T., Jocic, Z., Dansky, B., & Abbott, D. (1997). Relationship of childhood sexual abuse and eating disorders. *Journal of the American Academy of Child and Adolescent Psychiatry, 36,* 1107–1115.

Wonderlich, S., & Mitchell, J. (2001). The role of personality in the onset of eating disorders and treatment implications. *Psychiatric Clinics of North America, 24,* 249–258.

Woodside, D., & Garfinkel, P. (1992). Age of onset in eating disorders. *International Journal of Eating Disorders, 12,* 31–36.

CHAPTER 5

Antisocial Personality Disorder

Katherine A. Fowler • Scott O. Lilienfeld

WHAT IS ANTISOCIAL PERSONALITY DISORDER?

In DSM-IV (American Psychiatric Association, 1994), Antisocial Personality Disorder (APD) is operationalized as a pattern of disregard for, and violation of, the rights of others. Like other personality disorders, it is believed to be a stable and enduring pattern of behavior originating in childhood or adolescence. Indeed, conduct disorder is a prerequisite for the DSM-IV diagnosis of APD.

Individuals with APD fail to conform to societal norms, often resulting in repeated and varied illegal behaviors (e.g., stealing, assault, pursuing illegal occupations). Interpersonally, they disregard the rights and wishes of others, often deceiving and manipulating them for profit or pleasure (i.e., "conning" others). They tend to be impulsive, making many decisions without forethought or attention to consequences for self or others. This tendency is often manifested in such behaviors as sudden changes of jobs, relationships, and residences. Further, APD is often characterized by aggressiveness and irritability, defined as a proclivity toward physical assaults of others, including domestic violence. Individuals with APD are at heightened risk of causing indirect physical harm to others through reckless disregard for their safety and, in the case of childrearing, neglect.

Persons with this disorder tend to be consistently irresponsible (i.e., "reliably unreliable"). For example, they may be unemployed for significant periods of time despite job opportunities, quit jobs without a realistic plan for getting a new one, or be repeatedly absent from work for reasons other than personal or family illness. Furthermore, they typically lack a sense of personal responsibility for the adverse consequences of their actions, frequently blaming their victims and lacking remorse. In general, they fail to make amends for their misdeeds, at times offering superficial justifications such as "Life's unfair" or "I was just looking out for number one."

BASIC FACTS ABOUT ANTISOCIAL PERSONALITY DISORDER

Comorbidity. Individuals with APD complain frequently of dysphoria, depressed mood, boredom, restlessness, and tension. Disorders that commonly co-occur with APD include Anxiety Disorders, Depressive Disorders, Substance Use Disorders, Somatization Disorder, and Pathological Gambling and other impulse control disorders (APA, 2000).

Prevalence. In community samples, APD has been found to occur in 3% of males and 1% of females. Within clinical settings, prevalence estimates have ranged from 3% to 30%, depending on the characteristics of the sample. In substance abuse treatment and forensic settings, estimates have been higher.

Age at onset. As currently defined in the DSM, APD cannot be diagnosed prior to age 18.

Gender. APD is more prevalent in men than in women. It is diagnosed in about 3% of males compared with 1% of females in community samples.

Fowler, K. A., & Lilienfeld, S. O. (2006). Antisocial personality disorder. In Practitioner's J. E. Fisher & W. T. O'Donohue (Eds.), *Practitioner's Guide to evidence-based psychotherapy.* New York: Springer.

Course. APD often displays a chronic course, but may decline in severity or remit as the individual ages, particularly starting in the fourth decade of life. Although this "burn-out" phenomenon is particularly evident with respect to criminal behavior, a decline in behaviors comprising the full antisocial spectrum is often seen. Some authors have noted that the "character structure" underlying APD may not change with age, although the observable behaviors typically improve (Reid & Gacono, 2000). Indeed, longitudinal research on released prisoners confirms the suggestion that although the antisocial behaviors of such individuals tends to decline with age, many of their personality traits (e.g., lack of guilt, callousness) remains relatively constant with age (Hart, Kropp, & Hare, 1988). Individuals with APD are more likely than those in the general population to experience premature death by violent means (APA, 2000).

Impairment and other demographic characteristics. A small group of persistent male offenders (5–6%) has consistently been found to be responsible for a disproportionate amount of crime (approximately 50%) (see Farrington, Ohlin, & Wilson, 1986, for a review). Identification of this group of highest-risk offenders depends largely on two variables: early onset of criminal behavior and the persistence of that behavior (Skilling, Harris, Rice, & Quinsey, 2002). Several research groups have proposed variations on a general taxonomy of adolescence-limited vs. life-course persistent antisocial behavior (e.g., Loeber, 1982; Moffitt, 1993). Furthermore, they have noted the remarkable continuity of serious antisocial behavior across various samples (e.g., Loeber & Farrington, 1998) and even called age of onset of criminal behavior the "single best predictor of adult criminal outcomes" (Skilling et al., 2002, p. 27). Because APD includes criteria for early behavior problems and juvenile delinquency, as well as adult criminal behavior, it is not surprising that individuals with this condition are at heightened risk for criminality and incarceration.

Several authors have reported a small-to-medium association ($r = .15–.20$) between APD and general criminal recidivism (e.g., Glover, Nicholson, Hemmati, Bernfeld, & Quinsey, 2002; Hart et al., 1988). There is less consistency with relation to violent recidivism. Some authors (e.g., Harris, Rice, & Cornier, 1991) have reported moderate associations between APD and violent recidivism, whereas others (e.g., Glover, et al., 2002) have reported virtually no relation. Implementation of criteria from different DSM editions may contribute to some of this inconsistency, as may differential base rates of violence across studies.

APD tends to aggregate within families. It is more commonly found in first-degree biological relatives of those with APD than in the general population, and twin and adoption studies indicate that both genetic and environmental factors contribute to the risk of developing this disorder. Research indicates that biological relatives of females with the disorder are at greater risk than biological relatives of males with the disorder. This finding is consistent with a multifactorial threshold model of APD (see Cloninger, Christiansen, Reich, & Gottesman, 1978), whereby females both inherit and transmit a greater liability to APD than do males. Furthermore, when a family member has APD, female relatives are more likely to exhibit Somatization Disorder, whereas male relatives are more likely to develop APD and Substance Abuse disorders (see Lilienfeld, 1992). Individuals with an adoptive parent with APD also appear to be at increased risk for developing APD relative to the general population, although adopted-away children seem to resemble their biological parents more than their adoptive parents in terms of antisocial behavior (APA, 2000).

APD is associated with low socioeconomic status and is more prevalent in urban than rural settings. These findings have raised concerns that APD may be misapplied to some individuals in these settings, as antisocial behavior may occasionally serve as a protective strategy under such conditions. The DSM-IV accompanying text on APD urges the clinician to consider these factors when diagnosing the disorder. Alternatively, it is possible that (a) poverty may contribute to APD, (b) APD, which is often associated with occupational instability and failure, may lead to an increased risk for poverty, and/or (c) some of the same causal influences that give rise to poverty also give rise to APD.

ASSESSMENT

What should be ruled out?

When assessing APD, several important considerations must be borne in mind. First, if adult antisocial behaviors accompany a substance use disorder, a diagnosis of APD should be made only if features of APD were also present in childhood, and have continued into the adult years. Chronic antisocial behavior occurring only in the context of schizophrenia or during a manic episode should not be diagnosed as APD.

It is important to distinguish APD from other personality disorders with which it shares certain features. Like APD individuals, those with Narcissistic Personality Disorder (NPD) often present as glib, unempathic, and exploitative. However, individuals with NPD are not usually characterized by impulsivity and aggression. Individuals with Histrionic Personality Disorder may be reckless, seductive, and manipulative, as are those with APD. Nevertheless, individuals with Histrionic Personality Disorder do not necessarily engage in antisocial behaviors. Individuals with Borderline Personality Disorder are also often manipulative, but this manipulativeness usually appears to be motivated by attention- and nurturance-seeking rather by power or material gain, as it typically is in individuals with APD (APA, 2000).

The DSM-IV Text Revision (DSM-IV-TR; APA, 2000) asserts that APD is essentially synonymous with psychopathy, or psychopathic personality. The disorder known as APD, first seen in DSM-III, was intended to capture the same condition that had been known as psychopathy in former classification schemes and in the clinical literature (Cleckley, 1941). Psychopathy is characterized by a constellation of such personality traits as lack of guilt, callousness, dishonesty, manipulativeness, grandiosity, superficial charm, and poor impulse control. In an effort to circumvent the apparent subjectivity of these personality traits, the DSM-III diagnosis of APD focused largely or entirely on behavioral criteria, rather than personality features The resulting criteria have been highly controversial, as some authors argue that the criteria are overinclusive (e.g., Cunningham & Reidy, 1998; Hart & Hare, 1997; Lilienfeld, 1994), as there are most likely a wide array of etiological factors behind criminal behavior, only one of which is psychopathy (Lykken, 1995; Rogers & Dion, 1991). Still others have criticized APD criteria for being underinclusive (Millon, 1981; Widom, 1977), as these criteria may not adequately identify individuals who possess the core personality features of psychopathy, but do not manifest these traits in criminal behavior ("subclinical" or "successful" psychopaths). Moreover, there is compelling evidence that, contrary to DSM-IV-TR, APD and psychopathy are not synonymous, as only about 25–30% of individuals with APD in prison settings meet research criteria for psychopathy (Hare, 2003). As a consequence, *contra* DSM-IV-TR, there is good evidence that psychopathy and APD are separable conditions. In this chapter, we will report findings that pertain only to APD as defined by DSM criteria.

What is Involved in Effective Assessment?

Researchers and clinicians have typically attempted to assess APD using either self-report or interview-based measures. Although some instruments for assessing personality disorders have demonstrated acceptable reliability, low levels of agreement among instruments have been observed across studies, with some diagnoses exhibiting no higher than chance agreement levels across instruments (see Perry, 1992, for a review). For example, for APD, Perry (1992) reported Kappa coefficients ranging from .06 (SIDP vs. MCMI) to .59 (SCID vs. PDE) across different measures of APD. Although most of these findings were generated from research that employed DSM-III and DSM–III-R based instruments, this issue may well pertain to DSM-IV-based measures as well. In general, self-report measures of APD yield higher prevalence levels of the diagnosis than do structured interviews, perhaps because the former measures do not permit probing of responses. As a consequence, clinicians should bear in mind that diagnoses of APD derived from self-report measures may be overly liberal. For some of these measures, there are data on the reliability of APD per se, whereas for other measures there are only data on the reliability of DSM personality disorders in general. In cases in which there are reliability data specifically for APD, we report these data in the following sections.

Self-report measures. Although several instruments that assessed DSM-III and DSM-III-R PD criteria for APD exhibited adequate psychometric properties, little research pertaining to updated versions exists. We discuss four such instruments here: the Personality Diagnostic Questionnaire-4+ (PDQ-4+; Hyler, 1994), the Millon Clinial Multiaxial Inventory-III (MCMI; Millon, 1983,1987,1994), the Minnesota Multiphasic Personality Inventory-2 DSM-IV Personality Disorder scales (MMPI-2 DSM-IV PD scales), and the Wisconsin Personality Disorders Inventory (WISPI-IV; Klein & Benjamin, 1996) as well as one new instrument, the Assessment of DSM-IV Personality Disorders Questionnaire (ADP-IV; Schotte & De Doncker, 1996).

The PDQ-4+ is a self-report measure consisting of 99 true-false items that assess DSM-IV criteria for the 10 major personality disorders, and two personality disorders (passive-aggressive and depressive) designated for further study. Only one published study has examined the psychometric properties of the PDQ-4+. Fossati et al. (1998) administered the PDQ-4+ and Structured Clinical Interview for DSM-IV Personality Disorders, Version 2.0 (SCID-II) to a sample of 300 psychiatric inpatients and outpatients. Correlations among all PDQ-4+ and SCID-II scales were low to moderate, but significant (r = .19–.42). Additionally, PDQ-4+ scales exhibited mediocre internal consistencies. Only two scales (antisocial and dependent) showed strong powers of discrimination.

At one time, the MCMI was considered a well-researched instrument for use in personality disorder assessment. However, little research has been published regarding the latest revision of this instrument, the MCMI-III (Millon, 1994). As the MCMI-III has changed or replaced 95 of 175 items from the MCMI-II, it is essentially impossible to comment on the properties of this instrument until updated validation information is available. What is currently known about the MCMI-III will be reported here.

The MCMI-III was designed to assess the principal dimensions of Millon's biosocial theory of personality (see Millon, 2003). Like prior editions, it uses a true/false format. Millon (1994) reports test–retest reliability estimates of the MCMI-III PD scales, over periods from 5 to 14 days, ranging from ranging from .85 (Paranoia) to .93 (Antisocial, Borderline, and Depressive). Craig (1999) reports, however, that reliability estimates from Millon's group tend to be somewhat higher than those reported by other researchers.

Another set of scales once frequently used and researched has received little attention since the advent of DSM-IV. The MMPI DSM-III Personality Disorders (MMPI-PD) scales were developed by first asking psychologists to select MMPI items that appeared to assess each DSM-III personality disorder, and then refining the preliminary scales by eliminating items with low item-total correlations. Unlike the PDQ-4 items, the content of the MMPI items does not correspond directly to that of the DSM criteria for APD. The internal consistency of the MMPI DSM-III APD scale in a psychiatric sample was .78 (Morey, Waugh, & Blashfield, 1985), and its three-month test–retest reliability in a psychiatric sample was .82 (Trull, 1993). A revised set of personality disorder scales, including a scale for APD, has been developed for the MMPI-2 (Somwaru & Ben-Porath, 1995), although research concerning their psychometric properties is preliminary.

The WISPI-IV is the latest version of the Wisconsin Personality Disorders Inventory, a measure designed to assess personality disorders from an interpersonal perspective. It comprises 204 items, for which the individual is asked to rate statements on a 10-point scale from 0 (never or not at all true of you) to 10 (always or extremely true of you), to the degree that they describe one's "usual self" over the past five years. The items map onto 11 PD scales (10 primary DSM-IV personality disorders, and passive aggressive PD), and ten items are derived from the Marlowe-Crowne Scale for social desirability (Greenwald & Satow, 1970). Its scales have demonstrated good internal consistency, ranging from $\alpha = .74$ to $\alpha = .95$ in a mixed psychiatric and community sample (Klein & Benjamin, 1996; Smith, Klein, & Benjamin, 2003). Smith et al. (2003) reported a median correlation of .44 (range: .32–.60) between the WISPI-IV and a widely used semistructured interview, the SCID-II (see below), providing preliminary evidence of convergent validity.

The ADP-IV (Schotte & De Doncker, 1996) is a 94-item questionnaire that, like the PDQ-4+, assesses the criteria for the 10 DSM-IV personality disorders, plus those for the two designated for further study. Each item consists of a "trait question," which asks the individual to rate the degree to which he feels that a statement describes him on a 7-point Likert-type scale. If individuals agrees to some degree that the trait applies to them (i.e., rates it as a 5 "rather agree" or higher), then they he completes an additional item, rating the degree to which the trait in question has caused or causes distress in themselves or others on a scale from 1 ("not at all") to 3 ("definitely"). Schotte et al. (2004) reported that on average, 3–4 items on each individual's questionnaire are rated as present but not causing distress. The ADP-IV can be scored dimensionally, using trait scores, and categorically, using scoring algorithms that take into account both trait and distress cut-offs. The original version of the ADP-IV is in Dutch, but English, German, Japanese, and French versions are available.

Preliminary reports indicate promising psychometric properties for the ADP-IV. When scored dimensionally, the trait scales have demonstrated good internal consistency (median Cronbach's alpha: .76; range: .60–.84) (Schotte, De Doncker, Van Kerckhoven, Vertommen, & Cosyns, 1998), and adequate test–retest reliability and stability (median r=.82 over a six-month interval; Schotte et al., 2004). Furthermore, in a Flemish sample of $n = 487$ psychiatric inpatients, and $n = 659$ individuals from the general population, the ADP-IV was found to adequately discriminate those with and without a PD diagnosis in the psychiatric sample when scored both categorically and dimensionally. Additionally, at the dimensional level, the convergent correlations between the 12 PD scales and their corresponding scales on a widely used semistructured interview, the SCID-II (see below), ranged from .35 to .67, with a median of .52 (Schotte et al., 2004).

Structured interview measures Several structured and semistructured interview measures for the assessment of DSM-IV personality disorders are available, although as is the case for self-report measures, there is variation in the degree to which they are supported by research. We will discuss three widely used interview measures here: the Structured Clinical Interview for DSM-IV Axis II Personality Disorders (SCID-II; First, Gibbon, Spitzer, Williams, & Benjamin, 1997), the Diagnostic Interview for DSM-IV Personality Disorders (DIPD-IV; Zanarini, 1996), and the Structured Interview for DSM-IV Personality Disorders (SIDP-IV; Pfohl, Blum, & Zimmerman, 1997).

The SCID-II (First et al., 1997) is a semistructured diagnostic interview for assessment of the 10 DSM-IV Axis II personality disorders, as well as Depressive Personality Disorder and Passive-Aggressive Personality Disorders, which are included in Appendix B of DSM-IV as criteria sets for further study. Like the SCID-I, the SCID-II contains one item per criterion for each of the diagnoses, to be rated by the interview on a scale from 1 ("Absent or false") to 3 ("Threshold or true"). Most research on the SCID-II was conducted using its previous version, the DSM-III-R SCID-II (e.g., Renneberg, Chambless, Dowdall, Fauerbach, & Graceley, 1992; First, Spitzer, Gibbon, & Williams, 1995; Dreessen & Arntz, 1998), and indicates acceptable levels of interrater reliability and internal consistency. At least one study reports high levels of internal consistency for the SCID-II, and its inter-rater reliability is generally reported to be fair-to-excellent, with kappas ranging from .43 to .98, and intraclass correlations coefficients (ICCs) ranging from .61 to 1.00 for PD categories (Maffei et al., 1997). Findings from a recent study of the convergence of the WISPI-IV with the SCID-II indicate widely varying levels of internal consistency among the scales of the SCID-II, ranging from $\alpha = .30$ (histrionic) to $\alpha = .77$ (avoidant).

The DIPD is a semistructured diagnostic interview that assesses the presence of the 10 primary DSM-IV personality disorders, as well as the two for further research. It requires that the criteria for each PD must be "present and pervasive" (Grilo et al., 2001) for at least 2 years, and that they be characteristic of the person for most of his or her adult life. Adequate levels of inter-rater reliability (range: .52–1.0; APD = 1.0) and test–retest reliability (1–2 week interval; range .46–.85; APD = .84) have been reported for this measure (Zanarini et al., 2000), and internal consistencies within each of the diagnoses have been found to range from $\alpha = .47$ (Schizoid PD) to $\alpha = .87$ (APD) (Grilo et al., 2001).

The Structured Interview for DSM-IV Personality Disorders (SIDP-IV; Pfohl et al., 1997) is a 60- to 90-minute semistructured interview, in which the interview rates the presence or absence of DSM-IV PD criteria on a 4-point scale (0 = "not present," 1 = "subclinical presence," 2 = "present," 3 = "strongly present"). To be considered clinically present, a criterion must be rated 2 or 3. Past versions of the SIDP attained acceptable levels of inter-rater agreement when assessing the disorders categorically (joint interview $\kappa = .71$) (Stangl, Pfohl, Zimmerman, Bowers, & Corenthal, 1985), but psychometric properties of the current edition are not known.

What Assessments are Not Helpful?

There is no compelling evidence for the use of projective techniques in the detection of APD, although these instruments are often used to aid in the diagnosis of this condition. Although some authors (e.g., Gacono & Meloy, 1994) have maintained that certain Rorschach indices, such as an abnormally large number of reflection responses or an abnormally small number of texture responses, are associated with APD (and psychopathy), research has offered little support for these claims (Wood, Lilienfeld, Garb, & Nezworski, 2000). We are unaware of any evidence that the Thematic Apperception Test, human figure drawings, or other projective methods are helpful in the detection of APD. The MMPI-2 Psychopathic deviate (Pd) scale (Scale 4) is positively correlated with APD symptoms (Lilienfeld, 1999) and may be useful in the assessment of certain features of APD. Nevertheless, it should not be used by itself to generate diagnoses of APD because it does not map directly onto DSM-IV APD symptoms. Moreover, although certain Harris-Lingoes subscales of the Pd scale, especially Pd2 (Authority Problems) are moderately to highly associated with APD symptoms, other Pd subscales, particularly Pd3 (Social Imperturbability) and Pd4 (Social Alienation), appear to be negligibly associated with APD symptoms (Lilienfeld, 1999).

TREATMENT

What Treatments are Effective?

Considering the enormous toll that APD takes on the affected individual, the individual's family and friends, and society at large, it is unfortunate that there is little evidence of effective treatments for APD. Indeed, as Turkat (1990) observed, the treatment of APD is an "unpopular topic in psychiatry" (p. 60), probably because there is precious little evidence for efficacious treatments and because individuals with APD tend to be notoriously unpleasant to treat. Aside from a scattering of poorly controlled case studies, there is little treatment literature bearing on APD, and that which does exist discusses the benefits of treating such associated behaviors as substance abuse or violence, but says little about altering its underlying personality features.

Several studies have reporting encouraging findings regarding substance abuse treatment in individuals with APD. In a sample of patients with heroin addiction ($N = 183$), Darke, Finlay-Jones, Kaye, & Blatt (1996) found that APD patients were not significantly more likely to relapse, or to drop out or be removed from the treatment program, when compared to non-APD patients ($d = -.17$). In a sample of patients in treatment for alcohol addiction ($N = 309$), Verheul, van den Brink, Koeter, & Hartgers (1999) found no difference in post-treatment alcohol and social problems when comparing patients who met DSM-III-R criteria for APD and those who did not . The authors concluded that antisocial patients had benefited just as much as their nonantisocial counterparts from this program, which included detoxification, daycare and residential treatment, individual and group counseling, and relapse prevention. Goldstein et al. (2001) compared residential addiction treatment clients meeting DSM-III-R APD criteria with those displaying only adult antisocial behavior on several outcome variables. Although those meeting full criteria for APD were at slightly increased risk for first episode of relapse, the two groups did not differ in severity of relapse episode. Taken together, these findings provide preliminary indications that patients with co-occurring APD and substance abuse problems may sometimes fare as well in substance abuse treatment as patients without APD.

Nevertheless, other studies of substance abuse treatment report findings suggesting less improvement in individuals with APD than other individuals. For example, in a sample of inpatient alcoholics with co-occurring DSM-III personality disorders ($N = 102$), Poldrugo and Forti (1988) found significantly reduced compliance with group treatment and abstinence from alcohol in patients with APD ($n = 24$). Nevertheless, the comparison groups were quite small in this study, and that it was unclear (a) what criteria were used to determine treatment compliance and (b) whether the raters of this variable were blind to the patients' diagnoses. In a sample of low-SES methadone opiate dependent men enrolled in a methadone maintenance program at a VA hospital (N = 193), Alterman, Rutherford, Cacciola, McKay, and Boardman (1998) found that number of APD symptoms correlated negatively and moderately with treatment completion. Nevertheless, number of APD symptoms did not correlate significantly with other variables (e.g., presence of narcotic traces in urine; social, legal, or psychiatric problems), and was not a specific indicator, because conduct disorder scales, psychopathy scales, and an index of socialization predicted treatment completion equally well. The findings regarding the relation of APD to substance abuse treatment outcome are therefore inconsistent.

Additionally, there are preliminary indications that concurrent psychopathology can moderate treatment outcome in antisocial patients under some conditions. In a sample of opiate addicts (N = 63), receiving drug counseling plus professional psychotherapy (supportive or cognitive behavioral), Woody, McLellan, Luborsky, and O'Brien (1985) found that patients with opiate addiction plus APD (OP+APD) showed little improvement with treatment, whereas those with opiate addiction and APD plus depression (OP+APD+DEP) improved to a degree comparable to non-APD patients. Specifically, while OP+APD patients showed significant improvement on only 3 of 22 possible variables, confined to areas of drug use and legal status, OP+APD+DEP significantly improved on 11 variables, including days working, days using opiates, days using stimulants, illegal income, and symptom counts on the SCL-90, SADS anxiety and SADS depression. In terms of effect sizes representing overall improvement, OP+DEP+APD patients showed moderate improvement (d = .50), whereas OP+APD patients showed a small negative effect size (d = −.23), reflecting deterioration.

No group therapies, self-help treatments, or individual therapies (e.g., psychoanalysis, person-centered therapy) are known to be effective in treating APD. Although Turkat (1990) recommended that anger management and impulse control training strategies be used to minimize the problematic behaviors of individuals with APD, there is no controlled evidence for their efficacy. Other authors, such as Beck and Freeman (1990), have suggested a cognitive-behavioral approach to APD that addresses six self-serving beliefs and cognitive styles central to this condition: (1) Justification, (2) Thinking is believing, (3) Personal infallibility, (4) Feelings make facts, (5) The impotence of others, and (6) Low-impact consequences. In addition to addressing these dysfunctional beliefs, Beck and Freeman propose that therapists guide APD patients toward more abstract thinking and toward recognizing the effects of their behavior on others. Nevertheless, there are no known controlled studies of this treatment.

What is Effective Medical Treatment?

Although there is no controlled evidence that psychopharmacological treatment ameliorates APD features, a few studies suggest that drug treatment may minimize some of the destructive behaviors associated with APD. For example, some researchers have found an association between treatment with lithium carbonate (lithium) and carbamazepine (Tegretol) and decreased general violence, aggression, and impulsiveness (Tyrer, 1988). However, few controlled studies have demonstrated these effects. To our knowledge, no controlled studies have examined the effects of Tegretol on violent or antisocial behavior, and we located only one controlled clinical trial of this nature for lithium. Sheard, Marini, Bridges, and

Wagner (1976) treated 66 patients exhibiting serious assaultive and antisocial behavior, with Lithium or placebo for up to 3 months. They found a significant reduction in aggressive behavior in the Lithium group relative to placebo. Others have found that antisocial symptoms secondary to certain Axis I conditions (e.g., depression, paraphilias) may be effectively treated by means of pharmaceutical treatments traditionally prescribed for the treatment of those conditions (e.g., mood stabilizers, antiandrogens). In a double-blind, placebo-controlled trial of the selective serotonin-reuptake inhibitor fluoxetine hydrochloride (Prozac) conducted with 40 DSM-III-R personality-disordered individuals with histories of impulsive aggressive behavior and irritability, and no current major depression, bipolar disorder or schizophrenia, Coccaro and Kavoussi (1997) found that fluoxetine, but not placebo, resulted in a sustained reduction in self-reported irritability and aggression. Nevertheless, the relevance of these findings to the treatment of APD per se is unclear.

CONCLUDING REMARKS

In contrast to psychopathy, for which there are decades of clinical lore and research findings that contribute to a "therapeutic nihilism" (Reid & Gacono, 2000; but see Salekin, 2002), there is scant controlled intervention research on APD. As a consequence, it is difficult to offer definitive recommendations for the treatment of this condition. Although there are some indications that drug-addicted individuals with both APD and depression may be more likely to benefit from treatment than drug-addicted individuals with APD alone, these findings are preliminary and of unknown generalizability to individuals outside of substance abuse settings. Nevertheless, given evidence that APD (a) may in some cases be a negative treatment indicator and (b) is associated with increased risk for physical aggression, we advice clinicians who work in forensic settings, substance abuse settings, or both to incorporate well validated measures of APD into their assessment batteries. Because self-report measures of APD do not permit probing of responses and therefore may yield overly liberal diagnoses of this condition, we further recommend that these measures be supplemented with structured interviews. Hopefully, further controlled research on treatment outcome among APD patients will permit stronger conclusions to be drawn regarding the treatment implications of this diagnosis across various settings.

REFERENCES

Alterman, A. I., Rutherford, M. J., Cacciola, J. S., McKay, J. R., & Boardman, C. R. (1998). Prediction of 7 months methadone maintenance treatment response by four measures of antisociality. *Drug & Alcohol Dependence, 49,* 217–223.

American Psychiatric Association (1994). *Diagnostic and statistical manual of mental disorders* (4th ed.). Washington, DC: Author.

American Psychiatric Association (2000). *Diagnostic and statistical manual of mental disorders* (4th ed., text revision). Washington, DC: Author.

Beck, A. T., & Freeman, A. (1990). *Cognitive therapy of personality disorders.* London: The Guilford Press.

Cleckley, H. (1941). The mask of sanity: an attempt to reinterpret the so-called psychopathic personality. St. Louis: Mosby.

Cloninger, C. R., Christiansen, K. O., Reich, T., & Gottesman, I. I. (1978). Implications of sex differences in the prevalences of antisocial personality, alcoholism, and criminality for familial transmission. *Archives of General Psychiatry, 35,* 941–951.

Coccaro, E. F., & Kavoussi, R. J. (1997). Fluoxetine and impulsive aggressive behavior in personality-disordered subjects. *Archives of General Psychiatry, 54,* 1081–1088.

Craig, R. J. (1999). Testimony based on the Millon Clinical Multiaxial Inventory: Review, commentary, and guidelines. *Journal of Personality Assessment, 73,* 290–305.

Cunningham, M. D., & Reidy, T. J. (1999). Don't confuse me with the facts: Common errors in violence risk assessment at capital sentencing. *Criminal Justice & Behavior, 26*, 20–43.

Darke, S., Finlay-Jones, R., Kaye, S., & Blatt, T. (1996). Anti-social personality disorder and response to methadone maintenance treatment. *Drug and Alcohol Review, 15*, 271–276.

Dreessen, L., & Arntz, A. (1998). Short-interval test-retest interrater reliability of the Structured Clinical Interview for DSM-III-R Personality Disorders (SCID-II) in outpatients. *Journal of Personality Disorders, 12*, 138–148.

Farrington, D. P., Ohlin, L., & Wilson, J. Q. (1986). *Understanding and controlling crime.* New York: Springer Verlag.

First, M. B., Spitzer, R. L., Gibbon, M., & Williams, J. B. W. (1995). The Structured Clinical Interview for DSM-III-R Personality Disorders (SCID-II): I. Description. *Journal of Personality Disorders, 9*, 83–91.

First, M. B., Gibbon, M., Spitzer, R. L., Williams, J. B., & Benjamin, L. S. (1997). *User's guide for the Structured Clinical Interview for the DSM-IV Personality Disorders.* Washington, DC: American Psychiatric Press.

Fossati, A., Maffei, C., Bagnato, M., Donati, D., Donini, M., Fiorilli, M., Novella, L., & Ansoldi, M. (1998). Criterion validity of the Personality Diagnostic Questionnaire -4+ (PDQ-4+) in a mixed psychiatric sample. *Journal of Personality Disorders, 12*, 172–178.

Gacono, C. B., & Meloy, J. R. (1994). *The Rorschach assessment of aggressive and psychopathic personalities.* Hillsdale, NJ: Erlbaum.

Glover, A. J. J., Nicholson, D. E., Hemmati, T., Bernfeld, G. A., & Quinsey, V. L. (2002). A comparison of predictors of general and violent recidivism among high-risk federal offenders. *Criminal Justice and Behavior, 29*, 235–249.

Goldstein, R. B., Bigelow, C., McCusker, J., Lewis, B. F., Mundt, K. A., & Powers, S. I. (2001). Antisocial behavioral syndromes and return to drug use following residential relapse prevention/health education treatment. *American Journal of Drug and Alcohol Abuse, 27*, 453–482.

Greenwald, H. J. & Satow, Y. (1970). A short social desirability scale. *Psychological Reports, 27*, 131–135.

Grilo, C. M., McGlashan, T. H., Morey, L. C., Gunderson, J. G., Skodol, A. E., Tracie, S. M. et al. (2001). Internal consistency, intercriterion overlap and diagnostic efficiency of criteria sets for DSM-IV schizotypal, borderline, avoidant, and obsessive-compulsive personality disorders.

Hare, R. D. (2003). *Manual for the revised psychopathy checklist* (2nd ed.). Toronto, ON, Canada: Multi-Health Systems.

Harris, G. T., Rice, M. C., & Cornier, C. A. (1991). Psychopathy and violent recidivism. Law and Human Behavior, *15*, 625–637.

Hart, S. D., & Hare, R. D. (1997). Psychopathy: assessment and association with criminal conduct. In D. M. Stoff, J. Breiling, & J. D. Maser (Eds.), *Handbook of antisocial behavior,* (pp. 22–35). New York, NY: Wiley.

Hart, S. D., Kropp, P. R., & Hare, R. D. (1988). Performance of psychopaths following conditional release from prison. *Journal of Consulting and Clinical Psychology, 56*, 227–232.

Hyler, S. E. (1994). *The Personality Diagnostic Questionnaire 4+.* New York: New York State Psychiatric Institute.

Klein, M. H., & Benjamin, L. S. (1996). *The Wisconsin Personality Disorders Inventory-IV,* Madison, WI: University of Wisconsin, unpublished test.

Lilienfeld, S. O. (1992). The association between antisocial personality and somatization disorders: A review and integration of theoretical models. *Clinical Psychology Review, 12*, 641–662.

Lilienfeld, S. O. (1994). Conceptual problems in the assessment of psychopathy. *Clinical Psychology Review, 14*, 17–38.

Lilienfeld, S. O. (1999). The relation of the MMPI-2 Pd Harris–Lingoes subscales to psychopathy, psychopathy facets, and antisocial behavior: Implications for clinical practice. *Journal of Clinical Psychology, 55*, 241–255.

Loeber, R. (1982). The stability of antisocial and delinquent child behavior: A review. *Child Development, 53*, 1431–1466.

Loeber, R., & Farrington, D. O. (1998). *Serious and violent juvenile offenders: Risk factors and successful interventions.* Thousand Oaks, CA: Sage.

Lykken, D. T. (1995). The antisocial personalities. Hillsdale, NJ: Erlbaum.

Maffei, C., Fossati, A., Agostoni, I., Barraco, A., Bagnato, M., Donati, D., Namia, C., Novella, L., & Petrachi, M. (1997). Interrater reliability and internal consistency of the structured clinical interview for DSM-IV Axis II personality disorders (SCID-II), version 2.0. *Journal of Personality Disorders, 11*, 279–284.

Millon, T. (1981). *Disorders of personality DSM III Axis II.* New York: Wiley.

Millon, T. (1983). Millon Clinical Multiaxial Inventory manual. New York: Holt, Reinhart, & Winston.

Millon, T. (1987). Millon Clinical Multiaxial Inventory-II: Manual for the MCMI-II. Minneapolis, MN: National Computer Systems.

Millon, T. (1994). Millon Clinical Multiaxial Inventory-III: Manual. Minneapolis, MN: National Computer Systems.

Millon, T. (2003). Evolution: A generative source for conceptualizing the attributes of personality. In T. Millon & M. Lerner (Eds.), *Handbook of psychology: Personality and social psychology* (Vol. 5, pp. 3–30). New York: Wiley & Sons.

Moffitt, T. E. (1993). Adolescence-limited and life-course-persistent antisocial behavior: A developmental taxonomy. *Psychological Review, 100,* 674–701.

Morey, L. C., Waugh, M., & Blashfield, R. (1985). MMPI scales for the *DSM-III* personality disorders: Their derivation and correlates. *Journal of Personality Assessment, 49,* 245–251.

Perry, J. C. (1992). Problems and considerations in the valid assessment of personality disorders. *American Journal of Psychiatry, 149,* 1645–1653.

Pfohl, B., Blum, N., & Zimmerman, M. (1997). *Structured Interview for DSM-IV Personality.* Washington, DC: American Psychiatric Press.

Poldrugo, F., & Forti, B. (1988). Personality disorders and alcoholism treatment outcome. *Drug and Alcohol Dependence, 21,* 171–176.

Reid, W. H., & Gacono, C. (2000). Treatment of antisocial personality, psychopathy, and other characterologic antisocial syndromes. *Behavioral Sciences and the Law, 18,* 647–662.

Renneberg, B., Chambless, D. L., Dowdall, D. J., Fauerbach, J. A., & Graceley, E. J. (1992). The Structured Clinical Interview for DSM-III–R, Axis II and the Millon Clinical Multiaxial Inventory: A concurrent validity study of personality disorders among anxious outpatients. *Journal of Personality Disorders, 6,* 117–124.

Rogers, R., & Dion, K. (1991). Rethinking the DSM-III-R diagnosis of antisocial personality disorder. *Bulletin of the American Academy of Psychiatry and Law, 19,* 21–31.

Salekin, R. T. (2002). Psychopathy and therapeutic pessimism: Clinical lore or clinical reality? *Clinical Psychology Review, 22,* 79–112.

Schotte, C. K. W., & De Doncker, D. A. M. (1996). *ADP-IV Questionnaire: Manual and norms.* Antwerp, Belgium: University Hospital Antwerp.

Schotte, C. K. W., De Doncker, D., Vankerckhoven, C., Vertommen, H., & Cosyns, P. (1998). Self-report assessment of the DSM-IV personality disorders: Measurement of trait and distress characterstics: The ADP-IV. Psychological medicine, *28,* 1179–1188.

Schotte, C. K. W., De Doncker, D. A. M., DMitruk, D., Van Mulders, I., D'Haenan, H., & Cosyns, P. (2004). The ADP-IV questionnaire: Differential validity and concordance with the semistructured interview. *Journal of Personality Disorders, 18,* 405–419.

Sheard, M. H., Marini, J. L., Bridges, C. I., & Wagner, E. (1976). The effect of lithium on impulsive on impulsive aggressive behavior in man. *American Journal of Psychiatry, 133,* 1409–1413.

Skilling, T. A., Harris, G. T., Rice, M. E., & Quinsey, V. L. (2002). Identifying persistently antisocial offenders using the Hare Psychopathy Checklist and DSM Antisocial Personality Disorder Criteria. *Psychological Assessment, 14,* 27–38.

Smith, T. L., Klein, M. H., & Benjamin, L. S. (2003). Validation of the Wisconsin Personality Disorders Inventory-IV with the SCID-II. *Journal of Personality Disorders, 17,* 173–187.

Somwaru, D. P. & Ben-Porath, Y. S. (1995). Development and reliability of MMPI-2 based personality disorders. Presented at Annual Symposium on. Recent Developments in MMPI-2, MMPI-A, 30th, St. Petersburg Beach, FL.

Stangl, D., Pfohl, B., Zimmerman, M., Bowers, W., & Corenthal, C. (1985). A structured interview for the DSM-III personality disorders. *Archives of General Psychiatry, 42,* 591–596.

Trull, T. J. (1993). Temporal stability and validity of two personality disorder inventories. *Psychological Assessment: A Journal of Consulting and Clinical Psychology, 5,* 11–18.

Turkat, I. D. (1990). *The personality disorders: A psychological approach to clinical management.* Elmsford, New York: Pergamon Press.

Tyrer, P. (1988). *Personality disorders: Diagnosis, management, and course.* London: Wright.

Verheul, R., van den Brink, W., Koeter, M. W. J., & Hartgers, C. (1999). Antisocial alcoholic patients show as much improvement at 14-month follow-up as non-antisocial alcoholic patients. *American Journal on Addictions, 8,* 24–33.

Widom, C. S. (1977). A methodology for studying noninstitutionalized psychopaths. *Journal of Consulting and Clinical Psychology, 45,* 674–683.

Wood, J. M., Lilienfeld, S. O., Garb, H. N., & Nezworski, M. T. (2000). The Rorschach Test in clinical diagnosis: A critical review, with a backward look at Garfield (1947). *Journal of Clinical Psychology, 56,* 441–448.

Woody, G. E., McLellan, A. T., Luborsky, L., & O'Brien, C. P. (1985). Sociopathy and psychotherapy outcome. *Archives of General Psychiatry, 42,* 1081–1086.

Zanarini, M. C., Skodol, A. E., Bender, D., Dolan, R., Sanislow, C., Schaefer, E., Morey, L. C., Grilo, C. M., Shea, M. T., McGlashan, T. H., Gunderson, J. G. (2000). The collaborative longitudinal personality disorders study: reliability of Axis I and II diagnoses. *Journal of Personality Disorders, 14,* 291–299.

Asperger's Disorder

Christine E. Caselles

Asperger's disorder, more commonly referred to as Asperger's syndrome, is a chronic developmental disorder characterized by severe and pervasive social dysfunction and the presence of restricted, repetitive patterns of interests, behavior, and activities (American Psychiatric Association, 1994). Asperger's disorder is a pervasive developmental disorder distinguished from other such disorders by the presence of intact language and cognitive functions. Hans Asperger first described it in the literature in 1944 as a developmental disorder involving Aautistic psychopathy. Asperger's disorder was only officially recognized in the most recent revisions of the ICD-10 (World Health Organization, 1992) and DSM-IV (American Psychiatric Association, 1994). Impairment and abnormalities are quite pervasive in Asperger's disorder. In addition to the core characteristics, there are many other features that are common but not necessary for diagnosis.

Individuals with Asperger's disorder demonstrate severe impairment in reciprocal social interaction. This impairment may consist of an inability or a lack of desire to interact with peers, an inability to recognize social cues, and a lack of empathy or sensitivity. Although they may express interest in making friends, their approaches tend to be inappropriate and peculiar. They often appear to be unaware of social conventions and they rely on formalistic rules to govern their behavior. They are often perceived as socially awkward, eccentric, or strange. Because they have difficulty understanding the motivations of other people, individuals with Asperger's are socially naive and can be vicimtized by peers. These difficulties usually result in a lack of close peer relationships, social isolation, and peer rejection.

Individuals with Asperger's disorder have intense interests in unusual, circumscribed subject matter, such as elevators or movie schedules. Younger children with Asperger's may be preoccupied with parts of objects, such as wheels, and they may be overly interested in the mechanics of things. They spend large amounts of time engaged in activities related to their interests, such as amassing knowledge about the topic, collecting memorabilia, or talking unremittingly about their interests. They usually spend so much time involved in the topic which preoccupies them that there is little time to learn about more socially relevant topics. The actual subject matter often changes over time, but the intensity of their interest is an enduring characteristic.

DSM-IV and ICD-10 diagnostic criteria specifically exclude individuals from having Asperger's disorder if they had an early language delay (failure to use meaningful words by age 24 months and combined words and phrases by 36 months). However, various speech and communication abnormalities are noted in AS including idiosyncratic facial and gestural expressions, highly literal and concrete verbal expression and interpretations, extreme verbosity, a lack of conversational reciprocity, pedantic style of speaking, lack of eye-to-eye gaze, and poor modulation of volume, pace and tone of speech.

Individuals with Asperger's disorder often present with clumsy movement, unusual posture and gait, delayed acquisition of motor skills, and poor graphomotor

Caselles, C. E. (2006). Asperger's Disorder. In J.E. Fisher & W. T. O'Donohue (Eds.), *Practitioner's Guide to evidence-based psychotherapy*. New York: Springer.

abilities, although these characteristic are not necessary for diagnosis. Stereotypic movement may also be present, particularly in young children with Asperger's disorder.

BASIC FACTS ABOUT ASPERGER'S DISORDER

Prevalence. Few studies have examined the prevalence of Asperger's disorder and therefore epidemiological data are scarce. Prevalence estimates of Asperger's disorder vary widely resulting primarily from methodological differences among studies. The limited data suggest rates of ranging from .3 to 48.4 in 10,000 children. In a review of the epidemiological research, Fombonne and Tidmarsh (2003), concluded that the prevalence of AS is approximately 2 per 10,000 children.

Gender. Epidemiological data suggest that Asperger's disorder is more common in males than females with a male: female ratio of 4:1 (Khouzan, El-Gabalawi, Pirwani, & Priest, 2004).

Comorbidity. There has been little systematic research about comorbidity in Asperger's disorder. The limited available data and clinical reports suggest that it may coexist with several psychiatric disorders. It has been associated with obsessive-compulsive disorder (Thomsen, 1994). Clinically significant levels of depression and generalized anxiety occur at higher rates in populations of children with Asperger's disorder (Towbin, 2003; Kim, Szatmari, Bryson, Streiner, & Wilson, 2000). Problems with stress management and anger have also been reported in adolescents and young adults with Asperger's disorder (Ghaziuddin, Weidmar-Mikhail, & Ghaziuddin, 1998). Several earlier studies have found an association between Tourette's Syndrome and Asperger's disorder although more recent studies have not replicated this finding (Klin & Volkmar, 1997). Hyperactivity and inattention are common in children with Asperger's disorder (Towbin, 2003; Yoshida & Uchiyama, 2004). One study suggests that individuals with Asperger's disorder often received diagnoses of ADHD at some point during childhood (Martin, Scahill, Klin, & Volkmar, 1999) although it is unclear whether these diagnoses were accurate.

Onset. The symptoms of Asperger's disorder are usually apparent in preschool or grade school years. Wing (1981) suggested that abnormalities are apparent as early as the first two years of life including decreased interest in people, limited babbling, and reduced sharing of interests. Early fascination with letters and numbers and precocious decoding skills have also been noted as features of early development in children with Asperger's disorder (Klin & Volkmar, 1997). Delays in the development of motor skills, such as pedaling a bicycle, playing ball, and climbing, often occur in the preschool years (Khouzam et al., 2004) of children with Asperger's disorder. One study reported that the average age of diagnosis is 11 years, despite the fact that parents of these children begin to have concerns when their children are on average 30 months of age (Howlin & Asgharian, 1999). Although a clear pattern of difficulties in peer relationships and unusual, intense interests are present in the early school years, it has been estimated that 50% of children with Asperger's disorder reach adulthood without receiving a diagnosis or treatment (Szatmari, Archer, Fisman, Streiner, & Wilson, 1995).

Course. Asperger's disorder is a lifelong, enduring condition. The presentation of the disorder typically changes from childhood to adolescence and adulthood. Stereotypy, reduced sharing of interests, and preoccupation with parts of objects typically disappear by adolescence (Tantum, 2003). Adults with Asperger's disorder present with obsessive interests, a lack of empathy, social awkwardness and isolation, and illogical thinking. Anecdotal reports have demonstrated the ability of some individuals with Asperger's disorder to use special interests or talents in their vocational choices (Tsantsanis, 2003).

Associated features. Individuals with Asperger's syndrome usually have difficulty in tolerating changes in routine or previously laid plans. They may become upset by minor differences in their environment, such as moving the arrangement of furniture, or in the appearance of other people, such as a parent getting a new haircut. This inflexibility sometimes leads to tantrums, extreme anxiety, or aggression (Towbin, 2003). Individuals with Asperger's may also present with relative weaknesses in non-verbal cognitive abilities and may have highly concrete, "black-and-white" thinking.

ASSESSMENT OF ASPERGER'S DISORDER

Comprehensive Assessment

Asperger's disorder involves difficulties in multiple areas of functioning. Therefore, a thorough evaluation is necessary for diagnosis and prior to initiating treatment. In general, a comprehensive assessment of individuals with Asperger's disorder should include information related to the following:

- *Social skills and interactions with others.* Examination of quality of attachment to family members, the presence and quality of friendships and peer relationships, and awareness of social conventions, and behavior during social interactions.
- *Stereotyped behavior and special interests.* Examination of descriptions of special interests, amount of time spent engaging in topics, interference with other activities and with lives of family members, rituals and routines, stereotyped behaviors, and responses to interference with these activities.
- *Language and communication.* Examination of vocabulary development, use of grammar and syntax, speech content, use of nonverbal communication, tone, pace, and prosody of speech, and reciprocity in conversation.
- *Motor difficulties.* Examination of motor development and current gross and fine motor abilities.
- *Symptoms of comorbid conditions.* Examination for the presence of depressed mood, anxiety, compulsions and obsessions, and hyperactive behavior.
- *Cognitive and academic functioning.* Examination of general intelligence, intellectual strengths and weaknesses, and performance in academic subjects.
- *Affective functioning.* Examination of ability to understand affective responses other people, ability to identify one's own emotions, and responses to stress and anger.
- *Adaptive behaviour.* Examination of self-sufficiency in real-life situations.

Methods of Assessment

Developmental history. A careful developmental history is important in making an accurate diagnosis of Asperger's disorder. History should include information about early development and current characteristics and behaviors, medical history, and health history. The developmental history should be obtained from the child's primary caretaker as well as a review of medical, educational, and psychological records.

Diagnostic instruments. There are several well-standardized assessment instruments which can be included in a diagnostic evaluation of Asperger's disorder. The Autism Diagnostic Interview—Revised (ADI-R; Lord, 1995) is a semistructured, clinician-administered interview and is linked to DSM-IV and ICD-10 diagnostic criteria. The Autism Diagnostic Observation Scale-Generic (ADOS-G;

Lord et al., 2000) is a semistructured, behavior observation instrument and examines communication, social interaction, play, and imaginative behavior. Both the ADI-R and the ADOS-G require specialized training and are time consuming to administer. Hence, these instruments are rarely used in clinical settings.

Several screening tests have been developed to identify children who may have Asperger's disorder and other pervasive developmental disorders, including the Childhood Asperger Syndrome Test (CAST; Scott, Baron, Cohen, Bolton, & Bayne, 2002), the Pervasive Developmental Disorders Screening Test (PDDST; Seigel, 1998), and the Australian Scale for Asperger's Syndrome (Garnett & Attwood, 1998). However, these instruments are generally not well-standardized and little data exists to support their diagnostic utility.

Behavioral assessment. Behavioral assessment is important to plan and evaluate interventions for individuals with Asperger's disorder. Behavioral assessments involve directly observing the individual's behavior in order to establish target behaviors, perform a functional assessment of behavior, conduct task analyses, and determine the effectiveness of previous procedures (Haynes, O'Brien, & Hayes, 2000).

Developmental assessments. An evaluation of cognitive functioning is useful to select appropriate educational and psychological interventions, to assess prognosis, and to help families and individuals prepare for the future. An individually administered, standardized measure of intellectual functioning, such as the Wechsler scales or the Stanford-Binet, is appropriate for this purpose. A measure of adaptive behavior, such as the Vineland Adaptive Behavior Scales (Sparrow, et al., 1984), provides information about an individuals level of independence, social functioning, language and communication, motor skills, and the presence of maladaptive behaviors. An assessment of academic skills, such as the Wechsler Individual Achievement Test is useful to determine educational needs.

Rule out. Several conditions need to be ruled out in order to make a diagnosis of Asperger's disorder. An individual is excluded from having Asperger's if he or she has received a previous diagnosis of autism (precedence rule; American Psychiatric Association, 1994). According to DSM-IV criteria, the clear distinction between Asperger's disorder and autism is the presence of a language delay in autism during the first three years of life.

Differntial diagnosis of Asperger's disorder also involves ruling out obsessive-compulsive disorder which also presents with stereotyped behavior and resistance to change. Asperger's, however, also is characterized by severe, qualitative impairment in social functioning which is not typically characteristic of obsessive-compulsive disorder. Schizoid personality disorder also needs to be eliminated. Asperger's disorder is distinguished from schizoid personality disorder by intense, circumscribed interests and stereotyped behavior.

TREATMENT AND INTERVENTION

Although much has been written about the treatment of Asperger's disorder, there is a paucity of empirical data on the effectiveness of interventions. Numerous case studies (Ruberman, 2002; Cragar & Horvath, 2003; Frazier, Doyle, Chui, & Coyle, 2002) and descriptions of treatment protocols for children with Asperger's disorder (Attwood, 2000; 2003; Krasny, Williams, Provencal, & Ozonoff, 2003; Miles, 2003) have been published. Presently, however, there are no controlled, randomized studies that have evaluated the application of any treatment procedures for individuals diagnosed with Asperger's disorder. Research on treatment efficacy in Asperger's disorder has been complicated by the difficulty in establishing it as a discrete diagnostic entity distinguishable from other pervasive developmental disorders. Volkmar (2004) indicated that, in addition to the DSM-IV and ICD-10 criteria, there are at least five widely circulated definitions of Asperger's disorder.

Still, there has been a great deal of controversy regarding whether Asperger's disorder is a discrete diagnostic entity or whether it is a high-functioning form of autism. Currently there are scarce data to clarify this issue (Volkmar & Klin, 2001; Klin & Volkmar, 2003). Many researchers and authors use the label autistic spectrum disorders to include individuals with a broad range of clinical presentations and with diagnoses of autism, Pervasive Developmental Disorder, Not Otherwise Specified, and Asperger's disorder (Smith, Magyar, & Arnold-Saritepe, 2002; Paul, 2003; Constantino & Todd, 2003). Other researchers have used mixed groups of individuals who were labeled with high-functioning autism and Asperger's disorder (Baron-Cohen & Wheelwright, 2003). The classification and diagnostic discrepancies contribute to the difficulty in interpreting research on the application of interventions specifically for individuals with Asperger's disorder. Because Asperger's disorder involves severe and pervasive impairment across multiple areas of functioning, effective treatments are symptom based and tailored for the individual (Khourzan et al., 2004; Volkmar, 1997). The significant amount of symptom overlap between Asperger's disorder and other pervasive developmental disorders (Volkmar, 2003) makes it possible to draw from the literature on autism treatment to develop empirically supported, symptom-based interventions for Asperger's disorder.

Behavioral interventions. At present, behavioral treatments are the primary empirically supported interventions for pervasive developmental disorders as a whole. Behavioral interventions employ procedures derived from research on learning theory to increase adaptive behaviors and skills and to decrease inappropriate behavior (Newsom, 1998). Some investigators have reported that intensive behavioral intervention (20 hours or more per week for several years) results in increases in IQ scores, improved adaptive functioning, and less restrictive school placements in some cases (Lovaas 1987; 1993; 1995; Smith, 1999) although individual responses to these interventions vary widely. There is no evidence, however, that intensive interventions for individuals with Asperger's disorder are more effective than less intensive implementations.

For individuals with Asperger's, a *specific skills model* of behavioral intervention may be indicated (Smith et al., 2002). This model involves the use of behavioral techniques to teach specific social and adaptive skills to individuals with Asperger's disorder. Hundreds of studies have documented the effectiveness of specific behavioral procedures in treating autism. Many studies have reported success in using behavioral treatments to address specific behaviors and skill deficits that occur in Asperger's disorder. The majority of these studies are single-subject investigations or studies with relatively small sample sizes. However, because multiple investigations have documented the effectiveness of specific procedures, the evidence in support of these procedures is considerable (Bregman & Gerdtz, 1997).

Behavioral Procedures for Increasing Social Skills

A myriad of social difficulties comprise the hallmark symptoms of Asperger's disorder. Communication deficits and repetitive behaviors often lessen with age in individuals with Asperger's disorder (Piven, Harper, Palmer, & Arndt, 1996). Social difficulties are usually enduring and can be a severe impediment to progress and overall functioning (Howlin & Goode, 1998). Therefore, it is of primary importance that treatment plans for individuals with Asperger's disorder directly target social skills.

Behavioral procedures for improving social skills typically include modeling, direct instruction, prompting, rehearsal, and feedback and reinforcement from a practitioner, care giver, or peer. The efficacy of various behavioral procedures in improving social skills have been documented. Numerous recent studies demonstrated a positive effect of video modeling and positive reinforcement on various social abilities of children with autism, including their perspective taking skills (LeBlanc, Coates, Daneshvar, Charlop-Christy, & Lancaster, 2003), social initiations (Nikopolous & Keenan, 2004), conversational skills (Sherer, Pierce, Paredes, Kisacky, & Ingersoll, 2001; Charlop & Milstein, 1989) and developmental skills (Charlop-Christy, Le, & Freeman, 2000). One method of social skills training, called pivotal response training (PRT), targets behaviors thought to be crucial to social functioning using multiple cues and positive reinforcement (Koegel et al., 1989). Several studies have documented the effectiveness of this approach (Koegel & Frea, 1993; Peirce & Schriebman, 1997a,b).

In a recent review of the literature, Stahmer, Ingersoll, and Carter (2003) concluded that various behavioral approaches, including reciprocal imitation training, pivotal response training, differential reinforcement procedures, play scripts, and in vivo and video modeling, were effective in improving the play skills of children with autistic spectrum disorders.

Procedures involving social stories, or narratives describing social situations and appropriate behavior, have also been shown to be effective in improving social skills and reducing disruptive behavior (Thiemann & Goldstein, 2001; Swaggart et al., 1995).

Numerous studies have shown effects of behavioral interventions which utilize typically developing peers to model, instruct, prompt, and reinforce appropriate social behavior of children with pervasive developmental disorders (Krantz & McClannahan, 1998; Odom & Strain, 1984; 1986; Peirce & Schreibman, 1995; Peirce & Schreibman, 1997a,b; Strain, Kerr, & Ragland, 1979; Goldstein, Kaczmarek, Pennington, & Shafer, 1992; Thiemann & Goldstein, 2001). The research on peer-mediated interventions for children with autism is reviewed in an article by McConnell (2002).

Self-management procedures are behavioral strategies in which individuals are trained to monitor their own behavior and administer contingent rewards and consequences. A parent or instructional assistant is often involved in implementing self-management procedures, particularly during the introductory phase. Several studies have shown that self-management procedures are effective in improving the social behavior and reducing maladaptive behavior of individuals with pervasive developmental disorders (Koegel, Frea, & Surrat, 1994; Krantz, McDuff, & McClannahan, 1993; Krantz & McClannahan, 1998; Stahmer & Schreibman, 1992; Koegel, Koegel, Hurley, & Frea, 1992).

Behavioral Procedures for Reducing Repetitive, Circumscribed Interests and Activities

Many studies have demonstrated the efficacy of behaioral interventions in reducing repetitive and stereotypic behaviors of individuals with autism. Some of these interventions may be an appropriate component of symptom-based treatment plans for individuals with Asperger's disorder.

Interrption and redirection procedures involve directly blocking repetitive behavior and subsequently redirecting the individual to engage in another activity.

Several studies have demonstrated the effectiveness of interruption and redirection in reducing the repetitive behaviors of individuals with autism (Mulick & Meinhold, 1994; Maag, Wolchik, Rutherford, & Parks, 1986; Bebko & Lennox, 1988).

Reinforcement strategies involve rewarding appropriate behavior by following occurrences of the behavior with a desired consequence. Several reinforcement procedures may be appropriate to decrease circumscribed, excessive interests and activities of individuals with Asperger's disorder. Differential reinforcement techniques consist of reinforcing adaptive replacement behaviors or rewarding reduced rates of maladaptive behaviors. For example, in *differential reinforcement of other behavior (DRO)*, an individual is reinforced if the problem behavior has not occurred during an interval of time. Numerous studies have established differential reinforcement interventions as effective reductive procedures for individuals with autism (Bregman & Gerdtz, 1997).

Reinforcement-based interventions that employ the *Premack Principle* may also be appropriate for reducing the repetitive activities and interests of individuals with Asperger's disorder. Such interventions involve reinforcing an individual for completing a difficult or nonpreferred task by following it with an opportunity to engage in a preferred activity (Smith et al., 2002). For example, a child with Asperger's disorder might be rewarded for talking about a topic unrelated to their special interests by having time to read facts about that interest.

Self-management procedures, discussed previously in this chapter, have also been shown to be effective in reducing repetitive behaviors (Harchik, Sherman, & Sheldon, 1992) and inappropriate verbalizations (Mancina, Tankersley, Kamps, Kravits, & Parett, 2000) in individuals with autism. Self-management programs may be effective in reducing the amount of time spent talking about special interests and engaging in activities related to these interests.

Procedures for Managing Comorbid Anxiety and Depression

Mood disorders occur at a higher rate in individuals with Asperger's Disorder than in their nonafflicted peers. When present, these comorbid disorders need to be treated as part of the individuals overall intervention plan. Cognitive-behavioral therapy has been established through many empirical studies as the treatment of choice for both depression and anxiety disorders in children and adults (Compton, Marsh, Brent, Albano, & Weersing, 2004). These treatment may be adapted to become part of the symptom based treatment plan for individuals with Asperger's disorder. A single-subject study examined the use of cognitive-behavior therapy to treat social anxiety disorder and depression in an adult with Asperger's disorder. Standardized pre- and post-treatment measures indicated that the treatment was effective in reducing the symptoms of depression and social anxiety (Cardaciotto & Herbert, 2004).

Behavioral Procedures for Reducing Associated Tantrums and Aggression

Behavioral interventions for reducing disruptive behaviors generally involve conducting a functional assessment of behavior in order to determine the function the behavior serves for the individual. Modifications are made in the individual's environment to change the antecedent events that precipitate the behavior and the consequences that maintain it. Extinction, a procedure in which reinforcement is blocked or withheld following a previously reinforced behavior, has been shown to be an effective reductive procedure but does not teach appropriate alternative behaviors (Bregman & Gertz, 1997). There is a large amount of empirical support indicating that differential reinforcement procedures (discussed previously in this chapter) are effective in reducing disruptive behavior and increasing appropriate alternative behaviors in individuals with autistic spectrum disorders (Smith, et al., 2002).

Social skills treatment manuals. There are several manuals available which describe programs aimed at improving social adaptation of individuals with Asperger's Disorder and/or high functioning autism. Although there is no empirical data to support the effectiveness of these programs as a whole, many of the specific procedures included in the programs are empirically supported behavioral interventions. Following is a list of such treatments manuals.

- McAffee, J. (2001). *Navigating the social world: A curriculum for individuals with Asperger's syndrome, high functioning autism, and related disorders.* Arlington: Future Horizons.
- Krasny, L, Williams, BJ, Ozonoff, S. (in preparation). *Manual for the PROGRESS Curriculum: program for remediating and expanding social skills in children with autism spectrum disorders.*
- Quill, KA. *Do-watch-listen-say: Social and communication intervention for children with autism.* Baltimore: Paul H. Brooks.
- Gutstein, SG, Shelly, RK. (2002). *Relationship development intervention with young children: social and emotional development activities for Asperger syndrome, autism, PDD, and NLD.* London, England: Jessica Kingsley Publishers.
- Koegel, RL, Schreibman, L, Good, A, Cerniglia, L., Murphy, C., & Koegel, L.K. (1989). *How to teach pivotal behaviors to children with autism: A training manual.* Santa Barbara: University of California, Graduate School of Education, Counseling/Clinical/School Psychology Program.

Social skills groups. Participation in a social skills group is a common recommendation for children with Asperger's disorder. Although these groups are often anecdotally reported to be effective, only a few studies that have examined their efficacy. These studies, although limited in number and methodology, demonstrate a generally positive effect. One group of authors (Krasny, Williams, Provencal, & Ozonoff, 2003) reviewed extant research on social skills groups for children with autistic spectrum disorders. They concluded that there is a set of general principles that have been used in effective social skills group programs. These general principles or "key ingredients" include translating abstract social concepts into concrete, explicit rules, using a structured routine format for group meetings, selecting and prioritizing goals, fostering self-awareness and self-esteem, and targeting generalization and ongoing practice through homework assignments.

Parent training. Parent training is well-established as an effective intervention for treating children with autism and other pervasive developmental disorders. These interventions typically involve imparting didactic information related to the disorder, teaching parents to serve as social and communication coaches to their children, and training parents in behavior management strategies. Although there have been few randomized, controlled studies, the research on educational, cognitive-behavioral, and behavior modification parent training suggests positive effects on skills of children with autism as well as reduced parental stress and increases in parental self-efficacy (Marcus, Kunce, & Schopler, 1998). One study that examined parent training specifically for parents of children with Asperger's disorder found that parent training lead to improved self-efficacy in coping with problem behaviors (Sofroneff & Farbotko, 2002).

Pharmacological interventions. At the present time, there are no pharmacological agents that directly treat the core social deficits in Asperger's disorder (Smith, 1999; Towbin, 2003; Volkmar, Lord, Bailey, Schultz, & Klin, 2004). However, there are some data supporting the efficacy of some agents in reducing some of the "positive" or excessive behaviors in individuals with autistic spectrum disorders. The efficacy and safety of risperidone, an atypical neuroleptic, was investigated in a large multisite trial (RUPP, 2002). This study demonstrated that the drug was effective in reducing irritability, but had a side effect of significant weight gain. Other agents are commonly used to treat various symptoms of autistic spectrum disorders including serotonin reuptake inhibitors (SRI's) to treat comorbid mood problems, stereotypy, and behavioral rigidity, anti-anxiolytics to treat associated anxiety, and stimulant medications to treat hyperactivity and inattention. However, methodologically sound investigations of these agents, particularly for children, have been rare (Volkmar et al., 2004).

Selecting effective treatments. Asperger's disorder is a lifelong, pervasive disorder involving severe impairment in multiple areas of functioning. Effective treatments for Asperger's disorder are individually developed based on the presenting symptoms. In deciding on treatments, practitioners should assess and prioritize symptoms, including excessive behaviors and skill deficits. Symptoms should be prioritized based on the level of interference they impose on the individual's ability to function. Practitioner's should draw on the existing literature on Asperger's disorder, other pervasive developmental disorders, and symptom-related diagnostic entities to develop empirically derived treatment approaches.

REFERENCES

American Psychiatric Association (1994). *Diagnostic and statistical manual of mental disorders* (4th ed.). Washington, DC: Author.

Attwood, T. (2000). Strategies for improving the social integration of children with Asperger syndrome. *Special Issue Asperger Syndrome*, 85–100.

Attwood, T. (2003). Frameworks for behavioral interventions. *Child and Adolescent Psychiatric Clinics of North America, 12*, 65–86.

Baren-Cohen, S., Wheelwright, S. (2003). The Friendship Questionnaire: An investigation of adults with Asperger syndrome or high-functioning autism, and normal sex differences, *33*, 509–517.

Bebko, J. M., & Lennox, C. (1988). Teaching the control of diurnal bruxism to two children with autism using a simple cueing procedure. *Behavior therapy, 19*, 249–255.

Bregman, J. D., & Gerdtz, J. (1997). Behavioral interventions. In D. J. Cohen & F. R. Volkmar (Eds.), *Handbook of Autism and Pervasive Developmental Disorders* (2nd ed., pp. 606–630).

Cardaciotto, L. A., & Herbert, J. D. (2004). Cognitive-behavioral therapy for social anxiety disorder in the context of Asperger's syndrome: a single-subject report. *Cognitive and Behavioral Practice, 11*, 75–81.

Charlop-Christy, M. H., Le, L., & Freeman, K. A. (2000). A comparison of video modeling wiht in vivo modeling in teaching children with autism. *Journal of Autism and Developmental Disorders, 30(6)*, 537–552.

Charlop, M. H., & Milsteing, J. P. (1989). Teaching autistic children conversational speech suing video modeling. *Journal of Applied Behavior Analysis, 22(3)*, 275–285.

Compton, S. N., March, J. S., Brent, D., Albano, A. M., Weersing, J. (2004). Cognitive-behavioral psychotherapy for anxiety and depressive disorders in children and adolescents: An evidence-based medicine review. *Journal of the American Academy of Child and Adolescent Psychiatry, 43*, 930–959.

Constantino, J. N., & Todd, R. D. (2003). Autistic traits in the general population: A twin study. *Archives of General Psychiatry, 60*, 524–530.

Cragar, D. E., & Horvath, L. S. (2003). The application of social skills training in the treatment of a child with Asperger's disorder. *Clinical Case Studies, 2(1)*, 34–49.

Fombonne, E., & Tidmarsh, L. (2003). Epidemiological data on Asperger disorder. *Child and Adolescent Psychiatric Clinics of North America, 12*, 15–21.

Frazier, J. A., Doyle, R., Chiu, S., & Coyle, J. T. (2002). Treating a child with Asperger's disorder and comorbid bipolar disorder. *The American Journal of Psychiatry, 159*, 13–21.

Garnett, M. S., & Attwood, A. J. (1998). The Australian Scale for Aspergre's Syndrome. In Attwood (Ed.), *Asperger's Syndrome: A guide for parents and professionals* (pp. 17–19). London: Kingsley.

Ghaziuddin, M., Weidmar-Mikhail, E., & Ghaziuddin, N. (1998). Comorbidity of Asperger's syndrome: a preliminary report. *Autism, 42*, 279–283.

Goldstein, H., Kaczmarek, L., Pennington, R., & Shafer, K. (1992). Peer-mediated intervention: Attending to, commenting on, and acknowledging the behavior of preschoolers with autism. *Journal of Applied Behavior Analysis, 25*, 289–305.

Harchik, A. E., Sherman, J. A., & Sheldon, J. B. (1992). The use of self-management procedures by people with developmental disabilities: A brief review. *Research in Developmental Disabilities, 13(3),* 211–227.

Haynes, S. N., O'Brien, W. H., & Hayes, W. (2000). *Principles and practice of behavioral assessment.* New York: Plenum Press.

Howlin, P., & Asgharian, A. (1999). The diagnosis of autism and asperger's syndrome: Findings from a survey of 770 families. *Developmental Medicine and Child Neurology, 41,* 834–839.

Howlin, P., & Goode, S. (1998). Outcome in adult life for people with autism and Asperger syndrome. In F. Volkmar (Ed.), *Autism and pervasive developmental disorders.* New York: Cambridge University Press.

Khouzam, H. R., El-Gabalawi, F., Pirwani, N., & Preist, F. (2004). Asperger's disorder: A review of its diagnosis and treatment. *Comprehensive Psychiatry, 45(3),* 184–191.

Kim, J. A., Szatmari, P., Bryson, S. E., Steiner, D. L., & Wilson, F. J. (2000). The prevalence of anxiety an mood problems among children with autism and Apserger syndrome. *Autism, 4,* 117–132.

Klin, A., & Volkmar, F. R. (1997). Apserger's Syndrome. In D. J. Cohen, & F. R. Volkmar (Eds.), *Handbook of pervasive developmental disorders* (2nd ed.). New York: Wiley.

Klin, A., & Volkmar, F. R. (2003). Asperger syndrome: diagnosis and external validity. *Child and Adolescent Psychiatric Clinics of North America, 12,* 1–13.

Koegel, R. L., & Frea, W. D. (1993). Treatment of social behavior in autism through modification of pivotal social skills. *Journal of Applied Behavior Analysis, 26,* 369–377.

Koegel, R. L. Frea, W. D., & Surrat, A. V. (1994). Self-management in problematic social behavior. In E. Schopler & G. B. Mesibov (Eds.), *Behavioral issues in autism* (pp. 81–97). New York: Plenum Press.

Koegel, L. K., Koegel, R. L., Hurley, C., & Frea, W. D. (1992). Improving social skills and disruptive behavior in children with autism through self-managment. *Journal of Applied Behavior Analysis, 25,* 341–353.

Koegel, R. L., Schreibman, L., Good, A., Cerniglian, L., Murphy, C., Koegel, L. K. (1989). *How to teach pivotal behaviors to children with autism: A training manual.* Santa Barbar: University of Califormia, Graduate School of Education, Counseling/Clinical/School Psychology Program.

Krantz, P. J., & McClannahan, L. E., (1998). Social interaction skills for children with autism: A script-fading procedure for beginning readers. *Journal of Applied Behavior Analysis, 31,* 191–202.

Krantz, P. J., MacDuff, M. T., & McClannahan, L. E. (1993). Programming participation in family activities for children with autism: Parents' use of photographic activity schedules. Journal of Applied Behavior Analysis, 26, 137–138.

Krasny, L., Williams, B. J., Provencal, S., & Ozonoff, S. (2003). Social skills interventions for the autism spectrum: Essential ingredients and a model curriculum. *Child and Adolescent Psychiatry Clinics, 12,* 107–122.

LeBlanc, L. A., Coates, A. M., Daneshvar, S., Charlop-Christy, M. H. & Lancaster, B. M. (2003). *Journal of Applied Behavior Analysis, 36 (2),* 253–257.

Lord, C. (1995). Follow-up of two-year-olds referred for possible autism. *Journal of Child Psychology and Psychiatry, 36,* 1365–1382.

Lord, C., Risi, S., Lambrecht, L., Cook, E. H., Leventhal, B. L., DiLavore, P. C., Pickles, A., & Rutter, M. (2000). The Autism Diagnostic Observation Schedule-Generic: A standard measure of social and communication deficits associated with the spectrum of autism. *Journal of Autism and Developmental Disorders, 30,* 205–224.

Lovaas, O. I. (1987). Behavioral Treatment and Normal Educational and Intellectual Functioning in Young Autistic Children. *Journal of Consulting and Clinical Psychology, 55,* 3–9.

Lovaas, O. I. (1993). The development of a treatment-research project for developmentally disabled and autistic children. *Journal of Applied Behavior Analysis, 26,* 617–630.

Maag, J. W., Wolchik, S. A., Rutherford, J. B., & Parks, B. T. (1986). Response covariation on self-stimulatory behaviors during sensory extinction procedures. *Journal of Autism and Developmental Disorders, 16,* 145–154.

Mancina, C., Tankersley, M., Kamps, D., Kravits, T., & Parrett, J. (2000). Brief report: Reduction of inappropriate vocalizations in a child wiht autism using a self-management treatment program. *Journal of Autism and Developmental Disabilities, 30(6),* 599–606.

Marcus, L. M., Kunce, L. J., & Schopler, E. (2005). Working with families. In Handbook of autism and pervasive developmental disorders, Vol. 2: Assessment, interventions, and policy (3rd ed.) Volkmar, F., Paul, R., et al. US: John Wiley & Sons, Inc, 1055–1086.

Martin, A., Scahill, L., Klin, A., & Volkmar, F. R. (1999). Higher-functioning pervasive developmental disorders: rates and patterns of psychotropic drug use. *Journal of the American Academy of Child and Adolescent Psychiatry, 38,* 923–931.

McConnell, S. R. (2002). Interventions to facilitate social interaction for young children with autism: review of available research and recommendations for educational intervention and future research. *Journal of Autism and Developmental Disorders, 32,* 351–372.

Miles, B. S. (2003). Behavioral forms of stress management for individuals with Asperger syndrome. *Child and Adolescent Psychiatric Clinics of North America, 12,* 123–141.

Mulick, J. A., & Meinhold P. M. (1994). Developmental disorders and broad effects of the environment on learning and treatment effectiveness. In E. Schopler & G. B. Mesibov (Eds.), *Behavioral issues in autism* (pp. 99–128). New York: Plenum Press.

Newsome, C. B. (1998). Austistic disorder. In E. J. Marsh & R. A. Barkley (Eds.), *Treatment of childhood disorders* (2nd ed. pp. 416–467). New York: Guildfor Press.

Nikopoulos, C. K., & Keenan, M. (2004). Effects of video modeling on social initiations by with autism. *Journal of Applied Behavior Analysis, 37(1),* 93–96.

Odom, S. L., & Strain, P. S. (1984). Peer-mediated approaches to promoting children's social interaction: a review. *American Journal of Orthopsychiatry, 54,* 544–557.

Paul, R. (2003). Promoting social communication in high functioning individuals with autistic spectrum disorders. *Child and Adolescent Psychiatric Clinics of North America, 12,* 87–106.

Pierce, K., & Schreibman, L. (1997a). Increasing complex social behaviors in children with autism: Effects of peer-implemented pivotal response training. *Journal of Applied Behavior Analysis, 28,* 285–295.

Pierce, K., & Schreibman, L. (1997b). Multiple peer use of pivotal response training to increase social behaviors of classmates with autism: Results from trained and untrained peer. *Journal of Applied Behavior Analysis, 30(1),* 157–160.

Pierce, K., Schreibman, L. (1995). Increasing complex social behaviors in children with autism: Effects of peer-implemented pivoted response training. *Journal of Applied Behavior Analysis, 28,* 285–295.

Piven, J., Harper, J., Palmer, P., Arndt, S. (1996). Course of behavioral change in autism: A retrospective study of high-IQ adolescents and adults. *Journal of the american Academy of Child and Adolescent Psychiatry, 35,* 523–529.

Ruberman, L. (2002). Psychotherapy of children with pervasive developmental disorders. *American Journal of Psychotherapy, 56(2),* 262–275.

RUPP Autism Network. (2002). Risperidone in children with autism and serious behavioral problems. *New England Journal of Medicine, 347,* 314–321.

Scott, F. J., Baron, Cohen, S., Bolton, P., & Bayne, C. (2002). The CAST (Childhood asperger Syndrome Test): Preliminary development of a UK screen for mainstream-school-age children. *Autism, 6,* 9–31.

Sherer, M., Pierce, K. L., Paredes, S., Kisacky, K. L., & Ingersoll, B. (2001). Enhancing conversation skills in children with autism using video technology. Which is better, "self" or "other" as model? *Behavior Modification, 25(1),* 140–158.

Siegel, B. (1998). *Early screening and diagnosis in autism spectrum disorders: The Pervasive Developmental Disorders Screening Test (PDDST).* Invited address persnted at the NIH State of the Science in Austim Screeining and Diagnosis working Congerence, Bethesda, MD.

Smith, T. (1999). Outcome of early intervention for children with autism. *Clinical Psychology: Research and Practice, 6,* 33–49.

Smith, T., Magyar, C., Arnold-Saritepe, A. (2002). Autism spectrum disorders. In D. T. Marsh & M. A. Fristad (Eds.) *Handbook of serious emotional disturbance in children and adolescents.* (pp. 131–148). New York: John Wiley and Sons, Inc.

Sofroneff, K., & Farbotko, M. (2002). The effectiveness of parent management training to increase self-efficacy in parents of children with Asperger's syndrome. *Autism, 6,* 271–286.

Sparrow, S. S., & Cicchetti, D. V. (1984). The Behavior Inventory for Rating Development (BIRD): Assessments of reliability and factorial validity. Applied Research in Mental Retardation, *5,* 219–231.

Stahmer, A. C., Ingersoll, B., Carter, C. (2003). Behavioral approaches to promoting play. *Autism, 7(4),* 401–413.

Stahmer, A. C., & Schreibman, L. (1992). Teaching children with autism appropriate play in unsupervised environments using a self-management treatment package. *Journal of Applied Behavior Analysis, 25,* 447–259.

Strain, P. S., Kerr, M. M., & Ragland, E. U. (1979). Effects of peer-mediated social inititiations and prompting/reinforcement procedures on the social behavior of autistic children. *Journal of Autism and Developmental Disorders, 9,* 41–54.

Swaggait, B., Gagnon, E., & Bock, S. J. (1995). Using social stories to teach social and behavioral skills to children with autism. Focus on Autistic Behavior, *10(1),* 1–16.

Szatmari, P., Archer, L., Fisman, S., Streiner, D. L., & Wilson, F. (1995). Asperger's syndrome and autism: Differences in behaivor, cognition, and adaptive functioning. *Journal of the American Academy of Child and Adolescent Psychiatry, 34,* 1662–1671.

Tantum, D. (2003). The challenge of adolescents an adults with asperger syndrome. *Child and Adolescent Psychiatric Clinics of North America, 12,* 143–163.

Thiemann, K. S., & Goldstein, H. (2001). Social stories, written text cues, and video feedback: Enhancing social communication of children with autism. *Journal of Applied Behavior Analysis, 34(4),* 425–446.

Thomsen, P. H. (1994). Obsessive-compulsive disorder in children and adolescents: a 6-22-year follow-up study: Clinical descriptions of the course and continuity of obsesive-compulsive symptomatology. *European Child and Adolescent Psychiatry, 3(2),* 82–96.

Towbin, K. E. (2003). Strategies for pharmacological treatment of high functioning autism and Asperger syndrome. *Child and Adolescent Psychiatric Clinics of North America, 12,* 23–45.

Tsatsanis, K. D. (2003). Outcome research in asperger syndrome and autism. *Child and Adolescent Psychiatric Clinics of North America, 12,* 47–63.

Volkmar, F. R., & Klin, A. (2001). Asperger's disorder and higher functioning autism: Same or different? *International Review of Research in Mental Retardation, 23,* 83–109.

Volkmar, F. R., Lord, C., Bailey, A., Schultz, R. T., & Klin, A. (2004). Autism and pervasive developmental disorders. *Journal of Child Psychology and Psychiatry, 45(1),* 135–170.

Volkmar, F. R. & Woolston, J. C. (1997). Comorbidity of psychiatric disorders in children and adolescents. *Treatment strategies for patients with psychiatric comorbidity.* Wetzler, S., Sanderson, W. C., Hoboken, N. J., US: John Wiley & Sons, Inc, 307–322.

Volkmar, F. R. (2003), Autism. *Lancet, 362,* 1133–1141.

Wing, L. (1981). Asperger's syndrome: A clinical account. *Psychological Medicine, 11,* 115–129.

World Health Organization (1992). The ICD-10 classification of mental and behavioural disorders: clinical descriptions and diagnostic guidelines. Geneva, Switzerland: Author.

Yoshida, Y., & Uchiyama, T. (2004). The clinical necessity for assessing attention deficit/hyperactivity disorder (AD/HD) symptoms in children with high-functioning pervasive developmental disorder (PDD). *European Child and Adolescent Psychiatry, 13(5),* 307–314.

CHAPTER 7

Assertiveness Training

Melanie P. Duckworth • Victoria Mercer

WHAT IS ASSERTIVENESS?

Assertive behavior usually centers on making requests of others and refusing requests made by others that have been judged to be unreasonable. Assertive behavior also captures the communication of strong opinions and feelings. Assertive communication of personal opinions, needs and boundaries has been defined as communication that diminishes none of the individuals involved in the interaction, with emphasis placed on communication accuracy and respect for all persons engaged in the exchange.

Assertiveness is conceptualized as the behavioral middle ground, lying between ineffective passive and aggressive responses. Passiveness is characterized by an over-attention to the opinions and needs of others and the masking or restraining of personal opinions and needs. This over-attention to and compliance with the opinions and needs of others may serve as a strategy for conflict avoidance and/or maintenance of particular sources of social "reinforcement." Aggressiveness often involves the imposition of one's opinions and requirements on another individual. Implicit in the discussion of assertiveness is the suggestion that assertive behavior is the universally preferred behavioral alternative, and that assertive behavior necessarily leads to preferred outcomes. The degree to which assertive behaviors are to be considered superior to either a passive or an aggressive stance is determined by the situational context. The success of assertiveness does not always lie in tangible outcomes (e.g., request fulfillment). The success of assertiveness sometimes lies in the degree of personal control and personal respect that is achieved and maintained throughout the assertive exchange.

BASIC FACTS ABOUT ASSERTIVENESS TRAINING

The acquisition of assertiveness behavior is not specific to any discrete stage of childhood development but instead is a function of instruction, modeling, and rehearsal. Assertive behavior is acquired, practiced and refined as the individual develops. Problems with assertiveness can occur early in development in the form of overly shy or aggressive behavior, and later as social anxiety disorder and avoidant personality disorder. In outlining the facts about assertiveness, we have chosen to outline problem sets that can be conceptualized as due at least in part, to a deficit in assertiveness.

Prevalence. Low levels of assertive behavior, as evidenced by the presence of social anxiety disorder, is a highly prevalent problem. It is estimated that nearly 13.3% of all people in the US suffer from social anxiety at some point in their lives (Kessler et al., 1994). Social phobia is most prevalent amount people who are young (18–29 years of age), undereducated, single, and of lower socioeconomic status; social phobia is slightly less prevalent among the elderly (Magee, Eaton, Wittchen,

Duckworth, M. P. & Mercer, V. (2006). In J. E. Fisher & W. T. O'Donohue (Eds.), *Practitioner's guide to - evidence-based psychotherapy.* New York: Springer.

McConagle, & Kessler, 1996). Avoidant personality disorder occurs in less than 1% of the general population (Reich, Yates, & Nduaguba, 1989; Zimmerman, & Coryell, 1990). Displays of aggressive behavior may be relatively common, yet the prevalence of extreme aggression as evidenced by the presence of antisocial personality disorder is relatively rare, occurring in only about 1–3% of the general population (Sutker, Bugg, & West, 1993).

Age at onset. Extreme shyness is known to be present in a large percentage of children. The mean age at onset for social phobia is 16 years old. The age at onset for social phobia occurs later than the onset for simple phobias but earlier than the onset for agoraphobia (Öst, 1987). Studies have found that the number of children with social phobia is increasing (Magee, et al., 1996). Aggression also appears to be expressed in early adolescence. In a study of African-American and Hispanic adolescent males it was found that children who had high levels of externalized behavior problems also tended to assert themselves in a hostile manner (Florsheim, Tolan, & Gorman-Smith, 1996).

Gender. Although a larger percentage of men evidence assertive behavior than women men are also more likely to engage in aggressive behavior (Eagly & Steffen, 1986). Extreme aggression, as sometimes captured by antisocial personality disorder or psychopathy, is significantly more common in men (Dulit, Marin, & Frances, 1993; Sutker et al., 1993). Although women are represented more frequently among populations of persons experiencing anxiety disorders, social anxiety disorder occurs with relatively equal frequency across women and men. The gender ratio for social anxiety disorder is 1.4 to 1.0, females to males. Avoidant personality disorder also occurs equally across women and men. Taken together, these findings suggest that assertiveness may be an appropriate technique for men and women who engage in overly passive or overly aggressive behaviors.

Course. Extreme passivity, as captured by social phobia, begins in adolescence increases into the late 20s, and then declines in later life (Magee et al., 1996). Extreme aggression, as captured by antisocial personality disorder, begins in adolescence in the form of conduct disorder, increases through the 20s, and then decreases across the 40s (Hare, McPherson, & Forth, 1988).

Impairment and other demographic characteristics. Level of impairment is indicated by the problems experienced by people who are represented at the extremes of the assertiveness continuum. Problems associated with extreme passivity, can range from being bullied to experiencing repeat victimization by partners. Problems associated with aggression can range from suspension of privileges in childhood to serious negative legal consequences in adulthood.

There are differential finding for the impact of assertive behavior among ethnic groups, the impact seems entangled with socioeconomic status and culturally specific styles of communication (Malagady, Rogler, & Cortes, 1996; Zane, Sue, Hu, & Kwon, 1991). Social phobia is found to be equally prevalent among ethnic groups (Magee et al., 1996).

Given that assertive behavior occurs as a part of a broader interaction complex, the likelihood that an individual will engage in assertive behavior is a function of skill and performance competencies, reinforcement contingencies, motivational-affective and cognitive-evaluative factors. Behavioral explanations for the use of passive or aggressive strategies rather than assertive strategies emphasize opportunities for skills acquisition and mastery and reinforcement contingencies that have supported the use of passive or aggressive behaviors over time. Behavioral conceptualizations for passivity often emphasize early learning environments in which passive responding may have been modeled (e.g., care givers who were themselves anxious, shy, or in some other way less than assertive) or more assertive behavior punished (e.g., overly protective or dominating care givers). In the absence of opportunities for acquisition and reinforcement of other interaction strategies, passive behavior persists.

Important to any complete behavioral conceptualization of passive behavior would be an evaluation of the reinforcement that is associated with current displays of passive behavior, that is, how is passivity currently "working" for the individual? Behaviors that are reinforced are repeated. Repeated engagement in passive behavior suggests repeated reinforcement of such behavior. Passive responding may be reinforced through the avoidance of responsibility and decision-making. With what amount of attention, positive or negative, are passive responses met? The individual employing passive strategies may need to reconcile his or her "active" influence on situations with the alleged passivity.

Aggressive behaviors can be learned through the observation of aggressive models and reinforced through their instrumental effects. Even in the absence of overt goal attainment, aggressive behaviors may be experienced as intrinsically reinforcing by virtue of the autonomic discharge associated with such behaviors. Aggressive behavior may serve as a socially sanctioned interaction style (Tedeschi & Felson, 1994). Aggressive behavior may also be a consequence of the absence of opportunities to acquire alternative social interaction strategies.

Motivational-affective factors are important to patterned displays of passive and aggressive behavior. Although the affective experience of anger is not sufficient to explain aggressive behavior, feelings of anger do increase the likelihood that the actions of others will be experienced as aggressive and, thereby, elicit aggressive behavior. Cognitive explanations for passive and aggressive responding would posit that outcome expectations are primary in determining the passive or aggressive response. The passive individual may look to the history of failures in making and/or refusing requests in deciding whether to attempt the recommended assertive behavior. Outcome expectations may interfere with adoption of the "new" assertiveness. Such outcome expectations must be managed if the likelihood of assertive responding is to increase. The passive individual needs to be cautioned regarding the imperfect relationship between assertive responding and desired outcomes. Initially, assertive responses may not meet with desired outcomes. It is the *persistence* of the assertive response that will ensure that the probability of the desired outcome increases over time. In the short run, then, the measure of successful assertion may not be the occurrence of a desired outcome but the mere assertive communication of one's opinions, needs and/or limits.

ASSESSMENT

What should be Ruled Out?

Assertiveness appears to be of differential utility in the context of domestic violence. Some research suggests that battered women are potentially at increased risk as a result of assertive behavior in the context of ongoing domestic violence (O'Leary, Curley, Rosenbaum & Clarke, 1985). On the other hand, assertiveness training has been found to contribute to a woman's decision to leave a violent relationship (Meyers-Abell, & Jansen, 1980). Research addressing male batterers suggests that batterers have assertiveness deficits that may contribute to there use of aggression and violence to express their needs and manage the needs of their domestic partner (Maiuro, Cahn, & Vitiliano, 1986). In the context of female sexual victimization, assertiveness training appears to empower women and reduce their exposure to violence (Mac Greene & Navarro, 1998).

What is Involved in Effective Assessment?

Assessment of assertiveness skills and performance abilities should be broad enough to capture and distinguish among various explanations for performance failure. Traditionally, a hierarchical task analysis is used to determine the causal variable that accounts for the skill/performance deficit (Dow, 1994). Initially, assertiveness skills are evaluated in a nonthreatening (or less threatening) environment. Given that the client demonstrates adequate assertiveness skill in the non-threatening environment, assertiveness skills are evaluated in the context of more clinically relevant social situations. Given that skills are adequately performed in clinically relevant social situations, other contributions to response failure are evaluated including affective and cognitive variables that might mediate the skill–performance relation. Behavioral models of depression suggest that the pursuit of social interaction (and, thus, experience of reinforcement) may be limited by negative affective experiences that are present throughout the interaction (Lewinsohn, 1974). For example, anxiety that is experienced during an assertive interaction may be insufficient to impair performance but may be sufficient to render the interaction a punishing rather than reinforcing event.

Assertive behaviors presuppose the existence of adequate social skills. An assertive communication is measured not only by the content of the verbalization but also by the accompanying nonverbal behaviors. Appropriate posture and eye-contact are essential in executing an appropriately assertive response. An appropriately assertive posture would convey relaxed but focused attention, this posture contrasted with an overly rigid posture that might convey either anxiety or obstinacy. Other important nonverbal behaviors include facial expression and body movements and gestures. Affective displays should be congruent with the content of the assertive communication, not suggesting anxiety, false gaiety, or anger. Body movements that indicate nervousness and uncertainty (e.g. hand-wringing) should be avoided. Movements that convey anger or dominance (e.g., invasion of the other's personal space) should also be avoided. These nonverbal behaviors are included among behaviors identified by Dow (1985) as relevant to socially skilled behaving.

The content of the assertive communication is important in its clarity and form. The tone and fluidity of the request, command or refusal are also important. Generally, the assertive request is characterized by its reasonableness, its specificity regarding actions required to fulfill the request, and its inclusion of statements that convey the potential impact(s) of request fulfillment for both the individual making the request and the request recipient. The tone in which the request is delivered should convey the importance of the request; however, the tone should not imply some obligation on the part of the request recipient to comply with the request. The content and tone of assertive refusals share the quality of being even-handed and unwavering.

Assessment of skill sets and performance competencies is necessary prior to skills training and throughout the skills acquisition/practice process. Skills for assertive behaving are evaluated through the use of self-report instruments as well as behavioral observation in contrived and natural settings.

Clinician-administered measures. Generally evaluations of assertive behavior involve observations of skill displays (e.g., communication, social interactions) in clinical, analogue, and natural settings, rather than using clinically administered measures of assertiveness. Observational ratings of skill assets, deficits, and mastery made by the treating clinician can be formalized by systematically targeting all nonverbal and verbal behaviors considered relevant to assertive behaving. There are structured clinical interviews that assess diagnostic features of anxiety, the reader is referred to the social anxiety disorder chapter in this text for that information.

Self-report measures. Assertiveness skill evaluation and training often occurs in the broader context of social skill and social competence. The self-report instruments that purport to measure assertiveness range from actual measures of assertive behaviors to instruments that assess related constructs such as social avoidance, self-esteem, and locus of control. The most commonly used measure of assertiveness skills is the Rathus Assertiveness Scale (Rathus, 1973). Self-monitoring of social behaviors performed in the client's natural environment is essential to both assessment and treatment of potential skills and performance deficits. Monitoring instructions usually require that the client describe their social interactions with others along a number of dimensions. The client may be instructed to briefly describe interactions with males versus females, acquaintances versus intimate others, peers versus persons in authority, and in structured versus unstructured interactions. Although real world evaluation of skills is preferable, the office is the most common arena for skills evaluation and practice. Therefore it is essential that the client provide detailed accounts of problem interactions and that the content and cues of the experimental arena be as consistent with that real world as possible.

Behavioral assessment. Behavioral observation is considered the preferred strategy for evaluating assertiveness skills and performance competencies. Usually observations/evaluations of assertive performances are made in clinical or research settings rather than real world settings. Clinic and laboratory settings provide contexts for informal observation (waiting room behaviors and behaviors engaged in by the client during the clinical interview) and formal observation (social interaction tasks and role-plays) of an individual's behavior.

Clinical interview. In the clinical setting, the client's waiting room behavior (i.e., his/her interactions with other persons in the waiting room and with clinic staff) is available for observation. Exchanges had during initial assessment sessions also serve as data to be used in establishing the presence or absence of verbal and nonverbal communication skills considered essential to assertive displays as well as contextual/situational/interpersonal factors that may influence the likelihood of assertive behaving and the mastery with which assertive behaviors are performed.

Social interaction tasks in analog settings. In evaluating a client's social skill and comfort, the therapist may enlist confederates to engage the client in interactions that test the client's ability to initiate and participate in casual exchanges. These tasks are considered low demand tasks. Usually, these tasks do not contain any of the elements of identified problematic interactions.

Social interaction tasks in real-world settings. Of course, the optimal arena for evaluating assertive behavior is the client's natural environment. As often as possible, the real world context should be captured. For example, a male client reporting difficulty initiating social interactions with female peers might be observed in real world settings that are familiar to him and that present opportunities for contact with female peers (e.g., the college library, an undergraduate seminar, a scheduled, on-campus extracurricular event). Other local contact arenas are also acceptable for evaluation of skills including coffee houses, dance clubs, etc.

Role-plays. In the clinical context, a "true" observation of assertive behaviors is made through the use of role-playing. Based on the client's report of difficult interpersonal interactions/exchanges, interaction opportunities that mimic these difficult interpersonal interactions (to a lesser or greater degree) are engineered and the client's use of assertive behaviors observed. Typically, the therapist serves as the "relevant other" in such role play situations. Research participants or clients are asked to display their skills repertoire in the context of contrived interactions with the researcher/therapist or some confederate. In structuring the role play, the therapist aims to lessen the artificial quality of the role play and to strengthen the correlation/correspondence/reliability between the client's performance in artificial and natural settings. This is best achieved through the use of dialogue and contextual cues that most closely approximate the naturally occurring problematic interactions. Role-play confederates and scenarios are often selected with relevant contextual factors in mind.

What Assessments are Not Helpful?

In the context of assertiveness training, assessment capitalizes on the clinicians behavioral observation skills rather than some of the more traditional paper-and-pencil measures such as the MMPI or projective tests.

TREATMENT

What Treatments are Effective?

Assertiveness training, when employed as part of a more comprehensive cognitive-behavioral therapy package, is useful for the treatment of people whose lack of assertiveness skills manifests behavior appears as either passivity or aggression. When the absence of assertive behavior is explained by affective or cognitive factors rather than a skills deficit, other strategies are recommended as adjuncts to of assertiveness skills training and practice. Examples of such strategies include relaxation training to reduce performance inhibiting anxiety or anger, cognitive restructuring to challenge negative performance predictions and overgeneralizations regarding performance errors, and cognitive reframing with respect to performance goals and measures of performance success.

What are Effective Self-Help Treatments?

There are a plethora of self-help resources available to clients interested in self-initiated efforts towards assertive behaving. These resources are largely in the form of assertiveness training books and internet site targeted directly at the lay person. Although the effectiveness of any individual resource is generally not available to the client he or she may rely on the credentials of the authors or site hosts (e.g., authors who emphasize empirical research and universities as site hosts) to guide their selection of self-help materials.

Self-help books.

- Alberti, R. E. & Emmons, M. L. (2001). *Your perfect right: Assertiveness and equality in your life and relationships* (8th ed.). Atascadero, CA: Impact Publishers.
- Burton, S., & Shelton, N. (1993). *Assertiveness skills.* New York: McGraw-Hill.
- Davidson, J. (1997). *The complete idiot's guide to assertiveness* (1st ed.). Indianapolis, IN: Alpha Books.
- Dire, W. (1978). *Pulling your own strings: Dynamic techniques for dealing with other people and living your life as you choose.* New York: Harper Collins.
- Gabor, D. (2001). *How to start a conversation and make friends.* New York: Fireside.

- Magee, S, & Pachter, B. (2001). *The power of positive confrontation: The skills you need to know to handle conflicts at work, at home, and in life.* New York: Marlowe & Company.
- McKay, M., Rogers, P. D., & McKay, J. (2003). *When anger hurts: Quieting the storm within,* (2nd ed.) Oakland, CA: New Harbinger.
- Nay, W. R. (2004). *Taking charge of anger: How to resolve conflict, sustain relationships, and express yourself without losing control.* New York: The Guilford Press.
- Paterson, R. J. (2000). *The assertiveness workbook: How to express your idea and stand up for yourself at work and in relationships.* Oakland, CA: New Harbinger Publications.
- Petracek, L. J. (2004). *The anger workbook for women.* Oakland, CA: New Harbinger Press.
- Valentis, J., & Valentis, M. (2001). *Brave new you: 12 dynamic strategies for saying what you want and being who you are.* Oakland, CA: New Harbinger Publications.

Self help websites.

- http://www.couns.msu.edu/self-help/index.htm (Michigan State University Counseling Center)
- http://www.uiowa.edu/~ucs/asertcom.html (University of Iowa Counseling Services)
- http://www.uwec.edu/counsel/pubs/assertivecommunication.htm (University of Wisconsin-Eau Claire Counseling Center)
- http://www.couns.uiuc.edu/Brochures/assertiv.htm (University of Illinois Counseling Services)
- http://oregonstate.edu/dept/counsel/assertivenessskills.html (Oregon State University Counseling Department)
- http://www.utexas.edu/student/cmhc/booklets/assert/assertive.html (University of Texas at Austin Counseling and Mental Health Center)
- http://www.twu.edu/o-sl/counseling (Texas Woman's University Counseling Center)
- http://www.amanet.org/index.htm (American Management Association)

What are Effective Therapist-based Treatments?

When it has been established that a skills deficit explains performance failure it is often useful to begin at the beginning. In presenting the rationale for assertive communication, the therapist suggests that the honest and respectful communication of one's preferences and opinions maximizes the potential for achievement of relationship goals in both professional and intimate contexts. The therapist would begin the presentation of the rationale with a description of the three forms of communication that characterize most verbal exchanges.

People usually express their needs/desires and opinions in one of three ways: aggressively, passively or assertively.

The therapist follows this statement with descriptions of each of the three common form of communication.

(1) The aggressive expression of needs usually involves the goal of getting one's needs met or having one's opinion endorsed no matter the cost to the other individual or individuals participating in the exchange. Aggressive communication is often characterized by "shoulds" or "musts" or other language that suggests that the recipient is bound or required to meet the expressed need or agree with the expressed opinion. Aggressive communication is also characterized by nonverbal behaviors that are of the "in your face" quality. Aggressive communicators may ignore the boundaries of personal space, standing overly close to another individual. They may speak in loud, angry tones, and in a number of other ways convey

subtle pressure or even threat to the other individual or individuals participating in the communication exchange.

(2) Passive communication is problematic, not because of obvious demands placed on the recipient, but because passive communications often do not reflect the true needs or preferences of the speaker. Passive communications involve the use of acquiescent language. The passive communicator often responds to others' statements of preferences and opinions with statements such as "if you think so" or "whatever you want is fine" or "no problem, I can take care of that." In the short-term, the passive communicator may be seen as ensuring the pleasure and happiness of the recipients of such behavior. Passivity may also serve to assure the passive individual that relationships will be maintained. The problems with passive communications are usually experienced over time. The passive communicator begins to resent the fact that their true needs and opinions are not being honored within these relationships. The recipient of passive communications may feel that the passive individual is only half-heartedly participating in the relationship and is avoiding responsibility for making important decisions within the relationship.

(3) Assertive communication ensures that the needs and opinions of the speaker are honestly expressed and owned by the speaker. Opinions are expressed as opinions rather than as statements of inarguable fact. This allows other participants in the exchange to comfortably express similar or opposing opinions. In communicator presents the request in a manner that is at the same time clear but respectful of the recipient's right to refuse such a request. In refusing requests, the assertive communicator states the refusal clearly and unwaveringly while at the same time indicating appreciation for the other individual's circumstances. Again, assertive communication has the goal of mutual respect.

The goal, then, of assertiveness training is the communication needs and opinions in a mutually respectful manner, thereby increasing the probability of having needs met and opinions appreciated, as well as ensuring the maintenance of relationships. The therapist cannot reiterate this goal too often.

Prior to the practice of assertiveness skills, the client is made aware of certain content and procedural guidelines that govern assertive behavior. Content guidelines require that compliments, criticisms, and requests be made with a degree of reasonableness and with a degree of specificity. Procedural guidelines require that requests for behavior change be "sandwiched" between impact statements pertaining to the current behavior and the proposed behavior change. For example, in making a request for behavior change, the client would begin with a statement regarding the negative impact of the other's current behavior, then suggest a reasonable and specific behavioral alternative, and end with a statement suggesting the positive impact of the proposed behavioral alternative for both parties. The behavior change request is sandwiched between the two impact statements. In addition, Dow (1994) recommends that the assertive communicator refrain from making assumptions about the motivations driving others' behaviors, refrain from questioning others regarding their motives, and interject something positive about the individual with whom they are interacting.

In starting the practice of assertiveness skills, the therapist always begins with a review of the more basic elements of assertive communication and continues along a graded hierarchy of skills sets essential to assertive communication across contexts. Traditionally, assertiveness training packages have identified several skill sets as essential to assertive behaving, including nonverbal behavior as communication, giving and receiving compliments, giving and receiving criticism, and making and refusing requests. In addressing each of these skills sets, the therapist wishes to establish three things: (1) the presence and strength of a particular skill in the client's behavioral repertoire; (2) the situations in which the client competently and reliably displays the particular skill; and (3) the situations in which the client may be called upon to competently display the particular skill.

The presence and strength of a particular assertive skill or skill set may be established formally or informally. A client's nonverbal behaviors are immediately observable by the therapist. In the context of the therapeutic exchange, the therapist may observe nonverbal behaviors that are not at all consistent with the goals of assertive communication. This would signal that, at least within the context of the therapeutic exchange, direct training and practice of assertive nonverbal behavior is justified. When nonverbal behaviors have been observed to be sufficient in this context, the therapist may feel uncomfortable reviewing these more basic elements of assertive communication. In such situations the therapist is encouraged to (1) acknowledge the appropriateness of the client's nonverbal behavior in the therapeutic context and (2) suggest that the display of appropriately assertive nonverbal behavior is sometimes bound by context, that is, assertive nonverbal behaviors sometimes depend on how comfortable the person feels in a given situation or with a given individual. A review of nonverbal behaviors would be completed along with instructions that the client monitor and evaluate displays of appropriately assertive nonverbal behaviors in the natural environment.

The skills that characterize each level of the assertiveness hierarchy should be approached in a similar manner. For example, if in the ongoing context of therapy the client has evidenced skill in assertively requesting something of the therapist, this instance would be pointed to by the therapist and reinforced through praise. The therapist would then suggest that the display of even well-established skills can be influenced by situations and persons. The various aspects of request making would be reviewed, real-world instances of successful and unsuccessful request making attempts would be solicited, and the client would be instructed to monitor and practice assertive request making in the natural environment. The therapist will structure in-session role plays and homework assignments so that more common and less common request making situations are encountered over the course of such practice. Table 7.1 presents an eight-step guide to assertiveness skills training.

What is Effective Medical-based Treatment?

Assertiveness training is usually identified as an effective treatment strategy for problem sets that are characterized by either anxiety in social situations, or aggressive management of interpersonal interactions. In the context of social anxiety disorder, assertiveness training may be one component a multi-component treatment package. Another component of that package may be pharmacotherapy (Pollack, 1999). Although benzodiazepines work quickly and effectively, they are considered secondary due to a high risk of dependence (Stramek, et al., 2002). Beta-blockers were initially thought to be particularly well suited to the management of performance anxiety, however, there is a lack of evidence to support this claim (Turner, Beidel, & Jacob, 1994). There are many studies demonstrating the effectiveness of tricyclic antidepressants, compared to medication placebo in the treatment of social anxiety disorders (Liebowitz, et al., 1992). Currently, selective serotonin reuptake inhibitors (SSRIs) such as Paxil, Zoloft, and Effexo are approved by the Food and Drug Administration for pharmacological management of social anxiety disorder (Kaminer, & Stein, 2003; Stein, et al., 1998). There are two major studies that have compared antidepressant medications monoamine oxidase inhibitors

TABLE 7.1 *Key Components of an Assertiveness Training Protocol*

1. Assertiveness training usually begins with a didactic presentation of (a) the rationale for the use of assertive behavior; (b) definitions of assertiveness, passiveness and aggressiveness; and (c) the basic content and procedural guidelines that govern assertive behavior

2. Self-monitoring assignments are given and in-session role plays are undertaken to identify problematic interactions

3. For the particular skill set being targeted, the verbal content of a sufficiently assertive response is delineated and the appropriately assertive delivery of that verbal communication is modeled by the therapist or confederate

4. The client practices assertive behaviors in the context of in-session role-plays that are similar to the identified problematic interactions

5. The evaluation of the role-play performance should always begin with the solicitation of comments from the client. This strategy allows the therapist to (a) evaluate the client's understanding of the verbal and nonverbal behaviors that comprise the assertive response and (b) evaluate the accuracy and objectivity with which the client evaluates his or her performance. Evaluating one's performance subsequent to role-plays may be made difficult by recall burden. Videotaping role-plays is recommended to reduce recall burden and to provide specific, visual evidence for performance problems and performance gains over time

6. Feedback is provided by the therapist and/or confederate and instructions for further refinement of the assertive performance are provided. When there is a considerable discrepancy between the therapist-modeled assertive behavior and the client's performance, it is often useful to provide feedback in the form of a review of a videotape of the role-play

7. Real-world practice of assertive behavior is next. Again, the client provides a technical and affective evaluation of the assertive performance in the real-world situation

8. Reinforcement and reiteration of reasonable performance goals is essential throughout the assertiveness skills training process

[MAOIs and SSRIs] with psychological treatment of social anxiety disorder. Both studies found that while both medications and psychological treatments are highly effective, cognitive-therapy was associated with lower rates of relapse and better outcomes at all points measured across a 12 month follow-up (Liebowitz, et al., 1992; Clark, et al., 2003). For a more detailed exposition of effective medical management of social anxiety disorder the reader is referred to the social anxiety chapter in this text. Pharmacological management of aggressive behavior usually occurs when the overt aggression is a part of a larger psychiatric presentation. Medication, most typically antipscyhotics, have been found to be moderately effective in reducing aggression in referred psychiatric samples (Walker, Thomas, & Allen, 2003; Ruths, & Steiner, 2004). However, the effectiveness of medication in treating aggression in a nonreferred sample is not as well supported, suggesting the use of nonmedical interventions (Connor, Boone, Steingard, Lopez, & Melloni, 2003).

Combination Treatments

With the expectation of an additive effect of multiple treatment types, it may be tempting to combine pharmacological and psychological treatments for anxiety disorders. However, a review of the comparitive treatment efficacy of CBT versus CBT combined with pharmacologic monotherapies for anxiety disorders (obsessive compulsive, panic, social phobia, and generalized anxiety disorder) revealed no clear benefit or detriment of combined therapy compared to CBT alone; findings did suggest some benefit of combined therapy over pharmacotherapy alone (Foa, Franklin, & Moser, 2002; Rosser, Erskine, & Crino, 2004). Although research and clinical experience suggests that pharmacologic therapies be used as part of a multicomponent intervention package aimed at the treatment of severe aggression, there is little research that empirically establishes the contribution of combined therapies above and beyond the independent effectiveness of either monotherapy (Ziegler, 1996).

Other Issues in Management

Medical treatment. Of the pharmacotherapy treatments available for social anxiety disorder many have specific therapeutic windows and specified protocols needed for appropriate use. Eight to ten weeks is the minimum prescribed course for full efficacy of SSRIs to be evidenced (Sareen, & Stein, 2000). They are also contraindicated in combination with MAOIs. MAOIs are used when other drug treatments have been unsuccessful. Their use must be carefully monitored as they have adverse reactions with some foods and several common medications. Benzodiazapenes have addictive properties and must be titrated carefully when removing them form a patient's treatment plan in order to avoid withdrawal symptoms (Tajima, 2004). Beta-blockers are used for quick relief of physical symptoms (Sareen, & Stein, 2000).

Psychotherapy. When assertive behavior by an individual is lacking, there is often diminished accuracy and engagement of social communications. Therefore, within treatment for any of the psychological disorders involving problems of communication and social interaction such as major depressive disorder, dysthymic disorder, social anxiety disorder, panic disorder with agoraphobia, separation anxiety disorder, generalized anxiety disorder, pervasive developmental disorder, schizoid personality disorder, and avoidant personality disorder, the primacy of assertiveness training should be ascertained as a component of a comprehensive and empirically supported treatment appropriate for the specific psychological disorder.

Assertiveness in Specific Contexts

When assertive behavior is routinely absent in the context of a particular relationship or relationship set, an evaluation of the relationship history and implicit or explicit rules of the relationship is appropriate. This information may provide the therapist with clues as to the habit strength associated with the nonassertive behavior and the extent to which the pattern of habitual responding is reinforced by others. A realistic appraisal of the benefits and deficits of the relationship may need to be delineated along with an emphasis on the sufficiency of the self.

Intimate relationships. In the context of intimate relationships the greatest challenge to assertive behaving is often the long interaction history that has been established. Nonverbal and verbal components of intimate exchanges may have become habitual and less subject to immediate reinforcement contingencies. Intimate relationships are also unique with respect to the sensitivity of topics that may need to be addressed. The assertiveness skills forwarded for nonintimate interactions are applicable to intimate interactions. Particular attention may need to be given to acknowledging the degree to which a new interaction style is being forwarded. Sensitive behavior change requests (or request refusals) may involve family traditions, sexual behaving, or lifestyle behaviors. Sensitive topics such as changes in the frequency or type of sexual activities should be addressed in a manner that suggests an interest in experimentation rather than a permanent change to the couple's repertoire. It is also in such situations that the emphasis placed on overt reinforcement of satisfying aspects of current interactions cannot be too strong.

Business situations. Business situations are often replete individuals skilled in the art of persuasion. Because of the high level of assertiveness that often characterizes business interactions, specific techniques have been forwarded as helpful when making or refusing some business request. These include: the use of self-disclosure (suggestions of similarity in personal experiences or preferences are influential in "selling" an individual); repetition of request or request refusal (assuming a finite number of arguments for or against a given position, simple repetition of one's position suggests commitment to that stance and may wear down the resolve of the other individual); and singular focus (discussion of nonrelated or tangentially related topics may serve to distract the participants from the critical topic).

How Does One Select Among Treatments?

Assertiveness training can be an appropriate strategy for managing problem sets that encompass either passive behaviors or aggressive behaviors. When practiced as a component of psychological treatment for social anxiety disorder, assertiveness training requires that the client be willing to encounter anxiety. Provoking social situations and undergo a process of skills acquisition during which optimally assertive behavior is approximated with increasing success across practice trails. When practiced to manage aggression, assertiveness training requires that the client be willing to forego the emotional and instrumental "pay-offs" associated with aggressive behavior in favor of outcomes that are acceptable to all involved. Treatment selection is inextricably tied to the client's willingness to engage in the prescribed assertive behaviors.

In establishing the effectiveness of an assertive response, we often consider the outcome achieved. Although the ultimate goal of assertive communication may be influencing the behavior of others, the measure of assertiveness is the extent to which personal opinions, needs, and boundaries have been accurately and respectfully communicated and received. Competent performance of appropriately assertive behavior is best predicted when sufficient attention has been given to the interpersonal context in which the behavior is planned to occur. Treating professionals frequently fail to acknowledge consequences of assertive behaving that the client would consider negative (e.g., loss of perceived control for the formerly aggressive individual and loss of attachment figures for the formerly passive individual). In adopting an assertive stance, individuals are not merely engaging in a simple display of a new behavior set; They are often realigning and reordering relationship priorities.

REFERENCES

Clark, D. M., Ehlers, A., McManus, F., Hackmann, A., Fennell, M., Campbell, H. et al. (2003). Cognitive therapy versus fluoxetine in generalized social phobia: A randomized placebo-controlled trial. *Journal of Consulting and Clinical Psychology, 71,* 1058–1067.

Connor, D. F., Boone, R. T., Steingard, R. J., Lopez, I. D., & Melloni, R. H. (2003). Psychopharmacology and aggression: II. A meta-analysis of nonstimulant medication effects on overt aggression-related behaviors in youth with SED. *Journal of Emotional & Behavioral Disorders, 11*(3), 157–169.

Dow, M. G. (1985). Peer validation and idiographic analysis of social skill deficits. *Behavior Therapy, 16,* 76–86.

Dow, M. G. (1994). Social inadequacy and social skill. In L. W. Craighead, W. E. Craighead, A. E. Kazdin, and M. J. Mahoney, (Eds.), *Cognitive and behavioral interventions: An empirical approach to mental health problems,* (pp. 123–140). Boston, MA: Allyn and Bacon.

Dulit, R. A., Marin, D. B., & Frances, A. J. (1993). Cluster B personality disorders. In D. L. Dunner (Ed.), *Current psychiatric therapy* (pp. 405–411). Philadelphia: W. B. Saunders.

Eagly, A. H. & Steffen, V. J. (1986). Gender and aggressive behavior: A meta-analytic review of the social psychological literature. *Psychological Bulletin, 100*(3), 309–330.

Foa, E. B., Franklin, M. E., & Moser, J. (2002). Context in the clinic: How well do cognitive-behavioral therapies and medications work in combination. *Biological Psychiatry, 52*(10), 987–998.

Florsheim, P., Tolan, P. H., & Gorman-Smith, D. (1996). Family processes and risk for externalized behavior problems among African American and Hispanic boys. *Journal of Counseling and Clinical Psychology, 64*(6), 1222–1230.

Hare, R. D., McPherson, L. M., & Forth, A. E. (1998). Male psychopaths and their criminal careers. *Journal of Consulting and Clinical Psychology, 56*, 710–714.

Kaminer, D., & Stein, D. J. (2003). Social anxiety disorder. *World Journal of Biological Psychiatry, 4*, 103–110.

Kessler, R. C., McGonagle, K. A., Zhao, S., Nelson, C. B., Hughes, M., Eshleman, S., Wittchen, H. U., & Kendler, K. S. (1994). Lifetime and 12-month prevalence of DSM-III-R psychiatric disorders in the United Sates: Results from the National Comorbidity Survey. *Archives of General Psychiatry, 51*, 8–19.

Liebowitz, M. R., Schneier, F., Campeas, R., Hollander, E., Hatterer, J., Fyer, A., et al. (1992). Phenelzine vs. atenolol in social phobia: A placebo controlled comparison. *Archives of General Psychiatry, 49*, 290–300.

Lewinsohn, P. M. (1974). A behavioral approach to depression. In R. J. Friedman & M. M. Katz (Eds.), *The psychology of aggression: Contemporary theory and research*, (pp. 157–178). Washington, DC: Wiley.

MacGreene, D., & Navarro, R. L. (1998). Situation-specific assertiveness in the epidemiology of sexual victimization among university women: A progressive path analysis. *Psychology of Women Quarterly, 22*, 589–604.

Magee, W. J., Eaton, W. W., Wittchen, H.-U., McConagle, K. A., & Kessler, R. C. (1996). Agoraphobia, simple phobia, and social phobia in the National Comorbidity Study. *Archives of General Psychiatry, 53*, 159–168.

Maiuro, R. D., Cahn, T. S., & Vitaliano, P. P. (1986). Assertiveness deficits and hostility in domestically violent men. *Violence & Victims, 1*, 279–289.

Malagady, R. G., Rogler, L. H., & Cortes, D. E. (1996). Cultural expressions of psychiatric symptoms: Idioms of anger among Puerto Ricans. *Psychological Assessment, 8*(3), 265–268.

Millon, T. (1986). Schizoid and avoidant personality disorders in DSM-III. *American Journal of Psychiatry, 143*, 1321–1322.

Meyers-Abell, J. E. & Jansen, M. A. (1980). Assertiveness therapy for battered women: A case illustration. *Journal of Behavior Therapy & Experimental Psychiatry, 11*, 301–305.

O'Leary, K., Curley, A., Rosenbaum, A. & Clarke, C. (1985). Assertion training for abused wives: A potentially hazardous treatment. *Journal of Marital & Family Therapy, 11*, 319–322.

Öst, L. (1897). Age of onset in different phobias. *Journal of Abnormal Psychology, 96*(3), 223–229.

Pollack, M. H. (1999). Social anxiety disorder: Designing a pharmacologic treatment strategy. *Journal of Clinical Psychology, 6*(Suppl. 9), 20–26.

Rathus, S. A. (1973). A 30-item schedule for assessing assertive behavior. *Behavior Therapy, 4*, 398–406.

Reich, J., Yates, W., & Nduaguba, M. (1989). Prevalence of DSM-III personality disorders in the community. *Social Psychiatry and Psychiatric Epidemiology, 24*, 12–16.

Rosser, St., Erskine, A., & Crino, R. (2004). Pre-existing antidepressants and the outcome of group cognitive behavior therapy for social phobia. *Australian & New Zealand Journal of Psychiatry, 38*, 233–240.

Ruths, S., & Steiner, H. (2004). Psychopharmacologic treatment of aggression in children and adolescents. *Pediatric Annals, 33*, 318–327.

Sareen, L., & Stein, M. (2000). A review of the epidemiology and approaches to the treatment of social anxiety disorder. *Drugs, 59*, 497–509.

Stein, M. B., Liebowitz, M. R., Lydiard, R. B., Pitts, C. D., Bushnell, W., & Gergel, I. (1998). Paroxetine treatment of generalized social phobia (social anxiety disorder). A randomized clinical trial. *Journal of the American Medical Association, 280*, 708–713.

Stramek, J. J., Zarotsky, V., et al. (2002). Generalized anxiety disorder: Treatment options. *Drugs, 62*, 1635–1648.

Sutker, P. B., Bugg, F., & West, J. A. (1993). Antisocial personality disorder. In P. B. Sutker & H. E. Adams (Eds.), *Comprehensive handbook of psychopathology* (2nd ed., pp. 337–369). New York: Plenum Press.

Tedeschi, J. T., & Felson, R. B. (1994). *Violence, aggression, and coercive actions*. Washington, DC: American Psychological Association.

Tajima, O. (2004). Recent trends in pharmacotherapy for anxiety disorders. *Nihon Shinkei Seishin Yakurigaku Zasshi 24*, 133–136.

Truner, S. M., Beidel, D. C., & Jacob, R. G. (1994). Social phobia: A comparison of behavior therapy and atenolol. *Journal of Consulting Psychology, 62*, 350–358.

Walker, C., Thomas, J., & Allen, T. S. (2003). Treating impulsivity, irritability, and aggression of antisocial personality disorder with Quetiapine. *International Journal of Offender Therapy & Comparative Criminology, 47*, 556–567.

Zane, N. W. S., Sue, S., Hu, L., & Kwon, J. (1991). Asian-American assertion: A social learning analysis of cultural differences. *Journal of Counseling Psychology, 38*, 63–70.

Ziegler, R. G. (1996). Anxiety disorders in children: Applying a cognitive-behavioral technique that can be integrated with pharmacotherapy or other psychosocial interventions. In J. M. Ellison (Ed.), *Integrative Treatment of Anxiety Disorders* (pp. 199–247). Washington, DC: American Psychiatric Association.

Zimmerman, M., & Coryell, W. (1990). Diagnosing personality disorders in the community: A comparison of self-report and interview measures. *Archives of General Psychiatry, 47*, 527–531.

Attention-Deficit Hyperactivity Disorder (ADHD)

William E. Pelham, Jr • Daniel A. Waschbusch

WHAT IS ADHD?

The defining features of Attention-Deficit/Hyperactivity Disorder (ADHD) are inattention, hyperactivity and impulsivity (American Psychiatric Association, 2000). In individuals with ADHD, these behaviors are present for at least six months at levels higher than is typical for their stage of development, are present early in life (currently defined as before age 7), and cause impairment. Currently three subtypes of ADHD are recognized: primarily inattentive, primarily hyperactive/impulsive, and combined type. The inattentive subtype consists of individuals who exhibit inattentive behaviors but not hyperactive/impulsive behaviors, whereas the hyperactive/impulsive subtype consists of the reverse, and individuals with the combined subtype have both.

Children with ADHD have serious problems in multiple aspects of their lives. Children with ADHD typically experience more negative and hostile parenting styles, and mothers of children with ADHD experience greater stress and depression than do mothers of children without ADHD (Johnston & Mash, 2001). Children with ADHD tend to be actively rejected by their peers, often after just a few minutes of first meeting them (e.g., Pelham & Bender, 1982). Dozens of studies also demonstrate that children with ADHD perform less well at school, with lower daily productivity and accuracy on academic tasks and higher disruptiveness and off-task activity on measures on classroom behavior. These daily problems lead to lower academic achievement (DuPaul & Stoner, 2003).

The vast majority of ADHD research and treatment is directed at children. As a result, this review will focus primarily on children, with information on adolescents and adults included as appropriate.

BASIC FACTS ABOUT ADHD

Prevalence. ADHD is one of the most common mental health problems in children. Community based surveys suggest that approximately 3–5% of elementary age children meet criteria for ADHD, and that this is true across culture and across socioeconomic status (Lahey, Miller, Gordon, & Riley, 1999).

Gender. ADHD occurs more often in boys than in girls. The ratio of boys to girls with ADHD ranges from 3:1 to 9:1 (Gaub & Carlson, 1997).

Comorbidity. ADHD frequently occurs in conjunction with other disorders, the most common being oppositional defiant disorder (ODD) and conduct disorder (CD), with most studies reporting 30% (CD) to 75% (ODD) overlap (Lahey, et al., 1999). Mood and anxiety problems also overlap highly with ADHD, with most studies reporting a 10% to 25% rate of comorbidity (Angold, Costello, & Erkanli, 1999).

Pelham, W. E., & Waschbusch, D. A., (2006). In J. E. Fisher & W. T. O'Donohue (Eds.), *Practioner's guide to evidence-based psychotherapy.* New York: Springer.

Etiology. It is now clear that genetics play an important role in the development of ADHD. Approximately 15–25% of siblings and parents of children with ADHD have ADHD themselves. Conversely, rates of ADHD in offspring of adults with ADHD range from 20% to nearly 60%. In each case, these rates are significantly higher than in matched controls (Tannock, 1998). Twin studies suggest that 55–92% of identical (monozygotic) twins are concordant for ADHD, whereas the same rates for fraternal (dizygotic) twins are no different than between any other siblings. A number of environmental factors have also been associated with ADHD. Most notable are prenatal exposure to drugs (including alcohol and cigarettes), serious complications during prenatal development or delivery, postnatal head trauma, and exposure to lead and other toxins (Samudra & Cantwell, 1999). On the other hand, there are many claims about environmental factors causing ADHD that are unsupported, including dietary factors, allergies, socioeconomic variables, poor parenting, excessive television or video games, the culture or school climate of the 20th century, and parent/teacher intolerance.

Course. ADHD persists over development and is best conceptualized as a chronic disorder (Willoughby, 2003). Compared to controls, children with ADHD experience more negative outcomes when they become adolescents and adults. For example, data from recent longitudinal studies show that children with ADHD have a significantly greater risk than other children of becoming teenagers who fail academically, repeat grades, have worse social skills, fewer friends, and engage in risky behaviors such as poor driving and substance use (Barkley, Fisher, Edelbrock, & Smallish, 1990; Molina & Pelham, 2003).

ASSESSMENT

What Should Be Ruled Out?

The primary features of ADHD (inattention, hyperactivity, and impulsivity) are common behaviors in children with a variety of physical, emotional, and behavior problems. A diagnosis of ADHD is only assigned when they symptoms are not better accounted for by other health or mental health problems. Inattention, impulsivity and hyperactivity are also common in typically developing children; therefore, an important aspect of assessment is to determine whether the symptoms are present to a degree that is significantly greater than expected based on developmental norms, and whether the symptoms represent a pattern of behavior (i.e., multiple indicators of inattention, hyperactivity, or impulsivity are apprent) that is consistent across time (i.e., present for at least six months) and place (i.e., expressed in more than one place, such as home and school).

What Is Involved in Effective Assessment?

Effective assessment of ADHD involves evaluating the primary symptoms (inattention, impulsivity, and hyperactivity) and evaluating the functional deficits associated with ADHD. The former task is useful primarily for organizational purposes, such as communicating with insurance companies and linking the case with the research literature, whereas the latter task is useful for designing and implementing the intervention (Pelham, Fabiano, & Massetti, in press).

Assessment of defining features. Parents and teachers have been shown to be the optimal informants for the assessment of ADHD symptoms in children, whereas children's self-reports are not useful (Loeber, Green, Lahey, & Stouthamer-Loeber, 1989). Rating scales are particularly useful for gathering parent and teacher report on ADHD. Examples based on DSM criteria include the Disruptive Behaviour

Disorder (DBD) Rating Scale (Pelham, Gnagy, Greenslade, & Milich, 1992), the Swanson Nolan and Pelham-IV (Swanson, 1996), the Child and Adolescent Disruptive Behavior Inventory (Burns et al., 1997), the ADHD rating scale (DuPaul, 1991), and the Vanderbilt Rating Scale (Wolraich, Feurer, Hannah, Baumgaertel, & Pinnock, 1998). Scales that are not based on DSM criteria are also widely used for diagnosing ADHD (Pelham, Fabiano & Massetti, 2005) and relate well to DSM-based scles. Rating scales use a format that is well accepted by parents and teachers, have demonstrated reliability and validity, and provide normative information. Some of these must be purchased but others (DBD, SNAP, Vanderbilt) are available at no charge on the internet (Pelham, Fabiano & Massetti, 2005).

Structured interviews with parents (and sometimes teachers) are also used to assess ADHD symptoms. However, the main disadvantage of a structured interview is that they require considerably more time (for both the parent/teacher and the mental health professional) to complete than do rating scales and are therefore far more costly, and diagnosis based on interviews is predicted almost perfectly from rating scales (Pelham, Fabiano & Massetti, 2005).

Assessment of functional deficits. Functional analysis of ADHD involves gathering information from parents and teachers to determine what impairment the child with ADHD is experiencing and what can be done in treatment. Most functional analysis include an evaluation of the child's referring problems and the possible controlling environmental variables (antecedents and consequences), as well as the classroom and home management practices that have been employed with the target child and with other children. Evaluation of the effectiveness (if tried) of various interventions is also important to assess as well as the parent and teacher preferences regarding possible interventions that might be employed, and his or her opinion regarding the possible functions of the target behaviors (e.g., to gain peer attention, self-stimulation, to avoid tasks, etc.).

The clinician, along with parents and teachers, then formulate hypotheses regarding the functions of the target behaviors. Four primary functions have been suggested for behaviors expressed by children with ADHD (DuPaul & Eckert, 1997). ADHD behaviors may serve an escape or avoidance function (e.g., of academic tasks), a means of gaining attention from adults or peers (e.g., classroom clowning), a means to obtain a desired object or activity, or to regulate sensory stimulation. Based on the functional assessment, the consultant then assists the parent or teacher in manipulating antecedents or consequences to investigate whether the hypotheses regarding functions were correct. If such manipulations confirm the function of a given target behavior, then an intervention can be developed to change the behavior (Northup & Gulley, 2001). For example, if it can be established that peer attention is maintaining "classroom clowning", then an appropriate intervention might be a class-wide positive consequence for ignoring class clowning.

What Assessments Are Not Useful?

Commonly employed assessment procedures that are *not* useful for assessing ADHD include subscales on IQ tests such as the Freedom from Distractibility Index on the Wechsler scales, and such cognitive measures as continuous performance tasks. Careful research has failed to support the validity of such indices for the diagnosis and assessment of ADHD, and they are not recommended for use in school or clinical settings (American Academy of Pediatrics, 2001a). The same conclusion holds for the extensive list of neuropsychological tests that have been advocated for diagnosis of ADHD (Nichols & Waschbusch, 2004).

TREATMENT

What Treatments Are Effective?

Only behaviur therapy (BT), stimulant or related medication (MED), and the combination of BT and MED are empirically supported treatments for ADHD (AAP, 2001b).

What Treatments Are Not Effective?

There is a long list of treatments that have been tried for ADHD, including cognitive therapies, biofeedback, play therapy, herbal and dietary supplements or restrictions, and interactions with nature (i.e., playing with dolphins or walking in the woods). There is little or no empirical support for these treatments (AAP, 2001b; Waschbusch & Hill, 2001).

Medication Treatment

Efficacy. The most common medication treatment for ADHD is stimulant medication. Hundreds of studies have evaluated the use of stimulant medication for the treatment of ADHD (Swanson, McBurnett, Christian, & Wigal, 1995). Overall, this research demonstrates that stimulant medication treatment is effective as an acute treatment (i.e., improves classroom disruptiveness, on-task behavior, and compliance with adult requests), safe relative to other medications, and practical. Other types of medications for treatment of ADHD have been examined, but none has proven comparable to stimulants.

Limitations. At the same time, there are a number of limitations to the use of stimulants to treat ADHD. First, despite their clear beneficial effects in the short-term, there is currently no evidence that stimulants lead to improvements in long-term trajectories. Second, approximately one-quarter of children who are treated with stimulant medication show either an adverse response or no response, and only a minority of responders are normalized by medication. Third, medication has positive effects only when it is actively administered, with no generalization to unmedicated times or settings. Fourth, medication does not seem to adequately address all areas of children's functioning. For example, parenting behavior, peer relationships, and academic achievement are the key domains that medicate outcomes in children with disruptive behavior, and stimulants do not affect these keystone domains.

Behavior Therapy

Behavior therapy involves training parents to implement contingency-management programs with their children and consulting with the children's teachers with the same goal. In typical clinic-based programs, parents are given assigned readings and in a series of 8–16, weekly, group sessions are taught standard behavioral techniques such as time out, point systems, and contingent attention (Barkley, 1987; Anastopoulos, Shelton, & Barkley, 2005). Similarly, therapists work with teachers to develop: (1) classroom management strategies that can be implemented by the teacher with the target children, and (2) daily report cards that provide feedback to parents on the children's school performance, for which parents provide a consequence at home (DuPaul & Eckert, 1998). Numerous studies have found that standard, behaviorally based parent training and teacher consultation results in clinically important improvement on multiple measures in home and school settings for most children with ADHD who receive treatment (e.g., Pelham & Fabiano, in press; Pelham, Wheeler, & Chronis, 1998). There is some evidence that weekly social skills training groups combined with parent training can improve functioning with peers

(Pfiffner & McBurnett, 1997). Improvements that are obtained with these clinical behavioral interventions approximate those obtained with low to moderate doses of stimulant medication when medication is active. More intensive behavioral treatments or combined treatments (see below) are often required to maximize the impact of behavioral treatments on ADHD children. These techniques include components such as point/token economy reward systems, time out, and response–cost in school settings.

Efficacy studies of intensive behavior therapy have been conducted using a variety of methodologies, including both case studies and group studies. Both group studies (e.g., Carlson, Pelham, Milich, & Dixon, 1992) and case studies (e.g., Rapport, Murphy, & Bailey, 1980) are consistent in demonstrating clearly beneficial effects on both classroom work and classroom behavior. The effects of these more intensive treatments approximate relatively high doses of stimulants (Pelham et al., 2003). The evidence suggests that a substantial portion of ADHD children treated with behavior modification will function sufficiently well that medication is not needed (MTA Cooperative Group, 2004). More intensive behavioral treatments appear to be necessary to impact the peer domain in ADHD (Pelham et al., 2005).

Limitations of behavior therapy. The short-comings of behavioral interventions with ADHD children are nearly identical to those of psychostimulant medication (discussed above), with the addition that behavioral treatments are more costly than medication in the short-term.

Combined Treatment

The combination of behavior therapy and stimulant medication may be the optimal approach for treating many children with ADHD (American Academy of Pediatrics, 2001b; NIH Consensus Statement, 1998). Evidence suggests that behavior therapy and stimulant medication have complementary effects, with stimulants improving core DSM symptoms and behavior therapy impacting functional impairments in parents, children's academic functioning, and peer relationships (Pelham & Waschbusch, 1999) In addition, concurrent behavior therapy reduces the dose of medication needed to achieve a given level of functioning by 25–70% (e.g., MTA Cooperative Group, 1999; Pelham et al., 2003). Numerous studies have directly compared the combination of behavior therapy and stimulant medication (BT + MED) to behavior therapy alone (BT-only) and to medication only (MED-only), and these studies have generally shown that the combined treatment is superior to either treatment alone (Pelham & Waschbusch, 1999).

Also noteworthy are the results of the recent multi-modal treatment of ADHD (MTA) study funded by the National Institutes of Mental Health (MTA Cooperative Group, 1999). The primary purpose of the MTA study was to evaluate whether there is an incremental benefit of combining BT + MPH treatments over either alone. This study is especially important to consider because it enrolled a large number of participants (n = 579), used comprehensive measurement, and was implemented exceptionally well. Results showed that all three treatments produced clinically important improvements in multiple domains (MTA Cooperative Group, 1999). In general, the BT + Med groups showed greater improvement in ADHD symptoms and most functional domains, more excellent responders, a larger impact on comorbid children, and greater parental satisfaction with treatment (Conners et al., 2001; Jensen et al., 2001; MTA Cooperative Group, 1999; Pelham et al., (under review); Swanson et al., 2001).

How Does One Select Among Treatments?

A key question that remains unanswered concerns the sequence of delivering BT and/or MED. Currently, typical clinical practice is to first treat the child with medication, adding BT at a later date only when necessary. The arguments in support of this practice are that medication is substantially cheaper than BT, requires much less effort, and is at least as effective in reducing the symptoms of ADHD. Others argue that BT should almost always be administered prior to considering MED. The primary arguments in support of this approach are: (1) that BT is necessary to treat functional impairments; (2) that it will reduce the dose of medication needed, and most importantly; (3) that it reduces or eliminates the need for medication, and it is always desirable to avoid administering psychoactive substances to children.

SUMMARY AND FUTURE DIRECTIONS

Great progress has been made in the area of ADHD in terms of its etiology, development, and outcome; the disorder that was once thought by sceptics to be caused by sugar, bad parenting, and too much television, is now recognized as a legitimate mental health condition that is likely caused by a complex interplay of biological and environmental factors. Children suspected of having the disorder are now assessed using empirically valid and reliable tools and are subsequently treated with a variety of evidence-based treatments.

Despite the progress made in this field, there remains much research to be done to fully elucidate the development, course, outcome, and treatment of ADHD. First, more research is needed to address the impact of comorbidity on ADHD, and especially the interplay between comorbid conduct/oppositional problems and ADHD. Indeed, it has been suggested that children who have comorbid disorders fall into a separate diagnostic category than those who have either disorder alone, and that conduct problems can account for many of the problems thought to be associated with ADHD. Similarly, evaluating whether children with the inattentive subtype have the same disorder (i.e., causes, correlates, and outcomes) as those with combined type is in need of further research (Milich, Balentine, Lynam, 2001). Evaluating these issues is important for understanding the nature and interplay among disruptive behavior disorders.

Second, the role of gender in ADHD has been understudied. As a result, it remains unclear whether girls exhibit the same types of behaviors and developmental course of ADHD as do boys with ADHD. For example, the presence of the gender paradox in ADHD suggests that girls may not be identified as having the disorder unless the symptoms are especially severe.

Third, further research is needed regarding the developmental course across the lifespan of ADHD symptoms and impairment. Such research would allow for a more accurate conceptualization of the nature of the disorder and would help clarify the long-term effects (or lack thereof) of treatment on ameliorating ADHD symptoms and dysfunction.

Fourth, determining the most appropriate treatments for children with ADHD and their families is essential. Behavior therapy and stimulant medication have been shown to be effective in treating ADHD symptoms, but the evidence supporting these treatments have all been short-term. That is, there is currently no evidence that stimulant medication has a significant positive impact on children with ADHD over the long-term, and the long-term effect of behavior therapy has not been studied. Long-term studies of both modalities are needed. Further, even though children with ADHD show short-term improvement in response to behavior therapy, stimulant medication and their combination, these improvements typically do not lead to normalization. Instead, children with ADHD continue to be distinguished from their peers on numerous measures, especially in social functioning. Finally, research is needed on the main treatment issue facing families and practitioners—which treatment should be used first with a child and when should the other be added. Research on these topics is not only important for advancing science, it is also important for helping improve the lives of children, their families, and the societies in which they live.

REFERENCES

American Academy of Pediatrics. (2001a). Clinical practice guideline: Diagnosis and evaluation of a child with attention-deficit/hyperactivity disorder. *Pediatrics, 105*, 1158–1170.

American Academy of Pediatrics. (2001b). Clinical practice guideline: Treatment of the school-aged child with attention-deficit/hyperactivity disorder. *Pediatrics, 105*, 1033–1044.

American Psychiatric Association. (2000). *Diagnostic and statistical manual of mental disorders* (4th text revision ed.). Washington, DC: American Psychiatric Association.

Anastopoulos, A. D., Shelton, T. L., & Barkley, R. A. (2005). Family-based psychosocial treatments for children and adolescents with attention-deficit/hyperactivity disorder. In E. D. Hibbs & P. S. Jensen (Eds), *Psychosocial treatments for child and adolescent disorders: Empirically based strategies for clinical practice.* (pp. 327–350). Washington, DC: American Psychological Association.

Angold, A., Costello, E. J., & Erkanli, A. (1999). Comorbidity. *Journal of Child Psychology and Psychiatry, 40*, 57–87.

Barkley, R. A. (1987). *Defiant children: A clinician's manual for parent training.* New York, NY: Guilford Press.

Barkley, R. A., Fisher, M., Edelbrock, C. S., & Smallish, L. (1990). The adolescent outcome of hyperactive children diagnosed by research criteria: I. An 8-year prospective follow-up study. *Journal of the American Academy of Child and Adolescent Psychiatry, 29*, 546–557.

Burns, G. L., Walsh, J. A., Patterson, D. R., Holte, C. S., Sommers-Flanagan, R., & Parker, C. M. (1997). Internal validity of the disruptive behavior disorder symptoms: Implications from parent ratings for a dimensional approach to symptom validity. *Journal of Abnormal Child Psychology, 25*, 307–319.

Carlson, C. L., Pelham, W. E., Milich, R., & Dixon, M. J. (1992). Single and combined effects of methylphenidate and behavior therapy on the classroom behavior, academic performance and self-evaluations of children with attention deficit-hyperactivity disorder. *Journal of Abnormal Child Psychology, 20*, 213–232.

Conners, C. K., Epstein, J. N., March, J. S., Angold, A., Wells, K. C., Klaric, J., et al. (2001). Multimodal treatment of ADHD in the MTA: An alternative outcome analysis. *Journal of the American Academy of Child and Adolescent Psychiatry, 40*, 159–167.

DuPaul, G. J. (1991). Parent and teacher ratings of ADHD symptoms: Psychometric properties in a community-based sample. *Journal of Clinical Child Psychology, 20*, 245–253.

DuPaul, G. J., & Eckert, T. L. (1997). Interventions for students with attention-deficit/hyperactivity disorder: One size does not fit all. *School Psychology Review, 26*, 369–372.

DuPaul, G. J., & Eckert, T. L. (1998). Academic interventions for students with attention-deficit/hyperactivity disorder: A review of the literature. *Reading and Writing Quarterly, 14*, 59–83.

DuPaul, G. J., & Stoner, G. (2003). *ADHD in the schools: Assessment and intervention strategies.* New York: The Guilford Press.

Gaub, M., & Carlson, C. L. (1997). Gender differences in ADHD: A meta-analysis and critical review. *Journal of the American Academy of Child and Adolescent Psychiatry, 36*, 1036–1045.

Jensen, P. S., Hinshaw, S. P., Kraemer, H. C., Lenora, N., Newcorn, J. H., Abikoff, H. B., et al. (2001). ADHD comorbidity findings from the MTA study: New diagnostic subtypes and their optimal treatments. *Journal of American Academy of Child & Adolescent Psychiatry, 40*, 147–158.

Johnston, C., & Mash, E. J. (2001). Families of children with attention-deficit/hyperactivity disorder: Review and recommendations for future research. *Clinical Child and Adolescent Psychology Newsletter, 4*, 183–208.

Lahey, B. B., Miller, T. I., Gordon, R. A., & Riley, A. W. (1999). Developmental epidemiology of the disruptive behavior disorders. In H. C. Quay & A. E. Hogan (Eds.), *Handbook of disruptive behavior disorders* (pp. 23–48). New York: Kluwer Academic/Plenum Publishers.

Loeber, R., Green, S. M., Lahey, B. B., & Stouthamer-Loeber, M. (1989). Optimal informants on childhood disruptive behaviors. *Development and Psychopathology, 1*, 317–337.

Milich, R., Balentine, A. C., & Lynam, D. R. (2001). ADHD combined type and ADHD predominantly inattentive type are distinct and unrelated disorders. *Clinical Psychology: Science and Practice, 8*, 463–488.

Molina, B. S. G., & Pelham, W. E. (2003). Childhood predictors of adolescent substance use in a longitudinal study of children with ADHD. *Journal of Abnormal Psychology, 112*, 497–507.

MTA Cooperative Group. (1999). A 14-month randomized clinical trial of treatment strategies for attention-deficit/hyperactivity disorder. *Archives of General Psychiatry, 56*, 1073–1086.

MTA Cooperative Group (2004). National Institute of Mental Health multimodal treatment study of ADHD follow-up: Changes in effectiveness and growth after the end of treatment. *Pediatrics*, 113(4), 762–769.

Nichols, S., & Waschbusch, D. A. (2004). A review of the validity of laboratory cognitive tasks used to assess symptoms of ADHD. *Child Psychiatry and Human Development, 34*, 297–315.

NIH Consensus Statement. (1998). *Diagnosis and treatment of attention-deficit hyperactivity disorder*. Kensington, MD: National Institutes of Health Consensus Development Project.

Northup, J., & Gulley, V. (2001). Some contributions of functional analysis to the assessment of behaviors associated with attention deficit hyperactivity disorder and the effects of stimulant medication. *School Psychology Review, 30*, 227–238.

Pelham, W. E., & Bender, M. E. (1982). Peer relationships in hyperactive children: Description and treatment. In K. Gadow & I. Bailer (Eds.), *Advances in learning and behavioral disabilities* (Vol. 1, pp. 365–436). Greenwich, CT: JAI.

Pelham, W. E., Burrows-MacLean, L., Gnagy, E. M., Coles, E. K., Wymbs, B. T., Chacko, A., et al. (2003, November). *A dose ranging study of behavioral and pharmacological treatment for children with ADHD*. Poster presented at the 37th annual convention of the Association for Advancement of Behavior Therapy, Boston, MA.

Pelham, W. E., Erhardt, D., Gnagy, E. M., Greiner, A. R., Arnold, L. E., Abikoff, H. B., et al. Parent and teacher evaluation of treatment in the MTA: Consumer satisfaction and perceived effectiveness. Manuscript under review.

Pelham, W. E., & Fabiano, G. A. (in press). Evidence-based psychosocial treatment for attention-deficit/hyperactivity disorder: An update. *Journal of Clinical Child and Adolescent Psychology*.

Pelham, W. E., Fabiano, G. A., Gnagy, E. M., Greiner, A. R., Hoza, B., Manos, M., et al. (2005). The role of summer treatment programs in the context of comprehensive treatment for ADHD. In E. Hibbs & P. Jensen (Eds.), *Psychosocial treatments for child and adolescent disorders: Empirically based strategies for clinical practice* (pp. 377–410). New York: APA.

Pelham, W. E., Fabiano, G. A., & Massetti, G. M. (2005). Evidence-based assessment for Attention Deficit Hyperactivity Disorder in children and adolescents. *Journal of Clinical Child and Adolescent Psychology*, 34(3), 449–476.

Pelham, W. E., Gnagy, E. M., Greenslade, K. E., & Milich, R. (1992). Teacher ratings of DSM-III-R symptoms for the disruptive behavior disorders. *Journal of the American Academy of Child and Adolescent Psychiatry, 31*, 210–218.

Pelham, W. E., & Waschbusch, D. A. (1999). Behavioral intervention in ADHD. In H. C. Quay & A. E. Hogan (Eds.), *Handbook of disruptive behavior disorders* (pp. 255–278). New York: Plenum.

Pelham, W. E., Wheeler, T., & Chronis, A. M. (1998). Empirically supported psychosocial treatment for attention deficit hyperactivity disorder. *Journal of Clinical Child Psychology, 27*, 190–205.

Pfiffner, L. J., & McBurnett, K. (1997). Social skills training with parent generalization: Treatment effects for children with ADD/ADHD. *Journal of Consulting and Clinical Psychology, 65*, 749–757.

Rapport, M. D., Murphy, A., & Bailey, J. S. (1980). The effects of a response cost treatment tactic on hyperactive children. *Journal of School Psychology, 18*, 98–111.

Samudra, K., & Cantwell, D. P. (1999). Risk factors for attention-deficit/hyperactivity disorder. In H. C. Quay & A. E. Hogan (Eds.), *Handbook of disruptive behavior disorders* (pp. 199–220). New York: Plenum Press.

Swanson, J. M. (1996). The SNAP-IV teacher and parent rating scale, from *http://www.adhd. net/*

Swanson, J. M., Kraemer, H. C., Hinshaw, S. P., Arnold, L. E., Conners, C. K., Abikoff, H. B., et al. (2001). Clinical relevance of the primary findings of the MTA: Success rates based on severity of ADHD and ODD symptoms at the end of treatment. *Journal of the American Academy of Child and Adolescent Psychiatry, 40*, 168–179.

Swanson, J. M., McBurnett, K., Christian, D. L., & Wigal, T. (1995). Stimulant medications and the treatment of children with ADHD. In T. H. Ollendick & R. J. Prinz (Eds.), *Advances in clinical child psychology* (Vol. 17, pp. 265–322). New York: Plenum Press.

Tannock, R. (1998). Attention deficit hyperactivity disorder: Advances in cognitive, neurobiological, and genetic research. *Journal of Child Psychology and Psychiatry, 39*, 65–99.

Waschbusch, D. A., & Hill, G. P. (2001). Alternative treatments for children with attention-deficit/hyperactivity disorder (ADHD): What does the research say? *The Behavior Therapist, 24*, 161–171.

Willoughby, M. T. (2003). Developmental course of ADHD symptomatology during the transition from childhood to adolescence: A review with recommendations. *Journal of Child Psychology and Psychiatry, 44*, 88–106.

Wolraich, M. L., Feurer, I. D., Hannah, J. N., Baumgaertel, A., & Pinnock, T. Y. (1998). Obtaining systematic teacher reports of disruptive behavior disorders utilizing DSM-IV. *Journal of Abnormal Child Psychology, 26*, 141–152.

Autistic Disorder

O. Ivar Lovaas. • Scott Cross. Scott Revlin

WHAT IS AUTISTIC DISORDER?

Paul was only a baby when his parents became aware that he did not behave like his older sister when she was the same age. Unlike her, Paul stiffened when in his parents' arms and avoided eye contact by turning his face away from them when he was fed his bottle, seeming hard of hearing and actively resisted being held and cuddled. Unlike his peers at one year of age, Paul would not cry and seemed not to notice when his parents left the house. At two Paul's parents concerns grew as he still had not begun to speak and did not appear to understand what they said to him. He seemed lost in his own world. Instead of playing with toys like his peers, Paul engaged in seemingly meaningless and repetitive behaviors such as tapping objects, pacing back-and-forth across the floor, rocking his body while loudly vocalizing and gazing at lights. He seemed unaware of common dangers and had to be protected from sources such as hot surfaces, busy streets, and swimming pools. Tantrums and self-injurious behaviors often increased in response to changes in his environment as if he could not cope with it. Despite his parents' attempts to teach him, Paul had difficulties dressing himself, was not toilet trained and often failed to sleep through the night.

Paul illustrates a child who from infancy on exhibited behaviors signaling his parents that something was amiss and prompted them to seek professional help. Unlike Paul, some children appear to develop normally up to 18–24 months only to suddenly lose most or all acquired language and social skills within a period of two to three weeks for reasons no one as of yet understands.

Prevalence. The prevalence of autism is the subject of debate, as estimated rates of autism have increased in recent years. The Center for Disease Control (2004) is actively researching the prevalence of this disorder with current estimates ranging from 3.4 to 6.7 per 1,000. While the rate of autism appears to be rising, males are still four times as likely as females to be diagnosed.

Age at onset and course. The onset of autism is considered to occur prior to three years of age. According to DSM-IV (APA, 2000) only a small percent of individuals with autism are able to live and work independently as adults, instead requiring life-long protective care in specially designed treatment settings. Autism is conceptualized as falling on a continuum with Asperger's Disorder and Pervasive Development Disorder Not otherwise specified (PDD-NOS) and illustrates the variability in verbal communication, social relatedness, and cognitive functioning in this population.

WHAT ARE DIAGNOSTIC FEATURES?

According to DSM-IV-TR (APA, 2000) autism is described as a neurological disorder with a strong genetic link resulting in a wide range of developmental delays in the acquisition of verbal and non-verbal communication, social, cognitive, and self-help

Lovass, O. I., Cross, S., & Revlin, S. (2006). In J. E. Fisher & W. T. O'Donohue (Eds.), *Practitioner's guide to evidence-based psychotherapy.* New York: Springer.

skills. Approximately 75% of these children obtain scores within the retarded range on standardized tests of mental functioning. Behavioral excesses include tantrums, aggression, ritualistic, and self-stimulatory behaviors. Six or more diagnostic features are required by the American Psychiatric Association (APA) as set forth in their diagnostic criteria:

Social

1. marked delay in social behaviors (social referencing, eye to eye contact, social gestures)
2. delay in development of peer relations commensurate with chronological age
3. delay of social sharing (pointing, showing, bringing objects)
4. delay in social imitative/symbolic play

Language

5. delayed or devoid of receptive and expressive language without compensatory nonverbal communication
6. delays in initiating/sustaining conversations
7. stereotyped/repetitive use of language (echolalia)

Excessive behaviors

8. adherence to apparently non-functional routines and rituals
9. stereotypy (repetitive mannerisms such as body-rocking, hand-flapping, gazing at lights)
10. Preoccupation with parts of objects such as spinning the wheels of a toy car

HOW ARE DELAYED BEHAVIORS IDENTIFIED?

The behavioral delays in autism are identified by behavioral observation and often measurable by 18 months of age. Autism can be differentiated from other developmental disorders in the 20–26 month age range based upon the following delays (Lord, 1995; Baird et al., 2000):

- communicative use of eye contact
- orienting to one's name
- joint attention behaviors (i.e., pointing, showing, bringing, gaze monitoring, sharing)
- following another person's focus of attention through eye gaze or gesture
- pretend play
- imitation
- nonverbal communication
- language development

In a 2002 report on best practices for screening and diagnosis, The California Department of Developmental Disabilities, considers the following clinical signs to be "red flags" for children suspected to fall on the autism spectrum warranting immediate referral to a diagnostic team:

- by 12 months—absence of communicative gesture use (e.g., pointing)
- by 12 months failure to follow nonverbal communication (e.g., does not come when mom extends her arms)
- by 16 months absence of single words
- by 24 months absence of two-word phrases
- at any age loss of a social skill such as language

WHAT IS EFFECTIVE ASSESSMENT?

Assessments of cognitive, communicative, social, and adaptive behaviors provide information important for diagnosis and intervention planning. Given the multiple areas of delays, the contributions by several disciplines are likely to be needed (e.g., neurology and audiology). Note that a diagnosis alone is insufficient to guide intervention planning given the variability among children with autism.

Various diagnostic instruments have been helpful in discriminating autism from other developmental disorders. Two extensively researched and commonly used instruments are the Autism Diagnostic Interview-Revised (ADI-R) (Lord, Rutter, & Le Couteur, 1994) and the Autism Diagnostic Observation Scale (ADOS) (Lord, et al., 2000). To help establish reliability in the diagnosis it is recommended to seek agreement from independent certified assessors.

The National Research Council report (2001) and the California Best Practices Guidelines (2002) detail domains to be assessed as well as typical issues which a diagnostic team may confront while in the assessment process. It is recommended that readers refer to these documents. A diagnostic evaluation for identification and treatment of autism should contain the following six components:

- review of relevant background information
- parent/caregiver interview
- comprehensive medical evaluation
- behavioral observation
- cognitive assessment (e.g., Bayley Scales of Infant Development-Revised)
- measures of adaptive functioning (e.g., Vineland)

TREATMENT OF AUTISM

How was Autism Conceptualized in the Past?

Kanner's (1943) proposed that autism represents a distinct diagnostic category whereby behaviors (referred to as symptoms) were held together by a central dysfunction which he labeled Autism. Kanner further proposed that when this central dysfunction was located and treated, the various behavioral deviations would be normalized. Kanner invoked three distinct signs of autism. One, the child evidenced extreme isolation from the social environment and an inability to relate to others, including parents. Two, the child had a "pathological desire" to maintain sameness in his/her environment such a insisting on a parent's maintaining the same clothing, grooming, etc. Three, the child was mute but might evidence noncommunicative speech, as in echolalia (repeating the vocal utterances of others). Although there are a variety of manifestations of autism, the key elements reported by Kanner are present today in the DSM-IV-TR, APA, 2000. Although Kanner hinted that parenting practices might be causal in a child's development of autism, Bettleheim (1967) is best known for promoting the "cold mother" as the cause and advocating psychodynamic treatments, as Freud. Psychodynamic theories of etiology and treatment of autism maintained a stronghold for more than 40 years. Comprehensive reviews of the deleterious effect of psychoanalytic approaches have been presented in some detail in publications such as "Freudian-Fraud" (Torrey, 1992). The book presents numerous examples of how psychodynamic treatment has failed to be supported by scientific research and instead exercised a destructive influence on parents and others who have responsibility for teaching and caring for children diagnosed with autism and other special needs.

Given the failure of psychodynamic approaches in autism to generate effective treatment, the door was opened to introduce and test alternate approaches to treatment, using objective and data-based procedures. It is noteworthy that parents of children with autism helped stop psychodynamic treatments as they gained political influence by organizing groups such as The Autism Society of America (ASA). Rimland (1964) is the founding father of ASA and himself a parent of a child with autism.

PSYCHODYNAMIC TREATMENTS

It may be helpful to contrast traditional and behavioral approaches to research and treatment for children diagnosed with autism. Kanner's (1943) hypothesis generated a large variety of treatments with a common assumption, that by addressing one or a limited set of cardinal behaviors or processes for a limited period of time, and in clinical or segregated settings, comprehensive improvements are likely to generalize across most or all of the clients' behaviors and generalize across environments. Further, in the history of treatment for autism, almost every behavioral deviation (e.g., language, attention, social, cognition, emotional) as well as combinations of behaviors (e.g., social/emotional, language/cognitive), have been proposed as the cause of autism. There is as yet no published outcome research in peer-reviewed journals documenting the effectiveness of psychodynamic treatments.

How do Behaviorists Conceptualize and Treat Autism?

From a behavioral perspective, it may be more parsimonious and productive to consider the behavioral deviations in persons diagnosed with autism not as caused by a hypothetical disease like "Autism," but as variability across nervous systems. Although there is strength in variability (it is essential for survival), nature overshot her mark in most cases of autism. In behavioral treatment each behavioral delay and excess is measured and experimental manipulations are utilized to identify the environmental variables that control the separate behaviors. Treatment employs learning-based interventions which have been documented to be effective in earlier research (Lovaas, 2003).

Are Other Treatments Effective?

Smith (1996) wrote a critical review of a large number of interventions proposed to treat autism including Project TEACCH, Special Education, the Higashi School, sensory motor therapies such as Sensory Integration, Auditory Integration, Facilitated Communication, and psychotherapies such as Floor-Time, Holding Therapy, Option Method, and Gentle Teaching. It is distressing to note that, despite the wide use of these interventions, either outcome data are missing altogether or available data fail to support the effectiveness claimed by the originators of these programs. Likewise, many individuals with autism are provided with speech and language therapy, yet there appear to be no scientific studies demonstrating that speech and language therapy per se is effective with this population. The Natural Language Paradigm, Incidental Teaching, Pivotal Response Training, and FastForWord have similarly not been supported by objective data pertaining to long-term and comprehensive treatment outcomes.

Lovaas (1971) expressed his concerns about traditional treatment research in autism as follows: "The diagnosis of autism may lead to premature decisions about what it is we are studying. Children with autism present a whole set of behaviors and these different behaviors have different properties. The problem behaviors may not hang together" (p. 109). Rutter (1978) expressed similar concerns when he cautioned that "Kanner's use of the term autism was more than a simple label, and that is where the trouble really increases. It was also an hypothesis—a suggestion that behind the behavioral description lay a disease entity" (p. 3). A more basic problem centers on the possibility that autism is a social and not a scientific construct. Autism may be an arbitrary collection of low frequency behaviors, the diagnosis a myth in a way. Kuhn (1996) has cautioned that certain constructs are "social" and not based on scientific research. Social constructs can be modified and added to but cannot be rejected, and resists being improved upon in further research. Despite years of research and the expenditure of millions of dollars, we may be no closer to finding the cause and ultimate treatment of autism.

BEHAVIORAL TREATMENT RESEARCH

How does Behavioral Treatment Differ from Alternative Treatments?

For the last 100 years, starting with Thorndike's work at Columbia University, empirical research on learning processes has shown learning-based interventions to be successful in helping disadvantaged persons acquire many or most of the behaviors of typically developing persons as in the case of those diagnosed with autism (DeMyer, Hingtgen & Jackson, 1981; Rutter, 1985; Schreibman, 1988; Smith, 1993; Dawson & Osterling, 1997). This chapter attempts to describe the advances in treatment associated with learning-based behavioral treatment research as contrasted with traditional and unsupported approaches.

Knowledge about behavioral treatment was based on Skinner's (1957) research on operant conditioning and transferred from research laboratories into applied settings by Ayllon and Azrin (1968) and Goldiamond (1965), and extended into treatment of autism and other developmental disabilities in the early 1960s. With the support of Bijou (e.g., 1966) and Baer (e.g., Baer & Sherman, 1964), a behavioral group grew at the University of Washington and included, but was not limited to, Birnbrauer (e.g., Birnbrauer, Bijou, Wolf & Kidder, 1965), Risley (e.g., 1968), Hart (e.g., Risley, Reynolds & Hart, 1970), Sherman (e.g., 1964), Wahler (e.g., 1969), and Wolf (e.g., Wolf, Risley & Mees, 1964). All presented data-based interventions allowing for progress in an incremental manner helping individuals with autism and other developmental delays live more meaningful lives. It is a compliment to the field of Applied Behavior Analysis that literally hundreds of investigators have been able to generate hundreds of replicable studies that add in a cumulative manner to a large array of useful knowledge about treatment.

Three significant steps were involved in the development of behavioral treatment research.

1. The construct of autism was broken down into its separate behaviors to allow for accurate and sensitive measures of treatment outcomes.
2. Variables in the children's immediate environment were systematically manipulated (presented and withdrawn) to assess their effects on the various behaviors targeted for intervention.
3. It was assumed that the laws of learning, which are backed by explicit and empirical information about how behaviors of organisms could be manipulated to increase or decrease their strength serving as a basis for the selection and testing of treatment variables.

The ways in which these three steps facilitate research and optimize treatment outcome is briefly discussed below.

Measurement. Separate behaviors can be measured more reliably and precisely than the syndrome of autism as a whole. Sensitive and accurate measures of the various developmental delays and excesses provided opportunities to assess moment-to-moment fluctuations in the magnitude of each behavior in response to treatment variables, allowing the investigator immediate feedback regarding their effectiveness or lack thereof, helping guide future research. The use of precise and sensitive measures may be particularly important in the early stages of exploratory research, in part because smaller changes in behavior may be more frequently occurring than larger ones, hence, more likely to be detected. More or less "autism" will not yield sensitive measures as may be required to guide investigators in their future research.

Research on Modifying Separate Behaviors in Autism

Self-injury. There exists a large amount of experimental literature on the treatment of self-injury, a behavior which endangers persons with autism and other developmental delays. Treatment research directed at reducing self-injurious behavior illustrates the complexity of causes underlying a behavior with a common topography. Lovaas and Simmons (1969) found that self-injury can be increased by contingent social attention, Carr, Newsom, & Binkoff (1976) showed self-injurious behaviors to be strengthened (negatively reinforced) by the escape from environmental demands while Favell, McGimsey & Schell (1982) also reported that instances of self-injurious behavior could be controlled by sensory feedback created by the injurious behavior itself. In short, one behavioral topography appears to be maintained by three different kinds of functional relationships to the environment necessitating that treatment providers be competent in performing a functional analysis (isolating the cause–effect relationships) of self-injurious behavior so that appropriate kinds of treatment could be applied. A particular intervention that reduces one kind of self-injury may worsen another. To illustrate, placing children in "time out" (relative isolation) contingent on self-injury is likely to reduce self-injury if the behavior is based on positive reinforcement (such as delivery of attention). The same intervention may increase self-injury if based on negative reinforcement as in escape-avoidance behavior (Carr, Newsom, & Binkoff, 1976). Finally, self-injury based on sensory reinforcement would remain unaltered unless the sensory feedback generated by the injury was blocked or shifted to other behaviors (Favell et al., 1982). Matson and Taras (1989) have provided a review of a variety of behavioral procedures for reducing self-injury.

Self-stimulatory behavior. Persons with autism and other developmental delays may exhibit high rates of self-stimulatory behavior, such as repetitive hand-flapping and body-rocking. The major findings on self-stimulatory behavior can be summarized as follows:

(1) Self-stimulatory behavior can be observed to occur across many diagnostic categories and, in transient form, among typical individuals such as young children (Kravitz & Boehm, 1971; Thelen, 1979).

(2) Self-stimulatory behavior varies inversely with the magnitude of socially appropriate behavior and appears to be maintained by the sensory reinforcement generated by such behavior (Lovaas, Newsom, & Hickman, 1987).

(3) Access to self-stimulatory behavior can be used to reinforce (reward and strengthen) socially appropriate behavior (Rincover & Newsom, 1985).

(4) Effective treatment may consist of changing low-level forms of self-stimulatory behavior to socially appropriate forms (Epstein, Taubman, & Lovaas, 1985), examples

of which may be found in music, dance, card games such as solitaire, painting and photography, athletic performances such as basketball and golf and other behaviors involving lining and matching as reinforcement.

(5) Sensory feedback generated by self-stimulatory behavior may fulfill a biological need serving to maintain the afferent nervous system from deterioration. Treatment involving the direct suppression of self-stimulatory behaviors would be contraindicated unless alternate behaviors are established and reinforced (Sackett, 1966).

Attention. Children diagnosed with autism may act as if they are visually and/or hearing impaired. This may be evidenced by failing to respond to their parents calling their names, to people coming and going and to other significant environmental events. By contrast, they may respond to a barely audible noise from a fluorescent light fixture or the unwrapping of a candy bar. This phenomenon has been labeled "stimulus overselectivity" (overly narrow attention), referring to the experimental finding that only a small and restricted number of stimuli in a complex array control the behavior of a child diagnosed with autism (Lovaas, Koegel, & Schreibman, 1979). If a child is unable to concurrently process both visual and auditory stimuli (e.g., fail to attend to the parent's or instructor's concurrent facial and verbal expressions), it is likely that social, emotional and cognitive behaviors will be delayed as well. Overselective attention is greatly reduced or eliminated as a function of early and intensive behavioral treatment (McEachin, Smith, & Lovaas, 1993).

Imitation. Typical children learn countless new behaviors by imitating their peers (Bandura, 1969). The failure of those with autism to imitate has both practical and theoretical significance. Baer, Guess, and Sherman (1972) made initial and important progress toward identifying essential steps in teaching imitation through learning-based principles. Subsequently, discrete trial procedures were used to teach nonverbal imitation (Lovaas, Freitas, Gold, & Kassorla, 1967) and verbal imitation (Lovaas, Berberich, Perloff, & Schaeffer, 1966), both central skills in the establishment of language (Lovaas et al., 1966). For a detailed account of initial language acquisition refer to Teaching Individuals with Developmental Delays: Basic Intervention Techniques (Lovaas, 2003).

BEHAVIORAL TREATMENT RESEARCH

How did Comprehensive Treatment Originate?

In this portion of the chapter we attempt to illustrate how intensive and early behavioral treatment of individuals with autism evolved, and we do so by focusing on data from two treatment outcome studies conducted at the University of California, Los Angeles (UCLA) Young Autism Project (Lovaas, 1987). We also describe the criteria for appropriate treatment that resulted from the application of behavioral intervention. Note that major components of the treatment programs were not developed at UCLA but based on extensive research published in peer-reviewed journals by independent investigators. Most of the studies have been replicated. Also, note that none of the studies referred to have reported a major or sudden breakthrough. Rather, progress in treatment developed in an inductive, gradual and stepwise fashion, such as that done in the building of a pyramid where a solid foundation forms the basis for adding additional structure. Research projects by the UCLA Young Autism Project help to illustrate this development. Investigators have contended that the best way to know what aspects of a treatment make a treatment effective is by studying individual components of the treatment separately before performing an outcome study (Johnson, 1988).

The first comprehensive treatment study was started in 1964 and reflected many blind alleys in our own design (Lovaas, Koegel, Simmons, & Long, 1973). At present, more than 400 separate skill acquisition programs constitute the comprehensive intervention offered by UCLA and affiliated sites. The earlier treatment outcome data will be reviewed first to illustrate how weaknesses were identified and solutions sought. Treatment outcome data can be summarized as follows.

Positive findings.

(1) All children improved, though they evidenced marked individual differences in amounts of improvement.
(2) The longer the treatment lasted, the greater the improvement.
(3) Complex behaviors, such as language and toy play could be acquired.
(4) The children showed gains on standardized tests of intelligence and adaptive functioning.
(5) Maladaptive behaviors, such as self-stimulation and self-injury, could be decreased.

Negative findings.

(1) No child appeared to have achieved normal functioning.
(2) No child developed social interactions or played with other children.
(3) Treatment gains that were achieved in the clinic showed limited generalization to other environments or to behaviors that were not a focus of treatment.
(4) Children discharged to psychiatric institutions lost all their treatment gains while children discharged to their parents who had received parent training, continued to improve as evidenced by follow-up measures taken two to three years after discharge.

The 1987 UCLA Young Autism Project. The negative findings in the 1973 study (Lovaas et al., 1973) strongly influenced the design of the intervention strategies that formed the basis for the Lovaas (1987) report. Numerous studies by other investigators also suggested refinements (Smith, 1993). Four main changes were made:

1. The youngest children in the 1973 study had made the greatest progress. Treatment was therefore concentrated on very young children (mean chronological age of 34 months at intake).
2. In the 1987 study specific attempts were made to teach children peer play and to gradually and systematically include participants into normal preschool environments, programs which were not available in the 1973 study; neither did the social or legal basis for such mainstreaming exist.
3. The 1973 study had restricted intensive treatment to one year, while the 1987 study treated the clients intensively for two or more years, with 40 hours or more per week of one-to-one behavioral intervention combined with parent training which allowed for treatment most of the child's waking hours. This amount of treatment in the 1987 study did more closely approximate the opportunities available to average children, who appear to learn from their environments most of their waking hours.
4. Failure to observe significant transfer of treatment gains from the clinic to the home necessitated that treatment be conducted in the children's everyday environments such as home, school, and neighborhood.
5. Failure to find a pivotal response (i.e., limited response generalization) necessitated that most or all of a child's behaviors be addressed.

The 1987 study was comprised of three groups of children with comparable pretreatment data: (a) an experimental (intensive treatment) group (*n*=19); (b) a minimal treatment Control Group I (n=19); and (c) a no-treatment Control Group II (n=21). Post-treatment assessments were administered when the children were seven years old; 1–2 years after discharge. Children in the experimental group had gained an average of 20 IQ points and had made major advances in educational achievement. Only one of 40 children in the two control groups achieved such a favorable outcome. At a follow-up conducted at age 13, 8 of the 9 participants who achieved typical intellectual functioning ("best outcome") had retained their IQ gains and were indistinguishable compared to age-matched, typically developing peers assessed by psychologists blind as to the purpose of the study (McEachin et al., 1993).

CRITERIA FOR APPROPRIATE TREATMENT

It has been possible to formulate a consensus among many scientific researchers and practitioners that appropriate treatment contains the following elements (Simeonnson, Olley, & Rosenthal, 1987).

1. *A behavioral emphasis.* This involves not only imposing structure and rewarding appropriate behaviors when they occur, but also applying some more technical and data-based interventions such as discrete trials, shaping by successive approximations, producing shifts in stimulus control, establishing stimulus discriminations, and teaching imitation (Koegel and Koegel, 1988).
2. *Family participation.* Parents and other family members should be taught to participate in teaching the child who is developmentally delayed. Without such participation, gains made in professional settings such as in school environments, clinics or hospitals rarely lead to improved functioning in the home or community (Bartak, 1978; Lovaas et al., 1973).
3. *One-to-one instruction.* For approximately the first 12–18 months of treatment, instruction should be individualized rather than conducted in groups because children with autism and other developmental delays learn more readily in the delivery of one-to-one situations (Koegel, Rincover, and Egel, 1982). This training needs to be supervised by degreed professionals educated in Applied Behavior Analysis and extensively trained in behavioral treatment and program development. Thoroughly trained persons such as undergraduate students and family members may deliver the treatment (Lovaas and Smith, 1988).
4. *Integration.* Prior to integration in a group setting, usually a school environment, the child should be taught as many socially appropriate behaviors, including vocal speech as possible. The school environment should be carefully selected for integration, be directed by a cooperative and structured teacher and comprised of typically developing children. Children with autism benefit more when integrated with typically developing children than when placed with children of the same diagnosis (Strain, 1983). Children with autism require explicit instruction on how to interact with and learn from their typically developing peers, mere exposure is not sufficient to facilitate appropriate behavior. (Strain, 1983). In the presence of other children with autism, however, acquired social and language skills may disappear, presumably because appropriate/functional discriminative stimuli (SDs) are less likely to be available and such behaviors are not reinforced (Smith, Watthen-Lovaas, & Lovaas, 2002).
5. *Comprehensiveness.* Children with autism have few appropriate behaviors and new behaviors have to be taught one by one. For example, teaching language skills does not immediately lead to the emergence of social skills, and teaching one language skill, such as prepositions, does not lead directly to the emergence of other language skills, such as mastery of pronouns.

6. *Intensity.* Perhaps as a corollary for the need for comprehensiveness, an effective intervention requires a very large number of hours, 40 hours or more per week (Lovaas & Smith, 1988). Ten hours per week is inadequate (Lovaas & Smith, 1988), as is 20 hours (Anderson et al., 1987). Although increases in cognitive function (as reflected in IQ scores) may be observed, this should not be understood to mean that the student will be successfully integrated among typical peers, but rather that the student may regress unless treatment is continued. During the first nine months of intervention, the majority of the 40 hours should be dedicated to remedying language delays. Later, the 40 hours may be divided between programs promoting play with peers and other social and community skills so as to help increase meaningful speech and social interaction.

7. *Individual differences.* Large individual differences exist in children's responses to treatment. Under optimal conditions, a sizable minority of children acquires vocal imitation and can be taught to talk with additional treatment, achieving best-outcome (McEachin et al., 1993). These are children who can be labeled *auditory learners.* The remaining children *visual learners* learn to communicate using visual signs as in learning to read and write. Visual learners are not likely to reach normal functioning with behavioral treatment at this time but to require some form of support for the rest of their lives but are better able to benefit from less restrictive educational placements. Programs designed to facilitate communication for visual learners appear promising but are in need of further research and outcome data (Watthen-Lovaas and Lovaas, 1999).

8. *Quality control.* Given the visibility of the UCLA data, it is important to specify as many dimensions of the treatment as possible to facilitate replication. This becomes particularly important because almost anyone can falsely present oneself as qualified to deliver such treatment by, for example, having attended a short seminar and/or read the teaching manual Teaching individuals with developmental delays: Basic intervention techniques (Lovaas, 2003) or the ME Book (Lovaas, 1981) or through training as a one-to-one therapist but without training in designing comprehensive intervention curricula, in supervising treatment and in cooperating with parents. Given the complexity in teaching complex behaviors such as vocal language, time constructs, such as before and after, cause–effect relationships and social skills, the therapist or implementer, should be required to complete a nine-month full-time internship under the supervision of an experienced mentor at a site that is treating children with autism according to the UCLA treatment model.

REPLICATION AND FUTURE STEPS

The UCLA Young Autism Project would be of limited value if not replicated by independent investigators. Of concern was devising a way in which to quantify and replicate the quality of the initial study. To attempt to control for differences in the quality of services, each of the replicating directors completed a nine-month full time internship at the UCLA Young Autism Project or affiliated clinics. One replication project by Sallows and Graupner at the Wisconsin Early Autism Project in Madison, Wisconsin has been accepted for publication in the American Journal of Mental Retardation. Two other projects are currently pursuing publication; these are the Central Valley Autism Project, Modesto, California by M. A. Dickens, H. Cohen and T. Smith, and the Akershus College Project in Oslo, Norway by Eikeseth.

Outcome data from investigators not associated with the UCLA Young Autism Project have reported major improvements in children's cognitive growth following early and intensive behavioral intervention with treatment programs similar to those employed by the UCLA Young Autism Project (Fenske, Zalenski, Krantz, McClanahan, 1985; Harris, Handleman, Gordon, Kristoff, & Fuentes, 1991). Although these projects support replicability, long-term follow-up studies are needed, including data on the children's emotional and social post-treatment adjustment.

Much of the future focus for intervention will be placed on assisting children who fail to acquire vocal language. Preliminary evidence suggests this subgroup may make progress when presented with visual stimuli as in PECS (Frost and Bondy, 1994; Bondy and Frost, 2003) and in the Reading and Writing Program (Watthen-Lovaas and Lovaas, 1999). Observations from clinical practice suggest the facilitative progress in reading and writing skills on the acquisition of vocal language. The extent of such transfer merits further research.

Cost Effectiveness. Autism is the third most common childhood disorder after cerebral palsy and mental retardation, and occurs at a higher rate than childhood cancer, cystic fibrosis, and Down syndrome. Autism has been estimated to cost the United States in excess of $10 billion per year. Intensive early behavioral intervention is estimated at $5,000 per month (slightly over $30 per hour), or $60,000 per year per child. The average length of the intensive part of treatment for the 47% of children (Lovaas, 1987) who reached best-outcome (i.e., normal functioning) was 2 years, resulting in a total expense of $120,000 per child. Such persons will in all likelihood be employed and pay taxes, returning to society whatever expense they may have incurred. The estimated average cost per individual who needs lifelong protective and institutional care is at a minimum $40,000 per year or $2.4 million for the 60 or more years that such services will be rendered. Publication of the long-term follow-up in adulthood of clients from the Lovaas' 1987 study is projected for publication in 2006. The savings accrued from intensive behavioral treatment for those who do not achieve best-outcome yet benefit from less restrictive placements and an improved quality of life are also substantial (Jacobson, Mulick, & Green 1996).

CONCERNS ABOUT SHIFTS IN REINFORCEMENT CONTROL

Over the last 50 years behavioral psychologists have contributed significant data-based treatment helping optimize treatment outcome across several fields of psychopathology. As a result applied behavior analysis is today considered to provide the treatment of choice in many fields involving children diagnosed with autism. Consequently, there has been an increasing demand for such services, especially from parents of children with autism. As illustrated in this chapter, the success of behavioral treatment is based on the contributions of many investigators working together in a cumulative manner, reporting data helpful in optimizing treatment outcome.

The majority of the research activities in the past were facilitated and reinforced by universities who hired and promoted psychologists contingent on their scientific, data-based contributions to effective treatments. Anyone up for evaluation to tenure being promoted from assistant to full professor will remember the stress of such a peer review. Without data-based contributions the candidate was faced with dismissal and unemployment. As favorable treatment outcome became published and known to the public, the demand for persons providing behavioral treatment increased, a demand the universities could no longer meet. Over time funding shifted from universities to practitioners in the community who responded to parents' need for services. Funding for treatment was in many or most cases accompanied by an increase in clients and a decrease in peer-reviewed treatment outcome. Today, the majority of practitioners does not document their outcome data in peer-reviewed journals and to the best of my knowledge may be drifting off criterion given the shift in reinforcement control from peer-review to financial gain.

Resources

- http://www.autism-society.org (Autism Society of America)
- http://www.cdc.gov/ncbddd/autism/ (Centers for Disease Control)
- http://www.ddhealthinfo.org/ (California Department of Developmental Services)
- http://www.health.state.ny.us/nysdoh/eip/menu.htm (NY State Clinical Guidelines)
- http://www.surgeongeneral. gov/library/mentalhealth/chapter3/sec6.html# autism(US Surgeon General report on autism).
- http://www.abainternational.org/ (International Association for Behavior Analysis)
- http://www.behavior.org/ (Cambridge Center for Behavioral Studies)
- http://www.feat.org/ (Families for Effective Autism Treatment)
- http://www.lovaas.com (Official Lovaas Institute for Early Intervention website)

REFERENCES

American Psychiatric Association (2000). *Diagnostic and statistical manual of mental disorders—Text revised.* (4th ed.). Washington, DC: American Psychiatric Association.

Anderson, S. R., Avery, D. L., DiPietro, E. K., Edwards, G. L., & Christian, W. P. (1987). Intensive home-based early intervention with autistic children. *Education and Treatment of Children, 10,* 352–366.

Ayllon, T. & Azrin, N. (1968). Reinforcer sampling: A technique for increasing the behavior of mental patients. *Journal of Applied Behavior Analysis, 1,* 13–20.

Baer, D. M. (1993). Quasi-random assignment can be as convincing as random assignment. *American Journal on Mental Retardation, 97,* 373–375.

Baer, D. M., Guess, D., & Sherman, J. (1972). Adventures in Simplistic Grammar. In R. L. Schiefelbusch (Ed.) *Language of the mentally retarded.* Baltimore, MD: University Park.

Baer D. M. & Sherman, J. A. (1964). Reinforcement control of generalized imitation in young children. *Journal of Experimental Child Psychology, 1,* 37–49.

Baird, G., Charman, T., Baron-Cohen, S., Coz, A., Swettenham, J., Wheelwright, S., & Drew, A. (2000). A screening instrument for autism at 18 months of age: A 6-year follow-up study. *Journal of the American Academy of Child & Adolescent Psychiatry, 39,* 694–702.

Bartak, L. (1978). Educational approaches. In M. Rutter & E. Schopler (Eds.) Austin: A Reappraisal of Concepts and Treatment, New York, Plenum. (pp. 423–438).

Bettleheim, B. (1967). *The empty fortress: Infantile autism and the birth of the self.* New York: MacMillian Publishing Co.

Bijou, S. (1966). A functional analysis of retarded development. International Review of Research in Mental Retardation. *1,* 1–19.

Birnbrauer, J., Wolf, M. M., Kidder, J. M., & Tague, C. (1965). Classroom behavior of retarded pupils with token reinforcement. *Journal of Exceptional Child Psychology, 2:* 219–235.

Bondy, A., & Frost, L. (2003). Communication strategies for visual learners. In O. I. Lovaas (Ed.) *Individuals with developmental delays: Basic intervention techniques* (pp. 291–304). Austin, TX: PRO-ED, Inc.

California Department of Developmental Services (2002). *Autistic spectrum disorders: Best practice guidelines for screening, diagnosis, and assessment.* [On-line]. Available: www.ddhealthinfo. org.

Carr, E. G., Newsom, C. D., & Binkoff, J. A. (1976). Stimulus control of self-destructive behavior in a psychotic child. *Journal of Abnormal Child Psychology, 3,* 331–51.

Centers for Disease Control (2004). *How common is Autism Spectrum Disorder?* [On-line]. Available: http://www.cdc.gov/ncbddd/autism/asd common.htm.

Dawson, G., & Osterling, J. (1997). Early intervention in autism. In M. Guralnick (Ed.), The Effectiveness of early intervention (pp. 307–326). Baltimore, MD: Paul H. Brookes Pub. Co.

DeMyer, M., Hingtgen, J., & Jackson, R. (1981). Infantile autism reviewed: A decade of research. *Schizophrenia Bulletin, 7,* 388–451.

Epstein, L., Taubman, M., & Lovaas, O. I. (1985). Changes in self-stimulatory behaviors with treatment. *Journal of Abnormal Child Psychology, 13,* 281–94.

Favell, J., McGimsey, J., & Schell, R. (1982). Treatment of self-injury by providing alternative sensory activities. *Analysis and Intervention in Developmental Disabilities, 2,* 83–104.

Fenske, E., Zalenski, S., Krantz, P., & McClanahan, L. (1985). Age at intervention and treatment outcome for autistic children in a comprehensive intervention program. *Analysis and Intervention in Developmental Disabilities, 5,* 49–58.

Frost L., & Bondy, A. (1994). *The picture exchange communication system training manual.* Cherry Hill, NJ: PECS.

Goldiamond, I. (1965). Stuttering and fluency as manipulatable operant response classes. In L. Krasner & L. P. Ullman (Eds.) *Research in behavior modification,* New York: Holt, Rimehart, and Winston.

Harris, S. L., Handleman, J. S., Gordon, R., Kristoff, B., & Fuentes, F. (1991). Changes in cognitive and language functioning of preschool children with autism. *Journal of Autism and Developmental Disabilities, 21,* 281–290.

Jackobsen, J., Mulick, J., & Green G. (1998). Cost-benefit estimates for early intensive behavioral intervention for young children with autism: General model and single state case. *Behavioral Interventions, 13,* 201–226.

Johnson, J. M. (1988). Strategic and tactical limits of comparison studies. *The Behavior Analyst, 11,* 1–9.

Kanner, L. (1943). Autistic disturbances of affective contact. *The Nervous Child, 2,* 217–250.

Koegel, R. L. & Koegel, L. K. (1988). Generalized responsivity and pivotal behaviors. In R. H. Horner, G. Dunlap, & R. L. Koegel (Eds.), *Generalization and maintenance: Life-style changes in applied settings* (pp. 41–65). Baltimore: Brooks.

Koegel, R. L., Rincover, A. & Egel, A. L. (1982). Educating and understanding autistic children. San Diego, CA, College-Hill Press.

Kuhn, T. S. (1996). *The structure of scientific revolutions* (3rd ed.). Chicago & London: University of Chicago Press.

Kravitz, H. & Boehm, J. (1971). Rhythmic habit patterns in infancy: Their sequence, age of onset, and frequency. *Child Development, 42,* 399–413.

Lord, C. (1995). Follow-up of two-year-olds referred for possible autism. *Journal of Child Psychology and Psychiatry, 36,* 1365–1382.

Lord, C., Rutter, M. & LeCouteur, A. (1994). Autism diagnostic interview-revised: A revised version of a diagnostic interview for caregivers of individuals with pervasive developmental disorder. *Journal of Autism and Developmental Disorders, 24,* 659–685.

Lord, C., Risi, S., Lambrecht, L., Cook, E., Leventhal, B., DiLavore, P., et al. (2000). The Autism Diagnostic Observation Schedule—Generic: A standard measure of social and communication deficits associated with the spectrum of autism. *Journal of Autism and Developmental Disorders, 30,* 205–223.

Lovaas, O. I. (1971). Certain comparisons between psychodynamic and behavioristic approaches to treatment. *Psychotherapy: Theory, Research and Practice, 8,* 175–178.

Lovaas, O. I. (1981) (with Ackerman, A. B., Alexander, D., Firestone, P., Perkins, J., & Young, D.) (1981). *Teaching developmentally disabled children: The ME book.* Austin, TX: PRO-ED.

Lovaas, O. I. (1987). Behavioral treatment and normal educational and intellectual functioning in young autistic children. *Journal of Consulting and Clinical Psychology, 55,* 3–9.

Lovaas, O. I. (2003). *Teaching individuals with developmental delays: Basic intervention techniques.* Austin TX: PRO-ED, Inc.

Lovaas, O., Berberich, J., Perloff, B., & Schaeffer, B. (1966). Acquisition of imitative speech by schizophrenic children. *Science, 151,* 705–707.

Lovaas, O. I., Freitas, L., Nelson, K., & Whalen, C. (1967). The establishment of imitation and its use for the development of complex behavior in schizophrenic children. *Behavior Research and Therapy, 5,* 171–181.

Lovaas, O. I., Koegel, R. L., & Schreibman, L. (1979). Stimulus overselectivity in autism: A review of research. *Psychological Bulletin, 86,* 1236–1254.

Lovaas, O. I., Koegel, R. L., Simmons, J. Q., & Long, J. S. (1973). Some generalization and follow-up measures on autistic children in behavior therapy. *Journal of Applied Behavior Analysis, 6,* 131–165.

Lovaas, O. I., Newsom, C., & Hickman, C. (1987). Self-stimulatory behavior and perceptual reinforcement. Journal of Applied Behavior Analysis, 20, 45–68.

Lovaas, O. I. & Simmons, J. (1969). Manipulation of self-destruction in three retarded children. *Journal of Applied Behavior Analysis, 2,* 143–157.

Lovaas, O. I. & Smith, T. (1988). Intensive behavioral treatment with young autistic children. In B. B. Lahey, & A. E. Kazdin (Eds.) *Advances in Clinical Child Psychology, 11,* 285–324.

Matson, J., & Taras, M. (1989). A 20-year review of punishment and alternative methods to treat problem behaviors in developmentally delayed persons. *Research in Developmental Disabilities, 10,* 85–104.

McEachin, J., Smith, T., & Lovaas, O. I. (1993). Long-term outcome for children with autism who received early intensive behavioral treatment. *American Journal on Mental Retardation, 97,* 359–372.

National Research Council (2001) Educating children with autism. Committee on Educational Interventions for Children with Autism. In C. Lord, & J. P. McGee (Eds.), Division of Behavioral and Social Sciences and Education. Washington, DC: National Academy Press.

Rimland, B. (1964). Infantile autism. New York: Appleton-Century-Crofts.

Rincover, A., & Newsom, C. (1985). The relative motivational properties of sensory and edible reinforcers in teaching autistic children. *Journal of Applied Behavior Analysis 18,* 237–248.

Risley, T. (1968). The effects and side effects of punishing the autistic behaviors of a deviant child. *Journal of Applied Behavior Analysis, 1,* 21–34.

Risley, T. Reynolds, N. & Hart, B. (1970). Behavior modification with disadvantaged preschool children. In R. H. Bradfield (Ed.), Behavior modification: The human effort. San Rafael, CA: Dimensions.

Rutter, M. (1978). Diagnosis and definition. In M. Rutter, & E. Schopler (Eds.), *Autism: A reappraisal of concepts and treatment.* New York: Plenum Press.

Rutter, M. (1985). The treatment of autistic children. *Journal of Child Psychology & Psychiatry, 26,* 193–121.

Sackett, G. P. (1966). Monkeys reared in isolation with pictures as visual input: Evidence of an innate releasing mechanism. *Science, 154,* 1470–1473.

Schreibman, L. (1988). *Autism.* Beverly Hills, CA: Sage.

Sherman, J. (1964). Modification of nonverbal behavior through reinforcement of related verbal behavior. *Child Development, 35,* 717–723.

Simeonnson R. J., Olley, G., & Rosenthal, S. L. (1987). Early intervention for children with autism. In M. J. Guralnick & F. C. Bennett (Eds.), The effectiveness of early intervention for at-risk and handicapped children (pp. 275–296). Orlando, FL: Academic Press.

Skinner, B. F. (1957). *Verbal behavior.* New York: Appleton-Century-Crofts.

Smith, T. (1993). Autism. In T. Giles (Ed.), Effective psychotherapies. New York: Plenum.

Smith, T. (1996). Are other treatments effective? In C. Maurice (Ed.), *Behavioral treatment of autistic children.* Austin, TX: PRO-ED.

Smith, T., Watthen-Lovaas, N. & O. I. Lovaas (2002). Behaviors of children with high-functioning autism when paired with typically developing versus delayed peers: A preliminary study, *Behavioral Interventions, 17,* 129–143.

Strain, P. S. (1983). Generalization of autistic children's social behavior change: Effects of developmentally integrated an d segregated settings. *Analysis and Intervention in Developmental Disabilities, 3,* 23–34.

Thelen, E. (1979). Rhythmical stereotypes in normal human infants. *Animal Behaviour, 27,* 699–715.

Torrey, E. (1992). *Freudian fraud: The malignant effect of Freud's theory on American thought and culture.* New York, NY, US: Harper Collins Publishers.

Watthen-Lovaas, N., & Lovaas, E. (1999). *The reading & writing program: An alternative form of communication.* Austin, TX: PRO-ED, Inc.

Wahler, R. G. (1969). Oppositional children: A quest for parental reinforcement control. *Journal of Applied Behavior Analysis, 2,* 159.

Wolf, M. M., Risley, T., & Mees, H. (1964). Application of operant conditioning procedures to the behavior problems of an autistic child. *Behaviour Research and Therapy, 1,* 305–312.

Avoidant Personality Disorder

Lynn E. Alden • Judith M. Laposa • Charles T. Taylor

WHAT IS AVOIDANT PERSONALITY DISORDER?

Avoidant Personality Disorder (APD) is defined in the American Psychiatric Association Diagnostic and Statistical Manual (4th edition) as a "pervasive pattern of social inhibition, feelings of inadequacy, and hypersensitivity to negative evaluation" in which the person displays at least four of the following characteristics.

1. Avoids occupational activities that involve significant interpersonal contact because of fears of criticism, disapproval or rejection.
2. Unwilling to get socially involved unless certain of being liked.
3. Restrained in intimate relationships because of fear of being shamed or ridiculed.
4. Preoccupied with being criticized or rejected in social situations.
5. Inhibited in novel social situations because of feelings of inadequacy.
6. Views self as inept, unappealing or inferior to others.
7. Unusually reluctant to take personal risks or engage in new activities because they may prove embarrassing. (APA, 1994, p. 664).

The concept of the avoidant personality arose from Millon's (1969) theoretical depictions of people who habitually use social withdrawal and avoidance as a coping strategy to manage their hypersensitivity to rejection and shame. Millon was particularly interested in distinguishing the avoidant pattern from the schizoid personality for whom social withdrawal stemmed from indifference and apathy. APD was first included in the DSM system in 1980 as part of a larger effort to refine the diagnosis of personality disorders.

APD is estimated to occur in approximately 1% of the general population and in up to 25% of patients seeking treatment from mental health settings (Stuart et al., 1998). It occurs equally in men and women. APD causes significant life impairment, in particular, social isolation, failure to marry, and constricted school and work-related activities. APD has been shown to precede and increase the risk of developing depression as well as a variety of anxiety disorders.

PSYCHOBIOLOGICAL MODELS OF APD

Contemporary writers agree that APD arises from an interaction of innate biological vulnerabilities and adverse social developmental experiences, however, various writers focus on different features as the core of this disorder. Biological writers focus on the neurochemical processes associated with APD. Here, research shows that dopamine hypoactivity has been associated with trait detachment, social phobia, and incentive and reward function deficits, all of which are features of APD (Schneier, Blanco, Anita, & Liebowitz, 2002). Moreover, genetic research shows that certain features of dopamine receptors are associated with APD symptoms (Joyce et al., 2003). However, genetic research on APD is sparse, and twin studies and research examining neurophysiological correlates is lacking. More research is needed to identify biological contributors specific to APD.

Alden, L. E., Laposa, J. M., & Taylor, C. T., In J. E. Fisher & W. T. O'Donohue (Eds.), *Practitioner's guide to evidence-based psychotherapy*. New York: Springer.

Several psychological theories have also been developed. Beck and Freeman (1990), in their cognitive model, emphasize the role of cognitive beliefs, or schema, in the onset and maintenance of APD. According to those writers, the innate autonomic hypersensitivity found in people with APD is accompanied by the basic belief, "I may get hurt." Negative social experiences confirm that belief and lead to other fundamental beliefs about the self ("I am different, unlikable, defective") and others ("Others are critical, will reject me"). Those beliefs, in turn, produce negatively biased predictions and interpretations of social events, resulting in the use of dysfunctional behaviors to handle social situations, most notably, withdrawal and avoidance. In addition to social beliefs, Beck and Freeman proposed that people with APD hold dysfunctional beliefs about emotions ("I can't tolerate negative feelings") and as a result, seek to avoid negative internal experiences, such as feelings and cognitions. Thus, avoidance is triggered by internal as well as external cues. Few studies have examined the cognitive model, but those that have generally support the idea that people with APD hold a pattern of negative beliefs that distinguish them from some other personality disorders (e.g., Borderline Personality Disorder).

Widiger (2001) developed another prominent contemporary model of APD, which draws on the Five Factor Model (FFM) of personality. According to Widiger, APD is best viewed as a pathological extension of the general personality traits of neuroticism and introversion. In particular, people with APD are high on the neurotic facets of anxiety, vulnerability, and self-consciousness and low on the facets of gregariousness, assertiveness, activity, and excitement-seeking. Considerable research supports Widiger's view of APD as a combination of neuroticism and introversion. Moreover, twin studies reveal that both traits have heritability estimates of approximately 50%, i.e., are half attributable to inherited factors with the remainder apparently due to negative environmental events. Little work has addressed the nature of the life events responsible for the remaining 50% of APD symptoms.

ASSESSMENT

APD is most often diagnosed in clinical and research settings with semi structured interviews. The most frequently used interview is the Structured Clinical Interview for DSM-IV Personality Disorders (SCID II; First, Gibbon, Spitzer, Williams, & Benjamin, 1997). The interviewer rates each of the seven APD items on a scale of 1–3, where 3 = meets criteria for that item. The SCID-II has been shown to be a valid and reliable measure of personality disorders (e.g., Zanarini et al., 2000). Another popular interview measure is the Personality Disorders Examination (PDE, Loranger, 1988), which has been shown to have good interrater reliability. Researchers have also used interviews such as the Structured Interview for DSM-IV Personality (SIDP-R; Pfohl, Blum, & Zimmerman, 1995), the Personality Disorder Interview-IV (PDI-IV; Widiger, Mangine, Corbitt, Ellis, & Thomas 1995), the Diagnostic Interview for Personality Disorders (DIPD; Zanarini, Frankenburg, Chauncey, & Gunderson, 1987), or have simply asked about the seven DSM-IV criteria.

Several self-report measures also exist for assessing avoidant personality disorder and APD traits. The Millon Clinical Multiaxial Inventory III (MCMI III; Millon, 1994) and Personality Diagnostic Questionnaire for DSM-IV (PDQ-4; Hyler, 1994) are frequently used. These measures are typically found to have adequate reliability and internal consistency. Additional self-report measures include the Coolidge Axis II Inventory (CATI; Coolidge, 1993), or simply presenting the seven DSM-IV APD criteria in the form of questions. It is important to note that there is poor agreement between self-report and interview measures of personality disorders. Moreover, self-report measures often over-diagnose personality disorders, both in patient and nonpatient populations. For example, Hyler, Skodol, Kellman, Oldham, and Rosnick (1990) found that the PDQ-R self-report measure gave a prevalence rate of 24% for APD, whereas the PDE and SCID II interviews gave prevalence rates of 1%. On the whole, interviews work best for diagnosing APD.

DIAGNOSIS

APD, consisting as it does of an exaggeration of normal personality traits, suffers from high rates of overlap with other personality disorders. The most difficult Axis 11 diagnostic decision arises in distinguishing APD from Dependent Personality Disorder (DPD). Only the symptom of social withdrawal reliably discriminates the two conditions; the avoidant person has difficulty initiating social relationships, whereas the dependent person does not. That distinction notwithstanding, one study indicates that 43% of APD patients meet criteria for DPD and 59% of DPD patients meet criteria for APD. Although it may seem counterintuitive that patients could be avoiding other people at the same time as they are clinging to them, it may be that people with APD avoid most people but become overly dependent on the few people they trust.

In terms of Axis I conditions, APD shares many common features with Generalized Social Phobia (GSP). Considerable research has been conducted to determine whether the two constructs are in any way distinguishable. Although some studies indicated that people with APD received more comorbid diagnoses, displayed greater physiological arousal, or lacked social skills, other studies failed to replicate those findings (see Alden, Laposa, Taylor, & Ryder, 2002, for a review). Social phobia researchers tend to view APD as a more severe variant of GSP, a position that is reflected in the DSM-IV. In contrast, other researchers argue that the conceptual overlap between the two conditions is an artifact of the populations in which APD has been studied and misguided changes in the DSM system that increased the similarity in the diagnostic criteria of the two conditions (e.g., Arntz, 1999). Most work on APD has been conducted in samples of patients participating in treatment outcome studies for social phobia, which may increase the apparent overlap between the two disorders. Arntz (1999) began with a broad sample of outpatients that included many without social phobia, and found a 51% overlap, in contrast to the 88% or greater overlap found in social phobic populations. Nonetheless, it is clear that with the current DSM criteria, many APD patients will meet criteria for GSP and vice versa.

When conducting diagnostic assessments of APD, it is important to pay attention to the presence of depression. Approximately 40% of patients with APD also meet criteria for one of the mood disorders, and comorbid depression is believed to impede treatment response. Conversely, APD is one of the most frequent personality disorders associated with Major Depressive Disorder (MDD) and Dysthymic Disorder (DD). Comorbid APD was found in 12–28% of patients with MDD and between 12% and 32% of patients diagnosed with DD. Some work found that APD predicted greater social impairment and earlier onset of depressive episodes in depressed patients. Moreover, APD was found to predict the development of new cases of MDD in psychiatric outpatients followed over a six-year period. Finally, the presence of APD predicted poorer treatment response in a medication trial for patients with MDD (Papakostas et al., 2003). Thus, the combination of APD and depression has significant clinical implications.

TREATMENT

Most studies to address the effectiveness of psychosocial interventions examined the effect of APD on treatment outcome in patients with generalized social phobia (GSP). The majority of those studies evaluated various cognitive-behavioral treatment (CBT) regimens. Most studies found that GSP patients who obtain an APD diagnosis begin and end CBT more severely impaired than patients without APD but exhibit equivalent rates of change, which indicates that treatment strategies developed for GSP are useful for APD as well (e.g., Chambless, Tran & Glass, 1997). Notably, some work indicated that comorbid depression impeded treatment improvement.

A few studies have examined treatment effectiveness in patients directly selected on APD criteria. In terms of psychosocial regimens, both cognitive-behavioral regimens (CBT) and interpersonal psychotherapy (IPT) have been studied. To summarize those findings, patients with APD made significant gains in all treatment programs, and the improvements were maintained up to one year after termination (e.g., see Alden et al., 2002, for a review). However, a substantial number of patients completed treatment at the lower end or below the normative range for social avoidance. Those findings suggest that APD may require treatment of longer duration or the inclusion of additional elements to completely overcome the disorder. Several studies addressed differential treatment response and concluded that CBT was superior to IPT, both in APD and in MDD samples (e.g., Barber, Morse, Krakauer, Chittams & Critis-Christoph, 1997).

The central element of CBT for APD is graduated exposure to feared situations. Although some writers argue that social skills training augments the effects of exposure alone, empirical studies generally reveal no differences between exposure with and without skills training. In a similar vein, although the Beck and Freeman cognitive model of APD is influential, research has yet to demonstrate that cognitive techniques enhance treatment outcome beyond exposure. Thus, encouraging patients to repeatedly enter and remain in social situations is critical to reducing social anxiety and avoidance.

There have been few pharmacotherapy trials involving patients with APD. As with psychological outcome studies, research evaluating the effectiveness of pharmacological interventions for APD has been conducted primarily in the context of patients seeking treatment for social phobia. To summarize, avoidant personality features have been found to significantly decrease in GSP patients following treatment with the benzodiazepine alprazolam, the SRI venlafaxine, and a variety of MAOIs (see Alden et al., 2002, for a review). Additionally, one study found significant improvements in depressive symptomatology following SRI treatment. Some evidence suggests that patients with social phobia (without APD) demonstrate better overall improvement than those with APD, and that APD patients exhibit a slower treatment response. Finally, clinical researchers tend to agree that the SRIs may be the first-line pharmacological treatments of choice given that they are safer and better tolerated than alternative medications and that medications with less desirable side-effect profiles such as the MAOIs, should be reserved for treatment resistant patients (e.g., Blanco et al., 2003).

FUTURE RESEARCH

The literature reveals a number of fruitful lines for future research. One topic is the overlap between APD and Generalized Social Phobia. Various researchers have suggested different solutions. One proposal is that the diagnosis of social phobia should take precedence over APD, because this would encourage clinicians to use the pharmaceutical and psychological treatment strategies shown to be effective for APD in populations with social phobia (Liebowitz et al., 1998). Heimberg (1996) suggested that APD and social phobia be combined into Social Anxiety Disorder with APD treated as a more severe variant of this condition. The advantages of that approach are that it recognizes that social anxiety and avoidance fall along a continuum of severity and that APD and social phobia share many features. Widiger (2001) proposed that the Five Factor Model should be used in place of the current categorical system of personality disorders. In this scenario, APD would be measured in terms of ratings on the dimensions of neuroticism and introversion. Then, researchers could study the links between personality vulnerabilities and Axis I conditions, addressing such questions as why one person high on neuroticism and introversion would develop social phobia where another person with similar personality traits would develop depression. Finally, Arntz (1999) argued that definitions of APD should be re-written to return to the original concept of a broad-based pattern of avoidance, which that would include emotional and cognitive avoidance, as well as social avoidance. Which of these suggestions provides the best resolution for the DSM-V requires study.

A second topic for future work is to assess whether people with APD do indeed display the emotional, cognitive, and novelty avoidance suggested by Beck and Freeman (1990) and Arntz (1999). Preliminary research suggests that this is the case. A recent study in our lab indicated that, both in university and clinical samples, people with APD reported avoiding a wide range of emotions, including positive emotions (Taylor, Laposa, & Alden, 2004). They also displayed a preference for familiar routines and an avoidance of novel situations. Further investigation is necessary, however, before incorporating those features into diagnostic criteria for APD.

A third research area pertains to psychosocial contributors to APD. Although researchers have begun to identify the biological factors that increase vulnerability to APD, most writers believe that negative life events act in conjunction with that vulnerability to produce the full-blown condition. One study found that childhood abuse, as documented in legal records, significantly increased the risk of developing APD, and two other studies found that adults with APD reported negative childhood experiences. Work is needed to replicate and extend those findings.

Several key questions also remain regarding pharmacotherapy for APD. Some research revealed that GSP patients tended to relapse following medication discontinuation. Researchers have yet to determine whether people with a diagnosis of APD are at a greater risk of relapse, and if so to identify those factors that contribute to relapse. Additionally, no published studies on APD have examined whether a combined regimen of medication and psychological interventions enhances treatment response over each therapy alone. One possibility that requires study is that combination therapies might reduce the high dropout and relapse rates typically found in pharmacological outcome trials with avoidant patients. Research is also necessary to determine what factors predict treatment nonresponsiveness in patients with APD. For example, studies demonstrating the high occurrence of depression and other comorbid diagnoses in patients with APD highlight the possibility that pharmacological interventions that target multiple neurotransmitter systems (e.g., serotonin, dopamine, and norepinephrine) may have enhanced utility over single modality medications.

Finally, research is needed to develop new psychological treatment options for APD. Even studies of APD in carefully selected social phobic populations find that patients with APD begin and end treatment more severely impaired than those without the disorder, which suggests there is room for improvement in current treatment regimens. Beck and Freeman (1990) suggested that treatment for APD should involve techniques to overcome emotional and cognitive avoidance. In particular, they propose that these patients should be encouraged to experiment with allowing themselves to experience negative thoughts and emotions ("dysphoria training") in order to change their beliefs about being overwhelmed by distress. In light of recent work documenting novelty avoidance among people with APD, it may also be fruitful to determine whether encouraging patients to engage in unfamiliar activities and enter novel surroundings would be beneficial.

SUMMARY

APD is a prevalent personality disorder, one that causes moderate to severe life impairment. Despite its severity, effective treatment regimens have been developed that reduce social avoidance and help these individuals increase their quality of life. Although researchers have made some strides toward understanding the condition, much remains to be done, particularly in regards to the psychosocial factors that contribute to the disorder and may be key to treating it.

REFERENCES

American Psychiatric Association (1994). *Diagnostic and statistical manual of mental disorders* (4th ed.). Washington, DC: American Psychiatric Association.

Alden, L. E., Laposa, J. M., Taylor, C. T., & Ryder, R. G. (2002). Avoidant personality disorder: Current status and future directions. *Journal of Personality Disorders, 16*, 1–29.

Arntz, A. (1999). Do personality disorders exist? On the validity of the concept and its cognitive-behavioural formulation and treatment. *Behavior Research and Therapy, 37*, 97–134.

Barber, J. P., Morse, J. Q., Krakauer, I. D., Chittams, J., & Crits-Christoph, K. (1997). Change in obsessive-compulsive and avoidant personality disorders following Time-limited Supportive-Expressive Therapy. *Psychotherapy, 34*, 133–143.

Beck, A. T., & Freeman, A. (1990). *Cognitive therapy of personality disorders*. New York: The Guilford Press.

Blanco, C., Schneier, F. R., Schmidt, A., Blanco-Jerez, C. R., Marshall, R. D., Sanchez-Lacay, A., & Liebowitz, M. R. (2003). Pharmacological treatment of social anxiety disorder: A meta-analysis. *Depression and Anxiety, 18*, 29–40.

Chambless, D. L., Tran, G. Q., & Glass, C. R. (1997). Predictors of response to cognitive behavioral group therapy for social phobia. *Journal of Anxiety Disorders, 11*, 211–240.

Coolidge, F. L. (1993). *The Coolidge Axis II Inventory: Manual*. Colorado Springs, CO: Author.

First, M. B., Gibbon, M., Spitzer, R. L., Williams, B. W., & Benjamin, L. S. (1997). *User's guide for the Structured Clinical Interview for DSM-IV Axis II Personality Disorders*. Washington, DC.: American Psychiatric Press.

Heimberg, R. G. (1996). Social phobia, avoidant personality disorder and the multi-axial conceptualization of interpersonal anxiety. In P. M. Salkovskis (Ed.), Trends in cognitive and behavioural therapies (pp. 43–61). New York: John Wiley & Sons Ltd.

Hyler, S. E. (1994). *Personality Diagnostic Questionnaire - 4*. New York: New York State Psychiatric Institute.

Hyler, S. E., Skodol, A. E., Kellman, H. D., Oldham, J., & Rosnick, L. (1990). The validity of the Personality Diagnostic Questionnaire: A comparison with two structured interviews. *American Journal of Psychiatry, 147*, 1043–1048.

Joyce, P. R., Rogers, G. R., Miller, A. L., Mulder, R. T., Luty, S. E., & Kennedy, M. A. (2003). Polymorphisms of DRD4 and DRD3 and risk of avoidant and obsessive personality traits and disorders. *Psychiatry Research, 119*, 1–10.

Liebowitz, M. R., Barlow, D. H., Ballenger, J. C., Davidson, J., Foa, E. B., Fyer, A. J., Koopman, C., Kozak, M. J. & Speigel, D. (1998). DSM-IV anxiety disorders: Final overview. In T. A. Widiger, A. J. Frances, H. A. Pincus, R. Ross, M. B. First, W. Davis, & M. Kline (Eds.), *DSM-IV sourcebook* (Vol. 4, pp. 1047–1076). Washington, DC: American Psychiatric Association.

Loranger, A. E. (1988). *Personality Disorder Examination (PDE) manual*. White Plains, NY: Author.

Millon, T. (1969). *Modern psychopathology: A biosocial approach to maladaptive learning and functioning*. Philadelphia: W. B. Saunders.

Millon, T. (1994). *Manual for the Millon Clinical Multiaxial Inventory-III (MCMI-III)*. Minneapolis: National Computer Systems.

Papakostas, G. I., Petersen, T. J., Farabaugh, A. H., Murakami, J. L., Pava, J. A., Alpert, J. E., et al., (2003). Psychiatric comorbidity as a predictor of clinical response to nortriptyline in treatment-resistant major depressive disorder. *Journal of Clinical Psychiatry, 64*, 1357–1361.

Pfohl, B., Blum, N., & Zimmerman, M. (1995). *Structured Interview for DSM-IV Personality SIDP-IV.* Iowa City: University of Iowa, Department of Psychiatry.

Schneier, F. R., Blanco, C., Anita, S. X., & Liebowitz, M. R. (2002). The social anxiety spectrum. *Psychiatric Clinics of North America, 25*, 757–774.

Stuart, S., Pfohl, B., Battaglia, M., Bellodi, L., Grove, W., & Cadoret, R. (1998). The Co-occurence of DSM-III-R personality disorders. *Journal of Personality Disorders, 14*, 291–299.

Taylor, C. T, Laposa, J. M., & Alden, L. E. (2004). Is Avoidant Personality Disorder more than just social avoidance? *Journal of Personality Disorders, 18*, 573–597.

Widiger, T. A. (2001). Social anxiety, social phobia, and avoidant personality disorder. In R. Crozier & L. E. Alden (Eds.), *International handbook of social anxiety: Concepts, research and interventions relating to the self and shyness.* (pp. 335–356). United Kingdom: John Wiley & Sons.

Widiger, T. A., Mangine, S., Corbitt, E. M., Ellis, C. G., & Thomas, G. V. (1995). *Personality disorder interview-IV: A semistructured interview for the assessment of personality disorders.* Odessa, FL: Psychological Assessment Resources.

Zanarini, M. C., Frankenburg, F. R., Chauncey, D. L., & Gunderson, J. G. (1987). The Diagnostic Interview for Personality Disorders: Interrater and test–retest reliability. *Comprehensive Psychiatry, 28*, 467–480.

Zanarini, M. C., Skodol, A. E., Bender, D., Dolan, R., Sanislow, C., Schafer, E., et al. (2000). The collaborative longitudinal personality disorders study: Reliability of Axis I and II diagnoses. *Journal of Personality Disorders, 14*, 291–299.

Bereavement

Anthony D. Mancini • George A. Bonanno

WHAT IS GRIEF?

Grief is a healthy, normative response to the highly stressful experience of losing a loved one, and can consist of disruptions in functioning in a number of areas, including: (1) *dysphoric emotions*, including sadness, anger, anxiety, irritability, fear, hostility, loneliness, and guilt, as well as pining for the lost loved one; (2) *transient cognitive disorganization*, such as confusion and preoccupation with the deceased, identity disturbances ("a piece of me is missing"), feelings of uncertainty about the future, and a compromised sense of life's underlying meaning or purpose; (3) *health problems*, such as somatic difficulties, new or worsened illnesses, and additional or increased use of medications; and (4) *impaired social and occupational functioning*, including social withdrawal, difficulties meeting work and home obligations, and difficulties initiating and maintaining new intimate relationships (Bonanno & Kaltman, 2001).

Patterns of grief reaction. It should be emphasized that, as with acute stressors generally (e.g., Lucas, Clark, Georgellis, & Diener, 2003), bereaved persons vary greatly in the degree to which they experience such difficulties in reaction to loss (Bonanno & Kaltman, 1999, 2001; Wortman & Silver, 1989, 2001). A small minority of bereaved persons suffer from acute feelings of distress that can persist for years after the loss. However, others suffer less acutely and then gradually return to their former level of functioning, while still others show short-lived reactions and a relatively rapid return to their previous levels of functioning (Bonanno & Kaltman, 2001). The range of reactions people exhibit when a loved one dies has led to considerable controversy about what might be the "normal" course of bereavement, and who might need or benefit most from a grief-focused clinical intervention (Bonanno, 2004; Mancini, Pressman, & Bonanno, 2005).

Recent research has mapped these divergent grief reactions onto three primary trajectories or patterns (Bonanno, 2004; Bonanno, et al., 2002): *chronic or complicated grief* (acute and/or persistent and disabling grief symptoms), *recovery* (acute symptoms that gradually subside), and *minimal grief or resilience* (few, if any, symptoms that quickly resolve). The great majority of bereaved persons will demonstrate either a recovery pattern or a minimal grief pattern (for a review, see Bonanno & Kaltman, 2001) and regain psychological equilibrium relatively quickly after the loss (Bonanno, 2004). Such individuals are not likely to require and may even be harmed by clinical intervention (Jordan & Neimeyer, 2003; Raphael, Minkov, & Dobson, 2001). However, a small subset of bereaved persons experience severe and protracted symptoms that can endure for years after the loss. It is increasingly recognized that persons suffering from this chronic or complicated pattern of grief should be the principal focus of clinical concern (Jordan & Neimeyer, 2003; Mancini et al., 2005; Schut, Stroebe, van den Bout, & Terheggen, 2001).

Identifying chronic grief. Although investigators have developed diagnostic criteria for what has been variously described as chronic, complicated or pathologic

Mancini, A. D., & Bonanno (2006). In J. E. Fisher & W. T. O'Donohue (Eds.), *Practitioner's guide to evidence-based psychotherapy*. New York: Springer.

grief (e.g., Horowitz et al., 1997; Kim & Jacobs, 1991; Prigerson et al., 1995), these efforts have had substantial methodological limitations, so that no clear, empirically based criteria for chronic or complicated grief are widely endorsed in the field. Indeed, the DSM-IV classifies bereavement as a "V code," or a stressor that may be a focus of clinical concern but that is not considered a diagnosis in and of itself, even in its most severe or chronic forms (American Psychiatric Association, 1994).

How, then, should clinicians identify persons suffering from chronic grief? An obvious but perhaps principal difference between the conventional recovery pattern and chronic grief reactions is the duration of symptoms and their impact on functioning. However, duration of symptomatology does not appear to be the only factor to distinguish chronic reactions; severity of symptoms even in the initial months of bereavement also appears to inform such reactions. Recent research has shown, for example, that bereaved individuals who ultimately developed chronic reactions had more acute symptom levels in the early months of bereavement compared to bereaved individuals who evidenced a recovery pattern (Bonanno et al., 2002). Put another way, bereaved persons who show the recovery pattern may struggle with moderate levels of symptoms and experience difficulties carrying out their normal tasks at work or in the care of loved ones, but they somehow manage to struggle through these tasks and slowly but gradually begin to return to their preloss or baseline level of functioning, usually over a period of one or two years. By contrast, chronic grievers evidence substantial symptomatology and a reduced ability to perform well at work, to maintain relationships with friends or intimates, and to meet parenting obligations. These difficulties may persist for years after the loss, but, at a minimum, should endure for at least 1 year after bereavement to warrant the label chronic grief. One final consideration, not discussed in the DSM-IV, is that the apparent symptoms of chronic grief may, in fact, represent an unresolved depression that predated the loss, with important implications for treatment (Bonanno et al., 2002; Mancini et al., 2005). We will take up this issue of chronic grief vs. chronic depression in greater detail later in this chapter.

BASIC FACTS ABOUT BEREAVEMENT

Prevalence of types of grief reaction. Approximately 80–90% of bereaved persons will exhibit either a *recovery* or *minimal grief* pattern that will resolve on its own, while about 10–20% of persons will suffer from *chronic or complicated grief*, which, by its nature, can persist for years after the loss (Bonanno & Kaltman, 2001).

Clinical diagnosis and comorbidity. Available empirical evidence indicates that chronic or complicated grief is best understood in terms of symptoms associated with existing diagnostic categories for Generalized Anxiety Disorder, Major Depressive Disorder and, in some cases, Posttraumatic Stress Disorder (Bonanno & Kaltman, 2001). As mentioned, this typology is consistent with the DSM-IV's classification of bereavement as a "V code" (American Psychiatric Association, 1994). Some evidence also suggests that persons with chronic or complicated grief may be more likely to suffer from symptoms associated with Dependent Personality Disorder (Bonanno, et al., 2002; Bonanno, Wortman, & Nesse, 2004).

Hypothesized grief reactions. Other hypothesized grief reactions commonly invoked in the research and clinical literature on bereavement are *delayed grief* (a severe grief reaction years after loss) and *absent grief* (the pathological failure to grieve). However, these grief reactions have not been supported empirically. The relative absence of distress following the death of a loved one appears to be neither rare nor pathological; rather, as discussed, such a pattern has been observed with greater frequency than any other type of response (e.g., Bonanno, Keltner, Holen, & Horowitz, 1995; Bonanno, et al., 2002; Bonanno, Moskowitz, Papa, & Folkman, 2005). What is more, there has been no indication that these individuals are mal-adjusted or have less capacity for intimacy and social interaction (Bonanno et al., 2002; Bonanno et al., 2004, 2005). Finally, these studies have failed to uncover evidence in support of a delayed grief reaction years after loss (Bonanno & Field, 2001; Bonanno et al., 2002; Boerner, Wortman & Bonanno, 2005), even among studies where the researchers fully expected to demonstrate the phenomenon (e.g., Middleton, Burnett, Raphael, & Martinek, 1996).

Common assumptions about bereavement. One particularly widespread assumption is that active efforts are required to cope with loss, a process called "grief work" (W. Stroebe & Stroebe, 1991). Based on this perspective, traditional models for grief counseling frequently employ specific procedures to promote the bereaved person's efforts to work through the loss. For example, bereaved persons are implored to accept the reality of the loss, to review specific memories and express feelings (particularly negative ones) associated with the lost loved one, and to make active efforts to relinquish their attachment (e.g., Rando, 1993).

A related clinical assumption is that the absence of overt distress in response to bereavement is itself indicative of pathology, because it suggests that the person is inhibiting or dissociating from negative feelings (Middleton et al., 1993) or lacked a strong attachment to the deceased (Fraley & Shaver, 1999). When a person doesn't display overt distress, he or she may be presumed to be avoiding the "tasks" of grieving (Worden, 1991). Such responses to loss have often been thought to portend later and much more severe difficulties that could be avoided by engaging in "grief work" processes.

Despite widespread endorsement of the "grief work" perspective (and the concomitant pathologizing of those who fail to evince grief symptoms), startlingly little empirical evidence exists to support these assumptions about bereavement (Wortman & Silver, 1989). Indeed, there is increasing consensus among bereavement theorists that *traditional models of coping with loss are not supported by the empirical data* (Bonanno, 2001, 2004; Bonanno & Kaltman, 1999; Murphy, Johnson, & Lohan, 2003; Wortman & Silver, 1989, 2001). Of greater potential concern, there is growing evidence that not only is "grief work" incompatible with the evidence but engaging in practices that promote grief work may even exacerbate grief reactions (Bonanno & Kaltman, 1999). In our section on assessment and treatment, we discuss alternate conceptualizations of grief counseling that stand in contrast to traditional assumptions regarding the necessity for working through grief.

Age. Bereavement is generally associated with less severe grief reactions in old age (Lichtenstein, Gatz, Pedersen, Berg, & McClearn, 1996; Nolen-Hoeksma & Ahrens, 2002).

Gender. Men generally experience higher levels of distress, have more health problems, and have greater risk for mortality than women following spousal bereavement (Stroebe, Stroebe, & Schut, 2001), while mothers who lose children are at greater risk for developing chronic or complicated grief (Stroebe & Schut, 2001).

ASSESSMENT

What Should be Ruled Out?

Bereaved persons who exhibit symptoms of apparent chronic grief may instead be experiencing a chronic depression that existed before the loss (Bonanno, et al., 2002). And because the etiology of chronic depression and chronic grief are so divergent, interventions for each symptom pattern would address very different clinical issues, making it essential to distinguish chronic grief from chronic depression among bereaved persons before deciding on a course of treatment. Fortunately, a number of characteristics appear to distinguish chronic grievers from persons with chronic depression. For example, persons with chronic depression, when compared to chronic grievers, have been found to have greater perceived deficits in coping efficacy, more difficulty managing troubling feelings, and less positive affect (Bonanno, et al., 2004). In addition, those suffering from chronic depression experience, by definition, higher levels of preloss distress than chronic grievers. On the other hand, chronic grief, when compared to chronic depression, has been associated with more active efforts to understand the loss, including higher levels of processing and searching for meaning during the first six-months of bereavement (Bonanno et al., 2004).

What is Involved in Effective Assessment?

Thorough assessment of bereaved persons should include examination of the following areas:

Characteristics of loss	Clinical history	Current functioning	Personality variables
• Type of loss[*] • Nature of relationship to deceased • Degree of suddenness[*] • Traumatic aspects[*]	• Preloss functioning, esp. depressive symptoms[*] • Psychiatric or trauma history[*] • Past bereavements[*]	• Symptomatology (depression, anxiety, posttraumatic stress) • Social or occupational impairments • Level of preoccupation with loss • Support network	• Coping style (internalizing vs. externalizing) • Perceived coping deficits[*] • Dependency on deceased[*]

[*]Indicates potential risk factor for chronic or complicated grief.

Clinicians should also bear in mind risk factors, asterisked in the above chart, that may predispose bereaved persons to more adverse outcomes (Jordan & Neimeyer, 2003; Stroebe & Schut, 2001). Among the categorical risk factors are spousal loss for men, the loss of a child for mothers, and unexpected and/or traumatic loss for either gender. Other risk factors include preexisting psychopathology, trauma history, early or multiple losses, perceived coping deficits, and high levels of dependency on the lost loved one.

TREATMENT

What Treatments are Effective?

It should first be noted that *existing clinical interventions for bereavement have proven to be generally inefficacious* (Allumbaugh & Hoyt, 1999; Kato & Mann, 1999; Neimeyer, 2000). For example, two recent meta-analytic studies compared randomly assigned grief treatment and control groups. In contrast to the generally robust effect sizes typically observed for psychotherapeutic outcomes, grief-specific therapies in a range of formats produce only small and relatively inconsequential effects (Allumbaugh & Hoyt, 1999; Kato & Mann, 1999; Neimeyer, 2000). Importantly, in one of these analyses, an alarming 38% of the individuals receiving grief treatments grew worse relative to no-treatment controls (Neimeyer, 2000). As seems to be the case with psychotherapy generally, bereaved persons who self-selected grief therapy benefited more from the intervention than bereaved participants recruited by investigators (Allumbaugh & Hoyt, 1999). And the clearest benefits were evidenced with bereaved individuals experiencing chronic grief reactions, although the effect size in this case was still smaller than is normally observed for psychotherapy outcome (Neimeyer, 2000).

Why have grief therapies been so ineffective in controlled studies? One explanation is that the apparent symptoms of chronic grief may reflect a depressive disorder and other difficulties that preexisted the loss (Bonanno, et al., 2002). Indeed, because interventions in controlled studies usually occur at relatively late stages of grief (more than 2 years postloss, on average; Allumbaugh & Hoyt, 1999), it is likely that a sizable proportion of the participants identified as having chronic grief were in fact suffering from chronic depression. (One recent prospective study of spousal loss found that about 1/3 of the bereaved persons with a chronic symptom profile following loss had chronic depression; Bonanno, et al., 2002). It seems likely, and evidence strongly suggests, that a grief-focused intervention would prove particularly ineffective for persons whose chronic symptoms are less a function of grief than preexisting psychopathology (Bonanno et al., 2002; Bonanno et al., 2004; Mancini et al., 2005). Another and perhaps even more compelling explanation for the lack of efficacy found for grief therapies is the over-inclusion of bereaved individuals who have moderate or minimal symptoms and thus have no need for treatment (Bonanno, 2004; Jordan & Neimeyer, 2003). Because of the smaller scope for improvement for this group, the inclusion of persons with moderate or minimal symptomatology in efficacy studies of bereavement interventions would almost certainly diminish the overall effect size.

Because traditional grief counseling models, using both individual and group formats, have failed to generate convincing empirical support, investigators have increasingly emphasized treatment approaches that are responsive to individual differences in mourners, that selectively engage issues around grief, and that are consistent with broad principles of sound clinical practice (Jordan & Neimeyer, 200; Neimeyer, 2000; Zisook & Schuchter, 2001). Indeed, investigators have suggested that grief counseling should be derived from the broader literature on psychotherapy outcome, in which nonspecific, relational, and contextual aspects are widely regarded as the active ingredients in psychotherapy (Jordan & Neimeyer, 2003). However, as we discuss below, some provisional recommendations specific to the treatment of grief can be gleaned from recent research findings, although it should be borne in mind that these recommendations have not been directly tested in clinical trials.

What are Effective Self-Help Treatments?

There is a vast literature on self-help treatments for bereavement. Unfortunately, the great majority, if not virtually all, of these books are based on outmoded assumptions about the grief process, encouraging practices that lack empirical support and that have been found to be harmful, in some cases, when applied in a clinical setting. What's more, no evidence supports the effectiveness of self-help treatments for grief. For these reasons, we do not recommend any current self-help treatments. However, there is a user-friendly book on bereavement that combines a scholarly review of the bereavement literature with rich clinical accounts of loss. Though not strictly a self-help treatment, this book is useful as a compendium of information on loss and as a description of the grieving process (Nolen-Hoeksma & Larson, 1999).

Because some useful information is mixed in with inaccurate representations of the grief process, we recommend the following websites provisionally:

- http://www.nlm.nih.gov/medlineplus/bereavement.html#specificconditions
- http://www.nmha.org/infoctr/factsheets/42.cfm

- http://griefnet.org/
- http://familydoctor.org/079.xml
- http://www.centerforloss.com/default.asp

What are Effective Therapist Based Treatments?

As previously discussed, recent meta-analyses of grief therapies have found both individual and group modalities to be generally ineffective (Kato & Mann, 1999; Neimeyer, 2000). In the absence of clear findings for evidence-based treatment for bereavement, what recommendations can be gleaned from existing research? One such recommendation involves the role of emotional disclosure in the resolution of grief. Traditional grief therapies have emphasized the importance of expressing negative emotions associated with the loss, but research examining this question has found that expressing negative emotions (Bonanno & Keltner, 1997), confronting feelings of anger or sadness (Bonanno, Keltner, Holnen, & Horowitz, 1995), and focusing on emotions associated with the loss (Nolen-Hoeksema, Parker, & Larson, 1994) are associated with more persistent grief symptoms and worse outcomes. On the other hand, the expression of positive feelings, and the avoidance of negative ones, has been consistently associated with a more rapid improvement and reduction in grief symptoms (Keltner & Bonanno, 1997; Moskowitz, Folkman, & Acree, 2003; Ong, Bergman, & Bisconti, 2004).

One explanation for these findings on negative emotional expression can be derived from research on the benefits of verbal disclosure. For example, ample research has identified the adaptive consequences of talking about acute stressors or trauma (e.g., Pennebaker, 1993), a process that appears to promote important processes of cognitive integration and restructuring (Greenberg, Wortman, & Stone, 1996). In the context of bereavement, however, the positive effects have been less clear (Kelly & McKillop, 1996). Indeed, Stroebe, Stroebe, Schut, & van den Bout (2002) recently examined the effects of written and verbal forms of emotional disclosure during bereavement and found no evidence that the disclosure of grief-related emotion improved adjustment. Given such findings, it is worthwhile to consider an important moderating factor in disclosure, demonstrated by Lepore and colleagues (Lepore, Silver, Wortman, & Wayment, 1996): the extent to which others are seen as available and willing to listen to expressed feelings. Without a supportive environment, the benefits of disclosure are diluted (Lepore, Ragan, & Jones, 2000). These findings suggest that clinicians should not emphasize the expression of negative emotions, but should adopt a neutral, nondirective stance with regard to the content of the bereaved person's disclosures, focusing instead on providing a safe environment in which disclosure is supported and meaning construction is enhanced.

What is Effective Medical Treatment?

Although relatively few studies have directly examined medication treatment for bereavement, available evidence indicates that medications can be effective for chronic or complicated grief reactions that are associated with persistent or severe depressive symptoms (Zisook & Schuchter, 2001). SSRI's, TCAs, or MAOs may be used, and evidence does not favor one class or type of medication over another (Zisook & Schuchter, 2001). Rather, side-effect profiles and patient preferences should dictate medication choices. In addition, no evidence supports the effectiveness of benzodiazepines in the treatment of anxiety symptoms associated with chronic or complicated grief (Warner, Metcalfe, & King, 2001).

Other issues in management.

- Bereaved persons suffering from chronic depression are likely to have significant coping deficits and show minimal processing of the loss (Bonanno, et al., 2002). For this reason, chronically depressed bereaved persons appear most appropriate for a symptom- and skill-focused intervention, and may be particularly unresponsive to a grief-focused intervention.
- Severe levels of distress at early stages of bereavement may be prognostic of later difficulties. Thus, in cases where grief symptoms appear more severe than normal in the early stages, intervention may be indicated at early stages before the grief becomes chronic.
- In cases of traumatic grief events, evidence does not support global applications of critical incident debriefing for acute stressors (Rose, Brewin, Andres, & Kirk, 1999), which can impede natural recovery processes (Bisson, Jenkins, Alexander, & Bannister, 1997; Mayou, Ehlers, & Hobbs, 2000).

How Does One Select Among Treatments?

One critical issue in selecting an appropriate treatment is whether the bereaved person's symptoms are consistent with a pattern of chronic grief or chronic depression. As mentioned, evidence does not support a grief-focused interventions for bereaved persons with chronic depression. In the case of chronic or complicated grief, the relative focus on grief may depend on the bereaved person's level of preoccupation with the loss, the presence of significant functional impairments, and the patient's own preferences. In addition, depending on the presenting symptom profile, the treating clinician may also wish to consult treatment recommendations for Major Depressive Disorder, Generalized Anxiety Disorder, and Posttraumatic Stress Disorder (see this volume).

REFERENCES

Allumbaugh, D. L., & Hoyt, W. T. (1999). Effectiveness of grief therapy: A meta-analysis. *Journal of Counseling Psychology, 46,* 370–380.

American Psychiatric Association. (1994). *Diagnostic and statistical manual of mental disorders* (4th ed.). Washington, DC: Author.

Bisson, J., Jenkins, P. L., Alexander, J., & Bannister, C. (1997). Randomised controlled trial of psychological debriefing for victims of burn trauma. *The British Journal of Psychiatry, 171,* 78–81.

Boerner, K., Wortman, C. B., & Bonanno, G. A. (2005). Resilient or at risk?: A four-year study of older adults who initially showed high or low distress following conjugal loss. *Journal of Gerontology: Series B: Psychological Science and Social Sciences, 60B,* 67–73.

Bonanno, G. A. (2001). The crucial importance of empirical evidence in the development of bereavement theory: Reply to Archer (2001). *Psychological Bulletin, 127,* 561–564.

Bonanno, G. A. (2004). Loss, trauma, and human resilience: Have we underestimated the human capacity to thrive after extremely aversive events? *American Psychologist, 59,* 20–28.

Bonanno, G. A., & Field, N. P. (2001). Examining the delayed grief hypothesis across 5 years of bereavement. *American Behavioral Scientist, 44,* 798–816.

Bonanno, G. A., & Kaltman, S. (1999). Toward an integrative perspective on bereavement. *Psychological Bulletin, 125,* 760–776.

Bonanno, G. A., & Kaltman, S. (2001). The varieties of grief experience. *Clinical Psychology Review, 21,* 705–734.

Bonanno, G. A., & Keltner, D. (1997). Facial expressions of emotion and the course of conjugal bereavement. *Journal of Abnormal Psychology, 106,* 126–137.

Bonanno, G. A., Keltner, D., Holen, A., & Horowitz, M. J. (1995). When avoiding unpleasant emotions might not be such a bad thing: Verbal-autonomic response dissociation and midlife conjugal bereavement. *Journal of Personality & Social Psychology, 69,* 975–989.

Bonanno, G. A., Moskowitz, J. T., Papa, A., & Folkman, S. (2005). Resilience to loss in bereaved spouses, bereaved parents, and bereaved gay men. *Journal of Personality and Social Psychology, 88,* 827–843.

Bonanno, G. A., Wortman, C. B., Lehman, D. R., Tweed, R. G., Haring, M., Sonnega, J., et al. (2002). Resilience to loss and chronic grief: A prospective study from preloss to 18-months post-loss. *Journal of Personality & Social Psychology, 83,* 1150–1164.

Bonanno, G. A., Wortman, C. B., & Nesse, R. M. (2004). Prospective patterns of resilience and maladjustment in widowhood. *Psychology & Aging, 19,* 260–271.

Fraley, R. C., & Shaver, P. R. (1999). Loss and bereavement: Attachment theory and recent controversies concerning "grief work" and the nature of detachment. In J. Cassidy, & P. R. Shaver (Eds.), *Handbook of attachment: Theory, research, and clinical applications* (pp. 735–759). New York: Guilford Press.

Greenberg, M. A., Wortman, C. B., & Stone, A. A. (1996). Emotional expression and physical heath: Revising traumatic memories or fostering self-regulation? *Journal of Personality & Social Psychology, 71,* 588–602.

Horowitz, M. J., Siegel, B., Holen, A., Bonanno, G. A., Milbrath, C., & Stinson, C. H. (1997). Diagnostic criteria for complicated grief disorder. *American Journal of Psychiatry, 154,* 904–910.

Jordan, J. R., & Neimeyer, R. A. (2003). Does grief counseling work? *Death Studies, 27,* 765–786.

Kato, P. M., & Mann, T. (1999). A synthesis of psychological interventions for the bereaved. *Clinical Psychology Review, 19,* 275–296.

Kelly, A. E., & McKillop, K. J. (1996). Consequences of revealing personal secrets. *Psychological Bulletin, 120,* 450–465.

Keltner, D., & Bonanno, G. A. (1997). A study of laughter and dissociation: Distinct correlates of laughter and smiling during bereavement. *Journal of Personality & Social Psychology, 73,* 687–702.

Kim, K., & Jacobs, S. (1991). Pathologic grief and its relationship to other psychiatric disorders. *Journal of Affective Disorders, 21,* 257–263.

Lichtenstein, P., Gatz, M., Pedersen, N. Berg, S. & McClearn, G. (1996). A co-twin control study of response to widowhood. *Journals of Gerontology: Series B: Psychological Sciences and Social Sciences, 51,* P279–P289.

Lepore, S. J., Ragan, J. D., & Jones, S. (2000). Talking facilitates cognitive-emotional processes of adaptation to an acute stressor. *Journal of Personality & Social Psychology, 78,* 499–508.

Lepore, S. J., Silver, R. C., Wortman, C. B., & Wayment, H. A. (1996). Social constraints, intrusive thoughts, and depressive symptoms among bereaved mothers. *Journal of Personality & Social Psychology, 70,* 271–282.

Lucas, R. E., Clark, A. E., Georgellis, Y., & Diener, E. (2003). Reexamining adaptation and the set point model of happiness: Reactions to changes in marital status. *Journal of Personality & Social Psychology, 84,* 527–539.

Mancini, A. D., Pressman, D. L., & Bonanno, G. A. (2005). Clinical interventions with the bereaved: What clinicians and counselors can learn from the CLOC study. In D. Carr, R. M. Nesse, & C. B. Wortman (Eds.), *Late life widowhood: New directions in theory, research, and practice.* New York: Springer Publishing.

Mayou, R. A., Ehlers, A., & Hobbs, M. (2000). Psychological debriefing for road traffic accident victims. *British Journal of Psychiatry, 176,* 589–593.

Middleton, W., Burnett, P., Raphael, B., & Martinek, N. (1996). The bereavement response: A cluster analysis. *British Journal of Psychiatry, 169,* 167–171.

Middleton, W., Moylan, A., Raphael, B., Burnett, P., et al. (1993). An international perspective on bereavement related concepts. *Australian and New Zealand Journal of Psychiatry, 27,* 457–463.

Moskowitz, J. T., Folkman, S., & Acree, M. (2003). Do positive psychological states shed light on recovery from bereavement? Findings from a 3-year longitudinal study. *Death Studies, 27,* 471–500.

Murphy, S. A., Johnson, L. C., & Lohan, J. (2003). Challenging myths about parents' adjustment after the sudden, violent death of a child. *Journal of Nursing Scholarship, 35,* 359–364.

Neimeyer, R. A. (2000). Searching for the meaning of meaning: Grief therapy and the process of reconstruction. *Death Studies, 24,* 541–558.

Nolen-Hoeksma, S., & Ahrens, C. (2002). Age differences and similarities in correlates of depressive symptoms. *Psychology and Aging, 17,* 116–124.

Nolen-Hoeksma, S. & Larson, J. (1999). *Coping with loss.* Mahwah, NJ: Erlbaum.

Nolen-Hoeksma, S., Parker, L. E., & Larson, J. (1994). Ruminative coping with depressed mood following loss. *Journal of Personality & Social Psychology, 67,* 92–104.

Ong, A. D., Bergeman, C. S., & Bisconti, T. L. (2004). The role of daily positive emotions during conjugal bereavement. *Journal of Gerontology: Psychological Sciences, 59B,* 168–176.

Pennebaker, J. W. (1993). Social mechanisms of constraint. In D. Wegner & J. W. Pennebaker (Eds.), *Handbook of mental control. Century psychology series* (pp. 200–219). Englewood Cliffs, NJ: Prentice Hall.

Prigerson, H. G., Maciejewski, P. K., Reynolds, C. F., III, Bierhals, A. J., Newsom, J. T., Fasiczka, A., et al. (1995). Inventory of Complicated Grief: A scale to measure maladaptive symptoms of loss. *Psychiatry Research, 59,* 65–79.

Rando, T. A. (1993). *Treatment of complicated mourning.* Champaign, IL: Research Press.

Raphael, B., Minkov, C., & Dobson, M. (2001). Psychotherapeutic and pharmacological intervention for bereaved persons. In M. S. Stroebe, R. O. Hansson, W. Stroebe, & H. Schut (Eds.),

Handbook of bereavement research: Consequences, coping, and care (pp. 587–612). Washington, DC: American Psychological Association.

Rose, S., Brewin, C. R., Andrews, B., & Kirk, M. (1999). A randomized controlled trial of individual psychological debriefing for victims of violent crime. *Psychological Medicine, 29,* 793–799.

Schut, H. A., Stroebe, M. S., van den Bout, J., & Terheggen, M. (2001). The efficacy of bereavement interventions: Determining who benefits. In M. S. Stroebe, R. O. Hansson, W. Stroebe, & H. Schut (Eds.), *Handbook of bereavement research: Consequences, coping, and care* (pp. 705–738). Washington, D.C: American Psychological Association.

Stroebe, M, Stroebe, W., & Schut, H. (2001). Gender difference in adjustment to bereavement: An empirical and theoretical review. *Review of General Psychology, 5,* 62–83.

Stroebe, M. S., Stroebe, W., Schut, H., & van den Bout, J. (2002). Does disclosure of emotions facilitate recovery from bereavement? Evidence from two prospective studies. *Journal of Consulting & Clinical Psychology, 70,* 169–178.

Stroebe, W., & Schut, H. (2001). Risk factors in bereavement outcome: A methodological and empirical review. In M. S. Stroebe, R. O. Hansson, W. Stroebe, & H. Schut (Eds.), *Handbook of bereavement research: Consequences, coping, and care* (pp. 349–371). Washington, D.C: American Psychological Association.

Stroebe, W., & Stroebe, M. S. (1991). Does "grief work" work? *Journal of Consulting & Clinical Psychology, 59,* 479–482.

Warner, J., Metcalfe, C., & King, M. (2001). Evaluating the use of benzodiazepines following recent bereavement. *British Journal of Psychiatry, 178,* 36–41.

Worden, J. W. (1991). *Grief counseling and grief therapy: A handbook for the mental health practitioner* (2nd ed.). New York: Springer Publishing Company.

Wortman, C. B., & Silver, R. C. (1989). The myths of coping with loss. *Journal of Consulting & Clinical Psychology, 57,* 349–357.

Wortman, C. B., & Silver, R. C. (2001). The myths of coping with loss revisited. In M. S. Stroebe, R. O. Hansson, W. Stroebe, & H. Schut (Eds.), *Handbook of bereavement research: Consequences, coping, and care* (pp. 405–429). Washington, DC: American Psychological Association.

Zisook, S., & Schuchter, S. R. (2001). Treatment of the depressions of bereavement. *The American Behavioral Scientist, 44,* 782–797.

Bipolar Disorder

Michael W. Otto • David J. Miklowitz

WHAT IS BIPOLAR DISORDER?

Bipolar disorder, also known as manic-depressive disorder, is a prevalent, disabling, and chronic condition. Bipolar disorder is defined by periods of mood instability defined by the occurrence of at least one manic or hypomanic episode and commonly characterized by repeated episodes of major depression. A full manic episode is defined by a period (1 week unless interrupted by treatment or other factors) of feeling high, euphoric, or irritable, along with three (if mood is euphoric) or four (if mood is irritable) or more of the following symptoms: exaggerated feelings of importance, little need for sleep, racing thoughts, pressured speech, distractability, and reckless behavior (American Psychiatric Association, 1994). Hypomanic episodes represent a similar but less severe and impairing version of mania. The Bipolar I subtype of bipolar disorder is characterized by at least one episode of mania or mixed disorder (syndromal depression and mania simultaneously for at least one week), whereas the bipolar II subtype refers to individuals who have never had a full manic episode, but have had at least one hypomanic episode and one or more depressive episodes.

People with bipolar disorder differ with respect to their pattern of episodes, with some having a balance of episodes of depression and mania/hypomania, and others having mostly one type of episode. On average, however, depressive symptoms are present more often than manic/hypomanic symptoms, with Judd and associates finding that a sample of bipolar I patients had over 3.5 times as many weeks with symptoms of depression relative to manic or hypomanic symptoms (Judd et al., 2002), and bipolar II patients had depressive symptoms 38 times more frequently (50.3% of weeks vs. 1.3% of weeks) than hypomanic symptoms (Judd et al., 2003).

Bipolar patients experience significant functional impairments even when they are maintained on pharmacotherapy (Goldberg, Harrow, & Grossman, 1995; Coryell et al., 1993; Hammen, Gitlin, & Altshuler, 2000). For example, Coryell et al (1993) found that the functional deficits associated with manic episodes (i.e., poor work, relationship, and interpersonal functioning), were apparent five years after the episode had resolved. Dion et al. (1988) found that 30% of patients were unable to work at all, and only 21% worked at their expected level in the six months after an episode (Dion, Tohen, Anthony, & Waternaux, 1988). Only 35% of patients undergoing pharmacotherapy with lithium or lithium plus neuroleptics (see below) had good functioning over 41/2 years (Goldberg et al., 1995). In a longitudinal follow-up, Harrow et al. (1990) found that only 42% of manic patients showed steady work performance in the 1.7 years after hospitalization. In addition, bipolar disorder is associated with high rates of family or marital distress, dysfunction, separation, and divorce (Coryell et al., 1993; Simoneau, Miklowitz, Richards, Saleem, & George, 1998).

Otto, M. W., & Miklowitz, D. J. (2006). In J. E. Fisher & W. T. O'Donohue (Eds.), *Practitioner's guide to evidence-based psychotherapy*. New York: Springer Publishing Company.

BASIC FACTS ABOUT BIPOLAR DISORDER

Prevalence. Bipolar disorder has been estimated to affect between 1% and 2% of the population (Regier et al., 1988; Kessler et al., 1994), although higher rates have also been reported in select studies and for bipolar spectrum (e.g., cyclothymia) disorders (Akiskal, Bourgeois, & Angst, 2000; McIntyre & Konarski, 2004).

Age at onset. The average age of onset for clinical samples of patients with bipolar disorder is in the late-teens to early twenties (Kogan et al., 2004). Individuals with earlier onsets have greater anxiety and substance use comorbidity and a more chronic course marked by greater numbers of depressive episodes and an increased likelihood of suicidal behaviors among individuals with the earliest ages of onset (Perlis et al., 2004).

Gender. Women and men are equally likely to receive a diagnosis of bipolar disorder (Kessler et al., 1994). However, a sex difference has been detected for a rapid cycling (4 or more mood episodes a year), with more women meeting criteria for a rapid cycling subtype and for Bipolar II (Schneck et al., 2004).

Comorbidity. Comorbidity with other disorders is especially common in patients with bipolar disorder. The prevalence of comorbid anxiety disorders in clinical and epidemiologic studies range from 10.6% to 62.5% for panic disorder, 7.8% to 47.2% for social anxiety disorder, 7% to 40% for posttraumatic stress disorder, 3.2% to 35% for obsessive-compulsive disorder, and 7% to 32% for generalized anxiety disorder (for review see Simon et al., 2004). Likewise, studies of community samples (Kessler et al., 1997; Regier et al., 1990) and clinical populations (Brady, Castro, Lydiard, Malcolm, & Arana, 1991; Goldberg, Garno, Leon, Kocsis, & Portera, 1999) have documented high rates of substance use disorder (SUD) comorbidity, with estimates ranging from a prevalence of 21–45%. There is a sixfold increase in SUDs among individuals with bipolar disorder as compared to the general population. Elevated rates of eating disorders (McElroy et al., 2000) and childhood attention deficit disorder have also been reported for samples of bipolar patients (Nierenberg et al., in press).

COURSE

The most common clinical course of bipolar disorder is repeated episodes of depression and mania/hypomania that are disabling in their own right, but may be compounded by the financial, family, and social disruptions that may occur during or following severe episodes (Miklowitz & Goldstein, 1997). Over longer-term outcomes (4–5 years) three-quarters of patients can be expected to relapse, with approximately half of these relapses occurring in the first year (Gitlin, Swendsen, Heller, & Hammen, 1995; O'Connell, Mayo, Flatlow, Cuthbertson, & O'Brien, 1991; Tohen, Waternaux, & Tsuang, 1990). As noted, continued symptoms and role impairment is common between episodes.

A number of factors appear to play a significant role in the likelihood of a mood episode. Stressful life events are associated with delayed recovery and elevated relapse rates (Ellicott, Hammen, Gitlin, Brown, & Jamison, 1990; Johnson & Miller, 1997), and stressful family environments (as characterized by high levels of expressed emotion or negative interactional patterns) are linked with greater relapse rates (Miklowitz et al., 1988; see also Priebe et al., 1989).

Disorder comorbidity is linked with a poorer course (McElroy et al., 2000), and there is specific evidence for the prognostic significance of anxiety and substance use comorbidity. For example, anxiety comorbidity has been linked with a decreased likelihood of recovery from a mood episode, poorer role functioning and quality of life, less time euthymic, a greater likelihood of suicide attempts, and poorer response to at least one class of medications (Henry et al., 2003, Simon et al., 2004). Studies have also documented poorer recovery among bipolar patients with a comorbid SUD (Keller et al., 1986; Tohen et al., 1990), and a greater likelihood of medication non-compliance (Goldberg et al., 1999; Keck, McElroy, Strakowski, & Bourne, 1997), and hospitalization (Brady et al., 1991; Reich, Davies, & Himmelhoch, 1974). Psychotic features during depression are also associated with a poorer illness course (Tohen et al., 1990).

Suicide is also a particular concern for bipolar disorder. For example, Brown, Beck, Steer, and Grisham (2000) evaluated suicidal outcomes over the course of 20 years in nearly 7,000 psychiatric outpatients in Pennsylvania. Patients were diagnosed according to DSM-IV criteria, and among diagnoses, patients with bipolar disorder had the strongest risk for completed suicide, followed by major depression and personality disorders. As compared to the average psychiatric patients in the sample, bipolar patients were found to have a nearly four-fold increase in suicide risk, and major depression accounted for a three-fold increase in risk.

ASSESSMENT

Discriminating Bipolar Disorder from Other Conditions

Bipolar disorder is differentiated from unipolar major depression by the presence of manic, mixed, or hypomanic episodes. This process may be difficult, as mood instability may be characterized initially by depressive episodes alone, with the full bipolar pattern emerging later in life. For example, Goldberg et al. (2001) followed a sample of young adults selected on the basis of a hospitalization for severe unipolar depression. Over a 15-year follow-up period, 41% of this sample experienced a manic or hypomanic episode, thereby redefining their presumed unipolar depression as one pole of a bipolar disorder.

In individuals with a history of depression, the differential diagnosis of unipolar major depression vs. bipolar disorder involves the identification of manic or hypomanic episodes, including the discrimination of these episodes from other conditions. For example, loud or boisterous speech and actions as well as risky behaviors (e.g., unprotected sexual encounters, reckless driving, aggressive behavior) and their consequences (e.g., arrest, chaotic relationships) can be characteristic of alcohol or substance intoxication, and need to be differentiated from true hypomanic or manic symptoms, with sensitivity to the degree to which a substance use disorder and bipolar disorder may both be present. Likewise, Cluster B (borderline, antisocial, histrionic, and narcissistic) Axis II disorders co-occur with depression and may contribute symptoms (e.g., mood lability, irritability, interpersonal sensitivity, and risky behaviors) that may mimic those of hypomania, complicating diagnosis in individuals with the bipolar II subtype.

The presence of psychosis during manic episodes presents a diagnostic challenge: is it bipolar disorder, schizoaffective disorder, or schizophrenia? These questions are sometimes clarified only after acute recovery and review of the full history of mood instability, as well as information on past episodes, inter-episode functioning, and family history.

What is Involved in Effective Assessment?

Clinical assessment of bipolar disorder needs to include assessment of each pole of the disorder (manic and depressive symptoms), the history of the frequency and duration of episodes, potential biological causes of these episodes (e.g., drug use), family history of episodes, psychosocial stressors, support networks, and role functioning. Careful diagnostic assessment can be aided with the use of a structured interview such as the Structured Clinical Interview for DSM IV diagnosis (SCID; Spitzer, Williams, & Gibbon,1996). The Affective Disorder Evaluation (ADE; Sachs, 1990) utilizes a modified version of the mood and psychosis modules from the SCID while also assessing a wealth of clinical information including comorbidities, family history, number and length of prior episodes, periods of recovery, suicidal actions, and past treatments and response. The ADE has also been applied as a research tool in a large multicenter study of the course and treatment of bipolar disorder (Sachs et al., 2003). For these assessments, clarification of the history of mood episodes, particularly manic episodes, can be aided by including a family member in the assessment process. Because bipolar patients may underreport these episodes due to the judgment biases inherent in the episode (e.g., "sure I was hyped up, but things never got out of hand"), family members may be able to provide crucial information on the severity of these episodes. In addition, records from past providers or past hospitalizations may provide an index on the severity of mood episodes when they were occurring, instead of the bias that may occur when these episodes are recalled months or years later.

The assessment of individual symptom domains and the monitoring of symptoms over time can be aided by structured, clinician-administered interviews. For manic symptoms, the Young-Mania Rating Scale (YMRS; Young, Biggs, Ziegler, & Meyer, 1978) is used frequently in research settings. The Montgomery–Asberg Depression Rating Scale (MADRS; Montgomery & Asberg, 1979) or the Hamilton Rating Scale for Depression (HDRS; Hamilton, 1960) are frequently used for rating depression severity. As a clinical tool that has also been applied in research, the Clinical Monitoring Form (CMF; Sachs et al., 2002) is used by clinicians to document the symptom and treatment characteristics of patients at each clinical visit. It consists of modified versions of the SCID current mood modules, associated symptoms, medical problems and comorbid conditions, as well as fields to record selected mental status items, medications compliance, laboratory data, severity summary scores, and a written narrative and treatment plan.

Self-report screens for depressive symptoms and suicidal ideation, such as the Beck Depression Inventory-II (Beck, Steer, & Brown 1996) and the Beck Hopelessness Scale (Beck, Weissman, Lester, & Trexler 1974), can also be of use to track mood states over time.

What Assessments are Not Helpful?

Traditional psychological tests such as projective tests and the MMPI are not useful in diagnosing bipolar disorder. Neuropsychological tests have been used to characterize cognitive impairments associated with bipolar disorder, and may be of use in planning treatment (e.g., cognitive rehabilitation) or in evaluating the genesis of problems of poor motivation or adherence with treatment.

TREATMENT

Pharmacotherapy for Bipolar Disorder

For decades, pharmacotherapy alone has stood at the central treatment option for patients with bipolar disorder. Mood stabilizers (e.g., lithium, anticonvulsant medications, and atypical antipsychotics) as a primary treatment have been supplemented by a variety of antidepressant and antianxiety agents in attempts to provide acute care of mood episodes as well as longer-term maintenance treatment to prevent future episodes. The desired properties of a mood stabilizer are efficacy in the acute treatment of both depressive and manic episodes, and in the prevention of recurrence of both depressive and manic episodes, without increasing risk of mood cycling or switching into another mood state (Keck et al., 2004). Lithium (brand names Eskalith, Lithobid) most closely meets this definition of mood stabilizer, and in the United States has been used as a mood stabilizer for 30 years. Elements of mood stabilization are also offered by the anticonvulsants divalproex (brand name Depakote), carbamazepine (brand name Tegretol), and lamotrigine (brand name Lamictal), as well as a number of atypical antipsychotic medications: aripiprazole (Abilify), olanzapine (Zyprexa), quetiapine (Seroquel), risperidone (Risperdal), and ziprasidone(Geodon). Table 12.1 summarizes the medications that have Federal Drug Administration (FDA) indications for treatment of phases of bipolar disorder as of November 1, 2004.

Given the predominance of depressive symptoms in bipolar disorder (Judd et al., 2002, 2003), antidepressants are frequently combined with mood stabilizers. There is some danger of promoting a manic episode with the antidepressants. As evaluated in the context of acute antidepressant trials, this risk appears to be more specific to older agents (i.e., tryicyclics) than some of the newer, serotonin selective reuptake inhibitors (SSRIs (Gijsman, Geddes, Rendell, Nolen & Goodwin, 2004). A greater risk of conversion to mania (as defined as the emergence of a bipolar diagnosis in patients' records) was also seen more frequently among patients with mood or anxiety disorders treated with tricyclic antidepressants than SSRIs in a large scale (N = 87,920) pharmacoepidemiologic study. In this study, conversion rates also were significantly higher among patients with mood or anxiety disorders treated with SSRIs relative to similar patients without antidepressant exposure. Higher conversion rates were also seen among younger antidepressant users.

Benzodiazepines also are used as adjunctive pharmacotherapy for bipolar disorder (e.g., to reduce agitation or comorbid anxiety) (Regier et al., 1998), but the efficacy of these agents for broader mood stabilization in bipolar patients is generally lacking (e.g., Morishita & Aoki, 2002; Winkler et al., 2003).

Despite the clear benefits of pharmacotherapy for bipolar disorder, the most common course of bipolar disorder continues to be one of regular relapses to

TABLE 12.1 Agents with FDA Indications for the Treatment of Bipolar Disorder (as of 11/1/2004)

Generic name	Trade name	Acute Bipolar depression	Acute bipolar mania	Maintenance treatment of bipolar I disorder
Aripiprazole	Abilify		✓	
Chlorpromazine	Thorazine		✓	
Divalproex	Depakote		✓	
Lamotrigine	Lamictal			✓
Lithium	Eskalith		✓	✓
Olanzapine	Zyprexa		✓	✓
Quetiapine	Seroquel		✓	
Risperidone	Risperdal		✓	
Ziprasidone	Geodone		✓	
Olanzapine/fluoxetine combination	Symbyax	✓		

Figure adapted from Kahn, D. A., Keck, P. E., Perlis, R. H., Otto, M. W., & Ross, R. (2004). Treatment of bipolar disorder: A guide for patients and families. *A Postgraduate Medicine Special Report*, December, 1–108.

depression or mania/hypomania, with longitudinal studies indicating one-year relapse rates as high as 40% despite the use of mood stabilizers (Gitlin, Swendsen, Heller, & Hammen, 1995; see also O'Connell, et al., 1991). Medication adherence brings its own challenges, with inadequate medication use evident in one-half to two-thirds of patients within the first 12 months of treatment (Keck et al., 1998; Keck et al., 1996). Discontinuation of mood stabilizers brings with it the risk of relapse, particularly when medication is rapidly discontinued (Perlis et al., 2002). Brief psychosocial treatment has been successfully applied to the problem of adherence, and has been found to improve adherence and the course of bipolar disorder (Cochran, 1984), but as detailed below, psychosocial treatment also plays a broader role in the management of bipolar disorder.

What are Effective Therapist-Based Psychosocial Treatments?

An impressive trajectory of evidence over the last several years has provided increasing evidence that psychosocial treatments play a significant role in providing mood stability to bipolar patients. Used as an adjunct to ongoing medication treatment, cognitive-behavioral and family focused treatment strategies have been applied successfully to reduce relapse and intervene directly with episodes of depression and hypomania (see below). There is also recent evidence that these psychosocial interventions are becoming well-accepted by experts in bipolar disorder. In a recent survey (Keck et al., 2004), experts engaged in the research and treatment of bipolar disorder consistently recommended psychotherapy for those stages of the disorder when the patient is considered receptive to interventions, i.e., during the acute and maintenance treatment phases of episodes of depression and hypomania, but not during acute manic or psychotic episodes. Psychotherapy was also heartily endorsed for the treatment of comorbid conditions like anxiety, eating, or substance-use disorders, and as a first-choice option when pharmacotherapy is limited by medical 0conditions (e.g., heart disease, liver disease, renal conditions, obesity, or pregnancy). Overall, psychotherapy in combination with medication was recommended as a standard treatment strategy. Among psychotherapy options, the experts recommended the types of treatment that have received the most research in bipolar disorder.

Psychosocial interventions that have demonstrated strong treatment effects include specific relapse prevention protocols focusing on action plans to be implemented when prodromal symptoms are detected (Perry, Tarrier, Morriss, McCarthy, & Limb, 1999), comprehensive individual CBT designed to treat residual symptoms and prevent relapse (Lam et al., 2003; Scott, Garland, & Moorhead, 2001), individual treatment of bipolar depression with cognitive-behavioral protocols traditionally used in the treatment of unipolar depression (Zaretsky, Segal, & Gemar, 1999), comprehensive psychoeducational interventions offered in a group-therapy (Colom et al., 2003) and couples (Clarkin, Carpenter, Hull, Wilner, & Glick, 1998) settings, and family interventions designed to enhance the protective effects of family and social support systems (Miklowitz, George, Richards, Simoneau, & Suddath, 2003). Interpersonal therapy combined with interventions designed to balance sleep/wake and activity cycles has also been studied, although full determination of its efficacy is still pending (Frank et al., 1997, 1999; Frank, Swartz, & Kupfer, 2000).

These treatments tend to share in common a number of standard treatment elements including: (1) psychoeducation that provides patients with a model of their disorder, including the course of bipolar disorder and aggravating factors such as medication nonadherence and the role of sleep, lifestyle regularity, and stress management; (2) problem-solving and/or communication training to reduce family or external stress, and (3) strategies for early detection of and intervention for mood episodes (including the activation of increased support, more-frequent treatment sessions, or intensified pharmacotherapy). Depending on the protocol under study, these interventions may be combined with thought and activity monitoring, cognitive-restructuring, treatment contracting and other interventions in individual, group, and family settings (Otto & Miklowitz, 2004).

For example, a brief program of individual CBT (12–18 sessions within the first six months and two booster sessions in the second six months of care) relative to usual care alone was studied by Lam et al. (2003) in a sample of 103 patients. The patients had histories of frequent episodes (at least two episodes in the last 2 years, or three episodes in the last 5 years) despite use of mood stabilizers, but were not in an acute episode when they entered the study. The CBT included cognitive interventions for depression, sleep and routine management, life pacing (to try to reduce efforts to "make up for lost time" due to mood episodes), and mood monitoring with interventions for prodromal mood states. The results indicated strong protective effects for the CBT treatment, with a 43.8% relapse rate for CBT compared to a 75% rate for the control treatment. Benefits for CBT also included reduced days in episodes and fewer days spent hospitalized due to bipolar disorder.

Similarly, studies of Family Focused Treatment (FFT; Miklowitz & Goldstein, 1997) have documented the success of family interventions focusing on psychoeducation for patients and their families, communication enhancement training, and problem solving training. Interventions are particularly active, with frequent use of rehearsals (within and between sessions) and role-playing interventions. The psychoeducational interventions include not only discussions of risk and protective factors for mood episodes, but also rehearsal of relapse prevention efforts in response to prodromal symptoms. These interventions were evaluated in a randomized trial of 101 bipolar patients by Miklowitz et al. (2003). They found that 21 sessions (delivered over nine months) of FFT in combination with pharmacotherapy reduced both manic and depressive symptoms, and offered better protection against recurrences of mood episodes than a comparison condition that offered pharmacologic treatment in combination with two sessions of home-based family education and crisis intervention as needed over nine months.

A second trial (Rea et al., 2003), found that patients undergoing FFT and pharmacotherapy had longer delays prior to hospitalization or relapse than patients who received a comparably paced individual therapy consisting of psychoeducation, adherence monitoring, support, and problem-solving. In the year following delivery of the active psychosocial treatments, rates of rehospitalization in the FFT condition were 12%, compared to 60% in the individual therapy condition. Patients in FFT were also less likely to require hospitalization when they did relapse.

In summary, several treatments have emerged as efficacious adjuncts to pharmacotherapy in the maintenance treatment of bipolar disorder. Their adherents share the common belief that the outpatient treatment of bipolar disorder should be multi-modal, psychoeducational, and skill-based, and oriented toward long-term disorder management.

How Does One Select Among Treatments?

As compared to other Axis I conditions, where there is much more debate about whether psychosocial or pharmacologic treatment should be offered as an initial treatment option (see Otto, Smits, & Reese, in press), there is general agreement that combination treatment (pharmacologic and psychosocial) should be the

future standard for bipolar disorder, at least during the stabilization and maintenance phases (Kahn, Keck, Perlis, Otto, & Ross, 2004). However, even though psychosocial interventions are frequently offered in community settings as adjuncts to
pharmacologic treatment for bipolar disorder (Lembke et al., 2004), these interventions may correspond poorly to the treatment elements shown to be effective in
clinical trials. Because effective psychosocial treatment adjuncts for bipolar disorder have emerged only recently, individuals trained to offer these treatments tend
to be clustered in large academic centers. Nonetheless, it is clear that these psychosocial interventions are receiving increased acceptance in research and clinical
communities (Keck et al., 2004), an advance that augers well for increasing dissemination of these approaches.

What are Some Self-Help Resources?

Two self-help books are noteworthy for being written by individuals engaged in documenting the efficacy of psychosocial treatments for bipolar disorder.

- Miklowitz, D. J. (2002). The bipolar disorder survival guide. Guilford,
- Jones, S., Hayward, P., Lam, D. (2002). Coping with bipolar disorder: A guide to living with manic depression. Oneworld Publications: Oxford.

An informational handout for patients and their families is also provided by

- Kahn, D. A., Keck, P. E., Perlis, R. H., Otto, M. W., & Ross, R. (2004) Treatment of
  bipolar disorder: A guide for patients and families. A Postgraduate Medicine
  Special Report: Treatment of Bipolar Disorder 2004, December, 109–116.

Furthermore, personal accounts of bipolar disorder may be of use to patients or
family members seeking a personal perspective on the nature of the disorder.

- Jamison, K. R. (1996). An unquiet mind, a memoir of moods and madness. Vintage.
- Duke, P., Hockman G. A brilliant madness: living with manic-depressive illness.
  Bantam Books.

Finally, useful informational websites about bipolar disorder and other serious
depressive disorders incl ude the following.

- American Foundation for Suicide prevention. www.afsp.org
- Depression and Bipolar Support Alliance (DBSA) offering over 1,000 peer-run sup-
  port groups. www.DBSAlliance.org
- Madison Institute of Medicine offering information on mood stabilizers. www.mim-
  inc.org
- Massachusetts General Hospital Bipolar Clinic and Research Program (to which the
  authors have a research affiliation) offering information and resources for clinicians and patients. www.manicdepressive.org
- National Alliance for Mental Illness offering over 1,200 local affiliates. www.nami.org
- National Mental Health Association (NMHA) offering more than 340 affiliates.
  www.nmha.org

REFERENCES

(not including self-help resources unless otherwise cited)

American Psychiatric Association (1994). *Diagnostic an statistical manual of mental disorders* (4th
ed.). Washington, DC: Author.

Beck, A. T., Steer, R. A. & Brown, G. K. (1996). *Beck Depression Inventory manual* (2nd ed.). San
Antonio: The Psychological Corporation.

Beck, A. T., Weissman, A., Lester, D., & Trexler, L. (1974). The measurement of pessimism: The Hopelessness Scale. *Journal of Consulting and Clinical Psychology, 42*, 861–865.

Brady, K. T., Casto, S., Lydiard, R. B., Malcolm, R., & Arana, G. (1991). Substance abuse in an inpatient psychiatric sample. *American Journal of Drug and Alcohol Abuse, 17*, 389–397.

Brown, G. K., Beck, A. T., Steer, R. A., & Grisham, J. R. (2000). Risk factors for suicide in psychiatric outpatients: A 20-year prospective study. *Journal of Consulting and Clinical Psychology, 68*, 371–377.

Clarkin, J. F., Carpenter, D., Hull, J., Wilner, P., & Glick, I. (1998). Effects of psychoeducational intervention for married patients with bipolar disorder and their spouses. *Psychiatric Services, 49*, 531–533.

Cochran, S. (1984). Preventing medical noncompliance in the outpatient treatment of bipolar affective disorders. *Journal of Consulting and Clinical Psychology, 52*, 873–878.

Colom, G., Vieta, E., Martinez-Aran, A., Reinares, M., Goikolea, J. M., Benabarre, A., et al. (2003). A randomized trial on the efficacy of group psychoeducation in the prophylaxis of recurrences in boplar patients whose disease is in remission. *Archives of General Psychiatry, 60*, 402–407.

Coryell, W., Scheftner, W., Keller, M. (1993). The enduring psychosocial consequences of mania and depression. *American Journal of Psychiatry, 150*, 720–727.

Dion, G. L., Tohen, M., Anthony, W. A. (1998). Symptoms and functioning of patients with bipolar disorder six months after hospitalization. Hospital & Community Psychiatry, 39, 652–657.

Ellicott, A., Hammen, C., Gitlin, M., Brown, G., & Jamison, K. (1990). Life events and the course of bipolar disorder. *American Journal of Psychiatry, 147*, 1194–1198.

Frank, E., Hlastala, S., Ritenour A., Houck, P., Tu, X. M., Mark, T. H., et al. (1997). Inducing lifestyle regularity in recovering bipolar disorder patients. *Biological Psychiatry, 41*, 1165–1173.

Frank, E., Swartz, H. A., & Kupfer, D. J. (2000). Interpersonal and social rhythm therapy: Managing the chaos of bipolar disorder. *Biological Psychiatry, 48(6)*, 593–604.

Frank, E., Swartz, H. A., Mallinger, A. G., Thase, M. E., Weaver, E. V., Kupfer, D. J. (1999). Adjunctive psychotherapy for bipolar disorder: Effects of changing treatment modality. *Journal of Abnormal Psychology, 108*, 579–587.

Gijsman, H. M., Geddes, J. R., Rendell, J. M, Nolen, W. A., & Goodwin, G. M. (2004). Antidepressants for bipolar depression: A systematic review of randomized, controlled trials. *American Journal of Psychiatry, 161*, 1537–1547.

Gitlin, M. J., Swendsen, J., Heller, T. L., & Hammen, C. (1995). Relapse and impairment in bipolar disorder. *American Journal of Psychiatry, 152*, 1635–1640.

Goldberg, J. F., Harrow, M., & Whiteside, R. E. (2001). Risk for bipolar illness in patients initially hospitalized for unipolar depression. *American Journal of Psychiatry, 158*, 1265–1270.

Goldberg, J., Garno, J., Leon, A., Kocsis, J. & Portera, L. (1999). A history of substance abuse complicates remission from acute mania in bipolar disorder. *The Journal of Clinical Psychiatry, 60*, 733–740.

Hamilton M. A. (1960). A rating scale for depression. *Journal of Neurology, Neurosurgery, and Psychiatry, 23*, 56–62.

Hammen, C., Gitlin, M., Altshuler, L. (2000). Predictors of Work Adjustment in Bipolar I Patients: A Naturalistic Longitudinal Follow-Up. *Journal of Consulting and Clinical Psychology.* 68.

Henry, C., Van den Bulke, D., Bellivier, F., Etain, B., Rouillon, F., & Leboyer, M. (2003). Anxiety disorders in 318 bipolar patients: prevalence and impact on illness severity and response to mood stabilizer. *Journal of Clinical Psychiatry, 64*, 331–335.

Johnson, S. L., & Miller, I. (1997). Negative life events and time to recovery from episodes of bipolar disorder. *Journal of Abnormal Psychology, 106*, 449–457.

Judd, L. L., Akiskal, H. S., Schettler, P. J., Coryell, W., Endicott, J., Maser, J. D., et al. (2003). A prospective investigation of the natural history of the long-term weekly symptomatic status of bipolar II disorder. *Archives of General Psychiatry, 60*, 261–269.

Judd, L. L., Akiskal, H. S., Schettler, P. J., Endicott, J., Maser, J. D., Solomon, D. A. et al. (2002). The long-term natural history of the weekly symptomatic status of bipolar I disorder. *Archives of General Psychiatry, 59*, 530–537.

Kahn, D. A., Keck, P. E., Perlis, R. H., Otto, M. W., & Ross, R. (2004). Treatment of bipolar disorder: A guide for patients and families. *A Postgraduate Medicine Special Report, December*, 1–108.

Keck, P. E., McElroy, S. L., Strakwoski, S. M., & Bourne, M. L. (1997). Compliance with maintenance treatment in bipolar disorder. *Psychopharmacology Bulletin, 33(1)*, 87–91.

Keck, P. E., McElroy, S. L., Strakowski, S. M., Stanton, S. P., Kizer, D. L., Balistreri, T. M., et al. (1996). Factors associated with pharmacologic noncompliance in patients with mania. *Journal of Clinical Psychiatry, 57*, 292–297.

Keck, P. E., McElroy, S. L., Strakowski, S. M., West, S. A., Sax, K. W., Hawkins, et al. (1998). Twelve-month outcome of patients with bipolar disorder following hospitalization for a manic or mixed episode. *American Journal of Psychiatry, 155*, 646–652.

Keck, P. E., Perlis, R. H., Otto, M. W., Carpenter, D., Docherty, J. P., & Ross, R. (2004). Expert Consensus Guideline Series: Treatment of bipolar disorder. *A Postgraduate Medicine Special Report, December*, 1–108.

Keller, M. B., Lavori, P. W., Coryell, W., Andreasen, N. C., Endicott, J., Clayton, P. J., et al. (1986). Differential outcome of pure manic, mixed/cycling, and pure depressive episodes in patients with bipolar illness. *Journal of the American Medical Association, 255*, 3138–3142.

Kessler, R. C., Crum, R. C., Warner, L. A., Nelson, C. B., Schulenberg, J. & Anthony, J. C. (1997). Lifetime co-occurrence of DSM-III-R alcohol abuse and dependence with other psychiatric disorders in the National Comorbidity Survey. *Archives of General Psychiatry, 54,* 313–321.

Kessler, R. C., McGonagle, K. A., Zhao, S., Nelson, C. B., Hughes, M., Eshleman, S., et al. (1994). Lifetime and 12-month prevalence of DSM-III-R psychiatric disorders in the United States: Results from the National Comorbidity Survey. *Archives of General Psychiatry, 51,* 8–19.

Kogan, J. N., Otto, M. W., Bauer, M. W., Dennehy, E. B., Miklowitz, D. J., & Zhang H. (2004). Demographic and diagnostic characteristics of the first 1000 patients enrolled in the Systematic Treatment Enhancement Program for Bipolar Disorder (STEP-BD). *Bipolar Disorders, 6,* 460–469.

Lam, D. H., Watkins, E. R., Hayward, P., Bright, J., Wright, K., Kerr, et al. (2003). A randomized controlled study of cognitive therapy for relapse prevention for bipolar affective disorder: Outcome of the first year. *Archives of General Psychiatry, 60,* 145–152.

Lembke, A., Miklowitz, D. J., Otto, M. W., Zhang, H., Wisniewski, S. R., et al. (2004). Psychosocial service utilization by patients with bipolar disorders: Data from the first 500 participants in the Systematic Treatment Enhancement Program. *Journal of Psychiatric Practice, 10,* 81–87.

McElroy, S. L., Atshuler, L. L., Suppes, T., Keck, P. E., Frye, M. A., Denicoff, K. D., et al. (2000). Axis I psychiatric comorbidity and its relationship to historical illness variables in 288 patients with bipolar disorder. *American Journal of Psychiatry, 159,* 420–426.

McIntyre, R. S., & Konarski, J. Z. (2004). Bipolar disorder: A national health concern. *CNS Spectrums, 9(11),* 6–15.

Miklowitz, D. J., George, E. L., Richards, J. A., Simoneau, T. L., & Suddath, R. L. (2003). A randomized study of family-focused psychoeducation and pharmacotherapy in the outpatient management of bipolar disorder. *Archives of General Psychiatry, 60,* 904–912.

Miklowitz, D. R., & Goldstein, M. J. (1997). *Bipolar disorder: A family-focused treatment approach.* New York: Guilford Press.

Miklowitz, D. R., Goldstein, M. J., Nuechterlein, K. H., Snyder, K. S., & Mintz, J. (1988). Family factors and the course of bipolar affective disorder. *Archives of General Psychiatry, 45,* 225–231.

Montgomery, S. A., & Asberg, M. (1979). A new depression scale designed to be sensitive to change. British Journal of Psychiatry, 134, 382–389.

Morishita, S. &, Aoki, S. (2002). Clonazepam augmentation of antidepressants: does it distinguish unipolar from bipolar depression? *Journal of Affective Disorder, 71,* 217–220.

Nierenberg, A. A., Miyahara, S., Spencer, T., Wisniewski, S. R., Otto, M. W., Pollack, M. H., et al. (in press). Clinical and diagnostic implications of Lifetime ADHD Comorbidity in adults with bipolar disorder: Data from the first 1000 STEP-BD participants. *Biological Psychiatry.*

O'Connell, R. A., Mayo, J. A., Flatlow, L., Cuthbertson, B., & O'Brien, B. E. (1991). Outcome of bipolar disorder on long-term treatment with lithium. *British Journal of Psychiatry, 159,* 123–129.

Otto, M. W. & Miklowitz, D. J. (2004). The role and impact of psychotherapy in the management of bipolar disorder. *CNS Spectrums, 9 (11 Suppl 12),* 27–32.

Otto, M. W., Smits, J. A. J., & Reese, H. E. (2005). Combined psychotherapy and pharmacotherapy for mood and anxiety disorders in adults: Review and analysis. *Clinical Psychology: Science and Practice* 12, 72–86.

Perlis, R. H., Miyahara, S., Marangell, L. B., Wisniewski, S. R., Ostacher, M., DelBello, M. P., et al. (2004). Long-Term implications of early onset in bipolar disorder: Data from the first 1000 participants in the systematic treatment enhancement program for bipolar disorder (STEP-BD). *Biological Psychiatry, 55(9),* 875–881.

Perlis, R. H., Sachs, G. S., Lafer, B., Otto, M. W., Faraone, S. V., & Rosenbaum, J. F. (2002). Effect of abrupt change from standard to low serum lithium levels: A reanalysis of double-blind lithium maintenance data. *American Journal of Psychiatry, 159,* 1155–1159.

Perry, A., Tarrier, N., Morriss, R., McCarthy, E., & Limb, K. (1999). Randomised controlled trial of efficacy of teaching patients with bipolar disorder to identify early warning signs or relapse and obtain treatment. *British Medical Journal, 318,* 149–153.

Priebe, S., Wildgrube, C., & Muller-Oerlinghausen, B. (1989). Lithium prophylaxis and expressed emotion. *British Journal of Psychiatry, 154,* 396–399.

Rea, M. M., Tompson, M. C., Miklowitz, D. J., Goldstein, M. J., Hwang, S., & Mintz, J. (2003). Family-focused treatment versus individual treatment for bipolar disorder: Results of a randomized clinical trial. *Journal of Consulting and Clinical Psychology, 71,* 482–492.

Regier, D., Farmer, M., Rae, D., Locke, B., Keith, S., Judd, L., et al. (1990). Comorbidity of mental illness with alcohol and drug abuse: Results from the Epidemiologic Catchment Area (ECA) study. *Journal of the American Medical Association, 264,* 2511–2518.

Reich, L. H., Davies, R. K., & Himmelhoch, J. M. (1974). Excessive alcohol use in manic-depressive illness. *American Journal of Psychiatry, 131(1),* 83–86.

Sachs, G. S. (1990). Use of clonazepam for bipolar affective disorder. *Journal of Clinical Psychiatry, 51(5, Suppl.),* 31–34.

Sachs, G., Thase, M. E., Otto, M. W., Bauer, M., Miklowitz, D., Wisniewski, S. R. et al. (2003). Rationale, design, and methods of the systematic treatment enhancement program for bipolar disorder (STEP-BD). *Biological Psychiatry, 53,* 1028–1042.

Sachs, G. S., Guille, C., & McMurrich, S. (2002). A Clinical Monitoring Form for Mood Disorders. *Bipolar Disorders, 4*, 323–327.

Scott, J., Garland, A., Moorhead, S. (2001). A pilot study of cognitive therapy in bipolar disorders. *Psychological Medicine, 31*, 459–467.

Schneck, C. D., Miklowitz, D. J., Calabrese, J. R., Allen, M. H., Thomas, M. R., Wisniewski, S. R., et al. (2004). Phenomenology of rapid-cycling bipolar disorder: data from the first 500 participants in the Systematic Treatment Enhancement Program. *American Journal of Psychiatry, 161(10)*, 1902–1908.

Simon, N. M., Otto, M. W., Weiss, R., Bauer, M. S., Miyahara, S., Wisniewski, S. R., et al. (2004). Pharmacotherapy for bipolar disorder and comorbid conditions: Baseline data from STEP-BD. *Journal of Clinical Psychopharmacology, 24*, 512–520.

Simoneau, T. L., Miklowitz, D. J., Richards, J. A., Saleem, R., & George, E. L. (1999). Bipolar disorder and family communication: Effects of a psychoeducational treatment program. *Journal of Abnormal Psychology, 108*, 588–597.

Spitzer, R., Williams, J., & Gibbon, M. (1996). *Structured Clinical Interview for DSM-IV, Outpatient Version (SCID-OP)*. New York: Biometrics Research Department, New York State Psychiatric Institute.

Tohen, M., Waternaux, C. M., & Tsuang, M. T. (1990). Outcome in mania: A 4-year prospective follow-up of 75 patients utilizing survival analysis. *Archives of General Psychiatry, 47*, 1106–1111.

Winkler, D., Willeit, M., Wolf, R., Stamenkovic, M., Tauscher, J., Pjrek, E., et al. (2003). Clonazepam in the long-term treatment of patients with unipolar depression,bipolar and schizoaffective disorder. *European Neuropsychopharmacology, 13*, 129–134.

Young, R. C., Biggs, J. T., Ziegler, V. E., Meyer, D. A. (1978). A rating scale for mania: reliability, validity and sensitivity. *British Journal of Psychiatry, 133*, 429–435.

Zaretsky, A. E., Segal, Z. V., & Gemar, M. (1999). Cognitive therapy for bipolar depression: A pilot study. *Canadian Journal of Psychiatry, 44*, 491–494.

CHAPTER 13

Body Dysmorphic Disorder

Fugen Neziroglu • Sony Khemlani-Patel • Jose A. Yaryura-Tobias

WHAT IS BODY DYSMORPHIC DISORDER?

Body Dysmorphic Disorder (BDD) is an excessive preoccupation with an imagined or slight defect in one's physical appearance, not better accounted for by other disorders, such as Anorexia Nervosa (APA, 2000). BDD patients presenting with beliefs reaching delusional proportions receive an additional diagnosis of "Delusional Disorder, Somatic Type," although the need for dual diagnosis is questionable (Phillips, 2004). Current prevalence rates are estimated at 0.1–1% in the general population (Hollander & Wong, 1995), 3.2% in an outpatient clinical population (Zimmerman & Mattia, 1998) and up to 13% in an inpatient setting (Grant, Kim, & Crow, 2001).

BDD was first recognized in 1891 by an Italian psychiatrist by the name of Morselli. He described BDD as a fear of being/becoming deformed accompanied by much anxiety, calling it "dysmorphophobia." Interestingly, he noted many of the symptoms described in the current literature, including overvalued ideation and compulsive behavior.

Morselli's label "dysmorphphobia" was used until 1987 when the term "Body Dysmorphic Disorder" was introduced into the DSM nomenclature. The scant available literature on BDD vacillated between describing the disorder as a symptom of another disorder, as part of a personality disorder and eventually as a separate syndrome (Thomas, 1984, 1985) in the DSM-III-R in 1987. The major revision in the DSM-IV allowed for an additional diagnosis of Delusional Disorder, Somatic Type, to identify individuals whose beliefs reached delusional intensity.

Individuals with BDD can become preoccupied with any aspect of their physical appearance, although focus on the head area is the most common, such as excessive acne or facial blemishes, a large nose, or a receding hairline (Neziroglu & Yaryura-Tobias, 1993a; Phillips, 1996a,b; Phillips, McElroy, Keck, Pope, & Hudson, 1993). Research indicates that concern with more than one body part at the same time or shifting focus during the course of the illness is quite common. BDD involving the muscularity of the entire body is termed "muscle dysmorphia" (Phillips, O'Sullivan, & Pope, 1997; Pope, Gruber, Choi, Olivardia, & Phillips, 1997).

BDD patients present with a number of safety or avoidance behaviors typically aimed at checking and/or improving the defect (Perugi, Akiskal, Giannotti, Frare, DiVaio, & Cassano, 1997; Phillips, et al., 1993). Most frequently, patients engage in either excessive mirror checking or mirror avoidance, sometimes vacillating between the two extremes. Camouflaging behaviors are also quite common, using either clothing, make-up, as well as changing posture in order to hide or improve the body part of concern. Avoidance of public places and social situations occurs in almost all patients with BDD, with rates as high as 89% (Perugi, et al., 1997) to 97% of research participants (Phillips, et al., 1993). Patients may go to great lengths to function with accommodations to their daily life, such as saving daily errands for less crowded times, sitting

Neziroglu, F., Khemlani-Patel, S., & Yaryura-Tobias, J. A. (2006). In Fisher J. E. & W. T. O'Donohue (Eds.), *Practitioner's guide to evidence-based psychotherapy*. New York: Springer.

in the back of a classroom, and using drive-thru restaurants, which may eventually lead to individuals being housebound and isolated for years. Patients may also seek repeated consults with cosmetic and/or dermatological procedures and go to great lengths to find the financial resources to seek various appearance altering procedures. In extreme situations, patients have even engaged in "do it yourself" surgery (Veale, 2000), by purposely breaking one's nose or removing acne with sharp implements. Individuals preoccupied with skin blemishes may engage in skin picking or digging (Phillips & Taub, 1995), which ironically can lead to visible scars and in some cases, severe damage (O'Sullivan, Philips, Keuthen, & Wilhelm, 1999).

BASIC FACTS ABOUT BODY DYSMORPHIC DISORDER

Gender

Research has consistently shown that BDD occurs equally in men and women (Phillips, 1991, Phillips & Diaz, 1997, Perugi, et al., 1997).

Age

Individuals with BDD typically display symptoms in their teen years, with onset between the ages of 14–17 (Phillips, et al., 1993; Veale, et al., 1996), although earlier onset has been seen in clinical practice.

Classification

Although BDD is currently classified as a "Somatoform Disorder" within the DSM system, recent research indicates that it may be better classified within the "Obsessive Compulsive Spectrum Disorders" (Hollander, Liebowitz, Winchel, Klumer, & Klein, 1989; McElroy, Phillips, & Keck, 1994; McKay, Neziroglu, Yaryura-Tobias, 1997; Neziroglu & Yaryura-Tobias, 1993a; Phillips, et al., 1993). The "Obsessive Compulsive Spectrum" refers to a cluster of disorders which display similar features to OCD, such as obsessive thoughts, compulsive behaviors as well as similar course, demographics, family history, and response to psychological and pharmacological treatment (Hollander, 1993; Hollander & Wong, 1995; McElroy, et al., 1994). There is some debate regarding the inclusion of disorders within the spectrum. Currently, Body Dysmorphic Disorder, Hypochondriasis, Anorexia Nervosa, Trichotillomania, and Tourette's Syndrome are primarily included within the spectrum (Yaryura-Tobias & Neziroglu, 1997). Others (Cohen, Simeon, Hollander, & Stein, 1997) have proposed that disorders involving impulsive behaviors, such as repetitive self-injury, kleptomania, pyromania, sexual acting out behaviors, paraphilias, and pathological gambling as well as repetitive habit disorders, such as skin picking and nail biting should also be included.

Etiology

The etiology of BDD is multifaceted, similar to most psychological disorders. Sociocultural factors, such as exposure to unrealistic standards of beauty in the media may certainly have an impact similar to eating disorders. Psychological theories with psychodynamic theorists positing that BDD is a symbolic representation of unresolved conflicts (Bloch & Glue, 1988) and cognitive and behavioral therapists viewing it as a result of operant conditioning (Braddock, 1982), classical and operant conditioning (Neziroglu, 2004) and rehearsal of negative self-statements (Rosen, Reiter & Orosan, 1995). Traumatic incidents, such as abuse in childhood and adolescence (Neziroglu, Khemlani-Patel, Hsia, & Yaryura-Tobias, 2001; Neziroglu, Khemlani-Patel, Roberts, & Yaryura-Tobias, 2004) as well as accidents, teasing, family criticism, and operations have all been implicated (Rosen, 1995; Roskes, 1999).

Neurobiological theories consist of genetic, pathophysiological, and neuroanatomical explanations of BDD. Genetic studies with OC Spectrum disorders suggest a high rate of OCD in family members of BDD patients. In one study, 17% of the family members of 50 patients with BDD had OCD (Hollander, Cohen, & Simeon, 1993). BDD in first-degree relatives of OCD patients has also been noted (Bienvenu, et al., 2000).

Similar response of BDD and OCD to serotonin reuptake inhibitors suggests that a dysfunction in the serotonin system may be implicated in the etiology of BDD. Further evidence comes from case reports demonstrating worsening of BDD symptoms with low levels of tryptophan, which is the amino acid precursor of serotonin (Barr, Goodman, & Price, 1992) as well as with abuse of cyproheptadine, a serotonin antagonist (Craven & Rodin, 1987).

Neuroanatomical studies of BDD are quite scarce. Regional brain volumes were measured using morphometric magnetic resonance imaging in one preliminary case series of eight women with BDD (Rauch, et al., 2003). Results demonstrated that BDD patients exhibited a relative leftward shift in caudate symmetry and greater total white matter compared to healthy controls. Neuropsychological research has shown that BDD patient perform poorly on tests of executive functioning involving prefrontal lobe functioning (Hanes, 1998).

Since it is well known that body image distortions, such as agnosia, phantom limb phenomena and Gerstman's syndrome, are associated with lesions in the parietal lobe, it has been hypothesized that dysfunction in the somatosensory cortex may play a role in BDD (Yaryura-Tobias, Neziroglu, & Torres-Gallegos, 2002). Lesions in the somatosensory cortex, which borders the frontal and parietal lobes of the brain, can cause loss of perception or reception. Since an interdependence exists between the lobes of the brain via various pathways, it is difficult to localize BDD to one neuroanatomical area. It is possible that BDD may involve the basal ganglia, the prefrontal cortex, as well as the parietal lobe. Further research will certainly help clarify the issue.

Comorbidity

BDD patients are a challenge to treat due to a high degree of co-morbid conditions, including mood disorders (Phillips, 1991; Phillips, et al., 1993; Neziroglu & Yaryura-Tobias, 1993b), anxiety disorders (Brawman-Mintzer, et al., 1995; Phillips, et al., 1993; Wilhelm, Otto, Zucker, & Pollack, 1997) and personality disorders (Neziroglu, McKay, Todaro, & Yaryura-Tobias, 1996; Phillips & McElroy, 2000; Cohen, et al., 2000). Major depression seems to be the most common comorbid condition with BDD. Rates of depression range from 71% (Neziroglu, et al., 1996) to 78% for a lifetime occurrence (Gunstad & Phillips, 2003). Interestingly, one recent comorbidity study found that comorbid depression tended to occur after the onset of BDD, possibly suggesting that depression may be a complication of BDD (Gunstad & Phillips, 2003). Rates for comorbidity between OCD and BDD range from 16% (Bienvenu, et al., 2000) to 37% of OCD meeting criteria for BDD (Hollander, et al., 1993). Studies have also found that the lifetime incidence of OCD in a BDD population ranges around 30–37% (Gunstad & Phillips, 2003; Phillips, et al., 1993).

Associated Features

The primary associated feature with BDD is the presence of "overvalued ideation," which can be defined as a "fixed belief with doubting overtones that is unresponsive to challenges," with an underlying affective component (Neziroglu & Yaryura-Tobias, 1997). Overvalued ideation may fall on a continuum between rational thoughts and delusions, with patients fluctuating along this continuum during the course of their illness (Kozak & Foa, 1994). In other words, individuals with BDD believe quite strongly in the presence of their "defect." They are often not responsive to evidence that suggests the contrary and can be quite challenging to treat.

The disorder can lead to significant impairment in academics, occupation, and social life. Employment history and status is poor; most studies have reported that approximately 50% of participants are employed, with some working only part-time (Perugi, et al., 1997; Veale, et al., 1996). Low rates have also been found for marital status; approximately 75% of patients were single in one study (Phillips, et al., 1994). As a result, quality of life had been found to be worse than those suffering from diabetes or myocardial infarctions (Phillips, 2000). A high incidence of suicidal ideation and attempts, from 40% (Phillips, et al., 1993) to 45% (Perugi, et al., 1997) as well as a high incidence of BDD related hospitalizations (Khemlani-Patel, 2001; Phillips, et al., 1993) complicates the clinical picture.

Recent research also indicates that BDD individuals may place an excessive value assigned to attractiveness (Veale & Lambrou, 2001) that in addition to overvalued ideas contributes to low motivation to engage in psychological treatment.

ASSESSMENT

What Should Be Ruled Out?

There is much shame and secrecy in BDD, so much so that it often goes undiagnosed even when an individual is already seeking mental health services. In addition, BDD symptoms can often overlap with other mental health diagnoses, such as Social Anxiety Disorder, Obsessive Compulsive Disorder, Major Depression, Panic Disorder with Agoraphobia, Psychotic Disorders, and Avoidant Personality Disorder. Proper identification of the disorder and any comorbid conditions is crucial in proper treatment. If a patient displays any avoidance of social situations, has treatment resistant depression, obsessive thoughts, and picks his/her skin, it is worth probing for any body image disturbance, particularly BDD. Furthermore, patients who already present with an obsessive compulsive spectrum disorder should be screened for BDD since a high degree of comorbidity exists between these disorders and BDD (Brawman-Mintzer, et al., 1995; Phillips, et al., 1993; Wilhelm, et al., 1997).

What is Involved in Effective Assessment?

Identification of BDD can be straightforward with the help of proper self-report and interview tools. The Yale Brown Obsessive Compulsive Scale for BDD (YBOCS-BDD; Phillips, et al., 1997) and the Body Dysmorphic Disorder Exam (BDDE; Rosen & Reiter, 1996) were specifically designed for the assessment of BDD. In addition, simply asking a patient if they are particularly concerned about any part of their physical appearance along with related avoidance, checking, or appearance altering behaviors can indicate a possible diagnosis.

Other useful instruments include the Overvalued Ideas Scale (OVIS) (Neziroglu, McKay, Yaryura-Tobias, Stevens, & Todaro, 1999; Neziroglu, Stevens, & Yaryura-Tobias, 1999; Neziroglu, Stevens, McKay, & Yaryura-Tobias, 2001), the Brown Assessment of Beliefs (Eisen, et al., 1998) as well as depression and anxiety measures, such as the Beck Depression Inventory-II (Beck, Steer, & Brown, 1996) and the Beck Anxiety Inventory (Beck, Epstein, Brown, & Steer, 1988). Since there is significant impairment in daily functioning and a low quality of life, an instrument such as the "Quality of Life Inventory" (Frisch, 1994) can better assess BDD's impact on functioning. Since, BDD is often accompanied by a reluctance to engage and comply with treatment recommendations, a measure of readiness and or motivation to change should also be an integral component of an initial evaluation.

Clinicians should also be astute about suicidal ideation, since it is such a common occurrence in patients with BDD. A full lethality assessment may be helpful during initial sessions.

What are Effective Evidence-Based Psychological Treatments?

Based on current clinical and research evidence, cognitive and behavioral treatment seems to be the treatment of choice for BDD. The treatment for BDD is based on approaches for OCD and it is quite similar in nature, primarily involving in-vivo and/or imaginal exposure and response prevention (ERP) as well as cognitive therapy using either the Beck or Ellis approach.

Much of the current literature consists of case reports or case series with minimal control of treatment frequency, duration, and medication. Overall, results of studies indicate that in vivo or imaginal exposure and response prevention (ERP) (Braddock, 1982; Campisi, 1995; Marks & Mishan, 1988; McKay, et al., 1997; Munjack, 1978), cognitive therapy (Geremia & Neziroglu, 2001) as well as the combination is effective (Khemlani-Patel, 2001; Neziroglu & Yaryura-Tobias, 1993b; Schmidt & Harrington, 1995; Veale, et al., 1996). Studies reporting results with group treatment are also promising (Rosen, et al., 1995; Wilhelm, Otto, Lohr, & Deckersbach, 1999). In general, we have found with BDD an intensive treatment approach is more effective than weekly sessions. Family involvement can lead to quicker treatment gains as well. For a more complete review of the literature, see Neziroglu & Khemlani-Patel (2002).

In order for cognitive therapy to be effective, the appropriate core beliefs should be targeted in treatment rather than engaging the patient in a debate regarding the presence or absence of their perceived defect. Common BDD beliefs include: (1) happiness comes from looking good, (2) physical perfection is a necessary and achievable goal in life, and (3) one cannot succeed fully in life without beauty.

What are Effective Self-Help Treatments?

There are no known self-help treatment approaches for BDD. There is one workbook by Claiborn & Pedrick (2002) which offers some guidelines on changing attitudes and behaviors related to body image issues in general and for BDD.

Other Issues in Management

In general, patients with BDD are reluctant to be in psychological therapy. Why should one seek mental health services when the real problem is due to physical appearance? In fact, patients may wait up to nine years to seek the appropriate services (Perugi, et al., 1997). The initial phases of treatment, such as psycho-education and rapport building, may have to be lengthened for patients with BDD. In addition, motivational issues, suicidality, and/or comorbidity may have to be targeted first. If the patient is too depressed, is suicidal, or homebound, then hospitalization may be the initial treatment step.

The practitioner should also be aware that treating a patient with BDD may involve educating other medical and mental health professionals about the disorder, since it is still not that well known. Collaboration with dermatologists and cosmetic surgeons may be required, since patients commonly seek out those services during the course of psychological treatment. Of course getting such cooperation is not so easy, nor is it easy to convince patients that they should forgo cosmetic or dermatological interventions while they are engaging in cognitive and behavior therapy.

The key in treating BDD effectively is being flexible in one's treatment style. For example, BDD patients may require sessions late at night when the waiting room is empty, phone sessions if they are homebound, out of office sessions, as well being accompanied to their next cosmetic surgery consult. The latter we have found to be helpful in some instances because the patient often misinterprets the information given to them by the surgeon or dermatologist.

What is Effective Medical Treatment?

Pharmacological studies have demonstrated consistent results with the use of the newer generation of anti-depressants called the "selective serotonin reuptake inhibitors" (SSRIs) which have been successful in various diagnoses including OCD and Major Depression. SSRIs are known as "broad spectrum" drugs, effective in a variety of psychiatric disorders, including BDD (Phillips, 1996c). Case reports and open label studies have demonstrated success with fluoxetine (Brady, Austin, & Lydiard, 1990), and fluvoxamine (Kaplan & Lictenberg, 1995; Phillips, Dwight, & McElroy, 1998; Phillips, McElroy, Dwightman, Eisen, & Rasmussen, 2001). Recently, more controlled studies with BDD also corroborate earlier research with positive responses to fluoxetine (Phillips, Albertini, & Rasmussen, 2002). A positive treatment response has also been found with medications that are serotonin reuptake blockers, but not selective for serotonin alone, such as clomipramine (Hollander, et al., 1999). Response to SRI's seems to be positive even in cases of delusional BDD (Phillips, Dwightman, et al., 2001; Phillips, et al., 1994).

Augmentation strategies are often necessary for BDD, such as with buspirone (Phillips, 2002; Phillips, Albertini, Siniscalchi, Khan, & Robinson, 2001) and neuroleptics (Phillips, 1994; Yaryura-Tobias & Neziroglu, 1997). The general consensus indicates that higher SRI doses, augmentation strategies, and longer treatment trials lead to the most positive outcomes (Phillips, 2002).

How Does One Select Among Treatments?

Although the literature is so limited, there is consensus that a combination of cognitive, behavioral, and psychopharmacological approaches leads to the most positive outcome. In making a decision about which approach to implement first, therapists should consider the following: (1) is the patient too depressed or obsessional to engage in psychological treatment? If so, then a consultation with a psychopharmacologist may be the first step. (2) Is the patient at high risk for a suicide attempt or made previous attempts? If so, then hospitalization and medication may be the first step. (3) Is the patient's beliefs quite strong, highly overvalued, or are they too fearful to engage in ERP exercises? If so, then at least 12 sessions of cognitive therapy alone may be the first step in conjunction with medication.

In the authors' clinical experience, all BDD patients may benefit from initial cognitive therapy sessions as well as medication before proceeding with the more challenging behavioral therapy.

CONCLUSION

BDD is a very severe and chronic disorder that greatly impairs the individual. Many patients are unable to go to school or work, become homebound, suicidal and hospitalized. Most patients are secretive and do not reveal their symptoms unless asked.

They are more likely to talk about social anxiety or depression rather than preoccupation with their appearance. BDD is considered part of the obsessive compulsive spectrum disorders and is treated very similarly to OCD, although BDD patients tend to have more overvalued ideas and depression. They respond to cognitive and behavior therapy as well as psychopharmacological treatment with SSRI's. Usually a combination of all treatment modalities administered intensively, meaning several prolonged sessions is most effective.

REFERENCES

American Psychiatric Association. (2000). *Diagnostic and statistical manual of mental disorders: Fourth edition-text revision.* Washington, DC: American Psychiatric Association.

Barr, L. C., Goodman, W. K., & Price, L. H. (1992). Acute exacerbation of body dysmorphic disorder during tryptophan depletion. *American Journal of Psychiatry, 149,* 1406–1407.

Beck, A. T., Epstein, N., Brown, G., & Steer, R. A. (1988). The Beck Anxiety Inventory. San Antonio: Harcourt, Brace, Jovanovich, Inc.

Beck, A. T., Steer, R. A., & Brown, G. (1996). *The Beck Depression Inventory-Second Edition.* San Antonio: Harcourt, Brace, & Company.

Bienvenu, O. J., Samuels, J. F., Riddle, M. A., Hoehn-Saric, R., Liang, K-Y, Cullen, B. A. M., et al. (2000). The relationship of obsessive-compulsive disorder to possible spectrum disorders: Results from a family study.

Bloch, S., & Glue, P. (1988). Psychotherapy and dysmorphophobia: A case report. *British Journal of Psychiatry, 152,* 271–274.

Braddock, L. E. (1982). Dysmorphophobia in adolescence: A case report. *British Journal of Psychiatry, 140,* 199–201.

Brady, K. T., Austin, L., & Lydiard, R. B. (1990). Body dysmorphic disorder: The relationship to obsessive compulsive disorder. *Journal of Nervous and Mental Disease, 178,* 538–540.

Brawman-Mintzer, O., Lydiard, B., Phillips, K. A., Morton, A., Czepowicz, V., Emmanuel, N., et al. (1995). Body dysmorphic disorder in patients with anxiety disorders and major depression: A comorbidity study. *American Journal of Psychiatry, 152,* 1665–1667.

Campisi, T. A. (1995). Exposure and response prevention in the treatment of body dysmorphic disorder. Doctoral dissertation, Hofstra University, Hempstead, NY.

Claiborn, J., & Pedrick, C. (2002). The BDD Workbook: Overcome body dysmorphic disorder and end body image obsessions. New Harbinger Publications.

Cohen, L. J., Kingston, P., Bell, A., Kown, J., Aronowitz, B., & Hollander, E. (2000). Co-morbid personality impairment in body dysmorphic disorder. *Comprehensive Psychiatry, 41,* 4–12.

Cohen, L. J., Simeon, D., Hollander, E., Stein, D. J. (1997). In Hollander and D. J. Stein (Eds.) *Obsessive compulsive spectrum disorders in obsessive compulsive disorders: Diagnosis, etiology and treatment.* New York: Marcel Dekker, 1997.

Craven, J. L., & Rodin, G. M. (1987). Cyproheptadine dependence associated with an atypical somatoform disorder. *Canadian Journal of Psychiatry, 32,* 143–145.

Eisen, J. L., Phillips, K. A., Baer, L., Beer, D. A., Atala, K. D., & Rasmussen, S. A. (1998). The Brown Assessment of Beliefs Scale: Reliability and validity. *American Journal of Psychiatry, 155,* 102–108.

Frisch, M. B. (1994). *The quality of life inventory.* National Computer Systems, Inc.

Geremia, G. M., & Neziroglu, F. (2001). Cognitive therapy in the treatment of body dysmorphic disorder. *Clinical Psychology and Psychotherapy, 8,* 243–251.

Grant, J. E., Kim, S. W., & Crow, S. J. (2001). Prevalence and clinical features of body dysmorphic disorder in adolescent and adult psychiatric inpatients. *Journal of Clinical Psychiatry, 62,* 517–522.

Gunstad, J. & Phillips, K. A. (2003). Axis I comorbidity in body dysmorphic disorder. *Comprehensive Psychiatry, 44,* 270–276.

Hanes, K. R. (1998). Neuropsychological performance in body dysmorphic disorder. *Journal of the International Neuropsychological Society, 4,* 167–171.

Hollander, E. (1993). Obsessive-compulsive spectrum disorders: An overview. *Psychiatric Annals, 23,* 355–358.

Hollander, E., Allen, A., Kown, J., Aronowitz, B., Schmeidler, J., Wong, C., et al. (1999). Clomipramine vs. desipramine crossover trial in body dysmorphic disorder. *Archives of General Psychiatry, 56,* 1033–1039.

Hollander, E., Cohen, L., & Simeon, D. (1993) Body dysmorphic disorder. *Psychiatric Annals, 23,* 359–364.

Hollander, E, Liebowitz, M. R., Winchel, R., Klumker, A., & Klein, D. F. (1989). Treatment of body dysmorphic disorder with serotonin reuptake blockers. *American Journal of Psychiatry, 146,* 768–770.

Hollander, E., & Wong, C. M. (1995). Obsessive-compulsive spectrum disorders. *Journal of Clinical Psychiatry, 56 (Suppl. 4)*, 3–6.

Kaplan, Z., & Lictenberg, P. (1995). Delusional disorder, somatic subtype, treated with fluvoxamine. *European Journal of Psychiatry, 9*, 238–241.

Khemlani-Patel, S. (2001). Cognitive and behavioral therapy for body dysmorphic disorder: A comparative investigation. Doctoral Dissertation. Hofstra University: Hempstead, New York.

Kozak, M. J., & Foa, E. B. (1994). Obsessions, overvalued ideas and delusions in obsessive compulsive disorder. *Behavior Research and Therapy, 32*, 343–353.

Marks, I., & Mishan, J. (1988). Dysmorphic avoidance with disturbed bodily perception. A pilot study of exposure therapy. *British Journal of Psychiatry, 152*, 674–678.

McElroy, S. L., Phillips, K. A., & Keck, P. E. (1994). Obsessive compulsive spectrum disorders. *Journal of Clinical Psychiatry, 55*, 33–51.

McElroy, S. L., Phillips, K. A., Keck, P. E., Hudson, J. I., & Pope, H. G. (1993). Body dysmorphic disorder: Does it have a psychotic subtype? *Journal of Clinical Psychiatry, 54*, 389–395.

McKay, D., Neziroglu, F., & Yaryura-Tobias, J. A. (1997). Comparison of clinical characteristics in obsessive compulsive disorder and body dysmorphic disorder. *Journal of Anxiety Disorders, 11*, 447–454.

McKay, D., Todaro, J., Neziroglu, F., Campisi, T., Moritz, K., & Yaryura-Tobias, J. A. (1997). Body dysmorphic disorder: A preliminary evaluation of treatment and maintenance using exposure and response prevention. *Behavior Research and Therapy, 35*, 67–70.

Munjack, D. J. (1978). The behavioral treatment of dysmorphophobia. *Journal of Behavior Therapy and Experimental Psychiatry, 9*, 53–56.

Neziroglu F. (2004). How to apply cognitive and behavior therapy for body dysmorphic disorder. Symposium chair (Neziroglu). Body Dysmorphic Disorder: Is it a mind, body or socio-cultural problem and how do you treat it. Update. American Psychiatric Association Meeting, New York, May 2004.

Neziroglu, F., & Khemlani-Patel, S. (2002). A review of cognitive and behavior treatment of body dysmorphic disorder. *CNS Spectrums, 7*, 464–471.

Neziroglu, F., Khemlani-Patel, S., Hsia, C., & Yaryura-Tobias, J. A. (2001, July). *Incidence of abuse in body dysmorphic disorder*. Paper presented at the World Congress of Behavioral and Cognitive Therapies. Vancouver, BC, Canada.

Neziroglu, F., Khemlani-Patel, S., Roberts, M., & Yaryura-Tobias, J. A. (2004). Prevalence of abuse in body dysmorphic disorder and obsessive compulsive disorder. Unpublished manuscript.

Neziroglu, F., McKay, D., Todaro, J., & Yaryura-Tobias, J. A. (1996). Effect of cognitive behavior therapy on persons with body dysmorphic disorder and co-morbid axis II diagnoses. *Behavior Therapy, 27*, 67–77.

Neziroglu, F., McKay, D., Yaryura-Tobias, J. A. Stevens, K., & Todaro, J. (1999). The overvalued ideas scale: Development, reliability and validity in obsessive compulsive disorder. *Behavior Research and Therapy, 37*, 881–902.

Neziroglu, F., Stevens, K. P., McKay, D., Yaryura-Tobias, J. A. (2001). Predictive validity of the overvalued ideas scale: Outcome in obsessive-compulsive and body dysmorphic disorders. *Behavior Research and Therapy, 39*, 745–756.

Neziroglu, F., Stevens, K., Yaryura-Tobias, J. A. (1999). Overvalued ideas and their impact on treatment outcome. *Revista Brasileira de Psiquiatria, 21*, 209–216.

Neziroglu, F., & Yaryura-Tobias, J. A. (1993a). Body dysmorphic disorder: Phenomenology and case descriptions. *Behavioural Psychotherapy, 21*, 27–36.

Neziroglu, F., & Yaryura-Tobias, J. A. (1993b). Exposure, response prevention, and cognitive therapy in the treatment of body dysmorphic disorder. *Behavior Therapy, 1993, 24*, 431–438.

Neziroglu, F., & Yaryura-Tobias, J. A. (1997). A review of cognitive behavioral and pharmacological treatment of body dysmorphic disorder. *Behavior Modification, 21*, 324–340.

O'Sullivan, R. L., Phillips, K. A., Keuthen, N. J., & Wilhelm, S. (1999). Near fatal skin picking from delusional body dysmorphic disorder responsive to fluvoxamine. *Psychosomatics, 40*, 79–81.

Perugi, G., Akiskal, H. S., Giannotti, D., Frare, F., DiVaio, S., & Cassano, G. B. (1997). Gender related differences in body dysmorphic disorder (Dysmorphophobia). *Journal of Nervous and Mental Disease, 185*, 578–582.

Phillips, K. A. (1991). Body dysmorphic disorder: The distress of imagined ugliness. *American Journal of Psychiatry, 148*, 1138–1149.

Phillips, K. A. (1996a). *The Broken Mirror*. New York: Oxford University Press.

Phillips, K. A. (1996b). Body dysmorphic disorder: Diagnosis and treatment of imagined ugliness. *Journal of Clinical Psychiatry, 57 (Suppl. 8)*, 61–64.

Phillips, K. A. (1996c). Pharmacological treatment of body dysmorphic disorder. *Psychopharmacology Bulletin, 32*, 597–605.

Phillips, K. A. (2000). Quality of life for patients with body dysmorphic disorder. *Journal of Nervous and Mental Disease, 188*, 170–175.

Phillips, K. A. (2002). Pharmacologic treatment of body dysmorphic disorder: Review of the evidence and a recommended treatment approach. *CNS Spectrum, 7*, 453–463.

Phillips, K. A. (2004). Psychosis in body dysmorphic disorder. *Journal of Psychiatric Research, 38*, 63–72.

Phillips, K. A., Albertini, R. S., Siniscalchi, J. M., Khan, A., & Robinson, M. (2001). Effectiveness of pharmacotherapy for body dysmorphic disorder: A chart review study. *Journal of Clinical Psychiatry, 62,* 721–727.

Phillips, K. A., & Diaz, S. F. (1997). Gender differences in body dysmorphic disorder. *The Journal of Nervous and Mental Disease, 185,* 570–577.

Phillips, K. A., Dwight, M. M., & McElroy, S. L. (1998). Efficacy and safety of fluvoxamine in body dysmorphic disorder. *Journal of Clinical Psychiatry, 59,* 165–171.

Phillips, K. A., Hollander, E., Rasmussen, S. A., Aronowitz, B. R., DeCaria, C., & Goodman, W. K. (1997). A severity rating scale for body dysmorphic disorder: Development, reliability, and validity of a modified version of the Yale brown obsessive compulsive scale. *Psychopharmacology Bulletin, 33,* 17–22.

Phillips, K. A. & McElroy, S. (2000). Personality disorders and traits in patients with body dysmorphic disorder. *Comprehensive Psychiatry, 41,* 229–236.

Phillips, K. A., McElroy, S. L., Dwightmen, M. M., Eisen, J. L., & Rasmussen, S. A. (2001). Delusionality and response to open label fluvoxamine in body dysmorphic disorder. *Journal of Clinical Psychiatry, 62,* 87–91.

Phillips, K. A., McElroy, S. L., Keck, P. E., Pope, H. G., & Hudson, J. I. (1993). Body dysmorphic disorder: 30 cases of imagined ugliness. *American Journal of Psychiatry, 150,* 302–308.

Phillips, K. A., O'Sullivan, R. L., & Pope, H. G. (1997). Muscle dysmorphia. *Journal of Clinical Psychiatry, 58,* 361.

Phillips, K. A., McElroy, S. L., Keck, P. E. (1994). Psychopharmacology Bulletin, *30,* 179–186.

Phillips, K. A., Castle, D. J. (2002). In: Disorders of body image. Castle, D. J., Phillips, K. A. Petersfield, England: Wrightson Biomedical Publishing, Ltd, 101–120.

Phillips, K. A., & Taub, S. L. (1995). Skin picking as a symptom of body dysmorphic disorder. *Psychopharmacology Bulletin, 31,* 279–288.

Phillips, K. A., McElroy, S. L., Dwight, M. M. (2001). *Journal of Clinical Psychiatry, 62,* 87–91.

Pope, H. G., Gruber, A. J., Choi, P., Olivardia, R., & Phillips, K. A. (1997). Muscle dysmorphia: An under recognized form of body dysmorphic disorder. *Psychosomatics, 38,* 548–557.

Rauch, S. L., Phillips, K. A., Segal, E., Makris, N., Shin, L. M., Whalen, P. J., et al. (2003). A preliminary morphometric magnetic resonance imaging study of regional brain volumes in body dysmorphic disorder. *Psychiatry Research: Neuroimaging, 122,* 13–19.

Rosen, J. C. (1995). The nature of body dysmorphic disorder and treatment with cognitive behavior therapy. Behavioral Practices, *2*(1), 143–166.

Rosen, J. C., & Reiter, J. (1996). Development of the body dysmorphic disorder exam. *Behavior Research and Therapy, 34,* 755–766.

Rosen, J. C., Reiter, J., & Orosan, P. (1995). Cognitive-behavioral body image therapy for body dysmorphic disorder. *Journal of Consulting and Clinical Psychology, 63,* 263–269.

Roskes, E. (1999). Body dysmorphic disorder and a prosthesis. *Psychosomatics, 40,* 436–437.

Schmidt, N. B., & Harrington, P. (1995). Cognitive-behavioral treatment of body dysmorphic disorder: A case report. *Journal of Behavior Therapy and Experimental Psychiatry, 26,* 161–167.

Simeon, D., Hollander, E., Stein, D. J., Cohen, L., & Aronowitz, B. (1995). Body dysmorphic disorder in the DSM-IV field trial for obsessive compulsive disorder. *American Journal of Psychiatry, 152,* 1207–1209.

Thomas, C. S. (1984). Dysmorphophobia: A question of definition. *British Journal of Psychiatry, 144,* 513–516.

Thomas, C. S. (1985). Disorders with overvalued ideas. *British Journal of Psychiatry, 146,* 215.

Veale, D. (2000). Outcome of cosmetic surgery and "DIY" surgery in patients with body dysmorphic disorder. *Psychiatric Bulletin, 24,* 218–221.

Veale, D. M., Boocock, A., Gournay, K., Dryden, W., Shah, F., Willson, R., et al. (1996). Body dysmorphic disorder: A survey of fifty cases. *British Journal of Psychiatry, 169,* 196–201.

Veale, D., Gournay, K., Dryden, W., Boocock, A., Shah, F., Willson, R., et al. (1996). Body dysmorphic disorder: A cognitive behavioural model and pilot randomized controlled trial. *Behavior Research and Therapy, 34,* 717–729.

Veale, D. M., & Lambrou, C. (2002). The importance of aesthetics in body dysmorphic disorder. *CNS Spectrums, 7,* 429–431.

Wilhelm, S., Otto, M. L., Lohr, B., & Deckersbach, T. (1999). Cognitive behavioral group therapy for body dysmorphic disorder: A case series. *Behavior Research and Therapy, 37,* 71–75.

Wilhelm, S., Otto, M. W., Zucker, B. G., & Pollack, M. H. (1997). Prevalence of body dysmorphic disorder in patients with anxiety disorders. *Journal of Anxiety Disorders, 11,* 499–502.

Yaryura-Tobias, J. A., & Neziroglu, F. (1997). *Obsessive Compulsive Disorders Spectrum: Pathogenesis, Diagnosis, and Treatment.* Washington, DC: American Psychiatric Press, Inc.

Yaryura-Tobias, J. A., Neziroglu, F., & Torres-Gallegos, M. (2002). Neuroanatomical correlates and somatosensorial disturbances in body dysmorphic disorder. *CNS Spectrums, 7,* 432–434.

Zimmerman, M., & Mattia, J. I. (1998). Body dysmorphic disorder in psychiatric outpatients: Recognition, prevalence, comorbidity, demographic, and clinical correlates. *Comprehensive Psychiatry, 39,* 265–270.

Borderline Personality Disorder

Jennifer Sayrs • Ursula Whiteside

WHAT IS BORDERLINE PERSONALITY DISORDER?

Borderline personality disorder (BPD) is a serious mental disorder involving a pervasive dysfunction of the emotion regulation system. The hallmark features of this disorder include impulsive, self-destructive behavior (including self mutilation, suicide attempts, and suicide threats), as well as chaotic and stormy interpersonal relationships. This chronic and severely debilitating disorder is believed to have its roots in both biological and environmental factors. For a diagnosis of BPD as defined by the American Psychiatric Association's (APA) Diagnostic and Statistical Manual of Mental Disorders (DSM-IV-TR; APA, 2000), one must meet five of nine criteria which can be organized into four areas of problematic functioning (Lieb, Zanarini, Schmahl, Linehan, & Bohus, 2004; Linehan, 1993a). These patterns must be long-standing, be present in a number of contexts, and begin before or during early adulthood.

Affective criteria
- Inappropriate, intense anger or difficulty controlling anger (e.g., frequent displays of temper, constant anger, recurrent physical fights)
- Chronic feelings of emptiness
- Affective instability due to a marked reactivity of mood (e.g., intense episodic dysphoria, irritability, or anxiety usually lasting a few hours and only rarely more than a few days)

Cognitive criteria
- Transient, stress-related paranoid ideation or severe dissociative symptoms
- Identity disturbance: markedly and persistently unstable self-image or sense of self

Behavioral criteria (forms of impulsivity)
- Recurrent suicidal behavior, gestures, or threats, or self-mutilating behavior
- Impulsivity in at least two areas that are potentially self-damaging (e.g., spending, sex, substance abuse, reckless driving, binge eating) and do not include suicidal or self-mutilating behavior

Interpersonal criteria
- Frantic efforts to avoid real or imagined abandonment that do not include suicidal or self-mutilating
- A pattern of unstable and intense interpersonal relationships characterized by alternating between extremes of idealization and devaluation

The impulsive behavior that is characteristic of borderline personality disorder can be viewed as a solution to the problem of emotion dysregulation, as well as a consequence of that dysregulation (Linehan, 1993a).

Jennifer Sayrs, Evidence Based Treatment Centers of Seattle and University of Washington, Department of Psychology Ursula Whiteside, University of Washington, Department of Psychology

BASIC FACTS ABOUT BORDERLINE PERSONALITY DISORDER:

- BPD affects 1–2% of the general population (Torgersen, Kringlen & Cramer, 2001).
- 75% of those diagnosed with BPD are female (APA, 2000).
- BPD individuals are five times more likely to have a first degree biological relative with BPD than are individuals in the general population (APA, 2000).
- Despite its low prevalence, BPD individuals comprise 14–20% of mental health inpatients (Widiger & Frances, 1989; Widiger & Weissman, 1991) and 8–11% of outpatients (Widiger & Frances, 1989; Kroll, Sines, & Martin, 1981; Modestin, Abrecht, Tschaggelar, & Hoffman, 1997).
- BPD individuals make up 9–40% of high utilizers of psychiatric treatment (Widiger & Weissman, 1991; Geller, 1986; Surber et al. 1987; Swigar, Astrachan, Levine, Mayfield, & Radovich, 1991; Woogh, 1986).
- 30–60% of individuals diagnosed with a personality disorder meet BPD criteria (APA, 2000).
- Self-inflicted injury, defined as intentional and acute physical self-injurious behavior with or without the intent to die, is reported to be as high as 69–70% in individuals meeting criteria for BPD (Clarkin, Widiger, Francis, Hurt, & Gilmore, 1983; Cowdry, Pickar, & Davies, 1985).
- Individuals with BPD have a lifetime suicide rate of 8–10% (APA, 2000), constitute from 7–38% of all people who complete suicide, and are characterized by high rates of suicide attempts and nonsuicidal, intentional self-injury (Linehan, Rizvi, Welch, & Page, 1999).
- Although suicide rates in BPD are comparable to those for other diagnostic groups, more BPD individuals engage in self-mutilation, attempt suicide, and repeat parasuicide over time (Linehan & Heard, 1999; Tanney, 1992).

ASSESSMENT

What should be ruled out?

Individuals diagnosed with BPD often meet criteria for mood disorders, while individuals with mood disorders sometimes meet criteria for BPD. Both diagnoses may be given, but at times only one diagnosis is appropriate. While the presentation is often similar for mood disorders and BPD, the BPD diagnosis requires an onset in early adulthood and the presence of instability across a variety of contexts (APA, 2000).

There is significant overlap between BPD and other personality disorders. The DSM-IV-TR (APA, 2000) suggests the following guidelines for distinguishing between BPD and other personality disorders (PD):

- *Histrionic PD* does not generally include self-destructiveness, close relationships characterized with anger, and reports of emptiness and loneliness.
- *Schizotypal PD*-related paranoia is more stable and independent of changes in environmental variables.
- *Paranoid PD* and *Narcissistic PD* do not generally include the self destructiveness, impulsivity, instability of self, and fears of abandonment typical for BPD.
- *Antisocial PD* behavior may also be considered "manipulative," but is typically not engaged in as a means to gain the concern of others as can be the case with BPD.
- *Dependent PD* does not generally involve feelings of emptiness or anger in response to fears of abandonment, and does not usually involve a pattern of unstable, intense relationships.

Finally, BPD-like behavior may be the result of a general medical condition or of chronic substance use. Again, looking for early onset and the presence of problems in a variety of situations may help to make this distinction.

What is Involved in Effective Assessment?

Researchers use semistructured diagnostic interviews. These interviews have adequate reliability and are well-accepted in the research arena. They provide a comprehensive, detailed diagnosis. These interviews are, however, very lengthy to administer, require training to administer and score, and may not be feasible for some clinicians in traditional practice settings.

One of the most common semistructured interviews is the Structured Clinical Interview for DSM Personality Disorders (SCID-II; First, Spitzer, Gibbons, & Williams, 1997). Information regarding the SCID-II can be found at *http://www.scid4.org/scidupd. htm* and tapes can be ordered through the American Psychiatric Press, Inc., by calling 1-800-368-5777 or visiting *http://www.appi.org*.

There are also paper-and-pencil screening instruments for BPD. Many of these measures tend to over-diagnose BPD, but may be useful when followed by a clinical interview.

Common screening instruments include:

* Borderline Symptom List (BSL; Bohus et al., 2001; available at www.brtc.psych.washington.edu).
* McLean Screening Instrument for Borderline Personality Disorder (MSI-BPD; Zanarini et al., 2003).
* Personality Diagnostic Questionnaire 4th Edition + (PDQ-4+; Hyler, 1994).
* Wisconsin Personality Disorders Inventory IV (WISPI-IV; Klein & Benjamin, 1996).
* Borderline Features Scale of the Personality Assessment Inventory (PAI; Morey, 1991).

Many clinicians rely on unstructured clinical interviews to diagnose BPD. Focusing on the affective, cognitive, behavioral, and interpersonal patterns (as described earlier) can help to focus the assessment. Client records and information from informants are also important in establishing a long-standing pattern of pervasive emotion dysregulation.

To capture the changes within domains over time, many therapists turn to diary cards. Diary cards track emotional, interpersonal, behavioral, and cognitive variables, as well as any other relevant information (e.g., hours slept, hours worked, number of interactions with partner). The client completes the diary card daily and returns it to the therapist on a weekly basis. Diary cards can be created in any word processing program and tailored to a client's individual targets. When graphed, these data provide very clear, useful, specific information about fluctuations in the client's problematic and skillful behavior. See Figure 14.1 for a sample dialectical behavioral therapy (DBT; discussed in Effective Therapist Based Treatments section) diary card.

What Assessments are Not Helpful?
* Projective tests
* Nonspecific personality tests

TREATMENT

What Treatments are Effective?

Only two psychosocial treatments, dialectical behavior therapy (DBT; Linehan 1993a,b) and mentalization based treatment (MBT; Bateman & Fonagy, 2004), have

Dialectical Behavior Therapy Skills Diary Card					Initials		Filled out in Session? Y N (Circle)	How often did you fill out this side? ___ Daily ___ 2-3x ___ 4-6x ___ Once	Started: Date___/___/_
					ID #				

Circle Start Day	Highest Urge To:			Highest Rating for Each Day			Drugs/Medications							Actions					
Day Of Week	Comm it Suicid	Self Harm	Use Drugs	Emotio n. Misery	Physic al Misery	Joy	Alcohol		Illicit Drugs		Meds. As Prescribe d	PRN/Over the Counter		Self Harm	Lied	Skills	Rein- force		
	0-5	0-5	0-5	0-5	0-5	0-5	#	What?	#	What?	Y/N	#	What?	Y/N.	#	0-7	√		

Chain Analysis Notes

* USED

0 = Not thought about or used
1 = Thought about, not used, didn't want to
2 = Thought about, not used, wanted to
3 = Tried but couldn't use them

SKILLS:

4 = Tried, could do them but they didn't help
5 = Tried, could use them, helped
6 = Didn't try, used them, didn't help
7 = Didn't try, used them, helped

Urge to:	Before Session (0-5)	Ability to self-regulate/ self-control:	Before Session (0-5)
Quit Therapy		Emotions:	
Use Drugs		Action:	
Commit Suicide		Thoughts:	

Med Changes/Other:

© Behavioral Research and Training Clinic, University of Washington

FIGURE 14.1 Sample DBT Diary Card

randomized controlled trials supporting their efficacy. Pharmacotherapy is recommended as an adjunctive approach for specific problems (Soloff, 2000).

What are Effective Self-Help Treatments?

There are no empirically supported self-help treatments for borderline personality disorder. The following suggestions are popular with many clinicians, clients, and family members.

Books
- *Skills training manual for treating borderline personality disorder* by Marsha Linehan, 1993
- *New Hope for People with Borderline Personality Disorder: Your Friendly, Authoritative Guide to the Latest in Traditional and Complementary Solutions* by Neil R. Bockian, Nora Elizabeth Villagran, & Valerie Porr, 2002
- *Eclipses: Behind the Borderline Personality Disorder* by Melissa F. Thornton, 1997

Audiocassette/Videocassette The following DBT skills training tapes are available for clinicians and clients through *www.behavioraltech.org* or Guilford Press.

- *Crisis Survival Skills, Part One: Distracting and Self-Soothing: What Do You Do When a Crisis Comes?*

- *Crisis Survival Skills, Part Two: Improving the Moment and Pros & Cons: Making Choices That Help*
- *From Suffering to Freedom: Practicing Reality Acceptance: Alleviating Suffering Through Accepting the World As It Is*
- *Opposite Action: Changing Emotions You Want to Change: Dialectical Behavior Therapy Skills Training Video*
- *This One Moment: Skills for Everyday Mindfulness: Achieving Awareness of What Really Is*

Websites
- BPD Central: *http://www.bpdcentral.com/*
- Behavioral Research and Therapy Clinics *http://www.brtc.psych.washington.edu/*
- Behavioral Tech: *http://www.behavioraltech.org/*
- Borderline Personality Disorder Research Foundation: *http://borderlinepersonality disorder.com*
- Self-Injury: You are NOT the Only One: *http://www.palace.net/~llama/psych/ injury.html*
- Helen's World of BPD Resources: *http://www.bpdresources.com/*
- Treatment and Research Advancements for BPD: *http://www.tara4bpd.org*

What are Effective Therapist-Based Treatments?

Linehan, Davison, Lynch, & Sanderson (2005) analyzed the two empirically supported treatments for BPD, DBT (e.g., Linehan, Armstrong, Suarez, Allmon, & Heard, 1991; Linehan, Heard, & Armstrong, 1993; Linehan, Tutek, Heard & Armstrong, 1994; Linehan et al. 2002) and MBT (Bateman & Fonagy, 1999, 2001), and distilled several principles of effective treatment for BPD, including general principles, structural aspects, principles of changes, and strategies for enhancing collaboration:

General principles of treatment	• Balance between acceptance and specific behavior change is necessary
	• Therapists need a coherent theoretical approach (versus eclecticism)
	• Treatment is lengthy and intensive
	• Individualized analysis of *specific* behaviors and their functions is needed for treatment planning
	• Therapists should be honest and up front with clients about limits (e.g., "Our phone calls need to be more productive or I will start to feel burned out.")
	• Therapists should recognize the importance of intrapersonal and interpersonal issues and the relationship between the two
	• Insight should be the focus of treatment only once the client can tolerate the associated affect
	• Therapists should not assume clients already possess skills necessary for effective living
	• Discussion of historical events should not take place until client is well in control of current behaviors and emotions
	• Therapists need to be emotionally supportive of their clients
	• Agree upon treatment goals, format, modalities, and strategies at the outset
Structural principles	• Target client capabilities, skills, motivation, generalization, and arrange for reinforcement
	• Arrange for reinforcement for new behaviors and extinction of maladaptive behavior from the environment (e.g., family members)
	• Obtain consultation and supervision
	• Organize treatment targets according to hierarchy
Principles of change	• Use established principles of behavior change (e.g., reinforcement, extinction, behavioral rehearsal)

- Expose to the cue setting off maladaptive emotion while blocking escape behaviors; reinforce skillful opposite-to-action responses
- Focus on detailed analysis of antecedents, and consequences of problematic behavior
- Coach experiential acceptance as well as problem solving strategies for cognitive, emotional, and behavioral difficulties

Principles of motivation and collaboration
- Address client-therapist conflict with nonconfrontational strategies
- Keep flexible limits rather than rigid boundaries; become more available during crises
- Respond to clients in genuine, responsive manner
- Use self disclosure strategically
- Communicate an understanding of the difficulty of the treatment task

What is Effective Medical Treatment?

A summary of controlled medication trials was provided by Lieb et al. (2004; see Table 14.1 below). Again, pharmacotherapy should be implemented as a problem-specific treatment in conjunction with psychotherapy (Soloff, 2000).

Other Issues in Management

Contraindications for Psychotherapy DBT and MBT are comprehensive treatments. As such, no particular problematic behavior should preclude treatment. However, if a condition interferes with one's ability to benefit from treatment, that condition should be resolved prior to instigating treatment (e.g., acute psychosis; Linehan, 1993a).

Risk Management Risk management and the fear of legal action is a major concern of practitioners treating BPD, due to this population's high likelihood of suicide attempts and completions. Gutheil (2004), for example, argues that legally, it can be assumed that a successful suicide would have been prevented but for the clinician's negligence. This places the clinician in a very vulnerable position when treating individuals with BPD. That being said, liability does not stem from the suicide itself, but from the failure to thoroughly assess risk and document a treatment plan (Paris, 2004).

Gutheil (2004) argues for the following strategies to reduce the risk related to treating suicidal individuals:

- *Documentation.* Formal risk assessments, protective factors, crisis plans, and clients' commitment to the plan should be documented clearly. Assess risk directly and frequently.
- *Consultation.* Receiving consultation and supervision as needed can increase the likelihood the clinician will provide effective treatment.
- *Family members.* Make the risk clear to family members, preferably via the client (Linehan, 1993a). This may actually prevent the suicide, and can also reduce hostility towards the therapist following a completed suicide. In the unfortunate event of a client suicide, be available, responsive, and sympathetic toward the family. Do not avoid contact. (Be aware, however, that confidentiality may still need to be observed after a client's death.)
- *Establish the client's competency.* Gutheil recommends a competence assessment (Gutheil, Bursztajn, & Brodsky, 1986) that documents the ability to choose to avoid discussing suicidality (versus being incompetent to make that decision). This involves simple questions such as, "Do you understand I cannot help if you do not talk about your suicide urges?" Gutheil (2004) states that this can move the onus for the suicide to the client rather than the clinician.

TABLE 14.1 Summary of placebo-controlled trials in the treatment of BPD (from Lieb et al., 2004)

Drug	No. of patients Drug/ placebo	Mean dose/day	Weeks of treatment	Main effects	Reference
Amitriptyline	20/20	148 ± 14 mg	5	Depression	Soloff et al. (1986)
Tranylcypromine	16/16*	40 mg	6	Depression, anger, impulsivity, suicidality	Cowdry and Gardner (1988)
Phenelzine	38/34	60.5 ± 10 mg	5	Anger/hostility	Soloff et al. (1993)
Fluvoxamine	38/19	166 ± 27 mg	12	Rapid mood shifts	Rinne, van den Bink, Wouters & van Dyck (2002)
Fluoxetine	9/8	20–60 mg	12	Global measures, anger, anxiety	Markovitz (1995)
Fluoxetine	13/9	40 mg	13	anger	Salzman et al. (1995)
Trifluoperazine	16/16*	7.8 mg	6	Depression, anxiety, suicidality	Cowdry and Gardner (1988)
Thiothixene	25/25	8.7 mg	12	Psychotic cluster symptoms, anxiety, obsessive-compulsive symptoms	Goldberg et al. (1986)
Haloperidol	21/20	7.2 ± 3.2 mg	5	Depression, anxiety, hostility, psychotizism	Soloff et al. (1986)
Haloperidol	36/34	3.9 ± 0.7 mg	5	—	Soloff et al. (1993)
Olanzapine	19/9	5.3 ± 3.4 mg	26	Anxiety, anger/hostility, paranoia, interpersonal difficulties	Zanarini and Frankenburg (2001)
Carbamazepine	16/16*	820 mg	6	Behavioral dyscontrol	Cowdry and Gardner (1988)
Carbamazepine	10/10	Blood conc. range 6.4–7.1 μg/ml	4	—	De la Fuente and Lotstra (1994)
Valproic acid	12/4	n.d.	10	Global measures (CGI-I)	Hollander et al. (2001)
Valproic acid	20/10	850 ± 249 mg	26	Interpersonal sensitivity, aggression, anger/hostility	Frankenburg and Zanarini (2002)
Omega-3-fatty acid	20/10	1000 mg	8	Aggression, depression	Zanarini and Frankenburg (2003)

n.d., no data; *, double blind cross-over trial with placebo, tranylcypromine, trifluoperazine, carbamazepine, and alprazolam.

- *Assess and document any "dates with death".* Clients with non-imminent plans for death on a particular, distant date still mandate frequent assessment and documentation.

Hospitalization There is no evidence that hospitalization makes a suicidal individual safer (Paris, 2004). Hospitalization can, in fact, increase the likelihood of suicidal behavior (Linehan, 1993a). Unless the client is hospitalized for a particular treatment purpose, such as stabilization on a particular medication, hospitalization for chronic suicide threats, minor overdoses, and self-harm is not recommended (Paris, 2004).

Generalization of Therapeutic Gains Clients need to generalize changes into their own environments. The following can facilitate such generalization:

- Between-session phone contact (focused on skills coaching and risk management).
- Family skills training, where individuals in the client's environment learn skills along with the client. This is generally in conjunction with individual therapy.
- Family therapy.

Therapist Burn-out Therapist burn-out is a common complaint among those treating BPD. BPD clients' interpersonal dysregulation can often reduce therapists' motivation to treat them effectively. DBT requires a weekly consultation team meeting to address this problem. The team functions to support the therapist and ensure the treatment is delivered effectively. Therapists can be creative about how they engage in regular consultation; email, phone or video conference, or mailing videotapes are alternatives to a team meeting.

Cost-Effectiveness Both DBT and MBT have been found to be cost effective in comparison to treatment as usual (DBT: Linehan & Heard, 1999; Mental Health Center of Grater Manchester, 1998; MBT: Bateman & Fonagy, 2003).

How Does One Select Among Treatments?

DBT is empirically supported as an outpatient treatment. MBT is empirically supported as a partial hospitalization program.

KEY READINGS

Linehan, M. M. (1993). *Cognitive-behavioral treatment of borderline personality disorder.* New York: Guilford Press.
Linehan, M. M. (1993). *Skills training manual for treating borderline personality disorder.* New York: Guilford Press.
Bateman, A., & Fonagy, P. (2004). *Psychotherapy for borderline personality disorder: Mentalization based treatment.* New York: Oxford University Press.

REFERENCES

American Psychiatric Association. (2000). *Diagnostic and statistical manual of mental disorders* (4th ed., Text Revision). Washington, DC: APA.
Bateman, A., & Fonagy, P. (1999). Effectiveness of partial hospitalization in the treatment of borderline personality disorder: A randomized controlled trial. *American Journal of Psychiatry, 156,* 1563–1569.
Bateman, A., & Fonagy, P. (2001). Treatment of borderline personality disorder with psychoanalytically oriented partial hospitalization: An 18-month follow-up. *American Journal of Psychiatry, 158,* 36–42.
Bateman, A., & Fonagy, P. (2003). Health service utilization costs for borderline personality disorder patients treated with psychoanalytically oriented partial hospitalization versus general psychiatric care. *American Journal of Psychiatry, 160* (1), 169–171.
Bateman, A., & Fonagy, P. (2004). *Psychotherapy for borderline personality disorder: Mentalization based treatment.* New York: Oxford University Press.
Bockian, N. R., Villagran, N. E., & Porr, V. (2002). *New Hope for People with Borderline Personality Disorder: Your Friendly, Authoritative Guide to the Latest in Traditional and Complementary Solutions.* New York: Random House.
Bohus, M., Limberger, M. F., Frank, U., Sender, I., Gratwohl, T., & Stieglitz, R. (2001). Development of the Borderline Symptom List (BSL). *Psychotherapie Psychosomatik Medizinische Psychologie, 51* (5), 201–211. [Available in English at www.brtc.psych.washington.edu]

Clarkin, J., Widiger, T., Frances, A., Hurt, S., & Gilmore, M. (1983). Prototypic typology and the borderline personality disorder. *Journal of Abnormal Psychology, 92*, 263–275.

Cowdry, R. W., & Gardner, D. L. (1988). Pharmacotherapy of borderline personality disorder: Alprazolam, carbamezepine, trifluoperazine, and tranylcypromine. *Archives of General Psychiatry, 45*, 111–119.

Cowdry, R. W., Pickar, D., & Davies, R. (1985). Symptoms and EEG findings in the borderline syndrome. *International Journal of Psychiatry Medicine, 15*, 201–211.

De la Fuente, J. M., & Lotstra, F. (1994). A trial of carbamazepine in borderline personality disorder. *European Neuropsychopharmacology, 4*, 479–486.

First, M. B., Spitzer, R. L., Gibbon, M., & Williams, J. B. W. (1997). *Structured Clinical Interview for DSM-IV Personality Disorders, (SCID-II)*. Washington, DC: American Psychiatric Press, Inc.

Frankenburg, F. R., & Zanarini, M. C. (2002). Divalproex sodium treatment of women with borderline personality disorder and bipolar II disorder: A double-blind placebo-controlled pilot study. *Journal of Clinical Psychiatry, 63* (5), 442–446.

Geller, J. L. (1986). In again, out again: Preliminary evaluation of a state hospital's worst recidivists. *Hospital and Community Psychiatry, 37*, 386–390.

Goldberg, S. C., Schulz, S. C., Schulz, P. M., Resnick, R. J., Hamer, R. M., & Friedel, R. O. (1986). Borderline and schizotypal personality disorders treated with low-dose thiothixene vs placebo. *Archives of General Psychiatry, 43* (7), 680–686.

Gutheil, T. G. (2004). Suicide, suicide litigation, and borderline personality disorder. *Journal of Personality Disorders, 18* (3), 248–256.

Gutheil, T. G., Bursztajn, H., & Brodsky, A. (1986). A multi-dimensional assessment of dangerousness: Competence assessment and liability prevention. *Bulletin of the American Academy of Psychiatry Law, 14*, 123–129.

Hollander, E., Allen, A., Lopez, R. P., Bienstock, C. A., Grossman, R., Siever, L. J. et al. (2001). A preliminary double-blind, placebo-controlled trial of divalproex sodium in borderline personality disorder. *Journal of Clinical Psychiatry, 62* (3), 199–203.

Hyler, S. E. (1994). *Personality Questionnaire, PDQ-4+*. New York: New York State Psychiatric Institute.

Klein, M. H., & Benjamin, L. S. (1996). *The Wisconsin Personality Disorders Inventory-IV*. Madison, WI: University of Wisconsin, unpublished test. Available from Dr. M. H. Klein, Department of Psychiatry, Wisonsin Psychiatric Institute and Clinic, 6001 Research Park Blvd., Madison, WI 53719–1179.

Kroll, J. L., Sines, L. K., & Martin, K. (1981). Borderline personality disorder: Construct validity of the concept. *Archives of General Psychiatry, 39*, 60–63.

Lieb, K., Zanarini, M. C., Schmahl, C., Linehan, M. M., & Bohus, M. (2004). Borderline personality disorder. *The Lancet, 364*, 453–461.

Linehan, M. M. (1993a). *Cognitive-behavioral treatment of borderline personality disorder*. New York: Guilford Press.

Linehan, M. M. (1993b). *Skills training manual for treating borderline personality disorder*. New York: Guilford Press.

Linehan, M. M., Armstrong, H. E., Suarez, A., Allmon, D., & Heard, H. L. (1991). Cognitive-behavioral treatment of chronically parasuicidal borderline patients. *Archives of General Psychiatry, 48*, 1060–1064.

Linehan, M., Davison, G., Lynch, T., & Sanderson, C. (2005). Technique Factors in Treating Personality Disorders. In Castonguay, L., Beutler, L. (Eds.), *Principles of Therapeutic Change that Work*. Oxford University Press, pp. 239–252.

Linehan, M. M., Dimeff, L. A., Reynolds, S. K., Comtois, K. A., Welch, S. S., Heagerty, P., et al. (2002). Dialectical behavior therapy versus comprehensive validation therapy plus 12-step for the treatment of opiod dependent women meeting criteria for borderline personality disorder. *Drug & Alcohol Dependence, 67*, 13–26.

Linehan, M. M., & Heard, H. L. (1999). Borderline personality disorder: Costs, course, and treatment outcomes. In N. Miller & K. M. Magruder (Eds.), *Cost-effectiveness of psychotherapy* (pp. 291–305). New York: Oxford University Press.

Linehan, M. M., Heard, H. L., & Amstrong, H. E. (1993). Naturalistic follow-up of a behavioral treatment for chronically parasuicidal borderline patients. *Archives of General Psychiatry, 50*, 971–974.

Linehan, M. M., Rizvi, S. L., Welch, S., & Page, B. (1999). Suicide and personality disorders. In K. Hawton & K. van Heeringe (Eds.), *International handbook of suicide and attempted suicide*. Sussex, England: John Wiley & Sons, Ltd.

Linehan, M. M., Tutek, D. A., Heard, H. L., & Armstrong, H. E. (1994). Interpersonal outcome of cognitive behavioral treatment for chronically suicidal borderline patients. *American Journal of Psychiatry, 151*, 1771–1776.

Markovitz, P. J. (1995). Pharmacotherapy of impulsivity, aggression, and related disorders. In E. Hollander & D. J. Stein (Eds.). *Impulsivity and aggression* (pp. 263–287). Chichester, England: John Wiley & Sons.

Mental Health Center of Greater Manchester, NH. (1998). Gold Award: Integrating dialectical behavior therapy into a community mental health program. *Psychiatric Services, 49*, 1338–1340.

Modestin, J., Abrecht, I., Tschaggelar, W., & Hoffman, H. (1997). Diagnosing borderline: A contribution to the question of its conceptual validity. *Archives Psychiatrica Nervenkra, 233,* 359–370.

Morey, L. C. (1991). *The Personality Assessment Inventory professional manual.* Odessa, FL: Psychological Assessment Resources.

Paris, J. (2004). Is hospitalization useful for suicidal patients with borderline personality disorder? *Journal of Personality Disorders, 18* (3), 240–247.

Rinne, T., van den Brink, W., Wouters, L., van Dyck, R. (2002). SSRI treatment of borderline personality disorder: A randomized, placebo-controlled clinical trial for female patients with borderline personality disorder. *American Journal of Psychiatry, 159,* 2048–2054.

Salzman, C., Wolfson, A. N., Schatzberg, A., Looper, J., Henke, R., & Albanese, M., et al. (1995). Effect of fluoxetine on anger in symptomatic volunteers with borderline personality disorder. *Journal of Clinical Psychopharmacology, 15* (1), 23–29.

Soloff, P. H. (2000). Pharmacology of borderline personality disorder. *The Psychiatric Clinics of North America, 23* (1), 169–192.

Soloff, P. H., Cornelius, J. R., George, A., Nathan, R. S., Perel, J. M., & Ulrich, R. F. (1993). Efficacy of phenelzine and haloperidol in borderline personality disorder. *Archives of General Psychiatry, 50,* 377–385.

Soloff, P. H., George, A., Swami, N., Schulz, P. M. Ulrich, R. F., & Perel, J. M. (1986). Progress in pharmacotherapy of borderline disorders: A double-blind study of amitriptyline, haloperidol, and placebo. *Archives of General Psychiatry, 43,* 691–697.

Surber, R. W., Winkler, E. L., Monteleone, M., Havassy, B. E., Goldfinger, S. M., & Hopkin, J. T. (1987). Characteristics of high users of acute psychiatric inpatient services. *Hospital and Community Psychiatry, 38* (10), 1112–1114.

Swigar, M. E., Astrachan, B., Levine, M. A., Mayfield, V., & Radovich, C. (1991). Single and repeated admissions to a mental health center: Demographic, clinical and use of service characteristics. *International Journal of Social Psychiatry, 37* (4), 259–266.

Tanney, B. L. (1992). Mental disorders, psychiatric patients, and suicide. In R. W. Maris, A. L. Berman, & J. T. Maltsberger (Eds.), *Assessment and prediction of suicide.* (pp. 277–320). New York: Guilford Press.

Thornton, M. F. (1997). *Eclipses: Behind the borderline personality disorder.* Monte Sano Publishing.

Torgersen, S., Kringlen, E., Cramer, V. (2001). The prevalence of personality disorders in a community sample. *Archives of General Psychiatry 58,* 590–596.

Widiger, T. A., & Frances, A. J. (1989). Epidemiology, diagnosis, and comorbidity of borderline personality disorder. In A. Tasman, R. E. Hales, & A. J. Frances (Eds.), *American psychiatric press review of psychiatry,* (Vol. 8. pp. 8–24). D.C.: American Psychiatric Press.

Widiger, T. A., & Weissman, M. M. (1991). Epidemiology of borderline personality disorder. *Hospital and Community Psychiatry, 42,* 1015–1021.

Woogh, C. M. (1986). A cohort through the revolving door. *Canadian Journal of Psychiatry, 31* (3), 214–221.

Zanarini, M. C., & Frankenburg, F. R. (2001). Olanzapine treatment of female borderline personality disorder patients: a double-blind, placebo-controlled pilot study. *Journal of Clinical Psychiatry, 62* (11), 849–854.

Zanarini, M. C., & Frankenburg, F. R. (2003). Omega-3 fatty acid treatment of women with borderline personality disorder: A double-blind, placebo-controlled pilot study. *American Journal of Psychiatry, 160,* 167–169.

Zanarini, M. C., Vujanovic, A., Parachini, E. A., Boulanger, J. L., Frankenburg, & F. R. Hennen, J. (2003). A screening measure for BPD: The McLean Screening Instrument for Borderline Personality Disorder. *Journal of Personality Disorders, 17* (6), 568–573.

Bulimia Nervosa

James Lock • Ann M. Schapman

AN OVERVIEW OF BULIMIA NERVOSA

Bulimia Nervosa (BN) first entered the psychodiagnostic nomenclature in the 1970s and affects between 1 and 2 % of the population, primarily young women. It is hallmarked by recurrent binge eating, compensatory behavior, and an overemphasis on shape and weight in evaluating one's self-worth. In this chapter, the diagnostic criteria for Bulimia, as well as its associated features and medical sequelae, will be discussed. Next, etiological factors implicated in the onset of the disorder will be discussed, including biological, psychological, familial, and sociocultural variables. This chapter will then explicate assessment strategies for BN, focusing on clinical interviews and self-report inventories. Subsequently, empirically supported treatments for BN will be discussed, with an emphasis on Cognitive-Behavioral Therapy and Interpersonal Therapy. Finally, future directions for research will be delineated, underscoring the need for treatment studies with adolescent populations.

BULIMIA NERVOSA

The 1970s marked the first time that BN was recognized as a psychological disorder, although records indicated that it may have had its origins somewhere between the 1940s and 1960s (Russell, 1979). BN, which first has its onset in late adolescence or early adulthood and affects between 1% and 2% of the population (Flament et al., 1995), is a serious psychiatric condition that is hallmarked by three primary features: episodic overeating, compensatory behaviors, and an overemphasis on shape and weight in self-evaluation. This chapter reviews the current understanding of the nature and etiology of BN and will provide information on multimethod means of assessment, state-of-the-art treatment interventions, and future research directions for this debilitating disorder.

THE NATURE OF BN

Current DSM-IV Conceptualizations

Current *DSM-IV* (APA, 1994) criteria for BN include the following: recurrent binge eating and compensatory behaviors at least two times a week for at least three months, self-evaluation unduly influenced by weight and shape, and symptoms not occurring exclusively during an episode of Anorexia Nervosa. Binge eating is defined by the *DSM-IV* as eating within a discrete period of time, usually marked by any two-hour period, an amount more than other people would eat in a similar amount of time and under similar circumstances. Typical binge foods include those high in calories and easily consumed, such as ice cream, cakes, and candy. Another requirement for binge behavior is that the individual feels out of control while eating. Compensatory behaviors include self-induced vomiting (i.e., 80–90% of cases); laxative, diuretic, or enema use; fasting; or excessive exercise in order to prevent weight

Lock, J., & Schapman, A. M. (2006). Bulimia nervosa. In J. E. Fisher & W. T. O'Donohue (Eds.), *Practitioner's guide to evidence-based psychotherapy*. New York: Springer.

gain. Two specifiers accompany the DSM-IV diagnostic criteria for BN, including Purging Type, whereby the individual regularly engages in the self-induced vomiting or the misuse of laxatives, diuretics, or enemas; and Nonpurging Type, whereby the individual engages in other inappropriate compensatory behaviors (i.e., fasting or excessive exercise).

Associated Features

There are several characteristics of BN that are not diagnostic criteria but associated features. Such features include normal weight, impulsivity, interpersonal problems, substance use, and personality deficits (Beumont, 2002). In terms of associated psychopathologies, there is an increased rate of depressive and anxious symptoms among individuals with BN (Bulik, 2002), and such symptoms usually occur around the same time or subsequent to the onset of BN and remit following treatment. Other comorbid psychopathologies include Substance Abuse and Dependence (Wilson, 2002). In one-third of individuals, stimulant use first starts as a means to control appetite and weight. Personality Disorders are present in one-third to one-half of individuals with BN, and the population of individuals with BN is 90% female and primarily Caucasian (APA, 1994).

Medical Sequelae

BN is a serious and potentially fatal psychological condition in light of the multiple medical sequelae (see Pomeroy, 2004; Pomeroy & Mitchell, 2002, for reviews). A myriad of symptoms can result from purging, some of which include hypokalemia, hyponatremia, hypochloremia, metabolic alkalosis, and problems with teeth and gums. The use of ipecac to induce vomiting can lead to serious cardiac and skeletal myopathies. Frequent laxative use can cause metabolic acidosis and elevated serum amylase levels. Furthermore, it can lead to dependence on laxatives for bowel emptying. Amenorrhea, infertility, osteoporosis, and dehydration are other possible outcomes. Esophageal tears, gastric rupture, and cardiac arrhythmias and sudden cardiac death are rare but potentially fatal medical complications of BN.

ETIOLOGICAL FACTORS

The current understanding is that BN is a multiply-determined phenomenon, meaning biological, psychological, familial, and sociocultural factors have interacted to lead to the onset of the disorder.

Biological Bases

Studies have suggested a genetic basis to the disorder given that BN has been found to run in families and twin studies suggest that up to half of the variance in heritability is accounted for by genetic factors (i.e., Bulik, 2004; Kendler et al., 1991). Studies have implicated irregularities in the serotonergic system as well, namely finding reduced serotonin levels in individuals with BN. In particular, it has been suggested that people with BN have disturbances in the orbital–frontal serotonergic circuits, which are associated with behavioral dyscontrol (Kaye, 2002).

Psychological Factors

In terms of psychological factors, studies have suggested that BN may be related to low self-esteem and increased sensitivity to peer rejection (Pike, 1995). Impulsive tendencies, perfectionism, and interpersonal deficits are other psychological features implicated in the onset of BN.

Familial Profiles

Several familial factors have been linked to the development of BN as well (see Schmidt, 2002, and Vandereycken, 2002, for reviews). Studies have found that BN has been associated with exposure to parental obesity and familial criticisms about weight, shape, and eating. Families of individuals with BN appear to place greater importance on achievement and appearance. Patients with BN tend to view their families as unorganized, conflictual, and lacking in warmth and cohesion.

Sociocultural Influences

Sociocultural factors are believed to play a role in the onset of the disorder as well. Since the 1970s, there has been an increase in the number of BN cases presenting to clinics in the Western world. It has been suggested that sociocultural pressures for women to manifest a thin body, as portrayed via magazine and television advertisements, have led to increased rates of BN.

Integrational Models

Cognitive-behavioral model. The cognitive-behavioral model of BN-which incorporates psychological, physiological, and sociocultural factors-is perhaps the most widely espoused understanding of BN. This model suggests that the main factors involved in the maintenance of BN are dysfunctional attitudes toward body shape and weight and their various expressions. Such attitudes may be socioculturally or internally derived and lead to an overvaluation of thinness, bodily dissatisfaction, and attempts to control shape and weight by excessive dieting. This rigid and restrictive pattern results in both psychological and physiological deprivation. As a result of a variety of psychological and physiological processes, there is a vulnerability to intermittent but recurrent episodes of binge eating, particularly in response to adverse mood states (Waller, 2002). Because binge eating intensifies concerns about weight and shape, it is commonly followed by purging as an attempt to compensate for calories consumed during the binge (Agras & Apple, 1997; Fairburn, 1981). The model also suggests that self-esteem, overconcern with weight and shape, as well as dietary restraint are related constructs, because patients with BN tend to judge their self-worth largely in terms of shape and weight (Fairburn, 1997).

THE ASSESSMENT OF BN

Diagnostic Interviewing

The clinical interview. In assessing BN, clinicians should engage in typical clinical interviewing, assessing across social, academic, familial, and occupational domains, and investigating mental health, developmental, and medical history. In addition to these standard interview questions, clinicians should inquire about the history and current status of eating disorder pathology, such as restriction, binge eating, purging and other compensatory behaviors, and weight and shape concerns. Current and past information about associated features should be obtained as well, particularly regarding perfectionism, impulsivity, height and weight trends, history of weight control measures, and motivation for current treatment. Past experiences with teasing about weight and family culture around food, weight, and eating are important areas to assess. Associated medical symptoms should be assessed, such as fatigue, headaches, bloating and constipation, and irregular menstrual status. Associated psychopathologies should also be assessed, particularly depression, anxiety, substance abuse, and personality disorders, as they may be useful for conceptualizing the patient's global symptom presentation and planning treatment. For children and adolescents, data from multiple informants (i.e., parents and the youth) should be obtained.

Standardized interviews. Although unstructured clinical interviews are the most commonly used means of obtaining historical and diagnostic data, semistructured are also available for use and can be advantageous in terms of deciphering diagnostic status, understanding the severity of pathology, and measuring treatment progress over time. In the 1980s and 1990s, several standardized interviews for the assessment of eating disorders emerged (Crowther & Sherwood, 1997). These include the Clinical Eating Disorder Rating Instrument (CEDRI; Palmer, et al., 1987), the Interview for Diagnosis of Eating Disorders (IDED; Williamson, 1990), and the Structured Interview for Anorexia and Bulimia Nervosa (STAB; Fichter et al., 1991). The Eating Disorders Examination (EDE; Cooper & Fairburn, 1987; Cooper, Cooper, & Fairburn, 1989), however, is the semistructured interview that was subjected to the greatest empirical scrutiny, and therefore is most commonly utilized. The EDE allows one to decipher diagnostic status and derive scores to indicate the extent of dietary restraint and eating, weight, and shape concerns.

Self-Report Inventories

Several self-report inventories are available for the assessment of BN, and one of the most widely used measures is the *Eating Attitudes Test (EAT-26*; Garner, Olmsted, Bohr, & Garfinkel, 1982). The original EAT has shown good internal consistency, test–retest reliability, and concurrent and discriminant validity. The Eating Disorders Inventory-2 (*EDI-2*, Garner, 1991) is another popular self-report inventory of both AN and BN and allows for the derivation of Asceticism, Impulse Regulation, and Social Insecurity subscales. The *EDI-2* has been shown to have good convergent and predictive validity. A third commonly used self-report measure is the *Bulimia Test-Revised (BULIT-R*; Thelen, Farmer, Wonderlich, & Smith, 1991; see Anderson & Paulosky, 2004, for review of self-report measures).

Differential Diagnosis

Anorexia Nervosa. BN should be distinguished between other eating disorders that share some of the same symptoms. In particular, BN shares in common some food restriction that is also characteristic of Anorexia Nervosa (AN). In contrast to AN, however, individuals with BN tend to maintain a normal body weight. Furthermore, in contrast to AN, patients with BN tend to alternative between patterns of restriction and binge-eating, which is subsequently followed with compensatory behaviors. An irrational fear of gaining weight and amenorrhea are other criteria for AN that are not typically present in BN.

Eating Disorder, Not Otherwise Specified. Another disorder BN may resemble is Eating Disorder, Not Otherwise Specified (EDNOS). This disorder can occur when an individual manifests some eating disorder symptoms (i.e., restriction, binge eating, etc.), but not to the level of severity or frequency required for a BN or AN diagnosis. Furthermore, Binge-Eating Disorder, although not an official diagnostic category in the *DSM-IV*, is hallmarked by recurrent binge eating and for diagnostic purposes is subsumed under EDNOS.

THE TREATMENT OF BN

Given the multifaceted nature of BN, its treatment requires a multidisciplinary approach. Although it may vary based on an individual's presentation, multidisciplinary teams for the treatment of BN should generally include a psychologist, psychiatrist, nutritionist, and social worker. There are multiple levels of care in which a patient with BN can be treated, such as outpatient, partial day, residential, and inpatient treatment programs.

The main forms of treatment studied are Cognitive-Behavioral Therapy (CBT), Interpersonal Psychotherapy (IPT), and pharmacotherapy. In sum, CBT has been identified as the "treatment of choice" for BN, although IPT has also found substantial empirical support. Medication can be indicated if an individual is unresponsive to an initial trial of psychotherapy or when comorbid psychopathologies require intervention.

Cognitive-Behavioral Therapy (CBT)

CBT (Agras & Apple, 1997; Fairburn, 1981; Fairburn, Marcus, & Wilson, 1993) is a 20-session treatment consisting of three stages. In the first stage, the therapist and patient review the current cognitive-behavioral understanding of the etiology of BN and then tailor that understanding to fit with the patient's unique symptom presentation. Furthermore, in Stage One, the therapist and patient discuss structure, goals, and anticipated outcome of treatment; engage in psychoeducation about eating disorders, nutrition and weight regulation; establish self-monitoring of eating habits; and apply graded behavioral techniques for establishing a pattern for regular eating and reducing the frequency of overeating. Stage Two consists of identifying and challenging dysfunctional cognitions, confronting feared foods in a graduated exposure format, developing problem solving skills, addressing interpersonal issues related to the BN, and addressing weight and shape concerns. Finally, stage three involves relapse prevention, when the patient identifies stressful future situations that could elicit BN symptoms and delineates how she or he will cope with such experiences.

CBT used with adults with BN has been found to be more effective than other treatments (i.e., Agras et al., 2000; Walsh et al., 1997; Wilfley et al., 1993). Some 50% of patients with BN recover with CBT, while another 20% are much improved, and studies have found continued improvement at follow-ups. Fairburn and colleagues at Oxford University followed BN patients treated with CBT for six years posttreatment and found that nearly 60% of patients had no eating disorder and a further 20% had subclinical eating disorder symptoms (Fairburn et al., 1995).

Interpersonal Psychotherapy (IPT)

IPT, which was initially developed as a treatment for depression, was later modified as a treatment for BN. As applied to BN, IPT focuses on the interpersonal context within which the eating disorder developed and is maintained with the aim of helping the patient make specific changes in identified interpersonal problem areas. Little attention is paid to eating habits or attitudes toward weight and shape.

Several clinical trials and follow-up studies provide empirical support for the use of IPT to treat BN (i.e., Fairburn et al., 1991). Recently, CBT was compared to IPT in a large multisite trial involving 200 patients with BN (Agras et al., 2000). In this trial, CBT was superior to IPT at the end of treatment, but on 8–12 month follow-up, no differences were found between the two treatments.

Pharmacotherapy

Two studies found that antidepressants, when added to CBT, do not improve outcome in reducing binge eating (Agras et al., 1992; Mitchell et al., 1990). Mitchell et al. (1990), however, found that rates of depression decreased in those receiving medication, and dietary preoccupation was found to diminish in the combined medication and CBT group versus the CBT group alone (Agras et al., 1992). Overall, research on the use of antidepressants to treat BN has suggested that they are usually not sufficient as the sole treatment and are best used in conjunction with or as an adjunct to psychotherapy, particularly CBT (i.e., Hughes, Wells, & Cunningham, 1986; Hughes et al. (1986) Walsh et al., 1997).

Alternative Treatments

Dialectical behavior therapy (DBT). DBT is a form of therapy originally applied to Borderline Personality Disorder by Marsha Linehan (1993). It consists of an array of cognitive and behavioral techniques but adds components of dialectical philosophy, specifically a focus on achieving balance between acceptance and change (McCabe, LaVia, & Marcus, 2004). More recently, DBT is being adapted to treat Binge Eating Disorder in adults (Safer, Telch, & Agras, 2001; Telch, 1997; Wiser & Telch, 1999).

Family treatment. Many case studies attest to the efficacy of family therapy for BN in younger patients, however this type of treatment has not been systematically studied. Several studies have supported the use of family therapy for AN. Key components of this therapy include parental control over a youth's restrictive and dangerous eating patterns, reducing blame or guilt among the youth and family members by promoting understanding of AN as an illness for which no one is to blame, eliciting sibling support to help their brother or sister cope, and a gradual return of control over eating to the adolescent once medical stability is achieved (Lock, LeGrange, Agras, & Dare, 2001). Given that there are parallels between AN and BN, family treatment may be an effective approach to treating BN in adolescents as well (Dare & Eisler, 1995).

Developmental Considerations

As mentioned, all of the empirical studies of BN have been conducted with adult populations. Clinically, we can justify using CBT with an adolescent population given that theoretically it makes sense to do so, it has worked with adults, CBT for other disorders (i.e., namely anxiety and depression) has been helpful for children and adolescence. Furthermore, IPT can be justified for use with adolescents as well given that it has also been found effective with adults, has been used for adolescent depression, and theoretically it makes sense to do so, especially in light of the growing importance of interpersonal relationships during adolescence.

FUTURE DIRECTIONS FOR RESEARCH

Although many advances have occurred in the empirical study of BN, there is no paucity of areas for new research. There is a need for more randomized controlled clinical trials of new treatments of BN, given that up to 30–40% of patients do not respond well to existing treatments. There are needs for the assessment of moderating variables predicting treatment response, component analyses studies, increased generalizability of extant literature (i.e., which can be accomplished via effectiveness rather than efficacy studies), and studies of eating disorder prevention programs. Another need in the BN treatment outcome literature is studies of adolescent populations, as extant studies demonstrating effective psychological treatments for BN have been conducted exclusively among adult populations.

SUMMARY

BN is a severe and potentially fatal psychiatric illness that has primarily affected adolescent and young adult women. Although it is relatively new to the psychodiagnostic nomenclature, evidence of eating disorder presentations extend to ancient times. The etiology of BN is likely multifaceted, including biological, psychological, familial, and sociocultural mechanisms. In diagnosing BN, clinicians should look for converging evidence from multimethod and, in the case of younger patients, multiinformant means, including clinical and semistructured interviews and self-report measures. The current treatment of choice for BN is CBT, although IPT also appears to be effective. Medications (i.e., antidepressants) can be a helpful ancillary treatment to psychotherapy if there is an initial nonresponse to therapy or to address comorbid psychopathologies. Future research is imperative to further our understanding of BN, in particular in the realm of treatment outcome studies with younger patients.

REFERENCES

Agras, W. S., & Apple, R. F. (1997). *Overcoming eating disorders: A cognitive-behavioral treatment of bulimia nervosa and binge-eating disorder (Therapist guide).* San Antonio, TX: Graywind Publications.

Agras, W. S., Walsh, T., Fairburn, G., Wilson, G. T., & Kraemer, H. C. (2000). A multi-center comparison of cognitive-behavioral therapy and interpersonal psychotherapy for bulimia nervosa. *Archives of General Psychiatry, 57,* 459–466.

Agras, W. S., Rossiter, E. M., Arnow, B., Schneider, J., Telch, C. F., Raeburn, S. D., et al. (1992). Pharmacological and cognitive-behavioral treatment for bulimia nervosa: A controlled comparison. *American Journal of Psychiatry, 149(1),* 82–87.

American Psychiatric Association (1994). *Diagnostic and statistical manual of mental disorders* (4th ed.). Washington, DC: Author.

Anderson, D. A., & Paulosky, C. A. (2004). Psychological assessment of eating disorders and related features. In J. K. Thompson (Ed.). *Handbook of eating disorders and obesity.* New Jersey: John Wiley and Sons, Inc.

Beumont, P. J. V. (2002). Clinical presentation of anorexia nervosa and bulimia nervosa. In C. G. Fairburn & K. D. Brownell (Eds.). *Eating disorders and obesity* (2nd ed.): *A comprehensive handbook.* New York: Guilford Press.

Bulik, C. M. (2002). Anxiety, depression, and eating disorders. In C. G. Fairburn & K. D. Brownell (Eds). *Eating Disorders and Obesity* (2nd ed.): *A comprehensive handbook.* New York: Guilford Press.

Bulik, C. M. (2004). Genetic and biological risk factors. In J. K. Thompson (Ed.). *Handbook of eating disorders and obesity.* New Jersey: John Wiley and Sons.

Cooper, Z., Cooper, P. J., & Fairburn, C. G. (1989). The validity of the eating disorder examination and its subscales. *British Journal of Psychiatry, 154,* 807–812.

Cooper, Z. & Fairburn, C. G. (1987). The eating disorder examination: A semistructured interview for the assessment of the specific psychopathology of eating disorders. *International Journal of Eating Disorders, 6,* 1–8.

Crowther, J. H., & Sherwood, N. E. (1997). Assessment. In D. M. Garner & P. E. Garfinkel (Eds.). *Handbook of treatment for eating disorders* (2nd ed.). New York: Guilford Press.

Dare, C., & Eisler, I. (1995). Family therapy and eating disorders. In K. D. Brownell & C. G. Fairburn, (Eds.). *Eating disorders and obesity: A comprehensive handbook.* New York: Guilford.

Fairburn, C. G. (1981). A cognitive-behavioral approach to the treatment of bulimia. *Psychological Medicine, 11(4),* 707–711.

Fairburn, C. G. (1997). Eating disorders. In D. Clark, & C. G. Fairburn (Eds.). *Cognitive-behavioral therapy: Science and practice.* Oxford University Press: Oxford.

Fairburn, C. G., Jones, R. Peveler, R. C., Carr, S. J., et al. (1991). Three psychological treatments for bulimia nervosa: A comparative trial. *Archives of General Psychiatry, 48(5),* 463–469.

Fairburn, C. G., Marcus, M. D., & Wilson, G. T. (1993). *Cognitive-behavioral therapy for binge eating and bulimia nervosa: A comprehensive treatment manual.* In C. G. Fairburn, & G. T. Wilson (Eds.). *Binge eating: Nature, assessment, and treatment.* New York: Guilford Press.

Fairburn, C. G., Normal, P. A., Welch, S. L., O'Connor, M. E., et al. (1995). A prospective study of outcome in bulimia nervosa and long-term effects of three psychological treatments. *Archives of General Psychiatry, 52(4)*, 304–312.

Fichter, M. M., Elton, M., Engel, K., Meyer, A., et al. (1991). Structured interview for anorexia and bulimia nervosa. *International Journal of Eating Disorders, 10(5)*, 571–592.

Flament, M., et al. (1995). A population study of bulimia nervosa and subclinical eating disorders in adolescence. In H. Steinhausen (Ed.). *Eating disorders in adolescence: Anorexia and bulimia nervosa*. New York: Brunner/Mazel.

Garner, D. M. (1991). *Eating Disorder Inventory-2*. Odessa, FL: Psychological Assessment Resources.

Garner, D. M., Olmstead, M. P., Bohr, Y., & Garfinkel, P. E. (1982). The Eating Attitudes Test: Psychometric features and clinical correlates. *Psychological Medicine, 12*, 871–878.

Kaye, W. H. (2002). Central nervous system neurotransmitter activity in Anorexia Nervosa and Bulimia Nervosa. In C. G. Fairburn & K. D. Brownell (Eds.). *Eating disorders and obesity* (2nd ed.): *A comprehensive handbook*. New York: Guilford Press.

Kendler, K. S., MacLean, C., Neale, M., Kessler, R. C., et al. (1991). The genetic epidemiology of Bulimia Nervosa. *American Journal of Psychiatry, 148(12)*, 1627–1637.

Linehan, M. M. (1993). *Cognitive-behavioral treatment of borderline personality disorder*. New York: Guilford Press.

Lock, J., Le Grange, D., Agras, S., & Dare, C. (2001). *Treatment manual for Anorexia Nervosa: A family-based approach*. New York: Guilford.

McCabe, E. B., LaVia, M. C., & Marcus, M. D. (2004). Dialectical behavior therapy for eating disorders. In J. K. Thompson (Ed.). *Handbook of eating disorders and obesity*. New Jersey: John Wiley & Sons, Inc.

Mitchell, J. E., Pyle, R. L., Eckert, E. D., Hatsukami, D., Pomeroy, C., & Zimmerman, R. (1990). A comparison study of antidepressants and structured intensive group psychotherapy in the treatment of bulimia nervosa. *Archives in General Psychiatry, 47*, 149–157.

Palmer, R., Christie, M., Cordle, C., Davies, D., et al. (1987). A clinical eating disorders rating instrument (CEDRI): A preliminary description. *International Journal of Eating Disorders, 6(1)*, 9–16.

Pike, K. M. (1995). Bulimic symptomatology in high school girls: Toward a model of cumulative risk. *Psychology of Women Quarterly, 19(3)*, 373–396.

Pomeroy, C. (2004). Assessment of medical status and physical factors. In J. K. Thomspon (Ed.). *Handbook of eating disorders and obesity*. New Jersey: John Wiley and Sons, Inc.

Pomeroy, C., & Mitchell, J. E. (2002). Medical complications of Anorexia Nervosa and Bulimia Nervosa. In C. G. Fairburn, & K. D. Brownell, *Eating Disorders and Obesity* (2nd ed.): *A comprehensive handbook*. New York: Guilford Press.

Russel, G.(1979). Bulimia nervosa: an omnious variant of anorexia nervosa. *Psychological Medicine, 9*, 429-448.

Safer, D. L. C., Telch, F., & Agras, W. S. (2001). Dialectical behavior therapy for bulimia nervosa. *American Journal of Psychiatry, 158(4)*, 632–634.

Schmidt, U. (2002). Risk factors for eating disorders. In C. G. Fairburn & K. D. Brownell (Eds.). *Eating disorders and obesity* (2nd ed.): *A comprehensive handbook*. New York: Guilford Press.

Telch, C. F. (1997). Skills training treatment for adaptive affect regulation in a woman with binge-eating disorder. *International Journal of Eating Disorders, 22(1)*, 77–81.

Thelen, M. H., Farmer, J., Wonderlich, S., & Smith, M. (1991). A revision of the Bulimia Test: The BULIT-R. *Psychological Assessment, 3(1)*, 119–124.

Vandereycken, W. (2002). Families of patients with eating disorders. In C. G. Fairburn & K. D. Brownell (Eds). *Eating disorders and obesity* (2nd ed.): *A comprehensive handbook*. New York: Guilford Press.

Waller, G. (2002). The psychology of binge eating. In C. G. Fairburn, & K. D. Brownell (Eds.). *Eating disorders and obesity: A comprehensive handbook*. New York: Guilford Press.

Walsh, B. T., Wilson, G. T., Loeb, K. L., Devlin, M. J., et al. (1997). Medication and psychotherapy in the treatment of bulimia nervosa. *American Journal of Psychiatry, 154(4)*, 523–531.

Wilfley, D. E., Agras, W. S., Telch, C. F., Rossiter, E. M., et al. (1993). Group cognitive-behavioral therapy and group interpersonal psychotherapy for the non-purging bulimic individual: A controlled comparison. *Journal of Consulting and Clinical Psychology, 61(2)*, 296–305.

Williamson, D. A. (1990). *Assessment of eating disorders: Obesity, anorexia, and bulimia*. Elmsford, NY: Pergamon Press.

Wilson, G. T. (2002). Eating disorders and addictive disorders. In C. G. Fairburn & K. D. Brownell (Eds.). *Eating disorders and obesity* (2nd ed.): *A comprehensive handbook*. New York: Guilford Press.

Wiser, S., & Telch, C. F. (1999). Dialectical behavior therapy for binge-eating disorder. *Journal of Clinical Psychology, 55(6)*, 755–768.

Child Physical Abuse

Linda Anne Valle • John R. Lutzker

WHAT IS CHILD PHYSICAL ABUSE?

Child physical abuse (CPA) is generally defined as the nonaccidental physical injury of a child by a parent or other caregiver, which can include bruises, fractures, cuts, burns, welts, and other injuries. Unlike other disorders included in the *Diagnostic and Statistical Manual of Mental Disorders,* Fourth Edition (DSM-IV, American Psychiatric Association, 1994), there are no specific symptoms by which CPA is diagnosed other than the nature and history of the child's physical injury.

BASIC FACTS ABOUT CHILD PHYSICAL ABUSE

Incidence and Prevalence

In 2002, approximately 2.6 million reports of suspected child maltreatment were made to child protective services (CPS) in the United States. Of the 896,000 children who were determined to be maltreated following investigation, 8.6% experienced physical abuse (approximately 167,000). Approximately 1,400 children died in 2002 as a result of child maltreatment; 29.9% and 28.9% of the fatalities were due to CPA alone and combined types of maltreatment (including CPA), respectively (US Department of Health and Human Services, Administration on Children, Youth and Families, 2004). Official reports suggest less than 1% of children in the United States are physically abused annually, with rates remaining relatively stable over the past five years. However, official CPS data probably underestimate actual occurrences of child maltreatment because many incidents of child maltreatment, particularly less severe incidents, may never be recognized or reported. In addition, different CPS policies influence how cases are investigated and substantiated. For example, a report of CPA may not be officially substantiated but may not be ruled out. Children may also experience multiple forms of child maltreatment, and CPA may be subsumed under other categories in the official data. Estimates from sources other than CPS data suggest that over 600,000 children are physically abused a year, whereas general population survey research suggests that the prevalence of CPA may actually be as high as 10% (Kolko, 2002; Kolko & Swenson, 2002).

Age of Onset

There is limited empirical evidence suggesting a specific age of onset for CPA (but see sections on etiology and course below for age-related issues).

Gender

No clear patterns of gender differences in overall rates of CPA perpetration have emerged (e.g., Chaffin, Kelleher, & Hollenberg, 1996; Wolfner & Gelles, 1993), although fatal child abuse cases may more frequently involve male perpetrators (e.g., Bergman, Larsen, & Mueller, 1986; Lucas et al., 2002; Hicks & Gaughan, 1995; Jason & Andereck, 1983). In the majority of studies that have examined rates

Valle, L. A., & Lutzker, J. R. (2006). Child physical abuse. In J. E. Fisher & W. T. O'Donohue (Eds.), *Practitioner's guide to evidence-based psychotherapy.* New York: Springer.

of CPA victimization, boys appear to experience CPA at slightly higher rates than girls (e.g., Corliss, Cochran, & Mays, 2002; Trocme, Tourigny, MacLaurin, & Fallon, 2003; Wolfner & Gelles, 1993).

Etiology

Most theorists and researchers currently ascribe to some variation of a social ecological model (e.g., Belsky, 1980), which takes into account the combined effects of risk and protective factors in different levels of the family's social ecology, including individual parent and child characteristics, family characteristics, community factors, and societal factors. Despite increased knowledge of risk factors associated with CPA, causal factors that are necessary and sufficient for CPA to occur remain undetermined. In addition, although community and societal factors such as lack of support and resources for families, community violence and disorganization, and CPA-consistent cultural mores are believed to contribute to risk for CPA, psychotherapeutic approaches generally focus on individual and family characteristics associated with perpetration of CPA. However, it should be noted that some individual and family characteristics, such as demographic and historical variables, are not generally amenable to change using psychotherapy.

Individual characteristics associated with perpetration of CPA include demographic, cognitive, affective, behavioral, and biological factors. The following list is a brief summary of more comprehensive reviews (i.e., Kolko, 2002; Kolko & Swenson, 2002; Milner, 1998) of CPA risk factors and characteristics of families experiencing CPA.

- Demographic characteristics include being a single, young, or nonbiological parent; having low socioeconomic status and related factors (e.g., less formal education), and a parental history of family problems including receiving or observing maltreatment as a child.
- Cognitive characteristics include low self-esteem, external locus of control, high or rigid expectations for children's behavior, negative perceptions of one's children, poor problem-solving skills, and lack of empathy.
- Affective characteristics include personal distress, depression, negative affect, anxiety, anger, hostility, and loneliness.
- Behavioral characteristics include parental tendencies to greater use of harsh, inconsistent, or intrusive parenting and less use of discipline involving reasoning. Parental use or abuse of drugs or alcohol may be associated with some instances of CPA, such as fatal CPA.

- Biological characteristics include impulsivity, increased physiological arousal to child-related and other stimuli, and perceptions of physical handicaps and physical health problems. Increased physiological arousal and impulsivity may interact with cognitive and affective factors to increase the likelihood of physical abuse during disciplinary interactions.

Family characteristics associated with CPA include:

- many children in the home,
- family poverty, financial problems, and stressors associated with poverty,
- social isolation,
- family instability or disruptions,
- absence of positive parent–child interactions and communication,
- verbal and physical conflict or violence between parents or between parents and children.

Course

Children who experience CPA are at risk for adverse short- and long-term mental and physical health outcomes, many of which may persist into adulthood (e.g., Felitti et al., 1998; Williamson, Thompson, Anda, Dietz, & Felitti, 2002). Although evidence suggests that CPA that occurs during earlier developmental stages or is chronic throughout the child's life is more detrimental (Keiley, Howe, Dodge, Bates, & Pettit, 2001; Manly, Kim, Rogosch, & Cicchetti, 2001), considerable diversity in the types of problems attributed to experiencing CPA has been observed, suggesting a lack of uniform or universal effects. A substantial percentage of children appear to be resilient and demonstrate few, if any, known problems other than the physical injury. Variation in the type and severity of problems observed in children who have experienced CPA suggests that different characteristics of the CPA (e.g., severity, frequency, duration, child's developmental age at onset or occurrence), child (e.g., coping, gender, genetic predisposition to problems that may be triggered by the CPA), or environment (e.g., a supportive adult) may contribute to children's adaptation following CPA.

Impairment

Kolko (2002) and Kolko and Swenson (2002) provide more extensive reviews of the most commonly observed effects of CPA. These effects include:

- physical injuries and fatalities and physical health problems and related risk behaviors, including heart and lung disease, obesity, and smoking;
- left hemisphere neurological impairments that may be associated with impaired language development or other specific cognitive deficits related to attention and comprehension that impact academic and social performance;
- aggressive behavior and cognitive patterns and skills deficits associated with aggressive behavior, such as perceptions of others as hostile, difficulty with trust, and social problem-solving deficits;
- delinquency, conduct disorder, and substance use;
- low self-esteem, depression, suicidality, fears, and anxiety, including posttraumatic stress disorder (PTSD) or PTSD symptomatology;
- insecure attachment and difficulties in peer relationships, including social withdrawal, social skills deficits, and peer rejection.

ASSESSMENT

What Should Be Ruled Out?

A diagnosis of child physical abuse is not dependent on ruling out other conditions. DSM-IV classifies CPA as a "problem related to abuse or neglect" under the section "other conditions that may be a focus of clinical condition." CPA is classified as a V code for the relational unit/perpetrator (to note that there is insufficient information to determine if a presenting problem can be attributed to a mental disorder) and as 995.5 if the clinical focus is on the victim of the abuse (American Psychiatric Association, 1994).

What is Involved in Effective Assessment?

A thorough review of CPA indicators is beyond the scope of the current chapter, and interested readers should consult more comprehensive texts (e.g., Johnson, 2002; Helfer, Kempe, & Krugman, 1997). Briefly, child physical abuse is generally identified through injuries unusual in type (e.g., oddly shaped), location (e.g., back of the hands), severity (e.g., first-degree burns), or frequency (e.g., repeated fractures) for the child's developmental age. A thorough medical and social history may facilitate identification through documentation of past injuries and behaviors. Abrupt changes in children's behavior or academic performance, fears, depression, anxiety, and externalizing symptoms may indicate that children are experiencing stress or other adverse circumstances, but are not necessarily specific to CPA. Mandated child maltreatment reporting laws generally require only a reasonable suspicion or belief that a child has been maltreated prior to reporting. CPS then collects evidence to document whether or not maltreatment occurred.

In most families presenting for treatment, however, CPA has already been identified by CPS or other agencies through forensic evaluations, and families are referred or court ordered for services because of the CPA. Clinical assessment in therapy settings focuses on identifying the nature and severity of problems being experienced by the child and the family, so that appropriate services can be provided. Assessment guides psychotherapy treatment goals, as well as assists in identifying where consultation or collaboration with other professionals is necessary to coordinate services (e.g., CPS and other legal entities, child educational services; links to financial and other services; substance abuse services; medical services, including pharmacological interventions). A comprehensive overview of assessment is presented by Kolko and Swenson (2002).

Helpful assessment in physical abuse cases minimally includes:

- Assessment of child safety and risk for harm to guide safety planning and clinical intervention.
- Assessment of parent motivation for treatment and readiness to change. Because the majority of parents are mandated into services, they may be unaware of or unwilling to address problematic parent or child behaviors and may be unwilling or less likely to attend or participate in treatment.
- Given the heterogeneity of problems children may demonstrate following CPA, thorough assessment of the child, including the child's educational, emotional, cognitive, social, and physical problems and needs. Assessment should include a thorough history of trauma and assessment of CPA-specific cognitions and attributions (e.g., guilt, self-blame; hostile attributional biases), which have been associated with different symptomatic patterns and problems (e.g., Valle & Silovsky, 2002).
- Problems present in parents, including substance abuse, depression, other mental health issues, use of coercive discipline or other problematic parenting behaviors, and cognitions that may increase risk for CPA or interfere with parents' ability to participate in or benefit from psychotherapy.
- Family characteristics, including family strengths, stressors and supports, and intimate partner violence and the quality of parent–child relationships and interactions.

Relevant standardized instruments may be used to identify problems requiring intervention (e.g., parent or child depression; see other chapters in this volume for instruments). There presently are a limited number of instruments specific to assessing physical abuse risk factors or abuse-specific problems. However, Saunders, Berliner, and Hanson (2002) suggest existing relevant instruments and discuss additional issues related to assessment.

What Assessments Are Not Helpful?

Assessment unrelated to the issues listed in the previous section, such as the use of projective tests, are not generally useful in assessing CPA.

TREATMENT

What Treatments Are Effective?

Treatment of CPA perpetration Because the majority of CPA incidents tend to happen during disciplinary encounters, treatment historically has focused on teaching positive nonviolent child behavior management to parents. The focus on child management subsequently expanded to address other risk factors, including parents' distorted beliefs, attributions, and problem-solving skills, parent–child communication and relationships, and parents' anger and stress. Social ecological approaches may also include parental mental health and substance abuse services, vocational training, and interventions to improve parents' social support (e.g., Kolko, 2002). Although multicomponent interventions targeting multiple risk factors are intuitively appealing and may be necessary for families with severe concurrent problems, the relative gains of providing multi-component interventions over more focused parenting approaches for preventing recurrences of CPA in typical families referred for CPA has recently been questioned (e.g., Chaffin et al., 2004). Many programs have been developed and implemented, but relatively few have been rigorously evaluated for efficacy, particularly in preventing recurrences of CPA. A number of evaluations have shown pre- to posttreatment differences in parenting stress or attitudes, but such changes may or may not be related to actual risk for CPA (Chaffin & Valle, 2003).

Treatment of children, adolescents, and adults who experience CPA Wide-spread recognition of the need for treatment of children, adolescents, or adults who have experienced CPA is a recent development. It currently is recommended that psychotherapy with children and families who have experienced CPA focus on ameliorating any adverse effects of CPA on the child as well as preventing recurrences of abuse. Psychotherapy with the child who experienced CPA may be particularly important in addressing trauma-related symptoms, which may be less likely to diminish spontaneously or through the use of parenting interventions alone (e.g., Kolko & Swenson, 2002; Runyon, Deblinger, Ryan, & Thakkar-Kolar, 2004). Abuse-specific psychotherapy, which is similar to cognitive-behavioral approaches for PTSD related to other types of trauma, has been used to address trauma-related symptoms and includes exposure to the traumatic event, coping, stress management (e.g., relaxation training, emotional and behavioral self-control), and modifying maladaptive attributions and cognitions related to the CPA.

In addition, existing efficacious approaches for social skills deficits, depression, anxiety, and aggression may be adapted for use with children and adults who have experienced CPA. A special section in the May 2003 issue of *Child Maltreatment* (Chaffin, 2003) was devoted to diagnosis and treatment of less common sequelae that may follow maltreatment (i.e., bipolar disorder, dissociative disorder, borderline personality disorder, reactive attachment disorder, schizophrenia, and somatization disorder). In addition, therapeutic day treatment programs, milieu-based therapy, multisystemic therapy, and school-based interventions have also been suggested as beneficial approaches (e.g., Brunk, Henggeler, & Whelan, 1987; Fantuzzo, Sutton-Smith, Atkins, & Meyers, 1996, and see review by Kolko, 2002).

Combined parent–child approaches Family approaches that include parents and their children have been advocated for intact families (i.e., in which children have not been removed from the home for safety reasons) or for families in which the goal is family reunification (e.g., Runyon et al., 2004). For families without severe psychiatric disorders, sadistic CPA, or intellectual or other handicaps that may preclude learning or skills acquisition, there is evidence to suggest that family approaches, which provide opportunities for parents to learn and practice discipline, communication, and relationship skills while interacting with their children, are more beneficial than traditional educational approaches involving parents alone (see review by Runyon et al., 2004). Targets frequently include increased positive and decreased negative parent–child interactions, often through teaching parents to praise or reward positive child behaviors, communicate effectively, and implement nonviolent consequences (Saunders et al., 2003).

What are Effective Self-Help Treatments?

Currently, evidence supporting the use of self-help treatments for CPA perpetration or to ameliorate the effects of CPA victimization is lacking. However, educational and support groups for potentially abusive parents (*http://www.parentsanonymous.org*) and adult survivors of CPA (*http://wwwascasupport.org*) have been established. Additional websites providing information and resources for CPA include:

- *http://www.safechild.org*
- *http://www.be-free.info*
- *http://www.childhelpusa.org*

What are Effective Therapist-based Treatments?

Specific evidence-based approaches In a review of intervention approaches for CPA (i.e., Saunders et al., 2003), programs were identified that were theoretically sound, efficacious, accepted in the field, seen as having little danger of causing harm, and had written protocols for use. These specific evidence-based interventions for CPA are primarily cognitive-behavioral in theory, approach, and techniques. Duration of the interventions tends to range from 12 to 24 sessions, and practice and skill acquisition are emphasized. The following sections briefly summarize the recommended psychotherapeutic approaches specific to CPA.

Individual child and parent physical abuse-focused cognitive-behavioral therapy (Kolko, 1996; Kolko & Swenson, 2002). In this approach, intrapersonal and interpersonal skills are taught in parallel sessions for children and parents, using specific skills instructions, role playing, feedback, and home practice. Parents learn coping and self-control skills (e.g., anger and depression management) and nonphysical discipline techniques (e.g., time-out, praise). Attributions and expectations that may contribute to violence are addressed. The children's program focuses on modifying cognitions and attributions that support aggression and violence, coping and self-control skills (e.g., relaxation, safety planning, anger and stress management), and social skills training.

Physical abuse-informed family therapy (Kolko, 1996; Kolko & Swenson, 2002). In this approach, families' understanding of coercive behavior and acquisition of positive communication and problem-solving skills are used to enhance family functioning and relationships. Treatment consists of identifying the effects of physical force and clarifying attributions of responsibility for CPA, establishing no-violence contracts and safety plans, specific family problem-solving and communication skills training, and establishing problem-solving family routines to replace coercive family patterns.

Parent–child education program for physically abusive parents (Wolfe, 1991; Wolfe, Sandler, & Kaufman, 1981). In this approach, parents are linked to resources and support in the community. Parents are taught positive play and communication skills (e.g., praise, positive physical contact), appropriate limit setting and expectations, effective instruction and commands, and nonphysical discipline strategies. Parents also learn how to improve child compliance, attending, and communication and social skills. In addition, parents are taught anger and frustration management. Parents rehearse and practice skills and receive feedback.

Parent child interaction therapy (PCIT; Hembree-Kigin & McNeil, 1995). Although originally developed as an intervention for young oppositional children, PCIT has been modified for use with families with pre-adolescent children who are experiencing CPA (e.g., Chaffin et al., 2004; Urquiza & McNeil, 1996). PCIT consists of a relationship-building phase, in which parents are taught to use praise and other positive communication skills and reduce negative communications, and a discipline phase, in which parents are taught to give effective commands and use nonphysical discipline. Therapists provide live coaching and feedback to parents, who practice skills during actual parent–child interactions. Because this approach requires home practice and joint sessions with parents and children, it may be contraindicated when parents and children have no ongoing contact.

What is effective medical treatment?

Medical treatment generally addresses child injuries resulting from CPA. Although medication may be beneficial in addressing depression or other mental health problems (see other chapters in this book) that increase risk for CPA or symptoms resulting from CPA, there is no existing pharmacological treatment to address or prevent CPA.

Other issues in management

See the previous section on assessment with respect to issues related to collaboration and coordination of services and parent motivation.

How does one select among treatments?

Currently, the evidence suggests that therapist-based cognitive-behavioral approaches are most effective in preventing recurrences of CPA and addressing the most commonly observed symptoms of children who have experienced CPA. Provision of ancillary services or medication identified through assessment may be beneficial for some families who have experienced CPA.

REFERENCES

American Psychiatric Association. (1994). *Diagnostic and statistical manual of mental disorders* (4th ed.). Washington, DC: Author.

Belsky, J. (1980). Child maltreatment: An ecological integration. *American Psychologist, 35,* 320–335.

Bergman, A. B., Larsen, R. M., & Mueller, B. A. (1986). Changing spectrum of serious child abuse. *Pediatrics, 77,* 113–116.

Brunk, M., Henggeler, S. W., & Whelan, J. P. (1987). A comparison of multisystemic therapy and parent training in the brief treatment of child abuse and neglect. *Journal of Consulting and Clinical Psychology, 55,* 311–318.

Chaffin, M. (Ed). (2003). Recognizing and treating uncommon behavioral and emotional disorders in children and adolescents who have been severely maltreated [Special focus section]. *Child Maltreatment, 9,* 123–176.

Chaffin, M., Kelleher, K., & Hollenberg, J. (1996). Onset of physical abuse and neglect: Psychiatric, substance abuse, and social risk factors from prospective community data. *Child Abuse & Neglect, 20,* 191–203.

Chaffin, M., & Valle, L. A. (2003). Dynamic risk prediction characteristics of the Child Abuse Potential Inventory. *Child Abuse & Neglect, 27,* 463–481.

Chaffin, M., Silovsky, J. F., Funderburk, B., Valle, L. A., Brestan, E. V., Balachova, T., et al. (2004). Parent–child Interaction Therapy with physically abusive parents: Efficacy for reducing future abuse reports. *Journal of Consulting and Clinical Psychology, 72,* 500–510.

Corliss, H. L., Cochran, S. D., & Mays, V. M. (2002). Reports of parental maltreatment during childhood in a United States population-based survey of homosexual, bisexual, and heterosexual adults. *Child Abuse & Neglect, 26,* 1165–1178.

Fantuzzo, J. W., Sutton-Smith, B., Atkins, M., & Meyers, R. (1996). Community-based resilient peer treatment of withdrawn, maltreated preschool children. *Journal of Consulting and Clinical Psychology, 64,* 1377–1386.

Felitti, V. J., Anda, R. F., Nordenberg, D., Williamson, D. F., Spitz, A. M., Edwards, V., et al. (1998). Relationship of childhood abuse and household dysfunction to many of the leading causes of death in adults. *American Journal of Preventive Medicine, 14,* 245–258.

Helfer, M. E., Kempe, R. S., & Krugman, R. D. (Eds.). (1997). *The battered child* (5th ed.). Chicago: University of Chicago Press.

**Hembree-Kigin, T., & McNeil, C. B. (1995). *Parent–child Interaction Therapy.* New York: Plenum.

Hicks, R. A., & Gaughan, D. C. (1995). Understanding fatal child abuse. *Child Abuse & Neglect, 19,* 855–863.

Jason, J., & Andereck, N. D. (1983). Fatal child abuse in Georgia: The epidemiology of severe physical child abuse. *Child Abuse & Neglect, 7,* 1–9.

Johnson, C. F. (2002). Physical abuse: Accidental versus intentional trauma in children. In Myers, J. E. B., Berliner, L., Briere, J., Hendrix, C. T., Jenny, C., & Reid, T. A. (Eds.), *The APSAC handbook on child maltreatment* (2nd ed., pp. 249–268). Thousand Oaks, CA: Sage Publications.

Keiley, M. K., Howe, T. R., Dodge, K. A., Bates, J. E., & Pettit, G. S. (2001). The timing of child physical maltreatment: A cross-domain growth analysis of impact on adolescent externalizing and internalizing problems. *Development and Psychopathology, 13,* 891–912.

Kolko, D. J. (1996). Individual cognitive-behavioral treatment and family therapy for physically abused children and their offending parents. A comparison of clinical outcomes. *Child Maltreatment, 1,* 322–342.

Kolko, D. J. (2002). Child physical abuse. In Myers, J. E. B., Berliner, L., Briere, J., Hendrix, C. T., Jenny, C., & Reid, T. A. (Eds.), *The APSAC handbook on child maltreatment* (2nd ed., pp. 21–54). Thousand Oaks, CA: Sage Publications.

**Kolko, D. J., & Swenson, C. C. (2002). Assessing and treating physically abused children and their families: A cognitive-behavioral approach. Thousand Oaks, CA: Sage Publications.

Lucas, D. R., Wezner, K. C., Milner, J. S., McCanne, T. R., Harris, I. N., Monroe-Posey, C. et al. (2002). Victim, perpetrator, family, and incident characteristics of infant and child homicide in the United States Air Force. *Child Abuse & Neglect, 26,* 167–186.

Manly, J. T., Kim, J. E., Rogosch, F. A., & Cicchetti, D. (2001). Dimensions of child maltreatment and children's adjustment: Contributions of developmental timing and subtype. *Development and Psychopathology, 13,* 759–782.

Milner, J. S. (1998). Individual and family characteristics associated with intrafamilial child physical and sexual abuse. In P. K. Trickett & C. J. Schellenbach (Eds.), *Violence against children in the family and the community* (pp. 141–170). Washington, DC: American Psychological Association.

Runyon, M. K., Deblinger, E., Ryan, E. E., & Thakkar-Kolar, R. (2004). An overview of child physical abuse: Developing an integrated parent–child cognitive-behavioral treatment approach. *Trauma, Violence, & Abuse, 5,* 65–85.

Saunders, B. E., Berliner, L., & Hanson, R. F. (2003). *Child physical and sexual abuse: Guidelines for treatment (Final Report: January 15, 2003).* Charleston, SC: National Crime Victims Research and Treatment Center.

Trocme, N. M., Tourigny, M., MacLaurin, B., & Fallon, B. (2003). Major findings from the Canadian incidence study of reported child abuse and neglect. *Child Abuse & Neglect, 27,* 1427–1439.

Urquiza, A. J., & McNeil, C. B. (1996). Parent–child interaction therapy: An intensive dyadic intervention for physically abusive families. *Child Maltreatment, 1,* 134–144.

US Department of Health and Human Services, Administration on Children, Youth and Families. (2004). *Child Maltreatment 2002.* Washington, DC: US Government Printing Office.

Valle, L. A., & Silovsky, J. S. (2002). Attributions and adjustment following child sexual and physical abuse. *Child Maltreatment, 7,* 9–25.

Williamson, D. F., Thompson, T. J., Anda, R. F., Dietz, W. H., & Felitti, V. (2002). Body weight and obesity in adults and self-reported abuse in childhood. *International Journal of Obesity, 26,* 1075–1082.

**Wolfe, D. A. (1991). Preventing physical and emotional abuse of children. New York: Guildford Press.

Wolfe, D. A., Sandler, J., & Kaufman, K. (1981). A competency-based parent training program for child abusers. *Journal of Consulting and Clinical Psychology, 49,* 633–640.

Wolfner, G. D., & Gelles, R. J. (1993). A profile of violence toward children: A national study. *Child Abuse & Neglect, 17,* 197–212.

**Published manuals or written protocols for evidence-based programs.

Child Sexual Abuse

Amy Hoch-Espada • Erika Ryan • Esther Deblinger

WHAT IS CHILD SEXUAL ABUSE?

Child sexual abuse refers to sexual activity with a child where consent is not or cannot be given reflecting an unequal power relationship (Berliner, 2000; Finkelhor, 1994; Berliner & Elliott, 2002). This broad definition includes sexual contact such as direct genital touching, oral-genital contact, anal and/or vaginal penetration as well as noncontact abusive acts such as voyeurism, exposure, and involvement in or exposure to pornography.

BASIC FACTS ABOUT CHILD SEXUAL ABUSE

Finkelhor (1994) found that in a retrospective review of studies approximately 25% of women and 5–15% of men in the United States and Canada experienced contact sexual abuse as children. Additionally, Widom and Morris (1997) found that over 30% of adults with documented histories of sexual abuse failed to report those experiences when questioned, suggesting that Finkelhor's findings may be an underestimate of actual rates of childhood sexual abuse. Data on childmaltreatment is collected from Child Protective Services in each state and reported by the US Department of Health and Human Services. Sexual abuse reports made up 11.5% of 2.8 million reports of suspected abuse across the country (US Department of Health and Human Services, 2000). According to Kolko (2003) these figures are likely an underestimate of the prevalence of abuse given that they are based solely on cases reported to child protective agencies.

One reason these figures may be an underestimate of the prevalence of sexual abuse is that the definition of sexual abuse varies across states, agencies and researchers. The figures based on reports to child protection agencies are limited to those instances of abuse perpetrated by an individual in a caregiver role. Furthermore, it is unclear if estimates also include sexual abuse perpetrated by children and adolescents. There are alarming statistics that suggest that between 20% and 30% of sexual abuse is committed by adolescents and between 5% and 16% committed by children (Adler & Schutz, 1995, Bagley & Shewchuk-Dann, 1991; Margolin & Craft, 1990; Brown, 2004).

Research has examined the impact of sexual abuse in *primarily* two ways. One body of literature is retrospective in nature, often focusing on adult females, while the other reports examine the effects of child sexual abuse on children who have recently suffered sexual abuse. Studies with adult females have reported that a history of childhood sexual abuse is related to later psychological difficulties that include anxiety, depression, and substance use (Cunningham, Pearce & Pearce, 1988, Fry, 1993; Laws, 1993). A variety of sexual difficulties such as promiscuity, sexual dysfunctions, sexual dysphoria, and avoidance of sexual activity have also been reported by women with a history of sexual abuse (Thakkar, 2001; Finkelhor & Browne, 1985; Fry, 1993). Studies have also reported significant increased risk or

Hoch-Espada, A., Ryan, E., & Deblinger, E. (2006). Child sexual abuse. In J. E. Fisher & W. T. O'Donohue (Eds.), *Practitioner's guide to evidence-based psychotherapy.* New York: Springer.

revictimization in adulthood (Chewning-Korpach, 1993; Wyatt, Guthrie & Notgrass, 1992). Several investigators have also demonstrated a history of child sexual abuse impacting on adult physical health, including increased gynecological problems, digestive problems, pelvic pain, and headaches (Cunningham, Pearce & Pearce, 1988; Feltti, 1991; Walker, et al., 1992).

Children who have suffered sexual abuse appear to be at increased risk for experiencing PTSD, depression, sexually reactive behavior, and general behavior problems (Deblinger, Lippman & Steer, 1996; AACAP, 1998; Finkelhor & Browne, 1985; McCleer, Deblinger, Henry & Orvashel, 1992). Children also exhibit somatic problems, such as stomaches, headaches, and skin rashes (Dubowitz, Black, Harrington & Vershoore, 1993). Furthermore, recent research suggests that chronic PTSD experienced as a result of childhood abuse may have negative effects on brain development (DeBellis et al., 1999).

It should, however, be noted that a significant proportion of children who have suffered sexual abuse demonstrate highly resilient responses and experience minimal after effects (Kendall-Tackett, Williams & Finkelhor, 1993). As a result, researchers have actively examined factors that might explain the highly divergent impact of sexual abuse on the functioning and well being of children. While several studies have documented that the child's relationship to the perpetrator and the invasiveness and forcefulness of the abuse appears to have some bearing on the child's postabuse adjustment, these characteristics are not amenable to change, and may not be as significant in influencing recovery as the reaction and supportiveness of nonoffending parents. In fact, recent studies consistently suggest that greater levels of parental support and acceptance appear to be associated with more positive child outcomes (Cohen & Mannarino, 1998a,b; Deblinger, Steer & Lippmann, 1999a,b).

The expansive literature, documenting the potentially devastating emotional and behavioral impact sexual abuse may have on children, highlights the critical need for psychotherapeutic interventions for this population that are demonstrably effective. In fact, over the last decade, considerable progress has been made with respect to the development and evaluation of evidence-based interventions for children who have suffered sexual abuse. Since 1990, a series of pre–post investigations and randomized controlled trials have documented the efficacy of the trauma-focused cognitive behavioral therapy (CBT) approach to be described here in both individual and group therapy formats (Deblinger, McLeer & Henry, 1990; Deblinger, Stauffer & Steer, 2001; Deblinger et al., 1996; Cohen & Mannarino, 1996, 1998a,b; King et al., 2000). The findings of these investigations have not only demonstrated the superior benefits of trauma-focused CBT as compared to the nondirective supportive therapy, community-based treatments as well as the passage of time, but the results have also highlighted the important role nonoffending parents can play in the treatment process. Moreover, it should be noted that one and two year follow up studies have established that symptom improvements in response to trauma-focused CBT appear to be long lasting (Cohen & Mannarino, 1998a,b; Deblinger et al., 1996). More specifically, the findings of the most recent and only multi-site treatment outcome investigation in the field to date revealed that children randomly assigned to trauma-focused CBT as opposed to children assigned to client centered therapy showed greater improvement with respect to PTSD, depression, behavior problems, shame and feelings of perceived credibility and interpersonal trust (Cohen, Deblinger, Mannarino & Steer, 2004). Participating parents demonstrated similar superior benefits in response to trauma-focused CBT in terms of general levels of depression, abuse-specific distress, parental support, and skills in responding their childrens behavioral and emotional needs. Although there have been some outcome investigations examining alternative abuse-specific treatments, several recent critical reviews of the empirical literature have clearly established this trauma-focused CBT model as the treatment of choice at this time for children who have suffered sexual abuse and their families (Saunders, Berliner, & Hanson, 2003; *http://modelprograms.samhsa.gov.*)

ASSESSMENT

What is Involved in Effective Assessment?

Given the range of difficulties children may experience subsequent to sexual abuse, a thorough pretreatment assessment can better inform the course of treatment. However, this assessment should not serve as an investigative evaluation. A forensic evaluation is warranted when: children are unable to provide a clear disclosure; allegations emerge in a custody dispute; allegations are recanted; or sexual abuse is suspected but has not been substantiated (Lippmann, 2002). Please see references under *Key Readings* for a more comprehensive description of forensic evaluations of sexual abuse.

Before initiating a pretreatment assessment, clinicians should have clarity regarding the allegations of sexual abuse. This would include substantiation of the abuse through child protective services, law enforcement, medical examination or independent forensic evaluation. The pretreatment assessment should include both interview and self and other report standardized measures to assess symptomatology specific to the experience of sexual abuse including assessments of PTSD, depression, anxiety, behavior problems, sexualized behavior as well as feelings of shame, responsibility, and distrust of others. For adolescents you should also assess substance abuse, dissociation, suicidality, and self-injury.

Given the importance of caregiver involvement in treatment, one also needs to evaluate the caregiver's overall psychosocial adjustment with respect to depression, other severe psychopathology, substance abuse as well as their level of emotional distress specifically related to the child's sexual abuse. Other helpful areas to assess include parental feelings of guilt, fear, shame, embarrassment, and available resources for social support. Because the caregiver will be involved in implementing behavior management strategies at home, parenting skills should also be assessed.

Successful implementation of this model necessitates a level of child and caregiver stability in their own emotional and behavioral functioning as well as their external environment. For example, severe psychopathology, ongoing family violence, imminent placement change, and active suicidality should be taken into consideration prior to initiating trauma-focused treatment. When these difficulties are present, the clinician may recommend other courses of action and/or treatment so that the above difficulties can be addressed or stabilized prior to the initiation of trauma-focused treatment.

TREATMENT

What Treatments are Effective?

The expansive literature, documenting the potentially devastating emotional and behavioral impact sexual abuse may have on children, highlights the critical need for psychotherapeutic interventions for this population that are demonstrably effective. In fact, over the last decade, considerable progress has been made with respect to the development and evaluation of evidence-based interventions for children who have suffered sexual abuse. Since 1990, a series of pre–post investigations and randomized controlled trials have documented the efficacy of the trauma-focused cognitive behavioral therapy (CBT) approach to be described here in both individual and group therapy formats (Deblinger et al., 1990; Deblinger et al., 2001; Deblinger et al., 1996; Cohen & Mannarino, 1996, 1998a,b; King et al., 2000). The findings of these investigations have not only demonstrated the superior benefits of trauma-focused CBT as compared to the nondirective supportive therapy, community-based treatments as well as the passage of time, but the results have also highlighted the important role nonoffending parents can play in the treatment process. Moreover, it should be noted that one and two year follow up studies have established that symptom improvements in response to trauma-focused CBT appear to be long lasting (Cohen & Mannarino, 1998a,b; Deblinger et al., 1996). More specifically, the findings of the most recent and only multisite treatment outcome investigation in the field to date revealed that children randomly assigned to trauma-focused CBT as opposed to children assigned to client centered therapy showed greater improvement with respect to PTSD, depression, behavior problems, shame and feelings of perceived credibility, and interpersonal trust (Cohen, Deblinger, Mannarino & Steer, 2004). Participating parents demonstrated similar superior benefits in response to trauma-focused CBT in terms of general levels of depression, abuse-specific distress, parental support, and skills in responding their children's behavioral and emotional needs. Although there have been some outcome investigations examining other abuse-specific treatments, several recent critical reviews of the empirical literature have clearly established this trauma-focused CBT model as the treatment of choice at this time for children who have suffered sexual abuse and their families (Saunders, Berliner, & Hanson, 2003; *http://modelprograms.samhsa.gov.*) It is noteworthy that some of the basic elements found in the trauma-focused CBT interventions are incorporated in many of the treatment approaches described in the clinical literature. Authors from a variety of theoretical orientations report that some type of trauma-focused process is important to effective treatment with victims of trauma (Benedek, 1985; Terr, 1991; Pynoos & Nader, 1988; Friedrich, 1996).

What are Effective Therapist-Based Treatments?

TF-CBT consists of individual child and caregiver sessions and joint child–caregiver sessions over approximately 12 60–90 minute sessions. Generally, the model is considered short-term but it can be expanded based on the needs of the family. Legal involvement, reunification with the perpetrator, nonsupportive caregiver(s), active suicidality and self-injury might warrant extended treatment. However, difficulties such as family conflict, school problems, and diagnostic complexity can be addressed in a more general treatment approach.

The model is short-term because it reinforces a strength-based, success-focused approach to treatment. Often, clinicians feel that sexual abuse requires long-term treatment, especially when it coexists with other child and family problems. However, research has shown short-term treatment, that remains abuse-focused, is successful in alleviating significant PTSD, depression, and behavior problems. Additionally, a short-term, strength-based approach counteracts common attributions of self-blame, responsibility, and hopelessness (ruin), teaching children that the abuse was not their fault; that they can be successful and they can move beyond the sequalae of abuse, including therapy. A guiding principle of the model is to facilitate open communication between the child and caregiver. Therefore, in the first session, children and parents are informed of this approach and explained that information will be shared with one another unless specifically requested otherwise.

For ease of presentation, the model will be described as having separate components; however, in practice, implementation of the components (e.g. coping skills, gradual exposure, psychoeducation, sex education, personal safety) are integrated across sessions. Trauma-focused work (including gradual exposure) begins in session one with identification and discussion about feelings associated with the trauma. It is important to note the necessity for a collaborative relationship between the therapist and client. Despite a structured treatment format, the foundation of treatment is built on an empathic and empowering therapist–client relationship. This type of relationship may in and of itself be healing for children and caregivers who not only have been betrayed by the perpetrator of the abuse but also may feel helpless negotiating the larger legal and child protective systems. For a more comprehensive description of the treatment model, please see *Treating Sexually Abused Children and Their Nonoffending Parents* (Deblinger & Heflin, 1996) or *Trauma-Focused Cognitive Behavioral Therapy for Children and Parents* (Cohen, Mannarino & Deblinger, 2003).

Child sessions Individual child sessions begin by focusing on developing skills that will be necessary throughout the course of treatment. These skills include a variety of coping skills meant to address typical problem areas such as anxiety, anger, and interpersonal difficulties. It is often useful to start with a skill like emotional expression which provides a baseline of a child's ability to accurately identify, label, and communicate a range of both positive and negative feelings. This skill can be taught in a variety of ways including playing feeling charades, using feeling posters or cards, discussions and roleplays which facilitates rapport-building. Another key skill that every child should be taught is cognitive coping. The child is taught how feelings, thoughts and behaviors are connected. Clinicians can teach children that the way they talk to themselves can make them feel better or worse. Depending on a child's presenting problems, including sleep difficulties, fears, aggression or peer victimization, one would provide relaxation training, visualization, anger management, and/or assertiveness training.

After a sufficient skill base has been established, the next major goal of treatment is to continue the gradual exposure piece in a more structured way by creating a trauma narrative. A rationale for the importance of a trauma narrative should be provided to both children and caregivers. A common analogy one may use to illustrate this point is to compare developing a trauma narrative to cleaning out a painful wound. For example, if you fall off your bike and cut your leg you may be tempted to avoid cleaning and caring for the injury which may hurt and take time away from being with friends. If left untreated, the injury may become infected and even more bothersome. However, while it may be temporarily painful to open up the wound and clean it out, it will then be able to heal. Although there may be a scar which will occasionally remind one of the injury, it will no longer hurt.

The findings of field research conducted by Sternberg and colleagues (Sternberg et al., 1997; Sternberg, Lamb, Esplin, & Baradaran, 1999) demonstrated that when suspected victims of child sexual abuse are encouraged to provide detailed narratives about neutral events, this "practice" experience enhances their ability to provide detailed accounts of their abusive experiences. Building on this approach, therapists are encouraged to utilize this neutral event practice exercise to begin the gradual exposure process as it communicates an expectation for the child to provide detailed information about events from beginning to end. In addition, the therapist may encourage children to incorporate into these neutral narratives what they were feeling and saying to themselves during the event being described. By beginning the more structured GE process in this manner, children provide a baseline that reflects their developmental level in terms of their abilities to provide verbal detail and express feelings and thoughts, while also enhancing their skill in expressing abuse-related narratives. The therapist should create a preliminary hierarchy of abuse-related events ranging from least to most anxiety-provoking. Examples of common abuse-related events include: the first time the abuse happened, the last time, the first person they told, telling child protection/law enforcement, medical exam, counseling, and court and the worst experience. Therapists may enhance children's feelings of control by giving them a choice between two events to discuss or two activities to engage in during each session. Therapists should be careful not to assume what part of the sexual abuse experience is the most traumatizing for the child. It is possible that discussing the legal repercussions or the disclosure is more distressing than the physical act of abuse. More than one event may be discussed and processed in a session given the child's comfort level and time.

One approach that facilitates childrens' narratives is to create a "book" about their traumatic experience. Each abuse-related event can become a "chapter" in the book. The therapist should create a calm, quiet atmosphere, free of interruptions so the child can be "in the moment" as much as possible. The clinician should explain that he/she will be the secretary and record their words which facilitates the primary goal of allowing the child to tolerate and cope with his/her distress associated with remembering the event. Another advantage to the therapist recording the child's thoughts and feelings is to identify dysfunctional beliefs about the abuse. These abuse-related beliefs should be processed with the child after completion of the narrative.

Interrupting as little as possible, the therapist may need to prompt for thoughts, feelings, and sensations associated with the event. In addition, if the child stops talking and/or the narrative is very short, the therapist may need to use prompts such as "What happened next? Then what? I wasn't there so tell me more about that." The therapist should predict for the child that he/she will not be able to write as quickly as he/she thinks so the child will have to talk slowly to allow the therapist to keep up. Going slowly forces the child to tolerate his/her feelings longer and allows the therapist to repeat back what is said, facilitating desensitization to distressing thoughts, feelings, and memories. The child's narrative is reread on several occasions including after finishing each chapter; after writing additional chapters and at the book's completion.

In order to keep the child engaged, the development of the trauma narrative may take many forms. Therapists are encouraged to be creative and utilize children's strengths and interests. For example, narratives may take the form of drawings, poetry, songs, posters, audiotapes, puppet shows, and talk/radio shows.

The next treatment component is psychoeducation which includes general information about child sexual abuse, age-appropriate information about sex and sexuality and personal safety skills. Once again it should be noted that psychoeducation can precede GE and processing. For example, it may be particularly helpful to introduce general information about child sexual abuse prior to developing the trauma narrative. Children can use information they learned from this component to dispute dysfunctional beliefs about the abuse during the cognitive processing phase. Similarly, if a child is particularly avoidant discussing their abuse experience, providing age-appropriate sex education first may increase their comfort level regarding sexually explicit material.

Parent sessions The individual treatment with the caregivers mostly parallels the work done with the child. Thus, coping skills, including emotional expression/regulation, cognitive coping, relaxation, and anger management, provide a base for being able to process their child's sexual abuse experience. As the child is writing the trauma narrative, the therapist begins sharing it with the caregiver with the goal of helping them process their own thoughts and feelings about the experience.

Similar to the child's treatment, particular components are woven across sessions based on the family's need. Because children who have experienced trauma are at increased risk for developing behavioral and/or emotional problems, caregivers are provided education about behavior management. The therapist works with the caregivers to apply the behavior management strategies to the particular problems displayed by their child. For the majority of families, increasing the caregiver's use of global and specific praise is an effective behavioral tool for changing behavior as well as for improving the caregiver–child relationship.

Joint sessions In order to ensure successful joint sessions, the child and caregiver should be prepared in their individual session time by reviewing the task for the joint session and role playing praise and positive reinforcement. Although the activities for joint sessions will vary depending on the family and increase in difficulty as treatment progresses, the goals of open communication and positive interactions remain the same. Initial joint sessions may revolve around discussion about general sexual abuse information or sex education with the goal of later joint sessions progressing to discussing and processing the child's personal sexual abuse experience. The joint sessions should serve as a model for how caregivers and children can continue to discuss any difficult topic outside of the realm of treatment. It is important to note that joint sessions are counterindicated if a caregiver is unable to respond to the child's trauma narrative in a supportive manner. This therapist would make this determination based on the caregiver's response during individual sessions.

Challenges As mentioned previously, this approach is meant to be short in duration. It is unlikely that every challenge the family faces will be addressed. The goal is to provide skills to the family which are fine-tuned during the course of treatment so that they move beyond therapy and independently apply them to future challenges.

The involvement of a supportive caregiver is ideal, however, it is not always possible and children can complete this form of treatment alone assuming that the legal guardian has provided consent. If unavailable for participation, the legal guardian also may consent to the participation of another important individual in the child's life. Since children seem to greatly benefit from having a supportive adult participate, other individuals whose participation may be considered include older siblings, grandparents, foster parents, other relatives or close family friends. Nonoffending caregivers who express a desire to help the child but who also express ambivalence about the child's disclosure or who are struggling with ongoing feelings for the perpetrator may respond well to this approach with extended sessions.

The therapist's commitment to this treatment approach as well as their own level of discomfort may pose a challenge to treatment progress. It may seem counterintuitive to encourage a child to continue an activity that causes him/her visible distress, yet discontinuing trauma-focused work actually reinforces the child's avoidance. The success of gradual exposure is dependent on detailed and often graphic descriptions of the traumatic experience. Therefore, the therapist needs to be able to tolerate the child's distress and be aware of his/her own reactions to the descriptions and the impact they may place on the child. Ultimately, the most powerful motivator for therapists, initially adopting this approach, may be objective symptom improvements as well as the not uncommon spontaneous reports from children and parents who express that talking about the sexual abuse helped them feel stronger and closer as a family unit.

Conclusions There are two overarching premises to this treatment approach. First, several studies have demonstrated (Cohen et al., 2004) that children are not likely to initiate discussions about their abuse or focus on abuse-related difficulties without the structure and guidance of the therapist. Therefore, this approach requires the therapist to take a directive role with the caregiver and child to provide abuse-related information and focus on the family's traumatic experience. Part of this directive role necessitates modeling comfort and open communication about difficult topics such as sexual abuse and sexuality.

Second, the involvement of a nonoffending caregiver has been routinely demonstrated to positively impact outcome for children (Deblinger et al., 1996). The relationship the child has with their caregivers greatly outweighs the therapeutic relationship. Therefore, it is the role of the therapist to work collaboratively with the caregiver and empower them to act as a therapeutic and supportive resource for the child even after therapy is terminated.

Finally, it is recognized that the field is still very much in its infancy in terms of our understanding of how to best respond to the psychosocial needs of children and their families in the aftermath of trauma. Thus, continued research is needed to further clarify the critical ingredients of treatment and to increase the availability and accessibility of evidence-based models such as the one described above. In fact, efforts are underway to develop more effective means of disseminating trauma-focused CBT, while also adapting the model to enhance the growth and adjustment of children facing a wide array of traumatic experiences.

WHAT IS EFFECTIVE MEDICAL TREATMENT?

To treat PTSD symptomatology, the clinical literature describes the use of various medications (Famularo, et al., 1988; Harmon & Riggs, 1996). Yet, no psychopharmacological intervention in the literature has been rigorously evaluated for its efficacy. No controlled randomized trials addressing the impact of psychiatric medications on PTSD in children and adolescents have been done. It is recommended that professionals choose psychopharmacological interventions for children experiencing PTSD (e.g. SSRI's, imipramine) based on comorbid symptoms such as depression, anxiety and ADHD (AACP, 1998).

What are Effective Self-Help Resources?
- It Happened to Me: A Teen's Guide to Overcoming Sexual Abuse by Wm. Lee Carter, Ed.D.
- A Guide for Teen Survivors: The Me Nobody Knows by Barbara Bean & Shari Bennett
- How Long Does It Hurt? By Cynthia L. Mather
- An Educational Book About Body Safety by Lori Stauffer, Ph.D. & Esther Deblinger, Ph.D.
- My Body is Private by Linda Walvoord Girard
- Please Tell! Published by Hazelden
- When Your Child Has Been Molested: A Parent's Guide to Healing and Recovery, Revised Edition by Kathryn Brohl

Useful Websites

www.aacap.org/publications/facstfam/sexabuse.htm
www.ncptsd.org/facts/specific/fs_child_sexual_abuse.html
www.apa.org/html/ojjdp/jjbul2001_1_1/contents.html.
www.apsac.org
www.nccanch.acf.hhs.gov/
www.nctsnet.org
www.modelprograms.samhsa.gov/template_cf. cfm?page=model&pkProgramID=90

REFERENCES

Adler, N. A. & Schutz, J. (1995). Sibling incest offenders. *Child Abuse and Neglect, 19*, 811–819.

American Academy of Child and Adolescent Psychiatry (1998), Practice parameters for the Assessment and Treatment of children and Adolescents with Depressive Disorders. *J Am Acad Child Adolesc Psychiatry*, 37.

Bagley, C., & Shewchuck-Dann, D. (1991). Characteristics of 60 children and adolescents who have a history of sexual assault against others: Evidence from a controlled study. *Journal of Child and Youth Care, Special Issue*, 43–52.

Benedek, E. P. (1985). Children and psychic trauma: A brief review of contemporary thinking. In S. Eth & R. S. Pynoos (Eds.), *Posttraumatic stress disorder in children.* (pp. 1–16). Washington DC: American Psychiatric Press.

Berliner, L. (2000). What is sexual abuse? In H. Dubowitz & D. DePanfilis (Eds.), *Handbook for child protection* (pp. 18–22). Thousand Oaks, CA: Sage.

Barhiner, L. & Elliott, D. M. (2002). Sexual abuse of children. *The APSAC handbook on child maltreatment* (2nd ed.) Myers, John, E. B., Berliner, L. et al. Thousand Oaks, CA, US: Sage Publications, Inc, 55–78.

Brown, J. C. (2004). *Child on child sexual abuse. An investigation of behavioral and emotional sequelae.* Unpublished doctoral dissertation, University of Pennsylvania.

Chewning-Korpach, M. (1993). Sexual revictimization: A cautionary note. *Eating Disorders, 1,* 287–297.

Cunningham, J., Pearce, T., & Pearce, P. (1988). Childhood sexual abuse and medical complaints in adult women. *Journal of Interpersonal Violence, 3,* 131–144.

Cohen, J., Deblinger, E., Mannarino, A., & R. Steer (2004). A multisite, randomized controlled trial for children with sexual abuse-related PTSD symptoms. *Journal of the American Academy of Child Adolescent Psychiatry, 43*(4), 393–402.

Cohen, J. A., & Mannarino, A. P. (1996). A treatment outcome study for sexually abused preschool children: Initial findings. *Journal of the American Academy of Child and Adolescent Psychiatry 35*(1), 42–50.

Cohen, J. A., & Mannarino, A. P. (1998a). Factors that mediate treatment outcome in sexually abused preschool children: Six and 12-month follow-up. *Journal of the American Academy of Child and Adolescent Psychiatry 37*, 44–51.

Cohen, J. A., & Mannarino, A. P. (1998b). Interventions for sexually abused children: Initial treatment findings. *Child Maltreatment, 3*(1), 17–26.

Cohen, J. A., Mannarino, A. P., & Deblinger, E. (2003). Trauma-focused cognitive behavioral therapy for children and parents. Unpublished manuscript, Drexel University, College of Medicine, Allegheny General Hospital, Pittsburgh, PA.

DeBellis, M. D., Baum, A., Birmaher, B., Keshavan, M. S., Eccard, C. H., Boring, A. M. et al. (1999). Developmental traumatology part I: Biological stress systems. *Biological psychiatry, 45,* 1259–1270.

Deblinger, E., McLeer, S. V. & Henry, D. E. (1990) Cognitive/behavioral treatment for sexually abused children suffering Post-traumatic Stress: Preliminary findings: *Journal of the American Academy of Child and Adolescent Psychiatry, 29*(5), 747–752.

Deblinger, E., & Heflin, A. (1996). *Treating Sexually Abused Children and Their Nonoffending Parents.* Thousand Oaks, CA: Sage.

Deblinger, E., Lippmann, J., & Steer, R. (1996). Sexually abused children suffering posttraumatic stress symptoms: Initial treatment outcome findings. *Child Maltreatment, 1,* 310–321.

Deblinger, E., Steer, R. A., & Lippmann, J. (1999a). Two-year follow-up study of cognitive behavioral therapy for sexually abused children suffering post-traumatic-stress symptoms. *Child Abuse & Neglect, 23,* 1371–1378.

Deblinger, E., Steer, R., & Lippmann, J. (1999b). Maternal Factors Associated With Sexually Abused Children's Psychosocial Adjustment. *Child Maltreatment, 4*(1), 13–20.

Deblinger, E., Stauffer, L. B., & Steer, R. (2001). Comparative efficacies of supportive and cognitive-behavioral group therapies for young children who have been sexually abused and their non-offending mothers. *Child Maltreatment, 6,* 332–343.

Dubowitz, H., Black, M. Harrington, D. & Verschoore, A. (1993). A follow-up study of behavior problems associated with child sexual abuse. *Child Abuse and Neglect, 17,* 743–754.

Famularo, R., Spivak, G., Bunshaft, D. (1988). Advisability of substance abuse testing in patients who severely malreat their children: The issue of drug testing before the juvenile/family courts *Bulletin of the American Academy of Psychiatry & the Law, 1988,* 217–223.

Felitti, V. J. (1991). Long-term medical consequences of incest, rape, and molestation. *Southern Medical Journal, 84,* 328–331.

Finkelhor, D., & Browne, A. (1985). The traumatic impact of child sexual abuse: A conceptualization. *American Journal of Orthopsychiatry, 55,* 530–541.

Finkelhor, D. (1994). Current information on the scope and nature of child sexual abuse. *Future of Children, 4,* 31–53.

Friedrich, W. N. (1996). An integrated model of psychotherapy for abused children. In J. Briere, L. Berliner, J. A. Bulkley, C. Jenny, & Reid, T. (Eds.), *The APSAC handbook on child maltreatment.* (pp. 104–118). Thousand Oaks, CA, US: Sage Publications, Inc.

Fry, R. (1993). Adult physical illness and childhood sexual abuse. *Journal of Psychosomatic Research, 37,* 89–103.

Harmon, R. J., & Riggs, P. D. (1996). Clonidine for postraumatic strees disorder in preschool children, *Journal of the American Academy of Child & Addescent Psychiatry, 35,* 1247–1249.

Kendall-Tackett, K. A., Williams, L. M., & Finkelhor, D. (1993). Impact of sexual abuse on children: A review and synthesis of recent empirical studies. *Psychological Bulletin, 113*(1), 164–180.

King, N., Tonge, B. J., Mullen, P., Myerson, N., Heyne, D., Rollings, S., Martin, R., & Ollendick, T. H. (2000). Treating sexually abused children with post-traumatic stress symptoms: a randomized clinical trial. *Journal of the American Academy of Child and Adolescent Psychiatry 59*(11),1347–1355.

Kolko, D. J. (2003). Child physical abuse. In J. E. B. Myers, L. Berliner, J. Briere, C. T. Hendrix, C. Jenny, & T. A. Reed (Eds.), *The APSAC handbook on child maltreatment,* (2nd ed. pp. 21–54). Thousand Oaks, CA: Sage.

Laws, A. (1993). Does a history of sexual abuse in childhood play a role in women's Medical problems? A review. *Journal of Women's Health, 2,* 165–172.

Lippmann, J. (2002). Psychological issues. In M. A. Finkel & A. P. Giardino (Eds.). *Medical evaluation of child sexual abuse: A practical guide* (2nd ed. pp. 193–213). Thousand Oaks, CA: Sage.

Margolin, L. & Craft, J. L. (1990). Child abuse by adolescent caregivers. *Child Abuse and Neglect, 14,* 365–372.

McLeer, S. V., Deblinger, E., Henry, D. & Orvashel, H. (1992). Sexually abused children at high risk for PTSD. *Journal of the American Academy of Child and Adolescent Psychiatry, 31,* 875–879.

Pynoos, R. S., & Nader, K. (1988) Psychological first aid and treatment approach to children exposed to community violence: Research implications. *Journal of Traumatic Stress, 1,* 445–473.

Substance Abuse and Mental Health Services Administration (SAMHSA). Model Programs Web site. Available from: *http://modelprograms.samhsa.gov.* Accessed (2004).

Saunders, B. E., Berliner, L., & Hanson, R. F. (Eds.) (2003). Child physical and sexual abuse: Guidelines for treatment (revised report: April 26, 2004). Charleston, SC: National Crime Victims Research and Treatment Center. Available from: http://www.musc.edu/cvc/

Sternberg, K. J., Lamb, M. E., Esplin, P. W., & Baradaran, L. P. (1999). Using a scripted protocol in investigative interviews: A pilot study. *Applied Developmental Science, 3,* 70–76.

Sternberg, K. J., Lamb, M. E., Hershkowitz, I., Yudilevitch, L., Orbach, Y., Esplin, P. W. & Hovav, M. (1997). Effects of introductory style on children's abilities to describe experiences of sexual abuse. *Child Abuse and Neglect, 21,* 1133–1146.

Terr, L. C. (1991). Childhood trauma: An outline and overview. *American Journal of Psychiatry, 148,* 10–19.

Thakkar, R. R. (2001). *Daily stressors and physical health in women with and without a history of sexual abuse.* Unpublished doctoral dissertation, Northern Illinois University.

US Department of Human Services, Administration on Children, Youth, and Families. (2000). *Child Maltreatment, 1998: Reports from the States to the National Child Abuse and Neglect Data System.* Washington DC: Government Printing Office.

Walker, E. A., Katon, W. J., Hansom, J., Harrop-Griffiths, J., Holm, L., Jones, M. L., Hickok, L., & Jemelka, R. P. (1992). Medical and psychiatric symptoms in women with childhood sexual abuse. *Psychosomatic Medicine, 54,* 658–664.

Widom, C., & Morris, S. (1997). Accuracy of adult recollection of childhood victimization: Part 2. Childhood sexual abuse. *Psychological Assessment, 9,* 34–46.

Wyatt, G. E., Guthrie, D., & Notgrass, C. M. (1992). Differential effects of women's Child sexual abuse and subsequent sexual revictimization. *Journal of Consulting and Clinical Psychology, 60,* 167–173.

APPENDIX 1. Example of one 90-minute early session

	Goals	Activities	Time
Child–individual session	• Establish rapport	• General discussion about child's interests	30–40 minutes
	• Obtain a baseline narrative about the child's experience of a neutral or positive event	• First have child describe a neutral event in detail to set example, then explain why they are coming to treatment specific to the abuse	
	• Build emotional expression skills	• Feelings charades, feelings games, make a list of feelings, books, etc.	
	• Provide education about child sexual abuse	• Play a (question/answer) game about child sexual abuse and/or read a book about child sexual abuse	
Caregiver–individual session	• Provide treatment rationale – instill hope	• Highlight the importance of a supportive caregiver in outcome	30–40 minutes
	• Provide education about child sexual abuse	• Discuss factual information about child sexual abuse	
	• Introduce behavior management principle of praise	• Teach global and specific praise. Use examples and role plays	
Joint session	• Demonstrate open communication about child sexual abuse	• Card game (question/answer) about child sexual abuse information	10–15 minutes
	• Strengthen caregiver child relationship	• Mutual exchange of praise	

APPENDIX 2. Example of one 90-minute session from mid-treatment

	Goals	Activities	Time
Child–individual session	• Review rationale for gradual exposure	• Review child's gradual exposure work from prior sessions	30–40 minutes
	• Reduce distress associated with the abusive experience	• Continue to add additional "chapters" to child's book by providing choices of topics to focus on	
	• Elicit abuse related thoughts and feelings	• Reinforce education about child sexual abuse when disputing dysfunctional beliefs	
	• Process and dispute dysfunctional thoughts	• Prepare for joint session with caregiver. Help child generate questions for caregiver and practice praise for the caregiver	
Caregiver–individual session	• Reduce distress associated with the child's abusive experience	• Share the child's gradual exposure work	30–40 minutes
	• Elicit abuse related thoughts and feelings	• Assist in applying cognitive coping skills to combat dysfunctional beliefs	
	• Process and dispute dysfunctional thoughts	• Prepare for joint session with child. Role play caregiver's comments to the selected	

		"chapter" of the child's book as well as praise	
	• Assist caregiver in managing child's behavior at home		
Joint session	• Promote open communication about the child's experience of abuse	• Child shares a "chapter" from gradual exposure book	10–20 minutes
	• Provide an opportunity for the caregiver to model comfort when discussing the abuse	• Mutual exchange of praise	
	• Strengthen relationship		

APPENDIX 3. Example of one 90-minute session from mid-treatment

	Goals	*Activities*	*Time*
Child– individual session	• Review rationale for gradual exposure	• Review child's gradual exposure work from prior sessions	30–40 minutes
	• Reduce distress associated with the abusive experience	• Continue to add additional "chapters" to child's book by providing choices of topics to focus on	
	• Elicit abuse related thoughts and feelings	• Reinforce education about child sexual abuse when disputing dysfunctional beliefs	
	• Process and dispute dysfunctional thoughts	• Prepare for joint session with caregiver. Role play sharing the "chapter" from the child's book as well as praise for the caregiver	
Caregiver– individual session	• Reduce distress associated with the child's abusive experience	• Share the child's gradual exposure work	30–40 minutes
	• Elicit abuse related thoughts and feelings	• Assist in applying cognitive coping skills to combat dysfunctional beliefs	
	• Process and dispute dysfunctional thoughts	• Prepare for joint session with child. Role play caregiver's comments to the selected "chapter" of the child's book as well as praise	
	• Assist caregiver in managing child's behavior at home		
Joint session	• Promote open communication about the child's experience of abuse	• Child shares a "chapter" from gradual exposure book	
	• Provide an opportunity for the caregiver to model comfort when discussing the abuse	• Mutual exchange of praise	
	• Strengthen caregiver-child relationship		

CHAPTER 18

Psychotherapy with Chronic Pain Patients

Robert J. Gatchel • Richard C. Robinson • Anna Wright Stowell

INTRODUCTION

It is increasingly accepted among medical and mental health care providers that cognitions and emotions play a significant role in the perception of chronic pain and resulting disability. Though this seems an obvious point, it is a major leap considering that, as recently as 40 years ago, the primary thought was that all pain perception is directly related to the severity of injury (i.e., the worse it looks the worse it must be), as pain was believed to exist only in the presence of identifiable, causal, pathophysiology. This archaic, dualistic Cartesian style of thinking has since evolved considerably (Turk, 1996). In the 1950s, both (Bonica, 1953) and Engel (1959) described psychological factors as important contributors to the pain experience.

Melzack, a leader in the exploration of the etiology behind the perception and experience of pain, made an important early contribution to its understanding. In 1965, Melzack and Wall (1965) proposed the *gate control theory of pain*, which solidified the involvement of the central nervous system (CNS) as an essential component in the perception and processing of pain. The *gate control theory of pain* served to provide a scientific understanding of how brain-generated experiences, such as emotion, affected pain perception. This theory effectively narrowed the gap between the mental and physical health fields by tying together nociception and emotional experience. Following this, a proliferation of research arose aimed at identification of specific psychological and social factors believed to play a key role in the development, maintenance and perception of pain. Specifically, Gatchel and Epker (1999) and Turk (1996) discussed at length the various contributions of behavioral, affective, and cognitive factors, as well as psychosocial risk factors for pain. In sum, their research has served to further refute the previous dualistic view of pain—that pain patients were either legitimate medical patients with "real" physical etiology or that they were psychiatric patients whose pain experience was "all in their head."

Despite the incorrect assumption that chronic pain is an inherently psychological problem, chronic pain patients *do have* a higher prevalence of psychiatric disorders, such as depression and personality disorders, relative to the general population (Gatchel, Polatin, Mayer, & Garcy, 1994; Kinney, Gatchel, Polatin, Fogarty, & Mayer, 1993; Polatin, Kinney, Gatchel, Lillo, & Mayer, 1993). Specifically, Kinney et al. (1993) found that, among 200 chronic low back pain patients who were assessed with the Structured Clinical Interview for the Diagnostic and Statistical Manual of Mental Disorders-III-Revised, 70% met lifetime diagnostic criteria for Axis I disorders and 51% met criteria for Axis II diagnoses. In addition to significant psychiatric distress, patients with chronic pain often have a number of additional risk factors for increased difficulty in obtaining maximal treatment gains. Specific factors identified in the literature include: a patient's reliance on passive coping strategies (e.g., catastrophizing, hoping and praying, M. J. L. Sullivan et al., 2001)

Gatchel, R. J., Robinson, R. C., Stowell, A. W. (2006). Psychotherapy with chronic pain patients. In J. E. Fisher & W. T. O'Donohue (Eds.), *Practitioner's guide to evidence-based psychotherapy*. New York: Springer.

versus active ones (trying to distract oneself by getting together with friends or working on a hobby, etc., Truchon & Fillion, 2000); the presence of psychological distress, which is a barrier for positive patient outcomes through reduced treatment compliance (Proctor, Gatchel, & Robinson, 2000; Riley et al., 1999); vulnerability to stress-related increases in pain (e.g., as measured by elevations of certain Minnesota Multiphasic Personality Inventory (MMPI) profiles such as the "conversion V", Proctor et al., 2000); and depression (Proctor et al., 2000).

Gatchel (1996) has further described the complex interplay of pain, psychopathology, and personality in the form of a three-stage model of the progression from acute to subacute to chronic pain and disability. His model describes the emotional deconditioning that occurs over the progression of injury and illness. Specifically, in Stage 1, patients react to the pain stimulus with emotionality such as fear and anxiety. In Stage 2, pain extends past the normal expected duration of healing and patients begin to demonstrate psychosocial distress. This display of distress will likely depend on patients' premorbid personality characteristics and current stressors. In Stage 3, assumption of the "sick role" occurs when patients solely focus on the pain and resulting limitations. At this stage, they are unable to effectively cope and problem-solve appropriate pain management solutions without therapeutic assistance.

The above theories and models fit nicely with the currently well-accepted *biopsychosocial model* of pain, which has been relied upon heavily in the field of rehabilitation since the 1980's. Schultz (2000) traces the etiology of the *biopsychosocial model* 50 years ago to a meeting of the World Health Organization (WHO) in which health was defined as a multifaceted combination of biological/physical, emotional/psychological, and social well-being, as opposed to a mere absence of biological organic pathology. Thus, the WHO functionally recognized that health and, conversely, disability are defined by a complex interaction among a variety of factors. Further, Belar and Deardorff (1999) recount evidence dating back to the 1700s of individuals recognizing an interaction between the body and mind. The growing amount of evidence supporting a mind–body interaction eventually led to a model of pain and disability which, instead of exclusively focusing on either psychosocial or physical etiologies, conceptualizes pain and disability as a consequence of the *interaction* among biological, psychological and social phenomena. This model is a multifaceted model that considers biological, psychological, and social aspects (Crichton & Morley, 2002; Gatchel, 1996; Wright & Gatchel, 2002). Not only do these multiple factors contribute to the etiology of disability, they have a reciprocal effect of intensifying and perpetuating each other and, consequently, impacting the duration and intensity of pain and disability symptomatology (Crichton & Morley, 2002).

Within the biopsychosocial model, the patient is treated as a "whole" person, not just a body part or painful condition. Consequently, the treatment goals are aimed not exclusively at relieving the pain, but rather more importantly on improving the individual's quality of life and restoring his or her full functioning in physical, occupational, emotional, and social domains. Also, Kwan, Ferrari, and Friel (2001) stress that the *biopsychosocial model* of disability addresses all aspects of disability, including consideration of possible patient motivators such as secondary and tertiary gains. To date, the *biopsychosocial model* remains one of the most comprehensive ways of conceptualizing and treating chronic pain (Mayer, Gatchel, & Evans, 2002).

Though the biopsychosocial model is widely accepted and serves as the basis for the majority of interdisciplinary chronic pain treatment programs, scientific research of the mind–body relationship is ever evolving. Most recently, Melzack (1999) has built upon his previous *gate control theory of* pain and developed the *neuromatrix model of pain*. This model grew out of Melzack's work with patients who continued to experience pain following spinal cord resection (i.e., as in phantom limb pain). His new model proposes a complex interaction of neural inputs from within and outside of the brain. This latest model, the *neuromatrix model*, accounts for genetic contributions to the perception of pain, as well as the individual's recent past and present experience, and sensory inputs.

To address the multifactorial contributors to pain, including physical, psychological, and social phenomena, the most widely accepted and utilized method is the cognitive-behavioral therapeutic approach. Within the cognitive-behavioral model, patients are educated about the mind–body connection and then instructed in techniques to manage pain and related stress and disability for the purpose of increasing function *despite* pain. The key components of this approach are described below.

KEY CONCEPTUAL FACTORS

Physical Deconditioning

Physical deconditioning, involving the progressive lack of use of the body, generally accompanies patients during their progressing toward chronic disability. It produces a circular effect leading to increased mental deconditioning. The combined interaction of the symptoms negatively impacts the emotional well-being and self-esteem of an individual (Gatchel & Turk, 1996).

Pain versus Hurt

When patients engage in an activity that produces pain, they are likely to associate the pain with the initial hurt. This causes patients to fear and avoid pain and possible pain-producing situations. Unfortunately, pain often accompanies physical reconditioning and the additional steps needed in order to resume normal responsibilities and social obligations. Therefore, patients must be taught that hurt and harm are not the same (Fordyce, 1988).

Coping

The ways an individual manages and copes with general stressors help to determine who will become a chronic pain patient. Thus, assessment of coping styles and instructing patients on more adaptive coping skills is an important part of a cognitive behavioral approach to treatment. The Multidimensional Pain Inventory (MPI), formerly the West-Haven Yale Multidimensional Pain Inventory, developed by Kerns, Turk, and Rudy (1985), is one of the most widely used measures in the pain area. The MPI is a brief self-report instrument that examines the person's perception of pain and coping ability. The MPI helps to identify patients who have difficulty coping with their pain, and it can guide the implementation of pain reduction interventions. Turk and Rudy (1988) identified three coping styles, using a cluster analysis on the MPI scales with a heterogeneous group of chronic pain patients: *dysfunctional* (43%), *interpersonally distressed* (28%) and *adaptive copers* (29.5%). The dysfunctional group members reported that their pain, and the interference caused by their pain, was extreme. Patients in the interpersonally distressed group reported a lack of support, caring, and understanding from their family members and significant others. In contrast, individuals in the adaptive copers group reported high levels of activity and life control, as well as lower levels of pain intensity, perceived interference, and affective distress.

Catastrophizing

The role of catastrophizing in the prediction of chronic pain and disability has gained increased attention in recent years. Catastrophizing involves thinking negatively, and in an exaggerated fashion, about events and stimuli. This can be applied to how individuals perceive their pain or their ability to cope with their pain (Sullivan, Stanish, Waite, Sullivan, & Tripp, 1998). In one of the first studies to address this variable, Butler, Damarin, Beaulieu, Schwebel, and Thorn (1989) evaluated cognitive strategies and postoperative pain in a sample of general surgical patients, and they found that increased catastrophizing was associated with higher levels of postoperative pain intensity. Main and Waddell (1991) also looked at this variable and found a strong relationship between catastrophizing and depressive symptoms in a sample of low back pain patients. Furthermore, of the cognitive variables investigated by the authors, catastrophizing was determined to have the "greatest potential for understanding current low back symptoms" (Main & Waddell, 1991, p. 287). Fortunately, catastrophizing is amenable to, and especially suited for, cognitive-behavioral interventions.

COGNITIVE BEHAVIORAL THERAPY FOR CHRONIC PAIN

Turk and Gatchel (2002) succinctly describe five aims of cognitive behavior therapy (CBT) for chronic pain. The *first goal* is to help patients alter their perceptions of their pain, from something that is overwhelming to something that they can learn to manage. The *second goal* is to educate patients that CBT will provide them with the tools they need to manage their pain more adaptively. The *third goal* is to alter each patient's self-perception, from someone who is passive and helpless to someone who is active and has the ability to affect both self and environment. The *fourth goal* is to instruct patients on how to monitor thoughts, feelings, behaviors, and physiology so that they can develop and maintain an understanding of the relationship among these variables. Finally, the *fifth goal* is to teach patients to develop more adaptive responses to their chronic pain that can be used in a variety of settings, and that can be maintained over time.

With these goals in mind, treatment consists of four major components: (1) reconceptualization; (2) skills acquisition; (3) skills consolidation; and (4) generalization and maintenance (Turk & Gatchel, 2002). Each of the procedures that accompany these components will be briefly reviewed.

Reconceptualization

Reconceptualization of chronic pain has two major components. The first involves instructing patients on how to recognize problematic thoughts; the second is helping people restructure their thinking (a process termed *cognitive restructuring*). Using a pain diary that asks patient to record their pain and tension levels at various times throughout the day, as well as to record their thoughts and feelings before, during, and after those times when their pain increases, is a way of identifying maladaptive thoughts such as "The pain is killing me" or "If it hurts, I must be making it worse."

Once common negative thoughts have been identified, the therapist and the patient can work collaboratively to challenge the thoughts. This systematic questioning approach to previously unchallenged assumptions allows the patients to develop more objective, problem-solving, and therefore adaptive thoughts. For instance, a patient who thinks to herself, "I'll never travel again," can examine that thought objectively. It may be that the patient can travel, but that the physical cost of the pain would be unacceptable. However, with relaxation training, the cost of the pain could be decreased so that traveling is not something to be feared. Notice that the thought is not simply converted to a positive, "Pollyana-ish" thought, but to one that is more objective, active, and adaptive. Alteration of perceptions and long-standing beliefs does not happen during the sessions; rather, it happens when the patients practice more adaptive coping thoughts in their environment. When positive affective and behavioral changes occur, the therapist continuously draws the patients' attention to their accomplishments in an attempt to increase self-efficacy and reinforce adaptive change.

Skills Acquisition

Skills acquired in CBT for chronic pain can be roughly divided into self-regulatory skills and stress-management skills. *Self-regulatory skills* are techniques that allow patients to alter their physiological functioning in a manner that can decrease their pain, such as reducing muscle tension or autonomic arousal. The most common self-regulatory skills are relaxation training, distraction, self-hypnosis, and biofeedback. *Stress-management skills* entail teaching effective communication, planning, and time management strategies, as well as providing patients with a systematic approach to problem solving.

Two skills that are listed that may not be as recognizable to other CBT clinicians are attention diversion and pacing. With regard to *attention diversion*, also referred to as distraction techniques, the goal is to help the patient focus on other thoughts or feelings that are unrelated to his or her pain. One can easily imagine different distraction techniques, such as reading, conversing with a friend, or watching television.

Pacing is a deceptively simple-sounding concept that, in practice, can be challenging for patients without proper guidance and practice. The notion is that chronic pain patients will slowly begin to exercise and engage in physical activity that will increase adaptive beliefs and self-efficacy. The goal of pacing is for individuals to learn to be physically active to meet reasonable predetermined goals, rather than engaging in activity until the pain has overwhelmed them. For instance, if a patient can mow the yard for 30 min before his or her back begins to hurt, the patient may be instructed to mow the yard in 15 min increments.

Skills Consolidation

In the skill consolidation phase, patients continue to practice, refine, and rehearse the new skill they have acquired. Having the patient practice with the therapist in session, as well as beginning to have the patient more fully integrate the skill in his or her environment outside therapy, becomes increasingly important. Practitioners of CBT will often have patients imagine using the skills in different situations, or will role-play with the patient various different problems that may occur.

Generalization and Maintenance

Cognitive behavior therapy for chronic pain should not be thought of as a one-time treatment that leads to a definitive cure. It provides people with the tools to manage their pain, so that it has an appreciable impact on their ability to enjoy those things in their lives that they perceive as important. For CBT to be truly effective, patients must continue to practice even when they have completed their course of therapy. Follow-up appointments at 3- to 6-month intervals, or on an as-needed basis, insure that the patients' gains are maintained and reinforce the progress they have made. It should be noted that Marlatt and Gordon have written extensively on the issue of relapse prevention, and their ideas are easily translatable to pain patients (e.g., Marlatt & Gordon, 1985). That is to say, preparing the patients for inevitable setbacks does not make them more likely to occur. Instead, patients learn to reframe a setback as a temporary, manageable, and typical part of recovery. If a patient's pain flares up, and the patient has stopped practicing his or her relaxation skills, then the patient is well prepared to engage in objective examination of any irrational negative thoughts. Patients can begin to take the necessary steps to retrain their bodies to relax without interference from thoughts that the situation is "hopeless."

CONCLUSIONS

Cognitive behavior therapy for chronic pain incorporates techniques that are common for any CBT intervention. The slight adjustments to treatment involve educating patients about how psychosocial factors influence their pain. In addition, activity pacing and distraction are other techniques that are frequently used with chronic pain patients; they may not be as frequently used with nonchronic pain patients. Unfortunately, chronic pain has a ripple effect, and very few areas of a person's life are not impacted when his or her pain is severe enough, and when it has lasted for a long period of time. However, the techniques learned in CBT have a ripple effect as well, and they frequently impact areas of a person's life that are outside the treatment's immediate focus. Of course, it is also extremely important that therapists working with chronic pain patients have a thorough understanding of the biopsychosocial approach to pain assessment and treatment because of the often complex interaction among physical, psychological and socioeconomic factors that are underlying pathophysiology and pain behaviors (cf. Gatchel & Turk, 1996). Finally, for a more detailed review of material presented in this Chapter, the reader is referred to publications by Gatchel (2004) and Gatchel and Robinson (2003).

REFERENCES

Belar, C. D., & Deardorff, W. W. (1999). *Clinical health psychology in medical settings, revised.* Washington, DC: APA.

Bonica, J. J. (1953). *The management of pain.* Philadelphia: Lea & Febiger.

Butler, R. W., Damarin, F. L., Beaulieu, C., Schwebel, A. L., & Thorn, B. E. (1989). Assessing cognitive coping strategies for acute postsurgical. *Pain,* 139–153.

Crichton, P., & Morley, S. (2002). Treating pain in cancer patients. In D. C. Turk & R. J. Gatchel (Eds.), *Psychological approaches to pain management: A practitioner's handbook* (2nd ed.). New York: Guilford Press.

Engel, G. L. (1959). "Psychogenic" pain and the pain-prone patient. *American Journal of Medicine,* 899–918.

Fordyce, W. E. (1988). Pain and suffering: A reappraisal. *American Psychologist, 43,* 276–283.

Gatchel, R. J. (1996). Psychological disorders and chronic pain: Cause and effect relationships. In R. J. Gatchel & D. C. Turk (Eds.), *Psychological approaches to pain management: A practitioner's handbook* (pp. 33–52). New York: Guilford.

Gatchel, R. J. (2004). *Clinical essentials of pain management.* Washington, DC: American Psychological Association.

Gatchel, R. J., & Epker, J. T. (1999). Psychosocial predictors of chronic pain and response to treatment. In R. J. Gatchel & D. C. Turk (Eds.), *Psychosocial factors in pain: Critical perspectives* (pp. 412–434). New York: Guilford Publications, Inc.

Gatchel, R. J., Polatin, P. B., Mayer, T. G., & Garcy, P. D. (1994). Psychopathology and the rehabilitation of patients with chronic low back pain disability. *Archives of Physical Medicine & Rehabilitation, 75*(6), 666–670.

Gatchel, R. J., & Robinson, R. C. (2003). Pain management. In W. O'Donohue, J. E. Fisher & S. C. Hayes (Eds.), *Cognitive behavior therapy: Applying empirically supported techniques in your practice.* New York: John Wiley & Sons, Inc.

Gatchel, R. J., & Turk, D. C. (1996). *Psychological approaches to pain management: A practitioner's handbook*. New York: Guilford Publications, Inc.

Kerns, R. D., Turk, D. C., & Rudy, T. E. (1985). The West Haven-Yale multidimensional pain inventory. *Pain, 23*, 345–356.

Kinney, R. K., Gatchel, R. J., Polatin, P. B., Fogarty, W. J., & Mayer, T. G. (1993). Prevalence of psychopathology in acute and chronic low back pain patients. *Journal of Occupational Rehabilitation, 1993*, 95–103.

Kwan, O., Ferrari, R., & Friel, J. (2001). Tertiary gain and disability syndromes. *Medical Hypotheses, 57*(4), 459–464.

Main, C. J., & Waddell, G. (1991). A comparison of cognitive measures in low back pain: Statistical structure and clinical validity at initial assessment. *Pain, 56*, 287–298.

Marlatt, G. A., & Gordon, W. H. (1985). Relapse prevention: Introduction and overview of the model. *British Journal of Addiction, 79*, 261–273.

Mayer, T. G., Gatchel, R. J., & Evans, T. H. (2002). Chronic low back pain. In R. H. Fitzgerald, H. Kauger & A. L. Malkani (Eds.), *Orthopadics* (pp. 1192–1197). St. Louis: Mosby.

Melzack, R. (1999). Pain and stress: A new perspective. In R. J. Gatchel & D. C. Turk (Eds.), *Psychosocial factors in pain: Critical perspectives*. New York: Guilford Publications, Inc.

Melzack, R., & Wall, P. D. (1965). Pain mechanisms: A new theory. *Science, 50*, 971–979.

Polatin, P. B., Kinney, R., Gatchel, R. J., Lillo, E., & Mayer, T. G. (1993). Psychiatric Illness and Chronic Low Back Pain: The Mind and the Spine-Which Goes First? *Spine, 18*, 66–71.

Proctor, T., Gatchel, R. J., & Robinson, R. C. (2000). Psychosocial factors and risk of pain and disability. In D. C. Randolph & M. I. Ranavaya (Eds.), *Occupational Medicine: State of the Art Reviews* (Vol. 15, pp. 803–812). Philadelphia: Hanley and Belfus, Inc.

Riley, J., 3rd, Robinson, M., Wise, E., Campbell, L., Kashikar-Zuck, S., & Gremillion, H. (1999). Predicting treatment compliance following facial pain evaluation. *Cranio, 17*(1), 9–16.

Schultz, I. Z., Crook, J., Fraser, K., & Joy, P. W. (2000). Models of diagnosis and rehabilitation in musculoskeletal pain-related occupational disability. *Journal of Occupational Rehabiliation, 10*(4), 271–293.

Sullivan, M. J., Stanish, W., Waite, H., Sullivan, M., & Tripp, D. A. (1998). Catastophizing, pain and disability in patients with soft-tissue injury. *Pain, 77*, 253–260.

Sullivan, M. J. L., Thorn, B., Haythornthwaite, J. A., Keefe, F., Martin, M., Bradley, L. A., et al. (2001). Theoretical perspectives on the relation between catastrophizing and pain. *Clinical Journal of Pain, 17*(1), 52–64.

Truchon, M., & Fillion, L. (2000). Biopsychosocial determinants of chronic disability and low-back pain: A review. *Journal of Occupational Rehabilitation, 10*(2), 117–142.

Turk, D., & Rudy, T. (1988). Toward an empirically derived taxonomy of chronic pain patients: Integration of psychological assessment data. *Journal of Consulting & Clinical Psychology, 56*, 233–238.

Turk, D. C. (1996). Biopsychosocial perspective on chronic pain. In R. J. Gatchel & D. C. Turk (Eds.), *Psychological approaches to pain management* (pp. 3–32). New York: Guilford Press.

Turk, D. C., & Gatchel, R. J. (Eds.). (2002). *Psychological approaches to pain management: A practitioner's handbook* (2nd ed.). New York: Guilford.

Wright, A. R., & Gatchel, R. J. (2002). Occupational musculoskeletal pain and disability. In D. C. Turk & R. J. Gatchel (Eds.), *Psychological approaches to pain management: A practitioner's handbook, 2nd edition* (2nd ed., pp. 349–364). New York: Guilford.

Delirium

James A. D'Andrea

WHAT IS DELIRIUM?

Delirium is an acute disorder of cognition characterized primarily by a disturbance in attention. The DSM-IV criteria for delirium define it as the acute onset of a reduced ability to focus and sustain attention, disorganized thinking, with fluctuations over the course of a day, and with evidence of a neurologic or medical cause. The four disorders included in the DSM-IV delirium section all have similar disturbances in attention and cognition but are differentiated by their etiology: (1) delirium due to a general medical condition, (2) substance-induced delirium, (3) delirium due to multiple etiologies, and (4) delirium not otherwise specified. Delirium is reversible once the etiology is identified and appropriate treatment initiated.

The clinical presentation of most patients with delirium falls into two main categories: lethargic or agitated (Liptzin & Levkoff, 1992). In some patients the picture is consistent throughout the course of the acute episode, whereas in others, it can vary from lethargy to agitation during the same day. For example, the lethargic patient can become very anxious and agitated when the lights are turned off in the room at night, and the patient is left alone with reduced sensory stimulation. Disorientation in delirium with respect to time and place is common. Even when alertness is not altered, subtle changes in attention will be evident on traditional measures of attention (e.g., serial 7s or digit span tasks), and other continuous performance tasks (e.g., asking the patient to raise his hand each time to indicate when a word with the letter "A" is spoken in a sentence).

Delirium develops rapidly over hours or days, but rarely over more than a week. Besides decreased attention, other behavioral and neuropsychiatric symptoms are often associated with delirium including impairments in language, memory, visual-spatial ability, executive functioning, hallucinations, and delusions, alterations in mood, sleep cycle abnormalities, and autonomic dysfunction (Trzepacz et al., 2001).

The behavioral change most evident in delirium is an inability to sustain attention (Chedru & Geschwind, 1972a,b; Albert, 1988).

Language alterations in delirium include abnormal spontaneous speech, anomia, misnaming, and agraphia (Chedru & Geschwind, 1972a,b; Benson, 1979). The spontaneous speech content of delirious patients is rambling, incoherent, and can shift from topic to topic. Further, words can be slurred or mispronounced making it difficult to comprehend what is being verbalized. Anomia, may be observed in the course of spontaneous speech or observed on tasks of confrontational naming. The presence of paraphasias is rare in delirium and has stronger association with stroke or brain trauma than delirium. A wide range of handwriting abnormalities can be present in delirious patients including illegibility, poor spatial alignment, abbreviated agrammatical sentences, and spelling errors. Omissions, substitutions, and duplication errors are particularly common. As in writing, construction tasks are also affected in delirium. Line drawings of simple figures may be distorted, or unrecognizable. Three-dimensional aspects are lost, and lines and angles are omitted (Trezepacz, 1994).

D'Andrea, J. A. (2006). Delirium. In J. E. Fisher & W. T. O'Donohue (Eds.), *Practitioner's guide to evidence-based psychotherapy*. New York: Springer.

Memory and learning difficulties are virtually always present to some extent in delirium. Impairment in learning is attributed to poor registration caused by the attentional deficits caused by delirium. Memory deficits can be elicited when patients are asked to recall three words after a brief period of interpolated activity. Some patients may not be able to repeat the three words at all immediately after hearing them.

Executive functioning deficits in delirium are pervasive. Thinking becomes concrete, and abstraction and categorization skills are limited. Discrepancies do not trouble delirious patients even when they are pointed out. Errors in calculation occur on mathematical tasks that require sums to be "carried over" to adjacent columns. Perseveration is common in all aspects of behavior in patients with delirium. It contributes to repetition errors seen in writing, speaking, and construction. "Occupational delirium" (Wolff & Curran, 1935) refers to the repetitious behavior seen in patients who act as if they are continuing their usual occupation of driving, cooking, or working despite being in a hospital bed. They may pantomime activities of everyday life, such as removing nonexistent glasses, or take nonexistent pills.

Neuropsychiatric symptoms including hallucinations, delusions, and mood changes can exist in delirium. In some cases, they dominate the patient's presentation to such an extent that staff will call for mental health for consultation because it is believed the patient suffers from a psychiatric disorder. The hallucinations in delirium tend to be silent visual images such as people peering into the room through a window, or a dog walking through the room (Lipowski, 1990; Rummans, Evans, Krahn, & Fleming, 1995). Tactile hallucinations are not unusual, particularly in deliriums caused by withdrawal symptoms from illicit drug and alcohol abuse. Auditory hallucinations may also occur but are less likely to be found that visual hallucinations. The delusions occurring in delirium are wide ranging in their presentation. They can be simple, transient, or may be complex and rigidly held (Cummings, 1985; Nash, 1983). Occasionally, a specific type of delusion will occur called Capgras syndrome, the belief that significant others have been replaced by identical appearing imposters (Edelstyn & Oyebode, 1999). Delusions can cause patients to become combative, self-destructive, or paranoid in the behavior and be the most difficult aspect of delirium to manage.

A wide range of mood disturbances is frequently observed in delirious patients. Moods can range form euphoria to depression, and fearful paranoia to indifference, and apathy can occur (Chedru & Geschwind, 1972a,b; Lipowski, 1990; Trzepacz, 1994). The most common affective states in delirium are labile, perplexed, or excitable. Mood changes that accompany delusions are often congruent with the content of the delusions.

COURSE OF DELIRIUM

Strub and Black (1988) described the course of untreated delirium. In the early stages of delirium, patients are frequently restless, and have disturbed sleep patterns. Mild behavioral and affective changes are noted including anxiety or depressive feelings. Difficultly concentrating, conversation that tends to drift from the subject is observed. As they condition progresses, patients lose the ability to think clearly and efficiently. Their thoughts begin to lack coherence. Patients often lose track of time and the temporal sequence of recent events, describing events as having happened that day that actually occurred in the recent past. All these symptoms fluctuate but are usually accentuated at night.

In later states, these symptoms become more severe. Inattention and distractibility are more severe, speech is less coherent, and the patients appear confused and bewildered. They are unsure of the date and gradually show disorientation for place as well as time. Delirious patients exhibit changes in their activity level. Although restlessness may be accentuated to the point of agitation and hyperactivity, other patients can be observed to have decreased consciousness, psychomotor retardation, and lethargy. Furthermore, agitated patients may show swings from hyperactivity to lethargy within a 24-hour period. In this more severe stage, abnormalities in perception can occur, and patients may misperceive unfamiliar people in their environment as being familiar.

Eventually, delirious patients lose touch with reality, become grossly disoriented, incoherent, and hallucinatory. Fluctuations in level of awareness are more dramatic, and the patients are totally unable to sustain attention. At this point the behavioral symptoms can be classified as psychotic in degree. If the process is not reversed, the patients will rapidly become stuporous. Patients who have been grossly agitated may present with a muttering stupor (i.e., requiring vigorous stimulation to arouse, yet emitting constant muttering noises).

Statistically, the long-term prognosis for delirium is not good. Death is not an uncommon outcome because of the seriousness of many of the etiologic conditions. It has been shown that 35% of the patients who develop delirium die within one year of their confusional state (Rabins & Folstein, 1982). Although many of the patients in the terminal stages of metabolic disease or organ failure develop delirium, it does highlight the importance of identifying and treating the underlying causes of delirium in patients who exhibit a rapid decline in consciousness.

PREVALENCE AND ETIOLOGY OF DELIRIUM

Delirium is highly prevalent but often overlooked in medical settings perhaps because it can accompany so many different conditions, and because of the range of etiologies involved. Clinicians fail to diagnose delirium in about 32–67% of delirious patients (Inouye, 1994). Fifty one percent of postoperative patients develop delirium, and up to 80% of terminally ill patients will become delirious (Trzepacx, 1994; Tune, 1991). Delirium is particularly likely to occur in patients with preexisting intellectual impairment and in the elderly. Among hospitalized elderly, the prevalence of delirium is 10–40%. As many as one-half of hospitalized patients with delirium have an underlying dementia, and many of the remainder have some baseline cognitive impairment (Inouye, Viscoli, Horwitz, Hurst, & Tinetti, 1993). Moreover, the added presence of dementia greatly increases the susceptibility for developing a superimposed delirium (Pompeii et al., 1994). Thus, dementia patients who suddenly get worse or rapidly deteriorate should be evaluated for delirium (Macdonald & Treloar, 1996).

Delirium is an acute interruption of cognitive functioning that can have a large number of metabolic, toxic, and intracranial causes. The causes of delirium can be broadly divided into four general categories (Mendez & Cummings, 2003): (1) intoxication with exogenous substances including drugs and industrial agents; (2) systemic illness that affects cognitive functioning such as metabolic disorders, infections, and major organ failure; (3) primary cerebral disease including infection, tumors, trauma, epilepsy, and stroke; and (4) withdrawal from substances after dependency has developed such as delirium tremens from alcohol withdrawal. Among the elderly, the most common causes of delirium are metabolic disturbances, major organ failure, strokes, infections, and drugs (Mendez, 2000). Drug effects in the elderly are additive, and medications contribute to delirium in up to 40% of patients (Inouye, 1994; Inouye, 1996). The elderly are particularly sensitive to drugs with anticholiner-

gic effects that can lead to delirium including many over-the-counter cold preparations, antihistamines, antidepressants, and neuroleptics (Trzepacz, 1994).

In addition to specific causes of delirium, it is important to emphasize factors
that predispose patients to develop confusional behavior. Advancing age or existing
brain disease are by far the most prominent (Schor et al., 1992). The elderly and
particularly those patients showing evidence of early dementia are unusually susceptible to any physiologic or environmental disruption. A history of alcohol or
drug abuse or of recent sleep or sensory deprivation can all contribute. In fact,
sleep or sensory deprivation alone can cause concentration difficulties, perceptual
distortions, and decreased reasoning ability (Morris & Singer, 1966; Bruner, 1961).
In any confusional patient, sleep loss can be a major factor in perpetuating the confusional state even though the medical etiology was treated. Additional risk factors
for delirium the severity of the illness, the degree of physical impairment, hip or
bone fractures, infections or fevers, malnutrition, and recent surgeries especially
cardiac, orthopedic, prostate, and cataract surgeries (Inouye & Charpentier, 1996).

ASSESSMENT

What should be ruled out?

Many disorders have impaired attention associated with them. The differential
diagnosis of delirium includes dementia, amnesia, catatonic stupor, and hysterical
unresponsiveness. A frequent problem in distinguishing delirium from dementia is
that the both are characterized by a fluctuating disturbance in attention. Further,
delirium is the other neurobehavioral syndrome with multiple cognitive deficits
and is the most common neurobehavioral disorder seen in general hospitals
(Taylor & Lewis, 1993). Several characteristics help to distinguish delirium and
dementia. The main differentiating features of delirium compared to dementia are
the shorter time course and the presence of prominent fluctuating attentional disturbances. Delirium persists for hours and rarely for weeks, whereas dementia usually implies persistent deficits in intellectual does functioning that last for months
or more often years. Information from medical records, other caregivers, and family members may be helpful in determining whether a dementia was present before
the onset of a delirium. Visual hallucinations, changes in psychomotor activity, and
disturbed day–night cycles are typically more prominent in delirium than in
dementia. The acute fatality rate of delirium is greater for delirium than dementia
(Inouye, Schlesinger, Lydon, 1999; Inouye et al., 1999) but if the etiology of the
delirium is quickly identified and treated, the prognosis is usually better than for
dementia.

Amnesia enters the differential diagnosis of delirium because disorientation is
a prominent feature of both (Trzepacz, 1994). Amnesia refers to impairment in
new learning with intact attention and intellect. In contrast, delirium has prominent attentional deficits along with impairment of language, memory, cognition,
visuospatial skills, and personality. Disorientation in delirium is a product of inattention and is one among a host of other deficits. The amnesic patient is not "confused" as the disorientation accompanying amnesia is a product of the failure to
retain spatial and temporal information.

In addition to amnesia, another psychiatric condition that may be mistaken
for delirium is catatonia which can occur in thought disorders, mood disorders,
and in metabolic disturbances (Carol et al., 1994). Catatonic stupor in which
psychomotor slowing to the point of immobility occurs as part of a psychiatric disturbance usually lasts for a period of less than one week. Unlike in delirium,

patients with catatonic stupor and hysterical unresponsiveness have normal reflex functioning and EEG.

What is Involved in Effective Assessment

The diagnosis of delirium is often ruled in on the basis of clinical presentation alone and then confirmed with lab work and brief cognitive screening measures. If laboratory test results are already known and indicate the presence of a known cause of delirium and the patient develops an acute confusional state, then the diagnosis of delirium can also be ruled in on this basis. Since delirium has a medical cause, having laboratory results will often raise the probability of an accurate diagnosis though multiple etiologies can be present at any one time. In these cases the diagnosis can be made presumptively as each reversible cause for the acute confusional state is treated.

Patients with delirium require a comprehensive review of all systems due to the multiple etiologies including a careful history and chart review, physical examination, and laboratory tests. Laboratory tests to be performed and review include a complete blood panel for measurements of glucose, electrolytes, blood urea nitrogen, creatinine for kidney functioning, and liver enzymes. Lab work should also include tests for thyroid functioning, aterial blood gas studies, chest X-ray, electrocardiogram, urinalysis, and urine drug screening (Mendez & Cummings, 2003).

Neuroimaging is useful in diagnosing delirium when it can confirm subdural hematomas and other lesions that can occur in the elderly with few other signs or indications. However, routine neuroimaging in the absence of focal neurological findings often yields little. Due to its high cost and the availability of less expensive neuropsychological testing, neuroimaging is typically not done to diagnose delirium. Since electroencephalograph (EEG) changes are virtually always found in delirium, the presence of slowing brain wave activity particularly in the theta and delta range, and disorganization in brain wave activity can be used to diagnose delirium. However, in alcohol or sedative-hypnotic withdrawal, the EEG usually shows fast activity. EEG is currently considered experimental and should not be used alone in diagnosing delirium.

If careful mental status testing is carried out, most patients will demonstrate recent memory loss, difficulty writing poor calculating ability, and global problems with high-level abstract reasoning (Albert, 1988). With these cognitive changes, emotional abnormalities can also be observed including anxiety, fear, depression, paranoia, and delusions.

Brief cognitive testing is useful to obtain a baseline of impairment and then tracking attention deficits over the course of time. Rating the severity of delirium over time may be useful for monitoring the effect of an intervention. Several brief cognitive screening instruments are available when mental health is consulted in making a differential diagnosis of delirium. These scales have also been used to make the diagnosis by considering patients with scores above or a specified cutoff to have the diagnosis.

Several screening instruments exist to supplement the clinical examination and history in screening for screening delirium. These include the Clinical Assessment of Confusion-A (Vermeersch, 1990), Confusion Rating Scale (Williams, Ward, & Campbell, 1998), MCV Nursing Delirium Rating Scale (Rutherford, Sessler, Levenson, Hart, & Best, 1991), and NEECHAM Confusion Scale (Neelon, Champagne, Carlson, Funk, 1996). These tests were also designed so that nursing staff can administer them.

The most widely recognized test, the Mini-Mental Status Examination (MMSE) has been used widely in screening for delirium and dementia. It has advantage in that it takes approximately 15 minutes to administer. The MMSE is standardized and has norms adjusted for age and educational level (Crum, Anthony, Bassett, & Folstein, 1993). The MMSE covers five areas of functioning including orientation, attention, immediate and short-term verbal recall, language, and construction. Its disadvantage over other available tests is that 50% of items are related to orientation only. With respect to scoring orientation questions, the MMSE assigns one point for each correct response to the day, date, month, and year. However, an incorrect response to the year is a more critical error than responding with the incorrect day even though both are weighed the same in terms of scoring. There is also a high false positive rate with people with low education and advanced age, and it is not as comprehensive as other mental status examinations. Finally, the MMSE is a verbally weighted measure and could provide false positives especially in elderly who have hearing deficits or aphasias.

Another widely used measure in medical settings where brief mental status assessments are required is the Cognistat, formerly known as the Neurobehavioral Cognitive Screening Exam (Fields, Fulop, Sachs, Strain, Fillit, 1992). This cognitive screening measure is more comprehensive than the MMSE and therefore requires longer administering depending upon the severity of impairment. Average administration time is 20 minutes or more and scoring requires 10 minutes. The test provides a differentiated index of various cognitive domains with results summarized in profile format. Separate scores plotted for alertness, orientation, attention, language, memory, calculation, visuo-construction, and reasoning. It also addresses verbal fluency, immediate figural memory, and verbal registration. It avoids use of a single summary score, allowing the opportunity to examine level of performance in five cognitive domains. It is standardized on young, old, geriatric, and neurosurgical subjects. The test is well regarded for use in situations requiring consultation to medical staff. The Cognistat requires specific materials for testing (e.g., scoring form, colored tiles, stimulus booklet, etc.). The test does not assess reading, writing, and spelling.

Two other rating scales are the Delirium Rating Scale (DRS) (Trzepacz, Baker, & Greenhouse, 1988) and the Memorial Delirium Assessment Scale (Breitbart et al., 1997). The DRS is a 10-item scale developed as an attempt to objectify symptom severity when a confusional state/delirium is suspected. Scale items relate to symptomatology consistent with acute confusional state (e.g., sleep–wake cycle, cognitive status, psychomotor behavior, perceptual disturbance, fluctuation of symptoms) and severity ranking of each. It takes approximately 5 minutes to complete the test and the same to score it. The test is can be administered by a staff caregiver familiar with the patient. Its advantage over other available tests that assess the same area or category is that it is useful symptom checklist for structuring awareness of the clinical features of delirium, in monitoring severity, and in monitoring symptom resolution. Crossvalidation studies are needed before this scale can be recommended for diagnostic application.

Treatment

Treatment of delirium hinges upon recognition that acute confusional states are present in a wide variety of patient conditions. Many acutely confused patients go unrecognized and untreated because it is thought their behavior is the result of a chronic dementing or psychiatric illness. Those that are treated are likely to be those who are agitated and bring attention to themselves, and become management problems. Patients who are quietly confused are often overlooked because systematic documentation of their mental status is not done especially if they are admitted for medical reasons.

Two important avenues of treatment must be followed in the management of an acute confusional state: (1) the identification and correction of the underlying medical problem, and (2) the control of the abnormal and often disruptive behavior.

While acute confusion is a well-known clinical phenomenon, few systematic studies exist on how to treat it, and those that have been done are largely anecdotal. Inconsistent use of terms and use of well-defined diagnostic criteria have hampered also epidemiological studies of delirium. Evidence-based guidelines for treating delirium as a distinct disorder have only recently been created. However, evidence-based guidelines for treating other neurobehavioral conditions, especially dementia where the differential diagnosis between reversible (e.g., delirium and depression) and nonreversible causes of dementia nearly always includes guidelines for how to make the diagnosis.

Delirium has not received the same attention as dementia in the evidence-based literature, and empirically validated treatments for this disorder lag behind research done for other psychiatric illnesses. To address this, the American Psychiatric Association (APA) has published its Expert Consensus Guidelines and Treatment Guidelines for delirium (American Psychiatric Association, 1999). The guidelines from the APA cover three primary domains in the treatment of delirium: (1) psychiatric management, (2) environmental and supportive interventions, and (3) somatic interventions. Psychiatric management of delirium first includes coordinating care with other treatment providers because if the etiology is unknown it is treated as a medical emergency in which the patient is transferred to an acute medical setting to identify the causative factors. Within the acute care setting, consultation with psychiatry or psychology staff is usually done to assess the severity of the delirium. After the etiology is determined then the patient can be returned to a subacute setting and managed. Once the patient's delirium is identified and the severity assessed, the next step in good management is to determine the underlying cause of the acute confusional state. To determine the underlying cause, a complete workup must be performed including physical status, mental status, and laboratory tests ordered. Third, interventions for the acute confusional state are initiated. This can be done before the etiology is determined in life threatening situations. The mental health consultant can raise the awareness of reminding medical staff to the morbidity and mortality associated with delirium. Fourth, known reversible causes of delirium (e.g., hypoxia, hypoglycemia, poor nutritional status, hypothermia, and withdrawal) need to examined and ruled out. Fifth, ensuring patient and staff safety during the acute confusional state is done to keep the patient from accidentally hurting themselves or others. Behavioral manifestations and cognitive disturbances associated with delirium could lead to falls, wandering, and inadvertent suicide in response to hallucinations and delusions. Adequate monitoring and supervision by staff during the acute confusional state needs to be done to mitigate the risks of patient self-harm. The use of physical restraints is to be avoided whenever possible as research has shown that this can lead to increased agitation and carry further physical risks. If restraints are required proper documentation and adherence to legal regulations and institutional policies for the appropriate use of restraints must be done. Sixth, assessing the patient's mental status over time with one of the structured instruments previously reviewed is necessary due to the rapidly fluctuating course of the disturbance. Serial assessment allows for interventions to be monitored and tailored to changing behavioral presentations. Seventh, managing delirium involves reaching out to family members to assess their interpersonal dynamics and individual personality styles in dealing with their reactions to their loved ones with delirium. Eighth, establishing and maintaining therapeutic alliances with the patient, family members, and other treating providers is helpful in overall management of the delirious patient. Ninth, educating the family and patient (though patients will vary in their understanding due to their confusion) that delirium is temporary and usually part of their disease process can be reassuring. Finally, providing postdelirium management in the form of debriefing patients who have cleared from their delirium may be important, especially for those patients who recall hallucinations or are troubled by what they experienced.

Environmental and supportive interventions for delirium are underutilized in the treatment of delirium but are valued as being beneficial in based on clinical experience though there are only a few studies that have evaluated their effectiveness. Environmental interventions have support because environmental interventions they have few if any negative effects. Environmental interventions can be used effectively to counteract the effects of sensory deprivation and the disorienting effects of being on wards with artificial lighting throughout the day and night where there are no cues to time, or over-stimulation from constant noise of medical equipment. For example, by restoring a patient's glasses or hearing aid and ensuring that there is a clock and a calendar placed in the room facing the patient, one may substantially reduce the manifestations of delirium. Nursing staff can turn room lights on and off in the day and night respectively. Having familiar personal effects from the patient's home decorate the hospital room is reassuring and facilitates orientation. Supportive interventions for delirium include ensuring that the patient with delirium receives social stimulation from staff or family members, and providing education to family members who often have the same concerns as patients that delirium may represent a more severe psychiatric illness or brain injury.

Lastly, the use of somatic interventions to decrease agitation in some presentations of delirium can be highly effective. Medications have been used with varying degrees of success including antipsychotics, benzodiazepines, cholinergics, vitamins (for alcohol related delirium), morphine, and electroconvulsive therapy.

REFERENCES

Albert, M. S. (1988). Acute confusional states. In M. S. Albert, & M. B. Moss (Eds.), *Geriatric neuropsychology*. New York: The Guilford Press.

American Psychiatric Association (1999). Practice guideline for the treatment of patients with delirium. *American Journal of Psychiatry, 156*, 1–20.

American Psychiatric Association (1994). *Diagnostic and statistical manual of mental disorders* (4th ed.). Washington, DC: Author.

Benson, D. F. (1979). Aphasia, alexia, and agraphia. New York: Churchill Livingston.

Breitbart, W., Rosenfeld, B., Roth, F., Smith, M. J., Cohen, K., & Passik, S. (1997). The Memorial Delirium Assessment Scale. *Journal of Pain Symptom Management, 13*, 128–137.

Bruner, J. S. (1961). The cognitive consequences of early sensory deprivation. In Solomon, P., Kubzansky, P. E. Leiderman, P. H., Mendelson, J. H., Trumbull, R., & Wexler, D. (Eds.) *Sensory Deprivation: A Symposium held at Harvard Medical School*. Cambridge, MA: Harvard University Press.

Carroll, B. T., Anfinson, T. J., Kennedy, J. C., Yendrek, R., Boutros, M., & Bilon, A. (1994). Catatonic disorder due to general medical conditions. *Journal of Neuropsychiatry and Clinical Neurosciences, 6*, 122–133.

Chedru, F., & Geschwind, N. (1972a). Disorder of higher cortical functions in acute confusional states. *Cortex, 10*, 395–411.

Chedru, F., & Geschwind, N. (1972b). Writing disturbances in acute confusional states. *Neuropsychologia, 10*, 343–353.

Crum, R., Anthony, J., Bassett, S., & Folstein, M. (1993). Population-based norms for the Mini-Mental State Examination by age and educational level. *JAMA, 269*, 238–239.

Cummings, J. L. (1985). Organic delusions: phenomenology, anatomic correlations, and review. *British Journal of Psychiatry, 46*, 184–197.

Edelstyn, N. M. J., & Oyebode, F. (1999). A review of the phenomenology and cognitive neuropsychological origins of the Capgras syndrome. *International Journal of Geriatric Psychiatry, 14(1)*, 48–59.

Fields, S. D., Fulop, G., Sachs, C. J., Strain, J., & Fillit, H. (1992). Usefulness of the Neurobehavioral Cognitive Status Examination in the hospitalized elderly. *International Psychogeriatrics, 4(1)*, 93–102.

Inouye, S. K. (1994). The dilemma of delirium: Clinical and research controversies regarding diagnosis and evaluation of delirium in hospitalized elderly medical patients. *American Journal of Medicine, 97*, 278–288.

Inouye, S. K., Bogardus, S. T., Jr., Charpentier, P. A. Linda Leo-Summers, L., Acampora, D., Holford, T. R., et al. (1999). A multicomponent intervention to prevent delirium in hospitalized older patients. *New England Journal of Medicine, 340*, 669–676.

Inouye, S. K., & Charpentier, P. A. (1996). Precipitating factors for delirium in hospitalized elderly persons: Predictive model and interrelationship with baseline vulnerability. *JAMA, 275*, 852–857.

Inouye, S. K., Schlesinger, M. J., & Lydon, T. J. (1999). Delirium: A symptom of how hospital care is failing older persons and a window to improve quality of hospital care. *American Journal of Medicine, 44*, 1001–1002.

Inouye, S. K., Viscoli, C. M., Horwitz, R. I., Hurst, L. D., & Tinetti, M. E. (1993). A predictive model for delirium in hospitalized elderly medical patients based on admission characteristics. *Annals of Internal Medicine Archives of Internal Medicine, 119*, 474–481.

Lipowski, Z. J. (1990). Delirium: Acute confusional states. New York: Oxford University Press.

Liptzin, B. & Levkoff, S. E. (1992). An empirical study of delirium subtypes. *British Journal of Psychiatry, 161*, 843–845.

Macdonald, A. J., & Treloar, A. (1996). Delirium and dementia: Are they distinct? *Journal of the American Geriatrics Society 44*, 1001–1002.

Mendez, M. F., & Cummings, J. L. (2003). *Diagnosis of dementia.* In Dementia: A clinical approach. Philadelphia: Butterworth-Heinemann.

Mendez A. M. F. (2000). *Delirium.* In W. G. Bradley, R. B. Daroff, G. M. Fenichel, C. D. Marsden (Eds.) *Neurology in clinical practice* (3rd ed.). Boston: Butterworth-Heinemann.

Morris, G. O., & Singer, M. T. (1966). Sleep deprivation: The context of consciousness. *Journal of Nervous Mental Disorders, 143*, 291.

Nash, J. L. (1983). *Delusions.* Philadelphia: J. B. Lippincott.

Neelon, V., Champagne M. T., Carlson, J. R., & Funk, S. G. (1996). The NEECHAM Confusion Scale: Construction, validation, and clinical testing. *Nursing Research, 45*, 324–330.

O'Keefe, S., & Lavan, J. (1997). The prognostic significance of delirium in older hospital patients. *Journal of the American Geriatrics Society, 45*, 174–178.

Pompeii, P., Foreman, M., Rudberg, M. A., Inouye S. K., Braund, V., & Cassel, C. K. (1994). Delirium in hospitalized older persons: Outcomes and predictors. *Journal of the American Geriatrics Society, 42*, 809–815.

Rabins, P. V., & Folstein, M. F. (1982). Delirium and dementia. *British Journal of Psychiatry, 140*, 149.

Rummans, T., Evans, J. M., Krahn, L. E., & Fleming, K. C. (1995). Delirium in elderly patients: Evaluation and management. *Mayo Clinic Proceedings, 70*, 989–998.

Rutherford, L., Sessler, C., Levenson J. L., Hart, R., & Best, A. (1991). Prospective evaluation of delirium and agitation in a medical intensive care unit (abstract). *Critical Care Medicine, 19*, S81.

Schor, J. D., Levkoff, S. E. Lipsitz, L. A., Reilly, C. H., Cleary, P. D., Rowe, J. W., et al. (1992). Risk factors for delirium in hospitalized elderly. *JAMA, 267*, 827–831.

Strub, R. L., & Black, F. W. (1988). Acute confusional states (delirium). In *Neurobehavioral disorders*. Philadelphia: F. A. Davis Company.

Taylor, D., & Lewis, S. (1993). Delirium. *Journal or Neurology and Neurosurgical Psychiatry, 56*, 742–751.

Tombaugh, T. N., & McIntyre, N. J. (1992). The mini-mental state examination: A comprehensive review. *Journal of the American Geriatrics Society, 40*, 922–935.

Trzepacz, P. T. (1994). The neuropathogenesis of delirium: A need to focus our research. *Psychosomatics, 35*, 374–391.

Trzepacz, P., Baker, R., & Greenhouse, J. (1988). A symptom rating scale for delirium. *Psychiatry Research, 23*, 89–97.

Trzepacz, P. T., Mittal, D., Torres, R., Kanary, K., Norton, J., & Jimerson, N. (2001). Validation of the Delirium Rating Scale-Revised-98: Comparison with the Delirium Rating Scale and the Cognitive Test for Delirium. *Journal of Neuropsychiatry and Clinical Neuroscience, 13*, 229–242.

Tune, L. E. (1991). Post-operative delirium. *Psychogeriatrics, 3*, 325–332.

Vermeersch, P. E. (1990). The Clinical Assessment of Confusion-A. *Applied Nursing Research, 3*, 128–133.

Williams, M. A., Ward, S. E., & Campbell, E. B. (1988). Confusion: Testing versus observation. *Journal of Gerontological Nursing, 14*, 25–30.

Wolff, H. G., & Curran, D. (1935). Nature of delirium and allied states. *Archive of Neurology and Psychiatry, 33*, 1175–1215.

CHAPTER 20

Delusions

Daniel Freeman • Philippa A. Garety

INTRODUCTION

There has been a remarkable transformation in how delusions are viewed. The prevailing view had been that delusions are 'ununderstandable' in terms of normal psychological processes. Delusions were considered simply a symptom or epiphenomenon of an organic condition, schizophrenia. A consequence was that patients were discouraged from talking about their delusions. In the past ten years, however, this has changed. Empirical evidence indicates that delusions, though complex phenomena, can be understood in terms of psychological processes. Moreover, the new theoretical understanding has developed in tandem with cognitive-behavioural interventions for delusions. Together with medication, it is now recommended that most patients should be given time to talk about their experiences and that particular therapeutic techniques be used to reduce their distress. In this chapter we summarize the transformation in thinking about delusions.

WHAT IS A DELUSION?

In essence, a delusion is a fixed, false belief. In clinical settings the belief is likely to be distressing or disruptive for the individual. However, there has long been debate about such definitions, in that most proposed criteria do not apply to all delusions. A more sustainable position is that of Oltmanns (1988). Assessing the presence of a delusion may best be accomplished by considering a list of characteristics or dimensions, none of which is necessary or sufficient, that with increasing endorsement produces greater agreement on the presence of a delusion. For instance, the more a belief is implausible, unfounded, strongly held, not shared by others, distressing and preoccupying then the more likely it is to be considered a delusion. The practical importance of the debate about defining delusions is that it informs us that there is individual variability in the characteristics of delusional experience (see Table 20.1). Delusions are definitely not discrete discontinuous entities. They are complex, multi-dimensional phenomena (Garety & Hemsley, 1994). There also can be no simple answer to the question "What causes a delusion?". Instead, an understanding of each dimension of delusional experience is needed: what causes the content of a delusion? What causes the degree of belief conviction? What causes resistance to change? What causes the distress? And as clinicians we need to think with clients about the aspect of delusional experience that we are hoping will change during the course of an intervention.

HOW COMMON ARE DELUSIONS?

It is little discussed—though there is much evidence -that many people regularly have thoughts or ideas enter their mind of a delusional nature. For instance, questionnaire surveys have found that 20–30% of people regularly experience paranoid thoughts

Freeman, D., & Garety, P. A. (2006). Delusions. In J. E. Fisher & W. T. O'Donohue (Eds.), *Practitioner's guide to evidence-based psychotherapy*. New York: Springer.

TABLE 20.1 The multi-dimensional nature of delusions.

Characteristic of delusions	Variability in characteristic
Unfounded	For some individuals the delusions reflect a kernel of truth that has been exaggerated (eg. the person had a dispute with the neighbour but now believes that the whole neighbourhood is monitoring them and will harm them). It can be difficult to determine whether the person is actually delusional. For others the ideas are fantastic, impossible and clearly unfounded (eg. the person believes that she/he was present at the time of the Big Bang and is involved in battles across the universe and heavens)
Firmly held	Beliefs can vary from being held with 100% conviction to only occasionally being believed when the person is in a particular stressful situation
Resistant to change	An individual may be certain that they could not be mistaken and will not countenance any alternative explanation for their experiences. Others feel very confused and uncertain about their ideas and readily want to think about alternative accounts of their experiences
Preoccupying	Some people report that they can do nothing but think about their delusional concerns. For other people, although they firmly believe the delusion, such thoughts rarely come into their mind
Distressing	Many beliefs, especially those seen in clinical practice, are very distressing (e.g., persecutory delusions) but others (e.g., grandiose delusions) can actually be experienced positively
Interferes with social functioning	Delusions can stop people interacting with others and lead to great isolation and abandonment of activities. Other people can have a delusion and still function at a high level including maintaining relationships and employment
Involves personal reference	In many instances the patient is at the centre of the delusional system (e.g. "I have been singled out for persecution"). However friends and relatives can be involved (e.g., "They are targeting my whole family") and some people believe that everybody is affected equally (e.g., "Everybody is being experimented upon")

(e.g., Verdoux et al., 1998; Freeman et al., 2005). In approximately 10% of the general population these sorts of ideas are held at the level of a delusion (i.e., are firmly held and incorrect), though they mostly do not interfere with everyday functioning. An epidemiological study of seven thousand people in the Netherlands found that 3.3% had a "true," psychiatrist-rated delusion and 8.7% had a "not clinically relevant" delusion (van Os et al., 2000). In short, more people have delusions than receive a psychiatric diagnosis. This is consistent with a continuum view of delusional experience and indicates that delusions might indeed be understood in terms of normal psychological processes. Nevertheless, delusions are particularly prevalent in people with psychiatric diagnoses, especially psychotic disorders, and it is delusions in schizophrenia that have received by far the most research attention. In a World Health Organisation study in ten countries of first-in-lifetime contacts with services because of schizophrenia the frequencies of delusions were: delusions of reference (50%), delusion of persecution (50%), grandiose abilities (15%), religious delusions (10%), grandiose identity (5%) (Sartorius et al., 1986). In clinical services it is common to be dealing with delusions of reference and persecution because they are both the most distressing and most common delusions.

HOW ARE DELUSIONS UNDERSTOOD?

Delusions are complex phenomena that will not be explained by a single factor. Partly this is because, as we have seen, the experience contains many different elements. Many factors are implicated in delusion development, and the contribution of each in individual cases varies. In our summary of the evidence we will focus upon those factors that plausibly link to the subjective experiences that patients report and that have been the topic of research. These ideas can be used to help 'make sense' of delusions with clients seen in therapy. In Figure 20.1 how the factors may combine in delusional experience is summarized.

Explanations of experience

To understand delusions it is important to be clear about their function. In contemporary accounts, delusions are conceptualised as individuals' attempts to make sense of events. That is, delusions are explanations of experiences or personal narratives reflecting a search for meaning. This account was originally

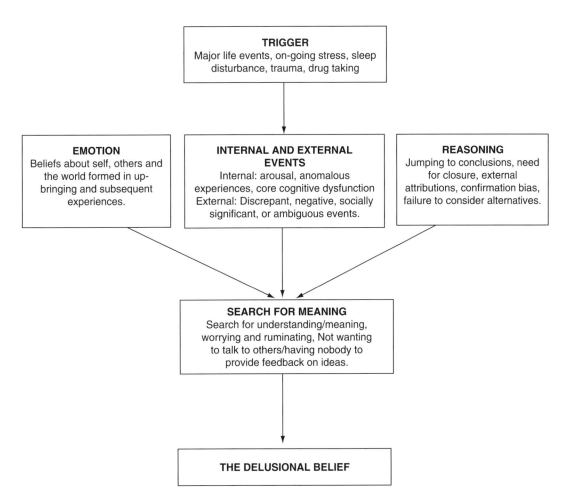

FIGURE 20.1 Outline of factors involved in delusion development

argued by the American psychologist Maher (1988). He particularly argues that delusions are explanations of unusual internal events, which includes hallucinations, perceptual anomalies, feelings of significance, depersonalisation, and arousal. The internal states may reflect a core cognitive dysfunction in psychosis that has an associated neurological disruption (e.g., Gray, Feldon, Rawlins, Hemsley, & Smith, 1991). Further, the cognitive dysfunction may arise from a proximal cause such as using certain illicit drugs or from distal causes such as a family history of psychosis or subtle deviance in brain development arising, for example, from obstetric complications (see Murray, Jones, Susser, van Os, & Cannon, 2003).

Crucially, rather than recognizing and correctly labeling unusual internal states, people with delusions instead take information from the external environment to form their explanation for their changed state. Typically, ambiguous social information, coincidences, and negative or irritating events are drawn in to the explanation. For example, a person may go outside feeling in an unusual state and rather than label this experience as such ("I'm feeling a little odd and anxious today, probably because I've not been sleeping well") the feelings are instead used as a source of evidence, together with the facial expressions of strangers in the street, that there is a threat ("People don't like me and may harm me"). Moreover, individuals with delusions have difficulties keeping in mind other (nondelusional) explanations for their experiences. In a recent study of 100 individuals with delusions it was found that only one-quarter had any alternative explanation for the experiences that their delusions were an attempt to explain (Freeman et al., 2004). Individuals who reported more internal events for their delusion found generating alternative explanations most difficult. This supports the idea that anomalous internal states may be crucial in leading to delusional explanations.

Emotion

The need for an explanation of experience may be caused by internal states but where does the particular delusional content arise from? Why a persecutory or grandiose explanation? It is likely that an important factor is emotion. Delusions build upon emotional concerns. There is evidence that anxiety, low self esteem, adverse events, victimisation, emigrating, isolation, and living in potentially difficult environments such as urban settings all raise the chances of later development of psychosis (e.g., Krabbendam, Janssen, Bijl, Vollebergh, & van Os, 2002). At an individual level such circumstances will influence beliefs about the self, others, and the world, and it is these sorts of beliefs that contribute to the delusional explanations. For example, having negative beliefs about the self (e.g., vulnerable, bad), others (e.g., untrustworthy, devious) and the world (e.g., unfair, punitive) will make persecutory ideation likely (e.g., Fowler et al., in press). Moreover, it is well established that psychosis often occurs at a time of stress. Life events, incidents that are threatening, stressful and arousing, are common in the 3-month period before symptom onset (Bebbington et al., 1993). This is likely to exacerbate long-standing emotional vulnerabilities. The emotion generated is likely to feed into the delusional explanations for experiences (see Table 20.2). Persecutory delusions may build on anxious concerns (there is a shared theme of the anticipation of danger), depressive delusions may build on depressive concerns (there is a shared theme of loss, guilt and shame), and grandiose delusions on elation (there is a shared theme of success and achievement).

TABLE 20.2 The themes of emotions and delusions. From Freeman & Garety (2004)

Emotions	Main theme of emotion	Delusion with shared theme
Anxiety	Anticipation of physical, social, or psychological threat	Reference ("People are watching me") Persecution ("People are saying negative things behind my back to get at me")
Depression	Loss, low self-esteem, guilt, shame	Guilt ("I've brought ruin to my family") Persecution ("I'm being persecuted because of what I've done in the past") Catastrophe ("The world is going to end and it's all my fault")
Anger	Deliberately wronged, frustration at not reaching goal	Persecution ("People are doing things to annoy me")
Happiness	Success, achievement, high self-esteem	Grandiose ("I've got special talents and am related to a famous person")
Disgust	Finding something offensive, revulsion, dislike	Persecutory ("My food is being poisoned") Hypochondriacal ("My insides are rotting") Appearance ("My body is ugly and misshapen")
Jealousy	Fear of losing another's affections	Jealousy ("My wife is sleeping with other men in our bed while I lie asleep")

Reasoning

It needs to be remembered that delusions are inherently a judgment, and therefore reasoning processes are also of central importance. Delusional ideation is most likely to become of delusional intensity when there are accompanying biases in reasoning. There is evidence for a number of reasoning biases in people with delusions. The most established finding has been of a "jumping to conclusions" bias in people with delusions (see review by Garety & Freeman, 1999). This reflects a data-gathering bias: on experimental tasks about half of people with delusions seek limited information before being certain of a decision. Making premature decisions is likely to lead to errors in belief formation, particularly when the experiences to be explained are inherently confusing. A further finding reported in the research literature is of people with delusions showing an externalising bias (that is, they are more likely to attribute blame to others rather than the self or situation) (Kinderman & Bentall, 1997). This is likely to make correct explanations for internal anomalous experiences less likely. There have also been preliminary findings of people with delusions not considering alternative explanations (Freeman et al., 2004) and having a high need for closure (Bentall & Swarbrick, 2003), which is a desire for an answer rather than tolerate uncertainty or ambiguity.

Maintenance Factors

Once formed, there is evidence for a number of factors that maintain delusions. The "confirmation bias" (Wason, 1960), the normal tendency to seek evidence that is consistent with beliefs rather than inconsistent, will provide a source of confirmatory evidence for delusions. Safety behaviors such as avoidance will prevent disconfirmatory evidence being processed in relation to persecutory delusions

(Freeman, Garety, & Kuipers, 2001). Rumination and worry will maintain delusion preoccupation and distress (Freeman & Garety, 1999). And difficulties with "belief flexibility," the meta-cognitive capacity of reflecting on one's own beliefs, changing them in the light of reflection and the evidence, and generating and considering alternatives, will lead to delusion persistence (Garety et al., 2005). Lastly, the person's interactions with others may become disturbed. The person may act upon their delusion in a way that elicits hostility or isolation (e.g. by being aggressive or treating others suspiciously), and they may suffer stigma, which will reinforce the delusional belief.

Summary

The study of delusions is a rapidly growing area of research. It is becoming clear that delusions are multidimensional phenomena that will need to be understood within multifactorial frameworks. A range of factors—anomalous experiences, emotional processes, reasoning biases, environmental factors, organic vulnerabilities—have now been shown to be associated with delusions. Such factors are incorporated into contemporary biopsychosocial models of delusions (Garety, Kuipers, Fowler, Freeman, & Bebbington, 2001; Freeman, Garety, Kuipers, Fowler, & Bebbington, 2002; Kapur, 2003). In essence, delusions are attempts by people to explain their experiences and these attempts to make sense are in line with previous experiences, knowledge, emotional state, memories, personality, and decision-making processes.

How can delusions be treated psychologically?

If delusions can be understood psychologically then it is likely they can be treated psychologically. In parallel with the development of the theoretical literature on delusions there have been repeated demonstrations of the efficacy of cognitive behavioural therapy for delusions (see review by Pilling et al., 2002). It is recommended for people with *distressing* delusions. Cognitive deficits are not a contraindication for treatment.

The evidence base is strongest concerning CBT for persistent positive symptoms such as delusions. Approximately 20% of patients with persistent symptoms do very well in treatment and another 40% show important improvements. Tarrier et al. (1998) report that receipt of CBT results in almost eight times greater odds of showing a reduction in psychotic symptoms of 50% or more in comparison with routine care alone. However, not all patients respond to this approach. Regarding acute groups, there is evidence that CBT can speed time to recovery (e.g., Drury, Birchwood, Cochrane, & MacMillan, 1996). Further, there is a small amount of evidence that forms of CBT for psychosis may be able to reduce relapse rates (Gumley et al., 2003). The intervention is certainly popular with clients and on the basis of the randomised controlled trials, CBT for psychosis is now a recommended intervention for schizophrenia in several countries including the US (Patient Outcomes Research Team; Lehman et al., 2004) and the UK (National Institute of Clinical Excellence, 2002).

It is important to note that at this stage of development CBT for delusions is not a brief treatment; typically it needs to be provided weekly for approximately 6–12 months. Although similar to CBT for other disorders clinicians should be aware that modifications to the approach are needed for delusions. CBT for psychosis therapists are often working with complex cases and need a good understanding of the psychology of psychosis, cognitive therapy skills, and regular supervision and support. It is also important to be aware that it is provided as part of a multimodal treatment that includes neuroleptic medication and, for example, assertive community treatment, rehabilitation, supported employment, and family intervention.

OUTLINE OF THE MAIN STRATEGIES OF CBT FOR DELUSIONAL BELIEFS

Engagement and Assessment

It is important to be flexible when working with people with delusions. Sessions are normally up to an hour but can be far briefer at the early stages of engagement. Basic engagement skills are crucial: being collaborative, warm, empathic, taking clients problems seriously, explaining what is happening in therapy, eliciting feedback, and not taking the stance of trying to prove that clients' beliefs are wrong. Ideally, clients and therapists should be on a "voyage of discovery" with the aim of understanding the clients' difficulties and taking steps to decrease their distress and increase their control. The aim of assessment is to derive a formulation based upon the factors that have been reviewed above. This occurs through detailed descriptions of delusional experiences and their development. Formal measures of symptoms should be taken to monitor the effectiveness of intervention (e.g., PSYRATS; Haddock, McCarron, Tarrier, & Faragher, 1999). The assessment should lead to the setting of clear therapeutic goals.

Individualised Formulation: "Making Sense of Psychosis"

The initial aim is to develop an individualised formulation that accounts for the delusion and the associated distress. This is a description based upon biopsychosocial models of clients' subjective experiences (e.g., Garety et al., 2001) and is not simply "education about illness." Sometimes all, or sometimes parts, of the formulation are shared with clients. There are a number of benefits to good formulation: a full description of clients' subjective experiences is made which is empathic, normalising, makes the experiences understandable and does not treat individuals as if they are "mad"; it enables clients to revisit their decision-making processes with the benefit of time and new information; it can provide an alternative nondelusional account of experiences; and it identifies targets of therapy.

Interventions After Formulation

Making sense of psychosis, and identifying the many factors and steps on the way to delusion development, illuminates many potential therapeutic paths. Thus, if anomalous experiences are assessed as central to delusion formation—for instance, the delusions are provoked by feelings of depersonalisation, a sense of reference, perceptual disturbances or hallucinations—therapy may aim to reduce the frequency of such experiences via a functional analysis, to change the interpretation of the anomalous experiences, or simply to enhance coping strategies. Where anxiety and worry processes contribute to the persistence of delusional ideas, other ways of dealing with thinking about fears can be introduced. In some cases it is possible to review with clients the evidence for and against different explanations for their experiences and to conduct behavioural experiments. In other cases, the therapist and client will be "working within" the delusion and distress may be reduced by, for example, focusing upon the interpretations associated with the most distressing aspects of the delusion, or by developing alternative ways of reacting to the threat. It is also the case that therapists often will work with clients to improve low self-esteem, reduce depression, increase activities, and structure time. Finally, the therapist and client may try to prevent relapse by identifying vulnerabilities and early warning signs and rehearsing compensatory strategies.

OVERALL SUMMARY

Delusions are complex phenomena that have started to be the focus of psychological research. Clearly, a number of factors combine in their formation and maintenance. This means that psychological therapy will draw upon a range of techniques that are applied on the basis of individual formulations of clients' difficulties. However, what unites the techniques is the underlying assumption that clients' subjective experiences should be taken seriously and that they can be helped to make delusional experiences less threatening, less interfering, and more controllable. This parallels the approaches taken to nonpsychotic disorders such as anxiety and depression.

FURTHER READING

Reviews of delusion theories: Garety & Freeman (1999); Winters and Neale (1983); Freeman & Garety (2004), Garety and Hemsley (1994).

Recent theoretical models of delusions: Garety et al. (2001); Freeman et al. (2002); Bentall et al. (2001); Kapur (2003).

CBT for psychosis manuals: Fowler et al. (1995); Chadwick et al (1996); Morrison (2002); Kingdon & Turkington (2002).

Website: British Psychological Society: *www.understandingpsychosis.com*

Self-help: Freeman et al. (2006).

REFERENCES

Bebbington, P. E., Wilkins, S., Jones, P., Forester, A., Murray, R. M., Toone, B., et al. (1993). Life events and psychosis: initial results from the Camberwell Collaborative Psychosis Study. *British Journal of Psychiatry, 162*, 72–79.

Bentall, R. P., Corcoran, R., Howard, R., Blackwood, N. & Kinderman, P. (2001).Persecutory delusions: A review and theoretical interpretation. *Clinical Psychology Review, 21*, 1143–1192.

Bentall, R. P., & Swarbrick, R. (2003). The best laid schemas of paranoid patients: autonomy, sociotropy, and need for closure. *Psychology and Psychotherapy, 76*, 163–171.

Chadwick, P. D. J., Birchwood, M. J., & Trower, P. (1996). *Cognitive therapy for delusions, voices and paranoia.* Chichester: Wiley.

Drury, V., Birchwood, M., Cochrane, R., & MacMillan, F. (1996). Cognitive therapy and recovery from acute psychosis: a controlled trial. I. Impact on psychotic symptoms. *British Journal of Psychiatry, 169*, 593–601.

Fowler, D., Freeman, D., Smith, B., Bebbington, P., Bashforth, H., Coker, S., Gracie, A., Dunn, G., & Garety, P. (in press). The Brief Core Schema Scales (BCSS): Psychometric properties and associations with paranoia and grandiosity in non-clinical and psychosis samples. *Psychological Medicine.*

Fowler, D., Garety, P. A., & Kuipers, L. (1995). *Cognitive behavior therapy for psychosis: Theory and practice.* Chichester: Wiley.

Freeman, D. & Garety, P. A. (1999). Worry, worry processes and dimensions of delusions: an exploratory investigation of a role for anxiety processes in the maintenance of delusional distress. *Behavioural & Cognitive Psychotherapy, 27*, 47–62.

Freeman, D. & Garety, P. A. (2004). *Paranoia: The Psychology of Persecutory Delusions.* Hove: Psychology Press.

Freeman, D., Garety, P. A., Bebbington, P. E., Smith, B., Rollinson, R., Fowler, D., et al. (2005). Psychological investigation of the structure of paranoia in a non-clinical population. *British Journal of Psychiatry, 186*, 427–435.

Freeman, D., Garety, P., Fowler, D., Kuipers, E., Bebbington, P., & Dunn, G. (2004). Why do people with delusions fail to choose more realistic explanations for their experiences? An empirical investigation. *Journal of Consulting and Clinical Psychology, 72*, 671–680.

Freeman, D., Garety, P. A., & Kuipers, E. (2001). Persecutory delusions: developing the understanding of belief maintenance and emotional distress. *Psychological Medicine, 31*, 1293–1306.

Freeman, D., Garety, P. A., Kuipers, E., Fowler, D., & Bebbington, P. E. (2002). A cognitive model of persecutory delusions. *British Journal of Clinical Psychology, 41*, 331–347.

Freeman, D., Freeman, J., & Garety, P.A. (2006). *Overcoming Paranoid and Suspicious Thoughts.* London: Robinson Constable

Garety, P. A. & Freeman, D. (1999). Cognitive approaches to delusions: a critical review of theories and evidence. *British Journal of Clinical Psychology, 38*, 113–154.

Garety, P. A. & Hemsley, D. R. (1994). *Delusions: Investigations into the Psychology of Delusional Reasoning.* Oxford: Oxford University Press.

Garety, P. A., Kuipers, E., Fowler, D., Freeman, D., & Bebbington, P. E. (2001). A cognitive model of the positive symptoms of psychosis. *Psychological Medicine, 31,* 189–195.

Garety, P. A., Freeman, D., Jolley, S., Dunn, G., Bebbington, P. E., Fowler, D., Kuipers, E., & Dudely, R., (2005) Reasoning, Emotions, and Delusional Conviction in Psychosis. *Journal of Abnormal Psychology.* 144, 373-384.

Gray, J. A., Feldon, J., Rawlins, J. P. N., Hemsley, D. R., & Smith, A. D. (1991). The neuropsychology of schizophrenia. *Behavioural and Brain Sciences, 14,* 1–20.

Gumley, A., O'Grady, M., McNay, L., et al. (2003). Early intervention for relapse in schizophrenia: results of a 12-month randomised controlled trial of cognitive behavioural therapy. *Psychological Medicine, 33,* 419–431.

Haddock, G., McCarron, J., Tarrier, N., & Faragher, E. B. (1999). Scales to measure dimensions of hallucinations and delusions: The psychotic symptom rating scales (PSYRATS). *Psychological Medicine, 29,* 879–889.

Kapur, S. (2003). Psychosis as a state of aberrant salience: a framework linking biology, phenomenology, and pharmacology. *American Journal of Psychiatry, 160,* 13–23.

Kinderman, P. & Bentall, R. P. (1997). Causal attributions in paranoia and depression: internal, personal and situational attributions for negative events. *Journal of Abnormal Psychology, 106,* 341–345.

Kingdon, D. & Turkington, D. (2002). *The case study guide to cognitive behavior therapy of psychosis.* Chichester: Wiley.

Krabbendam, L., Janssen, I., Bijl, R. V., Vollebergh, W. A. M., & van Os, J. (2002). Neuroticism and low self-esteem as risk factors for psychosis. *Social Psychiatry and Psychiatric Epidemiology, 37,* 1–6.

Maher, B. A. (1988). Anomalous experience and delusional thinking: the logic of explanations. In T. F. Oltmanns, & B. A. Maher (Eds.) *Delusional beliefs* (pp. 15–33). New York: Wiley.

Morrison, A. P. (2002). *A Casebook of Cognitive Therapy for Psychosis.* Hove: Brunner-Routledge.

Lehman, A. F., Kreyenbuhl, J., Buchanan, R. W., et al. (2004). The Schizophrenia Patient Outcomes Research Team (PORT): Updated treatment recommendations 2003. *Schizophrenia Bulletin, 30,* 193–217.

Murray, R. M., Jones, P. B., Susser, E., van Os, J., & Cannon, M. (2003). *The epidemiology of schizophrenia.* Cambridge: Cambridge University Press.

National Institute for Clinical Excellence (2002). *Schizophrenia: Core interventions in the treatment and management of schizophrenia in primary and secondary care.* London: NICE.

Oltmanns, T. F. (1988). Approaches to the definition and study of delusions. In T. F. Oltmanns, & B. A. Maher (Eds.) *Delusional beliefs* (pp. 3–12). New York: Wiley.

Pilling, S., Bebbington, P., Kuipers, E., et al. (2002). Psychological treatments in schizophrenia: I. Meta-analysis of family intervention and cognitive behavior therapy. *Psychological Medicine, 32,* 763–782.

Sartorius, N., Jablensky, A., Korten, A., et al. (1986). Early manifestations and first-contact incidence of schizophrenia in different cultures. *Psychological Medicine, 16,* 909–928.

Tarrier, N., Yusupoff, L., Kinney, C., et al. (1998). Randomised controlled trial of intensive cognitive behavioural therapy for patients with chronic schizophrenia, *British Medical Journal, 317,* 303–307.

Van Os, J., Hanssen, M, Bijl, R.V., V Ravelli, A. (2000). Strauss (1969) revisited: a psychosis continuum in the general population. Schizophrenia Research, 45, 11-20.

Verdoux, H., Maurice-Tison, S., Gay, B., et al. (1998). A survey of delusional ideation in primary-care patients. *Psychological Medicine, 28,* 127–134.

Wason, P. C. (1960). On the failure to eliminate hypotheses in a conceptual task. *Quarterly Journal of Experimental Psychology, 12,* 129–140.

Winters, K. C. & Neale, J. M. (1983). Delusions and delusional thinking in psychotics: a review of the literature. *Clinical Psychology Review, 3,* 227–253.

Dementia

Jane E. Fisher • Craig Yury • Jeffrey A. Buchanan

WHAT IS DEMENTIA?

"Dementia" is a descriptive term for a collection of symptoms that are caused by changes in brain function. Dementia is caused by many conditions; some can be reversed while others cannot. The two most common forms of degenerative dementia are *Alzheimer's disease* and *vascular dementia*. *Lewy body disease* and *frontotemporal* forms of dementia are the next most common forms of irreversible dementia. Reversible conditions that can cause symptoms of dementia include infection, high fever, drug reactions, dehydration, vitamin deficiency and poor nutrition, head injury, or normal pressure hydrocephalus (National Institute of Neurological Diseases and Stroke).

Degenerative forms of dementia such as Alzheimer's disease and vascular dementia have devastating effects on the lives of the affected person and their family. Over the course of a degenerative dementia, the affected person experiences progressive declines in all intellectual abilities. Patients eventually experience a complete loss of verbal abilities, memory function, and severe impairment in new learning. Those close to the person experience the cognitive declines as major changes in personality where the affected person is perceived as behaving in uncharacteristic ways such as showing poor judgment, recklessness in the management of finances and other responsibilities, or acting in uninhibited ways such as engaging in sexual acts in public.

In advanced dementia the development of difficult behaviors is common. These may include aggression (particularly during hands-on caregiving), disruptive vocalizations (e.g., screaming or calling out for hours, repeating same question hundreds of times per day), and wandering. During the course of a degenerative dementia the affected person will inevitably eventually require 24 hour supervision and become completely dependent on others for their care. In the end stage of a degenerative dementia the person loses motor control including the ability to walk and swallow.

The economic costs of dementia care are extraordinary. The cost of caring for persons with dementing illnesses is estimated to exceed $70 billion annually (National Institute on Aging, 2004). Much of this cost is associated with institutional long-term care and with the fact that patients often live for years while requiring 24 hour supervision.

Treatment planning for persons with dementia should be considered within the context of their social and physical environments. Caring for a person with dementia has considerable psychological and physical health consequences including impaired immune function, increased risk of mortality, severe depression, and suicidal ideation (Pinquart & Sorenson, 2003; Schulz, O'Brien, Bookwala, Fleissner, 1995). In designing treatment for a person with dementia, the dependent relationship of the patient on others requires that health care providers plan for the emotional and instrumental support of the caregiver.

Fisher, J. E., Cardinal, C., Yury, C., & Buchanan, J. A. (2006). Dementia. In J. E. Fisher & W. T. O'Donohue (Eds.), *Practitioner's guide to evidence-based psychotherapy*. New York: Springer.

Providing support to the caregiver will increase the likelihood that the patient will receive effective and safe care and the potentially debilitating effects of caregiving will be minimized. Given the critical role that family caregivers play in the treatment of persons with dementia, guidelines for the assessment and treatment of caregivers will also be reviewed.

BASIC FACTS ABOUT DEMENTIA

Comorbidity. Elderly persons with dementia experience the same risk for chronic illness as other elderly persons. Depression and anxiety are common in persons with dementia and appear to be associated with several factors including the person's recognition that his/her functioning is impaired and their exposure to increasingly confusing and aversive environmental stimuli. It is estimated that up to 50% of persons with dementia experience depression (Forsell & Wingblad, 1998). Diagnosis of comorbid conditions is a challenge as verbal abilities decline and reporting of symptoms becomes impossible for the patient. Conditions associated with pain can produce significant problems in the care of persons with dementia since moderately and severely impaired persons cannot effectively tact or describe their internal state.

Prevalence. The US Congress Office of Technology Assessment estimates that as many as 6.8 million Americans have dementia. Estimates of the prevalence among persons over the age of 65 affected with dementia range from 10% to 20%, with the number of people with the disease doubling every 5 years beyond age 65 (National Institute of Neurological Diseases and Stoke, 2005). Estimates of the prevalence of dementia among persons over age 85 are as high as 47% (Evans et al., 1989).

Age at onset. Age is the most important risk factor for dementia. The number of people with the disease doubles every 5 years beyond age 65. Dementia developing before the age of 65 is considered "early onset" dementia. The incidence of early onset dementia is quite low. Persons with early onset dementia account for 1–2% of cases (National Institute on Aging, 2005).

Gender. The number of women dying from dementia is greater than the number of men by a ratio of more than 2:1. The sex ratio reflects the larger number of women who live to older ages when the risk of death from dementia is more prevalent (Centers for Disease Control, 1999).

Course. The course and progression of decline varies significantly across patients. Efforts to describe the course of dementia as occurring in an orderly fashion through the application of stage models have not been supported by empirical research. On average, persons with AD live from 8 to 10 years after they are diagnosed, though the disease can last for as many as 20 years (National Institute on Aging, 2005).

WHAT ARE EFFECTIVE MEDICAL TREATMENTS FOR DEMENTIA?

Medical treatment for dementia is currently focused on two types of symptoms: cognitive symptoms and behavior problems.

What must be ruled out?

Before considering treatment for dementia-related problems, dementia must be properly diagnosed. The 1987 NIH Consensus Statement emphasizes a careful differentiation between progressive degenerative dementias (e.g., Alzheimer's type) and arrestable or reversible dementias due to delirium, infection, metabolic or nutritional disorders, vascular system or cardiac disease, lesions, normal pressure hydrocephalus, or affective disorders, particularly depression.

Because 75% of the elderly take at least one, and commonly several, prescription medications (Wood, 2002), for diagnostic purposes the NIH Consensus Statement (1987) recommends the withdrawal of all medications that are not absolutely necessary. Pharmacokinetic changes—associated with aging and lifestyle factors—and diminished homeostatic responses predispose elderly populations to adverse drug reactions (Katzung, 2001; Wood, 2002). Capable of producing cognitive impairment or of aggravating dementia is, as MacDonald (1998) points out, "the whole pharmacopeia" (p. 689), for example:

- neuroactive and psychoactive agents, such as
  - benzodiazepines
  - opioid analgesics
  - antipsychotics
  - antidepressants
- corticosteroids
- anticonvulsants
- anticholinergic preparations, e.g., for
  - movement disorders
  - allergic reactions
  - gastrointestinal disorders
- drugs used for cardiovascular purposes, such as
  - antihypertensives
  - antiarrhythmics
- antibiotics
- nonsteroidal anti-inflammatory drugs.

(NIH Consens Statement Online, 1987; Stewart & Fairweather, 2002; for a review of drug-induced cognition disorders in the elderly, see Gray, Lai, & Larson, 1999). Note that any combination of drugs may have nonlinear effects.

When progressive degenerative dementia has been diagnosed, the subtypes of dementia with Lewy body disease (LBD) and frontotemporal lobar dementia (FTLD) require special consideration. Dementia with Lewy body disease (LBD) must be ruled out if the use of atypical or typical antipsychotics (also called "neuroleptics") is considered. LBD is characterized by an increased risk of hypersensitivity to antipsychotic medication, such that the administration of such medication may result in delirium, neuromalignant syndrome, or death (Kaufer, 2004). There is also anecdotal evidence that the use of actylcholinesterase inhibitors, agents that may slow cognitive deterioration (details below), may lead to worsening of parkinsonian symptoms in individuals with LBD (Rozzini, Ghianda, Trabucchi, & Padovani, 2004).

Populations diagnosed with frontotemporal lobar degeneration (FTLD), the second most common type of early onset dementia, may also show relatively poor neuroleptic tolerance (medical record review by Pijnenburg, Sampson, Harvey, Fox, & Rossor, 2003).

PSYCHOTROPIC DRUGS FOR DEMENTIA

Psychotropic drug therapy refers to the prescription of medication with the explicit intent to alter cognitions, emotions, or behavior (Poling & Byrne, 2000). While the main goal in the development of psychotropic drugs for dementia is to halt or at least slow the rate with which deterioration progresses, psychotropic medication is also prescribed to reduce the frequency of challenging behaviors emitted by 60–80% of those diagnosed with dementia, with a lifetime prevalence of 100% (Lawlor, 2004; Profenno & Tariot, 2004). In April of 2005 the Federal Drug Administration issued a issued a public health advisory to alert health care providers, patients, and patient caregivers to new safety information concerning an unapproved (i.e., "off-label") use of atypical antipsychotic drugs. Clinical studies of these drugs to treat behavioral disorders in elderly patients with dementia have shown a higher death rate associated with their use compared to patients receiving a placebo. The advisory applies to antipsychotic drugs including Abilify (aripiprazole), Zyprexa (olanzapine), Seroquel (quetiapine), Risperdal (risperidone), Clozaril (clozapine), and Geodon (ziprasidone). Symbyax, which is approved for treatment of depressive episodes associated with bipolar disorder, is also included in the agency's advisory.

In analyses of seventeen placebo-controlled studies of four drugs in this class, the rate of death for those elderly patients with dementia was about 1.6–1.7 times that of placebo. Although the causes of death were varied, most seemed to be either heart-related (such as heart failure or sudden death) or from infections (pneumonia).

The atypical antipsychotics fall into three drug classes based on their chemical structure. Because the increase in mortality was seen with atypical antipsychotic medications in all three chemical classes, the FDA concluded that the effect is probably related to the common pharmacologic effects of all atypical antipsychotic medications, including those that have not been studied in the dementia population. The FDA is therefore considering adding a warning to the labeling of older antipsychotic medications because limited data also suggest a similar increase in mortality for these drugs. The review of the data on these older drugs, however, is still on-going.

Additional information concerning the advisory is available on FDA's Web site at: http://www.fda.gov/cder/drug/infopage/antipsychotics/default.htm and http://www.fda.gov/cder/drug/advisory/antipsychotics.htm.

FIRST-LINE MEDICATIONS

Currently, there is no treatment that can reverse progressive degenerative dementia. However, the US Food and Drug Administration approved the use of five prescription drugs, which fall into the functional categories of "acetylcholinesterase inhibitors" for mild to moderate or "N-methyl-D-asparate (NMDA) receptor antagonists" for moderate to severe dementia of the Alzheimer's type (Cummings, 2004). In randomized control trials, these drugs have been shown to improve performance on neuropsychological standardized tests relative to placebo controls (cognitive endpoint); to correlate with physicians' reports of relative symptom reduction and relatively lower rates of healthcare utilization (global endpoint); or to produce higher ratings by caregivers regarding mastery of activities of daily living (functional endpoint); or to produce higher ratings by caregivers regarding mastery of activities of daily living (functional endpoint). Generally, acetylcholinesterase inhibitors have demonstrated a positive influence on cognitive and functional endpoints, while the NMDA receptor antagonist memantine has positively affected global and functional endpoints.

Acetylcholinesterase Inhibitors

The main function of acetylcholinesterase inhibitors is to prevent the breakdown of acetylcholine and thereby to enhance cholinergic neurotransmission, but there is recent evidence that cholinergic drugs also affect dopaminergic systems (Zhang,

Zhou & Dani, 2004). The drugs listed below differ in the selectivity with which they can inhibit cholinesterases, and increased selectivity correlates with fewer peripheral adverse effects (Sonkusare, Kaul, & Ramarao, 2005). Ranked in terms of general tolerability, donepezil leads, followed by galantamine and by rivastigmine (Jones, 2003).

1. Tacrine (Cognex®, approved in 1993 and now rarely used; increased risk of hepatoxicity requires monitoring of liver transaminase)
2. Donepezil (Aricept®, approved in 1996)
3. Rivastigmine (Exelon®, approved in 2000)
4. Galantamine (Reminyl®, approved in 2001)

Acetylcholinesterase inhibitors have labeled indications for mild to moderate dementia of the Alzheime's type and off-label use for other dementia subtypes (e.g., vascular dementia, dementia with Lewy body disease) as well as for ADHD, autism, and schizophrenia (Medline search, November, 2004).

Effectiveness of acetylcholinesterase inhibitors. While the American Association for Geriatric Psychiatry, the Alzheimer's Association, the American Geriatrics Society, and the American Academy of Neurology recommend donepezil, galantamine, and rivastigmine as first-line pharmacological treatments of dementia, the effectiveness of acetylcholinesterase inhibitors, particularly of donepezil, is being questioned (AD 2000 Collaborative Group, 2004; Jones, 2004; Kaduzkiewicz, et al., 2004). Acetylcholinesterase inhibitors have consistently demonstrated their efficacy in industry-sponsored randomized clinical trials (Cummings, 2004); however, their effectiveness in community settings with less well-defined, "typical" patients with high rates of comorbidity is not clear (Schneider, 2004). Marginal benefit-to-risk ratios and a lack of globally and functionally relevant endpoints have recently shifted the hopes for decreasing rates of institutionalizations and of acute care hospitalizations to memantine (Sonkusare, Kaul, & Romarao, 2005).

General information for donepezil, rivastigmine, and galantamine

- *Hypothesis.* Neurodegeneration correlates with a cholinergic deficiency that can be temporarily remediated by the use of cholinergic agents.
- *Contraindications.* Hypersensitivity to cholinomimetic agents; severe hepatic impairment (galantamine)
- *Caution.* Bradycardia; cardiac arrhythmias; stomach or duodenal ulcers; concurrent use of nonsteroidal anti-inflammatory drugs; impaired intestinal peristaltic or sphincter function; asthma; chronic obstructive pulmonary disease; combination with anesthesia or muscle relaxers
- *General drug interactions.* Increase the effects of other cholinomimetic agents

Particular information on acetylcholinesterase inhibitors
Donepezil: www.aricept.com

- Dose Once/day before bedtime (5 mg/diem), possible increase to 10 mg/diem if there is a positive evaluation after four weeks
  - Most common side effects
  - 10–1%: Nausea, vomiting, diarrhea
  - >5%: Muscle spasms, fatigue, insomnia, headache, dizziness

  Galantamine: www.reminyl.com

- Contraindicated with severe hepatic impairment
- Dose:

- Twice daily with meals (2×4 mg/diem), possible increase to 2×8 mg/diem if there is a positive evaluation after four weeks; dependent upon individual evaluation, titration to 2×12 mg/diem is possible.
- If renal or hepatic impairment are present, the initial dose should not exceed 4 mg/diem; titration is limited to a daily dose of 16 mg/diem (2×8 mg/diem)
- Most common side effects:
  - 13–17%: Nausea, vomiting, diarrhea, abdominal pain, dyspepsia
  - >5%: Fatigue, dizziness, headaches, somnolence, anorexia
  - Behavioral changes, including agitation, and hallucination have been reported
- Drug–drug interactions: May increase the effect of muscle relaxers and decrease the effects of anticholinergic agents
- In 2004, the US Food and Drug administration issued a warning concerning the inappropriate dispensing and administration of "Amaryl®" (indicated for Type II diabetes mellitus) when "Reminyl®" (galantamine) had been prescribed. Various adverse events, including severe hypoglycemia and one death, resulted.

    http://www.fda.gov/medwatch/ SAFETY/2004/safety04.htm#Reminyl

    Rivastigmine: www.exelon.com

- Doses: Twice daily with meals (2×1.5 mg/diem), possible increase to 6–12 mg/diem (2×3 mg/diem to 2×6 mg/diem) if there is a positive evaluation after two weeks
- Most common side effects:
  - 27–35%: Nausea, vomiting, diarrhea
  - >5%: Somnolence, agitation, confusion, depression, and insomnia
- Drug–drug interactions: May increase the effect of muscle relaxers and decrease the effects of anticholinergic agents

N-methyl-d-asparate (NMDA) receptor antagonists

The NMDA receptor antagonist, memantine, has been available in Europe as Akatinol® for the treatment of CNS disorders, multiple sclerosis, and mild to moderate dementia since 1982. Merz, the patent holder for memantine, withdrew Akatinol® from the market on July 31, 2002, and reintroduced the identical substance one day later as Axura®. The name change and the new label indication for moderate to severe dementia were accompanied by a 74% increase in price (Schmitt-Feuerbach, 2002). Merz entered strategic licensing and cooperation agreements with Lundbeck (Denmark) and Forest Laboratories (US). The US Food and Drug Administration approved Nemantin® one year later, in 2003, and memantine is now marketed worldwide as Axura® (Merz), Ebixa® (Lundbeck), and Nemantin® (Forest Laboratories).

Memantine works on receptors that are specifically sensitive to the effects of N-methyl-D-aspartate (NMDA), a glutamate agonist. Under some circumstances (e.g., injury, seizures, or stroke), excessive calcium influx through channels activated by NMDA receptors can kill neurons ("excitotoxicity"). Memantine blocks the NMDA receptor when it is active, and thereby may protect the neuron without interfering with processes necessary for learning and memory. Indeed, memantine may enhance hippocampal synaptic transmission and memory, and it may also block serotonergic and nicotinic cholinergic receptors (for a detailed review, see Sonkusare, Kaul, & Ramarao, 2005).

Effectiveness of N-methyl-D-asparate (NMDA) Receptor Antagonists. Like the cholinesterase inhibitors, memantine has demonstrated its efficacy in randomized controlled trials (for a review of randomized control trials since 1991, see Möbius,

2003). Add-on therapy to acetylcholinesterase inhibitors has also been investi-
gated (Schmitt, Bernhardt, Moeller, Heuser, & Frölich, 2004). Sonkusare, Kaul, &
Ramarao (2005) conclude their review of the evidence by pointing out that meman-
tine might be able to prevent further neurodegeneration in dementia of the
Alzheimer's type. Current research focuses on building evidence for the applica-
tion of memantine to mixed dementia, mild to moderate vascular dementia,
Wernicke–Korsakoff syndrome, and mild cognitive impairment (Medline search,
November 2004).

General Information for Memantine (*www.namenda.com*)

- Hypothesis: Memantine decreases the probability of excitoxicity and enhances neu-
  rotransmission
- Contraindications: Hypersensitivity to memantine; seizure disorders; severe confu-
  sion; renal impairment
- Warnings: combination with anesthesia or NMDA antagonists, such as amantadine,
  ketamine or dextromethorphan
- Side effects are dose-dependent:
  - Most common: Hallucinations; dizziness; headache; confusion; fatigue; syncope
  - Less common: Cardiac failure; vertigo; akathisia; transient ischemic attacks;
    ataxia; hypokinesia; anaemia; increased alkaline phosphatase activity; skin rash;
    frequent micturition
- Drug interactions:
  - may increase the action and the toxicity of L-dopa, dopaminergic agonists, neuro-
    leptics, and anticholinergics;
  - may reduce the activity of barbiturates;
  - may potentiate the activity of anticonvulsants and morphine (Sonkusare, Kaul,
    & Ramarao, 2005)

Discontinue medication

- If adverse or side effects significantly decrease a person's quality of life.
- If, after three to six months of drug therapy, the progression of dementia is still con-
  tinuing its pre-drug course; if the deterioration is accelerated; or if there is an
  abrupt worsening of conditions.
- If a drug-free period shows that the medication does not make a difference in func-
  tioning or in the progression of deterioration.
- If a person becomes bedridden or is not able to communicate any more.
- If a person has reached the stage of severe dementia.

PSYCHOTROPIC MEDICATION FOR CHALLENGING BEHAVIORS

Recommendations for the management of challenging behaviors follow three steps:

1. First, caregivers must ensure optimal care. When people lose their ability to communicate, they may express their discomfort (e.g., from medication side effects or
   other physiological distress) through behaviors that are deemed inappropriate
   (Fisher, in press).
2. After a thorough and qualified assessment, nonpharmacological management of
   behavioral problems is the first-line approach.
3. Psychotropic medications may only be considered after behavioral interventions have
   failed, or in case of an emergency. The US Food and Drug Administration has not
   approved the use of any psychotropic medication for any challenging behaviors

correlated with dementia (Profenno & Tariot, 2004; Lawlor, 2004). The FDA (2005) has advised against the use of atypical antipsychotics for behavior problems occurring in dementia due to risk of death.

Given this lack of approval, one may consider each prescription of a drug an experiment if it has as its target a change in the behavior or mood of a person with dementia (Poling & Byrne, 2000). The experimental nature of the off-label use suggests empirically based strategies that have been explicitly developed for the use of psychotropic medication with other vulnerable, cognitively impaired populations (for the complete guidelines, see Kalachnik et al., 1998). At the heart of these strategies is the realization that the degree of cognitive impairment and possible physiological changes that accompany the degenerative process produce an "end-of-the-curve"-phenomenon: Populations with dementia do not fall into the median range of the bell-shaped distribution of normative or "typical" drug responses. They are, as elderly population generally and as a population with brain diseases specifically, more vulnerable to adverse effects of drug and thus have to be closely monitored while taking psychotropic medication (Gay, Lai, & Larson, 1999; Wood, 2002).

Questions that must be answered by caregivers

1. What are the frequency, intensity, and the quality of the problem behavior?
   a. Is the behavior dangerous to self or others, or is it annoying or embarrassing?
   b. Who is the main beneficiary of the drug intervention (i.e., the person with dementia or someone else)?
2. What constitutes a satisfactory outcome?
   a. Who is keeping track of whether the problem behavior actually decreases in rate?
   b. Will effects on other behaviors be assessed to prevent the risk of accelerating the loss of repertoires?
   c. If the problem behavior has decreased in rate, or if there is no change, when will the drug be discontinued? Is there a mechanism for a periodic review by health care professionals?
3. What is the rationale for choosing a particular drug over another? Is there literature on the off-label use of a particular drug with elderly dementia populations?
4. Is there a list of possible adverse effects? Who is monitoring the patient?
   a. Antipsychotics frequently induce akathisia. Caregivers must be trained to differentiate the restlessness and agitation that are side effects of the drug from a worsening of the behavioral problems. An increase in drug dose may lead to increased agitation (for a review, see Saltz, Robinson & Woerner, 2004).
   b. The risk of irreversible tardive dyskinesia from antipsychotic use increases with age (Wood, 2002).
   c. Atypical antipsychotics may increase the risk of metabolic syndrome (obesity, insulin resistance, impaired glucose regulation, etc.). They also may increase the risk of hyperglycemia and Type 2 diabetes. The US Food and Drug Administration issued warnings for all atypical antipsychotics in April of 2005. For a review, see Lieberman (2004a).
   d. Many drugs, including psychotropic drugs such as tricyclic antidepressants, have anticholinergic effects that may increase the risk of falls by producing confusion and an inability to concentrate. Other anticholinergic effects range from urinary retention and constipation to angina and myocardial infarction (for a review, see Lieberman, 2004b).
   e. Tricyclic antidepressants have cardiotropic side effects (Wood, 2002).

f. The use of anticonvulsant medication, such as carbamazepine, requires liver transaminase monitoring. Because of the high risk of toxicity when carbamazepine is combined with other medications, polypharmacy requires the periodic assessment of plasma concentrations of the prescribed drugs. Wood (2002) recommends looking out for signs of toxicity: "an increase in confusion, unsteadiness and falls, hypotension, constipation, urinary retention, and an ADH-like effect causing hyponatraemia" (p. 298).

g. Benzodiazepine use is accompanied by a high rate of side effects, such as "ataxia, falls, confusion, anterograde amnesia, sedation, light-headedness, and tolerance and withdrawal syndromes" (Profenno & Tariot, 2004, p. 70).

5. If drugs with known withdrawal effects are chosen, is there a plan for withdrawal and management of the correlated behavioral problems?

The systematic and informed implementation of drug therapy, including assessment, structured therapy, and periodical review, is more likely to reduce risk and to ascertain the focus on the person's quality of life.

PSYCHOLOGICAL ASSESSMENT AND TREATMENT STRATEGIES FOR PERSONS WITH DEMENTIA

What Assessments are Not Helpful?

Traditional psychological tests such as the MMPI and projective tests are not useful in assessing dementia. Self-report questionnaires normed on non-cognitively impaired elderly population may not be valid for use with a person with moderate or severe cognitive impairment. Neuropsychological assessment is useful for differential diagnosis and monitoring cognitive decline. It has limited utility for treatment planning.

What Psychological Treatments are Effective?

There is currently no treatment available for halting or reversing the deterioration in degenerative forms of dementia. Therefore, the goals of treatment should focus on maintaining the patient's repertoire and preventing or reducing *excess* disability (Fisher, in press). Excess disability is common in elderly persons with dementia. It is defined as impairment in function that is disproportionate to that directly attributable to the disease (Dawson, Wells, & Kline, 1993). Excess disability develops when the social and physical environments present inadequate support or excessive demands on the person with dementia. In a person with degenerative dementia, excess disability can be conceptualized as a premature reduction in behaviors that will inevitably be lost due to the disease process (Fisher, in press). For example, while persons with AD eventually lose all verbal abilities, a reduction in social interaction due to depression and social isolation may increase the risk of a premature reduction in verbal behavior (Ritchie, Touchon, & Ledesert, 1998).

Emotional symptoms. Early in the disease process, elderly persons with dementia may become hypervigilant in monitoring signs of their impairment and the response of others to the appearance of symptoms during social interactions. Social withdrawal and inactivity are common. Instruments designed for assessing emotional distress in persons with dementia have been developed (e.g., Cornell Scale for Depression in Dementia, Alexopoulos, Abrams, Young, & Shamoian, 1988). Cognitive behavior therapy is effective for the treatment of depression in mildly impaired persons with dementia (Gallagher-Thompson). Behavior activation interventions have also been found to be effective in reducing depression (Teri et al., 1999).

Behavioral symptoms. Behavioral problems such as aggression, wandering, repeated questions, and public displays of sexual behavior are common with over 50% of patients developing behaviors that warrant intervention (Chen, Borson, & Scanlan, 2000; Lyketsos, 2000). The occurrence of challenging behaviors is one of the primary reasons family caregivers decide to institutionalize the patient (Hope, Keene, Gedling, Fairburn, & Jacoby, 1998). Historically, these behaviors have been primarily managed by psychotropic medications, in particular antipsychotic and atypical antipsychotic medications (see FDA advisory described above). Federal legislation (Omnibus Reconcilation Act on Nursing Home Reform, OBRA, 1987) restricts the use of psychotropic medications for behavior management within nursing homes received Federal funds through Medicare and Medicaid programs. Interventions that do not involve chemical or mechanical "restraint" are now considered best practice in the field.

Behavioral interventions have been found to be effective in reducing and preventing behavior problems. Recent research suggests that the occurrence and maintenance of problem behaviors are highly influenced by environmental stimuli, even in advanced dementia (Bourgeois, Burgio, & Schultz, 1995; Buchanan & Fisher, 2002; Burgio et al., 1994; Fisher, in press). Recent data consistently indicate that problem behaviors that occur in degenerative dementia are adaptive in that they serve a purpose for the patient (e.g., accessing attention, occur under conditions of sensory deprivation or overstimulation, etc.) and that interventions based on the function of behavior may be more effective in reducing and preventing problem behavior (Fisher, in press). The results of this research suggest that *restraint free* interventions for persons with dementia should be based on the following principles: (1) behavioral disturbances are adaptive when examined in the context of the patient's declining competencies and the demands of the environment; (2) topographically similar behaviors may have different etiologies; (3) behavior problems are multiply determined; (4) The reasons a behavior occurs may change as dementia progresses; (5) the "reasons" a behavior occurs should determine the treatment; (6) treatment planning should be individualized; and (7) treatment goals should focus on promoting adaptive behavior and preventing problem behavior rather than eliminating behavior (and hence potentially contributing to excess disability).

What is involved in effective assessment of behavior problems?

1. *Rule out physical conditions* that might be causing or contributing to the problem. Conditions associated with pain (e.g., urinary tract infection, arthritis, indigestion, constipation), drug interactions and/or the side effects of commonly prescribed medications (e.g., nausea, sedation, dizziness, insomnia, agitation, tiredness, dry mouth, constipation, lightheadedness, headache, low blood pressure, blurred vision, and confusion) should be ruled out prior to implementing a behavioral intervention for a person with dementia.

2. *Behavioral description.* Develop a precise behavioral description (e.g., "repeats same question 20 times per hour" is more precise than "asks annoying questions"). Direct observation methods are the most effective assessment strategies for designing restraint free environments (see Bloom, Fischer, & Orme, 1995, for specific strategies). General points to consider in implementing a measurement system are: who will do the recording (e.g., professionals or family caregiver), the severity of the behavior (e.g., a dangerous behavior such as wandering or physical aggression may require a brief pretreatment assessment) at when behavior is to be observed, the observation interval (e.g., in one-minute blocks or hourly), and the specific

response dimensions are targeted (i.e., duration, frequency) (Bloom, Fischer, & Orme, 1995). Caregiver questionnaires such as the *Cohen-Mansfield Agitation Inventory* (Cohen-Mansfield & Billig, 1986) may be helpful for describing the topography and frequency of a problem behavior.

3. *Identify contingent relationships.* Two assessment strategies are used to identify the controlling environmental features of which behavior is a function; one is a descriptive (ABC) analysis, the other is an experimental or functional analysis (see Lerman, & Iwata, 1993).

4. *Monitor behavioral processes.* Treatment programs should be adjusted in accordance with prevailing contingencies of reinforcement. Are the antecedent stimuli too weak to evoke effective performance (e.g., due to sensory impairments)? Is the patient incapable of emitting the response in question? Is the reinforcement schedule too thin to support the target behavior? Are consequences delivered too late to effect the behavior of the person with severe short term memory impairment? Have previously effective reinforcers lost their potency (e.g., due to age-associated sensory or cognitive impairment or a comorbid health condition)? Within a restraint free model these factors are addressed by way of stimulus building, response building, contingency building, and consequence building, respectively.

   a. *Stimulus building.* The purpose of stimulus building techniques is to give weak or neutral antecedent stimuli the ability to evoke effective behavior (e.g., Hussian, 1981). For example, changing the intensity or size of discriminative stimuli (e.g., placing a picture of a toilet on a bathroom door) or combining antecedents, so as to increase overall valence (e.g., combining a verbal instruction with a physical gesture) (e.g., Nolan, Mathews, Truesdall-Todd, & VanDorp, 2002).

   b. *Response building.* Response building techniques employ movements that are regularly emitted but not currently in use to promote behavior (e.g., using physical guidance to promote feeding) (Lindsley, 1964a).

   c. *Contingency building.* Contingency building involves maintaining a response by increasing reinforcement density from richer schedules to thinner schedules of reinforcement. Initially, every response is followed by the delivery of the reinforcer. The reinforcer-to-response ratio is thus 1:1. Once a steady state of responding is achieved, gradually thin out reinforcement delivery to an intermittent schedule of reinforcement (e.g., every third response produces the reinforcer; Ferster & Skinner, 1957).

   d. *Consequence building.* Neutral events can become reinforces when they are frequently paired with powerful reinforcers. In general, the closer the temporal relationship between reinforcer and neutral stimulus increases the likelihood that neutral stimuli will acquire reinforcing functions.

INTERVENTIONS TO ENHANCE CAREGIVER FUNCTIONING

Caregivers' emotional coping and instrumental skill repertoires are directly related to negative health outcomes and therefore should be assessed. A family caregiver and their family member with dementia are likely to have had a decades long relationship history prior to the onset of the dementing illness. The nature of the relationship (e.g., affectionate vs. conflicted) will impact caregivers' attitude toward the person with dementia and his/her willingness to engage in the demands of the caregiving role. Four domains relevant for effective caregiver functioning should be assessed:

a. *Knowledge of the behavioral effects of dementia* and the caregiver's interpretation of patient's behavior (e.g., Are difficult behaviors perceived as intentional or due to the disease process?; Does the caregiver interpret patient's behavior as motivated by intention to harm or annoy the caregiver or as beyond the patient's control? Is the caregiver able to engage in perspective taking when they encounter problem behavior in the patient?).

b. *Emotion regulation and problem solving skills* for managing the emotional stressors (sleep deprivation, depression, anger, and frustration) associated with caregiving. Opportunity, practical and psychological barriers (e.g., repertoire deficits) for accessing pleasant experiences should also be assessed.

c. *Skill repertoire for managing instrumental tasks* associated with caregiving (e.g., bathing, feeding, managing medication, and housework; patient advocacy skills for effectively communicating with healthcare professionals and identifying and accessing relevant social services).

d. *Relationship quality* (historical and current factors that may impact the caregiver's willingness and emotional experience of engaging in demands of caregiving role).

Measures

The Revised-Ways of Coping Checklist (RWCCL) (Vitaliano, Russo, Carr, Maiuro, & Becker, 1985) is a 41-item scale that assesses emotional coping strategies in caregivers of persons with dementia. Subscales reflect the use of different coping strategies such as problem solving, support focused, avoidance, and blaming self. *Caregiver Task Checklist* (Gallagher-Thompson et al., 2000; assessment strategy developed by Poulshock & Deimling, 1984). The 29-item checklist assesses the basic and instrumental activities for which assistance is provided (e.g., grooming, toileting, metals, transportation, bathing, and finances) and whether the caregiver finds the task difficult, tiring, or upsetting to perform.

Revised Memory and Behavior Problem Checklist (RMBPC) (Teri, Zarit et al., 1992). A 24-item instrument that can be completed by a completed by a caregiver in 10 minutes to assess frequency and caregiver burden associated with patient's memory-related problems, disruptive behaviors, and depression. The subscale scores correlate with well-established indices of depression, cognitive impairment, and caregiver burden.

TREATMENT STRATEGIES FOR CAREGIVERS

Hundreds of books, websites, and support programs are available for family caregivers. Services include educational programs, support groups, respite services, individual counseling, and case management. Few of the products and services available had empirical support prior to their dissemination and this has contributed to a confusing array of options for a highly stressed consumer group. Given the myriad of resources available, clinicians should attempt to match services to the individual needs of the patient/caregiver dyad. This is particularly important given that caregiving demands on severely restrict caregivers' ability to access to services.

A meta-analysis of intervention for family caregivers indicated that psychoeducational interventions have a greater effect caregiver on outcomes (e.g., knowledge, burden, depression, etc.) compared to more traditional support group formats (Sorensen, Pinquart and Duberstein, 2002). Reviews of the dementia caregiver intervention literature (e.g., Schulz et al., 2002; Steffen & Mangum, in press) have found that psychoeducational interventions using behavioral and cognitive treatment strategies have the greatest impact on caregiver depressive symptoms and other indices of psychological health.

In 1995, the National Institute on Aging initiated Project REACH (Resources for Enhancing Alzheimer's Caregiver Health), a multisite intervention study aimed at designed to evaluate interventions for enhancing family caregiver psychological and physical health outcomes. Nine different social and behavioral interventions were tested. Investigators found that the combined effect of interventions alleviated caregiver burden, and that interventions that enhanced caregiver behavioral skills reduced depression.

In sum, research on caregiver distress has found that interventions involving structured, time-limited approaches that use guided mastery to teach behavioral, emotional, and cognitive self-regulation skills through direct instruction, in-session practice, and between-session assignments are most effective. Effective interventions include:

- "Coping with Caregiving"—Cognitive behavioral intervention designed to teach skills including relaxation, perspective taking, and goal setting for managing mood (Coon, Thompson, Steffen, Sorocco, & Gallagher-Thompson, 2003; Gallagher-Thompson et al., 2003).
- "Coping with Frustration"—Cognitive behavioral intervention for the treatment of anger and frustration related to caregiving. Components include relaxation training, techniques for challenging dysfunctional thoughts, and assertion training Gallagher-Thompson, & De Vries, 1994; Steffen, 2000).
- Training and intervention package for increasing caregivers' ability to manage behavior problems of the person receiving care and for improving problem solving skills (Burgio, Stevens, Guy, Roth, & Haley (in press).

What are Effective Self-Help Treatments?

Several self-help books and websites include information that is relevant for understanding the effects of dementia on the behavior of the patient and the experience of caregiving. There has been no empirical evaluation of these self-help books or websites as sole treatment interventions.

Alzheimer's Association. http://www.alz.org
Bell, V. & Troxel, D. (2002). *A dignified life: The best friends approach to Alzheimer's care, a guide for family caregivers.* Deerfield Beach, FL: Health Communications.

MEDline Plus.Alzheimer's disease. http://www.nlm.nih.gov/medlineplus/alzheimersdisease.html
National Institute on Aging (2005). *Alzheimer's Disease Education & Referral Center (ADEAR).* http://www.alzheimers.org/causes.htm
Werner, M. L. (2004). *The complete guide to Alzheimer's-proofing your home.* Lafayette, IN: Purdue University Press.

REFERENCES BY TOPIC, ALPHABETICALLY

ACETYLCHOLINESTERASE INHIBITORS

AD 2000 Collaborative Group. (2004). Long-term donepezil treatment in 565 patients with Alzheimer's disease (AD 2000): randomised double-blind trial. *Lancet, 363,* 2105–2115.
Cummings, J. L. (2004). Alzheimer's disease. *New England Journal of Medicine, 351,* 56–67.
Jones, R. W. (2003). Have cholinergic therapies reached their clinical boundary in Alzheimer's disease. *International Journal of Geriatric Psychiatry, 18,* S7–S13.
Kaduzkiewicz, H., Beck-Bornholdt, H. P., van den Bussche, H., & Zimmermann, T. (2004). Fragliche Evidenz fuer den Einsatz des Cholinesterasehemmers Donepezil bei Alzheimer-

Demenz—eine systematische Uebersichtsarbeit. *Fortschritte der Neurologischen Psychiatrie, 72*(10), 557–563.

Schneider, L. S. (2004). AD 2000: Donepezil in Alzheimer's disease. *Lancet, 363,* 2100–2101.

Zhang, L., Zhou, F., & Dani, J. A. (2004). Cholinergic drugs for Alzheimer's disease enhance in vitro dopamine release. *Molecular Pharmacology, 66*(3), 538–544.

ADVERSE MEDICATION EFFECTS

Gray, S. L., Lai, K. V., & Larson, E. B. (1999). Drug-induced cognition disorders in the elderly. *Drug Safety, 21*(2), 101–122.

Howard, R. L., Avery, A. J., Howard, P. D., & Partridge, M. (2003). Investigation into the reasons for preventable drug related admissions to a medical admission unit: observational study. *Quality and Safety in Health Care, 12,* 280–285.

Katzung, B. G. (2001). Special aspects of geriatric pharmacology. In B. G. Katzung (Ed.), *Basic and clinical pharmacology.* New York: McGraw-Hill.

Lieberman, J. A. (2004a). Metabolic changes associated with antipsychotic use. *Primary Care Companion to the Journal of Clinical Psychiatry, 6*(2), 8–13.

Lieberman, J. A. (2004b). Managing anticholinergic side effects. *Primary Care Companion to the Journal of Clinical Psychiatry, 6*(2), 20–23.

Kaufer, D. I. (2004). Pharmacologic treatment expectations in the management of dementia with Lewy bodies. *Dementia and Geriatric Cognitive Disorders, 17*(Suppl. 1), 32–39.

McDonald, A. J. D. (1998). Delirium. In R. Tallis & H. Fillit & J. C. Brocklehurst (Eds.), *Brocklehurst's textbook of geriatric medicine and gerontology* (5th ed., pp. 685–699). New York: Churchill Livingstone.

Pijnenburg, Y. A. L., Sampson, E. L., Harvey, R. J., Fox, N. C., & Rossor, M. N. (2003). Vulnerability to neuroleptic side effects in frontotemporal lobar degeneration. *International Journal of Geriatric Psychiatry, 18,* 67–72.

Rozzini, L., Ghianda, D., Trabucchi, M., & Padovani, A. (2004). Severe worsening of parkinsonism in Lewy body dementia due to donepezil. *Neurology, 63,* 1543–1544.

Saltz, B. L., Robinson, D. G., & Woerner, M. G. (2004). Recognizing and managing antipsychotic drug treatment side effects in the elderly. *Primary Care Companion to the Journal of Clinical Psychiatry, 6*(2), 14–19.

Stewart, N., & Fairweather, S. (2002). Delirium: The physician's perspective. In R. Jacoby & C. Oppenheimer (Eds.), *Psychiatry in the elderly* (3rd ed., pp. 592–615). Oxford, UK: Oxford University Press.

BEHAVIOR MANAGEMENT

Alexopoulos G. S., Abrams R. C., Young R. C., Shamoian C. A. (1988). Cornell Scale for Depression in Dementia. *Biological Psychiatry, 23*(3):271–84.

Buchanan, J. A., & Fisher, J. E. (2002). Noncontingent reinforcement as an intervention for disruptive vocalizations in Alzheimer's disease patients. *Journal of Applied Behavior Analysis, 35,* 99–103.

Burgio, L. D., Scilly, K., Hardin, J. M., Jankosky, J., Bonino, P., Slater, et al. (1994). Studying disruptive vocalization and contextual factors in the nursing home using computer-assisted real-time observation. *Journal of Gerontology: Psychological Sciences, 49,* P230–P235.

Burgio, L. D. & Stevens, A. B. (1999). Behavioral interventions and motivational systems in the nursing home. In R. Schultz, G. Maddox, & M. P. Lawton (Eds.), *Annual Review of Gerontology and Geriatrics* (pp. 284–320). New York: Springer.

Burgio, L., Stevens, A., Guy, D., Roth, D. L., & Haley, W. E. (in press). Impact of two psychosocial interventions on White and African American family caregivers of individuals with dementia. *The Gerontologist.*

Cohen-Mansfield J., Billig, N. (1986). Agitated behavior in the elderly: A conceptual review. *Journal of the American Geriatrics Society, 34,* 711–721.

Dawson, P., Wells, D. L., & Kline, K. (1993). *Enhancing the abilities of persons with Alzheimer's and related dementias: A nursing perspective.* New York: Springer Publishing Company.

Fisher, J. E., Harsin, C. M., & Hadden, J. E. (2000). Behavioral interventions for dementia patients in long term care facilities. *Professional Psychology in Long Term Care.* New York: Harleigh Co.

Fisher, J. E. (in press). Promoting adaptive behavior in elderly persons with dementia. *Clinical Gerontologist.*

Forsell, Y. & Wingblad, B. (1998). Major depression if a population of demented and non-demented older people: Prevalence and correlates. *Journal of the American Geriatrics Society, 46,* 27–30.

Hussian, R. A. (1981). *Geriatric psychology: A behavioral perspective.* New York: Van Nostrand Reinhold.

Hussian, R. A. & Davis, R. L. (1985). *Responsive care: Behavioral interventions with elderly people.* Champaign, IL: Research Press.

Lerman, D. C., & Iwata, B. A. (1993). Descriptive and experimental analyses of variables maintaining self-injurious behavior. *Journal of Applied Behavior Analysis, 26,* 293–319.

Nolan, B., Mathews, R. M., Truesdell-Todd, G., & Van Dorp, A. (2002). Evaluation of the effect of orientation cues on wayfinding in persons with dementia. *Alzheimer's Care Quarterly, 3*(1), 46–49.

Omnibus Reconciliation Act of Nursing Home Reform (OBRA) of 1987. P.L. 100–203.

Ritchie, K., Touchon, J., & Ledesert, B. (1998). Progressive disability in senile dementia is accelerated in the presence of depression. *International Journal of Geriatric Psychiatry, 13,* 459–461.

Sloane, P. & Barrick, A. (1998). Management of occasional and frequent problem behaviors in dementia: bathing and disruptive vocalizations. In M. Kaplan & S. Hoffman (Eds.), *Behaviors in dementia: best practices for successful management* (pp. 227–238). Baltimore, MD: Health Professions Press, Inc.

Teri, L., et al. (1999). Treatment of behavioral and mood disturbances in dementia. *Generations,* 50–56.

CAREGIVER ASSESSMENT AND INTERVENTION

Gallagher-Thompson, D. & DeVries, H. (1994). "Coping with Frustration" classes: Development and preliminary outcomes with women who care for relatives with dementia. *The Gerontologist, 34,* 548–552.

Gallagher-Thompson, D., Haley, W. E., Guy, D., Rubert, M., Arguelles, T., Tennstedt, S., et al. (2003). Tailoring psychosocial interventions for ethnically diverse dementia caregivers. *Clinical Psychology: Science and Practice, 10,* 423–438.

Gallagher-Thompson, D., Lovett, S., Rose, J., McKibbin, C., Coon, D., Futterman, A., & Thompson, L. W. (2000). Impact of psychoeducational interventions on distressed family caregivers. *Journal of Clinical Geropsychology, 6,* 91–110.

Pinquart, M., & Sorenson, S. (2003). Differences between caregivers and noncaregivers in psychological health and physical health: A meta-analysis. *Psychology and Aging, 18*(2), 250–267.

Schulz, R., Newsom, J. T., Mittelmark, M., Burton, L., Hirsch, C., & Jackson, S. (1997). Health effects of caregiving: The Caregiver Health Effects Study: An ancillary study of the Cardiovascular Health Study. *Annals of Behavioral Medicine, 19,* 110–116.

Schulz, R., O'Brien, A. T., Bookwala, J., & Fleissner, K. (1995). Psychiatric and physical morbidity effects of dementia caregiving: Prevalence, correlates, and causes. *Gerontologist, 36*(6), 771–791.

Steffen, A. M. (2000). Anger management for dementia caregivers: A preliminary study using video and telephone interventions. *Behavior Therapy, 31,* 281–299.

Steffen, A. M. (in press). Reducing psychosocial distress in family caregivers: The Case for behavioral and cognitive interventions. *Clinical Gerontology.*

Teri L., Truax P., Logsdon R., Uomoto J., Zarit S., Vitaliano, P. P. (1992). Assessment of behavioral problems in dementia: The revised memory and behavior problems checklist. *Psychology of Aging, 7,* 622–631.

DIFFERENTIAL DIAGNOSIS OF DEMENTIA

NIH Consensus Statement Online (1987). *Differential Diagnosis of Dementing Diseases.* Jul [cited 11/13/2004]; 6(11):1–27. *http://consensus.nih.gov/cons/063/063_statement.htm*

EMPIRICALLY BASED STRATEGIES FOR SINGLE-CASE CLINICAL ASSESSMENT

Collins, S. H., Ehrhardt, K., & Poling, A. (2000). Clinical drug assessment. In A. Poling & T. Byrne (Eds.), *Behavioral pharmacology* (pp. 191–218). Reno, NV: Context Press.

Kalachnik, J. E., Leventhal, B. L., James, D. H., Sovner, R., Kastner, T. A., Walsh, K. (1998). Guidelines for the use of psychotropic medications. In S. Reiss & M. Aman (Eds.), *Psychotropic medications and the developmental disabilities: The international consensus handbook* (pp. 45–72). Columbus, OH: Ohio State University, Nisonger Center for Developmental Disabilities.

Epidemiology of dementia

Centers for Disease Control and Prevention (1999). Mortality from Alzheimer's Disease: An update. *National Vital Statistics Reports, 47*(20).

Evans DA, Funkenstein H. H., Albert M. S., Scherr P. A., Cook N. R., Chown M. J., Hebert L. E., Hennekens C. H., Taylor J. O. (1989). Prevalence of Alzheimer's disease in a community population of older persons: Higher than previously reported," *Journal of the American Medical Association 262*, 2551.

MEMANTINE

Möbius, H. J. (2003). Memantine: update on the current evidence. *International Journal of Geriatric Psychiatry, 18*, S47–S54.

Sonkusare, S. K., Kaul, C. L., & Ramarao, P. (2005). Dementia of Alzheimer's disease and other neurodegenerative disorders—memantine, a new hope. *Pharmacological Research, 51*, 1–17.

Schmitt, B., Bernhardt, T., Moeller, H.-J., Heuser, I., & Frölich, L. (2004). Combination therapy in Alzheimer's disease: A review of the current evidence. *CNS Drugs, 18*(13), 827–844.

Schmitt-Feuerbach, B. (11/04/2002). Eine neue Karriere fuer den bewaehrten Wirkstoff Memantine. Aerzte Zeitung Online. (Retrieved on 11/14/04). *http://www.aerztezeitung.de/docs/ 2002/11/04/ 198a1401.asp?cat=/medizin/alzheimer*

Pharmacological behavioral management

Lawlor. (2004). Behavioral and psychological symptoms in dementia: The role of atypical antipsychotics. *Journal of Clinical Psychiatry, 65*(11), S5–S10.

Poling, A., & Byrne, T. (2000). Principles of pharmacology. In A. Poling & T. Byrne (Eds.), *Behavioral pharmacology* (pp. 43–63). Reno, NV: Context Press.

Profenno, L. A., & Tariot, P. N. (2004). Pharmacologic management of agitation in Alzheimer's disease. *Dementia and Geriatric Cognitive Disorders, 17*, 65–77.

Wood, P. (2002). Psychopharmacology in the elderly. In R. Jacoby & C. Oppenheimer (Eds.), *Psychiatry in the elderly* (3rd ed., pp. 286–314). Oxford, UK: Oxford University Press.

Dependent Personality Disorder

Kendra Beitz • Robert F. Bornstein

WHAT IS DEPENDENT PERSONALITY DISORDER?

Dependent personality disorder (DPD) is a personality disorder wherein the individual exhibits longstanding, inflexible, excessive dependency, which leads to difficulties in social, sexual, and occupational functioning. According to the DSM-IV-TR, the essential feature of DPD is a pervasive and excessive need to be taken care of that leads to submissive and clinging behavior and fears of separation, beginning by early adulthood and present in a variety of contexts (American Psychiatric Association, 2000). In addition to the essential feature, individuals with DPD have difficulties making everyday decisions without an excessive amount of advice and reassurance from others. They exhibit passivity and rely on others to assume responsibility for most major areas of life, such as living arrangements, career choices, and social relationships. Similarly, they have difficulties initiating projects or doing things on their own because they lack confidence in their judgment or abilities. Individuals with DPD have difficulties expressing disagreement because of a fear of loss of support or approval. Because of their perceived inability to function alone they will go to excessive lengths to obtain nurturance and support from others, to the point of volunteering to do things that are unpleasant. This includes submitting to demands that are unreasonable and tolerating various forms of abuse. In general, individuals with DPD have exaggerated fears about being unable to care for themselves and are unrealistically preoccupied with being alone. Therefore, they feel uncomfortable or helpless when alone and urgently seek another relationship as a source of care and support upon the dissolution of a close relationship (American Psychiatric Association, 2000).

Clinicians and clinical researchers conceptualize DPD in terms of four related components:

- *Cognitive.* A perception of oneself as powerless and ineffectual, coupled with the belief that other people are comparatively powerful and potent.
- *Motivational.* A desire to obtain and maintain relationships with protectors and caregivers.
- *Behavioral.* A pattern of relationship-facilitating behavior designed to strengthen interpersonal ties and minimize the possibility of abandonment and rejection.
- *Emotional.* Fear of abandonment, fear of rejection, and anxiety regarding evaluation by figures of authority.

These four core features lead to a pattern of self-defeating interpersonal functioning characterized by insecurity, low self-esteem, jealousy, clinginess, help-seeking, frequent requests for reassurance, and intolerance of separation (Pincus & Gurtman, 1995; Overholser, 1996). Although different patients express underlying dependency strivings in different ways, it is important to note that some expressions of dependency can involve behavior that is active and assertive—even quite aggressive (Bornstein, 1995). Thus, the clinician must take care not to equate dependency

Beitz, K., & Bornstein, R. F. (2006). Dependent personality disorder. In J. E. Fisher & W. T. O'Donohue (Eds.), *Practitioner's guide to evidence-based psychotherapy*. New York: Springer.

with passivity, and recognize that DPD can be characterized by a variety of active relationship-facilitating behaviors.

BASIC FACTS ABOUT DPD

Comorbidity. Comorbidity studies in inpatients, outpatients, and community samples suggest that DPD is in fact associated with a broader range of Axis I and Axis II syndromes than the DSM-IV-TR acknowledges. On Axis I, DPD is comorbid with mood disorders, anxiety disorders, eating disorders, adjustment disorder, and somatization disorder. On Axis II, DPD co-occurs with the majority of other PDs, including some (e.g., antisocial and schizoid) that bear little resemblance to DPD (Bornstein, 2005). These Axis II comorbidity patterns likely reflect the generalized, nonspecific nature of personality pathology, and the fact that patients who show PD symptoms in one category often show PD symptoms from an array of other categories as well.

Prevalence. According to a recent survey of 43,093 Americans, 0.49% of adults meet diagnostic criteria for DPD (National Epidemiologic Survey on Alcohol and Related Conditions (NESARC; Grant et al., 2004).

Age at onset. Like other personality disorders, DPD traits emerge in childhood or early adulthood, however individuals with DPD may not come to clinical attention until later in life (American Psychiatric Association, 2000). Results from the NESARC study suggest that 18- to 29-year-olds have a significantly higher risk of having DPD (Grant et al., 2004).

Gender. The prevalence of DPD in women is 0.6% and 0.4% in men (Grant et al., 2004). Thus, women are somewhat more likely than men to receive a DPD diagnosis.

Course. No studies have documented the pathways through which genetics alter DPD risk, but it is likely that inherited infantile temperament differences (e.g., high reactivity and low soothability) are involved. Overprotective and authoritarian parenting, alone or in combination, foster problematic dependency in offspring (Bornstein, 1992). In terms of gender role socialization, high levels of femininity and low levels of masculinity are associated with increased likelihood of a DPD diagnosis. These patterns hold for both men and women, although causal links between gender role and DPD risk have not been established (Bornstein, 1992). Children or adolescents who suffer from chronic physical illness or Separation Anxiety Disorder may be at greater risk to developing DPD (American Psychiatric Association, 2000).

Similar to other personality disorders, DPD is pervasive and persistent. Symptoms are not limited to particular developmental stages or Axis I or III disorders, however, and can be exacerbated by important losses (American Psychiatric Association, 2000).

Impairment and other demographic characteristics. DPD is associated with impairment in occupational functioning if independent initiative is required (American Psychiatric Association, 2000). Interpersonal problems are common in individuals with DPD. These individuals tend to feel inferior to others and are introverted, shy, self-critical, and socially anxious, which interferes with effective social functioning (Overholser, 1996). They are at increased risk for depression if they lack the requisite social skills needed to develop and maintain interpersonal relationships (Bornstein, 1993). In general, individuals with DPD may be at increased risk for mood, anxiety, and adjustment disorders.

Results from the NESARC study found no differences in risk of DPD among the race–ethic groups of the population (Grant et al., 2004). However, studies of trait dependency suggest that dependency levels may be somewhat lower in African

American than Caucasian adults in the United States (Bornstein, 1997). It also appears that the risk of DPD is higher for lower income, less educated, widowed, divorced, separated, or never married individuals (Grant et al., 2004).

ASSESSMENT

What Should be Ruled Out?

The DSM-IV-TR alerts clinicians to the fact that DPD must be distinguished from several Axis I and Axis II syndromes that often create an overlapping symptom picture and similar surface presentation. Differential diagnoses on Axis I include mood disorders, panic disorder, agoraphobia, and dependency arising from one or more general medical conditions. Differential diagnoses on Axis II include borderline, histrionic, and avoidant personality disorders.

Loss of an important relationship can temporarily increase dependency as the individual adjusts to loss (Overholser, 1990, 1992). Clinicians should be careful to distinguish an adjustment reaction from true DPD, which is associated with persistent dependency needs in the absence of a particular trigger (Overholser, 1996). In assigning a DPD diagnosis, it is important that the clinician ascertain that the patient's dependency does in fact cause difficulties in social, sexual, or occupational functioning. Research shows that many persons with relatively intense dependency needs actually function quite well (Bornstein & Languirand, 2003). Thus, intensity alone is insufficient to assign a DPD diagnosis, but when dependency is both *intense* and *maladaptive*, diagnosis may be warranted. Additionally, DPD should only be diagnosed when dependent behaviors (e.g., deferential treatment, passivity, or politeness) are in excess of the individual's cultural norms (American Psychiatric Association, 2000). To diagnose DPD, or any personality disorder, in an individual under 18, the features must be present for at least one year (American Psychiatric Association, 2000).

What is Involved in Effective Assessment?

In diagnosing DPD clinicians should be guided by three principles: (1) dependency is not always characterized by passivity. Dependent patients use a variety of self-presentation strategies to curry favor with others and preclude abandonment; some of these strategies (e.g., intimidation and breakdown threats) are quite active. (2) Self-reports do not always give a true picture. Because dependency is typically seen as a sign of weakness and immaturity, many adults—especially men—are reluctant to acknowledge dependent thoughts and feelings even if they experience them. Obtaining concurrent information from knowledgeable informants can be helpful in this regard. (3) Dependency levels vary over time and across situations. Increases in depression are associated with temporary increases in self-reported dependency, and even modest mood changes may have some impact on dependency levels.

When formal assessment is warranted the clinician should evaluate DSM-IV-TR diagnostic criteria and administer a validated instrument for quantifying DPD symptoms. Construct validity data for widely used DPD assessment tools are provided by Birtchnell (1991) and Bornstein (1999). Most of these instruments fall into one of two categories: clinician-administered and self-report measures.

Clinician-administered measures. The major advantage of diagnosing DPD via interview is the opportunity to follow up and obtain additional detail; the main disadvantage is the modest interdiagnostician reliability frequently obtained when Axis II disorders (including DPD) are diagnosed via interview. In recent years three interviews have been used most often to quantify DPD symptoms and diagnoses:

(1) the Structured Clinical Interview for DSM Personality Disorders (SCID-II; First, Gibbon, Spitzer, Williams, & Benjamin, 1997), (2) the International Personality Disorder Examination (IPDE; Loranger et al., 1994), and (3) the Structured Interview for DSM-IV Personality (SIDP-IV; Pfohl, Blum, & Zimmerman).

Self-report measures. Although paper-and-pencil measures do not allow the diagnostician to probe and follow up, they are relatively inexpensive and efficient, and they circumvent interdiagnostician reliability problems that characterize structured interviews. Two self-report instruments that have been used most frequently to diagnose DPD in recent years are the Millon Clinical Muliaxial Inventory-III (MCMI-III; Millon, 1994) and the Personality Diagnostic Questionnaire-4+ (PDQ-4+; Hyler, 1994a,b).

The Dependent Personality Questionnaire (DPQ) has recently been developed as a brief screening measure for DPD (Tyrer, Morgan, & Cicchetti, 2004). A strength of the DPQ is that it consists of eight items and requires 5–10 minutes for patients to complete. An initial study demonstrated that the DPQ predicts the diagnosis of DPD with predicted positive and negative accuracies of 87% (Tyrer et al., 2004). Given the recent development of this measure, further psychometric evaluation using larger samples is needed.

Behavioral assessment. Although behavioral observation may provide information about the range of dependent behaviors manifest in various situations in vivo, there are several limitations to this method. Direct observation can be difficult to perform, is limited to certain settings, and only provides information about overt behavior (Bornstein, 1993). Although observation systems have been developed to assess dependent behaviors in children, there are no specific direct observation systems for DPD.

What Assessments are Not Helpful?

There are no biological tests for DPD. The Rorschach Oral Dependency scale (ROD; Masling, Rabie, & Blondheim, 1967) and the Interpersonal Dependency Inventory (IDI; Hirschfeld et al., 1977) are good measures of trait dependency, but are not as useful for assessing DPD (Bornstein, 1994; Bornstein, 1999; Loas, Verrier, Gayant, & Guelfi, 1998).

TREATMENT

Recommendations for treatment of problematic dependency have been offered by cognitive (Overholser & Fine, 1994), psychodynamic (Coen, 1992), behavioral (Turkat, 1990) and experiential (Schneider & May, 1995) clinicians. A detailed review of these treatment strategies is provided by Bornstein (2005).

What Treatments are Effective?

There is no specific treatment for DPD that has consistently shown to be effective in well-designed studies. DPD is often studied in the context of other Axis I disorders, such as mood and anxiety disorders. Investigations typically evaluate the efficacy of empirically supported treatments for an Axis I condition with co-occurring DPD.

What are Effective Self-Help Treatments?

Currently there are no empirically supported self-help treatments for DPD. However, there are a number of websites that provide information about DPD and related resources:

- http://mentalhelp.net/poc/ view_doc.php?type=doc&id=477&cn=8 (Mental Help Net)
- http://www.nmha.org/ infoctr/factsheets/91.cfm (National Mental Health Association)
- http://www.mental health.com/rx/p23-pe09.html (Internet Mental Health)

What are Effective Therapist-Based Treatments?

Given the extensive clinical literature surrounding treatment of dependent patients, it is surprising that no studies have examined the impact of psychotherapy on DPD symptoms in psychiatric inpatients. Two clinical trials have assessed the effectiveness of psychotherapy in ameliorating DPD symptoms in outpatients, but these investigations produced contrasting results. Rathus, Sanderson, Miller, & Wetzler (1995) used cognitive-behavioral techniques to treat 18 DPD-diagnosed agoraphobic outpatients, finding a significant decrease in dependency levels during the 12-week course of therapy. Black, Monahan, Wesner, Gabel, & Bowers (1996) used cognitive intervention techniques to treat 44 DPD-diagnosed outpatients with cooccurring panic disorder, finding no change in dependency levels over 8 weeks of therapy.

What is Effective Medical Treatment?

Like studies of psychotherapy, clinical trials assessing the impact of pharmacological treatments on DPD symptoms have not produced promising findings. A broad range of medication classes have been assessed in these investigations (e.g., antidepressants, anxiolytics, and antipsychotics), and none have consistently fared better than placebo in reducing DPD symptoms. A review of these investigations is provided by Bornstein (2005).

Combination Treatments

Given the modest impact of traditional psychotherapeutic and pharmacological treatment regimens and the complex, multifaceted nature of dependency, the future of clinical work with DPD patients may lie in multimodal treatment. Intervention strategies aimed at altering multiple components of DPD—cognitive, motivational, behavioral, and emotional—will likely have stronger and more durable effects than intervention strategies aimed at altering a single dimension of functioning.

Other Issues in Management

In contrast to psychotherapy and pharmacotherapy outcome studies, studies examining the effect of DPD on treatment process and outcome have yielded consistent results, suggesting that in general, high levels of trait dependency and DPD are associated with a more positive treatment outcome when other disorders are the focus of treatment (e.g., depression and anxiety). Once engaged in treatment, DPD patients adhere more conscientiously than nondependent patients to psychotherapeutic and pharmacological treatment regimens, miss fewer therapy sessions than nondependent patients, and show higher rates of treatment completion in outpatient individual and group therapy (Bornstein, 1993).

Given the dynamics of DPD and the impact of dependency on psychotherapeutic process, several considerations are important in clinical management of DPD. Key guidelines include:

- *Set firm limits on after-hours contact early in treatment.* Unless firm limits are set at the outset of therapy, dependent patients tend to have a higher-than-average number of "pseudo-emergencies," and make frequent requests for between-session contact.

- *Gradually give the patient more responsibility for structuring treatment as therapy progresses.* By providing considerable structure early on and gradually requiring the patient to take increasing responsibility for structuring treatment, the therapist can help the patient experience autonomy within the therapeutic milieu.
- *Be aware of the potential for exploitation.* Many therapists infantilize dependent patients, and exploitation or abuse—usually financial or sexual—may follow. It is critical that the clinician acknowledges and confronts these problematic feelings, either in formal clinical supervision or in informal consultation with other mental health professionals.
- *Be alert for signs of patient deterioration or self-destructive behavior.* Dependent patients are at increased risk for perpetration of child and spouse abuse (Bornstein, 1993), and may be at increased risk for suicide as well (Bornstein & O'Neill, 2000); thus, the therapist must monitor continuously for negative indicators.
- *Work with the system, not just the person.* Because dependent people often construct interpersonal milieus that foster and propagate their dependency, concurrent marital and/or family therapy may be warranted to alter entrenched dysfunctional system patterns.

Although clinical work with dependent patients has traditionally focused on diminishing problematic dependency, recent research suggests that when dependency strivings are expressed in a flexible, modulated manner they can actually strengthen interpersonal ties and facilitate adaptation and healthy psychological functioning. Treatment of DPD should emphasize replacing unhealthy, maladaptive dependency with flexible, adaptive dependency.

How Does One Select Among Treatments

Given the lack of empirically supported treatments for DPD alone, the clinician should assess and provide empirically supported interventions for comorbid Axis I and II disorders when appropriate. Clinicians can follow our recommendations and recommendations made by other clinicians for treating DPD symptoms (e.g., Coen, 1992; Overholser & Fine, 1994; Schneider & May, 1995; Turkat, 1990). However, prior to beginning treatment the clinician should inform the patient about the empirical support, or lack thereof, for the intervention(s) they will be providing. If pharmacotherapy for a comorbid psychiatric disorder is indicated, side effects and possible contraindications should be considered and discussed with the patient. Given the nature of DPD, clinicians should evaluate their own strengths and liabilities and their willingness to treat this population. Because patients with DPD may be at increased risk for self-destructive behavior, ongoing risk assessment and management of that risk is necessary. By virtue of the diagnostic symptom presentation of DPD, these patients may at times be more taxing than other types of patients. Therefore, some clinicians may feel overwhelmed and easily burned out. Clinicians who do not feel able to effectively treat DPD should refer these patients elsewhere. Finally, it is important for clinicians to consider compliance issues when selecting among interventions. DPD patients may be hesitant to disagree with treatment recommendations, even if they are averse to engaging treatment or an aspect of treatment.

KEY READINGS

Abramson, P. R., Cloud, M. Y., Keese, N., & Keese, R. (1994). How much is too much? Dependency in a psychotherapeutic relationship. *American Journal of Psychotherapy, 48*, 294–301.

Baltes, M. M. (1996). *The many faces of dependency in old age.* Cambridge, UK: Cambridge University Press.

Bornstein, R. F. (1992). The dependent personality: Developmental, social, and clinical perspectives. *Psychological Bulletin, 112,* 3–23.

Head, S. B., Baker, J. D., & Williamson, D. A. (1991). Family environment characteristics and dependent personality disorder. *Journal of Personality Disorders, 5,* 256–263.

Livesley, W. K., & Jang, K. L. (2000). Toward an empirically based classification of personality disorder. *Journal of Personality Disorders, 14,* 137–151.

Millon, T. (1996). *Disorders of personality: DSM-IV and beyond.* New York: Wiley.

Nietzel, M. T., & Harris, M. J. (1990). Relationship of dependency and achievement/autonomy to depression. *Clinical Psychology Review, 10,* 279–297.

Pincus, A. L., & Wilson, K. R. (2001). Interpersonal variability in dependent personality. *Journal of Personality, 69,* 223–251.

Ryder, R. D., & Parry-Jones, W. L. (1982). Fear of dependence and its value in working with adolescents. *Journal of Adolescence, 5,* 71–81.

Tait, M. (1997). Dependence: A means or an impediment to growth? *British Journal of Guidance and Counselling, 25,* 17–26.

REFERENCES

American Psychiatric Association (2000). *Diagnostic and statistical manual of mental disorders, 4th edition, text revision.* Washington, DC: American Psychiatric Association.

Birtchnell, J. (1991). The measurement of dependence by questionnaire. *Journal of Personality Disorders, 5,* 281–295.

Black, D. W., Monahan, P., Wesner, R., Gabel, J., & Bowers, W. (1996). The effect of fluvoxamine, cognitive therapy, and placebo on abnormal personality traits in 44 patients with panic disorder. *Journal of Personality Disorders, 10,* 185–194.

Bornstein, R. F. (1992). The dependent personality: Developmental, social, and clinical perspectives. *Psychological Bulletin, 112, 1,* 3–23.

Bornstein, R. F. (1993). *The dependent personality.* New York: Guilford Press.

Bornstein, R. F. (1994). Construct validity of the Interpersonal Dependency Inventory: 1977–1992. *Journal of Personality Disorders, 8,* 65–77.

Bornstein, R. F. (1995). Active dependency. *Journal of Nervous and mental Disease, 183,* 64–77.

Bornstein, R. F. (1997). Dependent personality disorder in the DSM-IV and beyond. *Clinical Psychology: Science and Practice, 4,* 175–187.

Bornstein, R. F. (1999). Criterion validity of objective and projective dependency tests: A meta-analytic assessment of behavioral prediction. *Psychological Assessment, 11,* 48–57.

Bornstein, R. F. (2001). A meta-analysis of the dependency-eating disorders relationship: Strength, specificity, and temporal stability. *Journal of Psychopathology and Behavioral Assessment, 23,* 151–162.

Bornstein, R. F. (2005). *The dependent patient: A practitioner's guide.* Washington, DC: American Psychological Association.

Bornstein, R. F., & Languirand, M. A. (2003). *Healthy dependency.* New York: Newmarket Press.

Bornstein, R. F., & O'Neill, R. M. (2000). Dependency and suicidality in psychiatric inpatients. *Journal of Clinical Psychology, 56, 4,* 463–474.

Coen, S. J. (1992). *The misuse of persons: Analyzing pathological dependency.* Hillsdale, NJ: Analytic Press.

First, M. B., Gibbon, M., Spitzer, R., Williams, J. B. W, & Benjamin, L. S. (1997). *User's guide for the Structured Clinical Interview for the DSM-IV Axis II personality disorders.* Washington, DC: American Psychiatric Association.

Grant, B. F., Hasin, D. S., & Stinson, F. S. (2004). Prevalence, correlates, and disability of personality disorders in the United States: Results from the National Epidemiologic Survey on Alcohol and Related Conditions. *Journal of Clinical Psychiatry, 65,* 948–958.

Hirschfeld, R. M., Klerman, L., Gough, H. G., Barrett, J., Korchin, S. J., Chodoff, P. (1977). A measure of interpersonal dependency. *Journal of Personality Assessment, 41, 6,* 610–618.

Hyler, S. E. (1994a). The Personality Diagnostic Questionnaire 4+. New York, NY: New York State Psychiatric Institute.

Hyler, S. E. (1994b). *PDQ-4 and PDQ-4+ instructions for use.* New York, NY: New York State Psychiatric Institute.

Loas, G., Verrier, A., Gayant, C., & Guelfi, J. D. (1998). Depression and dependency: Distinct or overlapping constructs? *Journal of Affective Disorders, 47,* 81–85.

Loranger, A. W., Sartorius, N., Andreoli, A., Berger, P., Buchheim, P., Channabasavanna, et al. (1994). The International Personality Disorder Examination. *Archives of General Psychiatry, 51,* 215–224.

Masling, J. M., Rabie, L., & Blondheim, S. H. (1967). Obesity, level of aspiration, and the Rorschach and TAT measures of oral dependency. *Journal of Consulting Psychology, 31,* 233–239.

Millon, R. (1994). *Millon Clinical Multiaxial Inventory-III: Manual and scoring booklet.* Minneapolis, MN: National Computer Systems.

Overholser J. C. (1990). Emotional reliance and social loss: Effects on depressive symptomatology. *Journal of Personality Assessment, 55,* 618–629.

Overholser J. C. (1992). Interpersonal dependency and social loss. *Personality and Individual Differences, 13,* 17–23.

Overholser, J. C. (1996). The dependent personality and interpersonal problems. *Journal of Nervous and Mental Disease, 184,* 8–16.

Overholser, J. C., & Fine, M. A. (1994). Cognitive-behavioral treatment of excessive interpersonal dependency: A four-stage psychotherapy model. *Journal of Cognitive Psychotherapy, 8,* 55–70.

Pincus, A. L., & Gurtman, M. B. (1995). The three faces of interpersonal dependency: Structural analysis of self-report dependency measures. *Journal of Personality and Social Psychology, 69,* 744–758.

Pfohl, B. M., Blum, N., & Zimmerman, M. (1995). *Structured Interview for DSM-IV Personality: SIDP-IV.* Iowa City, IA: University of Iowa.

Rathus, J. H., Sanderson, W. C., Miller, A. L., & Wetzler, S. (1995). Impact of personality functioning on cognitive behavioral treatment of panic disorder: A preliminary report. *Journal of Personality Disorders, 9,* 160–168.

Schneider, K. J., & May, R. (1995). *The psychology of existence: An integrative, clinical perspective.* New York: McGraw-Hill.

Turkat, I. D. (1990). *The personality disorders: A psychological approach to clinical management.* New York: Pergamon Press.

Tyrer, P., Morgan, J., & Cicchetti, D. (2004). The Dependent Personality Questionnaire (DPQ): A screening instrument for dependent personality.

Depression

Keith S. Dobson • Martin C. Scherrer • Lauren C. Haubert

WHAT IS DEPRESSION?

Clinical depression is a disorder with various presentations and consequences. The term "depression" can be used to refer to sad mood, but clinical depression consists of a syndrome of at least five symptoms that have lasted for at least 2 weeks. These symptoms must represent a change from previous functioning, and must include at least one of the first two symptoms listed below (American Psychiatric Association, 2000):

1. Depressed or irritated mood
2. Diminished interest or pleasure in all or almost all activities
3. Significant weight loss or weight gain, or decrease or increase in appetite
4. Insomnia or hypersomnia
5. Psychomotor agitation or retardation
6. Fatigue or loss of energy
7. Feelings of worthlessness or excessive or inappropriate guilt
8. Diminished ability to think or concentrate, or indecisiveness
9. Recurrent thoughts of death, suicidal impulses or actions

The syndrome of depression, which is technically referred to as a Major Depressive Episode on its first occurrence, and Major Depressive Disorder if it recurs, can take many forms. Some persons only have five symptoms for a relatively brief period, but others may experience most of the above symptoms for years. Thus, the diagnosis of Major Depression is important, but also is the appreciation of its severity and duration.

BASIC FACTS ABOUT DEPRESSION

Comorbidity. Depression exhibits high rates of comorbidity with other Axis I and Axis II disorders. Some of these potentially comorbid conditions include dysthymia, cyclothymia, anxiety disorders, personality disorders (e.g., borderline, dependent, histrionic), eating disorders, as well as various medical conditions (e.g., hypothyroidism, myocardial infarct, and stroke), substance abuse, grief reactions, and adjustment disorders (see Stefanis & Stefanis, 1999).

Prevalence. Major depression is among the most common of all mental disorders, with an estimated annual incidence of 12.9% for women in the United States, a rate that was 1.7 times that for males (Kessler, Mcgonoale, Swartz, Blazer, & Nelson, 1993). Recent estimates indicate that nearly 20% of the US population will experience a clinically significant episode of depression during their lives. There is some suggestion that the global burden of illness is increasing in recent years, and that it may be as much as 50% more by the year 2050 than at present (Üstun, 2001).

Age at onset. The first onset of major depression typically occurs in mid- to late adolescence (Hammen, 2001), although a first episode of depression can occur at any point in the life span. It used to be argued that young children could not

Dobson, K. S., Scherrer, M. C., & Haubert, L. C. (2006). Depression. In J. Fisher & W. T. O'Donohue (Eds.), *Practitioner's guide to evidence-based psychotherapy.* New York: Springer.

experience clinical depression, but this viewpoint has given way to one that indicates that it is possible, although the symptom pattern may be somewhat different than for adults.

Gender. Beginning in early to middle adolescence and throughout adulthood, females are consistently twice as likely as males to develop depression (Garber & Flynn, 2001). Numerous explanations have been proposed to account for gender differences, including artifactual variables (e.g., reporting biases, differences in symptom presentation), hormonal differences, gender roles, differences in socialization, and differences in coping styles.

Course. In the absence of treatment, Major Depression typically lasts between four months and one year (American Psychiatric Association, 2000). Although some treatments have demonstrated effectiveness in treating depression (e.g., Chambless & Ollendick, 2001) it is increasingly recognized that Major Depression tends to be a chronic, recurrent disorder characterized by high relapse rates (Hammen, 2001; Kessler, et al., 1993). More severe and more enduring or recurrent patterns of Major Depression are likely more difficult to effectively treat than less severe or chronic forms.

Impairment and other demographic variables. Many individuals with depression experience significant levels of cognitive, behavioural, emotional, and physiological impairment that affects many areas of their daily functioning. For instance, many individuals experience disruption in occupational functioning (e.g., lost productivity) and school performance and difficulties in interpersonal relationships (e.g., with spouses and children).

WHAT SHOULD BE RULED OUT?

In order to make a formal diagnosis of Major Depression, the pattern of symptoms must not be attributable to either the direct effects of a substance (e.g. alcohol, CNS depressants) or a medical disorder (e.g. hypothyroidism). The diagnosis of Major Depression should not be made unless the symptoms last longer than two months following bereavement. Some other disorders share features of clinical depression (e.g., bipolar disorder, schizoaffective disorder), may present similarly to depression, and should be considered in the process of differential diagnosis.

WHAT IS INVOLVED IN EFFECTIVE ASSESSMENT?

By using several different types of measures (i.e., interviews, clinician ratings, and self-report inventories), clinicians can increase the reliability and validity of their assessment findings (Kellner, 1994). Ideally, information should also be gathered from several perspectives including the client, significant others (e.g., family members, employer), and the clinician or researcher, to yield the most valid and comprehensive picture of the client possible. Since severity plays a role in treatment planning and the monitoring of treatment outcome, it should be evaluated by either clinical interview or rating scales. The possibility of other psychiatric and medical conditions should also be addressed, since the assessment of associated and comorbid conditions may have implications for diagnosis and treatment planning. Consideration of the client's family, social, and occupational history is also advised, both for determining the degree of impairment resulting from the depression and for selecting targets for intervention and strategies for generalizing treatment change (Dozois & Dobson, 2002).

The decision to use specific procedures, inventories, methods, and questionnaires rests on several issues including the goals of the assessment, the amount of time one has to conduct an evaluation, and the nature of the population that is being assessed. Because so many assessment approaches and tools exist and each client's presentation and situation is unique, no definitive or universal assessment strategy exists. Effective decision-making is needed in the assessment of depression, related to the goals of assessment (Nezu, Nezu, & Foster, 2000). There are, however, guidelines that may be applied across clients and problem areas to assist in the formulation of an appropriate assessment plan (see Nezu, Nezu, McClure, & Zwick, 2002, and Nezu et al., 2000 for descriptions of a step-by-step decision making process).

Assessment instruments may be classified in a variety of different ways. For example, one broad distinction is between diagnostic and symptom severity measures, while another distinction exists among assessment tools that gather information through self-report or clinician ratings (Dozois & Dobson, 2002). A range of assessment techniques is presented here, with examples of several of the instruments that are extensively used by clinicians and researchers that have sound psychometric properties. The interested reader is referred to Nezu, Ronan, Meadows, and McClure (2000) for a review of over 90 depression-related measures.

Structured Diagnostic Interviews

The clinical interview is often viewed as the most effective method of detecting Major Depression in that it elicits the symptoms and the longitudinal course of the disorder. Examples of semistructured clinical interviews that have demonstrated strong reliability and validity include the Structured Clinical Interview for DSM-IV Axis I Disorders (SCID-I; First, Spitzer, Gibbons, & Williams, 1997), the Schedule for Affective Disorders and Schizophrenia (SADS; Endicott & Spitzer, 1978), and the Diagnostic Interview Schedule-IV (DIS-IV; Robins, Helzer, Croughan, & Ratcliff, 1981).

Benefits of the semistructured interview include its standardized format, which improves the reliability of longitudinal assessment and serves as a method of comparing information gathered by the clinical interview to normative data. In addition, the clinician may also choose to inquire further about inconsistent responses or supplement any missing information from other methods. The main disadvantages of the interview method is that they are time-intensive to administer, require extensive training, do not cover areas relevant to the formulation of a treatment plan (e.g., motivation for change, social support), and may lead to less rapport between the interviewer and the client.

Clinician-Rated Measures

Although clinician ratings may include questions that are similar to those on self-report measures, they are typically completed by the clinician following a clinical interview. Examples of widely used clinician-rated measures include the Hamilton Rating Scale for Depression (HRSD; Hamilton, 1960, 1967) and the Brief Psychiatric Rating Scale (BPRS; Overall & Gorman, 1962). These measures provide an index of symptom severity and overall impairment, and may also be used to identify problem areas to address in treatment, or symptom change during and following treatment. These clinician-completed rating scales may be more sensitive to improvement in the course of treatment and many have slightly greater specificity than do self-reports in detecting depression. Clinician ratings are likely to produce more reliable results than self-report inventories, but they do require more clinician time than other assessment techniques, and often require special training in the interviews that can accompany such procedures (Nezu et al., 2002).

Self-Report Measures

The self-report method of assessment involves obtaining an individual's answers to specific questions in the form of a questionnaire or inventory, typically using either a paper-and-pencil format or computer. Examples of self-report inventories include the Beck Depression Inventory-II (BDI-II; Beck, Steer, & Brown, 1996), Zung Self-Rating Depression Scale (ZSDS; Zung, 1965), Carroll Depression Scales-Revised (CDS-R; Carroll, 1998), and the Center for Epidemiological Studies Depression Scale (CES-D; Radloff, 1977).

Benefits of this assessment method include the fact that it may be completed by the client outside of the treatment session, may be relatively brief, and may be used as a form of periodic self-monitoring. Self-reports also have low cost relative to other assessment methods. Although client responses on these measures cannot be used to directly formulate a diagnosis of depression, a high score on one of these instruments may warrant a clinical interview for the purpose of diagnosis. A widely noted disadvantage of self-report methods is their vulnerability to response biases and misinterpretation. In addition, self-reports may not be appropriate for individuals who have difficulty with reality testing, have a thought disorder (e.g., schizophrenia), or have such severe depressive symptoms that their ability to concentrate is compromised (Dozois & Dobson, 2002). Under these circumstances, a clinician-rating measure may prove a more successful strategy.

Collateral Areas of Assessment

The measurement of related constructs may be helpful in the identification of potential mediators of depressive symptoms or other related phenomena (e.g., suicidal ideation). For example, it may be useful to assess interpersonal processes, social support, coping strategies, and life events (Dozois & Dobson, 2002), as these data can be beneficial for case conceptualization, formulating goals for therapy, identifying factors that contribute to the onset or maintenance of depression, or understanding problems that increase the risk of relapse or recurrence (Nezu et al., 2000). Some widely used instruments designed to assess these areas include the Beck Hopelessness Scale (BHS; Beck & Steer, 1988); the Dysfunctional Attitudes Scale (DAS; Weissman & Beck, 1978) and the Automatic Thoughts Questionnaires—Negative (ASQ-N; Hollon & Kendall, 1980).

The potential for suicide and a review of other areas of psychopathology, such as alcohol and/or substance abuse history, should also be considered during assessment. Psychometric instruments such as the BHS may be beneficial for detecting suicide risk; however, clinicians must also be cognizant of other potential risk factors (e.g., hopelessness, impulsivity, substance abuse, physical illness), resilience factors (e.g. social support, family, or moral considerations), and more immediate suicide indicators (e.g., specific plan, intent, and lethality of means). When there is evidence to suggest a medical disorder as a factor in the depression, physical examination, and laboratory tests to detect the specific disorders should be employed in the process of making a differential diagnosis (Agency for Health Care Policy and Research; AHCPR, 1993a). A number of laboratory tests, such as the sleep electroencephalogram or thyrotropin-releasing hormone stimulation test, may help to identify biological abnormalities characteristic of depression.

WHAT ASSESSMENTS ARE NOT HELPFUL?

Assessment for depression is likely the most practical and efficient when it focuses fairly specifically on the disorder, or related constructs. Omnibus or multidimensional tests of psychopathology, such as the Minnesota Multiphasic Personality Inventory-II, are not efficient for this purpose. Further, projective tests of personality, while appropriate for some forms of assessment, are not recommended for the assessment of depression, per se. Finally, it is important to note that no definitive medical or laboratory test for depression exists, and while medical assessment can help to evaluate the physiological aspects of specific symptoms, it cannot lead to a diagnosis or severity rating of Major Depression.

WHAT TREATMENTS ARE EFFECTIVE?

Significant advances have been made in the field of psychotherapy with the recent identification and advancement of empirically supported treatments (ESTs) and such advances have informed the treatment of depression in particular (Chambless et al., 1998; Chambless & Ollendick, 2001). Cognitive behavioral therapy (CBT), behavior therapy (BT), and interpersonal therapy (IPT) each have a sufficient database to warrant being considered empirically supported, while other therapies have also been identified as probably having efficacy and warranting further investigation, including: brief dynamic therapy, self-control therapy, and social problem solving therapy, as well as behavioral marital therapy for individuals with marital discord. The evidence also supports the use of cognitive therapy and reminiscence therapy in treating geriatric depression. This section reviews the major treatments identified above.

WHAT ARE EFFECTIVE THERAPIST BASED TREATMENTS?

Cognitive-Behavioral Therapy (CBT)

The dominant cognitive paradigm for depression has been the model originally proposed by Aaron T. Beck in the late 1960s (Dozois & Dobson, 2001). Cognitive therapy for depression attributes a central role to negatively biased information processing and dysfunctional beliefs in maintaining depression (Butler & Beck, 2001). Consequently, therapy aims to change the individual's maladaptive thinking which, in turn, is expected to be associated with improved affect, motivation, and behavior (Butler & Beck, 2001).

Cognitive therapy is delivered in a structured format and involves such elements as structured learning experiences, thought monitoring, instruction in adaptive coping skills, and Socratic questioning of maladaptive cognitions. A full course of treatment typically involves 14–16 sessions, and may include occasional booster sessions thereafter (see for example Clark, Beck, & Alford, 1999; Beck, 1995, for recent discussions of cognitive theory and therapy). Evidence supports the efficacy of CBT in treating depression (e.g., Gloaguen, Cottraux, Cucherat, & Blackburn, 1998), and outcome studies suggest that CBT is at least as effective as pharmacotherapy and may be more effective than pharmacotherapy alone in preventing relapse of the disorder (Butler & Beck, 2001). Finally, a recent development in the field of cognitive therapy that has garnered increasing attention is that of mindfulness-based cognitive therapy (MBCT), which incorporates the principles of mindfulness into the traditional CBT framework, in an attempt to prevent relapse (see, for example, Segal, Williams, & Teasdale, 2002).

Behavior Therapy (BT)

Predicated on the behavioral model of depression, which postulates a central role for decreased response contingent positive reinforcement in depressive symptomatology, BT aims to increase the frequency and quality of pleasant activities, which in turn is expected to improve mood (Hopko, Lejuez, Ruggiero, & Eifert, 2003). One structured treatment program based on this theoretical perspective is the Coping With Depression (CWD) Course. The CWD course typically takes the format of a psychoeducational group, consisting of 12 sessions over 8 weeks, and focuses on skills training, such as improving social skills, increasing pleasant activities, and relaxation training. Evidence suggests that the CWD course is at least as effective in the short term and perhaps more so in the long term than antidepressant medication in treating depression (Craighead & Craighead, 2003).

Interpersonal Therapy (IPT)

Interpersonal therapy (IPT) for depression was developed by Klerman, Weissman and colleagues in the early 1980s (Klerman & Weissman, 1986). IPT is based largely on the interpersonal school of psychiatry, which views depression as being caused, exacerbated, and/ or maintained by interpersonal difficulties (AHCPR, 1993b). Consequently, IPT centers on resolving one or more of a number of possible interpersonal difficulties, including delayed/incomplete grief, role transitions, role disputes, or interpersonal deficit.

IPT is delivered in a structured format and progresses through three phases (Weissman, Markowitz, & Klerman, 2000): (1) diagnosis, identification of the major interpersonal problem areas, and explanation of the approach; (2) resolution of the selected problem area(s); and (3) termination. IPT has been modified for use with a range of depressed populations, including adolescents and the elderly, and with other disorders as well. Finally, IPT has demonstrated efficacy as both an acute and maintenance therapy for major depression (Weissman et al., 2000).

WHAT ARE EFFECTIVE MEDICAL AND BIOLOGICAL TREATMENTS?

Pharmacotherapy

There are several classes of medication used in the treatment of depression, including the tricyclic antidepressants (TCAs), monoamine oxidase inhibitors (MAOIs), and the newer selective serotonin reuptake inhibitors (SSRIs; NIMH, 2004). Newer medications such as the SSRIs typically have fewer side effects than older classes such as the TCAs and are more specific in their action on neurotransmitters such as dopamine; however, all antidepressant medication are associated with side effects to varying degrees. Often, a variety of antidepressants and particular dosages are required in order to ascertain that which is most effective for a particular individual. Generally, medication must be taken for 3–4 weeks before its full therapeutic effect to begin.

Antidepressant medication is particularly indicated moderate to severe in cases of depression that involve psychotic, melancholic, or atypical features, and also in the event that psychotherapy delivered by a competent psychotherapist is not available (AHCPR, 1993b). Given the similar rate of efficacy across antidepressant medications and the fact that not all individuals respond to any one particular medication, a range of factors should be considered in medication selection including short- and long-term side effects, potential lethality of medication overdose, and prior response to the medication (AHCPR, 1993b). Individual response to a particular medication and dosage is continually monitored and adjusted as needed, and psychotherapy may be offered in conjunction with medication (AHCPR, 1993b). Medication may be continued following symptom remission in cases of recurrent depression in order to reduce the probability of recurrence, generally for a period of 4–9 months, and may typically be discontinued thereafter (AHCPR, 1993b).

Electroconvulsive Therapy (ECT)

ECT involves the controlled administration of electrical impulses to the brain (NIMH, 2002). Brief anesthesia and muscle relaxants are employed prior to the delivery of the electrical impulse, which causes a seizure within the brain lasting approximately 30 seconds. Typically, a series of treatments is required. The AHCPR Clinical Practice Guideline for the treatment of depression (1993) advises that ECT be used as a first-line treatment option only in cases that involve more severe or psychotic forms of depression that require rapid response, or else cases that have not responded to prior interventions. The AHCPR Guideline notes that very few clients require ECT and that this intervention can involve significant side effects (e.g., short-term retrograde and anterograde amnesia), yet there is considerable evidence for its efficacy, particularly in managing severe and/or psychotic depression. It is recommended, however, that ECT be employed in conjunction with other interventions, such as antidepressant medication.

Herbal Therapy

Roughly 30% of North Americans use complementary or alternative medicine, and recent years have witnessed increasing interest in the use of herbs in the treatment of depression (Brown & Gerberg, 2001). Some commonly used herbal supplements, such as ephedra, gingko biloba, Echinacea, and ginseng, have yet to be evaluated in large-scale clinical trials (NIMH, 2002). Others, including St. John's Wort (hypericum perforatum) and S-adenosyl-methionine (SAM-e), have received considerable research attention to date.

Early reports related to St. John's Wort (SJW) claimed efficacy rates comparable to, or exceeding those of, tricyclic antidepressants (TCAs), but with few associated side effects. More recent reviews have suggested that while SJW is similar to low-dose TCAs in efficacy when used to treat mild to moderate major depression, it may not be as efficacious in the treatment of moderate to severe forms of the disorder (Brown & Gerberg, 2001; NIMH, 2002). While its active components have yet to be identified, SJW exhibits a side effect profile and mechanism of action similar to the SSRI sertraline, and may be effective in as many as 50–70% of cases of mild depression (Brown & Gerberg, 2001).

SAM-e is a naturally occurring compound that is most concentrated in the liver and brain, and which increases levels of the neurotransmitters serotonin, dopamine, and norepinephrine by acting on a central metabolic pathway (Brown & Gerberg, 2001). Prior to its introduction to the US in the late 1980s, SAM-e was widely used in Europe for depression and a considerable body of evidence attests to its efficacy. In higher doses, SAM-e may be as effective as tricyclic antidepressants but with a faster onset of action and fewer side-effects (Brown & Gerberg, 2001). Such evidence is encouraging and both SJW and SAM-e may represent viable approaches, employed alone or in combination with traditional pharmacotherapy or psychotherapy, in the treatment of depression.

COMBINATION TREATMENTS

Most of the efficacy trials in the area of depression to date have been with single treatments, either alone or in comparison to each other. Specific trials that have combined medications and psychotherapy, do not typically find a statistically significant effect. Recent evidence from a combination of studies, however, (Pampallona, Bollini, Tibalbi, Kupelnick, & Munizza 2004), implies that the combination of psychotherapy and medications does increase the overall efficacy of treatment in comparison to medication alone.

WHAT ARE EFFECTIVE SELF-HELP TREATMENTS?

A number of self-help books are available that incorporate many of the elements of cognitive-behavioral treatment strategies that have been shown to be helpful in the treatment of depression. Self-help books include:

- Burns, D. D. (1999). *The feeling good handbook.* New York, NY: Plume.
- Copeland, M. E. (2001). *The depression workbook: A guide for living with depression and manic depression (2nd ed.).* Oakland, CA: New Harbinger Publications.
- Copeland, M. E., & Copans, S. (2002). *Recovering from depression: A workbook for teens.* Baltimore, MD: Paul H. Brookes Publishing.
- DePaulo, J. R., Jr., & Horvitz, L. A. (2002). *Understanding depression: What we know and what you can do about it.* New York, NY: John Wiley & Sons.
- Greenberger, D., & Padesky, C. A. (1995). *Mind over mood: Change how you feel by changing the way you think.* New York, NY: Guilford.
- McQuaid, J. R., & Carmona, P. E. (2004). *Peaceful mind: Using mindfulness and cognitive behavioral psychology to overcome depression.* New Harbinger Publications.
- Wright, J. H., & Basco, M. R. (2001). *Getting your life back: the complete guide to recovery from depression.* New York, NY: Free Press.

USEFUL WEBSITES

Useful informational websites about depression and related resources include:
- http://www.ahcpr. gov/clinic/deprsumm.htm (Agency for Health Care Policy and Research)
- http://www.apa.org/topics/topic_depress.html (American Psychological Association)
- http://www.ndmda.org (National Depressive and Manic-Depressive Association)
- http://www.depression.org/ (National Foundation for Depressive Illness)
- http://www.nimh.nih.gov/healthinformation/depressionmenu.cfm (National Institute of Mental Health)
- http://www.nmha. org/ccd/index.cfm (National Mental Health Association)
- http://www.obad.ca/depressioninfo.htm (Organization for Bipolar and Affective Disorders Society)

OTHER ISSUES IN MANAGEMENT

A significant factor in the clinical management of depression relates to the increased risk of hopelessness and suicide that accompany depression. Although it is certainly not true that all depressed persons have suicidal impulses, the increased risk of such concerns means that clinicians working in this area need to know how to assess, and effectively intervene, if suicidal risk dictates such response.

HOW DOES ONE SELECT AMONG TREATMENTS?

At present, there is no accepted algorithm for determining which treatment for depression ought to be considered a primary or secondary treatment, with the exception of electroconvulsive therapy, which is typically not considered as a first treatment option. Therapist training often plays a role in which treatment is offered, although patient preference should more typically be considered, given the roughly equal efficacy among treatments. Open communication with patients about the risks and benefits of treatment options represents good clinical care.

SUMMARY

Depression is a common and debilitating condition. In part due to these facts, it is fortunate that a number of viable alternative treatments have been developed that have demonstrated clinical efficacy. Careful assessment of Major Depression is always warranted in clinical practice, because of the possibility of medical and other conditions that simulate depression, and because of the common frequency of comorbid conditions. Treatment planning typically involves a therapist-delivered treatment, and several psychological, biological, and alternative health options exist for providing treatment. Unfortunately, because of these alternative treatment options, it is difficult to specify which treatment is best for any given person with depression. Often, treatment is related more to the availability of therapy, or in some cases personal preference, than any formulation of the person's problems, or which treatment(s) might best match those problems. Considerable research is needed to both develop and evaluate treatment guidelines for depression, although this work is beginning (cf. Beutler, Clarkin & Bongar, 2000).

REFERENCES

Agency for Health Care Policy and Research. (1993a). *Depression in primary care: Volume 1. Detection and diagnosis.* Rockville, MD: US Department of Health and Human Services.

Agency for Health Care Policy and Research. (1993b). *Depression in primary care: Volume 2. Treatment of major depression.* Rockville, MD: US Department of Health and Human Services.

American Psychiatric Association. (2000). *Diagnostic and Statistical Manual for Mental Disorders-Text Revision.* Washington, DC: American Psychiatric Association Press.

Beck, A. T., & Steer, R. A. (1988). *Beck Hopelessness Scale.* San Antonio, TX: Psychological Corporation.

Beck, A. T., Steer, R. A., & Brown, G. K. (1996). *Beck Depression Inventory Manual* (2nd ed.), San Antonio, TX: Psychological Corporation.

Beck, J. S. (1995). *Cognitive therapy: Basics and beyond.* New York: Guilford.

Beutler, L. E., Clarkin, J. F., & Bongar, B. (2000). *Guidelines for the systematic treatment of the depressed patient.* New York, NY: Oxford University Press.

Butler, A. C., & Beck, J. S. (2001) Cognitive therapy outcomes. A review of meta-analyses. *Tidsskrift for Norsk Psykologforening. 38,* 698–706.

Brown, R. P., & Gerbarg, P. L. (2001). Herbs and nutrients in the treatment of depression, anxiety, insomnia, migraine, and obesity. *Journal of Psychiatric Practice, 7,* 75–91.

Carroll, B. J. (1998). *Carroll Depression Scales-Revised (CDS-R): Technical manual.* Toronto: Multi-Health Systems, Inc.

Chambless, D. L., Baker, M. J., Baucom, D., et al. (1998). *Update on empirically validated therapies, II.* Retrieved August 11, 2004, from *http://pantheon.yale.edu/~tat22/est_docs/ValidatedTx.pdf*

Chambless, D. L., & Ollendick, T. H. (2001). Empirically supported psychological interventions: controversies and evidence. *Annual Review of Psychology, 52,* 685–716.

Clark, D. A., Beck, A. T., & Alford, B. A. (1999). *Scientific foundations of cognitive theory and therapy of depression.* Toronto: John Wiley & Sons.

Craighead, W. E., & Craighead, L. W. (2003). Behavioral and cognitive-behavioral psychotherapy. G. Stricker & T. Widiger, (Eds.) *Handbook of psychology: Clinical psychology,* (Vol. 8. pp. 279–299). New York, NY: John Wiley & Sons, Inc.

Dozois, D. J. A., & Dobson, K. S. (2002). Depression. In M. M. Antony & D. H. Barlow (Eds.), *Handbook of Assessment and Treatment Planning for Psychological Disorders* (pp. 259–299). New York: Guilford Press.

Dozois, D. J. A., & Dobson, K. S. (2001). Information processing and cognitive organization in unipolar depression: Specificity and comorbidity issues. *Journal of Abnormal Psychology, 110,* 236–246.

Endicott, J., & Spitzer, R. L. (1978). A diagnostic interview: The Schedule for Affective Disorders and Schizophrenia. *Archives of General Psychiatry, 35,* 837–844.

First, M. B., Spitzer, R. L., Gibbon, M., & Williams, J. B. W. (1997). *Structured Clinical Interview for DSM-IV Axis I Disorders–Clinician Version (SCID-CV).* Washington, DC: American Psychiatric Association Press.

Garber, J., & Flynn, C. (2001). Vulnerability to depression in childhood and adolescence. In R. E. Ingram & J. M. Price (Eds.), *Vulnerability to psychopathology: Risk across the lifespan* (pp. 175–225). New York: Guilford.

Gloaguen, V., Cottraux, J., Cucherat, M., & Blackburn, I. (1996). A meta-analysis of the effects of cognitive therapy in depressed patients. *Journal of Affective Disorders, 49,* 59–72.

Hamilton, M. (1960). A rating scale for depression. *Journal of Neurology, Neurosurgery and Psychiatry, 23,* 56–62.

Hamilton, M. (1967). Development of a rating scale for primary depressive illness. *British Journal of Social and Clinical Psychology, 6,* 278–296.

Hammen, C. (2001). Vulnerability to depression in adulthood. *Vulnerability to psychopathology: Risk across the lifespan* (pp. 175–225). New York: Guilford.

Hollon, S. D. & Kendall, P. C. (1980). Cognitive self-statements in depression: Development of an Automatic Thoughts Questionnaire. *Cognitive Therapy and Research, 4,* 383–395.

Hopko, D. R., Lejuez, C. W, Ruggiero, K. J., & Eifert, G. H. (2003). Contemporary behavioral activation treatments for depression: Procedures, principles and progress. *Clinical Psychology Review. 23,* 699–717.

Kellner, R. (1994). The measurement of depression and anxiety. In J. A. den Boer & J. M. Ad Sitsen (Eds.), *Handbook of depression and anxiety: A biological approach* (pp. 133–158). New York: Marcel Dekker.

Kessler, R. C., Mcgonaole, K. A., Swartz, M., Blazer, D. G., & Nelson, C. B. (1993). Sex and depression in the national comorbidity survey I: Lifetime prevalence, chronicity and recurrence. *Journal of Affective Disorders, 29,* 85–96.

Klerman, G. L., Weissman, M. M. (1986). The interpersonal approach to understanding depression. In T. E. Millon & G. L. Klerman (Eds) *Contemporary directions in psychopathology: Toward the DSM-IV.* (pp. 429–456). New York: Guilford Press.

National Institute of Mental Health. *Depression.* Bethesda (MD): National Institute of Mental Health, National Institutes of Health, US Department of Health and Human Services; 2002 [cited 2004 May 15]. (NIH Publication Number: 02-3561). 23p. Available from: http://www.nimh. nih.gov/publicat/index.cfm.

Nezu, A. M., Nezu, C. M., McClure, K. S., & Zwick, M. L. (2002). In I. H. Gotlib & C. L. Hammen (Eds), *Handbook of depression* (pp. 61–85). New York: Guilford Press.

Nezu, A. M., Ronan, G. F., Meadows, E. A., & McClure, K. S. (2000). *AABT Clinical assessment series: Practitioner's guide to empirically based measures of depression.* New York: Kluwer/Plenum.

Nezu, C. M., Nezu, A. M., & Foster, S. L. (2000). In A. M. Nezu, G. F. Ronan, E. A. Meadows, & K. S. McClure (Eds.), *Clinical assessment series: Vol. 1. Practitioner's guide to empirically-based measures of depression* (pp. 17–24). New York: Kluwer/Plenum.

Overall, J. E., & Gorman, D. R. (1962). *The Brief Psychiatric Rating Scale.* Psychological Reports, 10, 799–812.

Pampallona, S., Bollini, P., Tibalbi, G., Kupelnick, B., & Munizza, C. (2004). Combined pharmacotherapy and psychological treatment for depression: A systematic review. *Archives of General Psychiatry, 61,* 714–719.

Radloff, L. S. (1977). The CES-D Scale: A self-report depression scale for research in the general population. *Applied Psychological Measurement, 1,* 385–401.

Robins, L. N., Helzer, J. E., Croughan, J. L., & Ratcliff, K. S. (1981). National Institute of Mental Health Diagnostic Interview Schedule: Its history, characteristics, and validity. *Archives of General Psychiatry, 38,* 381–389.

Segal, Z. V., Williams, J. M. G., & Teasdale, J. D. (2002). *Mindfulness-based cognitive therapy for depression: A new approach to preventing relapse.* New York: Guilford.

Stefanis, C. N., & Stefanis, N. C. (1999). Diagnosis of depressive disorders: A review. In M. Maj & N. Sartorius (Eds.), *Depressive disorders* (pp. 1–51). New York: Wiley.

Üstun, T. B. (2001). The worldwide burden of depression in the 21st century. In M. M. Weissman (Ed.), *Treatment of depression: Bridging the 21st century.* Washington, DC: American Psychiatric Press, Inc. (pp. 35–46).

Weissman, A. N. & Beck, A. T. (1978). *Development and validation of the Dysfunctional Attitude Scale: A preliminary investigation.* Paper presented at the annual meeting of the Association for Advancement of Behavior Therapy, Chicago.

Weissman, M. M., Bland, R. C., Canino, G. J., et al. (1996). Cross-national epidemiology of major depression and bipolar disorder. *Journal of the American Medical Association, 276,* 293–299.

Weissman, M. M., Markowitz, J. C., & Klerman, G. L. (2000). *Comprehensive guide to interpersonal psychotherapy.* New York: Basic Books.

Zung, W. W. K. (1965). A self-rating depression scale. *Archives of General Psychology, 12,* 63–70.

CHAPTER 24

Dissociation and Dissociative Identity Disorder: Treatment Guidelines and Cautions

Steven Jay Lynn • Oliver Fassler • Joshua A. Knox • Scott O. Lilienfeld

WHAT IS DISSOCIATIVE IDENTITY DISORDER?

Interest in dissociation and dissociative disorders has waxed and waned from the time of Janet's (1889) landmark writings to contemporary attempts to understand dissociative phenomena in light of competing explanatory models and increasingly sophisticated experimental methods. From the eclipse of dissociation theory by early psychoanalytic theory, to the attack on dissociation by experimentalists later in the century (Rosenberg, 1959; White & Shevach, 1942), to the explosion of reports of cases of "multiple personality disorder" in the 1980's, to the ensuing skepticism regarding these reports in the 1990s and early 21st century, the study of dissociation has been permeated with conflict and controversy. Today, the most incapacitating and perplexing dissociative disorder—dissociative identity disorder (DID)—is among the most controversial of all psychiatric diagnoses. Accordingly, it is difficult for clinicians to chart a course through the welter of conflicting information on the topic and treat patients who present with vexing dissociative symptoms. Our goal is to provide a brief guide to scientifically based knowledge concerning DID by highlighting the tentative state of knowledge about this condition and the need for practitioners to appreciate the manifold sociocultural influences on the presentation of its symptoms.

According to DSM-IV [American Psychiatric Association (APA), 1994], DID is one of several dissociative disorders, all of which are marked by profound disturbances in memory, identity, consciousness, and/or perception of the external environment that "may be sudden or gradual, transient or chronic" (p. 477). Other dissociative disorders in DSM-IV include depersonalization disorder, dissociative fugue, and dissociative amnesia. According to DSM-IV, DID is characterized by the presence of two or more distinct personalities (i.e., relatively enduring pattern of perceiving, relating to, and thinking about the environment and self) or "personality states" (i.e., temporary patterns of behavior) that recurrently assume control over the individual's behavior. These alternate personalities or "alters" often exhibit psychological features that differ markedly from those of the primary or "host" personality and are identified by different names, ages, and genders. In addition, they can exhibit differences in vocabulary, general knowledge, and affect. In some cases, these features appear to be the opposite of those exhibited by the host personality. For example, if the host personality is shy and retiring, one or more alters may be outgoing or flamboyant. The number of alters has been reported to range from one (the so-called "split" personality) to hundreds or even thousands (Acocella, 1999). In general, women with DID tend to report more alters than men (APA, 1994).

Lynn, S. J., Fassler, O., Knox, J. A., & Lilienfeld, S. O. (2006). Dissociation and dissociative identity disorder: Treatment guidelines and cautions. In J. E. Fisher & W. T. O'Donohue (Eds.), *Practitioner's guide to evidence-based psychotherapy.* New York: Springer.

According to DSM-IV, individuals with DID report significant episodes of amnesia for important personal information that cannot be explained by "normal forgetfulness." For example, they may report frequent periods of "lost time" lasting hours or days in which they cannot recall where they were or what they were doing. This amnesia is often reported to be asymmetrical, whereby the host personality knows little about the behaviors of the alters, but not vice-versa (APA, 1994).

Basic Facts about Dissociative Identity Disorder

Prevalence. Until recently, it was widely assumed that DID was exceedingly uncommon. Although some authors (e.g., Piper, 1997) claim that genuine DID is very rare (see also Rifkin, Ghisalbert, Dimatou, & Sethi, 1998), others (e.g., Ross, 1997) maintain that DID is at least as common (1–2%) as schizophrenia. Recent estimates of the prevalence of DID in inpatient settings range from 1–9.6% (Rifkin, Ghisalbert, Dimatou, Jin, & Sethi, 1998; Ross, Duffy, & Ellason, 2002).

Gender differences. Virtually all prevalence studies reveal a marked female predominance, with most sex ratios ranging from 3 to 1 to 9 to 1 across clinical samples (APA, 1994). This imbalanced sex ratio may be an artifact of selection and referral biases. For example, a large proportion of males with DID may end up in prisons (or other forensic settings) rather than in clinical settings (Putnam & Loewenstein, 2000).

Is dissociation dimensional or taxonic? A longstanding assumption has been that dissociation is a continuous (dimensional) attribute, ranging from nonpathological mental activities such as daydreaming, "highway hypnosis" (the experience of periods of "lost time" while driving long distances), and being absorbed in a book, to more pathological manifestations, such as DID. However, at least some recent evidence suggests that DID is taxonic; that is, categorical in nature. Several studies (Waller, Putnam, & Carlson, 1996; Waller & Ross 1997) using sophisticated statistical procedures have reported that nonpathological dissociation appears to reflect a dissociative trait (Modestin & Erni, 2004), whereas pathological dissociation can best be described as a distinct "type" or latent class (taxon) that can be identified by eight items derived from the Dissociative Experiences Scale (DES; Bernstein & Putnam, 1986). Waller and Ross (1997) estimated that the population base rate of pathological dissociation is 3.3%. Because being classified as a taxon member cannot be equated with DID (Modestin & Erni, 2004), it is likely that the prevalence of DID in the general population is much lower than 3%. Nevertheless, because Watson (2003) found that scores on the hypothesized dissociative taxon are unstable over time, further research will be needed to verify the existence of this taxon.

Malingering. Factitious disorders may account for 2–10% of inpatient dissociative disorders (Friedl & Draijer, 2000). There is widespread agreement that DID can be successfully malingered. For example, Kenneth Bianchi, one of the two Hillside Stranger murderers, is widely believed to have faked DID to escape criminal responsibility (Orne, Dinges, & Orne, 1984). Nevertheless, outside of criminal settings, cases of malingered DID are believed to be rare, and the substantial majority of individuals with this condition do not appear to be intentionally producing their symptoms.

Familial clustering. The results of several controlled studies indicate that DID co-aggregates within biological families (APA, 1994). A recent study (Waller & Ross, 1997) of 280 identical twins and 148 fraternal twins revealed that approximately 45% of the variance on a measure of pathological dissociation was attributable to shared environmental influences, with the remaining variance due to nonshared environmental influences. Adoption studies would help to further clarify the extent to which familial clustering is due to genes, shared environment, or both.

Controversies. The primary controversy surrounding DID is the question of whether DID is a socially constructed and culturally influenced condition rather than a naturally occurring response to early trauma (Merskey, 1992). Proponents of the posttraumatic model (PTM; Gleaves, 1996, Gleaves, May, & Cardena, 2001; Ross, 1997) contend that DID is a posttraumatic condition that arises from a history of severe physical and/or sexual abuse in childhood that engenders the compartmentalization of the personality as a means of coping with intense emotional pain. Advocates of the PTM cite data suggesting that perhaps 90% or more of individuals with DID report a history of severe child abuse (Gleaves, 1996).

In contrast, proponents of the sociocognitive model (SCM; Spanos, 1994, 1996; see also Aldridge-Morris, 1989; Lilienfeld et al., 1999; Lynn & Pintar, 1997; McHugh, 1993; Merskey, 1992; Sarbin, 1995) contend that DID results from inadvertent therapist cueing (e.g., suggestive questioning regarding the existence of possible alters, hypnosis), media influences (e.g., television and film portrayals of DID such as "Sybil"), and broader sociocultural expectations regarding the presumed clinical features of DID. Proponents of the SCM (Lilienfeld et al., 1999; Lilienfeld & Lynn, 2003; Merckelbach & Muris, 2001) further note that significant questions can be raised concerning the child abuse-DID link for the following reasons: (a) Many ostensible confirmations of this association derive from studies that lack objective corroboration of child abuse (e.g. Coons, Bowman, & Milstein, 1988) or are plagued with methodological shortcomings (Coons, 1994; Lewis, Yaeger, Swica, Pincus, & Lewis, 1997). (b) The reported high levels of child abuse among DID patients may be attributable to selection and referral biases common in psychiatric samples (e.g., patients who are abused are more likely to enter treatment). (c) Correlations between abuse and psychopathology tend to decrease substantially or disappear when the person's perception of family pathology is statistically controlled. (d) It has not been established that early abuse plays a causal role in DID. These considerations do not exclude an etiological role for early trauma in DID, but they suggest the need for further controlled research before strong conclusions (e.g., Gleaves, 1996; Gleaves et al., 2001) can be drawn.

Advocates of the SCM cite the following findings (Lilienfeld & Lynn, 2003; Lilienfeld et al., 1999) as consistent with the SCM or as a challenge to the PTM: (1) the number of patients with DID has increased dramatically over the past few decades (Elzinga et al., 1998); (2) the number of alters per DID individual has similarly increased over the past few decades (North, Ryall, Ricci, & Wetzel, 1993), although the number of alters at the time of initial diagnosis appears to have remained constant (Ross, Norton, & Wozney, 1989); (3) both of these increases coincide with dramatically increased therapist and public awareness of the major features of DID (Fahy, 1988); (4) mainstream treatment techniques for DID appear to reinforce patients' displays of multiplicity, reify alters as distinct personalities, and encourage patients to establish contact with presumed latent alters (Spanos, 1994, 1996); (5) many or most DID patients show few or no clear-cut signs of this condition (e.g., alters) prior to psychotherapy (Kluft, 1984); (6) The number of alters per DID individual tends to increase substantially over the course of DID-oriented psychotherapy (Piper, 1997); (7) psychotherapists who use hypnosis tend to have more DID patients in their caseloads than do psychotherapists who do not use hypnosis (Powell & Gee, 1999); (8) the majority of diagnoses of DID derive from a relatively small number of psychotherapists, many of whom are specialists in DID (Mai, 1995); (9) laboratory studies suggest that nonclinical participants who are provided with appropriate cues and prompts can reproduce many of the overt features of DID (Stafford & Lynn, 2002; Spanos, Weekes, & Bertrand, 1985); (10) until fairly recently diagnoses of DID were limited largely to North America, where the condition has received widespread media publicity (Spanos, 1996), although DID is now being diagnosed with considerable frequency in some countries (e.g., Holland) in which it has recently become more widely publicized; and (11) laboratory research does not support the assertion that consciousness can be separated into multiple streams by amnesic barriers to form an independently functioning alter personality (Lynn, Knox, Fassler, Lilienfeld, & Loftus, 2004).

These 11 sources of evidence do not imply that DID can typically be created in vacuo by iatrogenic or sociocultural influences. It seems likely that iatrogenic and sociocultural influences often operate on a backdrop of preexisting psychopathology, and exert their impact primarily on individuals who are seeking a causal explanation for their instability, identity problems, and impulsive and seemingly inexplicable behaviors. Some important aspects of these two models may prove commensurable. For example, early trauma might predispose individuals to develop high levels of fantasy proneness (Lynn, Rhue, & Green, 1988), absorption (Tellegen & Atkinson, 1974), or related personality traits. In turn, such traits may render individuals susceptible to the iatrogenic and cultural influences posited by the SCM, thereby increasing the likelihood that they will develop DID following exposure to suggestive influences. This and even more sophisticated etiological models of DID have yet to be subjected to direct empirical tests.

ASSESSMENT

Who Should be Ruled Out?

Borderline personality disorder. According to DSM-IV, the presence of alters, as well as other features of DID, must not be attributable to either substance (e.g., alcohol) use or a medical condition (e.g., temporal lobe epilepsy). In children, the symptoms must not attributable to imaginary playmates or other fantasy play.

Ellason, Ross, and Fuchs (1992) reported that their sample of DID patients qualified for an average of 8 Axis I disorders and 4.5 Axis II disorders. A substantial proportion of DID patients (i.e., a half to two-thirds; Coons et al., 1988; Horevitz & Braun, 1984) meet criteria for borderline personality disorder (BPD). Kemp, Gilbertson, and Torem (1988) reported no significant differences between BPD and DID patients on measures of personality traits, cognitive and adaptive functioning, and clinician ratings. Histories of sexual and physical abuse are also reported frequently in both patient groups, and BPD patients score well above the norms for the general population on measures of dissociation (Lauer, Black, & Keane, 1993). Lauer et al., (1993) suggested that DID is an epiphenomenon of the combination of BPD and high suggestibility.

Schizoaffective disorder and schizophrenia. Many DID patients meet criteria for schizoaffective disorder (Lauer et al., 1993). The fact that as many as half of DID patients have received a previous diagnosis of schizophrenia (Ross & Norton, 1988) is not surprising given that auditory and visual hallucinations are common in both DID and schizophrenia. DID patients have been reported to endorse even more positive symptoms (e.g., delusions, hallucinations, and suspiciousness) and Schneiderian first rank symptoms, which involve themes of passivity, than schizophrenic patients (Ellason & Ross, 1995; Steinberg, Rounsaville, & Cichetti, 1990). Ellason and Ross (1995) argued that the presence of positive symptoms can be used to formulate an accurate differential diagnosis. Whereas DID patients report that the voices they hear seem to originate inside of their heads, schizophrenic patients tend to perceive the origin of voices outside of their heads and possess less insight regarding the nature of their symptoms (Kluft, 1993).

PTSD. PTSD is one of the most commonly comorbid conditions with DID (Loewenstein, 1991). Moreover, PTSD patients are more likely to present with symptoms of dissociation (e.g., numbing, amnesia, flashback phenomena) than patients with major depression, schizophrenia, and schizoaffective disorder (Bremner, Steinberg, Southwick, & Charney, 1993).

What is Involved in Effective Assessment

General considerations. Given the probable importance of sociocultural influences in the presentation of DID, the practitioner should conduct a thorough assessment of the patient's exposure to information about DID conveyed by movies, books, magazines, the internet, and, often most important, previous therapists. The use of suggestive procedures (e.g., dream interpretation, guided imagery, journaling of incidents of abuse) should be noted as part of an evaluation of the demand characteristics and cues inherent in previous therapies. As with any patient, historical information regarding abuse and neglect should be obtained during the course of routine assessment. However, serious questions have been raised about the veracity of recovered memories of childhood abuse among DID patients. Thus, the credibility of reported memories should be carefully evaluated. In particular, memories that are traumatic, highly implausible, or both (e.g., satanic ritual abuse), should be corroborated if at all possible. Measures of suggestibility (Stanford Scale of Hypnotic Susceptibility; Weitzenhoffer & Hilgard, 1962) and fantasy proneness (ICMI) can also provide valuable information insofar as dissociative individuals tend to score high on measures of hypnotic suggestibility (Covino, Jimerson, Wolfe, Franko, & Frankel, 1994) and fantasy proneness (Rauschenberger & Lynn, 1995). Both attributes predispose individuals to affirmative responses to leading questions and the creation of false memories (Eisen & Lynn, 2001).

Because of the association of DID symptoms with BPD as well as self-defeating and passive-aggressive (negativistic) personality disorders (Ellason, Ross, & Fuchs, 1995), a careful assessment of suicidality is warranted, along with an evaluation of self-mutilative behavior, which has also been linked with dissociation (Vanderhoff & Lynn, 2001).

Administer standardized measures. A comprehensive assessment of dissociative symptoms and experiences should include the administration of one or more widely used measures of dissociation. The Dissociative Experiences Scale (DES; Bernstein & Putnam, 1986) is a 28-item screening measure. Each item is scored from 0 to 100, and although a cutoff score of 30 or above is suggestive of a dissociative disorder (Carlson, Putnam, Ross, & Torem, 1993), the DES should not be used by itself to arrive at a diagnosis. Structured interviews including the Structured Clinical Interview for DSM-IV Dissociative Disorders (SCID-D) (Steinberg, Cicchetti, Buchanan, Hall, & Rounsaville, 1993) and the Dissociative Disorders Interview Schedule (DDIS, Ross, Heber, & Norton, 1989) can be used to formulate a diagnosis. The DDIS permits an evaluation of childhood physical and sexual abuse as well as BPD, somatization disorder, and major depression. Whereas the 131-item DDIS can typically be administered in 40 minutes, the 250-item SCID-D administration time can range from 10 to 180 minutes. However, the SCID-D affords the opportunity to rate patients' interview responses in terms of multiple dissociative symptoms (e. g., amnesia, depersonalization, identity alteration). The Clinician Administered Dissociative States Scale (Bremner et al., 1998), provides both the patient (19 items) and the therapist (8 items) with an opportunity to rate dissociative experiences (i.e., amnesia, depersonalization, and derealization). To avoid an undue emphasis on dissociative symptoms, and to glean valuable information across multiple domains of both abnormal and normal-range personality, we suggest that practitioners administer an omnibus personality measure such as the MMPI-2 or NEO-PI-R.

Conduct a functional analysis. We strongly recommend that practitioners conduct a functional analysis of the variables associated with the perception of the self as fragmented, and with the emergence of so-called alters. Questions for the practitioner to address are: (a) What thoughts, feelings, and actions are associated with the presentation of dissociative symptoms (e.g., amnesia, identity alterations)? (b) What personal and interpersonal variables are associated with the exacerbation, alleviation, and maintenance of dissociative symptoms? (c) What are the consequences and secondary gains associated with thinking of and presenting oneself as a "multiple?"

What Assessments are Not Helpful?

Assessment procedures that even subtly suggest a history of abuse or validate the manifestation of alters with separate histories (e.g., personality "system mapping" to establish contact with non-forthcoming alters, giving names to alters, prompting the emergence of alters) should be avoided. Therapists who repeatedly ask leading questions such as "Is it possible that there is another part of you with whom I haven't yet spoken?" may gradually elicit previously "latent alters" that ostensibly account for their clients' otherwise enigmatic behaviors (e.g., self-mutilation, rapid and intense mood shifts). Hypnosis has been associated with an increased risk of false memories, and should be not be used to recover ostensibly dissociated or repressed experiences. Repeated questioning about historical events is not helpful in that it can lead patients to believe that they have significant gaps (e.g., amnesia) in their autobiographical memories of childhood that they do not have (Belli, Winkielman, Read, Schwartz, & Lynn, 1998).

TREATMENT

What Treatments are Effective?

Individuals with DID are typically in treatment for an average of 6 to 7 years before being diagnosed with this condition (Gleaves, 1996). Such evidence raises the possibility that patients often develop unambiguous features of DID only after receiving unsuccessful psychotherapy. Anecdotal reports suggest that a panoply of treatments, ranging from hypnosis, to psychoanalysis, to family and couples therapy, to videotaped sodium amytal (so-called "truth serum") interviews, to cognitive-behavior therapy can be helpful in the treatment of DID (Caddy, 1985). Nevertheless, there is a dearth of systematic research on the treatment of DID, and controlled outcome studies are not available to inform recommendations regarding efficacious treatments.

What are Effective Self-Help Treatments?

To date, no self-treatment for DID is widely used or empirically supported.

Useful Websites

International Society for the Study of Dissociation: *www. issd.org*
International Society for Traumatic Stress Studies: *www.istss.org*
Society for Clinical and Experimental Hypnosis: *www.sceh.mspp.edu*
False Memory Syndrome Foundation: *www. fmsfonline.org*

What are Effective Therapist-Based Treatments?

As noted earlier, DID patients share many features with BPD patients. Accordingly, many of the tactics (e.g., cognitive-behavioral methods, mindfulness training, relaxation) found to be effective (Linehan,1993) with a borderline clientele would be expected to: (a) promote self-regulation (e.g., behavioral, affective, cognitive) and the acceptance of painful emotions in DID patients, and (b) minimize experiential avoidance, cognitive distortions, and the enactment of different "alters" to cope with conflicting emotions. We further suggest that education is essential to helping patients understand how they react to current stressors "as if" they have multiple personalities (e.g., sociocultural and suggestive influences in therapy, fantasy proneness and role enactment). However, it is imperative to underscore that dissociative and avoidant coping strategies are ineffective in the long term, and no matter how fragmented the personality seems to be, it is impossible for a person to truly possess more than "one personality" (Spiegel, 1993). For patients whose phenomenological experience of being a "multiple" is especially compelling, and who cannot be disabused of the erroneous idea that they harbor multiple personalities, images and metaphors that legitimize the "integration" of conflicting personalities (e.g., streams coming together and becoming a "strong" river) can be utilized. Kirsch and Barton (1988) suggested that when information gathering is rendered problematic by "shifting alters, "the metaphor of a "hidden observer" (i.e., "central switchboard," "executive center") can be used to obtain historical information. However, it is essential that the patient understand the metaphorical nature of this suggestion and not reify another "alter." A single "problem list" that does not confine specific issues and difficulties to discrete alters can be generated to create a viable treatment agenda. Exposure-based therapy, found to be efficacious in the treatment of posttraumatic stress disorder (Lohr, Hooke, Gist, & Tolin, 2003), along with cognitive-behavioral techniques, can be used to help patients cope with the lingering effects of traumatic experiences and dissociative symptoms that interfere with maintaining a present-centered, solution-oriented treatment focus.

What is Effective Medical Treatment?

Controlled outcome studies of the effects of pharmacological agents on DID are lacking. Accordingly, an empirical basis for medication guidelines has not been established. Pharmacological treatments generally focus on specific symptoms of dissociation and comorbid conditions, although different effects of medications have been reported across alters, and adverse effects following the use of neuroleptic medications have been reported (see Maldonaldo, Butler, & Spiegel, 2002).

Other Issues in Management

DID patients pose many of the same management problems as BPD patients. Practitioners should be prepared to set clear boundaries and limits in treatment and respond to suicidal crises, flamboyant displays of symptoms, challenges to the therapeutic alliance (e.g., "crises of trust," distortions of the practitioner's motives), and attempts to persuade the therapist of the "genuine" nature of the multiplicity and reported abuse history (e.g., "I can't work with you if you don't believe I was abused as an infant."). DID patients are likely to provoke strong and conflicting emotional reactions on the part of helpers, and attempts to challenge key aspects of the patient's presentation can be met with resistance.

How Does One Select Among Treatments?

There is no clear empirical basis for selecting among treatments. Nevertheless, we strongly recommend that practitioners avoid treatments that are suggestive in nature (e.g., hypnosis, journaling, guided imagery, dream interpretation), and use empirically supported methods to treat both comorbid conditions (e.g., depression, anxiety, PTSD) and symptoms within and across so-called alters.

REFERENCES

Acocella, Joan. (1999). *Creating hysteria: Women and multiple personality disorder.* San Francisco: Jossey-Bass.

Aldridge-Morris, R. (1989). *Multiple personality: An exercise in deception.* Hillsdale, NJ: Erlbaum.

American Psychiatric Association (1994). *Diagnostic and statistical manual of mental disorders* (4th ed.). Washington, DC: Author.

Belli, R. F., Winkielman, P., Read, J. D., Schwartz, N., & Lynn, S. J. (1998). Recalling more childhood events leads to judgments of poorer memory: Implications for the recovered/false memory debate. *Psychonomic Bulletin & Review, 5,* 318–323.

Bernstein, E. M., & Putnam, F. W. (1986). Development, reliability, and validity of a dissociation scale. *Journal of Nervous and Mental Disease, 174,* 727–735.

Bremner, J. D., Krystal, J. H., Putnam, F. W. Southwick, S. M., Marmar, C., Charney, D. S., & Mazure, C. M. (1998). Measurement of dissociative states with the Clinician Administered Dissociative States Scale (CADSS). *Journal of Traumatic Stress, 11,* 125–136.

Bremner, J. D., Steinberg, M., Southwick, S. M., Johnson, D. R., & Charney, D. S. (1993). Use of the structured clinical interview for DSM-IV dissociative disorders for systematic assessment of dissociative symptoms in posttraumatic stress disorder. *American Journal of Psychiatry, 150,* 1011–1014.

Caddy, G. R. (1985). Cognitive behavior therapy in the treatment of multiple personality. *Behavior Modification, 9,* 267–292.

Carlson, E. B., Putnam, F. W., Ross, C. A., & Torem, M. (1993). Validity of the Dissociative Experiences Scale in screening for multiple personality disorder: A multicenter study. *American Journal of Psychiatry, 150,* 1030–1036.

Coons, P. M. (1994). Confirmation of childhood abuse in child and adolescent cases of multiple personality disorder and dissociative identity disorder not otherwise specified. *Journal of Nervous and Mental Disease, 182,* 461–464.

Coons, P. M., Bowman, E. S., & Milstein, V. (1988). Multiple personality disorder: A clinical investigation of 50 cases. *Journal of Nervous and Mental Disease, 176,* 519–527.

Coons, P. M. (1984). The differential diagnosis of multiple personality disorder: A Comprehensive review Psychiatric Clinics of North America, 7, 51–67.

Covino, N. A., Jimerson, D. C., Wolfe, B. E., Franko, D. L., & Frankel, F. H. (1994). Hypnotizability, dissociation, and bulimia nervosa. *Journal of Abnormal Psychology, 103,* 455–459.

Eisen, M. L., & Lynn, S. J. (2001). Dissociation, memory and suggestibility in adults and children. *Applied Cognitive Psychology, 15,* S49–S73.

Ellason, J. W. & Ross, C. A. (1995) Positive and negative symptoms in dissociative identity disorder and schizophrenia: A comparative analysis. *Journal of Nervous & Mental Disease, 183,* 236–241.

Ellason, J. W., Ross, A., Fuchs, D. L. (1995). Assessment of dissociative identity with the Millon Clinical Multiaxial Inventory-II, Psychological Reports, Vol 76, Issue 3, p895, 11p, 2 charts.

Ellason, J. W., Ross, C. A., & Fuchs, D. L. (1996). Lifetime Axis I and Axis II comorbidity and childhood trauma history in dissociative identity disorder. *Psychiatry: Interpersonal and Biological Processes, 59,* 255–266.

Elzinga, B. M., van Dyck, R., & Spinhoven, P. (1998). Three controversies about dissociative identity disorder. *Clinical Psychology and Psychotherapy, 5,* 13–23.

Fahy, T. A. (1988). The diagnosis of multiple personality disorder: A critical review. *British Journal of Psychiatry, 153,* 597–606.

Friedl, M. C., & Draijer, N. (2000). Dissociative disorders in Dutch psychiatric inpatients. *American Journal of Psychiatry, 157,* 1012–1013.

Gleaves, D. H. (1996). The sociocognitive model of dissociative identity disorder: A reexamination of the evidence. *Psychological Bulletin, 120,* 42–59.

Gleaves, D. H., May, M. C., & Cardena, E. (2001). An examination of the diagnostic validity of dissociative identity disorder. *Clinical Psychology Review, 21,* 577–608.

Hilgard, E. R., Lauer, L. W. (1962). Lack of correlation between the California Psychological Inventory and hypnotic susceptibility. *Journal of Consulting Psychology, 26(4),* 331–335.

Horevitz, R. P. & Braun, B. G. (1984). Are multiple personalities borderline? *Psychiatric Clinics of North America, 7,* 69–87.

Janet, P. (1889). *L'automatisme psychologique.* Paris: Félix Alcan.

Kemp, K., Gilbertson, A. D., & Torem, M. (1988). The differential diagnosis of multiple personality disorder from borderline personality disorder. *Dissociation, 1,* 41–46.

Kirsch, I., & Barton, R. D. (1988). Hypnosis in the treatment of multiple personality: A cognitive-behavioural approach. *British Journal of Experimental & Clinical Hypnosis, 5,* 131–137.

Kluft, R. P. (1984). Treatment of multiple personality disorders: A study of 33 cases. *Psychiatric Clinics of North America, 7,* 9–29.

Kluft, R. P. (1993). Multiple personality disorders. In D. Spiegel (Ed.), *Dissociative disorders: A clinical review* (pp. 14–44). Lutherville, MD: Sidran Press.

Lauer, J., Black, D. W., & Keen, P. (1993). Multiple personality disorder and borderline personality disorder: Distinct entities or variations on a common theme? *Annals of Clinical Psychiatry, 5,* 129–134.

Lewis, D. O., Yeager, C. A., Swica, Y., Pincus, J. H., & Lewis, M. (1997). Objective documentation of child abuse and dissociation in 12 murderers with dissociative identity disorder. *American Journal of Psychiatry, 143,* 1703–1710.

Linehan, M. (1993). *Cognitive-behavioral treatment of borderline personality disorder.* New York: Guilford.

Lilienfeld, S. O. & Lynn, S. J. (2003). Dissociative identity disorder: Multiple personalities, multiple controversies. In S. O. Lilienfeld & S. J. Lynn (Eds.), *Science and pseudoscience in clinical psychology* (pp. 109–142). New York, NY: Guilford Press.

Lilienfeld, S. O., Lynn, S. J., Kirsch, I., Chaves, J. F., Sarbin, T. R., Ganaway, G. K., et al. (1999). Dissociative identity disorder and the sociocognitive model: Recalling the lessons of the past. *Psychological Bulletin, 125,* 507–523.

Loewenstein, R. J. (1991). Psychogenic amnesia and psychogenic fugue: A comprehensive review. In A. Tasman & S. M. Goldfinger (Eds.), *American Psychiatric Press Review of Psychiatry* (Vol. 10, pp. 189–222). Washington, DC: American Psychiatric Press.

Lohr, J. M., Hooke, W., Gist, R., Tolin, D. F. (2003). Novel and controversial treatments for trauma-related stress disorders. In S. O. Lilienfeld & S. J. Lynn (Eds.), *Science and pseudoscience in clinical psychology* (pp. 243–272). New York, NY: Guilford Press.

Lynn, S. J., Knox, J., Fassler, O., Lilienfeld, S. O., & Loftus, E. (2004). Trauma, dissociation, and memory. In J. Rosen (Ed.), *Posttraumatic stress disorder: Issues and controversies* (pp. 163–186). New York: Wiley.

Lynn, S. J., & Pintar, J. (1997). A social narrative model of dissociative identity disorder. *Australian Journal of Clinical and Experimental Hypnosis, 25,* 1–7.

Lynn, S. J., Rhue, J. W., & Green, J. P. (1988). Multiple personality and fantasy proneness: Is there an association or dissociation. *British Journal of Experimental and Clinical Hypnosis, 5,* 138–142.

McHugh, P. R. (1993). Multiple personality disorder. *Harvard Mental Health Newsletter, 10(3),* 4–6.

Mai, F. M. (1995). Psychiatrists attitudes to multiple personality disorder: A questionnaire study. *Canadian Journal of Psychiatry, 40,* 154–157.

Maldonaldo, J. R., Butler, L. D., & Spiegel D. (2002). Treatments for dissociative disorders. In P. E. Nathan & J. M. Gorman (Eds.), *A guide to treatments that work* (2nd ed.) (pp. 463–496). London: Oxford University Press.

Merckelback, H. & Muris, P. (2001). The causal link between self-reported trauma and dissociation: A critical review. *Behavior Research & Therapy, 39,* 245–254.

Merskey, H. (1992). The manufacture of personalities: The production of multiple personality disorder. *British Journal of Psychiatry, 160,* 327–340.

Modestin, J., Loetscher, K., & Erni, T. (2002). Dissociative experiences and their correlates in young non-patients. *Psychology and Psychotherapy: Theory, Research and Practice, 75,* 53–64.

North, C. S., Ryall, J-E. M., Ricci, D. A., & Wetzel, R. D. (1993). *Multiple personalities, multiple disorders.* New York: Oxford University Press.

Orne, M. T., Dinges, D. F., & Orne, E. C. (1984). On the differential diagnosis of multiple personality in the forensic context. *International Journal of Clinical and Experimental Hypnosis, 32,* 118–169.

Piper, A. (1997). *Hoax and reality: The bizarre world of multiple personality disorder.* Northvale, NJ: Jason Aronson.

Powell, R. A., & Gee, T. L. (1999). The effects of hypnosis on dissociative identity disorder: A reexamination of the evidence. *Canadian Journal of Psychiatry, 44,* 914–916.

Putnam, F. W., & Lowenstein, R. J. (2000). Dissociative identity disorder. In B. J. Sadock & V. A. Sadock (Eds.), *Kaplan and Sadockís Comprehensive Textbook of Psychiatry* (7th ed., Vol 1, pp. 1552–1564). Philadelphia: Lippincott, Williams, & Wilkins.

Rauschenberger, S. L., & Lynn, S. J. (1995). Fantasy proneness, DSM-III-R Axis 1 psychopathology, and dissociation. *Journal of Abnormal Psychology, 104,* 373–380.

Rifkin, A., Ghisalbert, D., Dimatou, S., Jin, C., & Sethi, M. (1998). Dissociative identity disorder in psychiatric inpatients. *American Journal of Psychiatry, 155,* 844–845.

Rosenberg, M. J. (1959). A disconfirmation of the descriptions of hypnosis as a dissociated state. *International Journal of Clinical & Experimental Hypnosis, 7,* 187–204.

Ross, C. A. (1997). *Dissociative identity disorder: Diagnosis, clinical features, and treatment of multiple personality.* New York: John Wiley & Sons.

Ross, C. A., Duffy, C. M. M., & Ellason, J. W. (2002). Prevalence, reliability and validity of dissociative disorders in an inpatient setting *Journal of Trauma & Dissociation, 3,* 7–17.

Ross, C. A., Heber, S., & Norton, G. R. (1989). The dissociative disorders interview schedule: A structured interview. *Dissociation, 2,* 169–189.

Ross, C. A., & Norton G. R. (1988). Multiple personality disorder patients with a prior diagnosis of schizophrenia. *Dissociation, 1,* 39–42.

Ross, C. A.., Norton, G. R., & Wozney, K. (1989). Multiple personality disorder: An analysis of 236 cases. *Canadian Journal of Psychiatry, 34,* 413–418.

Sarbin, T. R. (1995). On the belief that one body may be host to two or more personalities. *International Journal of Clinical and Experimental Hypnosis, 43,* 163–183.

Spanos, N. P. (1994). Multiple identity enactments and multiple personality disorder: A sociocognitive perspective. *Psychological Bulletin, 116,* 143–165.

Spanos, N. P. (1996). *Multiple identities and false memories: A sociocognitive perspective.* Washington, DC: American Psychological Association.

Spanos, N. P., Weekes, J. R., & Bertrand, L. D. (1985). Multiple personality: A social psychological perspective. *Journal of Abnormal Psychology, 94,* 362–376.

Spiegel, D. (1993, May 20th). Letter to the Executive Council, International Study for the Study of Multiple Personality and Dissociation. *News, International Society of the Study of Multiple Personality and Dissociation, 11,* 15.

Stafford, J., & Lynn, S. J. (2002). Cultural scripts, childhood abuse, and multiple identities: A study of role-played enactments. *International Journal of Clinical & Experimental Hypnosis, 50,* 67–85.

Steinberg, M., Cicchetti, D., Buchanan, J., Hall, P., & Rounsaville, B. (1993). Clinical assessment of dissociative symptoms and disorders: The Structured Clinical Interview for DSM-IV Dissociative Disorders. *Dissociation, 6,* 3–15.

Steinberg, M., Rounsaville, B., & Cichetti, D., (1990). The Structured Clinical Interview for DSM-III-R dissociative disorders: Preliminary report on a new diagnostic instrument. *American Journal of Psychiatry, 147,* 76–82.

Tellegen, A. & Atkinson, G. (1974). Openness to absorbing and self-altering experiences ("absorption"), a trait related to hypnotic susceptibility. *Journal of Abnormal Psychology, 83,* 268–277.

VanderHoff, H., & Lynn, S. J. (2001). The assessment of self-mutilation: Issues and clinical considerations. *Journal of Threat Assessment, 1,* 91–109.

Waller, N. G., Putnam, F. W., & Carlson, E. B. (1996). Types of dissociation and dissociation and dissociative types: A taxometric analysis of dissociative experiences. *Psychological Methods, 1,* 300–321.

Waller, N. G., & Ross, C. A. (1997). The prevalence and biometric structure of pathological dissociation in the general population: Taxometric and behavior genetic findings. *Journal of Abnormal Psychology, 106,* 499–510.

Watson, D. (2003). Investigating the construct validity of the dissociative taxon: Stability analyses of normal and pathological dissociation. *Journal of Abnormal Psychology, 112,* 298–305.

Weitzenhoffer, A. M., & Hilgard, E. R. (1962). *Stanford Hypnotic Susceptibility Scale: Form C.* Palo Alto, CA: Consulting Psychologists Press.

White, R. W. & Shevach, B. J. (1942). Hypnosis and the concept of dissociation. *Journal of Abnormal & Social Psychology, 37,* 309–328.

CHAPTER 25

Scientific Evidence for Domestic Violence Treatment

Jeffrey M. Lohr • L. Kevin Hamberger • Tricia H. Witte • Lisa M. Parker

INTRODUCTION

Transactional Context of Partner Violence

Domestic violence is a transaction between perpetrator and victim. It is defined not only by the perpetration of violence and abuse, but the fact that it occurs in an interpersonal relationship in which both parties actively participate. As such, the violence perpetrated is construed in more psychological terms than violence perpetrated upon strangers or on victims in other social roles, such as coworkers. There is little doubt that it represents a serious "relational problem." However, it is difficult to construe domestic violence as a psychiatric disorder in need of diagnostic criteria and formal classification.

Psychological Dysfunction vs. Diagnosis

Though domestic violence may not be a classifiable diagnosis, it certainly fits the definition of "mental disorder" as a harmful dysfunction (Wakefield, 1992). That is, it is a pattern of behavior that: (a) reflects a value-term based on social norms and (b) is a failure of a natural function having evolutionary significance or function. Moreover, research has revealed perpetrator typologies (Hamberger, Lohr, Bonge & Tolin, 1996; Holtzworth-Monroe & Stuart, 1994) that clearly indicate at substantial proportion of domestic violence perpetrators show serious forms of psychopathology, some of which conform to diagnostic characterization, such as Anti-Social and Borderline Personality Disorder (Hamberger et al., 1996; Dutton & Starzomski, 1993). The implications of these findings for the content of treatment are discussed below.

INTIMATE PARTNER VIOLENCE: DESCRIPTION AND DEFINITION

There is no universal agreement about what, exactly, constitutes partner violence. In fact, Pagelow (1984) states that the disagreement over definitions of partner violence is "fundamental" (p 27). Number of violent attacks contributes to the definition of some workers. For example, Pagelow differentiates primary battering, the first incident of violence in a relationship, from secondary battering; subsequent, repeated violent attacks. Other early conceptualizations of partner violence emphasized the degree of injury to the victim (Stewart & deBlois, 1981; Rounsaville & Weissman, 1978), as well as frequency of physical assault (Parker & Schumaker, 1977). Some researchers (e.g., Straus, 1977; Gelles & Straus, 1979) define violence as a continuum of acts ranging from relatively mild (e.g., push or shove) to severe and likely to cause injury (e.g., assault with or without a weapon). Barnett and Wilshire (1987) developed a type of frequency X severity algorithm whereby battering can include infrequent, severe violence (e.g., punching, multiple blows,

Lohr, J. M., Hamberger, L. K., Witte, T. H., & Parker, L. M. (2006). Scientific evidence for domestic violence treatment. In J. E. Fisher & W. T. O'Donohue (Eds.), *Practitioner's guide to evidence-based psychotherapy*. New York: Springer.

using a weapon) or less severe but more frequent violence (e.g., pushing, restraining, slapping).

Other scholars, such as Pagelow (1984) define violence within the family more broadly than the commission of specific acts and their frequency. Pagelow defines violence as the misuse of force or power to deny the rights and freedom of choice of another. Thus, intimate partner violence or abuse can include not only acts of physical violence but any type of act that interferes with the development and growth of another, deprives the right to make their own choices, or to exercise their human rights. Such behavior functions in the exercise of dominance by one partner over the other through fear induction (Adams, 1989; Barnett, Miller-Perrin, & Perrin, 1997; Pagelow, 1984). Pence (1989) focuses on the coercive, controlling functions of male violence toward female partners, as well as the interconnections between physical and sexual violence and other tactics of control and domination such as minimization and denial, intimidation and threats, economic control, using children as tools of coercion, and asserting male dominance and privilege.

PREDOMINANT MODELS OF BATTERER INTERVENTION

Feminist-Based Model

The Feminist-based model views battering as part and parcel of broader societal norms and practices that subordinate and oppress women within institutions and individual relationships. Within this model, battering is a *social* problem, and not an individual problem. Men learn, through male socialization processes, to oppress women through any means necessary, including violence. Psychological problems are not viewed as directly related to battering. Ending men's violence and oppression of women requires changing community and societal institutions and values in ways that both acknowledge and support the social and economic equality of women, and support the rights of women to live free from violence and oppression. As such, community systems are accountable to battered women for making appropriate changes. Intervention with batterers is primarily educational to increase awareness of oppressive, sexist attitudes and behaviors that function to dominate and control their partners. Subsequently, nonoppressive, egalitarian behaviors and attitudes are introduced and practiced. Intervention also emphasizes batterer accountability to his partner and his community for both his oppressive behavior and for making and maintaining appropriate changes. Hence, within treatment sessions, the client receives regular confrontation and feedback for both undesirable and desirable behaviors (Feder & Forde, 2000; Saunders, 1996).

Cognitive-Behavioral Model

Within the cognitive-behavioral model, battering behavior is analyzed as a complex combination of thought and attitudinal processes and overt behaviors that are acquired and serve particular psychosocial functions for the batterer (Hamberger & Lohr, 1989). In particular, batterers learn that certain behaviors lead to positive outcomes for them. For example, thoughts and actions that lead to sex are likely to be used again in future similar situations. Other behaviors lead to the ending of negative situations. For example, thoughts and actions that lead to ending a difficult argument are reinforced and likely to be used again in similar future situations. Battering behavior is maintained by rigid or limited problem-solving skills and limited, sexist attitudes and beliefs that set them up for oppressive and abusive behaviors (Holtzworth-Munroe & Hutchnson, 1993). In addition, the battering behavior represents a deficiency in behavioral skills for coping with interpersonal conflict and/or expression of personal needs, expectations and vulnerabilities (Holtzworth-Munroe & Anglin, 1994). Hence, responsibility for perpetrating violent and abusive behaviors, and for ending it, is placed with the perpetrator. Because it is the abuser's beliefs and actions lead to abuse and oppression, he alone, needs to change to end his abusiveness. Cognitive-behavioral treatment focuses on identification of deficient thought patterns and abusive behaviors, and their modification to nonabusive, noncontrolling skills. Treatment consists of in-session role-modeling and practice of appropriate skills, as well as feedback for the adequacy of the client's efforts and progress (Dunford, 2000b; Gondolf, 1999). Cognitive-behavioral treatments are consistent with psychoeducational interventions such as the Duluth model (Pence & Paymar, 1993) that focuses on the control and domination function of abuse and violence. They can also include feminist-based analysis of how particular attitudes and behaviors support violence, abuse and oppression (Saunders, 1996).

Psychodynamic/Trauma-Based Model

This model is based on the theory that domestic violence is a direct result of unresolved physical and emotional trauma to which batterers were exposed as children. Unresolved emotional sequela of trauma result in the development of a number of survival tactics to avoid negative emotions, including high-risk behaviors such as substance abuse, violence and controlling behaviors (Saunders, 1996; Stosny, 2002). Witnessed abuse, in combination with parental rejection, are presumed to shape disordered personality, particularly borderline and narcissistic personality disorder (Coleman, 2003; Dutton, 1998). In sum, adult intimate partner violence is functionally related to early, and pervasive negative childhood experiences that are potentiated by trauma. Intimate partner violence is but one aspect of personality problems and impaired interpersonal relationships.

The goal of psychodynamic/trauma-based treatment is to end violence by helping men to face their pain and its associated shame. Early phases of treatment work on helping clients to develop trust and safety within the group treatment context (Saunders, 1996). Once safety and trust are achieved, the men are assisted to identify and name the traumatic events of their childhood. Once the trauma has been resolved, violent and abusive behavior will no longer have the function of "covering" or avoiding the negative emotions. Hence, the behavior will end and be replaced by nonviolent, noncontrolling modes of relating to others.

EMPIRICAL EVIDENCE OF EFFICACY

Summary of Program Evaluation Research

Babcock, Green, and Robie (2004) conducted a meta-analysis of domestic violence treatment reports to quantitatively summarize the measured effects of batterer programs. Sixty-eight empirical studies were identified and classified according to methodology: experimental, quasi-experimental, and uncontrolled pre–post treatment assessments. The experimental studies randomly assigned participants to treatment or to no-treatment conditions. Quasi-experiments compared participants to complete treatment to matched participants who did not receive treatment or who dropped out of treatment. The treatment conditions included the psychoeducational Duluth Model, cognitive-behavioral treatment, or other types of intervention. The criterion variables included subsequent violence recidivism based on police records or partner report. The effect size was calculated with the d statistic, which is represented in standard deviation units. An effect size of .50 reflects improvement of one-half of a standard deviation as compared to no treatment. An effect size of .20 or less is considered "small," .50 is considered medium, and an effect size of .80 is considered large (Cohen, 1988).

Overall, Babcock et al. (2004) found that the effect size of treatment is within the "small" range. The effect sizes for method of reporting were equivalent (police report d = .18; partner report d = .18). Furthermore, there was no statistically significant difference in effect size among types of treatment for either police records or victim report of recidivism. Moreover, there was no statistically significant difference in effect size among quasi-experimental and experimental design studies. Thus, the results indicate that regardless of the reporting method, type of treatment, and methodological procedure, the effect size on recidivism is small. Given the apparently small statistical effect, it may be instructive to provide a qualitative review of the randomized controlled trials in greater detail.

Experimental Analysis of Treatment Efficacy

Published outcome studies

Experimental control of extraneous procedural factors is necessary to rule out the effects of passage of time, measurement reactivity, selection bias, and the effects of participant and researcher expectancy. It is through the use of increasingly rigorous procedural controls that confidence in the efficacy of the substantive features of treatment is maximized. To date, there are four randomized controlled trials that have examined the efficacy of batterer treatment. Palmer, Brown, and Barrera (1992) used a block randomized procedure to assign male batterers to either no treatment (probation-only) control group or an active treatment condition. The treatment condition involved 10 weekly sessions of psychoeducational content that included group discussion of beliefs about violence, coping with conflict and anger, self-esteem, and relationships with women. The results at 12-month follow-up indicated that perpetrators in the treatment group had lower police reports of reoffending than the perpetrators in the control condition, 10% and 31%, respectively.

Davis, Taylor, and Maxwell (1998) randomly assigned batterers to one of three treatment conditions: a 26-week psychoeducational group, a brief 8-week psychoeducational group, or community service. Group assignment was random except when a judge ordered re-assignment from the community service condition to psychoeducational treatment. Recidivism based on police records at 12 month follow-up was lower in the 26-week educational condition in comparison to the 8-week educational or community service conditions. There was no difference in recidivism between the 8-week condition and community service condition. However, when victim report of violence was used as the dependent variable, neither treatment condition was different from the community service condition.

Feder and Ford (2000) randomly assigned male batterers to either no treatment probation or feminist-oriented CBT group treatment that was administered once per week for 26 weeks. Dependent variables included recidivism based on police report and victim report. Statistical analyses showed no significant differences between the two conditions. As attrition rate in the treatment condition was high (60%), post hoc analyses were conducted on treatment completers which showed a statistically significant reduction for both measures of recidivism. The reduction, however, may be an artifact of self-selection.

Dunford (2000b) conducted perhaps the most rigorously controlled treatment outcome study using US Navy personnel stationed in San Diego, CA. The site-specific nature of the study maximized treatment fidelity, victim-report of recidivism and minimized cross-over assignments and treatment attrition. Eight hundred sixty-one male batterers were randomly assigned to either a 36-week cognitive-behavioral batterers group, a 26-week cognitive-behavioral couples therapy group, a rigorous monitoring-only group, or a no-treatment (victim safety planning) condition. Dependent variables included recidivism based on police and victim report. Statistical analyses showed no statistically significant differences between groups on either measure at 12-month follow-up.

Morrel, Elliot, Murphy, and Taft (2003) used a quasi-random procedure to assign male batterers to either supportive group therapy, or cognitive-behavioral group therapy. The latter included content to analyze motivations for violence, development of crisis management strategies, anger management techniques, and development of improved communication skills. Collateral partner reports of violence were assessed before and after treatment, and at 6-month follow-up. Criminal justice data were gathered 2–3 years after treatment. Statistical analyses of partner report of assault, psychological aggression, injuries, and sexual aggression showed reductions from pretreatment to post treatment and from post treatment to follow-up. However, neither partner report nor criminal data revealed statistically significant different differences among conditions. Though the apparent reductions in partner-reported recidivism are encouraging, the absence of a wait-list control condition with which to compare the treatment conditions makes it impossible to infer any specific effects of treatment. Though treatments may be followed by reductions in recidivism (Feder & Ford, 2000), when compared to no-treatment or wait-list controls, they have been shown to be no more effective (Davis et al., 1998; Dunford, 2000b). Indeed, Dunford (2000a) has observed without the inclusion of a no treatment control group in Dunford (2000b) he would have concluded that treatment had a beneficial effect when there was none. Therefore, we must interpret the apparent positive effects of cognitive-behavioral group therapy in Morrel et al. (2003) with caution. In sum, the weight of the findings thus suggest that the empirical demonstration of the specific beneficial effects of several different treatment modalities awaits more rigorous experimental analysis.

THE POTENTIAL OF TREATMENT MATCHING TO PERPETRATOR TYPE

The small effects of treatment in controlled outcome studies suggests a consideration the psychological and behavioral characteristics of the perpetrator which could be matched to the content of the treatment. Recent psychological research suggests the heterogeneity among perpetrators may be captured by empirically derived clusters or "typologies." Researchers have cluster-analyzed personality and psychopathological characteristics of large samples of adjudicated batterers and typically have found three subtypes. Holtzworth-Monroe and Stuart (1994) reviewed the descriptive research on batterers and theorized three identifiable subtypes. Hamberger et al. (1996) subsequently conducted a large sample cluster analysis of adjudicated batters and confirmed the prediction: (1) generally violent antisocial, (2) passive aggressive dependent, and nonpathological family-only. If the typology can be generalized to previous treatment outcome research, it is reasonable to infer that these subtypes have received the same content of treatment in randomized, quasi-randomized, and uncontrolled studies. If the content of treatment could be matched to batterer subtype, treatment outcome (such as effect size) might be enhanced (Beutler & Clarkin, 1990). Moreover, preliminary evidence suggests that the identification of cluster membership based on clinical assessment information is reliable and accurate (Lohr, Bonge, Witte, Hamberger, & Langhinrichsen-Rohling, 2005).

For example, White and Gondolf (2000) suggest that batterers who fit the anti-social subtype of Hamberger et al. (1996) would best respond to direct therapeutic challenge in group therapy. The therapist should enforce limits on behavior and frame the goal of treatment as a more pro-social means by which to attain desired goals. The development of team-oriented group cohesion might reduce the tendency of such individuals to strive for narcissistic superiority. The objective of treatment would be the containment and abatement of violent and abusive behavior rather than modification of personality characteristics.

White and Gondolf (2000) also suggest that the passive–aggressive dependent perpetrator may benefit most from treatment that is aimed at modifying interpersonal skills that may reduce fear of negative evaluation (interpersonal judgement). The use of imitation, role-play rehearsal, and positive social feedback could be used for social skill development. Cognitive-behavioral procedures could be applied to improving affect regulation, anger control, and modification of cognitive distortions that occur in the context of partner conflict.

For the nonpathological (family-only) subtype, the feminist cognitive-behavioral strategy (Pence & Paymar, 1993) might be most effective. The content of treatment would focus on violence and abuse as an instrumental means by which to assert power and control over the female partner. Treatment procedures would include exposure to prototypic violence scenarios involving such behavior as exemplars which are analyzed for such control functions. The purpose would be to improve the perpetrator's ability to self-monitor and self-regulate such behaviors and to initiate alternative adaptive means by which emotions are expressed and interpersonal influence is exercised.

In an outcome study addressing treatment matching, Saunders (1996) found that perpetrators with antisocial traits showed better outcome with the feminist cognitive-behavioral treatment, while those with dependent personality traits showed better outcome with psychodynamic treatment. It is important to note, however, that there were several methodological limitations that threaten the internal validity of the study; absence of a wait-list control condition, absence of fidelity assessment, and use of dependent variables with unknown reliability and validity. More important, the psychological variables that determine batterer subtype were not matched a priori to different treatment conditions.

CONCLUSIONS AND IMPLICATIONS

It is clear that methodological refinement of efficacy on batterer treatment is necessary (Babcock et al., 2004). Despite logistical and ethical challenges (Gondolf, 2001), experimental research methods must be applied to determine which treatments are efficacious, the nature of essential content and components, and whether some content is more effective with some types of perpetrators than others. The first two issues require control conditions for nonspecific factors of treatment in general, and component control conditions to identify "active ingredients" (Lohr, DeMaio, & McGlynn, 2003).

Research to determine the efficacy of matching perpetrator to treatment content will require the type of experimental research that has been brought to bear on treatment for alcohol and other substance related disorders (Project MATCH Research Group, 1997). Though Project MATCH failed to find reliable effects of matching variables on the efficacy of different treatments, the experimental strategy could serve as a guide for efficacy research on batterer treatment. One strategy would be to identify a priori batterers based on typology and then randomly assign them to either a wait-list control condition or active treatments as described above. Magnitude of change within each treatment condition could then be assessed for each type of perpetrator. If the results of such a study indicated a differential response to treatment, then subsequent studies providing for a priori matching of type to treatment content could be conducted to identify optimal treatment responsiveness. Prior to the conduct of such research, the informed clinician may be able to use such information in clinical assessments and apply this information in the implementation of different types of treatment on a case by case basis.

REFERENCES

Adams, D. (1989). Feminist-based interventions for battering men. In P. L. Caesar & L. K. Hamberger (Eds.), *Treating men who batter: Theory, practice, and programs* (pp. 3–23). New York: Springer.

Babcock, J. C., Green, C. E., & Robie, C. (2004). Does batterers' treatment work? A meta-analytic review of domestic violence treatment. *Clinical Psychology Review, 23,* 1023–1153.

Barnett, O. W., Miller-Perrin, C. J., & Perrin, R. D. (1997). *Family violence across the lifespan: An introduction.* Thousand Oaks, CA: Sage.

Barnett, O. W., & Wilshire, T. W. (July, 1987). *Forms and frequencies of wife abuse.* Paper presented at the Third National Family Violence Research Conference, Durham, NH.

Beutler, L. E., & Clarkin, J. (1990). *Systematic treatment selections: Toward targeted therapeutic interventions.* New York: Brunner/Mazel.

Cohen, J. (1988). *Statistical power analysis of the behavioral sciences.* Hillsdale, NJ: Lawrence Erlbaum.

Coleman, V. (2003).Treating the lesbian batterer: Theoretical ad clinical considerations – A contemporary psychoanalytic perspective. *Journal of Aggression, Maltreatment, and Trauma, 7,* 159–206.

Davis, R., Taylor, B., & Maxwell, C. (1998). Does batterers treatment reduce violence: A randomized experiment in Brooklyn. *Justice Quarterly, 18,* 171–201.

Dunford, F. W. (2000a). Determining program success: The importance of employing experimental research designs. *Crime and Delinquency, 46,* 425–434.

Dunford, F. W. (2000b). The San Diego Navy experiment: An assessment of interventions for men who assault their wives. *Journal of Consulting and Clinical Psychology, 68,* 468–476.

Dutton, D. G. (1998). *The abusive personality.* New York: Guilford.

Dutton, D. G., & Starzomski, A. J. (1993). Borderline personality factors in perpetrators of psychological and physical abuse. *Violence and Victims, 8,* 327–337.

Feder, L., & Forde, D. (2000). A test of the efficacy of court-mandated counseling for domestic violence offenders: The Broward experiment. Washington, DC: *National Institute of Justice.*

Gelles, R. J., & Straus, M. A. (1979). Determinants of violence in the family: Toward a theoretical integration. In W. R. Burr, R. Hill, F. Ivan Nye, & I. L. Reiss (Eds.), *Contemporary theories about the family* (Vol. 1, pp. 549–581). New York: Free Press.

Gondolf, E. W. (1999). A comparison of four batterer intervention systems: Do court referral, program length, and services matter? *Journal of Interpersonal Violence, 14,* 41–61.

Gondolf, E. W. (2001). Limitations of experimental evaluation of batterer programs. *Trauma, Violence, and Abuse, 2,* 79–88.

Hamberger, L. K., & Lohr, J. M. (1989). Proximal causes of spouse abuse: Theoretical analysis for cognitive-behavioral interventions. In P. L. Caesar and L. K. Hamberger (Eds.), *Treating men who batter: Theory, practice, and programs* (pp. 53–76). New York, Springer.

Hamberger, L. K., Lohr, J. M., Bonge, D., & Tolin, D. F. (1996). A large sample empirical typology of male spouse abusers an its relationship to dimensions of abuse. *Violence and Victims, 11,* 277–292.

Holtzworth-Munroe, A., & Anglin, K. (1991). The competency of responses given by maritally violent versus nonviolent men to problematic marital situations. *Violence and Victims, 6,* 257–269.

Holtzworth-Munroe, A., & Hutchinson, G. (1993). Attributing negative intent to wife behavior: The attributions of maritally violent versus nonviolent men. *Journal of Abnormal Psychology, 102,* 206–211.

Holtzworth-Monroe, A., & Stuart, G. L. (1994). Typologies of male batterers: Three subtypes and the differences among them. *Psychological Bulletin, 116,* 476–497.

Lohr, J. M., Bonge, D., Witte, T. H., Hamberger, L. K., & Langhinrichsen-Rohling, J. (2005). Consistency and accuracy of batterer typology identification. *Journal of Family Violence, 20,* 253–259.

Lohr, J. M., DeMaio, C., & McGlynn, F. D. (2003). Specific and nonspecific factors in the experimental analysis of behavioral treatment efficacy. *Behavior Modification, 27,* 322–368.

Morrel, T. M., Elliottt, J. D., Murphy, C. M., & Taft, C. T. (2003). Cognitive behavioral and supportive group treatments for partner-violent men. *Behavior Therapy, 34,* 77–95.

Pagelow, M. D. (1984). *Family Violence.* New York: Praeger.

Palmer, S. E., Brown, R. A., & Barrera, M. E. (1992). Group treatment program for abusive husbands: Long term evaluation. American Journal of Orthopsychiatry, 62, *276–283.*

Parker, B., & Schumaker, D. N. (1977). The battered wife syndrome and violence in the nuclear family of origin: A controlled pilot study. *American Journal of Public Health, 67,* 760–761.

Pence, E. (1989). Batterer programs: Shifting from community collusion to community confrontation. In P. L. Caesar, & L. K. Hamberger (Eds.), *Treating men who batter: Theory, practice, and programs* (pp. 24–50). New York: Springer.

Pence, E., & Paymar, M. (1993). *Education groups for men who batter: The Duluth Model.* New York: Springer.

Project MATCH Research Group. (1997). Matching alcohol treatments to client heterogeneity: Project Match posttreatment drinking outcomes. *Journal of Studies on Alcohol, 58,* 7–29.

Rounsaville, B. J., & Weisman, M. M. (1978). Battered women: A medical problem requiring detection. *International Journal of Psychiatry in Medicine, 8,* 191–202.

Saunders, D. (1996). Feminist-cognitive-behavioral and process-psychodynamic treatment for men who batter: Interaction of abuser traits and treatment model. *Violence and Victims, 11,* 393–414.

Stewart, M. A., & deBlois, C. S. (1981). Wife abuse among families attending a child psychiatry clinic. *Journal of the American Academy of Child Psychiatry, 20,* 845–862.

Stosny, S. (2002). Treating attachment abuse – The compassion workshop. In E. Aldarondo & F. Mederos (Eds.), *Programs for men who batter: Intervention and prevention strategies in a diverse society* (pp. 9-1–9-17). Kingston, NJ: Civic Research Institute.

Straus, M. A. (1977). Wife-beating: How common and why? *Victimology: An International Journal, 2,* 402–418.

Wakefield, J. C. (1992). The concept of mental disorder: On the boundary between biological facts and social values. *American Psychologist, 47,* 373–388.

White, R. J., & Gondolf, E. W. (2000). Implications of personality profiles for batterer treatment. *Journal of Interpersonal Violence, 15,* 467–488.

CHAPTER 26

Dysthymic Disorder

Rebecca S. Laptook • Daniel N. Klein

Depressive Disorders are among the most prevalent psychological disorders, affecting up to 20% of the US population at some point during each person's lifetime. Depression has traditionally been conceptualized as a condition with an episodic and remitting course. However, over the past 20 years, this view of depression as a more acute disorder has shifted to one which conceptualizes depression as often chronic in nature.

The Diagnostic and Statistical Manual of Mental Disorders (DSM-IV-TR; American Psychological Association, 2000) delineates two main categories of chronic depression: major depressive disorder (chronic type) and dysthymic disorder. Chronic major depression consists of major depressive episodes that continue to meet full criteria for a minimum of two years. Approximately 15–20% of patients who have a major depressive episode meet criteria for chronic major depression (Klein & Santiago, 2003). Dysthymic disorder is a less severe chronic condition that consists primarily of a depressed mood for most of the day, more days than not, and endures for at least two years.

The present chapter focuses on dysthymic disorder. The aim of the chapter is to discuss the classification and assessment of dysthymic disorder, address proposed etiological and maintaining variables, discuss empirically supported approaches to the treatment of the disorder, and, finally, comment on future directions in research on dysthymia.

DYSTHYMIC DISORDER

What is Dysthymic Disorder?

The DSM-IV defines dysthymic disorder as a chronic depressive condition lasting a minimum of two years in which the essential feature is a depressed mood that occurs for most of the day, more days than not. The symptoms must be persistent, in that the criteria require that the individual cannot be symptom-free for longer than two months during this two year period. In addition, the onset must be insidious, in that the criteria specify that there cannot be an occurrence of a major depressive episode within the first two years of dysthymia. In children, irritable mood may be present in place of depressed mood, and the minimum duration of symptoms is reduced to one year.

In addition to the core symptom of depressed mood, the DSM-IV requires the presence of at least two of the following six sets of symptoms: decreased energy or fatigue, insomnia or hypersomnia, increased or decreased appetite, low self-esteem, poor concentration or difficulty making decisions, and helplessness. People with dysthymic disorder often have more than the minimum requirement of criteria and may present with a full range of depressive symptoms. Cognitive (e.g., low self-esteem, hopelessness), affective (e.g., depressed mood), and social-motivational (e.g., loss of interest or pleasure, social withdrawal) symptoms are especially

Laptook, R. S., & Klein, D. N. (2006). Dysthymic disorder. In J. E. Fisher & W. T. O'Donohue (Eds.), *Practitioner's guide to evidence-based pyschotherapy*. New York: Springer.

common in dysthymia. Although dysthymic disorder is typically viewed as a milder form of depression, its chronic symptomatology results in significant impairment in social and vocational functioning. Indeed, the level of impairment in dysthymia equals or exceeds that associated with non-chronic major depressive disorder (Klein & Santiago, 2003).

Classification. Since the introduction of Dysthymia as a distinct category in the DSM-III (American Psychiatric Association, 1980), there has been controversy over whether it should be classified as a mood disorder or as a personality disorder. On the one hand, dysthymic disorder is characterized by depressive symptoms. On the other hand, its chronic course, and in many cases, childhood or adolescent onset, are suggestive of a personality disorder. As discussed below, there is now considerable evidence supporting a relationship between dysthymic disorder and the major mood disorders, including an elevated rate of mood disorders in first-degree relatives and a high risk for developing major depressive disorder. However, dysthymic disorder also overlaps with the personality disorders, as individuals with dysthymia have a high level of Axis II comorbidity and an elevated rate of personality disorders in their relatives.

Another issue concerns the boundaries between dysthymic disorder and other forms of chronic depression, such as "double depression" and chronic major depression. Recent studies comparing dysthymia, double depression, and chronic major depression have revealed few meaningful differences (Klein, Shankman, Lewinsohn, Rohde, & Seeley, 2004). These studies suggest that it may be possible to simplify the current classification of chronic depression by combining the various forms into a single category.

Despite the lack of differences between the existing categories of chronic depression, dysthymic disorder is probably heterogeneous, and includes multiple subtypes (Akiskal, 1983). One important source of heterogeneity appears to be age of onset. The DSM-IV divides dysthymia into early onset (i.e., before age 21) and late onset (i.e., after age 21) subtypes. This distinction has important implications. Early onset dysthymia is characterized by greater Axis I and II comorbidity and higher rates of mood disorders in relatives than late-onset dysthymia. Late-onset dysthymia may be more closely associated with stressful life events, such as losses and health problems (Klein & Santiago, 2003). Although the early–late onset distinction is formally applied only to dysthymic disorder, it cuts across most forms of depression, as it has similar correlates for both episodic and chronic major depression.

Basic Facts About Dysthymic Disorder

Prevalence. In the National Comorbidity Study, Kessler et al. (1994) reported that over 6% of the population experienced dysthymic disorder at some point in their lives, and that 3% suffer from dysthymia at any given point in time. The prevalence of dysthymic disorder is higher in clinical settings, with studies reporting rates of 22–36% in outpatient mental health clinics. Dysthymic disorder occurs equally as often in males and females during childhood; however, in adulthood, dysthymia occurs two to three times as often in women.

Comorbidity. Dysthymia frequently co-occurs with other Axis I and Axis II disorders. In a study of a large community sample of older adolescents and adults, Lewinsohn, Rohde, Seeley, and Hops (1991) found significantly higher rates of current and life-time comorbidity between dysthymia and major depression than was expected based each disorder's respective base rates. Moreover, the DSM-IV indicates that up to 75% of patients in clinical settings who have dysthymia will develop major depression within approximately five years. In addition to major depression, dysthymia is often comorbid with other Axis I disorders such as anxiety disorders and substance use. Regarding Axis II disorders, dysthymia most frequently co-occurs with borderline, histrionic, avoidant, and dependent personality disorders. Comorbid personality disorders are more common in dysthymia than in episodic major depression (Klein & Santiago, 2003).

Course. There are few long-term follow-up studies of the naturalistic course of dysthymic disorder. In a 10-year follow-up study of adult outpatients with dysthymia, we recently found that 74% eventually recovered, although the median time to recovery was 4½ years. In addition, there was a high risk of relapse: 74% of the patients who recovered experienced another episode of chronic depression. Over the course of the 10-year follow-up, patients with dysthymic disorder met criteria for a mood disorder for 61% of the follow-up period, compared to 21% for outpatients with episodic major depression.

Dysthymic disorder typically fluctuates in intensity over time, with the more intense periods often meeting criteria for a major depressive episode. Indeed, most individuals with dysthymia meet criteria for major depression at some point during their lives. Retrospective studies indicate that 75% of patients with dysthymic disorder have a history of major depressive disorder, and prospective studies suggest that the rate may be over 90%. The phenomenon of major depressive episodes superimposed on dysthymic disorder is referred to as "double depression" (Keller & Shapiro, 1982). The major depressive episodes may be triggered by stressful life events, and are often what leads patients with a long history of untreated dysthymia to seek help.

Etiological and maintaining variables. Recent theory and research has focused on six variables that may play an important role in predisposing to chronic depression and maintaining the disorder once it begins. These include family history, childhood adversity, temperament/personality, cognitive factors, interpersonal factors, and chronic stress. It is likely that biological variables, such as dysregulation of neurotransmitter, neuroendocrine, and sleep neurophysiology systems, also play important roles (Thase, Jindal, & Howland, 2002). However, research on biological factors in dysthymia is very limited, hence we will not consider these variables here.

Research has suggested that there is a link between the development of chronic forms of depression, such as dysthymia, and a family history of psychopathology. Unfortunately, we do not know whether this link results from genetic or environmental effects because twin and adoption studies of chronic depression are not available.

There are higher rates of dysthymia, major depression, and personality disorders in the first-degree relatives of persons with dysthymic disorder than in the relatives of persons with no history of mental illness (Klein et al., 1995; Klein, Shankman, et al., 2004). The relatives of individuals with dysthymic disorder also have higher rates of dysthymia and personality disorders, and similar or higher rates of major depression, than the relatives of individuals with episodic major depression. These data indicate that dysthymic disorder is transmitted within families. However, it is unclear whether the familial risk factors for dysthymic disorder are distinct from those that predispose to major depression, or whether dysthymic disorder and major depression share the same familial risk factors but that dysthymia reflects a greater familial liability.

Negative early experiences have been shown to influence the development of a wide variety of psychological disorders. Regarding mood disorders, the emergence of depression has been associated with experiences such as sexual and physical abuse and emotional maltreatment (Goodman, 2002). In a review of vulnerability factors in chronic depression, Riso and Klein (2004) note that a number of studies have found greater childhood adversity in cases of chronic depression compared to episodic depression, and that early adversity is one of the most robust predictors of a poor course and outcome of depression. As chronic depression often develops years after childhood adversity, it is likely that negative early experiences first influence a child's cognitive and interpersonal styles and neurobiological response to stress, which then lead to an increased risk for depression (Lara & Klein, 1999).

Certain types of temperament or personality have long been thought to be precursors to mood disorders (Klein, Durbin, Shankman, & Santiago, 2002). For example, Kraepelin hypothesized that the depressive temperament was often evident prior to the development of full-blown depressive episodes. Depressive personality shares many of the same traits as dysthymia, such as low self-esteem, pessimism/hopelessness, and gloominess; however, the two constructs are not identical (Klein & Vocisano, 1999). Depressive personality traits may be a specific risk factor for chronic depression, as there are higher levels of depressive personality traits in the relatives of patients with chronic than episodic depression. In addition, depressive personality traits predict the first onset of dysthymia, but not major depression (Klein et al., 2002).

The dimensions of low positive emotionality (PE) (low positive affect and engagement with the environment) and negative emotionality (NE) (increased sensitivity to negative stimuli, resulting in negative affects, such as sadness, fear, anxiety, and anger) have also been hypothesized to be precursors of, or predisposing factors for, the development of depressive disorders. These dimensions may play a particularly important role in chronic depression, as patients with chronic depression appear to have lower levels of PE and higher levels of NE than patients with episodic depression (Riso & Klein, 2004). To the degree that genetic factors are involved in the etiology of dysthymic disorder, it is reasonable to hypothesize that they are expressed at the behavioral level as temperament and personality traits rather than directly as depressive symptoms.

Patients with dysthymia often have dysfunctional or limited interpersonal relationships, and may continue to experience interpersonal difficulties even during periods of recovery. Interpersonal factors, such as low social support, family and marital discord, and difficulties relating to others, predict a poorer course and outcome of depression (Riso & Klein, 2004). James Coyne has hypothesized that depression is maintained through a vicious cycle in which the depressed individual drives those in his or her social environment away by engaging in excessive support seeking. Thomas Joiner has expanded this theory to include a number of self-propagating processes, such as stress generation, excessive reassurance and negative feedback seeking, and conflict avoidance, that possibly function to maintain the depression (see Lara & Klein, 1999 for a review).

Cognitive theories, such as those of John Teasdale and Susan Nolen-Hoeksema, have also been proposed to explain the chronicity of depression. In Teasdale's differential activation hypothesis, negative constructs are activated by depressed mood and then generate negative interpretations of new events. In Nolen-Hoeksema's response-style theory, depression is thought to be maintained by the rumination that occurs in response to depressed mood (Lara & Klein, 1999). Other cognitive variables, such as dysfunctional attitudes, attributional style, and an overly general autobiographical memory also predict a poorer course of depression (Riso & Klein, 2004).

While stressful life events appear to play an important role in the onset of depressive episodes (Monroe & Hadjiyannakis, 2002), chronic stress may be more important in the maintenance and chronicity of depression. Although there may be bidirectional influences, we recently found that chronic stress predicts increases in subsequent depression among outpatients with dysthymic disorder (Dougherty, Klein, & Davila, 2004). Interestingly, however, these effects were moderated by early adversity and family history of chronic depression. The association between chronic stress and subsequent depression was much greater among patients with a history of early adversity and patients with a lower familial loading for chronic depression. In contrast, chronic stress was not associated with depressive symptoms among patients with lower levels adversity and patients with a higher familial loading for chronic depression. Together with evidence of differential response to medication versus pharmacotherapy in chronically depressed patients with and without a history of childhood adversity (Nemeroff et al., 2003), these findings suggest that there may be several distinct pathways to chronic depression.

ASSESSMENT

What Should Be Ruled Out?

The diagnosis and assessment of dysthymic disorder can be challenging. The mild, chronic depressive symptoms are often perceived by both patients and clinicians as being part of the patient's personality or "usual self." Hence, patients may not bring these symptoms to the clinician's attention, and clinicians may overlook them while focusing on more florid Axis I syndromes (particularly superimposed major depressive episodes, but also anxiety disorders and other Axis I conditions). In addition, individuals with dysthymic disorder often have personality disorders. It is important not to overlook the dysthymia, which is a treatable condition, and focus exclusively on the personality disorder.

It may be particularly difficult to distinguish between dysthymic disorder and other chronic depressive disorders, such as chronic major depressive disorder, major depressive disorder in partial remission, and recurrent major depressive disorder with incomplete recovery between episodes. These differential diagnoses require a very careful and detailed history of the onset and shifts in the severity of depressive symptoms over the course of the disorder.

What is Involved in Effective Assessment?

In order to diagnose dysthymic disorder, clinicians must take a careful history of the patients' past depressive symptoms. If the patient has a history of major depressive episodes, it is critical to explore the presence of milder depression before and after the major episodes. It is often helpful to construct a life-chart or timeline with the patient that graphs their level of depression over time. It is also critical to explain to the patient that depression can exist at varying levels of severity, and that it is important to describe both the milder and more severe periods. When using semistructured diagnostic interviews (e.g., the Structured Clinical Interview for DSM-IV), it may be necessary to go beyond the standard interview probes in order to obtain sufficient information about course to distinguish dysthymic disorder from other chronic and highly recurrent depressive conditions.

What Assessments are Not Helpful?

Dysthymic disorder is diagnosed largely on the basis of its chronic course, not simply on the basis of mild depressive symptoms. Hence, measures that are limited to assessing the severity of depressive symptoms during a particular period of time, but do not include a detailed assessment of course, are not useful in diagnosing dysthymic disorder.

In monitoring and evaluating treatment, it may be necessary to modify some of the widely used assessment instruments for depression when applying them to dysthymia (e.g., the Hamilton Rating Scale for Depression). Many of these measures ask patients to describe their level of depression compared to a normal or usual baseline. However, for many patients with dysthymic disorder, their normal or usual state is depressed. Hence, symptoms may be overlooked if questions are phrased in terms of change or worsening from baseline.

TREATMENT

In this section, we will focus broadly on chronic depression, as most of the existing literature is based on patients with double depression or patients with a variety of forms of chronic depression.

What Treatments are Effective?

There are effective psychotherapies and pharmacotherapies for chronic depression, although it appears that the combination of psychotherapy and pharmacotherapy provides the maximum effectiveness. In addition, there is evidence that if patients fail to respond to one form of treatment, they will continue to have a good chance of responding to an alternative treatment. Finally, maintaining patients in treatment after they have achieved remission appears to significantly reduce the risk of relapse and recurrence.

What are Effective Self-Help Treatments?

Although effective self-help treatments (e.g., bibliotherapy) for depression are available, to our knowledge none have been tested for any forms of chronic depression. Given the persistent nature of dysthymia and the high level of associated comorbidity and psychosocial impairment, it may be hazardous to extrapolate from the outcome literature on self-help treatments on depression in general.

What are Effective Therapist-Based Treatments?

Of the various types of psychotherapy, the approach with the strongest empirical support for use with chronic depression at present is the Cognitive Behavioral Analysis System of Psychotherapy (CBASP) (McCullough, 2003). In a large multisite clinical trial, CBASP was found to be as effective as medication in treating patients with a variety of forms of chronic depression (Keller et al., 2000).

CBASP is one of the few approaches to psychotherapy that was specifically designed to treat chronic depression. It is structured and integrative, combining aspects of cognitive, behavioral, and interpersonal approaches to depression into one intervention. The core of the approach is a technique referred to as "Situational Analysis" (SA), which is designed to help patients to change their patterns of coping, improve their interpersonal skills, understand the consequences of their behavior, and interact more effectively with others. In SA, the patient identifies a recent, distressing interpersonal situation and examines it with the therapist. The process consists of three phases: elicitation, remediation, and generalization. In the elicitation phase, the patient describes: (1) the interpersonal event; (2) their behavior; (3) their interpretation of what occurred; (4) the outcome of the event; (5) what they would have liked the outcome to be (desired outcome); and (6) whether or not the desired outcome was achieved. In the remediation phase, the patient works with the therapist to revise their interpretations, behaviors, and/or goals during the situation to increase the probability of achieving a more desirable outcome. In the generalization phase, the patient and therapist review what has been learned, and explore how the patient's new understanding and skills can be applied to similar situations in the future (McCullough, 2003).

Recent data indicate that CBASP is effective even among patients who have failed to respond to antidepressant medication (conversely, pharmacotherapy is effective in patients who have failed to respond to CBASP). In addition, CBASP has proven effective as a maintenance phase treatment: patients who were randomly assigned to continue to receive one session of CBASP per month after recovering from chronic depression had a significantly lower recurrence rate over the course of a year than patients who were assigned to an assessment-only condition (Klein, Santiago, et al., 2004).

Other forms of psychotherapy have been used to treat chronic depression; however, little data exist to support their efficacy with this population. Interpersonal Psychotherapy (IPT) has demonstrated efficacy for acute major depression; however, there are few published data addressing the use of IPT with chronic depression. It can be difficult to apply the standard version of IPT to dysthymic disorder. Although the majority of chronically depressed patients experience substantial interpersonal difficulties, they tend to have fewer discrete life events to focus on in treatment than patients with episodic major depression. As a result, it has been necessary to modify IPT for use with Dysthymic Disorder (Markowitz, 2003). IPT may also be beneficial as a maintenance treatment for chronic depression, although this has not been examined in clinical trials.

Cognitive Therapy (CT) has also been modified to treat chronic forms of depression, although randomized clinical trials have not been reported. In adapting CT for use with dysthymic patients, the therapist places a greater emphasis on the patient's feelings of helplessness, hopelessness, and perfectionism. In addition, focus on the chronically depressed patient's maladaptive schemas and cognitive style is essential in addressing the deficits in problem solving that are often experienced by patients with chronic forms of depression. Components of CT for chronic depression do not differ from those included in the treatment of acute depression. However, the chronicity of disorders like dysthymia often requires the therapist to emphasize and focus on particular depressive features to a greater degree (Riso & Newman, 2003).

Supportive-Expressive therapy (SE) is a psychodynamic approach to the treatment of chronic depression. It may be particularly useful for a subgroup with a history of feeling misunderstood and lonely during childhood. SE therapy draws on Lester Luborsky's concepts of supportiveness, expressiveness, and the core conflictual relationship theme (CCRT). The CCRT is a method that describes a person's central relationship patterns or conflicts in terms of three components: (1) a person's wishes or needs, (2) the expected or actual responses from others, and (3) the person's own reactions to the responses of others. The CCRT is obtained by identifying these components across discrete relationship interactions or relationship episodes. Thus, the CCRT method can illuminate the dynamics that may underlie a dysthymic patient's interpersonal dysfunction. SE therapy also aims to provide a supportive context for a person to express his depressed self, thus allowing the patient to validate his experiences and learn from them. However, studies using SE therapy for chronically depressed patients have not yet been conducted (Mark, Barber, & Crits-Christoph, 2003).

What is Effective Medical Treatment?

In randomized, placebo-controlled clinical trials, a large number of antidepressant medications have been found to be efficacious in the acute-phase treatment of chronic depression. As indicated above, most of these studies have focused on patients with dysthymia and superimposed major depressive episodes, however, antidepressants have also demonstrated efficacy in patients with "pure" dysthymia.

Antidepressants in the tricyclic, selective serotonin re-uptake inhibitor, and atypical antidepressant classes appear to have similar efficacy for chronic depression, and all have been demonstrated to be superior to placebo. Despite these encouraging results, however, 40–50% of patients do not respond to a trial of antidepressant medication, and only about 25–30% have a full response (i.e., achieve remission). One problem is that patients with chronic depression appear to take longer to respond to medication. Therefore, it may be advisable to extend medication trials for longer than is customary in episodic major depression. Nonetheless, it is common to have to switch or augment medications for patients who cannot tolerate, fail to respond, or respond only partially to a drug. Fortunately, there are a large range of pharmacological options, and patients who fail to respond to one medication frequently respond to another (Kocsis, 2003).

Due to the high risk of relapse and recurrence, maintenance pharmacotherapy is an important consideration for patients with dysthymic disorder and other forms of chronic depression. Several double-blind placebo-discontinuation studies have demonstrated that maintaining patients who have recovered from chronic depression on medication is associated with a significantly lower risk of recurrence than placebo (Kocsis, 2003).

How Does One Select Among Treatments?

Few studies have directly compared medication to psychotherapy for chronic depression. In a recent review, Arnow and Constantino (2003) concluded that when all psychotherapies were considered, there was evidence of slightly greater efficacy for pharmacotherapy than psychotherapy. However, the two approaches may have similar efficacy when the form of psychotherapy is specifically tailored to chronic depression (Keller et al., 2000).

Few predictors of differential response to pharmacotherapy versus psychotherapy have been identified. However, Nemeroff et al. (2003) recently reported that psychotherapy was significantly more efficacious than medication for chronically depressed patients with a history of childhood adversity. In contrast, patients without a history of childhood adversity exhibited a nonsignficantly better response to pharmacotherapy.

Recent studies indicate that the combination of medication and psychotherapy is superior to either approach alone for the treatment of chronic depression (Arnow & Constantino, 2003). For example, in a 12-week trial with 681 patients with chronic depression, 73% responded to the combination of CBASP and nefazodone, compared to response rates of 48% to both CBASP alone and nefazodone alone (Keller et al., 2000). Thus, it appears that combination treatment may be the optimal treatment approach for chronic depression. However, because combination treatment is more costly than monotherapy, there is a need to explore the efficacy of sequenced approaches in which patients initially receive a single treatment and additional treatments are added if the patient does not have a full response to the initial treatment.

SUMMARY AND FUTURE DIRECTIONS

In summary, Dysthymic Disorder is a common condition that is associated with significant functional impairment. It has a chronic course, characterized by prolonged episodes and a high risk for recurrence. A history of early adversity, a family history of chronic depression, comorbid anxiety and personality disorders, and chronic stress are associated with a particularly poor course.

Patients with dysthymic disorder can be challenging to treat, as they exhibit high levels of comorbidity, interpersonal deficits, helplessness, and hopelessness. Nonetheless, there are a variety of psychopharmacological and psychotherapeutic treatments that are efficacious for both the acute and long-term treatment of dysthymic disorder, with the combination of medication and psychotherapy producing optimal outcomes.

A number of areas require further research in order to better understand the nature of dysthymic disorder and to develop better treatment strategies. Of particular importance is delineating the pathways involved in the development of dysthymic disorder. As dysthymia often has an onset in childhood or adolescence, this will require a developmental perspective. Moreover, as discussed above, dysthymia is probably etiologically heterogeneous, indicating that multiple pathways are likely to be involved. The current literature suggests that some of the key variables involved in these pathways include family history of mood disorders (particularly chronic depression), temperament, early adversity, and the development of neurobiological stress response systems.

With respect to treatment, a number of issues require further study. First, there are only limited data on the efficacy of psychotherapy for dysthymic disorder and chronic depression. Research is needed to determine the specificity and range of efficacious psychotherapeutic treatments and to identify the "active" ingredients and processes in order to develop optimal treatment packages. In addition, there are remarkably few data available to help determine the optimal parameters of psychosocial interventions, such as the frequency of sessions and the duration of treatment. Finally, despite the existence of efficacious treatments, only a minority of patients achieve a full response to a single medication or course of time-limited psychotherapy. Hence, there is a critical need for research that will help to develop algorithms for the optimal sequencing and combination of psychosocial and pharmacological treatments.

Recent research on chronic depression also has significant implications for revisions to the diagnostic nomenclature in DSM-V. This work indicates that there are clinically significant and etiologically relevant differences between chronic forms of depression and episodic major depression (Klein & Santiago, 2003). At the same time, there appear to be few meaningful differences between the various forms of chronic depression (Klein, Shankman, et al., 2004). These findings suggest that it may be possible to simplify the classification of depressive disorders by combining the various forms of chronic depression and introducing a distinction between chronic and episodic depression. As distinctions in severity are clinically important for treatment planning and monitoring, these groups could be subdivided by severity, producing a fourfold classification consisting of moderate-severe chronic (double depression and chronic major depression), mild chronic (dysthymia), moderate-severe acute (episodic major depression), and mild acute (minor depression) depressive conditions (Klein, Shankman, et al., 2004).

KEY READINGS

Akiskal, H. S. (1983). Dysthymic disorder: Psychopathology of proposed chronic depressive subtypes. *American Journal of Psychiatry, 140*, 11–20.

American Psychological Association. (1980). *Diagnostic and statistical manual of mental disorders third edition.* Washington, DC: American Psychological Association.

American Psychological Association. (2000). *Diagnostic and statistical manual of mental disorders fourth edition, text revision.* Washington, DC: American Psychological Association.

Arnow, B. A., & Constantino, M. J. (2003). Effectiveness of psychotherapy and combination treatment for chronic depression. *Journal of Clinical Psychology, 59*, 893–905.

Dougherty, L. R., Klein, D. N., & Davila, J. (in press). A growth curve analysis of the effects of chronic stress on the course of dysthymic disorder: Moderation by adverse parent–child relationships and family history. *Journal of Consulting and Clinical Psychology, 72*, 1012–1021.

Goodman, S. (2002). Depression and early adverse experiences. In I. H. Gotlib & C. L. Hammen. *Handbook of depression* (pp. 245–267). New York: Guilford Press.

Keller, M. B., McCullough, J. P., Klein, D. N., et al. (2000). A comparison of nefazodone, the cognitive behavioral-analysis system of psychotherapy, and their combination for the treatment of chronic depression. *New England Journal of Medicine, 342*, 1462–1470.

Keller, M. B., & Shapiro, R. W. (1982). "Double depression": Superimposition of acute depressive episodes on chronic depressive disorders. *American Journal of Psychiatry, 139*, 438–442.

Kessler, R. C., McGonagle, K. A., Zhao, S., Nelson, C. B., Hughes, M., Eshleman, S., et al. (1994). Lifetime and 12-month prevalence of DSM-III-R psychiatric disorders in the United States: Results from the National Comorbidity Survey. *Archives of General Psychiatry, 51*, 8–19.

Klein, D. N., Durbin, C. E., Shankman, S. A., & Santiago, N. J. (2002). Depression and personality. In I. H. Gotlib & C. L. Hammen. *Handbook of depression* (pp. 115–140). New York: Guilford Press.

Klein, D. N., Riso, L. P., Donaldson, S. K., Schwartz, J. E., Anderson, R. L., Ouimette, P. C., et al. (1995). Family study of early-onset dysthymia: Mood and personality disorders in relatives of outpatients with dysthymia and episodic major depression and normal controls. *Archives of General Psychiatry, 52*, 487–496.

Klein, D. N., & Santiago, N. J. (2003). Dysthymia and chronic depression: Introduction, classification, risk factors, and course. *Journal of Clinical Psychology, 59*, 807–816.

Klein, D. N., Santiago, N. J., Vivian, D., Arnow, B. A., Blalock, J. A., Dunner, D. L., et al. (2004). Cognitive-behavioral analysis system of psychotherapy as a maintenance treatment for chronic depression. *Journal of Consulting and Clinical Psychology, 72*, 681–688.

Klein, D. N., Shankman, S. A., Lewinsohn, P. M., Rohde, P., & Seeley, J. R. (2004). Family study of chronic depression in a community sample of young adults. *American Journal of Psychiatry, 161*, 646–653.

Klein, D. N., & Vocisano, C. (1999). Depressive and self-defeating (masochistic) personality disorders. In T. Millon, P. Blaney, & R. Davis (Eds.), *Oxford textbook of psychopathology* (pp. 653–673). New York: Oxford University Press.

Kocsis, J. H. (2003). Pharmacotherapy and chronic depression. *Journal of Clinical Psychology, 59*, 885–892.

Lara, M. E., & Klein, D. N. (1999). Psychological processes underlying the maintenance and persistence of depression: implications for understanding chronic depression. *Clinical Psychology Review, 19*, 553–570.

Lewinsohn, P. M., Rohde, P., Seeley, J. R., & Hops, H. (1991). Comorbidity of unipolar depression: I. Major depression with dysthymia. *Journal of Abnormal Psychology, 100*, 205–213.

Mark, D. G., Barber, J. P., & Crits-Christoph, P. (2003). Supportive-expressive therapy for chronic depression. *Journal of Clinical Psychology, 59*, 859–872.

Markowitz, J. C. (2003). Interpersonal psychotherapy for chronic depression. *Journal of Clinical Psychology, 59*, 847–858.

McCullough, J. (2003). Treatment for chronic depression using cognitive behavioral analysis system of psychotherapy. *Journal of Clinical Psychology, 59*, 833–846.

Monroe, S. M., & Hadjiyannakis, K. (2002). The social environment and depression: focusing on severe life stress. In I. H. Gotlib & C. L. Hammen (Eds.), *Handbook of depression* (pp. 314–340). New York: Guilford Press.

Nemeroff, C. B., Heim, C. M., Thase, M. E., Klein, D. N., Rush, A. J., Schatzberg, A. F., et al. (2003). Differential responses to psychotherapy versus pharmacotherapy in patients with chronic forms of major depression and childhood trauma. *Proceedings of the National Academy of Sciences, 100*, 14293–14296.

Riso, L. P. & Klein, D. N. (2004). Vulnerability to chronic depression: A review and preliminary model. In J. E. Alpert & M. Fava (Eds.), *Handbook of chronic depression* (pp. 49–71). New York: Marcel Dekker.

Riso, L. P. & Newman, C. F. (2003). Cognitive therapy for chronic depression. *Journal of Clinical Psychology, 59,* 817–831.

Thase, M. E., Jindal, R., & Howland, R. H. (2002). Biological aspects of depression. In I. H. Gotlib & C. L. Hammen. *Handbook of depression* (pp. 192–218). New York: The Guilford Press.

Encopresis

Clinton E. Field • Patrick C. Friman

ENCOPRESIS

What Is Encopresis?

Encopresis is generally defined as fecal incontinence, not resulting from physiological defect, among children with the developmental ability necessary to attain continence. Diagnostic criteria specified by the Diagnostic and Statistic Manual of Mental Disorders, 4th edition (DSM-IV) (American Psychiatric Association, 1994) include:

1. repeated passage of fecal matter into inappropriate places,
2. at least one episode of fecal incontinence per month for a minimum of three months,
3. four years of age or attainment of equivalent developmental level, and
4. incontinence not due to substances or physiological dysfunction.

Constipation is a physiological exception and is reflected by DSM-IV subtypes "with constipation and overflow incontinence" and "without constipation and overflow incontinence." An additional distinction is that of primary versus secondary encopresis. The primary subsample includes children that have not previously exhibited continence while the secondary subsample includes children that attained continence but subsequently became incontinent.

The etiology of encopresis remains unclear, in part due to the many variables that impact the elimination process (e.g., biological processes, diet, learning, emotion). It is likely that encopresis is the outcome of multiple aberrant pathways, not all of which are clearly understood. Nonetheless, several factors are known to play a causal role in the development of encopretic conditions including:

1. a congenital or acquired predisposition for constipation;
2. a diet insufficient in roughage, bulk, or quality fiber;
3. a diet excessively high in dairy products (this can reduce movement in the colon);
4. limited fluid intake or dehydration;
5. fecal retention or elimination avoidance;
6. side effects of medications; and
7. emotional states including level of motivation.

The prevailing etiological perspective is that some combination of these factors interact with a series of aversive biological events (e.g., painful bowel movements, constipation, abdominal pain) that negatively reinforce the child's tendency to avoid defecation and retain fecal matter, ultimately, resulting in subsequent biological events (e.g., increased constipation, incontinence, and fecal impaction) that represent significant health concerns (Friman, 2003).

Encopresis has been described as a "complex, multiply determined problem" (McGrath, Mellon, & Murphy, 2000) and as a "heterogeneous problem" (Schroeder & Gordon, 2002). Historically, incontinence has been construed as a psychological

Field, C. E., & Friman, P. C. (2006). Encopresis. In J. E. Fisher & W. T. O'Donohue (Eds.), *Practitioner's guide to evidence-based psychotherapy*. New York: Springer.

problem and framed as a symptom of problematic family background, a wrinkle in psychodynamic functioning, or a reflection of laziness or oppositionality. Such perspectives generated treatment that neglected the biological aspects of the condition and were often punitive or stigmatizing (e.g., Friman & Jones, 1998; Levine, 1982) in addition to being ineffective. Encopresis has been subjected to limited well-controlled research (e.g., McGrath et al., 2000), which is surprising since it is a highly frustrating, chronic, socially impairing condition linked to severe physiological consequences (Friman, 2003). Variability in problem presentation and the historical absence of a cogent conceptual framework may have suppressed initial attempts to investigate the problem. However, the defining clinical features of this condition are biological and a biobehavioral conceptualization of encopresis, widely acknowledged in recent years, has yielded an empirically informed clinical approach to the problem and a substantive scientific literature (e.g., Friman & Jones, 1998; Houts, 1991; Levine, 1982).

BASIC FACTS ABOUT ENCOPRESIS

1. Encopresis is often preceded or accompanied by constipation.
2. Encopresis is exhibited by 1–3% of the pediatric population (e.g., Bellman, 1966), although estimates as high as 7.5% have been reported (e.g., Doleys, 1983).
3. Encopretic concerns account for 3% of pediatric office visits and approximately 25% of referrals to pediatric gastroenterologists (Schroeder & Gordon, 2002).
4. Encopresis accounts for 3–6% of psychiatric office visits (e.g., Olatawura, 1973).
5. Encopresis is three to six times more likely to be experienced by males than females (Bellman, 1966).
6. Encopresis generally declines as children age with many children experiencing spontaneous recovery by early adolescence (e.g., Houts & Abramson, 1990).
7. Encopresis is not causally related to other child clinical problems or behavior concerns although such conditions may comorbidly exist and may impact treatment progress.
8. Significant physical health consequences can result from untreated or improperly treated encopretic conditions.

ASSESSMENT

What Should Be Ruled Out?

A thorough medical evaluation should investigate and rule out organic origins of incontinence. The presence of a disease process may preclude the need for further therapist involvement. A detailed review of differential diagnoses and associated medical conditions (e.g., imperforate anus, Hirschsprung's Disease, Hypothyroidism) is not feasible here. However, this information is readily available (e.g., Barr, Levine, & Watkins, 1979; Christopherson & Mortweet, 2001) and practitioners should be familiar with them.

What is Involved in Effective Assessment

There are two phases in the assessment of encopresis: medical evaluation and behavioral assessment. As a rule, behavioral assessment and treatment should not progress until a thorough medical evaluation has been completed.

The medical evaluation should assess the functioning of the external anal sphincter and whether surplus fecal matter has accumulated within the colon. As fecal matter accumulates, the colon becomes distended and serious medical concerns emerge (e.g., McGuire, Rothenberg, & Tyler, 1983). Typical medical assessment procedures include abdominal palpitation, rectal examination, and possibly X-ray evaluation (e.g., KUB [X-ray of kidneys, ureter, and bladder]).

A behavioral assessment can be conducted by a variety of trained health care providers and should include history of toilet training and encopresis development, associated treatment and results, and description of the context surrounding incontinence. Assessing reactions of the child and caregivers to incidents of fecal incontinence can also be valuable.

What Assessments are Not Helpful?

Data suggesting that aberrant psychological profiles are not related to elimination problems is mounting (e.g., Friman, Mathews, Finney, Christophersen, & Leibowitz, 1998). Thus, traditional psychological testing, especially when it focuses on personality, is of limited value.

TREATMENT

What Treatments are Effective?

A review by McGrath et al. (2000) categorized treatments as "well established," "probably efficacious," or a "promising intervention." Each of the treatments described included medical intervention, which is critical in treating encopresis. Reported cure rates ranged from approximately 55% (medical intervention plus positive reinforcement, medical intervention plus biofeedback) to approximately 82% (behavioral intervention plus medical management).

Consistent with this data, the treatment approach described here is biobehavioral and combines behavioral strategies (derived from established learning principles) and medical strategies (derived from the science of physiology) in resolving encopresis (e.g., Christopherson & Friman, 2004; Christopherson & Mortweet, 2001).

What are Effective Self-help Treatments?

Due to the biological nature of this condition and the potential for severe physiological consequences, self-help treatments are not recommended. Further, the effectiveness of such treatments has not been established.

Useful Websites

http://www.therapyadvisor.com/default.aspx. Biobehavioral treatment for functional encopresis: National Institute of Mental Health resource describing scientific approaches to treatment.

http://encopresistreatment.com. Encopresis Treatment Center: General information regarding the causes and treatment of encopresis.

http://ww.aboutencopresis.com/index.html. About Encopresis.com: Information regarding condition and treatment supported by eMedicine.

Useful Self-Help Manual

Owens-Stively, J., McCain, D., & Wynne, E. (1986). *Childhood constipation and soiling: A practical guide for parents and children.* Minneapolis, MN: Minneapolis Children's Medical Center.

What Are Effective Therapist-Based Treatments?

Biobehavioral approaches to treatment that include multiple treatment components (medical and behavioral) are associated with the best outcomes and lowest relapse rates. Primary healthcare providers (e.g., pediatrician, pediatric psychologist) function as the delivery agents of treatment and should be involved in treatment planning and implementation. Caregivers (e.g., parents) approaching treatment may be frustrated or pessimistic and empathic strategies can be used to encourage optimism and participation as treatment progresses.

Primary components of treatment include:

1. *Demystification.* Beginning early in treatment the provider should identify and correct faulty beliefs, misattributions, or stereotypes that may have been applied to the child as a result of incontinence. Intervention is flexible and may include data, metaphors, or analogies to invalidate faulty notions about the problem and replace with appropriate and accurate information.

2. *Bowel evacuation.* Central to treatment is the evacuation of retained fecal matter. Treatment should yield a clear colon and help establish regular bowel movements in the toilet. Enemas, suppositories, or medication (laxatives) may be used to promote bowel cleanout. Procedures are prescribed and monitored by the child's physician who is aided by the therapist. Cleanout procedures are implemented in the home setting by the child's caregivers except under extreme circumstances where it may occur in a primary medical setting. Caregivers may be required to implement similar procedures on a regular basis to prevent additional fecal retention.

3. *Medication adherence and fading.* A number of medical interventions may be prescribed to accomplish bowel evacuation and to increase motility of fecal matter within the colon. Therapists play a critical role in promoting medication adherence and in developing effective fading strategies. Clinical challenges related to adherence include helping parents remember to use medication, providing education regarding the necessity of medication and its appropriate use, and motivating children to participate in treatment. Most children will initially be prescribed a stool softener to aid in evacuation or to encourage regular bowel movements. The medication softens fecal matter considerably thereby decreasing the pain and increasing the frequency and ease of bowel movements.

Liberal doses of mineral oil may be used to soften stool although prescription laxatives, such as MiraLax, are prescribed extensively as well. Typical dosing of MiraLax calls for a tablespoon per day mixed with a preferred beverage, however, physician's instructions should be obtained and carefully followed (Physicians' Desk Reference, 2004). A bowel movement is expected within a few days of initiating use.

A more invasive but often necessary procedure is enema use. Enemas are utilized when laxatives are insufficient for colonic evacuation, especially at treatment onset. Ongoing use of enemas may be required in cases of treatment-resistant children or children that are highly retentive. Specific instructions for use will accompany the enema. Caregivers should prepare the bathroom by laying a towel on the floor and by gathering toys or materials to distract the child during the enema. A second enema is usually conducted approximately an hour after the first. The amount and consistency of evacuated contents should be monitored and reported to the prescribing physician.

It is preferable not to utilize enemas (or suppositories) when treating children for encopresis unless absolutely necessary. In contrast, oral medication such as mineral oil or MiraLax will be almost uniformly prescribed to aid in evacuation.

4. *Toileting schedule.* The child should regularly attempt bowel movements in a manner consistent with effective toileting practices. Bathroom trips are scheduled and the

child is required to sit on the toilet for five to ten minutes while attempting a bowel movement. Two sits per day is a typical schedule, although scheduling and frequency can be manipulated as necessary to provide for regular practice and bowel movements. Stimulation of the gastrocolonic reflex increases the chance of successful practice when practice is scheduled following a meal.

5. *Rewarding toileting effort.* This is especially important early in treatment while new skills and habits are being developed. Rewards can range from simple praise to potent reward systems. Simple strategies that may be used include sticker charts, dot-to-dot drawings (Friman & Jones, 1998), or picture coloring. Goal completion is associated with access to a grab bag or other reward. Potent rewards such as small prizes and special time should be reserved for successful bowel movements and less potent reinforcers used to encourage effort and compliance.

6. *Consequences of accidents.* Toileting accidents are typical during treatment and parents should not criticize or punish. Intervention should include a matter-of-fact cleanup process developmentally matched to the child's age. Consequences should be logically linked to cleanup of the accident and children should be praised for their compliance with cleanup activities. Children may have partial accidents and parents should be advised to require a toilet sit following accidents to ensure that the bowel movement is complete. Interruption of an inappropriate bowel movement and appropriate completion should yield praise and reward in a manner consistent with the strategies described previously. Children may be resistant to cleanup or required sitting on the toilet and mild aversive consequences may be used to modify this behavior. Such consequences are not designed to punish incontinence but rather to modify noncompliance with treatment. Aversive consequences may include positive practice (Christopherson & Mortweet, 2001), response cost procedures (Reimers, 1996), or a variety of other behavior modification practices (e.g., use of chair time-out, limited loss of play time or special activities).

7. *Cleanliness training.* Two aspects of cleanup are critical for children that have experienced bowel incontinence: wiping and flushing. Children receiving treatment often have not had extensive exposure to these practices and have been engaged in the practice of opposing habits. They have grown accustomed to circumstances devoid of proper hygiene and waste management practices. Such skills must be trained and practiced.

8. *Parental monitoring.* Caregivers must assess progress, provide praise and reward, and detect/manage accidents quickly. Parents should be trained to monitor their children via regular underwear checks to discern if accidents have occurred. Parents should also monitor progress by tracking toileting success and the amount and consistency of fecal matter.

9. *Dietary changes.* The guiding treatment objective is to establish bowel movement regularity and promote passage of fecal matter with a consistent and quality high-fiber diet. This will improve colonic motility and promote the presence of soft fecal matter that is easily passed. A variety of strategies for enhancing diet have been developed (e.g., Christopherson & Mortweet, 2001) and should be incorporated into treatment.

What is Effective Medical Treatment?

As mentioned previously, medical assessment and intervention are necessary components of biobehavioral treatment of encopresis. Alternative medical treatments and medical treatment alone (absent supportive behavioral strategies) have not been established as effective.

Other Issues in Management

1. Encopresis may be a preventable condition when risk and developmental factors are incorporated into standardized toilet training routines (e.g., Levine, 1982).
2. Healthcare providers that intend to treat encopresis should obtain a working understanding of the physiology related to fecal matter passage and evacuation.
3. The best-case scenario for treatment involves physicians and therapists partnering for implementing and monitoring treatment progress. The physician maintains responsibility for prescribing and titrating medication while therapists aid in promoting adherence, monitoring progress, and in fading medical interventions.
4. In many cases, treatment may progress over a period of weeks, and potentially months, requiring long-term follow up by the therapist.

How Does One Select Among Treatments?

As mentioned previously, McGrath et al. (2000) provide a review of empirically supported treatments. Biobehavioral approaches to treatment have produced best outcomes and should be prioritized unless individual circumstances preclude doing so.

KEY READINGS

Christopherson, E. R. & Friman, P. C. (2004). Elimination disorders. In R. Brown (Ed.), *Handbook of pediatric psychology in school settings* (pp. 467–487). Mahwah, NJ: Erlbaum.

Friman, P. C. (2003). Biobehavioral approach to bowel and toilet training treatment. In W. O'Donohue, J. E. Fisher, & S. C. Hayes (Eds.), *Cognitive behavior therapy: Applying empirically supported techniques in your practice* (pp. 51–58). Hoboken, NJ: John Wiley & Sons.

Friman, P. C. & Jones, K. M. (1998). Elimination disorders in children. In T. S. Watson & F. M. Gresham (Eds.), *Handbook of child behavior therapy* (pp. 239–260). New York: Plenum Press.

Levine, M. D. (1982). Encopresis: Its potentiation, evaluation, and alleviation. *Pediatric Clinics of North America, 29*, 315–330.

REFERENCES

American Psychiatric Association. (1994). *Diagnostic and statistical manual of mental disorders* (4th ed.). Washington, DC: Author.

Barr, R. G., Levine, M. D., & Watkins, J. B. (1979). Recurrent abdominal pain due to lactose intolerance. *New England Journal of Medicine, 300(26)*, 1449–1452.

Bellman, M. (1966). Studies on encopresis. *Acta Paediatrica Scandinavia, 55(Suppl. 170)*, 1–151.

Christopherson, E. R. & Friman, P. C. (2004). Elimination disorders. In R. Brown (Ed.), *Handbook of pediatric psychology in school settings* (pp. 467–487). Mahwah, NJ: Erlbaum.

Christopherson, E. R. & Mortweet, S. L. (2001). *Treatments that work with children: Empirically supported strategies for managing childhood problems*. Washington, DC: American Psychological Association.

Doleys, D. M. (1983). Enuresis and encopresis. In T. H. Ollendick & M. Hersen (Eds.), *Handbook of child psychopathology* (pp. 201–226). New York: Plenum Press.

Friman, P. C. (2003). Biobehavioral approach to bowel and toilet training treatment. In W. O'Donohue, J. E. Fisher, & S. C. Hayes (Eds.), *Cognitive behavior therapy: Applying empirically supported techniques in your practice* (pp. 51–58). Hoboken, NJ: John Wiley & Sons.

Friman, P. C. & Jones, K. M. (1998). Elimination disorders in children. In T. S. Watson & F. M. Gresham (Eds.), *Handbook of child behavior therapy* (pp. 239–260). New York: Plenum Press.

Friman, P. C., Mathews, J., Finney, J. W., Christophersen, E. R., & Leibowitz, J. M. (1988). Do encopretic children have clinically significant behavior problems? *Pediatrics, 82*, 407–409.

Houts, A. C. (1991). Nocturnal enuresis as a biobehavioral problem. *Behavior Therapy, 22*, 133–151.

Houts, A. M. & Abramson, H. (1990). Assessment and treatment for functional childhood enuresis and encopresis: Toward a partnership between health psychologists and physicians. In S. B. Morgan & T. M. Okwumabua (Eds.), *Child and adolescent disorders: Developmental and health psychology perspectives* (pp. 47–103). Hillsdale, NJ: Erlbaum.

Levine, M. D. (1982). Encopresis: Its potentiation, evaluation, and alleviation. *Pediatric Clinics of North America, 29*, 315–330.

McGrath, M. L., Mellon, M. W., & Murphy, L. (2000). Empirically supported treatments in pediatric psychology: Constipation and encopresis. *Journal of Pediatric Psychology, 25*, 225–254.

McGuire, T., Rothenberg, M., & Tyler, D. (1983). Profound shock following interventions for chronic untreated stool retention. *Clinical Pediatrics, 23,* 459–461.

Olatawura, M. O. (1973). Encopresis: A review of thirty-two cases. *Acta Paediatrica Scandinavia, 62,* 358–364.

Physicians' desk reference (58th ed.). (2004). Montvale, NJ: Thomson PDR.

Reimers, T. M. (1996). A biobehavioral approach toward managing encopresis. *Behavioral Modification, 20,* 469–479.

Schroeder, C. S. & Gordon, B. N. (2002). *Assessment and treatment of childhood problems: A clinician's guide* (3rd ed.). New York: Guilford Press.

CHAPTER 28

Treatment of Erectile Dysfunction

Nancy Gambescia • Gerald Weeks

WHAT IS MALE ERECTILE DISORDER?

Male Erectile Disorder or Erectile Dysfunction (ED) is the persistent or recurrent inability to attain, or to maintain until completion of the sexual activity, an adequate erection. The disturbance causes marked distress or interpersonal difficulty. The erectile dysfunction is not better accounted for by another Axis I disorder (other than a Sexual Dysfunction) and is not due exclusively to the direct physiological effects of a substance (e.g., a drug of abuse, a medication) or a general medical condition (APA, 1994).

- *Lifelong*. An extremely rare presentation in which the man has always had an erectile dysfunction.
- *Acquired*. This common form follows a period of normal sexual functioning that may have extended for years or decades.
- *Generalized*. A rarely reported variety that occurs in all situations, with a partner or during masturbation.
- *Situational*. The man has difficulty in certain situations or with some partners and not others. It is more common.

FACTS ABOUT ED

How Prevalent is ED?

ED is increasingly common with age (Feldman et. al, 1994; Lue, 2000). According to Bacon et al., (2003) healthy American men reported the following incidence:

- 4% between the ages of 40 and 49.
- 26% between 50 and 59,
- 40% between 60 and 69,
- 61% of men over 70.

What are the Causes of ED?

- *Organic*. ED is not necessarily a natural consequence of aging. Nevertheless, organic causes, such as diabetes or vascular disease, are clearly age dependent (Feldman et. al, 1994). These conditions interfere with erections by physically reducing the available blood supply to the penis.
- *Psychogenic*. Emotional factors, such as depression, anxiety, or relationship discord can adversely affect the physiological responses necessary for erectile capacity (Araujo, et al., 1998; Rosen, 2001).
- *Combined etiology*. Even in cases of organic etiology, if the man becomes anxious about diminished sexual performance, the residual erectile functioning can deteriorate.

Gambescia, N. & Weeks, G. (2006). Treatment of erectile dysfunction. In J. E. Fisher & W. T. O'Donohue (Eds.), *Practitioner's guide to evidence-based psychotherapy*. New York: Springer.

What are the Physical Risk Factors for ED?

Chronic diseases increase in prevalence with aging and contribute to ED (Feldman et al., 1994; Laumann, Paik & Rosen, 1999; Bacon et al., 2003).

- *Diabetes* causes atherosclerosis and nerve damage, affecting the blood vessels and impeding the nerve supply to the penis (Braun et al., 2000).
- *Hypertension* is a result of disease processes that obstruct circulation and can also cause ED (Feldman et al., 1994; Burchardt et al., 2000).
- *Parkinson's disease* affects erectile functioning by impairing the central nervous system processes needed to promote erection.
- *Cardiovascular disease* cause decreased oxygen supply to the arteries and organs including the penis (Meuleman, 2002; Sullivan, Keoghane, & Miller, 2002).
- *Other medical conditions* that have been associated with ED include thyroid problems, lung disease, and epilepsy.
- *Prostate cancer and its treatments* can damage nerves needed for erectile function.

Medications
- Many prescription drugs used to treat hypertension and other vascular and cardiac problems can adversely affect erectile capacity (Burchardt et al., 2000; Kloner, 2000).
- Psychotropic drugs for the treatment of anxiety, depression, and other psychological problems can impede erectile capacity (Labbate, Croft, & Oleshansky, 2003).

Modifiable physical risk factors
- *Smoking* may damage blood vessels that are needed for maintaining an erection (Condra et al., 1986; Sullivan, Keoghane, & Miller, 2002; Bacon et al., 2003).
- *Diet.* High cholesterol can harden, narrow, or block the arteries leading to the penis, resulting in ED (Feldman et al., 2000; Bacon et al., 2003).
- *Inactivity.* The absence of cardiovascular exercises increases the risk of heart disease, circulatory problems, and ED (Derby et al., 2000; Bacon et al., 2003).
- *Recreational drugs and alcohol* often decrease sexual performance (Bacon et al., 2003).
- Obesity is associated with increased risk of ED (Esposito et al., 2004; Saigal, 2004; Bacon et al., 2003).

Can a man Delay the Onset of ED?

Exercising, keeping the body lean, and not smoking can delay the onset of ED by approximately ten years according to Bacon et al. (2003).

What is the Prognosis Associated with ED?

Many cases of ED have medical causes that cannot be cured yet there are effective medical and psychological treatment options that will restore sexual functioning.

What Psychological Factors can Predispose a Man to Experience ED?

Risk factors are those issues within the individual, the relationship, or family background that predispose the man to experience sexual problems (Weeks & Gambescia, 2000).

The man's personal issues
- Performance anxiety is a specific type of anxiety that is sexually based. It stems from over-concern about being able to obtain and maintain an erection. The man worries and anticipates negative consequences, removing himself emotionally from the pleasurable feelings associated with sex play and intercourse.
- Depression and situational stressors such as career, financial, and family concerns can adversely affect a man's sexual functioning.

- Sexual ignorance and misinformation can limit or distort a man's sexual expectations and performance.
- Negative sexual cognitions and attitudes about sex can fuel performance anxiety.
- Body image concerns, fears of aging, apprehension about physical desirability can interfere with sexual enjoyment.

The man's relationship to his partner The following relationship issues can contribute to ED:

- communication problems,
- ineffective problem solving and conflict management,
- deficient sexual chemistry,
- incompatible sexual belief systems,
- a partner with a sexual dysfunction (such as the lack of desire or sexual pain),
- anger or resentment,
- life cycle changes such as fertility problems, having a baby, retirement, children leaving,
- fears of intimacy, dependency, rejection, losing or being controlled,
- lack of trust in his partner,
- infidelity.

Intergenerational and cultural dynamics

- Internalized negative attitudes about sexuality learned within the family of origin,
- gender-typed beliefs about sexuality such as performance oriented sex,
- faulty or rigid religious beliefs about sexual pleasure,
- internalized myths, legacies, secrets, and conflicts regarding sexuality,
- conflicted parental relationships,
- history of sexual abuse or covert incest.

ASSESSMENT

How can I Ask Specifically About Erectile Functioning?

The following questions will aid the clinician in determining the presence and severity of ED (Rosen, 1997; Rosen, Cappelleri, Smith, Lipsky, & Pena, 1999)

- How often are you able to get an erection during sexual activity?
- When you have erections with sexual stimulation, how often were your erections hard enough for penetration?
- When you attempt sexual intercourse, how often are you able to penetrate your partner?
- During sexual intercourse, how difficult was it to maintain your erection to completion of intercourse?
- Were you satisfied with the hardness of your erection?
- Were you satisfied with the overall sexual experience?
- Is sexual stimulation with your partner adequate?

What Questions can be Used to Distinguish Psychogenic from Organic ED?

Healthy men often have involuntary erections when awakening from sleep. Being unable to experience or maintain an erection upon awakening suggests that the problem is organic. Also, ED caused by organic factors occurs gradually but continuously over a period of time. Psychogenic ED tends have an abrupt onset and is often related to a recent situation. In addition, the man may be able to attain and sustain erections in some circumstances but not in others.

- Do you awaken from sleep with an erection? Describe the firmness of the erection. Has there been a change in the firmness of your erection over time when you awaken from sleep? Is so, when did you notice the difference?
- During self-stimulation as compared to intercourse, do you experience the same or similar erectile functioning?
- Can you get an erection at any time with any partner?
- Do you have difficulty in certain situations and not others?

What General Medical Information Should be Obtained?

The following questions will help the clinician to obtain a general medical history and have an idea of the level of medical attention the man has received.

- When did you notice the onset of your erectile difficulties?
- Did you discuss this problem with a physician?
- When was your last visit to a physician? Do you see other medical doctors for specific problems?
- Do you have any medical conditions involving circulation, the central nervous system, and hormonal balance?
- Do you have any physical abnormalities of the penis such as a curvature (Peyronie disease)?
- Please list all medications you are taking, including the dose and duration. Did you include prescribed, and over the counter, vitamins and other dietary supplements?
- Did you have prior surgeries, pelvic trauma, prostate surgery or radiation to the prostate?
- Generally, are you in good health? Do you exercise regularly, and eat a sensible diet?
- Do you smoke?
- How much alcohol do you consume in a week or month?
- Do you use recreational drugs?
- What remedies have you tried to correct the situation on your own?

TREATMENT

What Medical Treatments are Effective?

The man with ED and his partner can choose between noninvasive and invasive treatment modalities. Generally, invasive measures are recommended only when the man does not respond to medications. It is the responsibility of the therapist to review the advantages and risks associated with all medical treatments.

Oral Medications Phosphodiesterase type 5 (PDE5) inhibitors are mild systemic vasodilators that augment the blood supply to the genitals but do not increase libido or desire.

- Cialis® (tadalafil): effective for 36 hours (Cialis, 2003)
- Levitra® (vardenafil): effective for 4 hours (Levitra, 2003)
- Viagra® (sildenafil): effective for 4 hours (Viagra, 2003)
  - PDE5 inhibitors are contraindicated when taking Nitrates because the blood pressure could drop to an unsafe level.
  - Alcohol should be consumed in moderation when taking PDE5 inhibitors because of the increased vasodilatation.
  - Common side-effects of PDE5 inhibitors include headache, reddening of the face and neck (flushing), indigestion, and nasal congestion. Cialis® may cause muscle aches and back pain, which usually resolve 48 hours.

Vacuum constriction device This noninvasive device promotes erection through the insertion of the penis into a clear plastic cylinder. A hand or battery operated pump draws air from the cylinder and creates a vacuum. Reduced air pressure within the cylinder allows increased blood flow to the penis, causing an erection. Blood is trapped through the use of the tourniquet applied around the base of the penis that is removed after sexual relations. Although some men and their partners are satisfied with this appliance, few use it because of the mechanical issues, inconvenience, dampening of sexual spontaneity (Jardin et al., 2000).

Transurethral system A tiny pellet is inserted into the penile urethra with a thin plastic applicator approximately 15 minutes prior to sexual relations. The pellet contains a vasodilator which dissolves within the urethra and is absorbed into the, erectile tissue, promoting tumescence. Theoretically, a resulting erection can last for an hour, however, efficacy is often limited and many men experience burning after insertion (Mulhall Jahoda, Ahmed, & Parker, 2001).

Intracavernosal injection This direct delivery approach involves injecting a vasodilator directly into the erectile tissue of the penis roughly 20 minutes prior to anticipated sex. Essentially, the injection promotes an erection that can last for an hour by increasing the blood flow into the penis. Each man requires an individualized dosing regimen. Most men report successful erections, once the proper dose is found, although it cannot be used every day (Shabsigh et al., 2000).

Penile prosthesis Penile implants require a surgical procedure for insertion. Flexible rods or inflatable tubes are surgically inserted into the erectile tissue of the penis enabling tumescence sufficient for sexual relations. The flexible implant can be manipulated into different positions for sexual relations or for rest. The inflatable implant includes more working components. A pump is usually inserted into the abdomen with a reservoir of sterile liquid stored in the scrotum. When an erection is desired, the man pumps the fluid from the reservoir to the cylinders within the penis. The benefits must be carefully weighed against the associated risks of invasive surgery, anesthesia, and infection. Also, surgical, mechanical, and financial issues should be carefully considered (Carson, 2000).

What Psychological Treatment Options are Available?

Even if ED is caused by a physical problem, psychotherapy can help the man and his partner. For any medical treatment to be effective, the man's psychological reactions, and those of his partner need to be addressed (Weeks & Gambescia, 2000).

Individual psychotherapy Individual therapy utilizes a multiple modalities including:

- psychoeducation about normal sexual functioning and about ED;
- cognitive therapy to counter self-defeating sexual thoughts and substitute positive, reality-based cognitions;
- behavioral interventions for anxiety reduction and desensitization;
- guided self-stimulation homework to attain erectile control and desensitize against anxiety.

Couples counseling provides a format for the man and his partner to:

- discuss treatment options,
- address and reduce fear and anxiety,
- positively reframe the problem to combat pessimism and skepticism,
- increase their understanding of sexual functioning and ED,

- improve sexual communication and create realistic expectations for sex,
- receive sensate focus homework exercises intended to interrupt the cycle of avoidance and promote satisfying sensual and sexual interactions.

What Factors Should be Ruled Out?
- The presence of other sexual dysfunctions, such as premature ejaculation, must be ruled out. Ask if the ED followed another sexual difficulty or contributed to problems with sexual desire or orgasm.
- ED can be a psychological response to a sexual dysfunction in the partner.
- ED may be the first presenting symptom of a serious undiagnosed medical condition such as atherosclerosis, diabetes, and hypertension. Thus, a medical evaluation should always be performed (Sullivan, Keoghane & Miller, 2002; Kirby, Jackson, Betteridge, Friedli, 2002).
- Depression can predispose a man to ED and should be ruled out. Nonetheless, ED can have a devastating impact on a relationship and can cause depression, which may become chronic if not treated.

What Other Issues can Affect the Management of ED?
- *Pessimism and skepticism.* Often, men with ED and their partners have been dealing with the problem for months or years unsuccessfully. They have tried to remedy the difficulty on their own, hoped that it would go away, and found that the more they tried the more they failed. Frequently, the couple has avoided physical intimacy for months or years. The therapist must instill optimism, provide information, and recommend realistic treatments.
- *Noncompliance* to medical or psychological therapies sometimes occurs even if the treatment is successful. It is important to encourage the man and his partner to discuss the reasons for failing to use a particular treatment. Determine if thy need information, reassurance, or another strategy.

What Readings and Websites can I Recommend to Clients?
- Zilbergeld, B. (1992b). *The new male sexuality.* New York: Bantam.
- Barbach, L. (1983). *For each other: Sharing sexual intimacy.* Garden City, NY: Doubleday.
- Comfort, A. (1972). *The joy of sex.* New York: Crown.
- http://kidney.niddk.nih.gov/kudiseases/pubs/impotence/.
- http://www.erectile-dysfunction-impotence.org/.
- http://www.duj.com/erectile.html.
- http://www.mayoclinic.com/invoke.cfm?id=DS00162.
- http://www.docguide.com/news/content.nsf/PatientResAllCateg/Erectile%20Dysfunction?OpenDocument.

KEY READINGS

American Psychiatric Association. (1994). *Diagnostic and statistical manual of mental disorders* (DSM IV). Washington, DC: Author.

Araujo, A. B., Durante, R., Feldman, H. A., Goldstein, I., & McKinlay, J. B. (1998). The relationship between depressive symptoms and male erectile dysfunction: Cross-sectional results from the Massachusetts Male Aging Study. *Psychosomatic Medicine, 60(4),* 458–465.

Bacon, C., Mittleman, M., Kawachi, I., Giovannucci, E., et al. (2003). Sexual function in Men Older Than 50 Years of Age: Results from the Health Professionals Follow-up Study. *Annals of Internal Medicine, 139(3),* 161–168.

Braun, M., Wassmer, G., Klotz, T., Reifenrath B., et al. (2000). Epidemiology of erectile dysfunction: results of the Cologne male survey. *International Journal of Impotence Research, 12,* 305–311.

Burchardt, M., Burchardt, T., Baer, L., et al. (2000). Hypertension is associated with severe erectile dysfunction. *Journal of Urology, 164(4),* 1188–1191.

Carson, C. (2000). Penile prosthesis implantation in the treatment of Peyronie's disease and erectile dysfunction. *International Journal of Impotence Research, 4,* S122–S126.

Cialis® (tadalafil) (2003). *European Union prescribing information.* Brussels: Eli Lilly Benelux.

Condra, M., Morales, A., Owen, J. A., et al. (1986). Prevalence and significance of tobacco smoking in impotence. *Urology, 27,* 495–498.

Derby, C. A., Mohr, B. A., Goldstein, I., Feldman, H. A., et al. (2000). Modifiable risk factors and erectile dysfunction: Can lifestyle changes modify risk? *Urology, 56(2),* 302–306.

Esposito, K., Giugliano, F., Di Palo, C., Giugliano, G., et al. (2004). Effect of lifestyle changes on erectile dysfunction in obese men. *Journal of the American Medical Association, 291,* 2978–2984.

Feldman, H. A., Goldstein, I., Hatzichristou, G., Krane, R. J., & McKinlay, J. B. (1994). Impotence and its medical and psychosocial correlates: Results of the Massachusetts male aging study. *Journal of Urology, 151,* 54–61.

Jardin, A., Wagner, G., Khoury, S. et al., (Eds.) (2000). *Erectile dysfunction.* Plymouth, UK: Health Publication Ltd.

Kirby, M., Jackson, G., Betteridge, J., & Friedli, K. (2002). Is erectile dysfunction a marker for cardiovascular disease? *International Journal of Clinical Practice, 55(9),* 614–618.

Kloner, R. A. (2000). Hypertension as a risk factor for erectile dysfunction: Implications for sildenifil use. *Journal of Clinical Hypertension, 2,* 33–36.

Labbate, L. A., Croft, H. A., & Oleshansky, M. A. (2003). Antidepressant-related erectile dysfunction: Management via avoidance, switching antidepressants, antidotes, and adaptation. *Journal of Clinical Psychiatry. 10(64),* 11–19.

Laumann, E. O., Paik, A., & Rosen, R. C. (1999) The epidemiology of erectile dysfunction: results from the National Health and Social Life Survey. *International Journal of Impotence Research, 11,* 60–64.

Levitra® (vardenafil) (2003). *Prescribing information.* West Haven, CT: Bayer Phamaceuticals Corp.

Lue, T. F. (2000). Erectile dysfunction. *New England Journal of Medicine, 342,* 1802–1813.

Meuleman, E. J. (2002). Prevalence of erectile dysfunction: need for treatment? *International Journal of Impotence Research, 14,* S22–S28.

Mulhall, J. P., Jahoda, A. E., Ahmed, A. & Parker, M. (2001). Analysis of the consistency of intraurethral prostaglandin E(1) (MUSE) during at-home use. *Urology, 58(2),* 262–266.

Rosen, R. C., Cappelleri, J. C., Smith, M. D., Lipsky, J., Pena, B. M. (1999). Development and evaluation of an abridged, 5-item version of the International Index of Erectile Function (IIEF-5) as a diagnostic tool for erectile dysfunction. *International Journal of Impotence Research, 11,* 319–326.

Rosen, R. C., Riley, A., Wagner, G., Osterloh, I. H., et al. (1997). The international index of erectile function (IIEF): a multidimensional scale for assessment of erectile dysfunction. *Urology, 49(6),* 822–830.

Saigal, C. S. (2004). Obesity and erectile dysfunction: common problems, common solution? *Journal of the American Medical Association, 291,* 3011–3012.

Shabsigh, R., Padma-Nathan, H., Gittleman, M., McMurray, J., et al. (2000). Intracavernous alprostadil alfadex (EDEX/VIRIDAL) is effective and safe in patients with erectile dysfunction after failing sildenafil (Viagra). *Urology, 55(4),* 477–480.

Sullivan, M. E., Keoghane, S. R., Miller, M. A. (2002). Vascular risk factors and erectile dysfunction. *British Journal of Urology International, 87(9),* 838–845.

Viagra® (sildenafil) (2003). *Prescribing information.* New York: Pfizer Inc.

Weeks, G. R. & Gambescia, N. (2000). *Erectile dysfunction: Integrating couple therapy, sex therapy, and medical treatment.* New York: Norton.

Pathological Gambling

Lorne M. Korman • Tony Toneatto • Wayne Skinner

WHAT IS PATHOLOGICAL GAMBLING?

The diagnosis of pathological gambling first appeared in the third edition of the American Psychiatric Association's Diagnostic and Statistical Manual in 1980, and appears again in DSM-IV (APA, 1994). Although the DSM-IV categorizes pathological gambling as an impulse-control disorder not elsewhere categorized, the criteria specified for diagnosing this disorder are somewhat similar to those for alcohol and substance dependence disorders. Gambling can be defined as an attempt to win money by betting money on an uncertain event. The principal criterion for the diagnosis in the DSM-IV is persistent, recurring gambling behaviour that disrupts personal, family, and vocational pursuits. Similar to those features defining substance use disorders, other criteria for pathological gambling include preoccupation with gambling; betting increasingly larger amounts or taking greater risks to attain the same level of excitement; repeated, unsuccessful efforts to stop; restlessness or irritability when attempting to stop or reduce gambling; and jeopardizing relationships, work, and studies because of gambling. Gambling to escape dysphoric feelings, lying to others to conceal losses, "chasing losses," turning to family members and others for financial bailouts, and antisocial, criminal (typically nonviolent) behaviours like stealing and embezzlement (Lesieur, 1988) in order to generate money to gamble, are also common features of pathological gambling and are specified as criteria for the disorder in the DSM-IV.

BASIC FACTS ABOUT PATHOLOGICAL GAMBLING

Comorbidity

Comorbid psychiatric disorders are common among pathological gamblers. Substance use disorders may cooccur in as many as 50% of pathological gamblers (Cunningham-Williams, Cottler, Compton, & Spitznagel, 1998; Lesieur, Blume, & Zoppa, 1985; Ramirez, McCormick, & Russo, 1983). Depression is also common among pathological gamblers (Bergh & Kuhlhorn, 1994; Blaszczynski & McConaghy, 1989, McCormick, Russo, Ramirez, & Taber, 1984). In one sample of 25 Gamblers Anonymous participants, 72% met criteria for major depression, and 52% had recurrent major depressive episodes (Linden, Pope, & Jonas, 1986). In another study of 50 pathological gamblers, 76% were found to suffer from major depression, and 38% met criteria for hypomanic disorder (McCormick et al., 1984). Obsessive–compulsive disorder (Linden et al., 1986), bipolar disorder (Linden et al., 1986), hypomania (McCormick et al., 1984), attention-deficit disorder (Carlton, et al., 1987), and anxiety disorders such as agoraphobia and panic are also much more common among pathological gamblers (Blaszczynski & McConaghy, 1989; Linden et al., 1986; McCormick et al., 1984; Linden et al., 1986). Suicide is also more prevalent among pathological gamblers, with 13–20% attempting suicide (Frank, Lester, & Wexler, 1991), and 48–70%

Korman, L. M., Toneatto, T., & Skinner, W. (2006). Pathological gambling. In J. E. Fisher & W. T. O'Donohue (Eds.), *Practitioner's guide to evidence-based psychotherapy*. New York: Springer.

contemplate ending their lives (Lesieur & Anderson, 1995; Thompson, Gazel, & Rickman, 1996).

The DSM-IV (1994) makes reference to higher rates of a number of personality disorders and their possible associations to pathological gambling. Blaszczynski and Steel (1998) studied 82 individuals in treatment for pathological gamblers, and found that 93% met also met criteria for a personality disorder, with most participants meeting criteria for more than one personality disorder. Highest prevalence rates, by cluster, were: for Cluster A, paranoid (33%) and schizotypal (31%); for Cluster B, borderline (57%), histrionic (54%), and narcissistic (47%); and for Cluster C, dependent (40%), avoidant (30%), and passive–aggressive (29%). Black and Moyer assessed 30 individuals self-reporting problem gambling and found 87% meeting criteria for a personality disorder, with obsessive–compulsive (59%), avoidant (50%), schizoid (33%), schizotypal (30%), paranoid (26%), and borderline (23%) personality disorders the most common. However, in a sample of 40 individuals attending an outpatient treatment program for problem gambling, only 25% were found to meet criteria for a personality disorder, with 5% in Cluster A, 7% in Cluster B, and 17.5 % in Cluster C, with avoidant personality the most common disorder, diagnosed in 12.5% of participants (Specker, Carlson, Edmonson, Johnson, & Marcotte, 1996). Interestingly, none of Specker et al.'s participants met criteria for antisocial personality disorder, and overall, the sample did not differ from nonpsychiatric controls with regard to prevalence of Axis II disorders. Other studies of pathological gamblers have found rates of antisocial personality disorder ranging from 15% to 40% (Black & Moyer, 1998; Bland, Newman, Orn, & Stebelsky, 1993; Blaszcynski & McConaghy, 1992).

While there is some evidence that personality disorders negatively predict response to clinical interventions (Reich & Green, 1991), there is little research on how such disorders might influence clinical outcomes specifically related to pathological gambling (Blaszczynski & Steel, 1998). Blaszczynki and McConaghy (1992) did find that pathological gamblers who also met criteria for antisocial personality disorder tended to exhibit more dysfunction in a variety of psychosocial domains. In one study of substance-using individuals at a Veteran's Administration centre, those diagnosed with concurrent borderline personality also had higher scores on the South Oaks Gambling Screen, as well as higher levels of impulsivity (Kruedelbach, McCormick, Schulz, & Grueneich, 1993).

Prevalence

Prevalence rates for pathological gambling vary from 1% to 2% in the United States (Shaffer, Hall, & van der Bilt, 1997), Canada (Ladouceur, 1996), and Europe (Beconia, 1996). There is a positive relationship between the availability of gambling and rates of both nonpathological and pathological gambling (Custer, 1982; Dickerson, 1989), and the increased availability of gambling is expected to result in greater higher rates of pathological gambling problems (Toneatto & Ladouceur, 2003). In Canada, where the availability of casinos, online gaming, and video lottery terminals has increased, revenues have increased from $2.7 billion in 1992 to $11.3 billion in 2002 (Statistics Canada, 2003).

Demographics

Gambling problems may be more likely to occur in younger people and among those in lower socioeconomic groups, and such problems are more likely to be related to slot machines gaming, which is practiced equally by men and women (Blaszczynski, Walker, Sagris, & Dickerson, 1997; Crisp et al., 2000). Younger men are significantly more likely than older individuals and women to develop gambling problems with casino games and racing activities (Hraba & Lee, 1995).

ASSESSMENT OF PATHOLOGICAL GAMBLING

What Should be Ruled Out?

Pathological gambling is not diagnosed if the presence of a manic episode better accounts for an individual's gambling (APA, 1994). According to the DSM-IV, pathological gambling must also be distinguished from social gambling, which occurs with friends or acquaintances, and usually entails losses of time and money that are predetermined and not detrimental to the individual's overall functioning. Although gambling may be secondary to, or exacerbated by a personality disorder, depression, substance use, or other disorders, these do not preclude the diagnosis of pathological gambling.

What is Involved in Effective Assessment?

An assessment of pathological gambling should involve an evaluation of:

- DSM-IV criteria for pathological gambling.
- Severity of pathological gambling, including:
  - frequency and types of gambling,
  - amount of money typically spent and lost on gambling,
  - beliefs about gambling,
  - debt,
  - criminal behavior to support gambling.
- Overall functional impairment.
- Criminal history.
- Assessment of concurrent disorders, including substance use, antisocial personality, and manic episodes.
- When concurrent disorders present, assessment of functional relationships, if any between pathological gambling and other disorder(s).
- Social support/isolation.
- Current suicidality, and history of suicidal ideation, intent, and planning.

Diagnostic Tools

Several structured clinical interviews for assessing problem gambling have been recently developed (i.e., Diagnostic Interview for Gambling Severity (DIGS); Winters, Specker & Stinchfield, 1997; Diagnostic Interview Schedule (DIS) Pathological Gambling Module (GAM-IV)), with encouraging evidence for their reliability and validity (Govoni, Frisch, & Stinchfield, 2001). The DSM-IV diagnostic criteria for pathological gambling have also been operationalized into a 10-item self-report measure (Beaudoin & Cox, 1999).

The South Oaks Gambling Screen (SOGS; Lesieur & Blume, 1987), although not a diagnostic tool, continues to be a widely used self-report screening tool. According to Stinchfield (2002), the SOGS demonstrates excellent sensitivity and selectivity in clinical populations. The Canadian Problem Gambling Index (CPGI; Ferris & Wynne, 2001) consists of three main sections; gambling involvement, problem gambling assessment, and correlates of problem gambling (including familial history of gambling); and yields five categories of gambling behaviour (ranging from nongambling to problem gambling). Initial studies indicate the CPGI possesses good reliability and validity (Ferris & Wynne, 2001).

The two-item, Lie/Bet questionnaire (i.e., "Have you ever felt the need to bet more and more money?"; "Have you ever had to lie to people important to you about how much you gambled?") has been shown to possess good predictive validity (Johnson, Hamer, Nora, & Tan, 1997; Johnson, Hamer, & Nora, 1998).

Attitude and Belief Measures Several self-report measures of gambling related cognitive processes have been developed. The Gambling Attitudes Scale (GAS; Kassinove, 1998) measures attitudes that correlate with the development of disordered gambling. Initial findings showed the scale had adequate internal consistency and construct validity in samples of college students. Breen and Zuckerman (1999) have developed the Gambling Attitudes and Belief Survey (GABS) to assess cognitive biases and irrational beliefs. Steenbergh, Meyers, May and Whelan (2002) have developed the Gambler's Belief Questionnaire (GBQ), which assesses gambling-related cognitive distortions, specifically surrounding luck, perseverance and illusion of control, and the Gambling Self-Efficacy Questionnaire (GESQ), to assess perceived self-efficacy to control gambling behaviour. These instruments may be particularly useful in treatment planning and evaluating intervention efficacy, and appear to possess adequate reliability and validity. The Gambling-Related Cognitions Scale (GRCS; Raylu & Oei, 2004) is a well-validated measure of gambling-related beliefs, consisting of fived factors: interpretive control/bias, illusion of control, predictive control, gambling-related expectancies, and perceived inability to stop gambling. Cognitive distortions specific to video lottery terminal users can be measured by the Informational Biases Scale (IBS; Jefferson & Nicki, 2003).

TREATMENT

What Treatments are Effective?

The American Psychological Association has recommended that Empirically Validated Treatments (EVT; Chambless & Hollon, 1998, 2001) consist of interventions that have been evaluated in randomized clinical trials and shown to be efficacious in at least two studies by at least two independent research teams. Based on these minimal criteria, there are no gambling treatments that could be considered empirically-validated. However, there are several promising treatment approaches for which there is supportive evidence. The reader is referred to Toneatto and Ladouceur (2003) for a recent critical review of the controlled gambling treatment literature.

The most effective treatments generally can be classified as brief and cognitive-behavioral in orientation. The emphasis has been placed on modifying gambling-related behaviors and cognitions using practical problem-solving strategies and developing behavioral and cognitive coping skills to reduce gambling frequency, gambling expenditures, or urges. Gambling treatment has been strongly influenced by cognitive-behavioral treatment of addictions.

Cognitive-Behavioral Treatment Echeburua, Baez and Montalvo (1996) found higher abstinence rates for three cognitive-behavioral treatments (exposure–response prevention, group cognitive restructuring, and combined treatment) at six months post-treatment compared to a waiting list control group. The individually administered response–prevention treatment appeared to be superior to the group or combined treatment at the one-year follow-up. More recently, Echeburua, Fernandez- Montalvo, & Baez (2000) found that slot machine gamblers randomly assigned to individual or group relapse prevention (RP) groups did significantly better at the 12-month follow-up than those in the control condition. All gamblers had first received behavioral treatment (i.e., stimulus control, in vivo exposure/response prevention) to decrease their gambling.

Cognitive Treatment The most consistent evidence for the efficacy of cognitively oriented treatment has been reported by Ladouceur and his colleagues (e.g., Sylvain, Ladouceur, & Boisvert, 1997; Ladouceur, et al. 2001, 2003). This group of researchers have consistently found that gamblers treated with cognitively oriented therapy reduce their gambling behavior (e.g., frequency, hours spent gambling) and perform better on measures of diagnostic symptoms, desire to gamble, and perceived self-efficacy, compared to a waiting list control group. Gains were maintained throughout a 2-year follow-up in the study by Ladouceur et al. (2003).

Emotion-Based Treatments While cognitive and behavioral theories and treatments have received the most empirical support in the study of pathological gambling, more recently there has been increasing attention on the role of emotions in this disorder. Blaszczynski and Nower (2002) for example, have posited that one subgroup of pathological gamblers may be emotionally vulnerable, and that gambling among this group is motivated by the need to regulate affect. Korman, Collins, McMain, Skinner, Littman-Sharpe and Mercado (unpublished), recently completed a randomized control trial with a population of problem gamblers who also had anger problems. The study compared an integrative, skills-based treatment primarily targeting emotion dysregulation, with a cognitive behavioural treatment-as-usual (TAU). The integrative, emotion-focused treatment was significantly superior to the TAU in reducing gambling and anger, and in retaining participants in treatment. Though the study was limited to a specialized subpopulation of pathological gamblers who also had anger problems, the study suggests that targeting affect regulation might also be a helpful approach in the treatment of pathological gamblers, and warrants further study.

Improving Professionally Delivered Treatment Outcomes

Daughters, Lejuez, Lesieur, Strong and Zvolensky (2003) have suggested that gambling improving treatment outcomes could be improved by addressing the factors predicting treatment failure: gambling-related cognitive distortions and beliefs about randomness, impulsivity/ sensation-seeking (Castellani & Rugle, 1995; Blaszczynski, Steel, & McConaghy, 1997; Petry, 2001), biological vulnerabilities, and negative affect/mood symptoms. For example, significant comorbidity between gambling pathology and mental health disorders, especially substance use disorders, mood disorders, ADHD, and personality disorders has been well-established (e.g., Savron, Pilti, DeLuca & Guerreschi, 2001; Potenza, Kosten, & Rounsaville, 2001; Grant & Kim, 2001; Specker, et al. 1996). Ladd and Petry (2003), for example, found substance-abusing gamblers reported more depression, hallucinations, suicidal ideation and attempts, and difficulty controlling violent behaviour over their lifetime versus gamblers with no previous treatment for substance abuse. In addition, the role of cognitive factors within pathological gambling appears to be well-established (e.g., Gaboury & Ladouceur, 1989; Toneatto, 1999; Walker, 1992; Griffiths, 1996; Ladouceur & Dube, 1997; Delfabbro & Winefield, 2000) although there is less certainty as to whether such cognitions are causally related to the onset and maintenance of gambling. These moderating variables should be assessed and if necessary targeted in treatment in order to enhance treatment outcomes.

What are Effective Self-Help Treatments?

There is growing evidence that gamblers may respond to self-help interventions. Hodgins, Currie and el-Guebaly (2001) compared two versions of a cognitive-behaviorally based self-help manual (i.e., simply mailing the self-help manual versus preceding the mailing of the manual with a telephone motivational interview reviewing the assessment information and enhancing commitment to change) to a waiting list control. The study found significant reductions in gambling behavior by 84% of subjects in the self-help group over the one-year follow-up period.

Gamblers anonymous Founded in California in the late 1950s, Gamblers Anonymous (GA) adapted the 12 Steps for problem gamblers. Today, the GA website (http://www.gamblersanonymous.org/mtgdirTOP.html) lists groups in all 50 states in the USA, in all 10 provinces in Canada and in 35 other countries on every continent.

Despite a surge in interest in the late 1980s and early 1990s, there has been little research on GA since then, possibly due to the difficulties of researchers to gain access to a closed fellowship emphasizing the anonymity of its members (Ferentzy & Skinner, 2003). More recently there is evidence that GA is attracting more women to its fellowship, and that it is effecting a cultural shift towards a greater emphasis on the 12 Steps and a more supportive attitude to people engaged in recovery work (Ferentzy, Skinner, & Antze, 2004).

Brown (1987) found that those who quit GA were less concerned about their gambling problems than those who continued attending GA. This finding is consistent with the notion of "hitting bottom," which often is used to explain why people turn to 12 Step groups in general. While Blaszczynski (2000) suggests that those with more severe gambling problems need professional help, viewing self-help approaches like GA as appropriate for people with low severity problems, most researchers note that GA appears to be a last resort option for people with severe problems. Certainly the recovery trajectory required by GA makes it, like all 12 Step fellowships, the most arduous and extended of recovery approaches that are currently available (Blume 1987).

Currently there is little empirical evidence to support the efficacy of GA. Allcock (1986) estimated the percentage of newcomers who remain in GA for the long-term to be 10%. Carriocchi and Reinhart (1993) report a positive correlation between long-term abstinence and family environment for gamblers, but not for their spouses. Others criticize GA for its poor retention and success rates (Potenza, 2002). Nevertheless, the lack of empirical evidence does not mean that a recovery approach is not without merit. Findings from Project MATCH, for example, indicate that when evaluated against more formal therapeutic methods, 12 Step approaches may hold their own (Project MATCH, 1997). However, one evaluates the evidence for GA, it remains an enduring resource for people seeking recovery from gambling problems.

What are Effective Medical Treatments?

Disturbances in serotonergic neurotransmitter functioning among pathological gamblers have led to several medication studies in recent years (e.g., Carrasco, Saiz-Ruiz, Monero, Hollander, & Lopez-Ibor, 1994) and dopaminergic (e.g., Bergh, Eklund, Sodersten, & Nordin, 1997; Stojanov, et al., 2003). While several have shown promise, no medication has yet been approved for the treatment of pathological gambling.

Placebo-controlled trials of fluvoxamine (i.e., Hollander et al., 2000; Blanco, Petkova, Ibanez, & Saiz-Ruiz (2002), lithium and valproate (i.e., Pallanti, Quercioli, Sood, & Hollander, 2002), for example, have not yielded strong evidence in support of these medications. Paroxetine received support from one 8-week trial (i.e., Kim, Grant, Adson, Shin, & Zaninelli, 2002), but not in a subsequent 16-week trial (i.e., Grant et al., 2003). Kim, Grant, Adson, and Shin (2001) evaluated naltrexone in a 12-week double-blind randomized placebo-controlled study, and found the naltrexone group to show higher rates of very much/much improvement (75% of sample) compared to 24% of the placebo group.

With the exception of naltrexone, the evidence for the efficacy of any medication is modest. While improvement rates appear to favor the medication over placebo in many studies, statistical significance often is not attained. Thus, while there is reason to be optimistic that effective pharmacotherapy for problem gambling will be developed, much additional research is required. Readers are referred to Grant, Kim, & Potenza, (2003) for a comprehensive discussion of pharmacological treatments for gambling pathology.

How Does One Select Among Treatments?

The common prevalence of concurrent addictions and cognitive and psychiatric psychopathology among pathological gamblers has been well-established (e.g., Petry, 2002). Therefore, appropriate screening for comorbidity, and determination of the primary disorder should assist decisions about appropriate treatment (most likely a combination of psychological and pharmacological therapies). The treatment for gamblers who suffer from concurrent disorders should also take into account the functional relationship between gambling and other psychiatric and addiction symptoms in order to properly address the function of gambling.

For gamblers who do not possess a concurrent disorder, the initial intervention should strive to increase the individual's commitment to treatment and resolve treatment-disrupting ambivalence as much as possible. The relatively high rates of dropout and treatment non-completion suggest that more effort be made to strengthen the client's motivation to change. Interventions consistent with the stage of change of model would be appropriate.

Having strengthened motivation, the available empirical research suggests that cognitive-behavioral treatments, generally brief and delivered on an outpatient basis, are the most effective treatments to date. Concurrent pharmacotherapies (i.e., naltrexone, SSRIs) are promising adjuncts at the present time, although their use should be based on a consideration of particular scenarios rather than a general clinical practice.

WEBSITES OF INTEREST

http://www.camh.net/egambling/archive/index.html Journal of Gambling Issues
http://www.kluweronline.com/issn/1050-5350 Journal of Gambling Studies
http://www.ncpgambling.org/National Council on Problem Gaming (US)
http://www.easg.org/ European Association for the Study of Gambling
http://www.addiction.ucalgary.ca/ David Hodgins, University of Calgary
http://www.gamblingresearch.org/ Ontario Problem Gambling Research Centre
http://ess.ntu.ac.uk/griffiths/ Mark Griffiths, Nottingham Trent University
http://www.problemgambling.ca/ Gerry Cooper's Problem Gambling: A Canadian Perspective
http://www.cghub.homestead.com/index.html Compulsive Gamblers Hub

REFERENCES

Allcock, C. C. (1986). Pathological gambling. *Australian and New Zealand Journal of Psychiatry, 20*, 259–265.

American Psychiatric Association, (1994). *The diagnostic and statistical manual of the mental disorders (fourth ed.)*. Washington, DC: American Psychiatric Association.

Beaudoin, C., & Cox, B. (1999). Characteristics of problem gambling in a Canadian context: A preliminary study using a DSM-IV based questionnaire. *Canadian Journal of Psychiatry, 44*, 483–487.

Beconia, E. (1996). Prevalence surveys of problem and pathological gambling in Europe: The cases of Germany, Holland, and Spain. *Journal of Gambling Studies, 12*, 197–192.

Bergh, C., Eklund, T., Sodersten, P., & Nordin, C. (1997). Altered dopamine function in pathological gambling. *Psychological Medicine, 27*, 473–475.

Bergh, C., & Kuhlhorn, E. (1994). Social, psychological, and physical consequences of pathological gambling in Sweden. *Journal of Gambling Studies, 10*, 275–285.

Black, D. W., & Meyer, T. (1998). Clinical features and psychiatric comorbidity of subjects with pathological gambling behavior. *Psychiatric Services, 49(11)*, 1434–1439.

Blanco, C., Petkova, E., Ibanez, A., & Saiz-Ruiz, J. (2002). A pilot placebo-controlled study of fluvoxamine for pathological gambling. *Annals of Clinical Psychiatry, 14*, 9–15.

Bland, R. Newman, S., Orn, H., & Stebelsky, G. (1993). Epidemiology of pathological gamblers in Edmonton. *Canadian Journal of Psychiatry, 38*, 108–112.

Blaszczynski, A. P. (2000). Pathways to pathological gambling: Identifying typologies. *The Electronic Journal of Gambling Issues: eGambling, 1.* http://www.camh.net/egambling/issue1/feature/index.html

Blaszczynski A. P., & McConaghy, N. (1989). Anxiety and/or depression in the pathogenesis of pathological gambling. *International Journal of the Addictions 24*, 337–350.

Blaszczynski, A., & McConaghy, N. (1992). *Pathological gambling and criminal behaviours. Report to the Australian Institute of Criminology.* Canberra: Criminology Research Council.

Blaszczynski A, Walker, M. Sagris, A., & Dickerson, M. (1997). *Psychological aspects of gambling.* Position paper prepared for the Directorate of Social Issues, Australian Psychological Society. http://www.psychsociety.com.au/member/gambling/index.html.

Blaszczynski, A., & Steel, Z. (1998). Personality disorders among pathological gamblers. *Journal of Gambling Studies, 14*, 51–71.

Blaszczynski, A., Steel, Z., & McConaghy, N. (1997). Impulsivity in pathological gambling: The antisocial impulsivist. *Addiction Research, 92*, 75–87.

Blaszczynski, A., & Nower, L. (2002). A pathways model of problem and pathological gambling. *Addiction, 97*, 487–499.

Blume, S. B. (1987). Compulsive gambling and the medical model. *Journal of Gambling Behavior, 3*, 237–247.

Breen, R., & Zuckerman, M. (1999). Chasing in gambling behavior: Personality and cognitive determinants. *Personality and Individual Differences, 27*, 1097–1111.

Brown, R. I. F. (1987). Dropouts and continuers in Gamblers Anonymous: Part Four. Evaluation and Summary. *Journal of Gambling Behavior, 3*, 202–210.

Carlton P. L., Manowitz P., McBride H., Nora, R., Swartzburg, M., & Goldstein, L. (1987). Attention deficit disorder and pathological gambling. *Journal of Clinical Psychiatry, 48*, 487–488.

Carrasco, J., Saiz-Ruiz, J., Moreno, I., Hollander, E., & Lopez-Ibor, J. (1994). Low platelet MAO activity in pathological gambling. *Acta Psychiatrica Scandanavica, 90*, 427–431.

Castellani, B., & Rugle, L. (1995). A comparison of pathological gamblers to alcoholics and cocaine misusers on impulsivity, sensation seeking, and craving. *International Journal of the Addictions, 30*, 275–289.

Chambless, D. L., & Ollendick, T. H. (2001). Empirically supported psychological interventions: Controversies and evidence. *Annual Review of Psychology, 52*, 685–716.

Chambless, D. L., & Hollon, S. D. (1998). Defining empirically supported therapies. *Journal of Clinical and Consulting Psychology, 66*, 7–18.

Ciarrocchi, J. W., & Reinert, D. F. (1993). Family environment and length of recovery for married male members of Gamblers Anonymous and female members of GamAnon. *Journal of Gambling Studies, 9*, 341–351.

Crisp, B. R., Thomas, S. A., Jackson, A. C., Thomason, N., Smith, S., Borrell, J., et al. (2000). Sex differences in the treatment needs and outcomes of problem gamblers. *Research on Social Work Practice, 10*, 229–242.

Cunningham-Williams, R. M., Cottler, L. B., Compton, W. M., Spitznagel, E. L. (1998). Taking chances: Problem gamblers and mental health disorders–Results from the St. Louis ECA Study. *American Journal of Public Health, 88*, 1093–1096.

Custer, R. L. (1982). An overview of compulsive gambling. In P. Carone, S. Yoles, S. Keiffer, & L. Krinsky (Eds.), *Addictive disorders update* (pp. 107–124). New York: Human Sciences Press.

Daughters, S. B., Lejuez, C. W., Lesieur, H. R., Strong, D. R., & Zvolensky, M. J. (2003). Towards a better understanding of gambling treatment failure: implications of translational research. *Clinical Psychology Review, 23*, 573–586.

Delfabbro, P. H., & Winefield, A. H. (2000). Predictors of irrational thinking in regular slot machine gamblers. *Journal of Psychology, 134*, 117–128.

Dickerson, M. G. (1989). Gambling: A dependence without a drug. *International Review of Psychiatry, 1*, 157–172.

Echeburua, E., Baez, C., & Fernandez-Montalvo, J. (1996). Comparative effectiveness of three therapeutic modalities in the psychological treatment of pathological gambling. *Behavioral and Cognitive Psychotherapy, 24*, 51–72.

Echeburua, E., Fernandez-Montalvo, J. & Baez, C. (2000). Prevention in the treatment of slot-machine pathological gambling: Long-term out come. *Behavior Therapy, 31,* 351–364.

Ferentzy, P., & Skinner, W. (2003). "Gamblers Anonymous: A critical review of the literature." *Electronic Journal of Gambling Issues, 9.* Available from http://www.camh.net/egambling/issue9/index.html

Ferentzy, P., Skinner, W., & Antze, P. (2004). Evaluating mutual aid pathways to recovery from gambling problems. Research report prepared for the Ontario Problem Gambling Research Centre.

Ferris, J., & Wynne, H. (2001). *The Canadian Problem Gambling Index: User's manual.* Toronto, ON: Canadian Centre on Substance Abuse.

Frank, M. L., Lester, D., & Wexler, A. (1991). Suicidal behavior among members of Gamblers Anonymous. *Journal of Gambling Studies 7,* 249–254.

Gaboury, A., & Ladouceur, R. (1989). Erroneous perceptions and gambling. *Journal of Social Behavior and Personality, 4,* 411–420.

Govoni, R., Frisch, G., & Stinchfield, R. (2001). *A critical review of screening and assessment instruments for problem gambling.* Windsor, ON: University of Windsor, Problem Gambling Research Group.

Grant, J. E., Kim, S. W., Potenza, M. N. (2003). Advances in the pharmacological treatment of pathological gambling. *Journal of Gambling Studies, 19(1),* 85–109.

Grant, J. E., Kim, S. W., Potenza, M. N., Blanco, C., Ibanez, A., Stevens, L., et al., (2003). Paroxetine treatment of pathological gambling: a multi-centre randomized controlled trial. *International Clinical Psychopharmacology, 18,* 243–249.

Griffiths, M. (1996). *Adolescent gambling.* London: Routledge.

Hodgins, D. C., Currie, S. R., & el-Guebaly, N. (2001). Motivational enhancement and self-help treatments for problem gambling. *Journal of Consulting and Clinical Psychology, 69,* 50–57.

Hollander, E., DeCaria, C. M., Finkell, J. N., Begaz, T., Wong, C. M., & Cartwright, C. (2000). A randomized double-blind fluvoxamine/placebo crossover trial in pathologic gambling. *Biological Psychiatry, 47,* 813–817.

Hraba, J., & Lee, G. (1995). Gender, gambling and problem gambling. *Journal of Gambling Studies, 12,* 83–101.

Jefferson, S., & Nicki, R. (2003). A new instrument to measure cognitive distortions in video lottery terminal users: The Informational Biases Scale (IBS). *Journal of Gambling Studies, 19,* 387–403.

Johnson, E., Hamer, R., Nora, R., & Tan, R. (1997). The Lie/Bet questionnaire for screening pathological gamblers. *Psychological Reports, 80,* 83–88.

Johnson, E. Hamer, R. & Nora, R. (1998). The Lie/Best questionnaire for screening pathological gamblers: A follow-up study. *Psychological Reports, 83,* 1219–1224.

Kassinove, J. (1998). Development of the Gambling Attitude Scales: Preliminary Findings. *Journal of Clinical Psychology, 54,* 763–771.

Kim, S. W., Grant, J. E., Adson, D. E., & Shin, Y. C. (2001). A double-blind naltrexone and placebo comparison study in the treatment of pathological gambling. *Biological Psychiatry, 49,* 914–921.

Kim, S. W., Grant, J. E., Adson, D. E., Shin, Y. C., & Zaninelli, R. (2002). A double-blind placebo-controlled study of the efficacy and safety of paroxetine in the treatment of pathological gambling. *Journal of Clinical Psychiatry, 63,* 501–507.

Kruedelbach, N., McCormick, R., Schulz, S., & Grueneich, C. (1993). Impulsivity, coping styles and triggers for craving in substance abusers with borderline personality disorders. *Journal of Personality Disorders, 7,* 214–223.

Ladd, G. & Petry, N. (2003). A comparison of pathological gamblers with and without substance abuse treatment histories. *Experimental and Clinical Psychopharmacology, 11,* 202–209.

Ladoucer, R. (1996). The prevalence of pathological gambling in Canada. *Journal of Gambling Studies, 12,* 129–142.

Ladouceur, R., Sylvain, C., Boutin, S., Lachance, C., Doucet, C., & Leblond, J. (2003). Group therapy for pathological gamblers: a cognitive approach. *Behavior Research and Therapy, 41,* 587–596.

Ladouceur, R., Sylvain, C., Boutin, C., Lachance, S., Doucet, C., Leblond, J., et al. (2001). Cognitive treatment of pathological gambling. *Journal of Nervous and Mental Disease, 189,* 773–780.

Ladouceur, R., & Dube, D. (1997). Monetary incentive and erroneous perceptions in American roulette. *Psychology: A Journal of Human Behavior, 34,* 27–32.

Lesieur, H. R. (1988). *Pathological gambling in Canada: Golden goose or Trojan horse?* Vancouver: Simon Fraser University.

Lesieur, H. R., & Anderson, C. (1995). *Results of a survey of gamblers anonymous members in Illinois.* Park Ridge, IL: Illinois Council on Problem and Compulsive Gambling.

Lesieur, H. & Blume, S. (1987). The South Oaks Gambling Screen (SOGS): A new instrument for the identification of pathological gamblers, *American Journal of Psychiatry, 144,* 1184–1188.

Lesieur H. R., Blume, S. B., & Zoppa, R. M. (1985). Alcoholism, drug abuse, and gambling. *Alcoholism: Clinical and Experimental Research 10,* 33–38.

Linden, R. D., Pope, H. G., & Jonas, J. M. (1986). Pathological gambling and major affective disorder: Preliminary findings. *Journal of Clinical Psychology, 47(4),* 201–203.

McCormick, R. A. Russo, A. M., Ramirez, L. F., & Taber, J. I. (1984). Affective disorders among pathological gamblers in treatment. *American Journal of Psychiatry, 141,* 215–218.

Pallanti, S., Quercioli, L., Sood, E., & Hollander, E. (2002). Lithium and valproate treatment of pathological gambling: A randomized single-blind study. *Journal of Clinical Psychiatry, 63,* 559–564.

Petry, N. (2000). Psychiatric symptoms in problem gambling and non-problem gambling substance abusers. *American Journal on Addictions, 9,* 163–171.

Petry, N. M. (2001). Pathological Gamblers, With and Without Substance Use Disorders, Discount Delayed Rewards at High Rates. *Journal of Abnormal Psychology, 110(3),* 482–487.

Petry, N. M. (2002). How treatments for pathological gambling can be informed by treatments for substance use disorders. *Experimental and Clinical Psychopharmacology, 10,* 184–192.

Potenza, M. N. (2002). A Perspective on Future Directions in the Prevention, Treatment, and Research of Pathological Gambling. *Psychiatric Annals, 32,* 203–207.

Potenza, M. N., Kosten, T. R., & Rounsaville, B. J. (2001). Pathological Gambling. *Journal of the American Medical Association, 286,* 141–144.

Project MATCH Research Group (1997) Matching alcoholism treatments to client heterogeneity: Project MATCH post-treatment outcomes. *Journal of Studies in Alcohol, 59,* 631–639.

Ramirez, L. F., McCormick R. A., Russo A. M., (1983). Patterns of substance abuse in pathological gamblers undergoing treatment. *Addictive Behavior, 8,* 425–428.

Raylu, N. & Oei, T. (2004). The Gambling Related Cognitions Scale (GRCS): Development, confirmatory factor validation and psychometric properties. *Addiction, 99,* 757–769.

Reich, J., & Green, A. (1991). Effects of personality disorders on outcome of treatment. *Journal of Nervous and Mental Disease, 179,* 74–82.

Shaffer, H. Hall, M. N., & van der Bilt, J. (1997). *Estimating prevalence of disordered gambling behavior in the United States and Canada: A meta-analysis.* Boston: Havard Medical Division on Addictions.

Specker, S., Carlson, G., Edmonson, K., Johnson, P., & Marcotte, M. (1996). Psychopathology in pathological gamblers seeking treatment. *Journal of Gambling Studies, 12,* 67–81.

Statistics Canada (2003). *Perspectives on labour and income: Fact sheet on gambling, 4(4),* 75-001XIE.

Stinchfield, R. (2002). Reliability, validity and classification accuracy of the South Oaks Gambling Screen (SOGS). *Addictive Behaviors, 21,* 1–19.

Steenbergh, T., Meyers, A., May, R., & Whelan, J. (2002). Development and Validation of the Gamblers' Belief Questionnaire. *Psychology of Addictive Behaviors, 16,* 143–149.

Stojanov, W., Karayanidis, F., Johnston, P., Bailey, A., Carr, V., & Schall, U. (2003). Disrupted sensory gating in pathological gambling. *Biological Psychiatry,* 54, 474–484.

Sylvain, C., Ladouceur, R., & Bosivert, J. M. (1997). Cognitive and behavioral treatment of pathological gambling: A controlled study. *Journal of Consulting and Clinical Psychology, 65,* 727–732.

Thompson, W. N., Gazel, R., & Rickman, D. (1996). The social costs of gambling in Wisconsin. *Wisconsin Policy Research Institute Report, 9(6),* 1–44.

Toneatto, T., & Ladouceur, R. (2003). The treatment of pathological gambling: A critical review of the literature. *Psychology of Addictive Behaviors, 17,* 284–292.

Toneatto, T. (1999). Cognitive psychopathology of problem gambling. *Substance Use & Misuse, 34,* 1593–1604.

Walker, M. B. (1992). Irrational thinking among slot machine players. *Journal of Gambling Studies, 8(1),* 245–261.

Winters, K., Specker, S., & Stinchfield, R. (1997). *Brief manual for use of the diagnostic interview for gambling severity.* Minneapolis, MN: University of Minnesota Medical School.

Generalized Anxiety Disorder

Kristen H. Demertzis • Michelle G. Craske

WHAT IS GENERALIZED ANXIETY DISORDER?

The current version of the Diagnostic and Statistical Manual of Mental Disorders (DSM-IV-TR; American Psychiatric Association, 1994) defines GAD as a disorder characterized by excessive anxiety or apprehension over multiple issues (e.g., school, finances), experienced more days than not, for a period of at least six months. Furthermore, the worry is difficult to control and is associated with at least three of a prespecified cluster of six symptoms (i.e., restlessness, easily fatigued, concentration difficulties, irritability, muscle tension, and sleep disturbance). As with other Axis I disorders, the symptoms are associated with distress and/or impairment in functioning, are not attributable to the effects of a substance or medical condition, and do not occur exclusively during a mood, psychotic, or pervasive developmental disorder. Relative to younger groups, elderly individuals may express more health-(e.g., falling, death) and safety- (e.g., being burglarized) related worries, and suffer from a greater number of comorbid medical conditions that may contribute to realistic concerns (Kogan, Edelstein, & McKee, 1999).

Of all the anxiety disorders, GAD loads highest on neuroticism, or propensity to experience negative emotions (Mineka, Watson, & Clark, 1998). Negative affectivity is considered critical to the diminution of self-efficacy, as continuous experiences of negative affect are interpreted as evidence of failure in managing one's own emotions and situations in life (Craske, 2003). GAD is also associated with judgment and attentional biases believed to maintain anxiety, such as a tendency to interpret ambiguous situations in a threatening manner (e.g., Eysenck, Mogg, May, Richards, & Mathews, 1991) and to over-attend to threatening stimuli, even when not consciously perceived (e.g., Mathews & MacLeod, 1985). Also, relative to nonanxious controls, individuals with GAD judge self-referent negative events as more likely than positive events and other-referent negative events (Butler & Mathews, 1983).

Borkovec and colleagues suggest that the function of worry for persons with GAD is to suppress arousal elicited by emotionally charged images (Borkovec & Inz, 1990). The largely verbal, left-hemispheric act of worry is far less autonomically arousing than right-hemispheric, pictorial processing (e.g., worrying about the children's safety versus picturing them dead in a car accident) (Borkovec, 1994). By suppressing negatively charged images, habituation or correction to fear imagery does not occur in GAD patients, and a negative reinforcement cycle of worry is established. The fearful imagery reappears and motivates further worry to suppress the images. Purposeful suppression of thoughts is also ineffective as it has been shown to trigger worry and reinforce beliefs of uncontrollability of one's emotions (Purdon, 1999).

Also characteristic of GAD is low confidence in problem-solving abilities, partially due to worries over making the "wrong" decision. GAD patients prefer to acquire as much evidence as possible before making decisions, have a low tolerance

Demertzis, K. H., & Craske, M. G. (2006). Generalized anxiety disorder. In J. E. Fisher & W. T. O'Donohue (Eds.), *Practitioner's guide to evidence-based psychotherapy*. New York: Springer.

for ambiguity (Dugas et al., 2003), and engage in an iterative style of problem solving (Craske, 2003) compared to nonanxious controls. Such behavioral patterns contribute to distress over decision making and general anxiety.

Many GAD patients frequently engage in perfectionistic behaviors, excessive preparation (e.g., getting to an appointment an hour beforehand so as not to be late), or checking behaviors (e.g., making sure the children are safe when sleeping) as a means of alleviating distress (Wells & Mathews, 1994). These behaviors reinforce fears and further propagate the cycle of worry.

Wells and Matthews (1994) proposed a self-regulatory model that identifies positive and negative metacognitive beliefs about worry as mechanisms promoting further worry and rumination. Negative beliefs that worrying is uncontrollable and harmful (i.e., "I'm out of control to worry this excessively") appear to more strongly predict pathological worry compared to positive beliefs (Wells & Carter, 1999) by generating worry about worry, attempts to suppress further worry, avoidance behaviors, and reassurance seeking (Wells & Matthews, 1994).

In summary, the high loading of GAD on negative affectivity contributes to excessive, unpredictable, and uncontrollable worry and anxiety in a wide array of situations. Worry has different meanings for different individuals, but universally serves to suppress peaks in autonomic reactivity. Frequent experiences of negative affect and worry are interlaced with overestimations and catastrophizing of negative events, limited confidence in problem solving, requirement of additional evidence before making decisions, low tolerance of uncertainty, an iterative problem-solving style, worry about worry, and numerous behavioral and cognitive strategies that may actually be counterproductive and help maintain the self-perpetuating cycle of worry (Craske, 2003).

BASIC FACTS ABOUT GENERALIZED ANXIETY DISORDER

Prevalence. The lifetime prevalence estimate for GAD from the National Comorbidity Survey (NCS; Kessler, DuPont, Berglund, & Wittchen, 1994) was 5.1%. The 12-month prevalence rate ranged between 3.1% and 3.8%, and current prevalence was 1.6%. Additionally, numerous "subdiagnostic threshold" cases are estimated to be categorized as Anxiety Disorder NOS, Acute Stress Disorder, and Adjustment Disorder with Anxious Mood (Rickels & Rynn, 2002). GAD is also the second most frequent disorder identified in the primary care setting (e.g., Maier et al., 2000). GAD can be diagnosed in child, adolescent, adult, and elderly populations, although the majority of research on GAD has focused on younger to middle-aged adult samples. However, there is a growing literature highlighting the significant impact on and increased prevalence of GAD among the elderly (Blazer, 1997; Stanley & Beck, 2000).

Comorbidity. The majority (i.e., 66%) of persons with GAD also meet diagnostic criteria for at least one other Axis I disorder (Wittchen, Zhao, Kessler, & de Boer, 1994), and among anxiety disorders, GAD has one of the highest rates of cooccurrence with other disorders (Brown, Campbell, Lehman, Grisham, Mancill, 2001). Common comorbid disorders include major depression and social and specific phobias (Wittchen et al., 1994).

Age of Onset. Although age of onset for GAD varies, a large percentage of individuals with GAD report having the disorder most of their lives (Hoehn-Saris, Hazlett, & McLeod, 1991). Earlier onsets of GAD may be associated with stronger vulnerabilities (e.g., neuroticism) and greater reactivity to life stressors in individuals than later onsets (Craske, 1999).

Gender. Females are more likely than males to meet diagnostic criteria for GAD in epidemiological and clinical samples (e.g., Kessler et al., 1994).

Course and impairment. GAD is a chronic condition (Craske, 1999) that tends to wax and wane over the course of an individual's life, with less than 30% of individuals experiencing a spontaneous remission (Ballenger, Davidson, Lecrubier, et al., 2001). GAD is associated with significant functional impairment (e.g., Wittchen et al., 1994).

ASSESSMENT

What Should be Ruled Out?

Careful, differential diagnosis should be made to determine whether symptoms are better accounted for by another mental disorder (e.g., social phobia, unipolar depression). Regarding GAD assessment, some have argued that more important than worry or symptom *duration* is cognitive and physical symptom *severity* (e.g., Rickels & Rynn, 2001). Bienvenu, Nestadt and Eaton (1998) found that dividing up individuals by number of GAD symptoms reported, rather than symptom duration, yielded meaningful group differences in comorbidity and demographic profiles. Increasing the number of required symptoms while decreasing the duration requisite of the diagnostic nomenclature may result in individuals being captured diagnostically and provided appropriate treatments who do not meet the current duration criterion, but who report considerable symptoms and may represent as severe a population as more chronic cases.

What is Involved in Effective Assessment?

A comprehensive assessment of GAD should include:

- DSM-IV criteria for GAD
- Range of situations eliciting worry/anxiety
- Frequency and severity of avoidance behavior, behavior, perfectionistic behaviors, excessive preparation, or checking behaviors
- Substance use to self-medicate anxiety (e.g., to sleep)

- Severity of generalized worry and anxiety
- Severity of cognitive, emotional, and physical symptoms
- Functional impairment
- Social support network

- Controllability of worry
- Metacognitions about worry
- Comorbid psychological and medical conditions
- Suicidal ideation and past attempts

Clinician-administered measures. Diagnostic instruments include the DSM-IV Structured Clinical Interview for Mental Disorders (SCID; First, Spitzer, Gibbon, & Williams, 1997) and the Anxiety Disorders Interview Schedule for DSM-IV (ADIS-IV; Brown, DiNardo, & Barlow, 1994) which was designed to facilitate the differential diagnosis of anxiety disorders.

Self-report measures. Self-report measures specific to GAD include the Penn State Worry Questionnaire (Meyer, Miller, Metzger, & Borkovec, 1990). There are also self-report measures that tap into specific constructs, such as metacognitions about worry, which have been explored in the GAD literature and may prove quite useful for clinicians in conceptualization and treatment planning. Examples of such measures are the Thought Control Questionnaire (TCQ; Wells & Davies, 1994), the Anxious Thoughts Inventory (AnTI; Wells, 1994), and the Metacognitions Questionnaire (MCQ; Cartwright-Hatton & Wells, 1997), which is also available in a shortened form (MCQ-30; Wells & Cartwright-Hatton, 2004). The reader is referred to the respective references for a more detailed review of these assessment instruments.

What Assessments are Not Helpful?

The use of psychodiagnostic (e.g., MMPI, MCMI), projective, and medical tests is not particularly helpful for diagnostic purposes. However, psychodiagnostic and neuropsychological tests can enhance conceptualization comprehensiveness with respect to symptom pervasiveness, severity, and impact on cognitive functioning (e.g., attention/concentration, executive skills).

TREATMENT

What Treatments are Effective?

The chronic nature of the worry and anxiety associated with GAD often necessitates long-term treatment through medication and/or psychotherapy. Due to the pervasive and complex diagnostic profile of GAD, this is the least successfully treated of the anxiety disorders (Brown et al., 1994). To date, the efficacy of a number of pharmacological and psychosocial interventions has been tested in randomized controlled trials as treatments for GAD. Although data exist to support efficacy of a variety of classes of medications for treating GAD symptoms, paroxetine is the only medication approved for use for GAD patients by the US Food and Drug Administration. Of the psychosocial interventions, cognitive-behavioral therapy (CBT) has the most empirical support of randomized controlled trials.

What are Effective Self-Help Treatments?

Self-help treatment guides that incorporate principles of CBT as well as informational internet sites and palm-assisted computer aids for CBT are available to GAD patients. Although empirical support for self-help guides is lacking, a list of references for the reader is provided.

- Bourne, E. J. & Garano, L. (2003). *Coping with anxiety: 10 simple ways to relieve anxiety, fear, and worry.* Oakland, CA: New Harbinger Publications, Inc.
- Bourne, E. J., Brownstein, A., & Garano, L. (2004). *Natural relief for anxiety: Complementary strategies for easing fear, panic & worry.* Oakland, CA: New Harbinger Publications, Inc.
- Brantley, J. & Kabat-Zinn, J. (2003). *Calming your anxious mind: How mindfulness and compassion can free you from anxiety, fear, and panic.* Oakland, CA: New Harbinger Publications, Inc.
- Craske, M. G. & Barlow, D. H. (in press). *The Mastery of Your Anxiety and Worry.* New York, NY: Oxford Press.
- Davidson, J. & Dreher, H. (2003). *The anxiety book.* New York, NY: Riverhead Trade.
- Ellis, A. (1999). *How to control your anxiety before it controls you.* Secaucus, NJ: Carol Publishing Group.
- Hallowell, E. M. (1997). *Worry: Controlling it and using it wisely.* Pantheon Books.
- Hallowell, E. M. (1998). *Worry: Hope and help for a common condition.* Ballatine Books.
- Lark, S. M. (2000). *Dr. Susan Lark's anxiety & stress self help book: Effective solutions for nervous tension, emotional distress, anxiety, & panic.* Berkeley, CA: Celestial Arts.

- White, J. (1999). *Overcoming generalized anxiety disorder: Client manual: A relaxation, cognitive restructuring, and exposure-based protocol for the treatment of GAD (best practices for therapy).* Oakland, CA: New Harbinger Publications, Inc.
- *http://www.adaa.org/AnxietyDisorderInfor/GAD.cfm* (Anxiety Disorders Association of America)
- *http://www.anxietynetwork.com/gahome.html* (Anxiety Network)
- *http://www.mental-health-matters.com* (Mental Health Matters)
- *http://www.nmha.org/infoctr/factsheets/31.cfm* (National Mental Health Association)
- *http://www.mentalhealth. ucla.edu/projects/anxiety/behavioralanxietydisorders.htm* (UCLA - Department of Psychology—Anxiety Disorders Behavioral Research Program)
- *http://www.mentalhealth.ucla.edu/projects/anxiety/index.htm* (UCLA Anxiety Disorders Program)

What are Effective Therapist-Based Treatments?

The psychosocial intervention with the most empirical support for treating GAD is cognitivebehavioral therapy (CBT) (Borkovec & Ruscio, 2001), which includes: psychoeducation, self-monitoring (Overholser & Nasser, 2000), relaxation training (Öst, 1987), cognitive restructuring (e.g., Borkovec & Costello, 1993), and exposure to internal and external triggers of worry (e.g., Craske, Street, & Barlow, 1989). The goal of treatment is to interrupt the negative self-perpetuating cycles of worry and related behaviors.

CBT typically involves 10–15 sessions, but can contain additional sessions depending on patients' level of severity, the presence of comorbidity, patients' resistance to the treatment approach, therapists' competence, and the number of components incorporated into CBT (e.g., relaxation, imagery exposure). Individual and group CBT have been found to be more effective than waitlist control conditions (e.g., Dugas et al., 2003; Ladouceur et al., 2000), nondirective supportive therapy (e.g., Borkovec & Costello, 1993), and psychodynamic therapy (e.g., Durham, Fisher, et al., 1999). In a review of six randomized controlled psychotherapy trials for GAD, Fisher and Durham (1999) found that recovery rates for individual CBT and applied relaxation were 20–25% higher than for group CBT in an educational format and individual non-directive therapy. Low attrition rates have been reported for CBT and general maintenance of treatment effects has been demonstrated for up to 1 year (Borkovec & Ruscio, 2001). In addition, reductions in medication reliance following CBT interventions for GAD have been reported by many clients (e.g., Barlow, Rapee, & Brown, 1992; Öst & Breitholtz, 2000).

Conflicting data exist on which components are critical for optimal outcome (Arntz, 2003; Borkovec, Newman, Pincus, & Lytle, 2002), as some data indicate that multicomponent treatments are more effective than individual CBT components (e.g., Butler, Fennell, Robson, & Gelder, 1991) whereas other studies find the two comparable (e.g., Borkovec, 2002). These conflicting data likely emphasize the importance of tailoring treatment plans to address clients' individual profiles. The following is a brief description of core CBT components.

1. Psychoeducation. The main goals of psychoeducation are to inform and correct misconceptions regarding the functional roles of anxiety, worry, and associated symptoms; causative factors of pathological worry and anxiety; a model of factors that perpetuate GAD; and the provision of the treatment plan and rationale (i.e., not to eliminate anxiety, but help clients manage and cope with anxiety). Much of this information is integrated in presenting how a pathological cycle of worry and anxiety develops and is maintained in clients' lives.

2. Self-Monitoring involves the development of a personal-scientist model to observe one's reactions from an objective standpoint and examine episodes of worry regarding internal and external triggers, associated cognitions, feelings, behaviors, physiological sensations, images, and controllability. Also, self-monitoring allows patients to chart their progress in therapy.

3. Relaxation Training can be particularly meaningful for GAD clients as they often experience elevated muscle tension and reduced flexibility of autonomic functioning (e.g., Thayer, Friedman, & Borkovec, 1996). Relaxation training consists of progressive muscle relaxation (e.g., Bernstein, Borkovec, & Hazlett-Stevens, 2000) of all muscle groups of the body in a systematic manner. Breathing exercises may also be incorporated into relaxation training. In applied relaxation, relaxation is used as a coping tool for managing anxiety in response to a graduated hierarchy of anxiety-producing situations.

4. Cognitive Restructuring is a set of skills for identifying and modifying misappraisals that contribute to anxiety. Patients are shown how anxiety and maladaptive behaviors are generated by worrisome, catastrophic interpretations of events (Brown, O'Leary, & Barlow, 2001). Clients are helped to identify errors in thinking (e.g., probability overestimation) and rigid rules or beliefs that underlie dysfunctional thought patterns using various techniques (e.g., Socratic questioning). Patients then generate alternative interpretations or "hypotheses" to situations to be confirmed or disconfirmed through evidence gathered in exposure exercises. By accruing evidence that challenge clients' negative thoughts, underlying beliefs can be changed.

5. Imagery Exposure is designed to help clients tolerate negative affect; habituate to fearful images associated with their principle worries, which they often attempt to avoid through worry (e.g., Borkovec & Hu, 1990); and practice cognitive restructuring skills in high-distress situations. Clients generate hierarchies of fear images related to two or three main areas of worry, and are led through systematic exposure to these images. Mild anxiety elicited by an image is a signal to progress to the next image on the hierarchy. Two main versions of imagery exposure were developed by Craske, Barlow, and O'Leary (1992) and Borkovec and Costello (1993). In the former version, clients focus on a fearful image for 25–30 minutes, and then generate alternative outcomes to the scenario. In the latter version, called coping desensitization, clients are asked to utilize their cognitive restructuring and relaxation skills during imagery exercises.

6. Additional components that may be incorporated into CBT include problem-solving to combat indecisiveness and increase the ability to generate alternative solutions to problems (Meichenbaum & Jaremko, 1983); worry behavior prevention to reduce corrective, preventative, and ritualistic behaviors tied to worry that maintain anxiety (Craske et al., 1989); and time management training and goal setting to facilitate present task accomplishment instead of allowing worry to dominate (Brown, et al., 2001).

What is Effective Medical Treatment?

Benzodiazepines. The fast-acting, anxiolytic, and muscle relaxant properties of the benzodiazepines primarily work through reducing neural transmission of the γ-aminobutyric acid (GABA) system. Benzodiazepines are available in short-acting (e.g., alprazolam) and long-acting (e.g., clorazepate) forms, with both forms taking effect quite rapidly to reduce symptoms (e.g., Rickels, Downing, et al., 1993) as shown in randomized, double-blind, placebo-controlled trials (e.g., Rickels, DeMartinis, & Aufdembrinke, 2000). Some studies (e.g., Borkovec & Whisman, 1996) have cited failure of benzodiazepines to show effects that significantly differ from placebo beyond the first 4–6 weeks of treatment. Also, the physically addictive nature of benzodiazepines leads to dependence in some people and withdrawal symptoms upon discontinuation (Shader & Greenblatt, 1983). Other disadvantages include adverse side effects (e.g., motor impairment) (Shader & Greenblatt, 1983), which are particularly problematic for the elderly.

5-HT1A partial agonists. Buspirone (BuSpar), an azapirone, is postulated to operate through the serotonergic system (Taylor, 1990) and primarily targets the cognitive symptoms of GAD (Rickels, Wiseman, et al., 1982). Buspirone requires approximately 2 weeks for symptom reduction to be noted (e.g., Jacobson, Dominguez, Goldstein, & Steinbook, 1985). BuSpar is comparable in effectiveness to the benzodiazepines (e.g., Enkelmann, 1991; Laakmann et al., 1998), and patients may maintain treatment gains longer compared to benzodiazepine use (Rickels, Schweier, Csanalosi, Case, & Chung, 1988). Buspirone has few negative side effects and its discontinuation does not lead to withdrawal symptoms (e.g., Taylor, 1990).

Tricyclic antidepressants (TCAs). Randomized controlled clinical trials have demonstrated the efficacy of several of the tricyclic antidepressants, such as imipramine (Tofranil) (e.g., Rocca, Fonzo, Scotta, Zanalda, & Ravizza, 1997). The TCAs inhibit reuptake of serotonin and norepinephrine, and primarily affect the cognitive, rather than somatic, symptoms of GAD (e.g., Hoehn-Saric, McLeod, & Zimmeri, 1988), as well as reduce depressive symptoms. However, imipramine is associated with numerous, adverse side effects including edema, dry mouth, weight gain, blurred vision, constipation, and postural hypotension (Blackwell, 1981), which may reflect the drug's effects on additional receptor systems (e.g., histamine) (Richelson, 1994).

Selective serotonin reuptake inhibitors (SSRIs). The SSRIs are associated with mild adverse side-effects that include nausea, sexual dysfunction, and sleep disturbance. Currently, paroxetine (Paxil) is the only SSRI that has been approved for use for GAD patients by the US Food and Drug Administration, and again primarily reduces cognitive symptoms associated with GAD (Pollack et al., 2001). Paroxetine was found to be more effective than benzodiazepines and imipramine (Rocca et al., 1997), and yields remission rates of up to 73% and time to relapse up to 4.7 times longer than for placebo (Stochhi et al., 2003). Other SSRIs gathering empirical support for their efficacy in the treatment of GAD include fluvoxamine (Luvox) and sertraline (Zoloft), which are among the few medications that have been examined in the pediatric and adolescent populations, both showing promising results (Ryan, Siqueland, & Rickels, 2001).

Serotonin–norepinephrine reuptake inhibitors (SNRIs). Venlafaxine (Effexor) works primarily through its effects on the serotonin and norepinephrine systems, and yields both anxiolytic and antidepressant effects on GAD patients (e.g., Gelenberg et al., 2000). Venlafaxine is associated with generally mild side effects that include nausea, sexual dysfunction, dizziness, and dry mouth. A meta-analysis of five placebo-controlled trials of venlafaxine reported overall response rates of 67% compared to 44% in younger adults and 66% compared to 41% in older adults for venlafaxine versus placebo (Meoni, Salinas, Brault, & Hackett, 2001).

Combination Treatments

Generally, studies comparing pharmacotherapy and CBT alone or in combination show superior treatment outcome when CBT was incorporated (e.g., Power, Simpson, Swanson, & Wallace, 1990a;1990b). Although CBT appears to be associated with greater long-term effects on anxiety reduction than medication, the use of benzodiazepines (i.e., diazepam) in conjunction with CBT appears to result in earlier treatment gains than CBT alone (e.g., Power et al., 1990a;1990b). Some studies have noted higher attrition rates for patients assigned to medication (e.g., Buspirone) versus CBT treatment conditions (e.g., Bond, Wingrove, Curran, & Lader, 2002). Therefore, a combined approach of pharmacotherapy and CBT may be more effective in producing rapid symptom relief, although the knowledge and skills acquired through CBT may be instrumental in the long-term maintenance of treatment gains (Schweizer & Rickels, 1996).

What are Additional Psychosocial Treatments Being Explored for GAD?

Three alternative, psychosocial treatments are currently being evaluated for GAD. Mindfulness-based interventions have been shown to be efficacious in decreasing relapse following depression remission (Teasdale, Segal, & Williams, 1995) and anxiety symptoms in an uncontrolled study of individuals with GAD and panic disorder (Kabat-Zinn et al., 1992). Another approach is Acceptance and Commitment Therapy (ACT) that combines mindfulness with relinquishing control over internal states and orienting actions towards valued goals (Hayes, Strosahl, & Wilson, 1999). Finally, emotional regulation therapy (ERT) incorporates components of CBT such as psychoeducation and self-monitoring, as well as emotion-focused interventions that address emotion regulation deficits prominent in GAD, emotional avoidance, and interpersonal difficulties (through a psychodynamic framework) (see Mennin, 2004 for a detailed review of ERT and single case treatment for GAD using ERT).

Treatment Outcome and Special Issues for Child Clients

Outcome data are more optimistic for child studies compared to older age groups. Kendall, Kane, Howard, and Siqueland (1990) developed a highly successful and widely disseminated anxiety treatment program for children ages 7–16 who suffer from GAD, Separation Anxiety Disorder (SAD), and Social Phobia (SP) called the *Coping Cat Program*, which incorporates psychoeducation, somatic management, cognitive restructuring, problem-solving, exposure, and relapse prevention. Outcome data indicate a 64–70.3% success rate at post-treatment for children no longer meeting diagnostic criteria for GAD, SAD, or SP. Results are generally maintained at 12-month and 3-year follow ups (Kendall & Southam-Gerow, 1996). Combining family management training with CBT increased the success rate of this approach to 95.6% in a study conducted by Barrett, Dadds, & Rapee (1996). Barrett, Lowry-Webster, and Holmes (1998) developed the 10-week FRIENDS protocol suitable for children and adolescents. Continued research on child and adolescent treatments for GAD are warranted. Circumstances under which family involvement in treatment can be beneficial need to be explored further, as well as how cultural and ethnic variables may impact more family-oriented approaches.

Treatment Outcome and Special Issues for Elderly Clients

Although significant improvements have been noted in CBT-outcome studies conducted with elderly participants (e.g., Stanley, Beck, Novy, et al., 2003), generally the follow-up data are less optimistic for elderly compared to younger adults (e.g., Wetherell, Gatz, & Craske, 2003). Whether this is a reflection of a lower response to therapy or a higher rate of relapse is unclear. It is also unclear what factors contribute to the high attrition rates of elderly clients (e.g., 33%) (Stanley, Beck, & Glassco, 1996). Group treatment, where interactive experiences are encouraged and opportunities for self-disclosure and exploration of feelings are provided, may increase the efficacy of CBT in the elderly (e.g., Wetherell et al., 2003). Additional treatment considerations include the use of learning aids (e.g., acronyms for techniques) and memory enhancers (e.g., homework reminders, weekly reviews of techniques) to compensate for reduced short- and long-term memory abilities; reductions in homework assignments; and a slower pace of CBT sessions.

What are Predictors of Relapse?

Comorbid diagnoses and marital conflict may contribute to post-treatment relapse in GAD (e.g., Durham, Allan, & Hackett, 1997), as well as older age and history of mental health treatment (Wetherell et al., 2003). Failure to continue practicing CBT skills can also portend relapse (Newman, 2000). Booster sessions may be warranted when clients experience life stressors or setbacks that may cause reemergence or exacerbation of symptoms. Clients should generate a list of personal warning signs to circumvent relapses (Gorski & Miller, 1982).

How Does One Select Among Treatments?

With respect to considering pharmacological treatments for GAD, physicians should consider efficacy data of particular medications, symptom severity, duration of illness, comorbidity, patient's ability to tolerate side effects, and previous treatment history. For acute anxiety reactions, benzodiazepines are a good treatment option. However, for those patients who are in need of long-term treatment, particularly in the face of comorbid conditions, antidepressants, SSRIs, and possibly SNRIs should be considered. Regarding psychosocial interventions, CBT is the treatment of choice although clinicians should assess whether patients would be responsive to CBT and committed to engaging in the cognitive and behavioral components of the therapy despite possible initial increases in symptoms. Decisions on the appropriate treatment modality for patients should take into consideration multiple patient characteristics (e.g., patient age, severity of disorder, belief in treatment, comorbidity). The short- and long-term data are promising for the combination of CBT with medication as well.

REFERENCES (DOES NOT INCLUDE LIST OF SELF-HELP BOOKS UNLESS OTHERWISE CITED)

American Psychiatric Association. (1994). *Diagnostic and statistical manual of mental disorders (4th ed.)*. Washington, DC: Author.

Arntz, A. (2003). Cognitive therapy versus applied relaxation as treatment of generalized anxiety disorder. *Behaviour Research and Therapy, 41,* 633–646.

Barlow, D. H., Rapee, R. M., & Brown, T. A. (1992). Behavioral treatment of generalized anxiety disorder. *Behavior Therapy, 23,* 551–570.

Barrett, P. M., Dadds, M. R., & Rapee, R. M. (1996). Family treatment of childhood anxiety: A controlled trial. *Journal of Consulting and Clinical Psychology, 64,* 333–342.

Barrett, P. M., Lowry-Webster, H., & Holmes, J. (1998). *The friends program.* Brisbane, Australia: Australian Academic Press.

Bernstein, D. A., Borkovec, T. D., & Hazlett-Stevens, H. (2000). *New editions in progressive relaxation training: A guidebook for helping professionals.* Westport, CT: Praeger.

Bienvenu, J. O., Nestadt, M. B., & Eaton, W. W. (1998). Characterizing generalized anxiety: The symptomatic thresholds. *Journal of Nervous and Mental Disorders, 186,* 51–56.

Blackwell, B. (1981). Adverse effects of antidepressant drugs, Pt 1: Monoamine oxidase inhibitors and tricyclics. *Drugs, 21,* 201–219.

Blazer, D. (1997). Generalized anxiety disorder and panic disorder in the elderly: A review. *Harvard Review of Psychiatry, 5,* 18–27.

Bond, A. J., Wingrove, J., Curran, H. V., & Lader, M. H. (2002). Treatment of generalized anxiety disorder with a short course of psychological therapy, combined with buspirone or placebo. *Journal of Affective Disorders, 72,* 267–271.

Borkovec, T. D. (1994). The nature, functions, and origins of worry. In G. Davey & F. Tallis (Eds.), *Worrying: Perspectives on theory, assessment, and treatment* (pp. 5–33). New York: Wiley.

Borkovec, T. D. (2002). Training clinic research and the possibility of a National Training Clinics Practice Research Network. *The Behavior Therapist, 25,* 98–103.

Borkovec, T. D., & Costello, E. (1993). Efficacy of applied relaxation and cognitive-behavioral therapy in the treatment of generalized anxiety disorder. *Journal of Consulting and Clinical Psychology, 56*, 893–897.

Borkovec, T. D., & Hu, S. (1990). The effect of worry on cardiovascular response to phobic imagery. *Behaviour Research and Therapy, 28*, 69–73.

Borkovec, T. D., & Inz, J. (1990). The nature of worry in Generalised Anxiety Disorder: A predominance of thought activity. *Behaviour Research and Therapy, 28*, 153–158.

Borkovec, T. D., Newman, M. G., Pincus, A. L., & Ltle, R. (2002). A component analysis of cognitive-behavioral therapy for generalized anxiety disorder and the role of interpersonal problems. *Journal of Consulting and Clinical Psychology, 70*, 288–298.

Borkovec, T. D., & Ruscio, A. M. (2001). Psychotherapy for generalized anxiety disorder. *Journal of Clinical Psychiatry, 62(Suppl. 11)*, 37–42.

Borkovec, T. D., & Whisman, M. A. (1996). Psychosocial treatment for generalized anxiety disorder. In M. Mavissakalian & R. Prien (Eds.), *Long-term treatment for the anxiety disorders.* (pp. 171–199). Washington, DC: American Psychiatric Press.

Brown, T. A., Campbell, L. A., Lehman, C. L., Grisham, J. R., & Mancill, R. B. (2001). Current and lifetime comorbidity of the DSM-IV anxiety and mood disorders in a large clinical sample. *Journal of Abnormal Psychology, 110*, 585–599.

Brown, T. A., Di Nardo, P. A., & Barlow, D. H. (1994). *Anxiety disorders interview schedule for DSM-IV (ADIS-IV).* Boulder, CO: Graywind.

Brown, T. A., O'Leary, T. A., & Barlow, D. H. (2001). Generalized anxiety disorder. In D. H. Barlow (Ed.), *Clinical handbook of psychological disorders: A step-by-step treatment manual* (pp. 154–207). New York: Guilford.

Butler, G., Fennell, M., Robson, P., & Gelder, M. (1991). Comparison of behavior therapy and cognitive behavior therapy in the treatment of generalized anxiety disorder. *Journal of Consulting and Clinical Psychology, 59*, 167–175.

Butler, G. & Mathews, A. (1983). Anticipatory anxiety and risk prevention. *Cognitive Therapy Research, 11*, 551–565.

Cartwright-Hatton, S., & Wells, A. (1997). Beliefs about worry and intrusions: The Meta-cognitions Questionnaire. *Journal of Anxiety Disorders, 11*, 279–315.

Craske, M. G. (1999). *Anxiety Disorders.* Boulder, CO: Westview Press.

Craske, M. G. (2003). *Origins of phobias and anxiety disorders: Why more women than men.* Oxford: Elsevier.

Craske, M. G., Barlow, D. H., & O'Leary, T. A. (1992). *Mastery of your anxiety and worry.* Boulder, CO: Graywind.

Craske, M. G., Street, L., & Barlow, D. H. (1989). Instructions to focus upon or distract from internal cues during exposure treatment of agoraphobic avoidance. *Behaviour Research and Therapy, 27*, 663–672.

Dugas, M. J., Ladouceur, R., Leger, E., Freeston, M. H., Langlois, F., Provencher, M. D., et al. (2003). Group cognitive-behavioral therapy for generalized anxiety disorder: Treatment outcome and long-term follow-up. *Journal of Consulting and Clinical Psychology, 71(4)*, 821–825.

Durham, R. C., Allan, T., & Hackett, C. A. (1997). On predicting improvement and relapse in generalized anxiety disorder following psychotherapy. *British Journal of Clinical Psychology, 36*, 101–119.

Durham, R. C., Fisher, P. L., Treliving, L. R., Hau, C. M., Richard, K., & Stewart, J. B. (1999). One year follow-up of cognitive therapy, analytic psychotherapy and anxiety management training for generalized anxiety disorder: symptom change, medication usage and attitudes to treatment. *Behavioural and Cognitive Psychotherapy, 27*, 19–35.

Enkelmann, R. (1991). Alprazolam versus buspirone in the treatment of outpatients with generalized anxiety disorder. *Psychopharmacology, 105*, 428–432.

Eysenck, M. W., Mogg, K., May, J., Richards, A., & Mathews, A. (1991). Bias in interpretation of ambiguous sentences related to threat in anxiety. *Journal of Abnormal Psychology, 100(2)*, 144–150.

First, M. B., Spitzer, R. L., Gibbon, M., & Williams, J. B. W. (1997). Structured Clinical Interview for DSM-IV Axis I Disorders (SCID-I). American Psychiatric Publishing, Inc.

Fisher, P. L., & Durham, R. C. (1999). Recovery rates in generalized anxiety disorder following psychological therapy: An analysis of clinically significant change in the STAI-T across outcome studies since 1990. *Psychological Medicine, 29*, 1425–1434.

Gelenberg, A. J., Lydiard, R. B., Rudolph, R. L., Aguiar, L., Haskins, J. T., & Salinas, E. (2000). Efficacy of venlafaxine extended-release capsules in nondepressed outpatients with generalized anxiety disorder: A 6-month randomized controlled trial. *Journal of the American Medical Association, 283*, 3082–3088.

Gorski, T., & Miller, M. (1982). *Counseling for relapse prevention.* Independence, MO: Independence Press.

Hayes, S. C., Strosahl, K. D., & Wilson, K. G. (1999). *Acceptance and commitment therapy: An experiential approach to behavior change.* New York, NY: The Guilford Press.

Hoehn-Saric, R., McLeod, D. R., & Zimmerli, W. D. (1989). Somatic manifestations in women with generalized anxiety disorder: Psychophysiological responses to psychological stress. *Archives of General Psychiatry, 46*, 1113–1119.

GENERALIZED ANXIETY DISORDER

311

Jacobson, A. F., Dominguez, R. A., Goldstein, B. J., & Steinbook, R. M. (1985). Comparison of buspirone and diazepam in generalized anxiety disorder. *Pharmacotherapy*, 5, 290–296.

Kabat-Zinn, J., Massion, A. O., Kristeller, J., Peterson, L. G., Fletcher, K. E., Pbert, L., et al. (1992). Effectiveness of a meditation-based stress reduction program in the treatment of anxiety disorders. *American Journal of Psychiatry, 149(7)*, 936–943.

Kendall, P. C., Kane, M., Howard, B., & Siqueland, L. (1990). *Cognitive-behavioral treatment of anxious children: Treatment manual.* Temple University: Author.

Kendall, P. C., & Southam-Gerow, M. A. (1996). Long-term follow-up of a cognitive-behavioral therapy for anxiety disordered youth. *Journal of Consulting and Clinical Psychology, 64*, 724–730.

Kessler, R. C., DuPont, R. L., Berglund, P., & Wittchen, H. U. (1999). Impairment in pure and comorbid generalized anxiety disorder and depression at 12 months in two national surveys. *American Journal of Psychiatry, 156*, 1915–1923.

Kogan, J. N., Edelstein, B. A., & McKee, D. R. (1999). Assessment of anxiety in older adults: Current status. *Journal of Anxiety Disorders, 14*, 109–132.

Laakmann, G., Schule, C., Lorkowski, G., Baghai, T., Kuhn, K., & Ehrentraut, S. (1998). Buspirone and lorazepam in the treatment of generalized anxiety disorder in outpatients. *Psychopharmacology, 136*, 357–366.

Ladouceur, R., Dugas, M. J., Freeston, M. H., Leger, E., Gagnon, F., & Thibodeau, N. (2000). Efficacy of a cognitive-behavioral treatment for generalized anxiety disorder: Evaluation in a controlled clinical trial. *Journal of Consulting and Clinical Psychology, 68*, 957–964.

Lydiard, R. B., Ballenger, J. C., & Rickels, K. (1997). A double-blind evaluation of the safety and efficacy of abecarnil, alprazolam, and placebo in outpatients with generalized anxiety disorder. Abecarnil Work Group. *Journal of Clinical Psychiatry, 58(Suppl. 11)*, 11–18.

Mathews, A., & MacLeod, C. (1985). Selective processing of threat cues in anxiety states. *Behaviour Research and Therapy, 23(5)*, 17–22.

Meichenbaum, D. S., & Jaremko, M. E. (Eds.). (1983). *Stress reduction and prevention.* New York: Plenum Press.

Mennin, D. S. (2004). Emotion regulation therapy for generalized anxiety disorder. *Clinical Psychology and Psychotherapy, 11*, 17–29.

Meoni, P., Salinas, E., Brault, Y., & Hackett, D. (2001). Pattern of symptom improvement following treatment with venlafaxine XR in patients with generalized anxiety disorder. *Journal of Clinical Psychiatry, 62(11)*, 888–893.

Meyer, T. J., Miller, M. L., Metzger, R. L., & Borkovec, T. D. (1990). Development and validation of the Penn State Worry Questionnaire. *Behaviour Research and Therapy, 28*, 487–496.

Mineka, S., Watson, D., & Clark, L. A. (1998). Comorbidity of anxiety and unipolar mood disorders. *Annual Review of Psychology, 49*, 377–412.

Newman, M. G. (2000). Generalized anxiety disorder. In M. Hersen and M. Biaggio (Eds.), *Effective brief therapies: A clinician's guide* (pp. 158–178). San Diego, CA: Academic Press.

Öst, L. (1987). Applied relaxation: Description of a copying technique and review of controlled studies. *Behaviour Research and Therapy, 25*, 397–409.

Öst, L., & Breitholtz, E. (2000). Applied relaxation vs. cognitive therapy in the treatment of generalized anxiety disorder, *Behaviour Research and Therapy, 38*, 777–790.

Overholser, J. C., & Nasser, E. H. (2000). Cognitive-behavioral treatment of generalized anxiety disorder. *Journal of Contemporary Psychotherapy, 30*, 149–161.

Pollack, M. H., Zaninelli, R., Goddard, A., McCafferty, J. P., Bellew, K. M., Burnham, D. B., et al. (2001). Paroxetine in the treatment of generalized anxiety disorder: results of a placebo-controlled, flexible-dosage trial. *Journal of Clinical Psychiatry, 63*, 350–357.

Power, K. G., Simpson, R. J., Swanson, V., & Wallace, L. A. (1990a). A controlled comparison of cognitive-behaviour therapy, diazepam, and placebo, alone and in combination, for the treatment of generalised anxiety disorder. *Journal of Anxiety Disorders, 4*, 267–292.

Power, K. G., Simpson, R. J., Swanson, V., & Wallace, L. A. (1990b). Controlled comparison of pharmacological and psychological treatment of generalized anxiety disorder in primary care. *British Journal of General Practice, 40*, 289–294.

Purdon, C. (1999). Thought suppression and psychopathology. *Behavior Research and Therapy, 37*, 1029–1054.

Richelson, E. (1994). Pharmacology of antidepressants: characteristics of the ideal drug. *Mayo Clinical Proceedings, 69*, 1069–1081.

Rickels, K., DeMartinis, N., & Aufdembrinke, B. (2000). A double-blind, placebo-controlled trial of abecarnil and diazepam in the treatment of patients with generalized anxiety disorder. *Journal of Clinical Psychopharmacology, 20*, 12–18.

Rickels, K., Downing, R., Schweizer, E., et al. (1993). Antidepressants for the treatment of generalized anxiety disorder: a placebo-controlled comparison of imipramine, trazodone, and diazepam. *Archives of General Psychiatry, 50*, 884–895.

Rickels, K., & Rynn, M. (2001). Overview and clinical presentation of generalized anxiety disorder. *Psychiatric Clinic of North America, 24*, 1–17.

Rickels, K., & Rynn, M. (2002). Pharmacotherapy of generalized anxiety disorder. *Journal of Clinical Psychiatry, 63(Suppl. 14)*, 9–16.

Rickels, K., Schweier, E., Csanalosi, I., Case, W. G., & Chung, H. (1988). Long-term treatment of anxiety and risk of withdrawal: prospective comparison of clorazepate and buspirone. *Archieves of General Psychiatry, 45*, 444–450.

Rickels, K., Weisman, K., Norstad, N., Singer, M., Stoltz, D., Brown, A., et al. (1982). Buspirone and diazepam in anxiety: A controlled study. *Journal of Clinical Psychiatry, 43*, 81–86.

Rocca, P., Fonzo, V., Scotta, F., Zanalda, E., & Ravizza, L. (1997). Paroxetine efficacy in the treatment of generalized anxiety disorder. *Psychiatra Scandinavia, 95*, 444–450.

Ryan, M. A., Siqueland, L., & Rickels, K. (2001). Placebo-controlled trial of sertraline in the treatment of children with generalized anxiety disorder. *American Journal of Psychiatry, 158*, 2008–2015.

Schweizer, E., & Rickels, K. (1996). The long-term management of generalized anxiety disorder: Issues and dilemmas. *Journal of Clinical Psychiatry, 57(Suppl. 7)*, 9–12.

Shader, R. I., & Greenblatt, D. J. (1983). Some current treatment options for symptoms of anxiety. *Psychiatry, 44*, 21–30.

Stanley, M. A., & Beck, J. G. (2000). Anxiety Disorders. *Clinical Psychology Review, 20(6)*, 731–754.

Stanley, M. A., Beck, J. G., & Glassco, J. D. (1996). Treatment of generalized anxiety in older adults: A preliminary comparison of cognitive-behavioral and supportive approaches. *Behavior Therapy, 27*, 565–581.

Stanley, M. A., Beck, J. G., Novy, D. M., Averill, P. M., Swann, A. C., Diefenbach, G. J., et al. (2003). Cognitive-behavioral treatment of late-life generalized anxiety disorders. *Journal of Consulting and Clinical Psychology, 71(2)*, 309–319.

Stochhi, F., Nordera, G., Jokinen, R. H., Lepola, U. M., Hewett, K., Bryson, H., et al. (2003). Efficacy and tolerability of paroxetine for the treatment of generalized anxiety disorder. *Journal of Clinical Psychiatry, 64*, 250–258.

Taylor, D. P. (1990). Serotonin agents in anxiety. *Annual New York Academy of Science, 600*, 545–546.

Teasdale, J. D., Segal, Z., & Williams, J. M. (1995). How does cognitive therapy prevent depressive relapse and why should attentional control (mindfulness) training help? *Behaviour Research and Therapy, 33(1)*, 25–39.

Thayer, J. F., Friedman, B. H., & Borkovec, T. D. (1996). Autonomic characteristics of generalized anxiety disorder and worry. *Biological Psychiatry, 39*, 255–266.

Wells, A. (1994). Attention and the control of worry. In G. C. L. Davey & F. Tallis (Eds.), Worrying: Perspectives on theory, assessment and treatment. Chichester, UK: Wiley.

Wells, A., & Carter, K. (1999). Preliminary tests of a cognitive model of Generalised Anxiety Disorder. *Behaviour Research and Therapy, 37*, 585–594.

Wells, A., & Cartwright-Hatton, S. (2004). A short form of the metacognitions questionnaire: Properties of the MCQ-30. *Behaviour Research and Therapy, 42*, 385–396.

Wells, A., & Davies, M. (1994). The Thought Control Questionnaire: A measure of individual differences in the control of unwanted thoughts. *Behaviour Research and Therapy, 32*, 871–878.

Wells, A., & Matthews, G. (1994). *Attention and emotion: a clinical perspective.* Hove, UK: Erlbaum.

Wetherell, J. L., Gatz, M., & Craske, M. G. (2003). Treatment of generalized anxiety disorder in older adults. *Journal of Consulting and Clinical Psychology, 71*, 31–40.

Wittchen, H. U., Zhao, S., Kessler, R. C., & de Boer, A. G. (1994). DSM-III-R generalized anxiety disorder in the National Comorbidity Survey. *Archives of General Psychiatry, 51*, 355–364.

Hypochondriasis

Steven Taylor • Gordon J. G. Asmundson

WHAT HYPOCHONDRIASIS?

Hypochondriasis, as defined in the *Diagnostic and Statistical Manual of Mental Disorders—Fourth Edition Text Revision* (DSM-IV-TR; American Psychiatric Association [APA], 2000), is a somatoform disorder characterized by the following features. The primary feature is preoccupation with fears and beliefs about having a serious disease based on misinterpretation of bodily sensations. This preoccupation must persist despite appropriate medical evaluation and reassurance, disease-related beliefs cannot be of delusion intensity nor restricted to concerns about defects in appearance, there must be significant distress or impairment in important areas of functioning, and the preoccupation has to last at least six months. A diagnosis of hypochondrias is made when these criteria are met and disease preoccupation is not better accounted for by another disorder (e.g., obsessive compulsive disorder, major depressive disorder). DSM-IV-TR subtypes of hypochondriasis are defined according to insight. Hypochondriasis with poor insight is diagnosed when, for most of the time during the course of the disorder, the person does not recognize that their concern about having a serious disease is excessive or unreasonable.

There are two types of disease fear in hypochondriasis. These included the fear that one *currently* has a disease, and fear that one *might contract* a disease in the future. People with hypochondriasis usually fear that they have a disease, although they may also have future-oriented fears of contracting a disease. Fear of currently having a disease is associated with seeking reassurance from primary care physicians or family members that one's health is good, recurrent checking of one's body (e.g., frequent breast self-examinations), seeking out other sources of information on the dreaded disease (e.g., checking medical textbooks or the Internet), and trying various kinds of remedies such as herbal preparations (Côté et al., 1996; Taylor & Asmundson, 2004). Fear of contracting a disease is typically associated with phobic avoidance, such as staying away from crowded public places during influenza epidemics or not touching potentially germ-infested public door handles with bare hands.

The fear of currently having a disease tends to persist even though the person receives ample reassurance from physicians that there is no evidence of serious disease, and despite the fact that the frightening "symptoms" rarely become progressively worse (as might happen in the case of a serious physical condition). People with hypochondriasis typically resist the idea that they are suffering from a mental disorder. They tend to misinterpret the seriousness of harmless, natural bodily fluctuations, such as those that might arise during times of stress or other changes in daily routine, and to overestimate the seriousness of symptoms of general medical conditions (Côté et al., 1996). They may present with highly specific symptoms, or report symptoms that are vague, variable, and generalized (e.g., aching "all over"). Common specific symptoms include localized pain, bowel complaints (e.g., changes in bowel habits), and cardiorespiratory sensations (e.g., chest tightness) (Barsky & Klerman, 1983).

Taylor, S., & Asmundson, G. J. G. (2006). Hypochondriasis. In J. E. Fisher & W. T. O'Donohue (Eds.), *Practitioner's guide to evidence-based psychotherapy*. New York: Springer.

People with hypochondriasis may perpetually adopt a sick role, living as an invalid and avoiding all effortful occupational and home responsibilities (Barsky, 1992). In addition, they complain persistently about their health, discussing their concerns at length with anyone who will listen. This can lead to strained relationships with their family, friends, and physicians. Frustration and anger on the part of physician and patient are not uncommon (APA, 2000). "Doctor shopping"—visiting many different physicians in the hope of finding help (Kasteler et al., 1976; Sato et al., 1995)—is often the result. In seeing many different physicians, some people with hypochondriasis are at-risk of unnecessary or repeated medical and surgical treatments, some of which can produce troubling side effects or treatment complications (e.g., scarring, pain). Thus, hypochondriasis can be worsened by iatrogenic (physician-induced) factors.

BASIC FACTS ABOUT HYPOCHONDRIASIS

Comorbidity. Hypochondriasis frequently co-occurs with mood disorders, anxiety disorders, and somatization disorder (Asmundson Taylor, Sevgur, & Cox, 2001a; Noyes, 2001). Approximately 40% of patients with hypochondriasis assessed in primary care settings have concurrent major depression. This is much higher than the frequency of major depression in primary care patients without hypochondriasis (16–18%). Primary care patients with hypochondriasis are also more likely to have panic disorder (16–17%) than their counterparts without hypochondriasis (3–6%; Barsky, Barnett, & Cleary, 1994a; Noyes et al., 1994b). Hypochondriasis is also a common comorbid diagnosis in patients with other psychiatric disorders (Barsky, Wool, Barnett, & Cleary, 1994b).

Prevalence. Estimates suggest that hypochondriasis has a lifetime prevalence in the general population of 1–5% (APA, 2000). A recent review indicated that estimates of point prevalence (i.e., proportion of cases at the time of study) and 12-month prevalence (i.e., proportion of cases during a 12-month period) are also between 1% and 5% (Asmundson, Taylor, Wright, & Cox, 2001c). Prevalence estimates in medical settings vary considerably, ranging from 1% in specialty settings (e.g., cardiology clinics) to between 1% and 9% for primary care and general medical settings (Asmundson et al., 2001a). Thus, hypochondriasis is as common as many major psychiatric disorders, such as panic disorder and schizophrenia (APA, 2000).

Age at onset. Hypochondriasis can arise at any age, although it most commonly develops in early adulthood (APA, 2000). It typically arises when the person is under stress, seriously ill or recovering from a serious illness, or has suffered the loss of a family member (Barsky & Klerman, 1983). Excessive health anxiety also can occur when the person is exposed to disease-related media information, such as news reports about infectious outbreaks (Taylor & Asmundson, 2004).

Gender. Despite some inconsistencies in the literature, most studies have found that hypochondriasis is equally common in women and men (Asmundson et al., 2001a).

Course. The course of hypochondriasis is often chronic (APA, 2000), persisting for years in over 50% of cases (Barsky, Wyshak, Klerman, & Latham, 1990; Barsky, Fama, Bailey, & Ahern, 1998a; Barsky, Orav, Delamater, Clancy, & Hartley, 1998b; Robbins & Kirmayer, 1996). It is most likely to become chronic in people who (1) experience many unpleasant bodily sensations, (2) believe they have a serious medical condition, and (3) have a comorbid psychiatric disorder such as major depression (Barsky, Cleary, Sarnie, & Klerman, 1993; Noyes et al., 1994a,b).

Functional impairment. Hypochondriasis can significantly interfere with interpersonal relationships, work, and leisure activities. People with hypochondriasis, compared to those without the disorder, are less likely to be employed outside the home, have more days of bed rest, have greater physical limitations, and are more likely to be living on disability benefits (Barsky et al., 1990, 1998a,b; Escobar et al., 1998; Noyes et al., 1993). They also pay more visits to primary care physicians and specialists, have more medical laboratory tests and surgical procedures, and exert a greater economic burden on the health care system (Barsky, Ettner, Horsky, & Bates, 2001; Hollifield, Paine, Tuttle, & Kellner, 1999). There is also evidence to suggest that they may have a higher divorce rate (Cloninger, Sigvardsson, von Knorring & Bohman, 1984).

Other demographic characteristics. It is unclear whether health anxiety changes with age. The research so far has been based largely on cross-sectional (cohort) studies, which have yielded conflicting findings. Some studies suggest that health anxiety is greater in older than younger people (Altamura, Carta, Tacchini, Musazzi, & Pioli, 1998; Gureje, Üstün, & Simon, 1997), while other research has found no difference between age groups (Barsky, Frank, Cleary, Wyshak, & Klerman, 1991). Longitudinal studies are needed to further examine this issue. Cultural factors, such as societally transmitted values and expectations, can influence how a person interprets bodily changes and sensations, and whether treatment-seeking is initiated. There appear to be cross-cultural differences in which bodily changes and sensations tend to be feared the most (Escobar, Allen, Hoyos Nervi, & Gara, 2001). Some cultures appear to be more concerned about gastrointestinal sensations (e.g., excessive concern about constipation in the UK), while other cultures appear to be more concerned about cardiopulmonary symptoms (e.g., excessive concern about poor blood circulation and low blood pressure in Germany compared to other countries). The US and Canada appear to have particularly high concerns about immunologically based symptoms, such as those related to viruses, "sick building syndrome," and "multiple chemical sensitivity" (Escobar et al., 2001).

ASSESSMENT

What Should be Ruled Out?

A medical evaluation is needed to rule out any and all general medical conditions that might account for the patient's presenting concerns. By the time hypochondriasis is diagnosed, the patient typically has had numerous medical evaluations, usually at his or her own insistence, with the results failing to find a general medical condition that could account for the patient's concerns. In some cases a general medical condition may be diagnosed. In these cases, a diagnosis of hypochondriasis is made when the diagnosed medical condition does not fully account for the person's concerns about disease or for their bodily changes or sensations (APA, 2000). This is illustrated by the following examples (Schmidt, 1994).

- Hypochondriasis would be diagnosed when the person catastrophically misinterprets medical information about a general medical condition.
- When a person has a medical condition with a good prognosis, hypochondriasis would be diagnosed when she or he becomes excessively anxious about the prognosis and is unable to accept the physician's reassurance.
- Hypochondriasis would be diagnosed when disease fears or beliefs are based on bodily sensations or changes that have nothing to do with the diagnosed medical condition.
- Hypochondriasis would be diagnosed when there is evidence that it was present before the development of a general medical condition.

Because disease-related fears and beliefs are common in other psychiatric conditions—especially panic disorder, generalized anxiety disorder, obsessive compulsive disorder, mood disorders, and somatic type delusional disorder—these also need to be ruled out. Treatment of these conditions often leads to resolution of disease-related fears and beliefs.

What is Involved in Effective Assessment?

A thorough psychological assessment of hypochondriasis should include a general medical evaluation, assessment of current DSM-IV-TR axes I and II diagnoses (to assess for comorbid disorders), an evaluation of the patient's personal history, current living circumstances, specific features of hypochondriasis, and his or her reasons for seeking treatment for hypochondriasis. Some patients present for treatment because they have been pressured to do so by their doctor or family members. It is important to identify and address such issues because they can interfere with treatment adherence.

The patient's personal history is assessed in order to identify the learning experiences that may have contributed to the development of hypochondriasis (research suggests that environmental factors such as childhood experiences with illness may play an important role in hypochondriasis; Taylor & Asmundson, 2004). The patient's living circumstances are assessed in order to identify stressors (which may contribute to tension or anxiety-related bodily sensations that may be misinterpreted as indications of disease) and to assess the patient's relationship with her or his significant others (e.g., do family and friends provide excessive reassurance or take on many of the patient's responsibilities?).

The specific features of hypochondriasis that are assessed include the following: Troubling bodily changes (e.g., rashes, blemishes) or sensations (e.g., pains); disease fears; dysfunctional beliefs and strength of conviction (e.g., beliefs such as "Healthy people never experience bodily sensations"); and avoidance or "safety" behaviors that the patient engages in (e.g., remaining in close proximity of hospitals "just in case" of illness).

Clinician-administered measures. The Structured Clinical Interview for DSM-IV (First, Spitzer, Gibbon, Williams, & Lorna, 1994) provides a comprehensive assessment of the more common disorders, along with an assessment of hypochondriasis. For clinicians desiring a more detailed assessment of hypochondriasis, the Health Anxiety Interview (Taylor & Asmundson, 2004) provides a comprehensive evaluation of the nature and history of the patient's health concerns.

Self-report measures. There are numerous self-report measures of hypochondriasis and related constructs. The most widely used of these are reproduced in an appendix in Taylor and Asmundson (2004). The questionnaires differ in several ways, including breadth of assessment, time required for administration and scoring, availability of norms, and the amount of research on their reliability and validity. The choice of scale depends partly on the purpose of the assessment. If the clinician requires a quick assessment of health anxiety, then the Whiteley Index (Pilowsky, 1967) is a particularly good choice because, unlike other brief measures, norms and screening cut-off scores are available. The Whiteley Index is short enough for periodic re-administration throughout treatment to monitor progress. If a more detailed assessment of the various facets of health anxiety are desired, then the Illness Attitude Scales (Kellner, 1986, 1987) would be a good choice, particularly because it is easy to score, there are a good deal of data on its reliability and validity, and norms are available.

Behavioral assessment. Direct observation methods are rarely used in the assessment and treatment of hypochondriasis. Prospective monitoring methods are more often used, and likely to be more informative. Prospective monitoring involves the use of a daily diary or checklist (e.g., see the appendix of Taylor & Asmundson, 2004). Patients can be asked to complete the diary each day for one or two weeks prior to treatment. This provides a wealth of information about daily episodes the patient's health concerns and health behaviors.

What Assessments are Not Helpful?

Patients with hypochondriasis may request extensive medical evaluations. Some doctors try to placate the patient by providing these medically unnecessary assessments. Such tests are not helpful, and may perpetuate hypochondriasis, because repeated testing can have iatrogenic effects (e.g., scarring and pain due to repeated exploratory surgeries), and can reinforce the patient's mistaken belief that she or he has a serious disease (e.g., "I must have something seriously wrong with me because the doctor has agreed to conduct more tests") (Taylor & Asmundson, 2004).

Projective tests and neuropsychological tests are not useful in assessing hypochondriasis. Although the MMPI and MMPI-2 are widely used psychological tests, the "hypochondriasis" scales in these tests have been widely criticized; these scales measure the experience of physical symptoms rather than the fear that one has, or might acquire, a disease (Asmundson, Taylor, & Cox, 2001b).

TREATMENT

What Treatments are Effective?

A small but steadily growing number of studies have evaluated pharmacologic and psychosocial treatments for hypochondriasis. A recent meta-analysis examined 25 treatment trials of full-blown or subclinical hypochondriasis (Taylor, Asmundson, & Coons, 2005). Although there were not a large number of studies for inclusion, the meta-analytic findings provided some suggestive results, which were consistent with the results of individual studies that compared two or more interventions, and with the results of narrative reviews (e.g., Asmundson et al., 2001b). The medications examined were various types of selective serotonin reuptake inhibitors (SSRIs; e.g., paroxetine, fluvoxamine, fluoxetine) and the most commonly examined psychosocial interventions were cognitive-behavioral interventions (e.g., psychoeducation, exposure and response prevention, cognitive therapy, cognitive-behavior therapy, behavioral stress management). The meta-analyses suggested that effect sizes were larger for all psychosocial interventions and SSRI interventions than for wait-lists. There was some suggestion that a combination of cognitive and behavioral interventions was more effective than either intervention alone, with treatment gains maintained at 12-month follow-up. The most promising medication was fluoxetine.

Despite the pessimism about treating hypochondriasis expressed by some clinical practitioners (e.g., Gelder, Gath & Mayou, 1983; Martin & Yutz, 1994; Nemiah, 1985), the empirical evidence indicates that there are effective pharmacologic and cognitive-behavioral interventions. The meta-analysis also indicated that for mild (subclinical) hypochondriasis, psychoeducation alone is an effective intervention, compared to no-treatment controls. Psychoeducation involves the provision of information about the roles of dysfunctional beliefs and maladaptive behaviors, such as checking and reassurance-seeking, in the maintenance of hypochondriasis. Patients receiving psychoeducation are given information about methods that they can use to challenge dysfunctional beliefs and eliminate maladaptive behaviors (for details, see Asmundson & Taylor, 2005).

What are Effective Self-Help Treatments?

Although there are a number of informative books written by people who have struggled with, and to some degree overcome hypochondriasis (e.g., Cantor, 1996), there are very few self-help books and, to our knowledge, only one empirically supported self-help treatment for hypochondriasis. Cognitive-behavioral self-help programs are described in books by Zgourides (2002) and Asmundson and Taylor (2005). The usefulness of these books, either as adjuncts to therapist-based treatments or as stand-alone interventions for hypochondriasis, remain to be evaluated; however, results from a controlled trial comparing 4-weeks of cognitive-behavioral self-help (as outlined in a brief, unpublished booklet from Warnford Hospital, Oxford, UK) to waitlist in patients with mild health anxiety indicated that the treatment group showed less anxiety at post-test than did the controls (Jones, 2002). This, combined with evidence of the merits of therapist-administered psychoeducation for subclinical hypochondriasis (Taylor et al., 2005), provides encouraging evidence that self-help treatments may be useful for people with this mild health anxiety.

What are Effective Therapist-Based Treatments?

The meta-analytic findings, along with the results of the individual studies, suggest that various cognitive-behavioral interventions are effective, particularly multi-component interventions such as cognitive-behavior therapy and behavioral stress management. Both types of intervention begin with psychoeducation. The "noisy body" analogy is a useful psychoeducational tool for introducing patients to a cognitive-behavioral approach. Here, troubling sensations are re-labeled as harmless "bodily noise" rather than indications of physical dysfunction. The behavioral stress management approach emphasizes the role of stress in producing harmless, but unpleasant bodily sensations. The patient is encouraged to practice various stress management exercises (e.g., relaxation training, time management skills, problem solving exercises) as a means of managing stress, and thereby reducing the bodily sensations that fuel hypochondriacal concerns.

Although this latter approach has been found to be effective (Clark et al., 1998), a conceptually more elegant approach is to teach patients that they do not even need to try to rid themselves of stress-related bodily sensations, because the sensations are not harmful. This is the approach taken by cognitive-behavior therapy. This involves cognitive restructuring, to examine beliefs about the meaning of bodily sensations, and behavioral exercises to further test beliefs and to examine the effects of hypochondriacal behavior patterns. For example, to test the effects of reassurance-seeking, the patient could be encouraged to refrain from this behavior for a period of time. Often, patients discover that reassurance-seeking drives their disease fears and feelings of vulnerability. Once patients refrain from reassurance-seeking they often find that they are less preoccupied with their health, and feel less vulnerable, because they are not exposed to daily reminders of morbidity and mortality.

What is Effective Medical Treatment?

Case studies suggest that tricyclic antidepressants, such as imipramine, can reduce hypochondriasis, although most of the empirical research has focused on SSRIs (Taylor & Asmundson, 2004; Taylor et al., 2005). SSRI medications such as paroxetine, fluoxetine, fluvoxamine, and nefazadone all appear to be useful, although preliminary evidence suggests that fluoxetine is especially promising (Taylor et al., 2005). Little is currently known about the long-term efficacy of various medications for treating hypochondriasis, or about the relapse rates once the medications are discontinued. In comparison, studies have shown that the gains from cognitive-behavioral interventions are generally maintained after treatment has been discontinued, as assessed at follow-up intervals up to 12 months (Taylor et al., 2005).

Combination Treatments

No information is currently available about the efficacy of combining cognitive-behavioral interventions with psychotropic medications.

Other Issues in Management

Medical treatment Treatment for hypochondriasis, whether psychosocial or pharmacologic, is conducted in the context of good medical management. Primary care physicians play an important role in encouraging patients to try a course of cognitive-behavioral therapy for their fears and beliefs about having a serious disease (Visser & Bouman, 2001). Patients referred for such treatment are typically those that have failed to respond to simpler interventions, such as physician assurance that their health is fine. To avoid unnecessary medical evaluations, the patient, cognitive-behavioral practitioner, and the patient's primary care physician can generate a tailored list of guidelines for when a physician should be consulted. Specific guidelines for seeking medical care will depend on the nature of the patient's physical health. For elderly or infirm patients, it may be medically necessary for frequent (e.g., monthly) medical check-ups.

Psychotherapy A typical course of cognitive-behavioral therapy consists of 12–16 weekly individual sessions. Little is known about the predictors of treatment response, although patients are likely to prematurely terminate treatment if they perceive that it lacks credibility or if they perceive that the therapist is not taking the patient's health concerns seriously (Wells, 1997). Accordingly, treatment engagement strategies are important, particularly at the beginning of treatment. There are various forms of engagement strategies, including ones using a motivational enhancement approach (Taylor & Asmundson, 2004). These approaches involve various means of encouraging the patient to consider a psychosocial approach to their problems, while not dismissing or trivializing the distressing nature of their health fears.

Websites The Internet is a vast source of health-related information and misinformation. With the widespread availability of the Internet, people suffering from hypochondriasis have been increasingly searching medical web sites to learn about feared symptoms and diseases, such as on-line medical reference sites, medical school research sites, health-related websites set up by lay people or private companies, and bulletin boards devoted to the discussion of symptoms and diseases. Often web searches make the person's health anxiety much worse. Thus, Internet checking can induce or perpetuate what the media has dubbed "cyberchondria."

Some websites contain bulletin boards devoted primarily to hypochondriasis. These boards and their associated websites are intended for people who realize that their health anxiety is excessive, or have significant others with this problem. The goal of these Internet resources is to provide support and helpful information to health-anxious people. However, a review of the postings on these boards reveals that people are all too often using them for the purpose of reassurance seeking. Some people place weekly postings, with concerns about a different "symptom" each week. They receive temporary reassurance from other people, until the next troubling "symptom" arises. Thus, these bulletin boards may inadvertently perpetuate health anxiety.

There are numerous website providing basic information about hypochondriasis for clinical practitioners. However, there is little available in terms of other web-based resources for therapists.

How Does One Select Among Treatments?

Is one form of treatment more acceptable than others? Walker, Vincent, Furer, Cox, and Kjernisted (1999) presented balanced written descriptions of cognitive-behavior therapy and pharmacotherapy for "intense illness worries" to a community-based sample of 23 people with hypochondriasis interested in seeking treatment for their concerns. The written descriptions outlined the time commitment and the major advantages and disadvantages of each treatment. Most preferred cognitive-behavioral therapy. Indeed, it was the first choice of 74% of participants and, or these, 48% said they would only accept this treatment. Given that cognitive-behavior therapy and some medications may be roughly equivalent in efficacy, at least in the short-term, and that there is no evidence that one treatment works any faster than another, some clinicians let the patient choose between the two (Enns, Kjernisted, & Lander, 2001). The availability of choices might enhance treatment acceptability and adherence. Patients failing to benefit from one intervention could be placed on another.

There is little evidence that specific characteristics of hypochondriasis indicate that specific treatments should be used. Patients with a strong preference for one type of treatment (e.g., cognitive-behavior therapy) may have a worse prognosis if offered some other type of treatment (e.g., medications) because the odds of dropping out may be higher if they receive a non-preferred treatment. Otherwise, the bulk of useful prognostic factors appear to predict outcome for a range of treatments, including medications and psychosocial interventions. Good prognostic signs, as identified by various sources (APA, 2000; Barsky, 1996; Barsky et al., 1998; Fallon et al., 1993; House, 1989; Kellner, 1983; Noyes et al., 1994a; Pilowsky, 1968; Speckens, Spinhoven, van Hemert, Bolk, & Hawton, 1997) are hypochondriasis that is mild, short-lived, and not associated with complicating factors such as personality disorders, comorbid general medical conditions, or contingencies ("secondary gains") that reinforce health anxiety or sick-role behavior.

Little is known about how treatment protocols need to be adapted or modified for special populations of patients with hypochondriasis, such as particular age groups, cultural groups, or groups with severe general medical conditions. Such individuals need to be considered on a case-by-case basis. For children, interventions should be consistent with the child's developmental level (e.g., cognitive restructuring exercises would be simplified or omitted). For cognitively impaired (e.g., dementing) patients, simple behavioral programs might be most effective, such as contingency management programs (Williamson, 1984) where patients are reinforced for adaptive behaviors (e.g., engaging in health activities, talking about topics other than their health), and not rewarded for maladaptive behaviors (e.g., complaining about symptoms). For the cognitively intact elderly it is our impression, and that of others (e.g., Logsdon & Hyer, 1999; Snyder & Stanley, 2001) that cognitive-behavioral interventions can be useful in treating hypochondriasis.

FUTURE RESEARCH DIRECTIONS

There are numerous directions for future research that will improve our understanding of the mechanisms that underlie hypochondriasis and thereby facilitate our ability to provide accurate assessment and effective intervention. Some of the most important issues, presented in greater detail elsewhere (Asmundson et al.,

2001c), include: (1) better understanding the causal relationship between hypochondriasis and individual difference factors that increase vulnerability to psychopathology (e.g., neuroticism), (2) determining and understanding environmental and genetic influences on preoccupation with disease-related fears and beliefs, (3) exploring biological mechanisms that may be involved in hypochondriasis, (4) establishing whether there are subtypes of hypochondriasis that differ in phenomenology, mechanisms, and response to treatments, and (5) resolving debate regarding whether hypochondriasis should remain a somatoform disorder or be reclassified as either an anxiety disorder or and axis II (personality) disorder with empirically supported recommendations. Clearly, as evidenced in the preceding pages, additional research on the efficacy of various treatment strategies, alone and in combination, are also required. Likewise, further controlled trials of self-help approaches are warranted. Given the prevalence of hypochondriasis, there is a need to develop and make available a variety of effective interventions for those who may, for various reasons (e.g., geographic isolation, disability), be unable to gain in-person access to a cognitive-behavior therapist.

REFERENCES

Altamura, A. C., Carta, M. G., Tacchini, G., Musazzi, A., & Pioli, M. R. (1998). Prevalence of somatoform disorders in a psychiatric population: An Italian nationwide survey. *European Archives of Psychiatry and Clinical Neuroscience, 248,* 267–271.

American Psychiatric Association. (2000). *Diagnostic and statistical manual of mental disorders* (4th ed. text revision). Washington, DC: Author.

Asmundson, G. J. G., & Taylor, S. (2005). *It's not all in your head: How worrying about your health could be making you sick—and what you can do about it.* New York: Guilford.

Asmundson, G. J. G., Taylor, S., & Cox, B. J. (2001b). *Health anxiety: Clinical and research perspectives on hypochondriasis and related disorders.* New York: Wiley.

Asmundson, G. J. G., Taylor, S., Sevgur, S., & Cox, B. J. (2001a). Health anxiety: Classificiation and clinical features. In G. J. G. Asmundson, S. Taylor, & B. J. Cox (Eds.) *Health anxiety: Clinical and research perspectives on hypochondriasis and related disorders* (pp. 3–21). New York: Wiley.

Asmundson, G. J. G., Taylor, S., Wright, K. D., & Cox, B. J. (2001c). Future directions and challenges in assessment, treatment, and investigation. In G. J. G. Asmundson, S. Taylor, & B. J. Cox (Eds.), *Health anxiety: Clinical and research perspectives on hypochondriasis and related disorders* (pp. 365–382). New York: Wiley.

Barsky, A. J. (1992). Amplification, somatization, and the somatoform disorders. *Psychosomatics, 33,* 28–34.

Barsky, A. J. (1996). Hypochondriasis: Medical management and psychiatric treatment. *Psychosomatics, 37,* 48–56.

Barsky, A. J., Barnett, M. C., & Cleary, P. D. (1994a). Hypochondriasis and panic disorder: Boundary and overlap. *Archives of General Psychiatry, 51,* 918–925.

Barsky, A. J., Cleary, P. D., Sarnie, M. K., & Klerman, G. L. (1993). The course of transient hypochondriasis. *American Journal of Psychiatry, 150,* 484–488.

Barsky, A. J., Ettner, S. L., Horsky, J., & Bates, D. W. (2001). Resource utilization of patients with hypochondriacal health anxiety and somatization. *Medical Care, 39,* 705–715.

Barsky, A. J., Fama, J. M., Bailey, E. D., & Ahern, D. K. (1998a). A prospective 4- to 5-year study of DSM-III-R hypochondriasis. *Archives of General Psychiatry, 55,* 737–744.

Barsky, A. J., Frank, C. B., Cleary, P. D., Wyshak, G., & Klerman, G. L. (1991). The relation between hypochondriasis and age. *American Journal of Psychiatry, 148,* 923–928.

Barsky, A. J., & Klerman, G. L. (1983). Overview: Hypochondriasis, bodily complaints, and somatic styles. *American Journal of Psychiatry, 140,* 273–283.

Barsky, A. J., Orav, J. E., Delamater, B. A., Clancy, S. A., & Hartley, L. H. (1998b). Cardiorespiratory symptoms in response to physiological arousal. *Psychosomatic Medicine, 60,* 604–609.

Barsky, A. J., Wool, C., Barnett, M. C., & Cleary, P. D. (1994b). Histories of childhood trauma in adult hypochondriacal patients. *American Journal of Psychiatry, 151,* 397–401.

Barsky, A. J., Wyshak, G., Klerman, G. L., & Latham, K. S. (1990). The prevalence of hypochondriasis in medical outpatients. *Social Psychiatry and Psychiatric Epidemiology, 25,* 89–94.

Cantor, C. (1996). *Phantom illness: Shattering the myth of hypochondria.* New York: Houghton Mifflin.

Clark, D. M., Salkovskis, P. M., Hackmann, A., Wells, A., Fennell, M., Ludgate, J., et al. (1998). Two psychological treatments for hypochondriasis: A randomised controlled trial. *British Journal of Psychiatry, 173,* 218–225.

Cloninger, C. R., Sigvardsson, S., von Knorring, A.-L., & Bohman, M. (1984). An adoption study of somatoform disorders: II. Identification of two discrete somatoform disorders. *Archives of General Psychiatry, 41*, 863–871.

Côté, G., O'Leary, T., Barlow, D. H., Strain, J. J., Salkovskis, P. M., & Warwick, H. M. C., (1996). Hypochondriasis. In T. A. Widiger, A. J. Frances, H. A. Pincus, R. Ross, M. B. First, & W. W. Davis (Eds.), *DSM-IV sourcebook*, (Vol. 2 pp. 933–947). Washington, DC: American Psychiatric Association.

Enns, M. W., Kjernisted, K., & Lander, M. (2001). Pharmacological management of hypochondriasis and related disorders. In G. J. G. Asmundson, S. Taylor, & B. J. Cox (Eds.), *Health anxiety: Clinical and research perspectives on hypochondriasis and related conditions* (pp. 193–219). New York: Wiley.

Escobar, J. I., Allen, L. A., Hoyos Nervi, C., & Gara, M. A. (2001). General and cross-cultural considerations in a medical setting for patients presenting with medically unexplained symptoms. In G. J. G. Asmundson, S. Taylor, & B. J. Cox (Eds.), *Health anxiety: Clinical and research perspectives on hypochondriasis and related conditions* (pp. 220–245). New York: Wiley.

Escobar, J. I., Gara, M., Waitzkin, H., Silver, R. C., Holman, A., & Compton, W. (1998). DSM-IV hypochondriasis in primary care. *General Hospital Psychiatry, 20*, 155–159.

Fallon, B. A., Liebowitz, M. R., Salman, E., Schneier, F. R., Insino, C., Hollander, E., et al. (1993). Fluoxetine for hypochondriacal patients without major depression. *Journal of Clinical Psychopharmacology, 13*, 438–441.

First, M. B., Spitzer, R. L., Gibbon, M., Williams, J. B. W., & Lorna, B. (1994). *Structured Clinical Interview for DSM-IV Axis II personality disorders (SCID-II) (Version 2.0)*. New York: Biometrics Research Department, New York State Psychiatric Institute.

Gelder, M. G., Gath, D., & Mayou, R. A. (1983). *Oxford textbook of psychiatry*. Oxford: Oxford University Press.

Gureje, O., Üstün, T. B., & Simon, G. E. (1997). The syndrome of hypochondriasis: A cross-national study in primary care. *Psychological Medicine, 27*, 1001–1010.

Hollifield, M., Paine, S., Tuttle, L., & Kellner, R. (1999). Hypochondriasis, somatization, and perceived health and utilization of health care services. *Psychosomatics, 40*, 380–386.

House, A. (1989). Hypochondriasis and related disorders: Assessment and management of patients referred for a psychiatric opinion. *General Hospital Psychiatry, 11*, 156–165.

Jones, F. A. (2002). The role of bibliotherapy in health anxiety: An experimental study. *British Journal of Community Nursing, 7*, 498–504.

Kasteler, J., Kane, R. L., Olsen, D. M., & Thetford, C. (1976). Issues underlying prevalence of "doctor shopping" behavior. *Journal of Health and Social Behavior, 17*, 328–339.

Kellner, R. (1983). Prognosis of treated hypochondriasis: A clinical study. *Acta Psychiatrica Scandinavica, 67*, 69–79.

Kellner, R. (1986). *Somatization and hypochondriasis*. New York: Praeger.

Kellner, R. (1987). *Abridged manual of the Illness Attitudes Scale*. Unpublished manual, Department of Psychiatry, School of Medicine, University of New Mexico, Albuquerque.

Logsdon, C. D., & Hyer, L. (1999). Treating hypochondria in later life: Personality and health factors. In M. Duffy (Ed.), *Handbook of counseling and psychotherapy with older adults* (pp. 414–435). New York: Wiley.

Martin, R. L., & Yutzy, S. H. (1994). Somatoform disorders. In R. E. Hales, S. C. Yudofsky, & J. A. Talbott (Eds.), *American Psychiatric Press textbook of psychiatry (2nd ed.)* (pp. 591–622). Washington, DC: American Psychiatric Press.

Nemiah, J. C. (1985). Somatoform disorders. In H. I. Kaplan & B. J. Sadock (Eds.), *Comprehensive textbook of psychiatry (4th ed.)*, (pp. 924–942). Baltimore, MD: Williams & Wilkins.

Noyes, R. (2001). Hypochondriasis: Boundaries and comorbidities. In G. J. G. Asmundson, S. Taylor, & B. J. Cox (Eds.), *Health anxiety: Clinical and research perspectives on hypochondriasis and related conditions* (pp. 132–160). New York: Wiley.

Noyes, R., Kathol, R. G., Fisher, M. M., Phillips, B. M., Suelzer, M., & Woodman, C. L. (1994a). One-year follow-up of medical outpatients with hypochondriasis. *Psychosomatics, 35*, 533–545.

Noyes, R., Kathol, R. G., Fisher, M. M., Phillips, B. M., Suelzer, M., & Woodman, C. L. (1994b). Psychiatric comorbidity among patients with hypochondriasis. *General Hospital Psychiatry, 16*, 78–87.

Noyes, R., Roger, G., Fisher, M. M., Phillips, B. M., Suelzer, M. T., & Holt, C. S. (1993). The validity of DSM-III–R hypochondriasis. *Archives of General Psychiatry, 50*, 961–970.

Pilowsky, I. (1967). Dimensions of hypochondriasis. *British Journal of Psychiatry, 113*, 89–93.

Pilowsky, I. (1968). The response to treatment in hypochondriacal disorders. *Australian and New Zealand Journal of Psychiatry, 2*, 88–94.

Robbins, J. M., & Kirmayer, L. J. (1996). Transient and persistent hypochondriacal worry in primary care. *Psychological Medicine, 26*, 575–589.

Sato, T., Takeichi, M., Shirahama, M., Fukui T., & Gude, J. K. (1995). Doctor shopping patients and users of alternative medicine among Japanese primary care patients. *General Hospital Psychiatry, 17*, 115–125.

Schmidt, A. J. M. (1994). Bottlenecks in the diagnosis of hypochondriasis. *Comprehensive Psychiatry, 35*, 306–315.

Snyder, A. G., & Stanley, M. A. (2001). Hypochondriasis and health anxiety in the elderly. In G. J. G. Asmundson, S. Taylor, & B. J. Cox (Eds.), *Health anxiety: Clinical and research perspectives on hypochondriasis and related conditions* (pp. 246–274). New York: Wiley.

Speckens, A. E. M., Spinhoven, P., van Hemert, A. M., Bolk, J. H., & Hawton, K. E. (1997). Cognitive behavioural therapy for unexplained physical symptoms: Process and prognostic factors. *Behavioural and Cognitive Psychotherapy, 25,* 291–294.

Taylor, S., & Asmundson, G. J. G. (2004). *Treating health anxiety: A cognitive-behavioral approach.* New York: Guilford.

Taylor, S., Asmundson, G. J. G., & Coons, M. J. (2005). Current directions in the treatment of hypochondriasis. *Journal of Cognitive Psychotherapy, 19,* 291–310.

Visser, S., & Bouman, T. K. (2001). The treatment of hypochondriasis: Exposure plus response prevention vs cognitive therapy. *Behaviour Research and Therapy, 39,* 423–442.

Walker, J., Vincent, N., Furer, P., Cox, B., & Kjernisted, K. (1999). Treatment preference in hypochondriasis. *Journal of Behavior Therapy and Experimental Psychiatry, 30,* 251–258.

Wells, A. (1997). *Cognitive therapy of anxiety disorders.* New York: Wiley.

Williamson, P. N. (1984). An intervention for hypochondriacal complaints. *Clinical Gerontologist, 3,* 64–68.

Zgourides, G. (2002). *Stop worrying about your health! How to quit obsessing about symptoms and feel better now.* Oakland, CA: New Harbinger.

Insomnia

Christina S. McCrae • Sidney D. Nau • Daniel J. Taylor • Kenneth L. Lichstein

WHAT IS INSOMNIA?

Insomnia is a complaint of nonrestorative or inadequate sleep. Individuals with insomnia have difficulty with one or more of the following:

- initiating sleep
- maintaining sleep
    - awakening frequently during the night with difficulty returning to sleep
    - awakening too early in the morning with difficulty returning to sleep
- unrefreshing sleep (restless, light, or poor quality)

Insomnia is not defined by the total number of hours an individual sleeps each night. Although '8 hours' is commonly considered 'ideal', individuals have varying needs.

The most common form of insomnia is *acute or transient,* lasting for one month or less. *Persistent* insomnia lasts for more than four weeks, and *chronic* insomnia for more than six months.

Insomnia is not a single disorder. Insomnia is the general term for a person with difficulty sleeping; it is also a *clinical symptom* associated with over 30 sleep disorders, many of which are not insomnia disorders.

BASIC FACTS ABOUT INSOMNIA

Prevalence

Approximately 30% of all adults experience transient insomnia each year, with 15% reporting chronic insomnia.

Evidence suggests 60–64% of chronic insomnia cases go unrecognized in primary care offices.

Sleep difficulties occur in 40–60% of depressed outpatients and up to 90% of depressed inpatients.

Age and Gender

Insomnia increases with age and is more common in females (especially after menopause). In middle-age samples, the frequency of chronic insomnia is about 10% and estimates rise to 25% or higher in older adults.

Racial Differences

Very few studies have examined racial differences. Best available evidence indicates similar insomnia prevalence in African Americans and Caucasian Americans. However, where Caucasian Americans show gradual increases in prevalence, African Americans show a bimodal pattern, with peaks in middle age and late-life. Rates of insomnia in Asian populations (Japanese American, Korean) are comparable to those of Caucasian populations.

McCrae, C. S., Nau, S. D., Taylor, D. J., & Lichstein, K. L. (2006). Insomnia In J. E. Fisher & W. T. O'Donohue (Eds.), *Practitioner's guide to evidence-based psychotherapy.* New York: Springer.

Daytime Functioning

Daytime consequences include impaired psychosocial, occupational, and physical functioning. Specific adverse daytime effects include depressed mood, anxiety, fatigue, irritability, social discomfort, impaired motor skills, reduced concentration, memory complaints, and nonspecific physical symptoms.

Common causes of Insomnia

Circadian disruption (jet lag, shift work, sleep scheduling).

Psychiatric symptomatology (mood disorders, anxiety disorders, stress).

Medications/alcohol/drugs of abuse (the acute effects, plus tolerance and withdrawal).

Medical/neurological illness (e.g., apnea, periodic limb movements, pain, reflux, COPD).

Predisposing psychological characteristics (subclinical anxiety or depression).

Periods of intense stress.

Psychophysiological reactivity:

- Physiological arousal (tense muscles, restlessness)
- Cognitive arousal ('think too much', 'mind won't turn off', 'thoughts jump from topic to topic')
- Sensitivity to stimuli (environmental sounds, temperature, light)

Insomnia that begins due to one of these causes often leads to:

Sleep-preventing behaviors

- Spending too much time in bed—causes more fragmentation and allows more time in bed to ruminate, thus increasing anxiety/depression and decreasing sleep drive.
- Sleeping in on mornings after insomnia—disrupts circadian rhythm, pushing back the body's actual sleep onset, while the patient often fails to adjust expected sleep onset.
- "Trying too hard to sleep" in reaction to insomnia—increases sleep-related performance anxiety that makes sleep more difficult.
- Daytime naps—satisfies some of next night's sleep needs, making a sleep onset delay more likely.
- Increased caffeine or other stimulant intake—decreases sleep need and often delays sleep onset.
- Alcohol—decreases quality of sleep and increases fragmentation.
- Hypnotic/sedative medications—result in psychological or physical dependence and tolerance.

Sleep-preventing associations

- Anticipatory anxiety—thoughts of bedtime and anticipated insomnia become associated with anxiety, which over time causes bedtime to trigger anxious feelings and increased arousal.
- Conditioned fear—when a person with insomnia awakens normally during the night, conditioned fear of insomnia causes increased arousal, thus reducing the likelihood of returning to sleep and increasing the likelihood of anxious rumination.
- Conditioned arousal—entering the bedroom and getting into bed for the night (as well as behaviors that lead up to bedtime) can trigger conditioned arousal because of the repeated associations between bedtime, the bed and not sleeping.

Over time, as negative experiences with difficulty sleeping are repeatedly paired with psychophysiological reactions to the difficulty, sleep-preventing associations are gradually established and strengthened. (These associations are in addition to the original cause for the bout of insomnia.)

Sleep-preventing behaviors and associations are important because although they develop as consequences of acute or transient insomnia, they often serve to perpetuate an insomnia that had its origins in a medical, psychiatric, or circadian disturbance.

Behavioral therapies for insomnia (see Section "Effective Therapist-Based Treatments", below) are designed to reverse both sleep-preventing associations and behaviors as well as reduce psychophysiological arousal.

Primary vs. secondary

When insomnia is the core of the disorder or persists in times when another disorder (e.g., depression) is absent, it is considered *primary*. When insomnia is precipitated by another disorder (medical or psychiatric) or substance (medication/drug/alcohol), it is considered *secondary*. Secondary insomnia is the most common form of insomnia, accounting for approximately 75% of cases seen in patient populations.

Types of Disorders that Present with Insomnia

Transient or short-term factors (most frequent cause of insomnia)
Adjustment sleep disorder. Identifiable stress or environmental change produces emotional arousal at night (beginning a new school year, facing work, or personal problems).

Insomnia related to psychophysiological reactivity and/or conditioning factors
Psychophysiological insomnia (Classic 'pure' insomnia). Persistent or chronic disorder of somatized tension, maintained by learned sleep-preventing associations, characterized by "trying too hard" to sleep and conditioned arousal to bedroom.

Idiopathic insomnia. Rare, lifelong inability to obtain adequate sleep; presumably due to an abnormality in the neurological regulation of sleep (the sleep-wake system).

Sleep state misperception. Subjective complaint of insomnia occurs, but is unsubstantiated by objective sleep laboratory results.

Inadequate sleep hygiene. Habits inconsistent with obtaining good quality sleep and maintaining full daytime alertness (daytime napping, irregular sleep schedule, excessive time in bed, stimulant intake, etc.).

Sleep disorders associated with mental disorders
Psychoses associated with sleep disturbance. Schizophrenia, schizophreniform disorder, and other functional psychoses.

Mood disorders associated with sleep disturbance. Major depression, dysthymia, mania, hypomania, and other mood disorders.

Anxiety disorders associated with sleep disturbance. Generalized anxiety disorder, simple phobias, obsessive-compulsive disorder, and posttraumatic stress disorder.

Panic disorder associated with sleep disturbance. Panic episodes can be associated with sudden awakenings, followed by persistent arousal and difficulty returning to sleep.

Alcoholism associated with sleep disturbance. Insomnia is a common consequence of chronic excessive alcohol intake.

Insomnia related to medications, drugs, and alcohol
Hypnotic-dependent sleep disorder. Occurs in association with tolerance to or withdrawal from sedative/hypnotic medications.

Stimulant-dependent sleep disorder. Reduction of sleepiness or suppression of sleep by central nervous system stimulants.

Alcohol-dependent sleep disorder. Regular ingestion of ethanol in the evening as a hypnotic.

Insomnia associated with circadian rhythm disorders

Delayed sleep phase syndrome. Daily major sleep episode delayed (shifted to a later time period) in relation to the desired clock times for retiring and arising.

Advanced sleep phase syndrome. Daily major sleep episode advanced (shifted to an earlier time period) in relation to the desired clock times for retiring and arising.

Shift work sleep disorder. Transient symptoms of insomnia and excessive sleepiness that recur in relation to work schedule.

Irregular sleep–wake pattern. Circadian disorganization with variable timing of sleep and wake episodes; sleep broken into three or more short periods in each 24 hour period.

Insomnia secondary to sleep-related physiological disorders

Periodic limb movement disorder. Frequent, rhythmic limb twitches or movements during sleep.

Restless legs syndrome. Uncomfortable leg sensations and the ability of voluntary leg movement to temporarily relieve the discomfort; usually occur prior to sleep onset.

Central sleep apnea. Sleep-related respiration shows intervals with marked decrease or cessation of ventilatory effort.

Obstructive Sleep Apnea. Repetitive episodes of upper airway obstruction during sleep, usually associated with brief oxygen desaturations; characteristic snoring pattern.

Narcolepsy. Severe excessive daytime sleepiness, typically associated with three REM-related symptoms (cataplexy, hypnagogic hallucinations, and sleep paralysis).

Insomnia related to neurological illness Cerebral degenerative disorders, dementia, and parkinsonism.

Insomnia associated with other medical illness Common disorders include fibrositis syndrome, sleep-related gastroesophageal reflux, hyperthyroidism, pain, cancer, and COPD.

Insomnia associated with situational factors Sleep disturbance due to physiological response to environmental factors (environmental sleep disorder, altitude-related insomnia).

ASSESSMENT

What Should be Ruled Out?

- Other sleep disorders
  - sleep apnea and periodic limb movements can also produce insomnia symptoms
- Medical/neurological/psychiatric disorders that can cause insomnia symptoms
  - Depression
  - Anxiety
  - Substance use disorders
- Medications
  - Several antidepressants (e.g., SSRIs) as well as beta antagonistic antihypertensives, pseudoephedrine, theophylline and stimulants can cause insomnia.

What is Involved in Effective Assessment?

- The large number of disorders that present with insomnia provides an opportunity for specificity in diagnosis and treatment recommendations; however, it also presents a potentially lengthy assessment task.

- Most insomnia complaints are first seen by primary care physicians, who generally do not have time to perform lengthy clinical evaluations.
- Consequently, an assessment of insomnia often involves two levels:
  1. *Limited assessment.* Less time-consuming evaluation for nonspecialists.
  2. *Comprehensive assessment.* More exhaustive evaluations for sleep specialists.
- *Limited assessments* are suitable for the *initial* insomnia evaluation and treatment selection. Recent onset and less severe cases can be successfully treated by nonspecialists.
- *Comprehensive assessments* are indicated for chronic, severe, or complicated (e.g., patient also has pain, depression, cancer, etc.) cases.

> *Limited assessment.* At a minimum, effective assessment involves a *brief sleep history* (see below), and completion of a *brief medical/psychiatric history.*
>
> *Comprehensive assessment.* To evaluate more severe and more complex cases, sleep specialists perform an *extended sleep history, an extended medical/psychiatric history, and frequently a physical examination. Additional assessment procedures* are often performed (e.g., sleep diaries, psychological testing). Such thorough assessment is often needed with persistent insomnia, allowing treatment to be more reliably tailored to the specific cause or causes of the sleep disturbance.

Parts of an Assessment

Brief sleep history

- Primary sleep complaint(s). May include difficulty falling asleep, difficulty staying asleep, early morning awakenings, decreased total sleep time, poor quality sleep and/or daytime fatigue.
- Antecedents. What factor(s) does the patient believe may have caused the insomnia? (e.g., acute stress, medical or psychiatric illness, time zone change, abrupt sleep schedule change, substance use or withdrawal, other identifiable stressor).
- Duration. Less than four weeks-acute or short-term insomnia; more than four weeks-persistent insomnia; more than six months-chronic; episodes occur from time to time-intermittent.
- Type, duration and judged effectiveness of past treatment. If ineffective, ask why? (side-effects, poor compliance).
- Nocturnal symptoms and events. Increased arousal at bedtime (suggesting conditioned arousal), restless legs symptoms, periodic leg movements, respiratory distress (including dyspnea, choking and gasping), nocturnal panic attacks, pain, gastroesophageal reflux, nocturnal urination, and environmental noise.
- Bed partner report. Ask about loudness of snoring, frequency of pauses in breathing or leg jerks during sleep. Ask about daytime consequences of insomnia.
- Daytime consequences. A complaint of insomnia, in the absence of negative daytime effects does not indicate significant insomnia.
- Excessive daytime sleepiness. People with insomnia do not typically exhibit severe daytime sleepiness. If excessive sleepiness is present, consider referral for sleep disorders center consultation.
- Consider need for treatment. Acute or transient insomnia often resolves without treatment. To determine whether to treat, consider: Severity?, Distress?, Consequences?, Likelihood will resolve soon without treatment?, Comorbidity? (e.g., depression, anxiety disorder). If do not treat, schedule a re-evaluation 1–4 weeks later.

Comprehensive insomnia evaluation. In order to perform an extended sleep history and extended medical/psychiatric evaluations, sleep specialists add the following steps:

- Additional sleep pattern information. Sleep habits, nighttime sleep pattern, daytime functioning, sleep-wake schedule, beliefs about sleep.
- Sleep diary. The patient records estimated bedtime, sleep onset, wake time after sleep onset, final wake time, final arise time, nap time, etc. every day for two weeks (see example at: *www.sleepfoundation.org*).
- Consistency. Are there periods when the insomnia has been less of a problem? Does it appear to cycle with anything else, such as mood, season, medications, illness, etc. (can help judge primary vs. secondary insomnia).
- Expanded physical/mental health assessment.

During all insomnia evaluations (whether limited assessments or comprehensive sleep specialist evaluations), screen for etiologies of persistent insomnia

- Other sleep disorders
  - sleep apnea, periodic limb movements, and circadian rhythm disorders can all present as insomnia.
- Psychiatric disorders (see above).
- Medical disorders (see above).
  - Lab work should always be considered, as hyperthyroidism can cause insomnia
- Medications
  - Several anti-depressants (e.g., SSRIs) as well as beta antagonistic antihypertensives, pseudoephedrine, theophylline and stimulants can cause insomnia.

If insomnia is *secondary* to one or more of the above, consider treatment for primary disorder and referral as appropriate. Also, consider direct treatment for insomnia to prevent chronicity.

If insomnia is *primary*, screen for type:

- Inadequate sleep hygiene—Negative sleep habits?
- Idiopathic insomnia—Long-standing insomnia; childhood onset?
- Sleep state misperception—normal quantity of sleep?
- Psychophysiological insomnia—conditioned arousal to bedroom? Tension/ arousal before bedtime? Excessive concern? Trying too hard to sleep?

Model for a sleep history interview is available in the American Academy of Sleep Medicine's (AASM) report on insomnia evaluation, which is posted on the website, aasmnet.org (Table 13.3 of the publication).

What Assessments are Not Consistently Helpful?

Sleep laboratory studies involving polysomnography are recommended only if an undiagnosed physiological sleep disorder (e.g., sleep apnea, narcolepsy) is suspected, or the initial treatment for insomnia has been unsuccessful.

TREATMENT

What Treatments are Effective?

All types of insomnia may benefit from basic education about normal sleep (may reduce patient's anxiety about sleep) and sleep hygiene (activities that interfere with sleep).

Effectiveness of other treatments varies by type of insomnia:

Acute or short-term insomnia. Often resolves on its own. If decide to treat, consider trial (1–4 weeks) of hypnotic medication (followed by supervised withdrawal), or a trial of cognitive-behavioral treatment.,

Persistent or Chronic Primary Insomnia. Consider hypnotic medication, cognitive-behavioral therapy (e.g., a treatment package containing stimulus control and/or sleep restriction plus relaxation training), or cognitive-behavioral therapy combined with hypnotic medication (for acute relief of symptoms), followed by supervised hypnotic withdrawal.

Persistent or Chronic Secondary Insomnia. Consider treatment for primary disorder; possible referral to sleep specialist. Cognitive-behavioral treatment of insomnia has been shown useful in this population even when the primary disorder was not addressed.

Basic sleep education

- Sleep needs vary from person to person.
- Sleep needs vary from night to night.
- Taking 30 minutes or less to fall asleep is normal.
- Waking up for 30 minutes or less during the night is normal.
- The average person wakes up 1–4 times a night.

Sleep hygiene-activities that interfere with sleep

- Frequent napping.
- Variable bedtimes or morning wake-up times.
- Frequently spending an excessive length of time in bed.
- Use of sleep-disruptive substances near bedtime (alcohol, tobacco, caffeine).
- Exercise or hot bath too near bedtime.
- Stimulating activities too close to bedtime.
- Use of the bed for nonsleep-related activities (such as watching television, reading, snacking).
- Uncomfortable bed.
- Poor bedroom environment (e.g., too much light, heat, cold, or noise).
- Performing activities that demand strong concentration before bed.
- Working, paying bills, or talking about stressful topics before bed.
- Consuming excessive liquids (>8 oz.) within 2 hours of bed.
- Allowing oneself to persist in sleep-preventing mental activities while in bed, such as, thinking, planning, reminiscing, etc. (When these mental activities persist, it is best to get out of bed for a while to do something relaxing until sleepy).

What are Effective Self-Help Treatments?

No More Sleepless Nights by Peter Hauri and Shirley Linde (1996).
Get a Good Night's Sleep by Katherine A. Albert (1997).
Goodbye Insomnia, Hello Sleep by Samuel Dunkell (1994).

Useful Websites

These sites contain a wide-variety of sleep information for both practitioners and patients:

American Academy of Sleep Medicine: www.aasmnet.org
American Insomnia Association: www.americaninsomniaassociation.org
National Sleep Foundation: www.sleepfoundation.org
National Heart, Lung, and Blood Institute: www.nhlbi.nih.gov/health/public/sleep/insomnia.htm
National Institute of Neurological Disorders and Stroke: www.ninds.nih.gov
Sepracor: www.getsomesleep.com
Help Guide: http://www.helpguide.org/aging/sleep_disorders.htm

To find an accredited sleep disorders center
American Academy of Sleep Medicine: www.aasmnet.org

What are Effective Therapist -Based Treatments?

Cognitive-behavioral treatments are designed to reverse the behavioral/conditioning and psychophysiological factors that can be the key perpetuating factors for a chronic insomnia.

Cognitive-behavioral treatments present no physical tolerance or dependency risks and are rated as more appropriate and acceptable than medications.

Length of treatment. Typically 6–8 weekly or bi-weekly, 1 to 1½ hour treatment sessions.

Most widely used include:

Relaxation. Goal is to teach patient how to be relaxed at bedtime and during awakenings. Consists of multiple techniques, including progressive muscle relaxation, passive relaxation, biofeedback, meditation, imagery training, autogenic training, and diaphragmatic breathing.

Stimulus control. Based upon the idea that insomnia is caused by the association of the bed/bedroom and bedtime with wakefulness and non-sleep activities (e.g.., watching TV, worrying); *goal* is to break sleep incompatible associations and strengthen the association of the bed/bedroom and bedtime with sleep.

Sleep Restriction and Sleep Compression. Based upon observation that many patients with insomnia spend too much time awake in bed; *goal* is to consolidate sleep by restricting the time the patient is allowed to spend in bed, thus breaking the association between being in bed and being awake.

Cognitive restructuring. Goal is to interrupt vicious cycle of distress over poor sleep that provokes dysfunctional cognitions which lead to more distress and more sleep disturbance; faulty beliefs and attitudes about sleep are replaced with more adaptive beliefs and attitudes.

Cognitive-behavioral therapy. Behavioral treatments are compatible and are often combined to create multi-component treatment packages; *goal* is to increase benefits by adding interventions.

Less widely used (but effective) include:

Paradoxical intention. Patient is instructed to "try to stay awake" at night; *goal* is to prevent the anxiety associated with *trying too hard to sleep.*

Biofeedback. Goal is to teach patient to use physiological arousal information to increase own ability to lower general level of arousal

For therapist manuals see:

Lichstein, K. L. & Perlis, M. L. (2003). *Treating sleep disorders: Principles and practice of behavioral sleep medicine.* New York, NY: John Wiley & Sons, Inc.

Lichstein, K. L. & Morin, C. M. (2000). *Treatment of late-life insomnia.* Thousand Oaks, CA: Sage Publications, Inc.

Morin, C. M. (1996). *Insomnia: Psychological assessment and management.* New York, NY: Guilford Press.

Morin, C. M, & Espie, C. A. (2003). *Insomnia: A clinical guide to assessment and treatment.* New York, NY: Kluwer Academic/Plenum Publishers.

What is Effective Medical Treatment?

Hypnotic medications are typically effective for the brief treatment of acute primary insomnia, but become less effective over time. Medications commonly used include benzodiazepines, the newer nonbenzodiazepine hypnotics, sedating antidepressants (TCAs), antiepileptics, and neuroleptics.

Other Issues in Management

For chronic insomnia, behavioral treatment may be the best option. Both behavioral treatment and hypnotic medication provide effective short-term management of insomnia. Unfortunately, hypnotic medications lose effectiveness over time, but maintain their dependence characteristics. Thus, there is always the issue of rebound insomnia (increase in insomnia and anxiety) when hypnotics are used intermittently and when withdrawing from the medication, which could cause difficulties when a combination approach is used.

Withdrawal from hypnotic medications should be done gradually to reduce withdrawal side effects.

Secondary insomnia *does not* consistently resolve following treatment of the primary disorder. Secondary insomnia also responds to cognitive-behavioral treatment, even when the primary disorder is not addressed. Thus, early consideration of direct treatment for the insomnia should always be considered.

If cognitive-behavioral treatment is ineffective after 6–8 sessions, a sleep disorders center evaluation is recommended.

Cognitive-behavioral treatment may take a few weeks to produce improvement, but is more effective in the long-run than hypnotic medications.

Potential side-effects of hypnotic medications are an important consideration. Use of benzodiazepines, particularly with older patients, carries increased risks of falls, fractures, hospitalizations, and automobile accidents.

Hypnotic-dependence (physical and psychological) Although physical addiction to sedatives is often a concern, this is rare in patients with insomnia. Physical tolerance to the drug and eventual ineffectiveness, as well as psychological dependence, however, are both common. *Hypnotic-dependent insomnia* is a significant problem, which includes drug dependency and a history of withdrawal symptoms; in addition to tolerance and loss of effectiveness for the drug.

Nonetheless, chronic hypnotic use is a reasonable treatment option when *the following conditions have been met*:

1. behavioral treatments are unsuccessful or unwanted;
2. sleep laboratory studies have ruled out untreated physiological causes for insomnia;
3. medication is provided by a single provider.

Evaluate potential for drug interactions and arousing/sleep interfering effects of other medications (particularly for elderly patients for whom polypharmacy is common).

How Does One Select Among Treatments?

- Patient preference.
- Previous response to treatment.
- Patient characteristics (the elderly, patients with history of addiction-may wish to avoid hypnotic medication).
- Other medications being taken.
- Cause(s) of insomnia.
- Determining whether insomnia is transient or persistent, primary vs. secondary.
- When initiating cognitive-behavioral treatment for primary insomnia, stimulus control or sleep restriction alone, or a CBT treatment package is recommended.

KEY READINGS

Albert, K. A. (1997). *Get a good night's sleep*. New York: Simon & Shuster.
American Academy of Sleep Medicine. (1999). Practice parameters for the nonpharmacologic treatment of chronic insomnia. *Sleep, 22*, 1128–1133.

American Psychiatric Association. (1994). *Diagnostic and statistical manual of mental disorders* (4th ed.), Washington, DC: Author.

American Sleep Disorders Association. (1997). *The international classification of sleep disorders-revised.* Rochester, MN: Author.

Babar, S. I., Enright, P. L., Boyle, P., Foley, D., Sharp, D. S., Petrovitch, H., et al. (2000). Sleep disturbances and their correlates in elderly Japanese American men residing in Hawaii. *Journal of Gerontology, 55A(7),* M406–M411.

Bootzin, R. R. (1972). A stimulus control treatment for insomnia. *Proceedings of the American Psychological Association,* 395–396.

Bootzin, R. R., & Epstein, D. R. (2000). Stimulus control. In K. L. Lichstein & C. M. Morin (Eds.), *Treatment of late-life insomnia* (pp. 167–184). Thousand Oaks, CA: Sage.

Bradley, T. D., McNicholas, W. T., Rutherford, R., Popkin, J., & Zamel, N. (1986). Clinical and physiologic heterogeneity of the central sleep apnea syndrome. *The American Review of Respiratory Disease, 134,* 217–221.

Buysse, D. J., & Reynolds, C. F. (1990). Insomnia. In M. J. Thorpy (Ed.), *Handbook of sleep disorders* (pp. 375–433). New York: Marcel Dekker.

Carskadon, M. A., Dement, W.C., & Mitler, M. M. (1976). Self-reports versus sleep laboratory findings in 122 drug-free subjects with complaints of chronic insomnia. *American Journal of Psychiatry, 133,* 1382–1388.

Coleman, R. M. (1982). Periodic movements in sleep (nocturnal myoclonus) and restless legs syndrome. In C. Guilleminault (Ed.), *Sleeping and waking disorders: Indications and techniques* (pp. 265–295). Menlo Park, CA: Addison-Wesley.

Czeisler, C. A., Richardson, G. S., Coleman, R. M., Zimmerman, J. C., Moore-Ede, M. C., Dement, W. C., et al. (1981). Chronotherapy: Resetting the circadian clock of patients with delayed sleep phase insomnia. *Sleep, 4,* 1–21.

Dunkell, S. (1994). *Goodbye insomnia, hello sleep.* New York: Birch Lane Press.

Foley, D. J., Monjan, A. A., Izmirlian, G., Hays, J. C., & Blazer, D. G. (1999). Incidence and remission of insomnia among elderly adults in a biracial cohort. *Sleep, 22(Suppl. 2),* S373–S378.

Guilleminault, C., & Anagnos, A. (2000). Narcolepsy syndrome. In M. H. Kryger, T. Roth, & W. C. Dement (Eds.), *Principles and practice of sleep medicine* (3rd ed. pp. 676–686). Philadelphia, PA: WB Saunders.

Guilleminault, C., & Bassiri, A.G. Clinical features and evaluation of obstructive sleep apnea. In M. H. Kryger, T. Roth, & W. C. Dement (Eds.), *Principles and practice of sleep medicine* (3rd ed. pp. 869–878). Philadelphia, PA: WB Saunders.

Hauri, P. & Linde, S. (1996) *No more sleepless nights.* New York: John Wiley & Sons.

Hauri, P. J., & Olmstead, E. M.(1980). Childhood onset insomnia. *Sleep, 3,* 59–65.

Hauri, P. J., Friedman, M., & Ravaris, C. L. (1989). Sleep in patients with spontaneous panic attacks. *Sleep, 12,* 323–337.

Hauri, P. J., & Fisher, J. (1986). Persistent psychophysiologic (learned) insomnia. *Sleep, 9(1),* 38–53.

Kales, A., Bixler, E. O., Tan, T. L., Scharf, M. B., & Kales, J. D. (1974). Chronic hypnotic-drug use: Ineffectiveness, drug-withdrawal insomnia, and dependence. *JAMA, 227,* 513–517.

Kamei, R., Hughes, L., Miles, L., & Dement, W. (1979). Advanced-sleep-phase syndrome studied in a time isolation facility. *Chronobiologia, 6,* 115.

Lichstein, K. L. (1988). *Clinical relaxation strategies.* New York: Wiley.

Lichstein, K. L., McCrae, C. S., Wilson, N. M., Nau, S. D., Aguillard, R. N., Lester, K. W., et al. (2003). Treatment of hypnotic dependence in older adults. *Sleep, 26,* A290.

Lichstein, K. L. & Morin, C. M. (Eds.) (2000). *Treatment of late-life insomnia.* Thousand Oaks, CA: Sage Publications, Inc.

Lugaresi, E., Cirignotta, F., Coccagna, G., & Montagna, P. (1986). Nocturnal myoclonus and restless legs syndrome. *Advances in Neurology, 43,* 295–307.

McCrae, C. S., & Lichstein, K. L. (2001). Secondary insomnia: Diagnostic challenges and intervention opportunities. *Sleep Medicine Reviews, 5(1),* 47–61.

Morin, C. M., Culbert, J. P., & Schwartz, S. M. (1994). Nonpharmacological interventions for insomnia: A meta-analysis of treatment efficacy. *American Journal of Psychiatry, 151,* 1172–1180.

Morin, C. M., Gaulier, B., Barry, T., & Kowatch, R. A. (1992). Patients' acceptance of psychological and pharmacological therapies for insomnia. *Sleep,15,* 302–305.

Nau, S. D., & Lichstein, K. L. (2004). Insomnia: Causes and treatments. In P. R. Carney, R. B. Berry, and J. D. Geyer (Eds), *Clinical Sleep Disorders.* Philadelphia: Lippincott, Williams & Wilkins, 157–190.

Ohayon, M. M. (2002). Epidemiology of insomnia: What we know and what we still need to learn. *Sleep Medicine Reviews, 6(2),* 97–111.

Ohayon, M. M., Caulet, M., & Lemoine, P. (1998). Comorbidity of mental and insomnia disorders in the general population. *Comprehensive Psychiatry, 39,* 185–197.

Ohayon, M. M., & Hong, S. (2002). Prevalence of insomnia and associated factors in South Korea. *Journal of Psychosomatic Research, 53,* 593–600.

Roehrs, T., & Roth, T. (2000). Hypnotics: efficacy and adverse effects. In M. H. Kryger, T. Roth, W. C. Dement (Eds.), *Principles and practice of sleep medicine* (3rd ed. pp. 414–418). Philadelphia, PA: WB Saunders.

Spielman, A. J., Saskin, P., & Thorpy, M. J. (1987). Treatment of chronic insomnia by restriction of time in bed, *Sleep, 10,* 45–56.

Walsh, J. K., Tepas, D. I., & Moss, P. D. (1981). The EEG sleep of night and rotating shift workers. In L. C. Johnson, D. I. Tepas, W. P. Colquhoun, M. J. Colligan (Eds.), *Biological rhythms, sleep and shift work* (pp. 347–356). New York: SP Medical & Scientific Books.

Zarcone, V. P. (1982). Sleep and alcoholism. In E. D. Weitzman (Ed.), *Sleep disorders: Intersections of basic and clinical research: Vol 8. Advances in sleep research* (pp. 125–135). New York: Spectrum Press.

CHAPTER 33

Intermittent Explosive Disorder

Kyle E. Ferguson

WHAT IS INTERMITTENT EXPLOSIVE DISORDER?

Intermittent Explosive Disorder (IED) falls under the category of Impulse-Control Disorders Not Elsewhere Classified (APA, 1994).[1] In addition to IED, kleptomania, pyromania, pathological gambling, Trichotillomania and Impulse-Control Disorders Not Otherwise Specified are also included in this category. The essential feature of all Impulse-Control Disorders is "the failure to resist an impulse, drive, or temptation to perform an act that is harmful to the person or others" (APA, 1994, p. 609). In most cases, individuals feel an overwhelming sense of arousal and a release of that arousal upon committing the act. After committing the act, individuals may or may not feel a sense of guilt or remorse (see Figure 33.1).

The only diagnostic criteria in the DSM that describes nonpsychotic, nonbipolar aggressive disorders is IED (Coccaro, Kavoussi, Berman, & Lish,1998).[2] To receive the diagnosis of IED, three criteria must be met (APA, 2000, p. 281). These are:

a. Several discrete episodes of failure to resist aggressive impulses that result in serious assaultive acts or destruction of property.
b. The degree of aggressiveness expressed during the episode is grossly out of proportion to any precipitating psychosocial stressors.
c. The aggressive episodes are not better accounted for by another mental disorder and are not due to direct physiological effects of a substance or a general medical condition.

FIGURE 33.1 Arousal increases until the impulsive act. Tension is released; arousal dissipates, dropping below normal levels. Modeled after McElroy et al. (1998) Figure 1, p. 208.

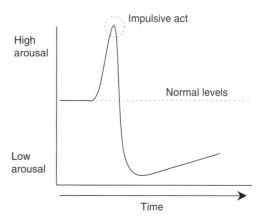

---

[1] The ICD-10's equivalent category is "Habit and Impulse Disorders" (Code F63) (World Health Organization, 1992).
[2] See Coccaro et al. (1998) for revised diagnostic criteria for IED (IED-R), which may, ultimately, bolster reliability (e.g., their IED-R had a $\kappa = 0.92$). The most significant addition is a frequency criterion: "Aggressive outbursts occur twice in a week, on average, for at least a period of 1 month" (p. 369).

Ferguson, K. E. (2006). Intermittent explosive disorder. In J. E. Fisher & W. T. O'Donohue (Eds.), *Practitioner's guide to evidenced-based psycotherapy.* New York: Springer.

335

Episodes of violence, which start and stop abruptly, typically last several minutes, though have been known to continue for hours (Maxmen & Ward, 1995). Infrequently, both prodromal physiological or mood symptoms and partial amnesia are reported after the aggressive act (Meyer & Deitsch, 1996). Individuals, who met the diagnostic criteria for IED, often describe these aggressive impulses as the "need to attack", the "need to strike out", an "adrenaline rush", "seeing red", or the "urge to kill someone" (McElroy, Soutullo, Beckman, Taylor, & Keck, 1998, p. 205).

Let us turn next to an example of IED, showcasing the diagnostic criteria. No example paints a clearer picture of IED than that of "road rage".

An Example of IED

"Road rage" has attracted much media attention as of late. Road age is an incident in which an angry or impatient motorist or passenger intentionally injures or kills another motorist, passenger, or pedestrian (Rathbone & Huckabee, 1999). It should be noted that road rage and aggressive driving are not one and the same. "Road rage" is uncontrolled anger that results in a violent act or the threat of violence; it is criminal behavior. Aggressive driving, such as tailgating or abrupt lane changes are certainly dangerous behaviors, however, do not rise to the level of criminal behavior.

Some researchers argue that road rage can be characterized as IED, because both share the essential feature, "discrete episodes of failure to resist aggressive impulses in serious assaultive acts or destruction of property" (Galovski, Blanchard, & Veazey, 2002, p. 642). For the purpose of illustration, let us consider a recent story that made the news in the writer's community, where a man followed a woman after she cut him off on the Interstate. After both motorists pulled over, an altercation ensued. It ended in the man reaching into the cab of her vehicle, pulling out her small dog, and hurling it in front of vehicles traveling at highway speeds. After an investigation, it was discovered that the man had allegedly been getting in trouble at work for "blowing up" at coworkers.

This incident presents a convincing case for IED. Conceivably, the aggressive motorist (1) could not "resist" the "aggressive impulse" that resulted in a "serious assaultive act". Certainly (2) the "degree of aggressiveness expressed during the episode (was) grossly out of proportion to any precipitating psychosocial stressors," as the dog was not attacking him and the other motorist had not engaged in physical aggression (i.e., he was not acting out of self-defense). This and previous aggressive episodes (3) "(could) not be better accounted for by another mental disorder," as he had no recent or longstanding psychiatric history, apart from an "explosive temper." Likewise, he was not under the influence of a substance during the time of the episode (and presumably at work, as he had been gainfully employed at the same place of business for some time). Nor was it uncovered that he had a "direct physiological or medical condition" that could account for his "explosive temper."

IS IED A SEPARATE ENTITY?

Despite the fact that IED has been discussed in the literature for several decades and has been included in several editions of the *Diagnostics and Statistics Manual* (though it almost did not make it into the fourth edition), there is still much debate among researchers and practitioners about the existence of IED as a separate entity (Hucker, 2004). Rather, IED is seen as a nonspecific symptom that coincides with a wide range of psychiatric and medical disorders (McElroy, 1999).

Proponents against the idea that IED is an independent phenomenon argue that anger and aggressive behavior is extremely common across many psychiatric conditions. For example, in a sample of 1,300 psychiatric outpatients, Posternak and Zimmerman (2002) reported that half had significant problems with anger and aggressive behavior in the previous week. Moreover, in preparing for the *DSM-IV*, Bradford, Geller, Lesieur, Rosenthal, & Wise (1994) reviewed 800 probable cases of IED. Given that so many of the cases overlapped with other psychiatric conditions, only 17 cases (about 2%) were identified.

PROBLEMS WITH DIAGNOSTIC CRITERIA

There are several inherent problems in the diagnostic criteria that are worthy of mention; these are: the use of the term "impulse"; the problem with the criterion of "serious assaultive acts" or "destruction of property"; and the criterion to rule out IED when the aggressive behavior is due to the "direct physiological effects of a diagnosable medical condition." Of course, due to page limitations, every weakness will not be discussed here. Interested readers are referred to *Rethinking the DSM: A Psychological Perspective* (2002) for an in-depth discussion on these and other limitations of the DSM-IV.

The first problem with IED is the use of the term "impulse." Unfortunately, the DSM-IV provides no elaboration on this term. It is therefore open to many interpretations. Let us consider several variants; the emphasis of which has major interpretive implications. In a vernacular sense, "impulse" is an intense feeling or emotion that immediately precedes an action. From a psychoanalytic point of view, it entails a "psychic" or "unconscious drive." According to a sociobiological perspective, it means "instinctual urge," as in the case of "instinctual" or "territorial aggression." From a biomedical orientation, an "impulse" refers to the excitation of a neuron. All of these interpretations are admissible because the DSM's authors fail to elucidate what they mean by "impulse."

A second problem with IED is the fact that there has to be "serious assaultive acts" or "destruction of property" to warrant a psychiatric diagnosis. Because the diagnosis is only allowable in those who commit "serious" acts of aggression (again the word "serious" is open to interpretation), many individuals with significant impulsive-aggressive behaviors fall by the wayside (Coccaro et al., 1998). Indeed, many individuals who commit less "serious" acts of aggression also have considerable functional impairment (i.e., cannot hold a job) and/or legal problems (e.g., misdemeanor for smashing a neighbor's garden gnome). Thus, even though both groups of individuals are *functionally* the same (i.e., significant impulse-control difficulties), because they differ somewhat *topographically* (e.g., one group destroys more expensive property), one group meets the criteria for IED and the other does not.

A third problem with IED concerns the criterion, rule out IED when the "pattern of aggressive episodes is judged to be due to the *direct* physiological effects of a diagnosable general medical condition" (APA, 1994, p. 611, italics added). How is it even possible to determine "direct" from the implied "indirect physiological effects" of the medical condition during an episode of aggression? All medical conditions have "*direct* physiological effects" on the entire organism, all the time. Take Type I Diabetes, for example. A faulty pancreas has "direct physiological" effects on all organ systems. Poorly managed diabetes, for example, results in cardiovascular disease, retinopathy (eye disease), nephropathy (kidney disease), and neuropathy (nerve disease). Behaviorally, individuals are moody, lethargic, have difficulties with concentration, and can behave "impulsively." Accordingly, at what point are clinicians able to determine "direct" from "indirect" effects of diabetes?

BASIC FACTS ABOUT INTERMITTENT EXPLOSIVE DISORDER

Comorbidity

Apart from McElroy et al.'s (1998) study, no research has been conducted on IED using DSM-IV criteria (McElroy, 1999). McElroy et al. (1998) examined 27 individuals with IED. Many participants were convicted felons or had been referred by a healthcare provider. Comorbidity with other psychiatric disorders was highly prevalent in this sample: 93% ($N = 25$) of the participants had lifetime DSM-IV diagnoses of mood disorders; 48% ($N = 13$) with substance use disorders; 48% ($N = 13$) with anxiety disorders; and 37% ($N = 10$) with major depressive disorder. While these data are informative, caution is in order in interpreting these findings. Namely, as noted by Galovski et al. (2002), there were no patient controls, no normal controls, and no dimensional psychological tests were employed.

Prevalence

Reliable prevalence data are not available. However, the received view is that IED is extremely rare (APA, 1994). For example, data taken from clinical surveys of psychiatric patients and patients undergoing treatment for IED, suggest that rates with IED in psychiatric settings ranges from 1% to 2% (Coccaro, Schmidt, Samuels, & Nesadt, 2004; Monopolis, & Lion, 1983). Thus, the prevalence of IED is likely comparable to that of schizophrenia.

Age of Onset and Course

Based on limited data, this disorder usually begins in late adolescence or early childhood and continues until individuals reach 30 years of age (APA, 1994; McElroy et al., 1998; Meyer & Deitsch, 1996).

Gender

IED is more prevalent in males than females. Previous studies suggest that the gender ratio is about three males for every female (Coccario et al., 1998; McElroy et al., 1998).

Impairment and other characteristics

IED is associated with significant impairment in day-to-day functioning. In McElroy et al.'s (1998) study, for example, most participants reported problems with chronic anger and frequent episodes where they experienced aggressive impulses, though resisted the urge or engaged in less destructive behavior. While not addressed in the literature on IED, chronic anger is related to a host of chronic health problems, particularly difficulties with cardiovascular health. For decades, hostility, anger, and aggression have been highly correlated with hypertension, coronary heart disease, and coronary arterial disease (Robins & Novaco, 2000).

Another area where individuals with IED are sure to be impacted is driving. Driving is frustrating for everyone, and can elicit much anger in persons with IED. Many individuals get into motor vehicle accidents (MVA) due to aggressive driving (Galovski & Blanchard, 2002). The Assistant General Counsel of the American Insurance Association estimated that about half of all MVA crashes involve aggressive driving (Snyder, 1997, as cited in Galovski & Blanchard, 2002).

Individuals with IED also experience regret, remorse, and embarrassment over their aggressive displays, and often isolate themselves so as to avoid coming into contact with situations that evoke aggression (McElroy, 1999). Accordingly, due to the nature of the disorder (i.e., "aggressive impulses that result in serious assaultive acts or destruction of property"), many individuals become "loners" or suffer from interpersonal and/or work problems. In more extreme cases, such individuals get in trouble with the law (McElroy et al., 1998).

ASSESSMENT

What Should be Ruled Out?

Aggressive episodes better accounted for by another mental disorder This is the hardest decision that clinicians face, as the diagnostic criteria for IED overlap with so many other disorders, particularly Cluster B Personality Disorders. Antisocial Personality Disorder (APD) is arguably the most closely related disorder in the DSM. Consider the following diagnostic criteria.

> They may repeatedly perform acts that are grounds for arrest . . . such as destroying property . . . A pattern of impulsivity may be manifested by a failure to plan ahead . . . Decisions are made on the spur the moment, without forethought, and without consideration for the consequences to self or others; this may lead to sudden changes of jobs, residences, or relationships. Individuals with Antisocial Personality Disorder tend to be irritable and aggressive and may repeatedly get into physical fights or commit acts of physical assault (APA, 1994, p. 646).

Likewise, APD also begins in childhood or early adolescence and continues into adulthood.

In deciding whether a client meets the diagnostic criteria for APD or IED, clinicians should orient to the essential feature of APD, that being, "a pervasive pattern of disregard for, and violation of, the rights of others" (APA, 1994, p. 646). Specifically, does the pattern of behavior suggest psychopathy or sociopathy? Does the client "disregard the wishes, rights, or feelings of others" (APA, 1994, p. 646)? Is the client "frequently deceitful and manipulative" (APA, 1994, p. 646)? Of course, "a pervasive pattern of disregard for, and violation of, the rights of others" would entail other situations in addition to just those involving aggressive acts. With IED, an individual would only have "disregard for, and violation of, the rights of others" during aggressive outbursts, not at other times. Individuals with APD also do not express remorse for their aggressive actions, which often is not the case for individuals with IED. Moreover, individuals with IED probably would not evidence patterns of behavior frequently deemed "deceitful and manipulative".

Borderline Personality Disorder (BPD) also entails episodes of inappropriate anger and impulsive–aggressive behavior. However, with BPD, there is "a pervasive pattern of instability of interpersonal relationships (and) self-image" (APA, 1994, p. 654, parenthesis added). Moreover, clients with BPD usually vacillate between "extremes of idealization and evaluation" in all relationships, including that with the therapist (APA, 1994, p. 654). They also frequently report feelings of "emptiness", lack a sense of "self," and make recurrent threats or engage in suicidal and/or parasuicidal behavior (APA, 1994, p. 654). Neither of these is associated with IED.

Anger and impulsive–aggressive behavior also occurs during episodes of psychosis and mania (APA, 1994). Delusions (e.g., persecutory type), hallucinations, and disorganized or incoherent speech are associated with psychotic and manic episodes, not IED. Should a client present with a thought disorder, therefore, rule out IED.

Direct effects of a general medical condition. Rule out IED if the aggressive behavior is likely due to the "direct effects" of a general medication (APA, 1994, p. 611). Impulsive aggression due to severe traumatic brain injury (particularly in the orbital-frontal region) and Tourette's syndrome are obvious examples (Budman, Rockmore, Stokes, & Sossin, 2003). Other examples include: psychomotor seizures; acute metabolic derangements, due to hypoglycemia; and certain types of brain tumors (e.g., involving the temporal lobes) (Victor & Ropper, 2002, p. 205).

Substance intoxication or withdrawal. Rule out IED if aggressive act(s) occurred in association with substance intoxication or substance withdrawal. Certain psychomotor stimulants (e.g., cocaine and amphetamines), for example, potentiate attack behaviors, while other drugs (e.g., alcohol) interfere with the cognitive functioning that underlies planning and impulse-control (Hoaken & Stewart, 2003; Pihl & Hoaken, 2002; Pihl & Peterson, 1995).

Substance related aggressive behavior is best determined by way of a blood or urine screen. Should plencyclidine, cocaine, barbiturates, inhalants, and/or high levels of alcohol turn up on the screen, rule out IED (APA, 1994, p. 611).

Delirium

Rule out IED if aggressive behavior occurs exclusively during an episode of delirium. Delirium is an acute confusional state that usually involves agitation, problems with perception, vivid hallucinations, intense emotional experiences, and overactivity of psychomotor and autonomic nervous system functions (Victor & Ropper, 2002). Delirium can be induced by sudden withdrawal of ethanol in alcohol–dependent persons (e.g., delirium tremens), drug intoxication, electrolyte imbalance, and infection (e.g., meningitis).

Dementia

Rule out IED if the aggressive behavior occurs in individuals with suspected dementia. Dementia is an acquired, usually a progressive impairment in cognitive functioning (Greenberg, Aminoff, & Simon, 2002). In addition to problems with memory function, other cognitive spheres might also be affected, such as language, concentration, and the ability to plan routine activities. Alzheimer's disease, Parkinson's disease, Hunington's disease, vascular dementia (stroke), and general medical conditions like HIV are common examples. Treatable causes of dementia include normal pressure hydrocephalus, vitamin B_{12} deficiency, and hypothyroidism.

Malingering

Rule out IED for suspected malingering. Malingering is the intentional production of false or grossly exaggerated physical and/or psychological symptoms, motivated by external incentives such as avoiding military duty or work, obtaining financial compensation, evading criminal prosecution or obtaining drugs (APA, 2000, p. 309). Given the nature of the diagnosis (i.e., "serious assaultive acts or destruction of property"), many individuals encounter legal problems and as such, are motivated to malinger. Although winning a criminal case by pleading "not guilty by reason of insanity" is rare (given court reform after the assassination attempt on President Reagan's life), individuals and their attorneys may argue for "diminished capacity"; namely, pleading guilty to a lesser crime due to mental retardation, a psychiatric disorder and/or health condition (e.g., severe brain injury), that affects a person's ability of knowing right from wrong. While pleading "not guilty by reason of insanity" refers to whether or not a person is culpable, "diminished capacity" pertains to the *degree to which* a defendant should be held responsible for a crime (Brogdon, Adams, & Bahri, 2004). For example rather than plead guilty to first-degree murder (i.e., intent to do harm with deliberation or premeditation), due to "diminished capacity" a defendant may plead guilty to second-degree murder (i.e., intent to do harm without deliberation or premeditation) or manslaughter (i.e. murder without express or implied intent to do harm). Of course, impulsive behavior by its very nature concerns acting without forethought, with little or no regard about the consequences. Accordingly, should a defendant meet the criteria for IED, this can constitute "diminished capacity" in a court of law.

As a general rule, malingering is especially suspect with the convergence of two or more of the following (APA, 2000, pp. 309–310):

1. the client is referred by an attorney
2. there are marketed discrepancies in test data
3. the client extends little effort or is uncooperative during the evaluation

What is Involved in Effective Assessment?

The diagnosis of IED should be made only after a thorough medical work-up. Once medical conditions are ruled out, a comprehensive assessment of IED should include an examination of the following variables (Coccaro et al., 1998).

- DSM criteria for IED
- degree of aggressive behavior
- frequency of failure to resist aggressive impulses
- extent of premeditation
- psychiatric comorbidity
- functional impairment
- substance use

Anger is inherently a multidimensional construct, which consists of physiological (e.g., sympathetic arousal), cognitive (e.g., automatic thoughts), phenomological (e.g., subjective experience), and behavioral (e.g., facial expression) variables (Eckhardt, Norlander, Deffernbacher, 2004, p. 20). As such, how the case is conceptualized and the clinician's theoretical orientation will have bearing on what instruments are employed in the assessment proper. In assessing IED, there are no hard and fast rules, as is the case with other disorders (e.g., use the Beck Depression Inventory-II for clients who meet criteria for major depression; Beck, Steer, Ball, & Ranieri., 1996). Be that as it may, the literature on IED and impulsive-aggressive behavior, more generally, provide guidance in what instruments are and are not useful when working with clients who present with IED. Apart from those instruments reviewed here, see Eckhardt et al. (2004) for an extensive review of the various types of brief assessment devices that are currently in use and readily available; many of which are psychometrically sound and cost-effective.

Clinician-administered measures Because of the wide array of Axis I disorders that need to be ruled out before making a diagnosis of IED, it is important that clinicians cover all clinically-relevant variables during the interview. The Structured Clinical Interview for DSM-IV Axis I Disorders (SCID-I) was designed with this aim in mind; to guide clinicians through the differential diagnosis process, by asking questions pertaining to each major diagnostic category (First et al., 1996).

The Module for Intermittent Explosive Disorder (M-IED), based on the SCID, attempts to refine the diagnosis by focusing on frequency of outbursts, level of aggression, and level of social impairment (Coccaro et al. 1998). This approach augments the SCID, providing precise inclusionary and exclusionary criteria for making the diagnosis of IED. For example, aggressive behavior is assessed for premeditation (i.e., it is not committed "in order to achieve some tangible objective"); aggressive behavior causes marked distress; and the aggressive behavior occurs twice weekly, for one month, or the individual has had three episodes of impulsive-aggressive behavior, that resulted in physical assault or destruction of property, over a one year period (Coccaro et al., 2004, p. 821).

Self-report measures The most popular measure of the construct hostility is the Buss–Durkee Hostility Inventory (BDHI; Buss & Burkee, 1957; Eckhardt et al., 2004). This 75-item instrument consists of eight subscales: assault, indirect hostility, verbal hostility, irritability, negativism, resentment, suspicion, and guilt.

Although popular, there are various conceptual and psychometric inadequacies that mitigate against using the BDHI (e.g., poor reliability coefficients; see Biaggio, 1980). In lieu of the BDHI, a comparable measure, the Aggression Questionnaire (AQ), which corrected for these, is recommended (Buss & Perry, 1992).

The Aggressive Questionnaire (AQ) measures respondents' propensity for aggressive behaviors and their ability to resist engaging in destructive behavior (Buss & Perry, 1992). This 34-item, Likert-type, measure consists of five scales: physical aggression, verbal aggression, anger, hostility, and indirect aggression (i.e., expression of anger in the absence of confrontation). The AQ is superior to the BDHI in terms of "psychometric adequacy, conceptual clarity, and practical utility" (Eckhardt et al., 2004, p. 24).

The Novaco Anger Scale (NAS) is a measure of anger from an information-processing approach (Jones, Thomas-Peter, & Trout, 1999; Novaco, 1994). Respondents endorse statements about themselves that describe their experience of anger. The NAS is a two-part instrument. Part A consists of 48 items, rated on a three-part scale, that assess cognitive (e.g., hostile attitudes), arousal (e.g., feelings of tension), and behavioral indices (e.g., physical aggression). Part B, comprising 25 items, describes circumstances in which an individual becomes angry (e.g. being treated disrespectfully). Among other strengths, the NAS possesses excellent internal consistency (0.95, in both parts) and is highly accurate (94%) in discriminating between individuals referred for anger management treatment and nonclinical comparisons (Eckhardt et al., 2004; Jones, Thomas-Peter, & Trout, 1999).

The State-Trait Anger Expression Inventory (STAXI) is a measure of anger from a state-trait personality theoretical perspective (Spielberger, 1988). This Likert scale is comprised of 44 items. It assesses the intensity of the experience of anger and the extent to which hostility is a personality attribute. The STAXI has impressive psychometric properties and is useful in discriminating between violent and nonviolent groups (see Eckhardt et al., 2004, p. 28ff).

Behavioral assessment Research indicates that self-monitoring episodes of anger and aggressive behavior helps distinguish between individuals with problematic anger and those who experience less problematic, lower levels of anger (Deffenbacher, Demm, & Brandon, 1986; Deffenbacher & Sabadell, 1992). One of the simplest self-monitoring devices is a variant of that developed by Bijou and colleagues (Bijou, Peterson, & Ault, 1968). It consists of three columns: (1) antecedent, (2) behavior, and (3) consequence (see Figure 33.2). The Antecedent column is reserved for recording situations that trigger impulsive-aggressive behavior. Behavioral descriptions of what the impulsive-behavior looks like, is recorded under the Behavior column. Aggressive thoughts and self-statements are also recorded here. The interpersonal,

FIGURE 33.2 A self-monitoring form commonly used in assessing anger. Modeled after Bijou et al. (1968).

Antecedent	Behavior	Consequence
- guy cut me off in traffic	-I thought, "This f****** ***hole has no right!" - I fingered him and honked my horn	- he pulled over - we both got out - I punched him before he punched me - he went down and I kicked him in the back a few times - the cops came and I got arrested!

legal, and/or emotional consequences (e.g., guilt, remorse, embarrassment) are recorded under the column titled Consequence. See Heidt & Marx, 2003, for step-by-step guidelines in providing clients with the rationale of self-monitoring; how to operationally define behavioral targets; and how to instruct clients in recording instances of behavior and its consequences.

What Assessments are Not Helpful?

Projective tests, such as the Rorshach and Thematic Apperception Test (TAT) should not be used in assessing IED. They are simply not valid assessment instruments.

TREATMENT

What are Effective Self-Help Treatments?

Due to financial problems, unstable living arrangements, substance abuse, as well as other factors, attrition rates among male batterers ranges from 50% to as high as 90% (DeHart, Kennerly, Burke, & Follingstad, 1999; Grusznski & Carrillo, 1988; Rooney & Hanson, 2001). Many male batterers, of course, meet the diagnostic criteria for IED. While the above factors do not necessarily overlap with other groups that also meet these criteria (e.g., individuals who experience recurrent road rage), both groups share one thing in common: help-seeking is probably instigated by others (Howells & Day, 2003). As such, one might expect a certain degree of defensiveness and resistance on the part of clients who feel forced to undergo treatment (e.g., court-mandated therapy).

As it turns out, there is some evidence to suggest that highly resistant individuals tend to do better with self-directed versus therapist-directed activities (Beutler, 1991). One approach to overcoming resistance, therefore, is to employ self-directed bibliotherapy.

There are dozens of anger management self-help books on the market today. Several of these appear below. While based on cognitive-behavioral principles, readers should note that neither of these has been empirically validated, independently, or as part of a treatment package. Additionally, self-directed, relaxation exercises, on-line training, and home study programs are also included.

- Benson, H. (1975). *The relaxation response.* New York: Avan Books.
- Davis, M., Eshelman, E. R., & McKay, M. (1995). *The relaxation & stress reduction workbook* (4th ed.). Oakland, California: New Harbinger Publications.
- Ellis, A. (1994). *Anger: How to live with and without it.* New York: Carol Publishing Group.

- Ellis, A., & Tafrate, R. C. (1998). *How to control your anger before it controls you.* New York: Citadel Press.
- McKay, M., & Rogers, P. (2000). *The anger control workbook.* Oakland, CA: New Harbinger Publications.
- Nhat Hanh. Hanh, T. N. (2002). *Anger: Wisdom for cooling the flames.* New York: Penguin USA (a mindfulness approach to anger management).
- Potter-Efron, R. (1994). *Angry all the time: An emergency guide to anger control.* Oakland, CA: New Harbinger Publications.
- Schiraldi, G. R., & Kerr, M. H. (2002). *The anger management sourcebook.* New York: McGraw-Hill.
- William, D. (2001). *Overcoming anger and irritability.* New York: New York University Press.

Useful Informational Websites about Anger and Related Resources:

- http://www.apa.org/pubinfo/anger.html
- http://mentalhelp.net/psyhelp/chap7/
- http://www.services.unimelb.edu.au/counsel/issues/anger.html
- http://www.pe2000.com/anger.htm
- http://www.state.sc.us/dmh/bryan/webanger.htm
- http://www.apahelpcenter.org/featuredtopics/feature.php?id=38 (teen violence)
- http://www.long-beach.med.va.gov/Our_Services/Patient_Care/cpmpbook/cpmp-15.html (anger and chronic pain)
- http://www.anger-management-techniques.org/ (mindfulness approach to anger management)
- http://www.angerclass.com/ (online classes)
- http://www.angeronline.com/ (online classes)
- http://angermanagementonline.com/ (online classes)
- http://angermgmt.com/ (home study options available)
- http://www.ajnovickgroup.com/ (home study options available)

What Treatments are Effective?

Several meta-analytic reviews of anger management programs (i.e., cognitive therapy, cognitive-behavioral therapy, social skills training, and relaxation therapy—group and individual modes of delivery) have been published (Beck & Fernandez, 1998; Edmondson & Conger, 1996; Tufrate, 1995; Vecchio & O'Leary, 2004). All reviews demonstrated medium to large effect sizes for some aspects of anger, while small for others. Regarding explosive anger, cognitive-behavioral therapy (CBT), coupled with relaxation, appears to be the treatment of choice for anger expression problems (Edmondson & Conger, 1996; Vecchio & O'Leary, 2004). Moreover, as an added bonus, there is some evidence to suggest that combining relaxation with cognitive-behavioral therapies lowers attrition rates (Deffenbacher & Stark, 1992).

What is CBT?

CBT employs both cognitive and behavioral techniques in designing treatments. There are several assumptions underlying all CBT interventions. First, thoughts or beliefs, emotions, and behavior are interrelated. Behavior thus affects thoughts and feelings and thoughts and feelings affect behavior; they are inexplicably tied. Second, changing thoughts, beliefs, and/or behavior alters mood. Identifying and modifying negative or dysfunctional beliefs and/or engaging in more adaptive behavior, therefore, improves mood. Three, all CBT interventions employ similar techniques; the emphasis of which is on cognitive restructuring (Edmondson & Conger, 1996).

Cognitive restructuring. Cognitive restructuring (CR) is the core strategy in cognitive therapy and many cognitive-behavior therapies (Mahoney, 1977). It is a treatment technique aimed at directly modifying specific thoughts or beliefs that purportedly mediate maladaptive behavioral and emotional responding (Foa & Rothbaum, 1998; Last, 1989). According to several of these models, each emotion is believed to be associated with a particular thought or belief (e.g., Beck, 1995):

- Perceived danger or threat = *anxiety*
- Perceived loss of something crucial in one's life = *depression*
- Perceiving the actions of others as wrong or unfair = *anger*
- Perceiving the actions of oneself as wrong or unfair = *guilt*

The four major cognitive and cognitive-behavioral approaches, based on CR, are Beck's (1976) Cognitive Therapy (CT), Ellis's Rational-Emotive Therapy (RET; 1962; more recently, Rational-Emotive Behavior Therapy; REBT), Meichenbaum's (1977) Self-Instructional Training, and Burns's popular "Feeling Good" Therapy (1989). Let us turn to Ellis's Rational Emotive Therapy as an illustration of a CBT program that has been successfully used in treating anger and anger-related issues.

Rational-Emotive Therapy. Ellis's (1962, 1994) Rational Emotive Therapy (RET) "concentrates on people's current beliefs, attitudes and self-statements as contributing to or 'causing' and maintaining their emotional and behavioral disturbances" (Ellis et al., 1988, pp. 1–2). What logically follows, therefore, is the notion that *appropriate emotions* are preceded by *rational beliefs* and *inappropriate emotions* like hostility are preceded by *irrational beliefs* (Ellis, 1971). While the list of potentially irrational beliefs would seem endless, Ellis, McInerney, DiGiuseppe, & Yeager (1988) have narrowed it down to four, demandingness, awfulizing, human worth ratings, and low frustration tolerance (Ellis, 1994; Ellis et al., 1988):

1. *Demandingness*—the tendency to substitute demands for wishes, as mirrored in word choices such as "should," "ought," "must," and "have to" (e.g., "I must control my anger at all times").
2. *Awfulizing*—extreme and exaggerated negative evaluations of events—colloquially, blowing the situation way out of proportion (e.g., "My life is over if I don't get into college").
3. *Human worth ratings*—evaluations or denigrations of people including oneself (e.g., "Not being able to control myself makes me worthless to everyone in my life").
4. *Low frustration tolerance*—the perceived inability to withstand the discomfort of an activating event—activating events evoke emotional and behavioral responding (e.g., "I can't live another day").

From an Ellisian perspective irrational core beliefs ought to be disputed rationally. Cognitive disputations are attempts at changing the client's erroneous beliefs through persuasion, didactic presentations, Socratic dialogue, vicarious experiences, and other forms of verbally-mediated approaches (Ellis, 1962, 1971, 1994). In what follows are four major techniques, upon which irrational beliefs are disputed (Walen, DiGiuseppe, & Dryden, 1992):

- *Logical disputation questions*—(getting clients to evaluate the logical consistency or semantic clarity in their thinking) (p. 159). Example: Just because a person knows right from wrong does not *logically* follow that he or she must behave in accordance with these.
- *Reality-testing disputation questions*—(asking whether their beliefs are consistent with empirical reality). Example: Awfulizing beliefs can be challenged by asking such questions as (p. 161):

1. Where's the evidence . . . "that you blow every interaction?"
2. What would happen if . . . "you started to lose it and then caught yourself mid-stream?"
3. Let's be scientists. What do the data show?
4. What is the probability of a bad consequence, is it 2 to 1, 200 to 1, 2,000 to 1, etc.?

- *Pragmatic disputation questions*—(getting clients to assess the "hedonic" value—i.e., desire for pleasure and avoidance of pain—of their belief systems) (pp. 161–162). Example: The belief is used to regulate emotional upset.

Relaxation Many CBT anger management programs involve some form of relaxation. The rationale for employing relaxation is based on reciprocal inhibition theory (Wolpe, 1958). Namely, arousal is inhibited after pairing relaxation with anger-provoking stimuli. One simply cannot feel aroused and relaxed at the same time. Thus, on future occasions, there is a better chance that such stimuli will prompt a relaxation response versus intense anger.

Progressive muscle relaxation (PMR), using Bernstein and Borkovec's (1973) standardized protocol, and diaphragmatic breathing are recommended. PMR teaches clients how to discriminate between feelings of relaxation and arousal, by having them notice the physiological sensations as they systematically tense and release various muscle groups of their bodies. By improving self-awareness, clients are better able to recognize nascent arousal and employ self-soothing techniques before arousal escalates into an outburst. The following is the training sequence by which clients are taught to tense and release the various muscle groups (Bernstein & Borkovec, 1973, p. 25):

1. dominant hand and forearm,
2. dominant biceps,
3. nondominant hand and forearm,
4. nondominant biceps,
5. forehead,
6. upper cheeks and nose,
7. lower cheeks and jaws,
8. neck and throat,
9. chest, shoulders, and upper back,
10. abdominal or stomach region,
11. dominant thigh,
12. dominant calf,
13. dominant foot,
14. nondominant thigh,
15. nondominant calf,
16. nondominant foot.

Diaphragmatic breathing (DB) is also recommended, as it lends itself well to most situations and is relatively easy to learn (see Hazelett-Stevens & Craske, 2003, for a review of breathing techniques). For example, clients can employ DB when on the road or waiting in line—even during a potential altercation, before the situation gets out of hand.

The Structure of CBT-Relaxation-Augmented Therapies[3]

- *Sessions 1 and 2*: First, provide the rationale for CBT (e.g., how thoughts and behavior are related to mood), anger management, and relaxation (see below). Second,

---

[3] Recommendations are extrapolated from Deffenbacher and Stark (1992), Deffenbacher, McNamara, Stark, & Sabadell (1990), and Deffenbacher, Story, Brandon, Hogg, & Hazaleus (1988).

teach progressive muscle relaxation and diaphragmatic breathing. Third, instruct clients in how to elicit relaxing imagery, as they relax on their own. Fourth, homework involves self-monitoring anger-provoking situations (use the Antecedent-Behavior-Consequence form discussed earlier) and daily relaxation exercises. Review homework during the first half of the second session.

Sample anger management rationale script:

. . . earlier you told me that you often do impulsive things that have resulted in trouble for you . . . Many people say they do things like this because they react before they've had a chance to think about how the action will affect themselves or others. They also say that anger makes it harder to prevent them from doing impulsive behaviors that will get them in trouble . . . You will learn to recognize these feelings and thoughts early, when they are not as strong. This should enable you to do other behaviors that will keep you out of trouble. Do you have any questions? (Donohue & Cavenagh, 2003, p. 12).

Sample relaxation rationale script:

. . . relaxation training consists of learning to sequentially . . . relax various groups of muscles all through the body, while at the same time paying very close and careful attention to the feelings of . . . relaxation . . . in addition to teaching you how to relax, I will also be encouraging you to learn to recognize and pinpoint tension and relaxation as they appear in everyday situations . . . You should understand quite clearly that learning relaxation skills is very much like learning any other kind of skill such as swimming, or golfing, or riding a bicycle; thus in order for you to get better at relaxing you will have to practice doing it just as you would have to practice other skills. It is very important that you realize that . . . relaxation training involves learning on your part; there is nothing magical about the procedures. I will not be doing anything *to* you; I will merely be introducing you to the technique and directing your attention to various aspects of it, such as the presence of certain feelings in the muscles. Thus, without your active cooperation and regular practicing of the things you will learn today, the procedures are of little use . . . The goal of . . . relaxation training is to help you learn to reduce muscle tension in your body far below your adaptation level at any time you wish to do so . . . Do you have any questions about what I've said so far? (Bernstein & Borkovec, 1973, pp. 19–20, italics in original).

- *Session 3.* This session focuses on cognitive-restructuring. After reviewing homework assigned during the second session, follow Beck's (1995) or Ellis's (1962, 1994) cognitive-restructuring guidelines.
- *Sessions 4–8.* These sessions focus on the application of cognitive-restructuring and relaxation by having the client visualize difficult situations, depicting anger-provoking scenes. The techniques are used to reduce anger. Problem-solve with clients in preparing for angering events outside of the therapist's office. In vivo homework is also assigned, where clients place themselves in increasingly difficult, though manageable situations. Additionally, always review homework from the previous session. This sends the message that work outside the therapist's office is as important as what transpires in session.

What is Effective Medical Treatment?

The first-line of medical-pharmacological approaches to managing impulsive-aggressive behaviors is selective serotonin reuptake inhibitors (SSRI). In particular, fluoxetine (e.g., prozac) is gaining currency in primary care settings. SSRIs have been show to have an "antiaggressive" effect (i.e., reduction in violent behavior) on impulsive aggressive adults (Coccario & Kavoussi, 1997; Coccaro et al.,

1997). SSRIs typically take several weeks to take effect and remain in the body several weeks after discontinuing use (Silverman, 1998).

Patients who do not respond to an SSRI may respond to a mood stabilizer. An antiaggressive response in impulsive-aggressive adults and children has been reported for antipsychotic medications like lithium and quetiapine (Sheard, Marini, Bridges, & Wapner, 1976; Siassi, 1982), and several anticonvulsants (Barratt, 1993; Barratt, Stanford, Felthous, & Kent, 1997; Cowdry & Gardner, 1988; Donovan et al., 2000; Kavoussi & Coccaro, 1998; Walker, Thomas, & Allen, 2003). To a lesser extent, the β-adrenergic blocking agent, propranolol, has been used to treat episodic sudden outbursts of verbal abuse and physical violence (Jenkins & Maruta, 1987; Mattes, 2003).

Readers should note that alprazolam and amitriptyline are contraindicated in managing impulsive-aggressive behavior, as these have been shown to increase agitation (Gardner & Cowdry, 1985; Soloff, George, Nathan, Schulz, & Perel, 1986).

Many of the results from these and other drug studies should be interpreted with caution, as methodological concerns remain. Given that many experiments are case studies, subjects are not randomized to treatment conditions. Lack of randomized control trials limits internal validity. Moreover, sample sizes are often too small to make reasonable assumptions from the populations from which they were sampled. As such, small sample sizes place limits on external validity.

How Does One Select Among Treatments?

Patients should be well-informed about the extant evidence-based treatment options available, including psychological and medical interventions. Should clinicians elect to use medication treatment, possible side effects and drug interactions should be discussed with patients. If individual treatment is prohibitive, consider anger-management groups or bibliotherapy. In addition to a wealth of self-help books, there are a number of discrete, on-line options readily available. However, readers should not that, while bibliotherapy can be based on empirical principles, none of these has empirical support.

REFERENCES

American Psychiatric Association. (1994). *Diagnostic and statistical manual of mental disorders* (4th ed.). Washington, DC: Author.

American Psychiatric Association. (2000). *Quick reference to the diagnostic criteria from DSM-IV-TR.* Washington, DC: Author.

Biaggio, M. K. (1980). Assessment of anger arousal. *Journal of Personality Assessment, 44,* 289–298.

Barratt, E. S. (1993). The use of anticonvulsants in aggression and violence. *Psychopharmac. Bull., 29,* 75–81.

Barratt, E. S., Stanford, M. S., Felthous, A. R., & Kent, T. A. (1997). The effects of phenytoin on impulsive and premeditated aggression: a controlled study. *Journal of Clinical Psychopharmacology, 17,* 341–349.

Beck, A. T. (1976). *Cognitive therapy and the emotional disorders.* New York: International Universities Press.

Beck, A. T., Steer, R. A., Ball, R., & Ranieri, W. F. (1996). Comparison of Beck Depression Inventories-IA and –II in psychiatric outpatients. *Journal of Personality Assessment, 67,* 588–597.

Beck, J. S. (1995). *Cognitive therapy: Basics and beyond.* New York: The Guilford Press.

Beck, R., & Fernandez, E. (1998). Cognitive-behavioral therapy in the treatment of anger: A meta-analysis. *Cognitive Therapy and Research, 22,* 63–74.

Bernstein, D. A., & Borkovec, T. D. (1973). *Progressive relaxation training: A manual for the helping professions.* Champaign, IL: Research Press.

Beutler, L. E. (1991). Predictors of differential response to cognitive, experiential, and self-directed psychotherapeutic procedures. *Journal of Consulting and Clinical Psychology, 59,* 333–340.

Bijou, S. W., Peterson, R. F., & Ault, M. H. (1968). A method to integrate descriptive and experimental field studies at the level of data and empirical concepts. *Journal of Applied Behavior Analysis, 1,* 175–191.

Bradford, J., Geller, J., Lesieur, H., Rosenthal, R., & Wise, M. (1994). Impulse control disorders. In T. A. Witiger, A. J. Frances, H. A. Pincus, M. B. First, R. Ross, & W. Davis (Eds.), *DSM-IV sourcebook*. Washington, DC: American Psychiatric Press.

Brogdon, M. G., Adams, J. H., & Bahri, R. (2004). Psychology and the law. In W. T. O'Donohue & E. R. Levensky (Eds.), *Handbook of forensic psychology* (pp. 3–26). New York: Academic Press.

Budman, C. L., Rockmore, L., Stokes, J., & Sossin, M. (2003). Clinical phenomenology of episodic rage in children with Tourette syndrome. *Journal of Psychosomatic Research, 55*, 59–65.

Burns, D. D. (1989). *The feeling good handbook*. New York: A Plume Book.

Buss, A. H., & Durkee, A. (1957). An inventory for assessing different kinds of hostility. *Journal of Consulting Psychology, 21,*343–349.

Buss, A. H., & Perry, M. (1992). The aggression questionnaire. *Journal of Personality and Social Psychology, 59*, 73–81.

Coccario, E. F., Kavoussi, R. J. (1997). Fluoxetine and impulsive aggressive behavior in personality-disordered subjects. *Archives of General Psychiatry, 54,*1081–1088.

Coccari, E. F., Kavoussi, R. J., Berman, M. E., & Lish, J. D. (1998). Intermittent Explosive Disorder-Revised: Development, reliability, and validity of research criteria. *Comprehensive Psychiatry, 39*, 368–376.

Coccaro, E. F., Kavoussi, R. J., & Hauger, R. L. (1997). Serotonin function and antiaggressive response to fluoxetine: A pilot study. *Biological Psychiatry, 42*, 546–552.

Coccario, E. F., Scmidt, C. A., Samuels, J. F., & Nestadt, G. (2004). Lifetime and 1-month prevalence rates of Intermittent Explosive Disorder-Revised in a community sample. *Journal of Clinical Psychiatry, 65*, 820–824.

Cowdry, R. W., & Gardner, D. L. (1988). Pharmacotherapy of borderline personality disorder: alprazolam, carbamazepine, trifluoperazine, and tranylcypromine. *Archives of General Psychiatry, 45*, 111–119.

Deffenbacher, J. L., Demm, P. M., & Brandon, A. D. (1986). High general anger: Correlates in treatment. *Behavior Research and Therapy, 24*, 481–489.

Deffenbacher, J. L., McNamara, K., Stark, R. S., & Sabadell, P. M. (1990). A comparison of cognitive-behavioral and process oriented group counseling for general anger reduction. *Journal of Counseling and Development, 69*, 167–172.

Deffenbacher, J. L., & Sabadell, P. M. (1992). Comparing high trait anger individuals with low trait anger individuals. In M. Muller (Ed.), *Anger and aggression in cardiovascular disease*. Burn, Switzerland: Hans Huber.

Deffenbacher, J. L., & Stark, R. S. (1992). Relaxation and cognitive-relaxation treatments of general anger. *Journal of Counseling Psychology, 39*, 158–167.

Deffenbacher, J. L., Story, D. A., Brandon, A. D., Hogg, J. A., & Hazaleus, S. L. (1988). Cognitive and cognitive-relaxation treatments for anger. *Cognitive Therapy and Research, 12*, 167–184.

DeHart, D. D., Kennerly, R. J., Burke, L. K., & Follingstad, D. R. (1999). Predictors of attrition in a treatment program for battering men. Journal *of Family Violence, 14*, 20–34.

Donohue, B., & Cavenagh, N. (2003). Anger (negative impulse) management. O'Donohue, J. E. Fisher, & S. C. Hayes (Eds.), *Cognitive behavior therapy* (pp. 10–15). Hoboken, New Jersey: John Wiley & Sons, Inc.

Donovan, S. J., Stewart, J. W., Nunes, E. V., Quitkin, F. M., Parides, M., Daniel W., et al. (2000). Divalproex treatment for youth with explosive temper and mood lability: A double-blind, placebo-controlled crossover design. *American Journal of Psychiatry, 157,*1038.

Eckhardt, C., Norlander, B., & Deffernbacher, J. (2004). The assessment of anger and hostility: A critical review. *Aggression and Violent Behavior, 9*, 17–43.

Edmondson, C. B., & Conger, J. C. (1996). A review of treatment efficacy for individuals with anger problems: Conceptual, assessment, and methodological issues. *Clinical Psychology Review, 16*, 251–275.

Ellis, A. (1962). *Reason and emotion in psychotherapy*. New York: Lyle Stuart.

Ellis, A. (1971). *Growth through reason*. North Hollywood, CA: Wilshire.

Ellis, A., McInerney, J. F., DiGiuseppe, R., & Yeager, R. J. (1988). *Rational-emotive therapy with alcoholics and substance abusers*. Boston: Allyn and Bacon.

Ellis, A. (1994). *Anger: How to live with and without it*. New York: Carol Publishing Group.

First, M. B., Spitzer, R. L., Gibbon, M., et al. (1996). *Structured Clinical Interview for Axis I DSM-IV Disorders–Patient Edition (with psychotic screen) (SCID-I/P) (Version 2.0)*. New York, NY: Biometric Research, New York State Psychiatric Institute.

Foa, E., B., & Rothbaum, B. O. (1998). *Treating the trauma of rape: Cognitive-behavioral therapy for PTSD*. New York: The Guilford Press.

Galovski, T. E., & Blanchard, E. B. (2002). The effectiveness of a brief psychological intervention on court-referred and self-referred aggressive drivers. *Behaviour Research and Therapy, 40*, 1385–1402.

Galovski. T., Blanchard, E. B., & Veazey, C. (2002). Intermittent explosive disorder and other psychiatric comorbidity among court-referred and self-referred aggressive drivers. *Behaviour Research and Therapy, 40*, 641–651.

Gardner, D. I., Cowdry, R. W. (1985). Alprazolam-induced dyscontrol in Borderline Personality Disorder. *American Journal of Psychiatry, 142*, 98–100.

Greenberg, D. A., Aminoff, M. J., & Simon, R. P. (2002). *Clinical neurology.* New York: McGraw-Hill.

Grusznski, R. J., & Carrillo, T. P. (1988). Who completes batterer's treatment groups? An empirical investigation. *Journal of Family Violence, 3,* 141–150.

Hazelett-Stevens, H., & Craske, M. G. (2003). Breathing retraining and diaphragmatic breathing techniques. In W. O'Donohue, J. E. Fisher, & S. C. Hayes (Eds.), *Cognitive behavior therapy: Applying in empirically supported techniques in your practice* (pp. 59–64). New York: John Wiley & Sons.

Heidt, J. M., & Marx, B. P. (2003). Self-monitoring as a treatment vehicle. In W. O'Donohue, J. E. Fisher, & S. C. Hayes (Eds.), *Cognitive behavior therapy* (pp. 361–367). Hoboken, New Jersey: John Wiley & Sons, Inc.

Hoaken, P. N. S., & Stewart, S. H. (2003). Drugs of abuse and the elicitation of human aggressive behavior. *Addictive Behaviors, 28,* 1533–1554.

Howells, K., & Day, A. (2003). Readiness for anger management: Clinical and theoretical issues. *Clinical Psychology Review, 23,* 319–337.

Hucker, S. J. (2004). Disorders of impulse control. In W. T. O'Donohue & E. R. Levensky (Eds.), *Handbook of forensic psychology* (pp.471–487). New York: Academic Press.

Jenkins, S. C., & Maruta, T. (1987). *Therapeutic use of propranolol for intermittent explosive disorder.* Mayo Clinical Proceedings, 62, 204–214.

Jones, J. P., Thomas-Peter, B. A., & Trout, A. (1999). Brief report Normative data for the Novaco Anger Scale from a non-clinical sample and implications for clinical use. *British Journal of Clinical Psychology, 38,*417–424.

Kavoussi, R. J., & Coccaro, E. F. (1998). Divalproex sodium for impulsive aggressive behavior in patients with personality disorder. *Journal of Clinical Psychiatry, 59,* 676–680.

Last, C. G. (1985). Cognitive restructuring. In A. S. Bellack & M. Hersen (Eds.), *Dictionary of behavior therapy techniques* (pp. 59–60). New York: Pergamon.

Mahoney, M. J. (1977). Reflections on the cognitive learning trend in psychotherapy. *American Psychologist, 32,* 5–13.

Mattes, J. A. (2003). Comparative effectiveness of carbamazepine and propranolol for rage outbursts. *Journal of Neuropsychiatry and clinical Neuroscience, 2,* 159–164.

Maxmen, J. S., & Ward, N. G. (1995). *Essential psychopathology and its treatment.* New York: W. W. Norton & Company.

McElory, S. L. (1999). Recognition in treatment of DSM-IV Intermittent Explosive Disorder. *Journal of Clinical Psychiatry, 60,* 12–16.

McElory, S. L., Soutullo, C. A., Beckman, D. A., Taylor, Jr., P., & Keck, Jr., P. E. (1998). DSM-IV Intermittent Explosive Disorder: A report of 27 cases. *Journal of Clinical Psychiatry, 59,* 203–210.

Meyer, R. G., & Deitsch, S. E. (1996). *The clinician's handbook: Integrated diagnostics, assessment, and intervention in adult and adolescent psychopathology* (4th ed.). Boston: Allyn and Bacon.

Meichenbaum, D. (1977). *Cognitive-behavior modification: An integrative approach.* New York: Plenum Press.

Monopolis, S., & Lion, J. R. (1983). Problems in the diagnosis of intermittent explosive disorder. *American Journal of Psychiatry, 140,* 1200–1202

Novaco, R. W. (1994). Anger as a risk factor for violence among the mentally disordered. In J. Monahan & H. Steadman (Eds.), *Violence and mental disorder: Developments in risk assessment* (pp. 21–60). Chicago: University of Chicago Press.

Pihl, R. O., & Hoaken P. N. S., (2002). Biological bases to addiction and aggression in close relationships. In C. Wekerle & A. M. Wall (Eds.), *The violence and addiction equation: Theoretical and clinical issues in substance abuse and relationship violence* (pp. 25–43). Brunner/Mazel: Philadelphia, PA.

Pihl, R. O., & Peterson, J. B. (1995). Drugs and aggression: Correlations, crime and human manipulative studies and some proposed mechanisms. *Journal of Psychiatry & Neuroscience, 20,* 141–149.

Posternak, M. A., & Zimmerman, M. (2002). Partial validation of the atypical features subtype of major depressive disorder. *Archives of General Psychiatry, 59,* 70–76.

Rathbone, D. B., & Huckabee, J. C. (1999). *Controlling road rage: A literature review and pilot study.* The AAA Foundation for Traffic Safety.

Robins, S., & Novaco, R. W. (2000). Anger control as a health promotion mechanism. In D. I. Mostofsky & D. H. Barlow (Eds.), *The management of stress and anxiety in medical disorders* (pp. 361–377). Boston: Allyn and Bacon.

Rooney, J., & Hanson, R. K. (2001). Predicting attrition from treatment programs for abusive men. *Journal of Family Violence, 16,* 131–149.

Sheard, M., Marini, J., Bridges, C., & Wapner, A. (1976). The effect of lithium on impulsive aggressive behavior in man. *American Journal of Psychiatry, 133,* 1409–1413.

Siassi, I. (1982). Lithium treatment of impulsive behavior in children. *Journal of Clinical Psychiatry, 43,* 482–484.

Silverman, H. M. (Ed.). (1998). *The pill book* (8th ed.). New York: Bantam Books.

Soloff, P. H., George, A., Nathan, R. S., Schulz, P. M., & Perel, J. M. (1986). Paradoxical effects of amitriptyline in borderline patients. *American Journal of Psychiatry, 143,* 1603–1605.

Spielberger, C. D. (1988). *State-Trait anger expression inventory professional manual.* Odessa, FL: Psychological Assessment Resources.

Tafrate, R. C. (1995). Evaluation of treatment strategies for adult anger disorders. In H. Kassinove (Ed.), *Anger disorders: Definition, diagnosis, and treatment* (pp. 109–129. Washington, D.C.: Taylor & Francis.

Vecchio, T. D., & O'Leary, K. D. (2004). Effectiveness of anger treatments for specific anger problems: A meta-analytic review. *Clinical Psychology Review, 24,* 15–34.

Victor, M., & Ropper, A. H. (2002). *Adam and Victor's Manual of Neurology* (7th ed.). New York: McGraw-Hill.

Walen, S. R., DiGiuseppe, R., & Dryden, W. (1992). *A practitioner's guide to Rational-Emotive Therapy* (2nd ed.). Oxford: Oxford University Press.

Walker, C., Thomas, J., & Allen, T. S. (2003). Treating impulsivity, irritability, and aggression of Antisocial Personality Disorder with quetiapine. *International Journal of Offender Therapy and Comparative Criminology, 47,* 556–567.

Wolpe, J. (1958). *Psychotherapy by reciprocal inhibition.* Stanford, CA: Stanford University Press.

World Health Organization. (1992). *The ICD-10 Classification of Mental and Behavioral Disorders: Clinical descriptions and diagnostic guidelines.* World Health Organization: Geneva.

Irritable Bowel Syndrome

Laurie Keefer • Edward B. Blanchard

ABSTRACT

Irritable Bowel Syndrome (IBS) is a chronic and fluctuating functional gastrointestinal disorder characterized by abdominal pain and discomfort and accompanying altered bowel habit. The prevalence of IBS is estimated at about 10–13% in the United States. The etiology of IBS is poorly understood, but the relations noted between stress, heightened sensitivity to stimuli and gastrointestinal symptoms has been labeled by gastroenterologists and psychologists alike as the "brain-gut axis," and has increasingly allowed for the acceptance of psychological interventions for IBS. This chapter attempts to offer the clinician some general, evidence-based guidelines for the assessment and treatment of irritable bowel syndrome. Special emphasis is given to the use of hypnotherapy and cognitive-behavioral therapy in treating these disorders.

IRRITABLE BOWEL SYNDROME: DEFINITIONS AND EPIDEMIOLOGY

Irritable Bowel Syndrome (IBS) is a chronic and fluctuating functional gastrointestinal disorder characterized by abdominal pain and discomfort and accompanying altered bowel habit. The prevalence of IBS is estimated at about 10–13% (Drossman et al., 1993; Saito et al., 2000) in the United States, and fairly similar around the world (Thompson, 2002). In the United States, surveys suggest that the prevalence may be similar in whites and blacks and slightly lower in Hispanics (AGA, 2002), although others have suggested that IBS is up to five times more common in whites than blacks (Sandler, 1990). The prevalence of diarrhea-predominant IBS and constipation-predominant IBS is about equivalent (Saito, Schoenfeld, & Locke, 2002). When compared to the prevalence of other diseases such as asthma (5%), diabetes (3%), heart disease (9%), and hypertension (11%) in the United States, however, the occurrence of IBS in the population is significant (Wells, Hahn & Whorwell, 1997).

IBS is the seventh most commonly diagnosed digestive disease in the United States and accounts for up to 50% of referrals to gastroenterologists (Wells et al., 1997). Women appear to be more commonly afflicted than men, with some reports suggesting a 2:1 female to male ratio (Drossman et al., 1993; Talley, Boyce, & Jones, 1997); this estimate may be biased by higher health care utilization among women in general, and changes in the definition of IBS over time. Constipation, bloating and nausea appear to be more common in women (Thompson, 1997), and some studies suggest that symptoms can be linked to the menstrual cycle (Houghton, Lea, Jackson, & Whorwell, 2002).

IBS accounts for almost $19 billion a year in medical costs and lost productivity (Talley, Gabriel, Harmsen, Zinsmeister, & Evans, 1995; Talley, Fett, & Zinsmeister,

Keffer, L., Blanchard, E. B. (2006). Irritable bowel syndrome. In J. E. Fisher & W. T. O'Donohue (Eds.), *Practitioner's guide to evidence-based psychotherapy*. New York: Springer.

1995b). People with IBS have been shown to miss up to three times as much work as healthy controls (Drossman et al., 1993), and are more likely to undergo surgery (Saito et al., 2002). A recent study suggested that IBS is one of the most significant financial burdens on employers, both with respect to direct and indirect costs (Leong et al., 2003).

Onset is common in the teen years (Hyams et al., 1996) and may peak in the 30s and 40s (Ehlin, Montgomery, Ekbom, Pounder, & Wakefield, 2003). Less is known about the role of familial aggregation in IBS. However, familial aggregation has been shown to occur, even after family patterns of somatization have been accounted for, supporting some level of genetic or shared environmental component of the disease (Kalantar, Locke, Zinsmeister, Beighley, & Talley, 2003).

ETIOLOGY: THE BRAIN-GUT AXIS

The etiology of IBS is poorly understood. IBS is considered a *functional* bowel disorder because it represents *disturbed colonic motility* (or function), rather than a structural problem such as a polyp or other anomaly usually found in Inflammatory Bowel Disease (Crohn's Disease or Ulcerative Colitis). Intestinal luminal irritants, post-infective and post-inflammatory processes and stress have all been proposed to be underlying mechanisms in the onset and maintenance of the disorder (Collins Vallance, Barbara, & Borgaonkar, 1999; Camilleri & Prather, 1992). Patients with IBS have also been shown to have altered gastrointestinal motility. Studies have found that IBS patients exhibit an exaggerated response to stimuli such as meals, stress, distention, and corticotropin-hormone injections (AGA, 2002), and increased sensitivity to rectal distension (Naliboff et al., 1997; Mertz et al., 1995). The relations noted between stress, heightened sensitivity to stimuli and gastrointestinal symptoms has been labeled by gastroenterologists and psychologists alike as the "brain-gut axis." This conceptualization provides a useful framework for introducing psychological interventions as a treatment option for IBS.

OBTAINING A DIAGNOSIS

The most widely accepted criteria for diagnosing IBS is the Rome II criteria (Figure 34.1). Many gastroenterologists now support the notion that, in the absence of symptoms such as weight loss, fever and blood in the stool, and in the presence of a normal

At least 12 weeks, which need not be consecutive, in the preceding 12 months of abdominal discomfort or pain that has two of three features:
1. Relieved with defecation; and/or,
2. onset associated with a change in frequency of stool; and/or
3. onset associated with a change in form (appearance) of stool.
Symptoms that cumulatively support the diagnosis of IBS:
1. Abnormal stool frequency (for research purposes, "abnormal" may be defined as greater than three bowel movements per day and less than three bowel movements per week);
2. abnormal stool form (lumpy/hard or loose/watery stool);
3. abnormal stool passage (straining, urgency, or feeling of incomplete evacuation);
4. passage of mucous;
5. bloating or feeling of abdominal distention.

FIGURE 34.1. Rome II Diagnostic Criteria for Irritable Bowel Syndrome[1]

---

[1] Drossman, D.A., Corrazziari, E., Talley, N.J., Thompson, W.G., and Whitehead, W.E. (Eds). (2000). *Rome II: The Functional Gastrointestinal Disorders (2nd ed.).* McLean, VA: Degnon, 351–96.

physical exam, the new criteria can be highly predictive of IBS (Thompson et al., 2000). Nevertheless, IBS remains a disorder of exclusion. In other words, to meet criteria for IBS, all other gastrointestinal diseases must be ruled out. Blood tests and medical procedures such as flexible sigmoidocsopy or colonoscopy may be required to obtain proper diagnosis.

THE PSYCHOLOGICAL INTERVIEW

Once IBS has been diagnosed, the psychologist should spend time helping the patient carefully characterize the nature of the symptoms, including their primary symptoms (diarrhea-predominant, constipation-predominant, mixed type), the frequency and intensity of symptoms, the context of the onset of symptoms, factors that worsen symptoms, including food and stress, and the patient's fears and concerns about their diagnosis. For example, diarrhea is often associated with urgency, fear of accidents or actual fecal incontinence, or avoidance of places where a toilet is not available. Constipation can result in bloating, nausea and altered body image. The Albany IBS History[2] is a useful tool for the initial assessment, and takes about 45 minutes to administer.

IBS patients often report impaired quality of life (Creed et al., 2001; Gralnek, Hats, Kilbourne, Naliboff, & Mayer, 2000). One well-validated measure of quality of life in IBS patients that can be used as a therapeutic endpoint in clinical work is the IBS-QOL (Drossman, Patrick, Whitehead, & Tener 2000).

A good assessment should also include asking the patient about a history of physical, sexual or emotional abuse. A history of sexual and/or physical abuse has been known to occur in 20–60% of treatment-seeking IBS patients (e.g. Leserman et al., 1996; Talley et al., 1995a,b) and has been proposed to be a risk factor for refractory symptoms and higher health care utilization, and may even be linked to the development of the disease (Mayer, Naliboff, Chang and Coutinho, 2001). Emotional abuse may also be common (Ali et al., 2000). The view that abuse is linked to the onset of IBS is somewhat controversial, and several studies have suggested that IBS patients do not differ significantly from patients with other gastrointestinal diseases with respect to abuse (Drossman et al., 1997; Talley et al., 1995a,b). Supporters of an abuse model of IBS suggest that abuse may (1) reduce the threshold of gastrointestinal symptom experience or increase intestinal motility; (2) modify one's appraisal of bodily sensations through an inability to control symptoms; and (3) lead to feelings of guilt and internal responsibility, making disclosure of symptoms unlikely (Drossman et al., 2000, p. 178; Drossman et al., 1997).

Given the high rate of psychiatric disorders in the treatment-seeking IBS population, it is also important to assess for the presence of co-morbid psychopathology, especially emphasizing mood, anxiety and somatization. Only about 40% of people with IBS seek treatment for their symptoms (Drossman et al., 1993). Research has been inconsistent with respect to identifying differences between treatment-seekers and nontreatment seekers with respect to symptom severity and psychopathology. It is commonly believed, however, that patients who seek treatment for their IBS tend

---

[2] The Albany IBS History includes a gastrointestinal symptom history, a method for identifying the antecedents, behaviors and consequences associated with IBS symptoms, a psychosocial history covering the history of gastrointestinal problems in the family, problem areas in the patient's lives, especially as it relates to their IBS and a mental status exam (optional based on the population). Published in Blanchard, E.B. (2001). *Irritable Bowel Syndrome: Psychosocial Assessment and Treatment.* Washington, DC: American Psychological Association.

to be more psychologically distressed, with as many as 60% of treatment-seeking patients with IBS meeting criteria for a psychiatric disorder (Blanchard, 2001; Walker, Roy-Byrne, & Katon, 1990). Mood and anxiety disorders (Lydiard, 1992, Walker, 1990), particularly Generalized Anxiety Disorder and, to a lesser extent, Social Phobia appear to be the most common (Blanchard, 2001). Some research suggests that treating the underlying psychopathology can facilitate an improvement of IBS symptoms directly (Lydiard, Laraia, How I, & Ballenger, 1986; Noyes, Cook, Garvey, & Summers, 1990).

Less is known about personality variables and IBS. Studies using the Eysenck Personality Inventory (EPI; Eysenck and Eysenck, 1968), and the Minnesota Multiphasic Personality Inventory (MMPI; Hathaway and McKinley, 1967) have revealed inconclusive findings with respect to whether personality traits such as "neuroticism" differentiate patients with IBS from controls or those with other gastrointestinal (GI) diseases (Blanchard, Radnitz, Schwarz, Neff, & Geraldi 1987; Latimer et al., 1981).

The first study to look at the presence of DSM-IV personality disorders in IBS patients found that 30% of a treatment-seeking sample of IBS patients met criteria for an Axis II disorder (Blanchard et al., 2004), as determined by the Structured Clinical Interview for DSM-IV, Axis II Disorders (First, Gibben, Spitzer, & Williams, 1996). The most common personality disorder found in the sample was Obsessive–Compulsive Personality Disorder (12%), followed by Avoidant Personality Disorder (5%). However, these findings are only preliminary and more extensive research is needed.

ASSOCIATED DISORDERS

Eating Disorders

The research on the relations between eating disorders and IBS is limited. However, both disorders seem to share some similarities, including a higher prevalence of women, a history of sexual abuse, restriction of foods, and perfectionistic ideals. Women with IBS who reported vomiting as a primary IBS symptom admitted to bulimic-type symptoms, as measured by the Eating Disorders Inventory in one small study (Tang et al., 1998). While IBS patients did not actively engage in self-induced vomiting, they did report thoughts of vomiting as a means of weight control. IBS patients also scored more pathologically than inflammatory bowel disease patients and healthy controls on an Eating Attitudes Test, but scored lower than patients with known eating disorders (Sullivan, Blewett, Jenkins, & Allison, 1997).

Bowel Obsessions

Psychologists should be careful to differentiate between individuals who have obsessions and compulsions related to the bowel habits and those who have IBS. While the delineation between an obsessive–compulsive disorder and IBS is not clear-cut, "bowel obsession," a form of obsessive–compulsive disorder, is characterized by an overwhelming and irrational fear of fecal incontinence such that the person begins to avoid situations where toilets are not available and/or restricts their food intake (Jenike, Baer & Minichello, 1990). Individuals may also spend inordinate amounts of time on the toilet to ensure complete evacuation of stool. While IBS patients may have maladaptive behaviors and/or cognitions around their bowel habits, bowel obsessions are likely to be more specific in their theme and more severe in presentation. If OCD/bowel obsession seems to be the primary disorder, treatment with behavioral interventions (Hatch, 1997) and/or antidepressant medications (Ramachandi, 1990) has been shown to be modestly effective.

Panic Attacks

Bowel symptoms such as diarrhea, vomiting and/or nausea should not occur exclusively during a panic attack (Lydiard et al., 1986).

THE ROLE OF PSYCHOLOGICAL INTERVENTIONS

A recent metaanalysis has suggested that psychological treatments are an effective class of interventions and seem to be superior to control conditions in reducing symptoms (Lackner, Morley, Dowzer, Mesmer, & Hamilton, in press, JCCP). This seems to be especially the case for the more severely afflicted patients (Drossman, Patrick, Whitehead, & Toner, 2000). While most psychological interventions have been shown to be effective, the mechanism by which they work remains unclear.

Hypnotherapy

The use of hypnotherapy for IBS has shown considerable promise, with up to 80% of patients exhibiting and retaining improvement in intestinal symptoms and general well being for up to 1 year (Gonsalkorale, Houghton, & Whorwell, 2002). Hypnotherapy has been proposed to work by altering the patient's focus of attention and changing meaning about sensations arising from the gastrointestinal tract (Palsson, Turner, Johnson, Burnett, & Whitehead, 2002), and by encouraging the body to restore itself to normal (Gonsalkorale, 1998).

Peter Whorwell pioneered the use of hypnosis for this population in the early 1980s with severe, refractory IBS patients (Whorwell, Prior, & Faragher, 1984) and his protocol has been successfully replicated and extended in both the United Kingdom and the United States (e.g. Gonsalkorale et al., 2002; Houghton et al., 2002; Galovski and Blanchard, 1998). It is now believed that verbatim delivery of hypnosis through the use of written scripts, such as the 7-session protocol offered by Palsson's group (2002) or the 12-session protocol offered by Whorwell's group (Whorwell, Prior, & Colgan 1984; Whorewell et al. 1987) can be effective when provided by licensed clinicians who have undergone basic training in clinical hypnosis (Palsson, Turner, Johnson, Burnett, & Whitehead, 2002). In the future, home-hypnosis protocols, which are beginning to be tested empirically (Forbes, MacAuley, & Chiotakakou-Faliakou, 2000), may help to make this form of treatment the most cost-effective.

Cognitive-Behavioral Therapy

One of the most widely evaluated psychological interventions is cognitive-behavioral therapy (CBT). The behavioral component of these treatments serve to modulate arousal through relaxation training, teach skills such as assertiveness to improve interpersonal functioning (Toner, Zindel, Emmott, & Myran, 1998) and modify the environment to reduce behaviors and contingencies that reinforce IBS symptoms (Bennett & Wilkinson, 1985). Cognitive aspects of treatment address appraisal of symptoms and underlying patterns of thinking that affect ones reactions to IBS symptoms (Payne & Blanchard, 1995).

Cognitive-behavioral treatment has been shown to be effective in a few studies out of the Albany group. In one larger-scale study, treatment included education about IBS and normal bowel functioning, progressive muscle relaxation, thermal biofeedback and cognitive therapy. This treatment was effective and improvements seemed to hold up well over 4 years of follow-up (Blanchard, Schwarz et al., 1992)

It is possible that cognitive therapy alone may be effective in treating IBS. A series of randomized controlled trials (RCT), primarily out of the Albany group has suggested that cognitive therapy is an engaging and effective treatment in both individual (Greene & Blanchard, 1994) and small-group format (Vollmer & Blanchard, 1998). Most importantly, this treatment seems to be superior to a psychoeducational support group (Payne & Blanchard, 1995). The Albany Cognitive Therapy Manual has been published and is available for use by clinicians with a background in CBT (Blanchard, 2001).

While a few recent studies have attempted to test CBT with other established interventions, such as the tricyclic desipiramine (Drossman et al., 2003) or routine clinical care (Boyce, Talley, Balaam, Koloski & Truman, 2003), these studies have methodological problems that do not allow for comparisons to be made regarding the effectiveness of CBT over antidepressant medication or other standard gastroenterological treatments. This is also an important area for future research.

Other treatments

While hypnotherapy and CBT have been the most commonly used interventions for IBS, a few other forms of treatment have been met with some success. Short-term psychodynamic therapy has also been shown to be effective, and is generally offered over 7–10 sessions and emphasizes insight and exploration of feelings about having an illness (Svedlund, Sjodin, Ottosson, & Dotevall, 1983; Guthrie, Creed, Dawson, & Tomenson, 1991). Interpersonal psychotherapy, based on the short-term psychodynamic therapy described by Guthrie and colleagues, when combined with the selective serotonin reuptake inhibitor (SSRI) paroxetine, was superior to both SSRI alone and standard care over the long-term with respect to *health care costs* (Creed et al., 2003). One small study has also suggested that Relaxation Response Meditation (as described by Benson, 1975) can be effective in both the short-term (Keefer and Blanchard, 2001) and at one-year follow-up (Keefer and Blanchard, 2002). Similar results were found when progressive muscle relaxation alone was used (Blanchard Greene, Scharff, & Schwarz-McMorris, 1993), although this form of treatment had an unusually high dropout rate and may not be well-tolerated by patients.

Future Directions

While IBS research has continued to expand, there are still a few significant gaps in the literature that should be addressed. One of the most significant gaps in knowledge is how the psychological interventions hold up against each other. We have considerable data to support the use of psychological interventions, but no studies comparing, for example, hypnotherapy to cognitive therapy have been performed. This type of research would assist us with better understanding the mechanism of action of psychological interventions. Similarly, antidepressant medication is often the treatment of choice by gastroenterologists, despite limited empirical support (Jackson et al., 2000)—it would be interesting to compare antidepressant medications against some of the established psychological interventions to determine whether the combination of antidepressants and psychotherapy can augment treatment, as has been shown to be the case with depression (Keller et al., 2001).

SELF-HELP BOOKS

Bolen, B. B. (2000). *"Breaking the Bonds of Irritable Bowel Syndrome: A Psychological Approach to Regaining Control of your Life."* Oakland, CA: New Harbinger Publications.

KEY READINGS

Blanchard, E. B. (2001). *Irritable Bowel Syndrome: Psychosocial Assessment and Treatment.* Washington, D.C: American Psychological Association.

Toner, B. B., Segal, Z. V., Emmott, S. D., & Myran, D. (1999). *Cognitive-Behavioral Treatment of Irritable Bowel Syndrome: The Brain-Gut Connection.* New York; Guilford Press.

Drossman, D. A., Corazziari, E., Talley, N. J., Thompson, W. G., & Whitehead, W. E. (Eds). (2000). *Rome II: The functional gastrointestinal disorders (2nd ed.).* McLean, VA: Degnon, 351–396.

REFERENCES

Ali, A., Toner, B. B., Stuckless, N., Gallop, R., Diamant, N. E., Gould, M. I., & Vidins, E. I. (2000). Emotional abuse, self-blame, and self-silencing in women with irritable bowel syndrome. *Psychosomatic Medicine 62(1),* 76–82.

American Gastroenterological Association (2002). AGA Technical Review on Irritable Bowel Syndrome. *Gastroenterology 123,* 2108–2131.

Bennett, P., & Wilkinson, S. (1985). A comparison of psychological and medical treatment of the irritable bowel syndrome. *British Journal of Clinical Psychology 24,* 215–216.

Benson, H. (1975). *The Relaxation Response.* New York, William Morrow and Company, Inc.

Blanchard, E. B., & Schwarz, S. P. (1987). Adaptation of a multicomponent treatment for irritable bowel syndrome to a small-group format. *Biofeedback and self-regulation 12(1),* 63–69.

Blanchard, E. B., Radnitz, C., Schwarz, S. P., Neff, D. F., & Geraldi, M. A. (1987). Psychological changes associated with self-regulatory treatment of irritable bowel syndrome. *Biofeedback and Self-Regulation 12,* 31–37.

Blanchard, E. B., Schwarz, S. P., Suls, J. M., Gerardi, M. A., Scharff, L., Greene, B., (1992). Two controlled evaluations of multicomponent psychological treatment of irritable bowel syndrome. *Behavior Research and Therapy 30(2),* 175–189.

Blanchard, E. B., Greene, B., Scharff, L., & Schwarz-McMorris, S. P. (1993). Relaxation training as a treatment for irritable bowel syndrome. *Biofeedback and Self-Regulation 18(3),* 125–132.

Blanchard, E. B. (2001). *Irritable bowel syndrome: Psychosocial assessment and treatment.* Washington, DC: American Psychological Association.

Blanchard, E. B., Keefer, L., Lackner, J. M., Galovski, T. E., Krasner, S., & Sykes, M. A. (2004). The role of childhood abuse in Axis I and Axis II psychiatric disorders and medical disorders of unknown origin among irritable bowel syndrome patients. *Journal of Psychosomatic Research 56,* 431–436.

Bolen, B. B. (2000). *Breaking the bonds of irritable bowel syndrome: A psychological approach to regaining control of your life.* Oakland, CA, New Harbinger Publications.

Boyce, P. M., Talley, N. J., Balaam, B., Koloski, N. A., & Truman, G. (2003). A randomized controlled trial of cognitive behavior therapy, relaxation training and routine clinical care for the irritable bowel syndrome. *The American Journal of Gastroenterology 98(10),* 2209–2218.

Camilleri, M., & Prather, C. M. (1992). The irritable bowel syndrome: Mechanisms and a practical approach to management. *Annals of Internal Medicine 116,* 1001–1008.

Collins, S. M., Vallance, B., Barbara, G., & Borgaonkar, M. (1999). Putative inflammatory mechanisms and immunological mechanisms in functional bowel disorders. *Balliere's Best Practices in Research and Clinical Gastroenterology 13(3),* 429–436.

Creed, F., Ratcliffe, J., Fernandez, L., Tomenson, B., Palmer, S., Rigby, C., et al. (2001). Health-related quality of life and health care costs in severe, refractory irritable bowel syndrome. *Annals of Internal Medicine 134,* 860–868.

Creed, F., Fernandes, L., Guthrie, E., Palmer, S., Ratcliffe, J., Read, N., et al. (2003). The Cost-effectiveness of psychotherapy and paroxetine for severe irritable bowel syndrome. *Gastroenterology 124,* 303–317.

Drossman, D. A. (1997). Irritable bowel syndrome and sexual/physical abuse history. *9,* 327–330.

Drossman, D. A., Li, Z., Andruzzi, E., Temple, R. D., Talley, N. J., Thompson, W. G., et al. (1993). US Householder Survey of Functional Gastrointestinal Disorders: Prevalence, sociodemography, and health impact. *Digestive Diseases and Sciences 38,* 1569–1580.

Drossman, D. A., Patrick, D. L., Whitehead, W. E., & Toner, B. B. (2000). Further validation of the IBS-QOL: A disease specific quality of life questionnaire. *American Journal of Gastroenterology 95,* 999–1007.

Drossman, D. A., Toner, B. B., Whitehead, W. E., Diamant, N. E., Dalton, C. B., Duncan, S., et al. (2003). Cognitive-behavioral therapy versus education and desipramine versus placebo for moderate to severe functional bowel disorders. *Gastroenterology 125,* 19–31.

Drossman, D. A. S. E., Corazziari, E., Talley, N. J., Thompson, W. G., & Whitehead, W. E. (Eds.) (2000). *The Functional Gastrointestinal Disorders.* McLean, VA, Degnon Associates.

Ehlin, A. G. C., Montgomery, S. M., Ekbom, A., Pounder, R. E., & Wakefield, A. J. (2003). Prevalence of gastrointestinal diseases in two British national birth cohorts. *Gut, 52,* 1117–1121.

Eysenck, H. J., & Eysenck, S. B. G. (1968). *Eysenck Personality Inventory.* San Diego, Educational Testing Service.

First, M. B., Gibbon, M., Spitzer, R. L., & Williams, J. B. W. (1996). *Structured Clinical Interview for DSM-IV.* New York, Biometrics Research Department, New York State Psychiatric Institute.

Forbes, A., MacAuley, S., & Chiotakakou-Faliakou, E. (2000). Hypnotherapy and therapeutic audiotape: Effective in a previously unsuccessfully treated irritable bowel syndrome? *International Journal of Colorectal Disease 15(5–6)*, 328–334.

Galovski, T. E., & Blanchard, E. B. (1998). The treatment of irritable bowel syndrome with hypnotherapy. *Applied Psychophysiology and Biofeedback, 23*, 219–32.

Gonsalkorale, W. M., Houghton, L. A., & Whorwell, P. J. (2002). Hypnotherapy in irritable bowel syndrome: A large-scale audit of a clinical service with examination of factors influencing responsiveness. *The American Journal of Gastroenterology 97(4)*, 954–961.

Gralnek, I. M., Hats, R. D., Kilbourne, A., Naliboff, B., & Mayer, E. (2000). The impact of irritable bowel syndrome on health-related quality of life. *Gastroenterology 119*, 655–60.

Greene, B., & Blanchard, E. B. (1994). Cognitive therapy for irritable bowel syndrome. *Journal of Consulting and Clinical Psychology 62(3)*, 576–782.

Guthrie, E., Creed, F., Dawson, D., & Tomenson, B. (1991). A controlled trial of psychological treatment for irritable bowel syndrome. *Gastroenterology 100*(450–457).

Hatch, M. L. (1997). Conceptualization and treatment of bowel obsessions: two case reports. *Behavior Research and Therapy 35(3)*, 253–257.

Hathaway, S. R., & McKinley, J. C. (1967). *Minnesota Multiphasic Personality Inventory: Manual for Administration and scoring*. New York, Psychological Corporation.

Houghton, L. A., Lea, R., Jackson, N., & Whorwell, P. J. (2002). The menstrual cycle affects rectal sensitivity in patients with irritable bowel syndrome but not healthy volunteers. *Gut 50*, 471–474.

Hyams, J. S., Burke, G., Davis, P. M., et al. (1996). Abdominal pain and irritable bowel syndrome in adolescents: A community-based study. *Journal of Pediatrics 129*, 220.

Jackson, J. L., O'Malley, P. G., Tomkins, G., Balden, E., Santoro, J., & Kroenke, K. (2000). Treatment of functional gastrointestinal disorders with anti-depressants: A meta-analysis. *American Journal of Medicine 108*: 65–72.

Jenike, M. A., Baer, L., & Minichiello, W. E. (1990). *Obsessive–Compulsive Disorders; Theory and Management*. Chicago, IL, Year Book Medical.

Kalantar, J. S., Locke, G. R., Zinsmeister, A. R., Beighley, C. M., & Talley, N. J. (2003). Familial aggregation of irritable bowel syndrome: a prospective study. *Gut 52*, 1703–1707.

Keefer, L., & Blanchard, E. B. (2001). The effects of relaxation response meditation on the symptoms of irritable bowel syndrome: Results of a controlled treatment study. *Behaviour Research and Therapy 39*, 801–811.

Keefer, L., & Blanchard, E. B. (2002). A one year follow-up of relaxation response meditation on the symptoms of irritable bowel syndrome: Results of a controlled treatment study. *Behaviour Research and Therapy 40*, 541–546.

Keller, M. B., McCullough, J. P., Klein, D. N., Arnow, B., Dunner, D. L., Gelenberg, A. J., et al. (2001). A comparison of nefazadone, the cognitive-behavioral analysis system of psychotherapy, and their combination for the treatment of chronic depression. *New England Journal of Medicine 345(3)*, 232.

Lackner, J. M., Morley, S., Dowzer, C., Mesmer, C., & Hamilton, S. (in press). Psychological treatments for irritable bowel syndrome: A systematic review and meta-analysis. *Journal of Consulting and Clinical Psychology*.

Latimer, P., Sarna, S., Campbell, D., Latimer, M., Waterfall, W., & Daniel, E. E. (1981). Colonic motor and myoelctrical activity: A comparative study of normal subjects, psychoneurotic patients and patients with irritable bowel syndrome. *Gastroenterology 80*, 893–901.

Leong, S. A., Barghout, V., Birnbaum, H. G., Thibeault, C. E., Ben-Hamadi, R., Frech, F., et al. (2003). The economic consequences of irritable bowel syndrome: A US employer perspective. *Archives of Internal Medicine 163*, 929–935.

Leserman, J., Drossman, D. A., Zhiming, L., Toomey, T. C., Nachman, G., & Glogau, L. (1996). Sexual and physical abuse history in gastroenterology practice: How types of abuse impact health status. *Psychosomatic Medicine 58*, 4–15.

Lydiard, R. B., Laraia, M. T., Howell, E. F., & Ballenger, J. C. (1986). Can panic-disorder present as irritable bowel syndrome. *Journal of Clinical Psychiatry 47*, 470–473.

Lydiard, R. B. (1992). Anxiety and the irritable bowel syndrome. *Psychiatric Annals 22*, 612–618.

Mayer, E. A., Naliboff, B. D., Chang, L., & Coutinho, S. V. (2001). Stress and irritable bowel syndrome. *American Journal of Physiology: Gastrointestinal and Liver Physiology 280(4)*: G519–G524.

Mertz, H. R. (2003). Irritable Bowel Syndrome. *The New England Journal of Medicine 349*, 2136–2146.

Noyes, R., Cook, B., Garvey, M., & Summers, R. (1990). Reduction of gastrointestinal symptoms following treatment for panic disorder. *Psychosomatics 31*, 75–79.

Palsson, O. S., Turner, M. J., Johnson, D. A., Burnett, C. K., & Whitehead, W. E. (2002). Hypnosis treatment for severe irritable bowel syndrome: Investigation of mechanism and effects on symptoms. *Digestive Diseases and Sciences 47(11)*, 2605–2614.mkh

Payne, A., & Blanchard, E. B. (1995). A controlled comparison of cognitive therapy and self-help support groups in the treatment of irritable bowel syndrome. *Journal of Consulting and Clinical Psychology 63(5)*, 779–786.

Ramchandani, D. (1990). Trazadone for bowel obsessions. *American Journal of Psychiatry 147*, 124.

Saito, Y. A., Locke, G. R., Talley, N. J. et al. (2000). A comparison of the Rome and Manning criteria for case identification in epidemiological investigations of irritable bowel syndrome. *American Journal of Gastroenterology 95*, 2816–2824.

Saito, Y. A., Schoenfeld, P., & Locke, G. R. (2002). The epidemiology of irritable bowel syndrome in North America: A systematic review. *The American Journal of Gastroenterology 97(8)*, 1910–1915.

Sandler, R. S. (1990). Epidemiology of irritable bowel syndrome in the United States. *Gastroenterology 99(2)*, 409–415.

Sullivan, G., Blewett, A. E., Jenkins, P. L., & Allison, M. C. (1997). Eating attitudes and the irritable bowel syndrome. *General Hospital Psychiatry 19*, 62–64.

Svedlund, J., Sjodin, I., Ottosson, J. O., & Dotevall, G. (1983). Controlled study of psychotherapy in irritable bowel syndrome. *The Lancet*: 589–591.

Talley, N. J., Gabriel, S. E., Harmsen, W. S., Zinsmeister, A. R., & Evans, R. W. (1995a). Medical costs in community subjects with irritable bowel syndrome. *Gastroenterology 109*(1736–1741).

Talley, N. J., Fett, S. L., & Zinsmeister, A. R. (1995b). Self-reported abuse and gastrointestinal disease in outpatients: Association with irritable bowel-type symptoms. *The American Journal of Gastroenterology 90(3)*, 366–371.

Talley, N. J., Boyce, P. M., & Jones, M. (1997). Predictors of health care seeking for irritable bowel syndrome: A population based study. *Gut 41*, 394–398.

Tang, T. N., Toner, B. B., Stuckless, N., Dion, K. L., Kaplan, A. S., & Ali, A. (1998). Features of eating disorders in patients with irritable bowel syndrome. *Journal of Psychosomatic Research 45(2)*, 171–178.

Thompson, W. G. (1997). Gender differences in irritable bowel symptoms. *European Journal of Gastroenterology and Hepatology 9*, 299–302.

Thompson, W. G., Longstreth, G. F., Drossman, D., Heaton, K. W., Irvine, E. J., & Mueller-Lissner, S. A. (2000). Functional bowel disorders and functional bowel pain. *Rome II: Functional gastrointestinal disorders: Diagnosis, pathophysiology, and treatment.* D. A. Drossman, N. J., Talley, W. G. Thompson, W. E. Whitehead, & McLean, E. Corrazziari, (Eds.), VA: Degnon Associates, Inc: 351–432.

Thompson, W. G., Irvine, E. J., Pare, P., Ferrazzi, S., & Rance, L. (2002). Functional gastrointestinal disorders in Canada: first population based survey using Rome II criteria with suggestions for improving the questionnaire. *Digestive Diseases and Sciences 96*, 1072–1079.

Toner, B. B., Zindel, V. S., Emmott, S. D., & Myran, D. (1999). *Cognitive-Behavioral Treatment of Irritable Bowel Syndrome: The Brain-Gut Connection*. New York, Guilford Press.

Vollmer, A., & Blanchard, E. B. (1998). Controlled comparison of individual versus group cognitive therapy for irritable bowel syndrome. *Behavior Therapy, 29*, 19–33.

Walker, E. A., Roy-Byrne, P. P, & Katon, W. J. (1990). Irritable bowel syndrome and psychiatric illness. *American Journal of Psychiatry 147*, 565–572.

Wells, N. E. J., Hahn, B. A., & Whorwell, P. J. (1997). Clinical economics review: Irritable bowel syndrome. *Aliment Pharmacological Therapy 11*, 1019–1030.

Whorwell, P. J., Prior, A., & Faragher, E. B. (1984). Controlled trial of hypnotherapy in the treatment of severe refractory irritable bowel syndrome. *Lancet*: 1232–1234.

Whorwell, P. J., Prior, A., & Colgan, S. M. (1987). Hypnotherapy in severe irritable bowel syndrome: Further experience. *Gut 28*, 423–425.

Kleptomania

Carolynn S. Kohn • David M. Kalal • Karla Kastell • Joann Viera

A consensus about the origins and development of kleptomania has remained elusive to the field of psychology. Although this is due in part to the usual theoretical differences in perspective, it is exacerbated by a paucity of research into the disorder and because kleptomania appears to be a relatively rare problem, with an estimated prevalence rate ranging from 0.6% to 0.8% (Dannon, 2002; Goldman, 1992; Lepkifker et al., 1999). Different researchers have concluded that from none to a quarter of all shoplifters may suffer from kleptomania (Bradford & Balmaceda, 1983; Goldman, 1991; McElroy, Hudson, Pope, & Keck, 1991; Schleuter, O'Neal, & Hickey, 1989). Others suggest that kleptomania may be more common than previously thought, but is underdiagnosed due to secrecy, bias, or constricted diagnostic criteria (Abelson, 1989; Kohn & Antonuccio, 2002; McElroy, Pope, Hudson, Keck, & White, 1991; McElroy, Keck, & Phillips, 1995; Murray, 1992). As so little research exists on the disorder, past theories about the etiology of kleptomania have been based largely on individual case or small group studies using mostly psychoanalytic models. However, as interest has grown in this disorder, cognitive-behavioral and biological models have become the most current and cited perspectives.

PSYCHOANALYTIC MODELS OF ETIOLOGY

Many psychoanalytic theorists believe that kleptomania is an attempt by the person "to obtain symbolic compensation for an actual or anticipated loss," and feel that the key to understanding the etiology lies in the symbolic meaning of the stolen items (Cupchik & Atcheson, 1983, as cited in McNeilly, 1997, p. 119). Other psychoanalytic perspectives have used drive theory to hypothesize that the act of stealing is a defense mechanism, possibly against early traumatic experiences, in which stealing serves to modulate or keep undesirable feelings or emotions from being expressed (Goldman, 1991, 1992).

COGNITIVE-BEHAVIORAL MODELS OF ETIOLOGY

In recent years cognitive-behavioral models have largely replaced psychoanalytic models in providing an explanation for the development of kleptomania. Cognitive-behavioral practitioners often conceptualize the disorders as being the result of operant conditioning, behavioral chaining, distorted cognitions, and poor coping mechanisms (e.g., Gauthier & Pellerin, 1982; Kohn & Antonuccio, 2002). Cognitive-behavioral models posit that after a person steals some item, for various reasons, the behavior is positively reinforced. If this individual experiences minimal or no negative consequences (punishment), then the likelihood that the behavior will reoccur is increased. As the behavior continues to occur, stronger antecedents or cues become contingently linked with it, in what ultimately becomes a powerful behavioral chain. According to cognitive-behavioral theory both antecedents and consequences may either be in the environment or in the mind, as cognitions. For example, Kohn

Kohn, C. S., Kalal, D. M., Kastell, K., & Viera, J. (2006). Kleptomania. In J. E. Fisher & W. T. O'Donohue (Eds.), *Practitioner's guide to evidence-based psychotherapy*. New York: Springer.

and Antonuccio (2002) describe a client's antecedent cognitions, which include thoughts such as "I'm smarter than others and can get away with it"; "they deserve it"; "I want to prove to myself that I can do it"; and "my family deserves to have better things." These thoughts were strong cues to stealing behaviors. All of these thoughts were precipitated by additional antecedents which were thoughts about family, financial, and work stressors or feelings of depression. "Maintaining" cognitions provided additional reinforcement for stealing behaviors and included feelings of vindication and pride, for example: "score one for the 'little guy' against the big corporations"; "I knew I could get away with it." Although those thoughts were often afterward accompanied by feelings of remorse, this came too late in the operant sequence to serve as a viable punisher. Eventually, individuals with kleptomania come to rely upon stealing as a way of coping with stressful situations and distressing feelings, which serve to further maintain the behavior and decrease the number of available alternative coping strategies.

BIOLOGICAL MODELS OF ETIOLOGY

Biological models that seek to explain the origins of kleptomania have been based mostly on pharmacotherapy treatment studies that used selective serotonin reuptake inhibitors (SSRIs), mood stabilizers, and opioid receptor antagonists (see Dannon, 2002 for a review of the literature; Grant & Kim, 2002b). These studies suggest that kleptomania is caused by poor regulation of serotonin, dopamine, and/or natural opioids within the brain. More specifically, explanations based on SSRI studies suggest that kleptomania is akin to impulse control or affective disorders, in that it is mediated by poor regulation of serotonin levels in the brain. Explanations based on opioid antagonist studies suggest that kleptomania is caused by poor regulation of serotonin and/or dopamine. This is because opioid antagonists appear to reduce some people's urges to steal and mute the "rush" typically experienced immediately after stealing (Dannon, 2002; Goldman, 1991; Grant & Kim, 2002b). An alternative explanation also based on opioid antagonist studies states that kleptomania is similar to the "self-medication" model, such that stealing serves as a means for stimulating the person's natural opioid system. "The opioid release 'soothes' the patients, treats their sadness, or reduces their anxiety. Thus, stealing is a mechanism to relieve oneself from a chronic state of hyperarousal, perhaps produced by prior stressful or traumatic events, and thereby modulate affective states" (Grant & Kim, 2002b, p. 354).

SUMMARY

The common thread that ties each of the above-mentioned models appears to be that the stealing behavior, indicative of kleptomania, is a reflection of some other underlying problem, whether it be a defense mechanism, a chain of antecedents and consequences paired with poor coping skills, or poor regulation of neurotransmitters in the brain. Regardless, it is clear that our knowledge regarding the etiology of kleptomania is as conflicted as our understanding about the assessment and, and to a lesser extent, the treatment for individuals with this disorder.

DIAGNOSIS

Controversy also surrounds the manner in which kleptomania is assessed and diagnosed. At one extreme some researchers believe that kleptomania is simply theft and refute the notion that there are psychological components involved (Abelson, 1989; Bresser, 1979 as cited in Wiedemann, 1998), while others view kleptomania as part of a substance-related addiction (Gross, 1990). Others view kleptomania as an "affective spectrum disorder," citing research linking it to depression and anxiety (McElroy Hudson et al., 1991). Still others classify kleptomania as a variant of an impulse control disorder, such as obsessive compulsive disorder or eating disorders. For example Tynes, White, and Steketee (1990) state that persons with eating disorders often display kleptomania symptoms. Additionally, first degree relatives of individuals with kleptomania are more likely to be diagnosed with comorbid impulse control disorders (Grant, 2003). To further complicate matters, throughout much of the literature the terms "compulsive shoplifting" or "compulsive stealing" have been used interchangeably with "kleptomania" (e.g., McElroy, 1991; Hudson, et al. McElroy, Pope et al. 1991; Murray, 1992), resulting in some confusion about the diagnostic criteria used in various studies.

Although there is currently no consensus on this issue, recent research by Grant and Kim (2002a) suggests that kleptomania falls into the spectrum of impulse control disorders, or to a lesser degree, among affective-spectrum disorders. The Diagnostic and Statistical Manual of Mental Disorders, Fourth Edition, Text Revision (DSM-IV-TR: American Psychiatric Association, 2000) classifies kleptomania under the umbrella of impulse control disorders. The essential feature is a recurring failure to resist impulses to steal, even though those items stolen are not needed for personal use or monetary value (Criterion A). The individual must also experience an increasing sense of tension just prior to the theft (Criterion B) and feel pleasure, gratification, or relief when committing the theft (Criterion C). The stealing is not committed in order to express anger or vengeance, is not done in response to a delusion or hallucination (Criterion D), and, finally, is not better accounted for by conduct disorder, a manic episode, or antisocial personality disorder (Criterion E).

Persons diagnosed with kleptomania often have comorbid diagnoses of disorders involving mood, anxiety, eating, impulse control, and substance use (Grant & Kim, 2002a; McElroy, Pope, et al., 1991; Sarasalo, Bergman, & Toth, 1996; Weidemann, 1998). High levels of perceived stress, guilt, shame, and secrecy are associated with the stealing behaviors (Grant, Kim, & Grosz, 2003). These emotions are believed to either cause or exacerbate common comorbid disorders (Grant & Kim, 2002a; Kohn & Antonuccio, 2002; McNeilly & Burke, 1997). The ego-dystonic nature of the stealing behaviors can lead to other problems as well, including social isolation and substance abuse, further exacerbating existing comorbid disorders (Kohn & Antonuccio, 2002; McNeilly & Burke, 1997). The variety of other disorders commonly co-occuring with kleptomania often makes differential diagnosis problematic. This is further complicated by the overlap with characteristics from some Axis II personality disorders, particularly antisocial personality (Kohn & Antonuccio, 2002; Sarasalo et al. 1996), although this personality type can often be ruled out by self-initiated (i.e., nonmandated) presentation for treatment.

ASSESSMENT

Given the high comorbidity of affective disorders and substance use disorders with kleptomania, a thorough assessment of current symptoms and history of symptoms is crucial. Measures such as the Beck Depression Inventory-II (BDI-II; Beck, Steer, & Brown, 1996) and the Beck Anxiety Inventory (BAI; Beck & Steer, 1993) can help identify the severity (i.e., dimensional aspects) of depressive and anxiety symptoms;

whereas the Structured Clinic Interview (SCID-CV; SCID-II) for DSM-IV (First, Spitzer, Gibbon, & Williams, 1996, 1997) and DSM-IV-TR criteria (APA, 2000) can help identify the categorical occurrence of mood and affective disorders. Additionally, given the high rate of comorbidity with other impulse control disorders and, to a lesser degree, personality disorders, these should also be assessed for and documented.

A client's initial treatment gains can be assessed using Improvement Scaling (IMS), a versatile self-report measure tailored to each client's treatment goals that has been successfully utilized in the assessment and treatment of kleptomania (Kohn & Antonuccio, 2002). The Kleptomania Symptom Assessment Scale (K-SAS; Grant & Kim, 2002b) is a self-report measure designed to assess change in cognitions, behaviors, and urges during treatment, and has shown preliminary adequate psychometric properties. Measures of impulsiveness have also been used to assess kleptomania, although they have not shown adequate divergent validity to be considered useful (e.g., Grant & Kim, 2002b).

TREATMENT

Currently there have been no controlled treatment studies for kleptomania, although a review of the extant literature suggests that pharmacotherapy and cognitive-behavior therapy have been used to sucesssfully treat kleptomania.

SSRIs, antiepileptics, and opioid antagonists have all been used to treat kleptomania with varying results (Burstein, 1992; Dannon, 2003; Dannon, Iancu, & Grunhaus, 1999; Kraus, 1999; Grant & Kim, 2002b). However, pharmacological interventions are frequently accompanied by side effects (e.g., Antonuccio, et al., 1999; Dalfan & Stewart, 2001; Grant & Kim, 2002b; Kindler, Dannon, Iancu, et al., 1997), which clients can find disagreeable, leading to poor compliance with the medication (e.g., Dannon, 2003; Dannon et al. 1999).

A fair number of uncontrolled studies have demonstrated the effectiveness of using cognitive-behavior therapy (CBT) to treat kleptomania (e.g., Gauthier & Pellerin, 1982; Glover, 1985; Kohn & Antonuccio, 2002; Murray, 1992; Weidmann, 1998). Each utilize several fundamental components typical of cognitive-behavioral approaches, and include covert sensitization, behavioral chaining, problem-solving, cognitive restructuring, and homework (e.g., O'Donohue, Hayes, & Fisher, 2003). Although all of these components have been used successfully on individuals with kleptomania, the completion of a thorough functional analysis will dictate the unique implementation, format, and structure of each of these techniques for each individual (Kanfer & Saslow, 1965; Kohn & Antonuccio, 2002; Weidemann, 1998). For example, covert sensitization, the "pairing of imagined consequences of stealing with the desire to steal" (Goldman, 1991, p. 993), can use kleptomania-specific consequences (e.g., getting arrested, going to jail), rather than the commonly used images of nausea or vomiting as the aversive event to facilitate treatment goals (Gauthier & Pellerin, 1982; Kohn & Antonuccio, 2002). In this approach clients describe the scenario aloud, in vivid detail, allowing their anxiety to increase until they reach a predetermined end-point, such as spending time in jail or the conclusion of a court trial. Due to the anxiety provoking nature of this exercise, it is important to leave several minutes at the end of the session for a debriefing and "cooling off" period. In addition to covert sensitization, clinicians should discuss with clients the Abstinence Violation Effect (AVE; e.g., Larimer, Palmer, & Marlatt, 1999). Research indicates that among shoplifters, individuals who experience stable, global feelings of shame (e.g., "I'm a bad person") are more likely to continue stealing;

whereas those who experience situation-specific feelings of shame (e.g., imagining getting caught stealing when one is an otherwise "good" person) are more likely to stop (Tibbetts, 1997). One explanation is that global feelings of shame that are replaced with situation-specific feelings are more conducive to increased self esteem (Abramson, Metalsky, & Alloy, 1989). Finally, given the high comorbidity of mood disorders and the correspondingly high rate of using SSRIs to treat either kleptomania symptoms and comorbid depressive symptoms (e.g., Fishbain, 1987; Grant & Kim, 2002a), clinicians should educate clients regarding the potential for Discontinuation Effects of SSRIs (Coupland, Bell, & Potokar, 1996). Such warning can prevent a belief that a relapse of depression or anxiety is occurring (Kohn & Antonuccio, 2002).

CONCLUSIONS

As stated above, a diagnosis of kleptomania is rarely made in isolation. Rather, it is usually accompanied by a multitude of comorbid conditions, most commoningly affective, impulse control, and substance use disorders. Additionally, there exist higher rates of affective and substance use disorders in first-order family members of indivudals with kleptomania (Grant & Kim, 2002a) and reports of social isolation, dysfunctional cognitions, and high levels of perceived stress are also associated with increased frequency and/or intensity of kleptomania behaviors (Grant, et al. 2003; Kohn & Antonuccio, 2002). Grant and Kim's (2002b) proposed psychobiological model attempts to explain the genesis of kleptomania in a manner that combines neurochemistry with behavioral theories of classical and operant conditioning. They posit that certain individuals become conditioned to react to certain stimuli or cues (e.g., desired items) or to crave or desire stealing because of the rewarding sensation that follows it, both of which cause changes in the brain. These changes subsequently lead to increased motivation (e.g., urges or cravings) to steal again. Based on this model it is possible that a pre-existing disorder, such as depression, combined with positive reinforcement and lack of punishment for stealing behavior increases the risk for kleptomania. Conversely, individuals without pre-existing disorders who are punished for stealing early on are less likely to develop kleptomania. In fact, research suggesting "evidence of metabolic changes associated with improvement in psychotherapy that are similar to those seen with antidepressants" (Antonuccio, et al., 2002, p. 7) provide support for this combined biobehavioral model.

Although research has provided us with more information regarding kleptomania, our knowledge may be hindered by our preconceived notions. Historically, kleptomania has been considered a disorder mainly seen in white, upper- and upper middle-class women (Abelson, 1989; Goldman, 1991; McElroy, Hudson et al. 1991). Aside from some isolated research (Bergman & Toth, 1996; Grant & Kim, 2002a, 2002b; Weidemann, 1998) comparatively little is known about males or individuals of lower economic status with kleptomania and how treatment may differ due to these variables (e.g., Goldman, 1991, 1992; Murray, 1992). The necessity to meet *Criterion A* from the DSM-IV is an example of how examining mainly those in the upper economic status may bias both diagnosis and treatment of kleptomania. *Criterion A* presumes that the individual would otherwise have adequate income to pay for the stolen items and, as such, may be an artifact of studying mainly upper-class clients. For example, a report of 20 cases of kleptomania found that 90% of kleptomania patients, all of whom were of lower economic status, did use the stolen items (McElroy, Pope et al. 1991). Moreover, there is some research which suggests there are gender differences in controlling shoplifting behaviors (Tibbetts & Herz, 1996);

thus, it is plausible that there may also be gender differences in the treatment of kleptomania. It is possible that the current criteria for kleptomania only capture a limited segment of the population (e.g., upper middle class, white women) and ostensibly ignore others that may be suffering from kleptomania, but instead are labeled as criminals (e.g., lower SES, males). Therefore, we suggest that researchers continue to examine the characteristics of those diagnosed with kleptomania, while not constraining themselves to the current, commonly accepted criteria. Including kleptomania in future Catchment or large population studies can help to provide more information about the disorder in an empirical, less self-selected manner. Moreover, although psychotropic interventions have shown some success, to date cognitive-behavioral interventions appear credible, effective, and safer, due of their lack of side effects, and thus should be considered the first line of treatment for kleptomania.

REFERENCES

Abelson, E. S. (1989). The invention of kleptomania. *Signs: Journal of Women in Culture and Society, 15,* 123–143.

Abramson, L. Y., Metalsky, G. I., & Alloy, L. B. (1989). Hopelessness depression: A theory-based subtype of depression. *Psychological Review, 96,* 358–372.

American Psychiatric Association (2000). *Diagnostic and Statistical Manual of Mental Disorders* (4th ed.). Washington DC: American Psychiatric Association.

Antonuccio, D. O., Burns, D. D., & Danton, W. G. (2002). Antidepressants: A triumph of marketing over science? *Prevention & Treatment, 5,* Article 3. Available on the World Wide Web: http://journals.apa.org/prevention/volume5/pre0050025c.html.

Antonuccio, D. O., Danton, W. G., DeNelsky, G. Y., Greenberg, R. P., & Gordon, J. S. (1999). Raising questions about antidepressants. *Psychotherapy and Psychosomatics, 68,* 3–14.

Bradford, J. M., & Balmaceda, R. (1983). Shoplifting: Is there a specific psychiatric syndrome? *Canadian Journal of Psychiatry, 28,* 248–254.

Burstein, A. (1992). Fluoxetine-lithium treatment for kleptomania. *Journal of Clinical Psychiatry, 53,* 28–29.

Cautela, J. R. (1966). Treatment of compulsive behavior by covert sensitization. *Psychological Record, 86,* 33–81.

Coupland, N. J., Bell, C. J., & Potokar, J. P. (1996). Serotonin reuptake inhibitor withdrawal. *Journal of Clinical Psychopharmacology, 16,* 356–362.

Cupchik, W. (1992). Kleptomania and shoplifting. *American Journal of Psychiatry, 149,* 1119.

Dalfen, A. K., & Stewart, D. E. (2001). Who develops stable or fatal adverse drug reactions to selective serotonin reuptake inhibitors? *Canadian Journal of Psychiatry, 46,* 258–262.

Dannon, P. (2002). Kleptomania: An impulse control disorder? *International Journal of Psychiatry in Clinical Practice, 6,* 3–7.

Dannon, P. (2003). Topiramate for the treatment of kleptomania: A case series and review of the literature. *Clinical Neuropharmacology, 26,* 1–4.

Dannon, P., Iancu, I., & Grunhaus, L. (1999). Naltrexone treatment in kleptomanic patients. *Human Psychopharmacology: Clinical & Experimental, 14,* 583–585.

First, M. B., Spitzer, R. L, Gibbon M., & Williams, J. B. W. (1996). *Structured Clinical Interview for DSM-IV Axis I Disorders, Clinician Version (SCID-CV).* Washington, DC: American Psychiatric Press.

First, M. B., Spitzer, R. L, Gibbon M., & Williams, J. B. W. (1997). *Structured Clinical Interview for DSM-IV Personality Disorders, (SCID-II).* Washington, DC: American Psychiatric Press.

Fishbain, D. A. (1987). Kleptomania as risk-taking behavior in response to depression. *American Journal of Psychotherapy, 41,* 598–603.

Gauthier, J., & Pellerin, D. (1982). Management of compulsive shoplifting through covert sensitization. *Journal of Behavior Therapy and Experimental Psychiatry, 13,* 73–75.

Glover, J. H. (1985). A case of kleptomania treated by covert sensitization. *British Journal of Clinical Psychology, 24,* 213–214.

Goldman, M. J. (1991). Kleptomania: Making sense of the nonsensical. *American Journal of Psychiatry, 148,* 986–996.

Goldman, M. J. (1992). Kleptomania: An overview. *Psychiatric Annals, 22,* 68–71.

Grant, J. E. & Grosz, R. (2004). Pharmacotherapy outcome in older pathological gamblers: A preliminary investigation. *Journal of Geriatric Psychiatry & Neurology, 17,* 9–12.

Grant, J. E., Kim, S. W., & Grosz, R. L. (2003). Percieved stress in kleptomania. *Psychiatric Quarterly, 74,* 251–258.

Grant, J. E. & Kim, S. W. (2002a). Clinical characteristics and associated psychopathology of 22 patients with kleptomania. *Comprehensive Psychiatry, 43,* 378–384.

Grant, J. E. Kim, S. W. (2002b). An open-label study of naltrexone in the treatment of kleptomania. *Journal of Clinical Psychiatry, 63,* 349–356.

Kanfer, F. H., & Saslow, G. (1965). Behavioral analysis: An alternative to diagnostic classification. *Archives of General Psychiatry, 12,* 529–538.

Kindler, S., Dannon, P. N., Iancu, I., et al. (1997). Emergence of kleptomania during treatment for depression with serotonin selective reuptake inhibits. *Clinical Neuropharmacology, 20,* 126–129.

Kohn, C. S., & Antonuccio, D. O. (2002). Treatment of kleptomania using cognitive and behavioral strategies. *Clinical Case Studies, 1,* 25–38.

Kraus, J. E. (1999). Treatment of kleptomania with paroxetine. *Journal of Clinical Psychiatry, 60,* 793.

Larimer, M. E., Palmer, R. S., & Marlatt, G. A. (1999). Relapse prevention. An overview of Marlatt's cognitive-behavioral model. *Alcohol Research and Health, 23,* 151–160.

Lepkifker, E., Dannon, P. N. Ziv, R., et al. (1999). The treatment of kleptomania with serotonine reuptake inhibitors. *Clinical Neuropharmacology, 22,* 40–43.

McConaghy, N., & Blaszczynaski, A. (1988). Imaginal Desensitization: a cost-effective treatment in two shop-lifters and a binge-eater resistant to previous therapy. *Australian and New Zealand Journal of Psychiatry, 22,* 78–82.

McElroy, S. L., Hudson, J. I., Pope, H. G., & Keck, P. E. (1991). Kleptomania: Clinical characteristics and associated psychopathology. *Psychological Medicine, 21,* 93–108.

McElroy, S. L., Keck, P. E., & Phillips, K. A. (1995). Kleptomania, compulsive buying, and binge-eating disorder. *Journal of Clinical Psychiatry, 56,* 14–26.

McElroy, S. L., Pope, H. G., Hudson, J. I., Keck, P. E., & White, K. L. (1991). Kleptomania: A report of 20 cases. *American Journal of Psychiatry, 148,* 652–657.

McNeilly, D. P., & Burke, W. J. (1998). Stealing Lately: A case of late-onset kleptomania. *International Journal of Geriatric Psychiatry, 13,* 116–121.

Murray, J. B. (1992). Kleptomania: A review of the research. *The Journal of Psychology, 126,* 131–138.

O'Donohue, W. T., Hayes, S. C., & Fisher, J. E. (2003). Cognitive Behavior Therapy: Applying Empirically Supported Techniques in your Practice. PLACE: Wiley & Sons.

Sarasalo, E., Bergman, B., & Toth, J. (1996). Personality Traits and psychiatric and somatic morbidity among kleptomaniacs. *Acta Psychiatrica Scandinavica, 94,* 358–364.

Smith, A., Cardillo, J. E., Smith, S. C., & Amezaga, A. M. (1998). Improvement Scaling (rehabilitation version): A new approach to measuring progress of patients in achieving their individual rehabilitation goals. *Medical Care, 36,* 333–347.

Tibbetts, S. G. (1997). Shame and rational choice in offending decisions. *Criminal Justice and Behavior, 24,* 234–255.

Tibbetts, S. G., & Herz, D. C. (1996). Gender differences in factors of social control and rational choice. *Deviant Behavior: An Interdisciplinary Journal, 17,* 183–208.

Tynes, L. L., White, K. & Steketee, G. S. (1990). Toward a new nosology of obsessive compulsive disorder, *Comprehensive Psychiatry, 31,* 465–480.

Wiedemann, G. (1998). Kleptomania: Characteristics of 12 cases. *European Psychiatry, 13,* 67–77.

Learning Disorders

Steven G. Little • Angeleque Akin-Little • Teresa L. Richards

WHAT ARE LEARNING DISORDERS?

Learning Disorders/Learning Disabilities (LD) comprise a relatively heterogeneous grouping of disorders involving difficulties in academic performance. Numerous definitions of LD have been proposed but there is no universally accepted definition (Heward, 2003). The most commonly accepted definitions are those in the Individuals With Disabilities Education Act (IDEA), National Joint Committee on Learning Disabilities (NJCLD), and the *DSM-IV-TR* (APA, 2000). There is no one single perspective on the etiology, diagnosis, or treatment of LD but perspectives can usually be grouped in three general areas: biological, cognitive, and contextual (Sternberg & Spear-Swerling, 1999). The biological perspective encompasses explanations involving brain damage or central nervous system dysfunction, genetics, or biochemical disturbances. The cognitive perspective focuses on information-processing functions and how they contribute to the development of learning difficulties. Contextual perspectives focus on the environment and its role in the development of learning problems.

IDEA definition. The Individuals with Disabilities Act (formerly the Education for All Handicapped Children's Act of 1975) has maintained the same definition of LD since first conceptualized. This definition has been preserved through all incarnations of the law from 1975 to the Individuals with Disabilities Education Improvement Act of 2004 (HR 1350, May 13, 2004). That definition is as follows:

The term 'specific learning disability' means a disorder in one or more of the basic psychological processes involved in understanding or in using language, spoken or written, which may manifest itself in imperfect ability to listen, think, speak, read, write, spell, or do mathematical calculations. Such term includes such conditions as perceptual disabilities, brain injury, minimal brain dysfunction, dyslexia, and developmental aphasia. Such term does not include a learning problem that is primarily the result of visual, hearing, or motor disabilities, of mental retardation, of emotional disturbance, or of environmental, cultural, or economic disadvantage. (USOE, 1977, p. 65083)

NJCLD definition. The National Joint Committee on Learning Disabilities (NJCLD) is a group composed of official representatives of 10 professional organizations that are involved with students with learning disabilities. Their definition of LD is as follows:

Learning disabilities is a general term that refers to a heterogeneous group of disorders manifested by significant difficulties in the acquisition and use of listening, speaking, reading, writing, reasoning, or mathematical abilities. These disorders are intrinsic to the individual, presumed to be due to a central nervous system dysfunction, and may occur across the life span. Problems in self-regulatory behaviors, social perception, and social interaction may exist with learning disabilities, but do not by themselves constitute a learning disability. Although learning disabilities may occur concomitantly with other disabilities (for example,

Little, S. G., Akin-Little, A., & Richards, T. L. (2006). Learning disorders. In J.E. Fisher & W. T. O'Donohue (Eds.), *Practitioner's guide to evidence-based psychotherapy*. New York: Springer.

sensory impairment, mental retardation, serious emotional disturbances) or extrinsic influences (such as cultural differences, insufficient or inappropriate instruction), they are not the result of those conditions or influences (NJCLD, 1989, p. 1).

The NJCLD criticizes the federal definition of LD as it appears in IDEA for several weaknesses. These include the fact that the IDEA definition refers only to school-age children and LD can occur at any age, the use of the term "basic psychological processes," inclusion of spelling as a learning disability, and the use of obsolete terms (e.g., dyslexia, minimal brain dysfunction, developmental aphasia) (Heward, 2003).

DSM-IV-TR. Learning Disorders fall under Disorders Usually First Diagnosed in Infancy, Childhood, or Adolescence (Axis I). The general description is "Learning Disorders are diagnosed when the individual's achievement on individually administered achievement tests in reading, mathematics, or written expression is substantially below that expected for age, schooling, and level of intelligence" (APA, 2000; p. 49). Substantially below is defined as two standard deviations between IQ and achievement. Learning Disorders are further divided into Reading Disorder (315.00), Mathematics Disorder (315.1), and Disorder of Written Expression (315.2). There is also a category for Learning Disorder Not Otherwise Specified (315.9) for "disorders in learning that do not meet criteria for any specific Learning Disorder" (p. 56).

Operational definitions. Kavale and Forness (2000) conclude that the IDEA and NJCLD definitions of LD fail to provide much understanding of the true nature of the condition and provide little assistance in diagnosis. While the DSM-IV-TR definition includes specific diagnostic parameters, it is not used in most schools, and it is school children who are most likely to receive this diagnosis. The US Office of Education issued an operational definition of LD in 1976 and the general concept is still the most commonly used criterion for defining learning disability in practice (Kavale, 2002). It states

A specific learning disability may be found if a child has a severe discrepancy in achievement and intellectual ability in one or more of several areas: oral expression, written expression, listening comprehension or reading comprehension, basic reading skills, mathematics calculation, mathematics reasoning, or spelling" (p. 52405).

How this severe discrepancy is operationalized varies from state to state. Reschly (2004) conducted a survey of states regarding LD policies, practices, and prevalence. A severe discrepancy between ability and achievement was found in 48 of 50 states with only Iowa and Louisiana not using an IQ—achievement discrepancy model at this time. Ten states required a standard score of standard deviation difference with a range of from 15 points in Idaho, Mississippi, North Carolina, and Texas to 30 points in Montana. The most common discrepancy needed is 23 points which is found in nine states. Twenty states required a regression method in which the magnitude of the discrepancy varies depending on the individual's IQ. Twenty states either do not specify how the discrepancy is to be calculated or use an idiosyncratic method. Further, 13 states require the identification of a processing deficit in conjunction with the IQ—achievement discrepancy to diagnose LD. It is important that a psychologist conducting an LD assessment on a school-age child outside of the school be aware of and conform to their state's Department of Education guidelines for the diagnosis of LD so that the school can use the results in making special education eligibility decisions.

Questions regarding the reliability and validity of the ability-achievement discrepancy model of LD determination have appeared consistently since it was first proposed in 1976 (e.g., Cruickshank, 1979, Fletcher et al., 1998; Gresham, 2002; Lyon, 1996; Lyon et al., 2001; Siegel, 1989, 2003; Stage, Abbot, Jenkins, & Berninger, 2003; Stuebing et al., 2002; Vellutino, Scanlon, & Lyon, 2000). There are many problems associated with the IQ-achievement discrepancy model. The use of this model means that children must fall below a predicted level of achievement before being eligible for an LD designation and related services and these levels are not easy to achieve at the lower grades making early identification of LD difficult with this model. Lyon et al. (2001) report that it is not until about age 9 that psychologists can reliably measure an IQ-achievement discrepancy, therefore, the IQ-achievement discrepancy becomes a "wait-to-fail" model. Given that children with reading disabilities (the most common form of LD) are likely to continue to have reading problems into adulthood (Shaywitz et al., 1999), failure to identify problems early and provide effective intervention may result in a lifetime of learning difficulties. Concern about the discrepancy model has led Congress to propose options in the 2004 IDEA reauthorization bill (HR 1350 as amended by the Senate on May 13, 2004). Section 164 (b) states:

Notwithstanding section 607(b), when determining whether a child has a specific learning disability as defined in section 602(29), a local educational agency *shall not be required* (emphasis added) to take into consideration whether a child has a severe discrepancy between achievement and intellectual ability in oral expression, listening comprehension, written expression, basic reading skill, reading comprehension, mathematical calculation, or mathematical reasoning . . . . . In determining whether a child has a specific learning disability, a local educational agency may use a process that determines if the child responds to scientific, research-based intervention as a part of the evaluation procedures described in paragraphs (2) and (3). (p. 154)

Gresham (2002) is the prime advocate of the responsiveness to intervention (RTI) approach to the identification of learning disabilities. The RTI approach identifies students as having a learning disability only if their academic performance in relevant areas does not change in response to an empirically validated intervention implemented with integrity. Many questions arise when considering an RTI approach to LD eligibility determination. First and foremost is that, while Congress appears to be advocating this approach, they are not requiring it and the decision on whether to adopt RTI or continue using a discrepancy model lies with each local education agency (school district). Gresham identifies additional concerns including (a) selection of the best intervention available, (b) determination of the optimal length and intensity of the intervention, (c) ensuring the integrity of interventions, and (d) determining the rules of how to define adequate responsiveness to the intervention. It is safe to say that additional research needs to be conducted on the RTI model before it sees widespread acceptance in the schools.

BASIC FACTS ABOUT LEARNING DISORDERS

Prevalence. Many different estimates of the number of children with learning disabilities have appeared in the literature with a range of from 1% to 30% of the population (Folse, 2004). The US Department of Education reports that approximately half of all students served in special education fall into the LD category. This corresponds to about 5% of the school-age population and represents a 28% increase in the last 10 years (Klotz, Feinberg, & Nealis, 2004). Reading difficulties characterize the majority of individuals with learning disabilities (Bender, 2004). According to the *DSM-IV-TR* (APA, 2000) reading disorders comprise 80% of Learning Disorders and have a prevalence of 4% of school-age children. Mathematics Disorder (when not comorbid with other learning disorders) comprises the other approximate 20% of individuals with a Learning Disorder, representing about 1% of school-age children (APA). It may, however, also occur in combination with Reading Disorder. Disorder of Written language is rare as a singular condition and is usually associated with other learning disorders, particularly reading disorder (APA).

Comorbidity. A high rate of comorbidity has been found between LD and ADHD with LD being reported in 25% to 61% of individuals with ADHD (Swanson, Harris, & Graham, 2003). It should be stressed, however, that ADHD is not synonymous with LD (Heward, 2003). High rates of comorbidity are also found with Tourette Syndrome (approximated 33%) and Neurofibromatosis Type I (25–61%) (Cutting & Denckla, 2003). Individuals with emotional and behavioral difficulties may also be more likely to be diagnosed LD.

Age at onset. Although signs of LD may be present as early as kindergarten, diagnosis seldom occurs until formal instruction, particularly in reading, begins in first grade. As was mentioned previously, the IQ-achievement discrepancy model of diagnosis may result in under diagnosis in the early grades.

Gender. According to the *DSM-IV-TR* (APA, 2000) males comprise the vast majority of individuals diagnosed with reading disorder (60–80%) although it is noted that the overrepresentation of males may be due in part to a higher rate of disruptive behavior in boys.

Course. Because LD is so heterogeneous, it is difficult to chart a particular course for individuals diagnosed with LD. Those identified are usually diagnosed in the schools and provided with some form of special education services but this may not occur until after they have demonstrated a pattern of failure in academic activities. Children with reading difficulties typically enter school lacking adequate phonological skills which limits their word reading skills (Lyon et al., 2001). A cycle of failure develops as a result of their slow and laborious reading leads to poor comprehension and limited reinforcement for reading activities. Without adequate instruction reading difficulties remain throughout the lifespan. Early intervention is essential if this course is to be altered as children diagnosed with reading disorder after Grade 2 rarely catch up to the reading level of their peers (Lyon et al.)

ASSESSMENT

What Should be Ruled Out?

LD, by definition, must be differentiated from academic deficits that are primarily the result of visual, hearing, or motor disabilities, mental retardation, emotional disturbance, or environmental, cultural, or economic disadvantage. The *DSM-IV-TR* (APA, 2000) further states that LD must be "differentiated from normal variations in academic attainment and from scholastic difficulties due to lack of opportunity, poor teaching, or cultural factors" (p. 51). Making such determinations can be difficult. However, factors that should definitely be taken into consideration include individuals for whom English is not the primary language and those whose have an inconsistent educational background (i.e., absenteeism problem, frequent changes in academic placement).

What is Involved in Effective Assessment?

As mentioned, there have been numerous calls to eliminate the ability-achievement discrepancy model for the diagnosis of LD. At some point, the RTI model may supplant the discrepancy model as the dominant method for LD diagnosis but at this time even the IDEA reauthorization is only offering RTI as a possible alternative model and the *DSM-IV-TR* (APA, 2000) continues to use a discrepancy definition in their diagnostic criteria. It is unlikely that the ability-achievement discrepancy model will become rare any time soon. For this reason, the National Association of School Psychologists (NASP) recommends that a comprehensive evaluation may include: (a) indirect sources of information such as parent, teacher, and student interviews; work products; review of pertinent records, (b) direct observation, (c) documentation of response to general education interventions, and (d) individual assessment, as prescribed by the evaluation team that may include norm-referenced and criterion-referenced measures of cognitive and academic skills as well as direct sources of data (Cantor & Klotz, 2004)

As mentioned previously, diagnosis in schools in most states requires the documentation of an ability-achievement discrepancy as does the *DSM-IV-TR* (APA, 2000) which is more likely to be used with adult LD assessment. Regardless of the deficiencies with this model, psychologists assessing either children or adults for a learning disorder must be familiar with the most appropriate procedures for using norm-referenced tests to determine if a discrepancy exists. We recommend the following general outline to follow in the assessment of an individual suspected of LD.

1. Preassessment screening, which should include:
   a. Operationalization of the problem with teacher and/or parent for child or the individual him/herself for adult.
   b. Evaluate and exclude alternative hypotheses. Including:
      * Educational History (numerous school placements, attendance, etc.)
      * Social Functioning and Behavior
      * Environmental and cultural factors
      * Motor Functioning
      * Speech and Language Functioning
      * Health, Medical History, and Physical Status
      * Hearing and Vision Screening
2. Document response to intervention. This can be conducted by the psychologist or documented by the classroom teacher. However, it is important that the intervention be empirically validated.
3. Obtain an accurate measure of general intelligence. If an ability-achievement discrepancy is to be used, the instrument's measure of "g" is the most appropriate measure to use unless there is a documented reason for using a scale of the test (e.g., speech or language difficulties, motor difficulties, spoiled subtests). It is inappropriate to use a subtest score as a measure of ability in any situation.
4. Obtain measures of achievement from a norm-referenced test. Recognize that you are looking for low achievement in the areas of reading, written language, or mathematics. The appropriate score to compare to IQ is the cluster score that represents performance in one of these areas, not an individual subtest score.
5. Use state or *DSM-IV-TR* (APA, 2000) guidelines to determine if there is a significant discrepancy. If the state requires documentation of a processing deficit you may also need to determine if this can be documented. There is very little agreement as to what constitutes a processing deficit or how to determine if a processing deficit

exists so it would be best to consult someone with experience in this field in your state.

6. Follow-up with curriculum-based assessment. Norm-referenced achievement tests give you information about how the individual is functioning relative to a national norm group. It provides little information that is relevant to the materials on which the individual is being instructed. In order to make valid recommendations you must be familiar with how the child is functioning with his/her current curriculum.

What Assessments are Not Helpful?

Personality tests, projective tests, and neuropsychological tests are not useful in assessing for a learning disability. Standard measures of perceptual-motor ability such as the *Bender* or *Developmental Test of Visual-Motor Integration* (VMI) also have limited utility due to psychometric deficiencies in these instruments.

TREATMENT

What Treatments are Effective?

The fact is, psychologists are most likely not going to be the primary treatment agent for an individual diagnosed with a learning disorder. As the majority of individuals with LD are children, treatment is most likely to be completed by a teacher (either special or regular education) in the classroom. That does not, however, mean that psychologists do not have a great deal to offer with regard to treatment. There is little doubt that the field of education has a long history of advocating teaching practices that have little or no empirical support. One consistent finding, however, has been that Direct Instruction programs have been demonstrated to be superior to other programs in achieving academic success (Adams & Carnine, 2003). The formal term Direct Instruction (DI) refers to a published curricula that has been field tested with students using a three-stage curriculum-testing process (Adams & Engelmann, 1996). Unless a school has adopted this curriculum it will not be a part of the individual's education. What the psychologist can recommend to teachers, however, is to incorporate certain elements of DI into her/his teaching practices for the individual with LD. This starts by recognizing that instruction needs to teacher-directed. This does not mean the teacher simply lectures to the student or that the teacher does not recognize the needs of the students. It does mean that the teacher organizes instructional materials and methods based on the needs of the individual student. The teacher also should use techniques such as pacing, have students respond verbally, cuing, frequent reinforcement, etc. Recommendations for teachers should also stress the importance for explicit instruction. This involves using carefully designed materials and activities that provide a great deal of structure and support so that students can make sense of new information and concepts (Heward, 2003). Heward further recommends that teachers (a) use a number of examples to illustrate concepts or strategies, (b) provide step-by-step strategies as well as broad questions, (c) having students explain their decision making process, (d) providing frequent, positive feedback on student performance, and (e) providing students with adequate practice opportunities with interesting curricular materials. Others have found that teachers who use content enhancements (e.g., guided notes, graphic organizers, visual displays, mnemonic instruction) may increase success in the classroom for both disabled and nondisabled peers (Brigham & Brigham, 2001; Bulgren, Deshler, Schumaker, & Lenz, 2000; Dye, 2000; Lazarus, 1996).

What are Effective Self-Help Treatments?

Self-help treatments are generally not widely used in the treatment of individuals with a learning disorder. Parents may assist teachers in developing a child's academic capabilities by consulting with the teacher and working with their child on homework and other teacher assigned tasks. Reading to a child and having the child read orally to the parents can also facilitate reading acquisition. In addition, many organizations have information on their websites to aid parents in extending educational activities to the home.

Useful Websites

http://www.ldonline.org/
http://www.air.org/ldsummit/ (Learning Disabilities Summit)
http://www.nrcld.org/index.html (National Research Center on Learning Disabilities)
http://www.ld.org/ ((National Center for Learning Disabilities)
http://www.teachingld.org/ (Division of Learning Disabilities, Council for Exceptional Children)

What are Effective Therapist-Based Treatments?

When psychologists are working directly with a client or parent to help improve academic competencies, there are a range of behavioral programs that have been developed that have been demonstrated efficacious. Programs such as Reading to Read (Tingstrom, Edwards, & Olmi, 1995) or various applied behavior analytic approaches (i.e., functional assessment of academic problems) (e.g., Daly, Witt, Martens, & Dool, 1997; Eckert, Ardoin, Daly, & Martens,. 2002; VanAuken, Chafouleas, Bradley, & Martens, 2002) may be useful for clinicians.

What is Effective Medical Treatment?

There are no medical treatments that have a direct effect on learning disorders. If the individual has comorbid ADHD, psychostimulent medication has been consistently demonstrated to enhance behavioral, academic, and social functioning (DuPaul & Stoner, 2003).

Other Issues in Management

Children who experience academic difficulties are likely to develop deficits in self-esteem and social skills (APA, 2000). Therefore, in addition to addressing academic deficiencies, emotional and behavioral factors may also need to be a focus of treatment. LD is a very heterogeneous disorder and so are the emotional and behavioral manifestations of individual with LD. The appropriate behavioral or cognitive behavior techniques to use will therefore vary greatly depending on the age and the needs of the individual.

How Does One Select Among Treatments?

If treatment is to be administered by a parent, the parents capability to administer the treatment must be considered. If it is determined that the parent lacks sufficient skills to assist in academic remediation, intervention may need to be solely school-based.

REFERENCES

Adams, G. L., & Engelmann, S. (1996). *Research on direct instruction: 25 years beyond DISTAR.* Portland, OR: Educational Achievement Systems.

Adams, G., & Carnine, D. (2003) Direct instruction. In H. L. Swanson, K. R. Harris, & S. Graham (Eds.), *Handbook of learning disabilities* (pp. 403–416). New York: Guilford Press.

American Psychiatric Association (2000). *Diagnostic and statistical manual of mental disorders* (4th ed., text revision). Washington, DC: Author.

Bender, W. N. (2004). *Learning disabilities: Characteristics, identification, and teaching strategies.* Boston: Pearson Education.

Brigham R., & Brigham, M. (2001). *Current practice alerts: Mnemonic instruction.* Reston, VA: Division for Learning disabilities and Division for Research of the Council for Exceptional Children.

Bulgren, J. A., Deshler, D. D., Schumaker, J. B., & Lenz, B. K. (2000). The use and effectiveness of analogical instruction in diverse secondary content classrooms. *Journal of Educational Psychology, 16,* 426–441.

Cantor, A., & Klotz, M. B. (2004). NASP's recommendation for LD identification: The importance of comprehensive assessment. *Communiqué, 32(8),* 37,

Cruickshank, W. M. (1979). Learning disabilities: Perceptual or other? *ACLD Newsbriefs, 125,* 7–10.

Cutting, L. E., & Denckla, M. B. (2003). Attention: Relationship between attention-deficit hyperactivity disorder and learning disabilities.. In H. L. Swanson, K. R. Harris, & S. Graham (Eds.), *Handbook of learning disabilities* (pp. 3–15). New York: Guilford Press.

Daly, E. J., Witt, J. C., Martens, B. K., & Dool, E. J. (1997). A model for conducting a functional analysis of academic performance problems. *School Psychology Review, 26,* 554–574.

DuPaul, G. J., & Stoner, G. (2003). *ADHD in the schools: Assessment and intervention strategies.* New York: Guilford.

Dye, G. A. (2000). Graphic organizers to the rescue! Helping students link- and remember-information. *Teaching Exceptional Children, 32(3),* 72–76.

Eckert, T. L., Ardoin, S. P., Daly, E. J., & Martens, B. K. (2002). Improving oral reading fluency: A brief experimental analysis of combining and antecedent intervention with consequences,. *Journal of Applied Behavior Analysis, 35,* 271–281.

Fletcher, J. M., Francis, D. J, Shaywitz, S. E., Lyon, G. R., Foorman, B. R., Stuebing, K. K, et al. (1998). Intelligent testing and the discrepancy model for children with learning disabilities. *Learning Disabilities Research and Practice, 13,* 186–203.

Folse, R. T. (2004). *Learning disabilities.* Retrieved September 30, 2004 from http://www.childpsychologist.com/ld/learning.htm.

Gresham, F. M. (2002). Responsiveness to intervention: An alternative approach to the identification of learning disabilities. In R. Bradley, L. Danielson, & D. P. Hallahan (Eds.) *Identification of learning disabilities: Research to practice* (pp. 467–519). Mahwah, NJ: Lawrence Erlbaum.

Heward, W. L. (2003). *Exceptional children: An introduction to special education.* Upper Saddle River, NJ: Merrill Prentice Hall.

Kavale, K. A. (2002). Discrepancy models in the identification of learning disability. In R. Bradley, L. Danielson, & D. P. Hallahan, (Eds.), *Identification of learning disabilities: Research to practice* (pp. 369–426. Mahwah, NJ: Lawrence Erlbaum.

Kavale, K. A., & Forness, S. R. (2000). What definitions of learning disability say and don't say: A critical analysis. *Journal of Learning Disabilities, 33,* 239–256.

Klotz, M. B., Feinberg, T., & Nealis, L. K. (2004). Learning disability identification and eligibility: A NASP forum for discussion. *Communiqué, 33(1),* 1, 4–5.

Lazarus, B. D. (1996). Flexible skeletons: Guided notes for adolescents with mild disabilities. *Teaching Exceptional Children, 28(3),* 37–40.

Lyon, G. R, Fletcher, J. M., Shaywitz, S. E., Shaywitz, B. A., Wood, F. B., Schulte, A., et al. (2001). Rethinking learning disabilities. In C. E. Finn, Jr., A. J. Rotherham, & C. R. Hokanson, Jr. (Eds.). *Rethinking special education for a new century* (pp. 259–287). Washington, DC: Thomas B. Fordham Foundation and Progressive Policy Institute.

Lyon, G. R. (1996). Learning disabilities. *The Future of Children: Special Education for Students with Disabilities, 6,* 56–76.

National Joint Committee on Learning Disabilities (1989, September 18). *Letter from NJCLD to member organizations. Topic: Modifications to the NJCLD definition of learning disabilities.*

Reschly, D. J. (2004, April). *Goal 2: State and local LD identification policies, practices, and prevalence.* Paper presented at the annual meeting of the Council for Exceptional Children, New Orleans.

Shaywitz, S. E., Fletcher, J. M., Holahan, A. E., Schneider, K. E., Marchione, K. E., Steubing, K. K., et al. (1999). Persistence of dyslexia: The Connecticut longitudinal study at adolescence. *Pediatrics, 104,* 1351–1359.

Siegel, L. S. (1989). IQ is irrelevant to the definition of learning disabilities. *Journal of Learning Disabilities, 22,* 469–479.

Siegel, L. S. (2003). IQ discrepancy definitions and the diagnosis of LD. *Journal of Learning Disabilities, 36,* 2–3.

Stage, S. A., Abbott, R. D., Jenkins, J. R., & Berninger, V. W. (2003). Predicting response to early reading intervention from verbal IQ, reading-related language abilities, attention ratings, and verbal IQ-word reading discrepancy: Failure to validate discrepancy method. *Journal of Learning Disabilities, 36,* 24–33.

Sternberg, R. J., & Spear-Swerling, L. (Eds.) (1999). *Perspectives on learning disabilities: Biological, cognitive, contextual.* Boulder, CO: Westview Press.

Stuebing, K. K., Fletcher, J. M., LeDoux, J. M., Lyon, G. R., Shaywitz, S. E., & Shaywitz, B. A. (2002). Validity of IQ-discrepancy classifications of reading disabilities: A meta-analysis. *American Educational Research Journal, 39*, 469–518.

Swanson, H. L., Harris, K. R., & Graham, S. (2003). Overview of foundations, causes, instruction, and methodology in the filed of learning disabilities. In H. L. Swanson, K. R. Harris, & S. Graham (Eds.), *Handbook of learning disabilities* (pp. 3–15). New York: Guilford Press.

Tingstrom, D. H, Edwards, R. P, & Olmi, D J. (1995). Listening previewing in reading to read: Relative effects on oral reading fluency, *Psychology in the Schools, 32*, 318–327.

US Office of Education (1977). Procedures for evaluating specific learning disabilities. *Federal Register, 42*, 65082–65085.

vanAuken, T. L., Chafouleas, S. M., Bradley, T. A., & Martens, B. K. (2002). Using brief experimental analysis to select oral reading interventions: An investigation of treatment utility. *Journal of Behavioral Education, 11*, 163–169.

Vellutino, F. R., Scanlon, D M., & Lyon, G. R. (2000). Differentiating between difficult-to-remediate and readily remediated poor readers: More evidence against the IQ-achievement discrepancy definition of reading disability. *Journal of Learning Disabilities, 33*, 223–238.

CHAPTER 37

Low Sexual Desire

Lisa G. Regev • Antonette Zeiss • Joel P. Schmidt

WHAT IS LOW SEXUAL DESIRE (A.K.A. HYPOACTIVE SEXUAL DESIRE DISORDER)?

Sexual desire refers to desire associated with a wide-range of sexual activity, including urges, fantasies, dreams, masturbation, and partnered sexual activity, such as oral/anal sex, manual stimulation of partner, or intercourse.

According to DSM-IV-TR (APA, 2000), low desire is diagnosed when an individual is experiencing "persistently or recurrently deficient or absent sexual fantasies and desire for sexual activity" that causes "marked distress or interpersonal difficulty." However, defining "deficient" is often difficult because there is no standard for a "sufficient" amount of desire, and desire levels vary considerably from person to person. Therefore we recommend assessing desire ideographically by comparing the individual's level of desire to their baseline level (i.e., before the sexual problem began). Additionally, desire is influenced by a wide variety of contextual factors related to sexuality, such as interpersonal conflict or loss, the cultural setting, and competing demands for energy and attention. Such factors are important to consider prior to diagnosing low desire.

BASIC FACTS ABOUT LOW SEXUAL DESIRE

Low desire stemming from psychological factors can be clinically challenging to treat because it can be caused by a number of factors and the appropriate treatment target can be difficult to isolate (Leiblum & Rosen, 1988). Most often, there are multiple determinants and relationship factors play a significant role.

Prevalence. Up to 17% of men and 40% of women in the general population experience low desire lasting at least 1 month in a given year, however, whether they view the low desire as problematic is less clear (Mercer et al., 2003).

Age. Younger women and older men are more likely to experience low desire than older women and younger men, respectively (Laumann, Paik, & Rosen, 1999).

Partner status. The availability of a consistent, committed sexual partner is associated with enhanced desire (Laumann et al., 1999).

Ethnicity. African American women report higher rates of low desire and Hispanic women report lower rates of low desire (Laumann et al., 1999). However, caution must be exercised in interpreting these findings because they are based on relatively small sample sizes.

Etiology. There are many medical and psychological conditions that influence a person's level of desire. These include:

- Medical conditions that directly reduce desire:
  - low testosterone—both males and females with low levels of testosterone experience low desire
  - hypothyroidism

Regev, L. G., Zeiss, A., & Schmidt, J. P. (2006). Low sexual desire. In J. E. Fisher & W. T. O'Donohue (Eds.), *Practitioner's guide to evidence-based psychotherapy.* New York: Springer.

- Medical conditions that indirectly reduce desire
  - general medical conditions that result in negative physical and emotional states, such as weakness, pain, concerns related to body image, and fear of death (e.g., heart attack, infertility, cancer treatment)
  - medications
    - antidepressant (especially SSRIs), neuroleptic, anticonvulsant, antihypertensive (diuretics, beta-blockers), antineoplastic, and antiarrhythmic medications and chemotherapy are associated with low desire
- Psychological Factors that influence desire
  - another sexual dysfunction, such as problems of arousal, orgasm, or genital pain
    - up to 35% of those with low desire also experience another sexual dysfunction (Mercer et al., 2003)
  - depression
    - Generalized loss of interest in pleasurable activities can manifest in lower sexual desire
  - anxiety
    - Individuals who are anxious about having sex may be likely to avoid sexual activity. Also, anxiety related to life stressors can disrupt sexual thoughts and interests
  - PTSD/previous sexual assault
    - Previous traumatic experiences can interfere with interpersonal trust and intimacy, thus making sex scary or aversive, which can masquerade as low desire
  - relationship difficulties
    - decreased physical affection (nonsexual)
    - increased distress
    - poor communication/problem-solving skills
    - power imbalance
    - marital boredom
    - physical and/or emotional abuse
    - extramarital affair
    - diminished partner attractiveness
  - situational problems—e.g., insufficient privacy for partners who are parents or who have others living with them
  - partner's development of a sexual dysfunction
  - partner's development of a chronic illness
  - sexual orientation dissatisfaction—e.g., someone who avoids sex because he or she is disturbed by being attracted to same-sex individuals
  - substance use/abuse
    - low doses of alcohol, cocaine, marijuana, heroin, and PCP can increase sexual desire
      - temporarily disinhibits and reduces anxiety, fear, and guilt and increases receptivity to sexual activity
    - higher doses and chronic use of these substances can result in diminished desire (due to diffusely impaired higher cortical functions and limbic system and changes in production and metabolism of testosterone)
  - Sexual myths—there are also numerous sexual myths that may inhibit individuals' desire (see Zilbergeld, 1999)
    - all touching is sexual and should lead to sex
    - a man is always interested in and always ready for sex
    - good sex is spontaneous, with no planning or talking

- most couples have sex daily
- men have stronger sexual urges than women
- older adults do not or should not experience sexual desire
- people with disabilities do not experience sexual desire
- sexual activity can be hazardous to your health
- erectile dysfunction means having low desire

Related disorder. Many people who experience low desire may not seek treatment because it is not bothersome to them. Low desire often becomes a problem when there is a *desire discrepancy* between partners.

What is a Desire Discrepancy (see Leiblum & Rosen, 1988)?
- When one partner experiences either more desire for sexual activity or different forms of sexual activity than the other partner there is a desire discrepancy
- Assess both partners to determine whether one partner's desire is low, the other partner's desire is high, or both (see assessment section below)
- One partner may pressure the other to engage in more sexual activity:
  - one partner's demand for sexual activity can lead the other partner to withdraw and thereby desire sexual activity less frequently
  - can cause relationship difficulties
  - can lead to more sexual activity than desired by one partner, making the actual frequency of sexual activity an inaccurate measure of the underlying sexual desire

ASSESSMENT

What is involved in effective assessment (see Wincze & Carey, 2001; Zeiss, Zeiss, & Davies, 1999)?
- Assess both partners' sexual functioning where relevant and possible (as delineated below)
- Build rapport – sexuality is a sensitive and private issue and can be embarrassing for people to talk about. Some techniques for enhancing rapport/openness to discuss sexual issues include:
  - asking permission to talk explicitly about sex
  - discussing confidentiality
  - asking more general questions first to help establish rapport and to give the client time to become comfortable in the session
  - keeping a nonjudgmental tone
  - using precise, clear terms
  Assessing low desire can be difficult for a number of reasons. For example:
- When there is a desire discrepancy, the low desire partner may engage in treatment under duress, rather than personal interest in pursuing treatment
  - Using frequency of sexually activity as a way to diagnose low desire may lead you down the wrong path. Be sure to ask about frequency of desire, urges, fantasies, dreams, masturbation, too
- Persons with low desire may not have engaged in sexual activity in a long period of time, thereby making it difficult to assess for other associated sexual dysfunctions
  - Ask about their sexual functioning during the last few months they did engage in sexual activity
- Some people confuse arousal and desire, assuming that, for example, if the male cannot get an erection then he is experiencing low desire
  - Distinguish between these by asking about desire regardless of ability to obtain an erection

- Some people experience a desire for desire and as a result mistakenly state that they do not experience low desire, thereby resulting in a false negative assessment
    - Ask specific questions about their sexual desire, including the frequency of sexual activity (masturbation and partner sex), wet dreams for males, urges, and fantasies to help determine whether they experience low desire.
    A step-by-step assessment.
- Medical evaluation
    - endocrine lab panel review—especially hormonal functioning (testosterone, bioavailable testosterone, FSH, LH)
    - genital functioning
    - health problems/conditions, including menopausal status
    - medications
- Psychological factors to assess
    - Life situation—people's level of stress and whether or not they have time to think about or engage in sexual activity will be an important aspect to consider when assessing their level of desire. Assess the following areas:
        - relationship status
        - children
        - living situation
        - work
        - current stressors
    - Comorbid mental disorders
        - depression
        - anxiety (e.g., panic disorder, obsessive-compulsive disorder, performance anxiety),
        - posttraumatic Stress Disorder (PTSD)
    - Substance use
        - alcohol
        - tobacco
        - caffeine
        - illicit drugs
    - Sexual functioning in the past month
        - *Desire*: frequency of sexual interest, thoughts, urges, feelings; frequency of engaging in sexual activity (including masturbation), contextual factors that enhance or inhibit desire
        - *Arousal*: % erection/lubrication–swelling response typically and maximally, with partner and/or in masturbation (male clients: also assess morning erections)
        - *Orgasm*: presence, timing, amount of foreplay, with a partner and/or in masturbation
        - *Genital pain*: presence, intensity, during which type of sexual activity
    - Baseline sexual functioning (prior to time their sexual difficulties began):
        - *Desire*: frequency of sexual interest, thoughts, urges, feelings; frequency of engaging in sexual activity (including masturbation)
        - *Arousal*: % erection/lubrication-swelling response typically and maximally, with partner and/or in masturbation (male clients: also assess morning erections)
        - *Orgasm*: presence, timing, amount of foreplay, with a partner and/or in masturbation

- *Genital pain*: presence, intensity, during which type of sexual activity
- Onset—when did the sexual problem begin?
    - Did the problem develop gradually or abruptly?
    - Did the problem start around the same time as any of the psychological factors assessed above (e.g., life stressors, mental disorders)?
    - Did the problem start around the time of beginning a new medication, giving birth, or other event that could have led to biological changes?
- Context – global versus situational
    - Does the person experience low desire with all partners and during all sexual activities (e.g., intercourse, masturbation) or is only occur in certain situations (e.g., with a specific partner or a specific sexual activity)?
    - Are there thoughts/fears related to sexual activity that might be affecting desire?
    - E.g., fears of STDs, pregnancy, loss of control, failure, closeness, feelings of vulnerability, disgust or that sex is morally wrong
- Relationship issues
    - Quality of emotional intimacy/communication
    - Do the sexual difficulties adversely impact the overall relationship?
    - If a desire discrepancy is noted, do partners' differing levels of desire result in other sexual or relationship problems?
    - Communication patterns regarding sex in general and their sexual difficulties
- Causal beliefs
    - What do they think is causing the problem?
- Goals for treatment
    - Realistic?

What should be ruled out?

- Another Axis I disorder (except another sexual dysfunction) that better accounts for the problem, such as depression or PTSD resulting from sexual assault
- Physiological effects of a substance that exclusively account for the problem, including prescription and street drugs
- Unrealistic expectations regarding how much desire a person "should" have According to DSM-IV-TR (APA, 2000), specify:
- Onset
    - Whether the person never experienced sufficient desire ("lifelong") or the disorder was "acquired" at some point
- Context
    - Whether low desire is true in all situations ("generalized") or only some situations ("situational")
        - E.g., experiences low desire with all sexual activities or only intercourse; experiences low desire with all potential sexual partners or only with a specific partner
- Etiological factors
    - Whether low desire is due to "psychological factors" (e.g., relationship distress, anxiety, depression), "physiological factors," or "combined factors" (including both psychological and physiological factors)
    - According to DSM-IV-TR (APA, 2000), when low desire is due exclusively to the physiological effects of a general medical condition, the appropriate diagnosis is "Sexual dysfunction due to a general medical condition"

TREATMENTS

What treatments are effective (see Leiblum and Rosen, 1988)?

Historically, Masters and Johnson's (1970) 2-week intensive therapy was considered the standard of care. However, research has found that one therapist is as effective as two therapists (LoPiccolo, Heiman, Hogan, & Roberts, 1985), longer-term therapy is as effective as intensive therapy (about 12 weeks; Ulrich-Clement & Schmidt, 1983), and group and bibliotherapy (with minimal therapist contact; Libman, Fichten, & Brender, 1985; van Lankveld, 1998) formats are as effective as full-therapist contact conditions.

Despite continual interest in developing aphrodisiacs throughout history, there are no substances scientifically demonstrated to increase sexual desire (however, see below for testosterone replacement therapy for men and women with low testosterone levels). While there is limited research focusing specifically on the effectiveness of treatments for low desire, treatment should generally focus on the factors that caused and are maintaining the low desire. Often times, low desire may be due to a combination of factors and a multidimensional approach is warranted. This often involves effective interprofessional collaboration between a physician, often an endocrinologist, and a psychologist or other mental health provider. Consider the following treatment components:

- Medical interventions
  - testosterone replacement therapy (TRT) for people with low testosterone (especially bioavailable testosterone)
    - TRT will not enhance desire if testosterone is within normal range
  - discuss the possibility of changing the dose or type of medication that is causing low desire with the prescribing physician
  - discuss treatment of the medical condition causing low desire with the treating physician, encourage compliance with treatment
  - discuss treatment of the medical condition that may be indirectly causing low desire with the treating physician
    - e.g., while treating the cardiac condition may not directly increase the individual's desire, it may indirectly increase desire because the person feels more confident and safe
- Psychological interventions (see Leiblum & Rosen, 1988; Wincze & Carey, 2001)
  - have client self-monitor desire and the conditions that produce desire
  - provide psychoeducation about the following (as appropriate):
    - debunk myths related to sexual desire (see Zilbergeld, 1999)
    - discuss realistic goals
    - discuss the impact of medical conditions/medications on sexual desire
    - describe normal age-related changes in sexual functioning (see Zeiss & Zeiss, 1999)
    - talk about relationship issues as they pertain to low desire
    - discuss other psychological factors that influence desire, such as energy, time, etc.
  - enhance motivation for treatment by discussing pros and cons of enhanced desire for the couple and the individual
  - encourage physical affection, without the performance demands of sexual activity. Activities such as kissing, hugging and holding can allow for conditions in which desire might increase without the anxiety associated with sexual performance.
  - encourage client to actively seek out desirous situations

- read/view erotica
- smell erotic scents
- wear erotic clothing
- help clients plan for intimacy/sexual activity
  - set aside time, go out on a date
- maximize emotional health/energy
  - exercise, stay active
  - engage in other pleasurable activities
  - relaxation exercises
- facilitate enjoyment of sexual activity
  - for women with low desire, learning to consistently reach orgasm results in increased sexual assertiveness, sexual arousal, and sexual satisfaction (Hurlbert, 1993)
- treat the desire discrepancy (see Leiblum & Rosen, 1988)
  - help the couple communicate and negotiate their sexual activity
  - discuss and destigmatize the use of masturbation for the more desirous partner
- treat the sexual dysfunction causing low desire
  - aversion, arousal, orgasm, and pain disorders (see Leiblum & Rosen, 2000; Wincze & Carey, 2001)
- treat the relationship issues causing low desire
  - teach communication and problem-solving skills (see Gottman & Silver, 2000)
- treat the psychological condition causing low desire
  - e.g., depression, PTSD, substance abuse, negative body image

Use the PLISSIT Model—a step-care approach (see Annon, 1976):
- Permission
  - help clients give themselves permission to engage in sexual activity
- Limited Information
  - provide psychoeducation regarding their sexual concerns
- Specific suggestions
  - provide specific suggestions on how they can improve their sexual functioning (as delineated above)
  - Intensive treatment
  - when necessary, provide or refer for more intensive treatment

Therapist Manuals

There are a variety of therapist manuals that address sexual dysfunction in general and low desire more specifically. Recommended manuals include:

Annon, J. (1976). *Behavioral treatment of sexual problems* (vol 1 & 2). Harper Collins.

Kaplan, H. (1995). *The sexual desire disorders: Dysfunctional regulation of sexual motivation.* New York: Brunner/Mazel.

Leiblum, S., & Rosen, R. (Eds.) (1988). *Sexual desire disorders.* New York: Guildford Press.

Leiblum, S., & Rosen, R. (Eds.) (2000). *Principles and practice of sex therapy.* (3rd ed.). New York: Guildford Press.

O'Donohue, W., & Geer, J. (Eds.) (1993). *Handbook of assessment and treatment of sexual dysfunctions.* Boston: Allyn & Bacon.

Wincze, J., & Carey, M. (2001). *Sexual dysfunction: A guide for assessment and treatment.* (2nd ed.). New York: Guilford Press.

Self-Help Alternatives

Self-help can be an effective way to treat low desire, especially with periodic follow-up to maintain motivation to follow-through with readings and homework exercises. Recommended self-help books include:

Barbach, L. (1984). *Pleasures: Women write erotica.* New York: Doubleday & Co. (a sexual fantasy guide) $13.95.

Friday, N. (1991). *Women on top.* New York: Pocket Books (a sexual fantasy guide) $7.99.

Gottman, J. & Silver, N. (2000). *The seven principles for making marriage work.* Three Rivers Press (to treat relationship distress) $13.95.

McCarthy, B., & McCarthy, E. (2003). *Rekindling desire: A step-by-step program to help low sex and no sex marriages.* New York: Brunner-Routledge. $16.95.

Reichman, J. (1998). *I'm not in the mood: What every woman should know about improving her libido.* New York: Quill. $12.00 (primarily biological bases of low desire).

Zilbergeld, B. (1999) *The new male sexuality* (2nd ed.). New York: Bantam Books. $14.95.

Websites

Websites related to sexual health are plentiful. Here are a few that are particularly useful:

To purchase sexual materials, such as videos, books and intimacy aids:

The Sinclair Intimacy Institute's professional library at www.intimacyinstitute.com/library/professional/index.html includes a variety of instructive videos developed by human sexuality professionals for clinical and educational purposes.

Good Vibrations at www.goodvibes.com also provides a selection of videos and books that may appeal to a wide variety of viewers, including lesbian, gay, and bisexual individuals.

For General sexual information: www.sexualhealth.com, www.siecus.org, and www.sexuality.org.

For medical information: www.gettingwell.com and www.webmd.com

People can get their sexual health questions answered at www.goaskalice.columbia.edu

Additional Research

Low desire can be a particularly difficult problem to treat, which is not surprising considering the multitude of psychological and relationship variables that can influence the experience of sexual desire. Unfortunately, our current knowledge base is limited both in terms of conceptualizing and effectively treating low desire.

Regarding the conceptualization of low desire, DSM nosology emphasizes the difficulties males and females experience based on the sexual response cycle, which was physiologically determined. Psychological aspects of desire are inadequately addressed using this model (see Kaschak and Tiefer's, 2002 new view of women's sexual problems for a more contextual approach to problem definition). Additionally, the high prevalence of low desire in women may suggest that low levels of desire are merely a variant of normal female sexual functioning rather than pathological in nature. Additional research investigating the multidimensional processes (i.e., endocrine, other physical, psychological, and relational processes) underlying male and female desire may produce a clearer, more comprehensive conceptualization that can offer appropriate treatment recommendations.

To date, there is a paucity of controlled clinical trials testing the effectiveness of treatments for low desire. This is true for medical, psychological, and combined treatment approaches. Additional research investigating the effects of the various treatment components individually and in combination would substantially contribute to the field.

KEY READINGS

Hurlbert, D. (1993). A comparative study using orgasm consistency training in the treatment of women reporting hypoactive sexual desire disorder. *Journal of Sex and Marital Therapy, 19,* 41–55.

Kaplan, H. (1977). Hypoactive sexual desire. *Journal of Sex and Marital Therapy, 3,* 3–9.

Kaschak, E., & Tiefer, L. (Eds.) (2002). *A new view of women's sexual problems.* Haworth.

Lief, H. (1977). What's new in sex research? Inhibited sexual desire. *Medical Aspects of Human Sexuality, 11*(7), 94–95.

Schover, L., & LoPiccolo, J. (1982). Treatment effectiveness for dysfunctions of sexual desire. *Journal of Sex and Marital Therapy, 8,* 179–197.

Zeiss, A, & Zeiss, R. (1999). Sexual dysfunction: Using an interdisciplinary team to combine cognitive-behavioral and medical approaches. In M. Duffy's (Ed.) *Handbook of counseling and psychotherapy with older adults.* (pp. 294–313). New York: Wiley.

Zeiss, A., Zeiss, R., & Davies, H. (1999). Assessment of sexual function and dysfunction in older adults. In P. Lichtenberg's (Ed) *Handbook of assessment in clinical gerontology.* (pp. 270–296). New York: Wiley.

REFERENCES

American Psychiatric Association (2000). *Diagnostic and statistical manual of mental disorders,* fourth edition, text revision. Washington, DC: Author.

Annon, J. (1976). *Behavioral treatment of sexual problems* (vol 1 & 2). Harper Collins.

Gottman, J., & Silver, N. (2000). *The seven principles for making marriage work.* Three Rivers Press.

Hurlbert, D. (1993). A comparative study using orgasm consistency training in the treatment of women reporting hypoactive sexual desire disorder. *Journal of Sex and Marital Therapy, 19,* 41–55.

Laumann, E. O., Paik, A., & Rosen, R. C. (1999). Sexual dysfunction in the United States: Prevalence and predictors. *Journal of the American Medical Association, 281,* 537–544.

Leiblum, S., & Rosen, R. (Eds.) (1988). *Sexual desire disorders.* New York: Guildford Press.

Leiblum, S., & Rosen, R. (Eds.) (2000). *Principles and practice of sex therapy.* (3rd ed.). New York: Guildford Press.

Libman, E., Fichten, C. S., & Brender, W. (1985). The role of therapeutic format in the treatment of sexual dysfunction: A review. *Clinical Psychology Review, 5,* 103–117.

LoPiccolo, J., Heiman, J., Hogan, D., & Roberts, C. (1985). Effectiveness of single therapists versus cotherapy teams in sex therapy. *Journal of Consulting and Clinical Psychology, 53,* 287–294.

Masters, W., & Johnson, V. (1970). *Human sexual inadequacy.* Boston: Little, Brown.

Mercer, C. H., Fenton, K. A., Johnson, A. M., Wellings, K., Macdowall, W., McMannus, S., Nanchahal, K., and Erens, B. (2003). Sexual function problems and help seeking behaviour in Britain: National probability sample survey. *British Medical Journal, 327,* 426–427.

Ulrich-Clement, D., & Schmidt, G. (1983). The outcome of couple therapy for sexual dysfunctions using three different formats. *Journal of Sex and Marital Therapy, 9*(1), 67–78.

van Lankveld, J. J. D. M. (1998). Bibliotherapy in the Treatment of Sexual Dysfunctions: A Meta-Analysis. *Journal of Consulting and Clinical Psychology, 66(4),* 702–708.

Wincze, J., & Carey, M. (2001). *Sexual dysfunction: A guide for assessment and treatment.* (2nd ed.). New York: Guilford Press.

Zeiss, A., & Zeiss, R. (1999). Sexual dysfunction: Using an interdisciplinary team to combine cognitive-behavioral and medical approaches. In M. Duffy's (Ed.) *Handbook of counseling and psychotherapy with older adults.* (pp. 294–313). New York: Wiley.

Zilbergeld, B. (1999). *The new male sexuality* (2nd ed.). New York: Bantam Books.

CHAPTER 38

Malingering

Allan Gerson • David Fox

For the treating therapist the concept of malingering may be foreign, and may not seem to apply to daily use. Malingering does not occur often in atypical therapeutic setting because people come in for help. However, there are circumstances where this could occur and the therapist needs to be aware. It is the intent of this chapter to demonstrate the applicability of the concept to therapy. At first glance malingering may not seem to apply because we are trained not to doubt our patients. We understand, believe and have the same agenda—getting them better. But there are a small percentage of cases where people do not want to get better. This is not always about money. Malingering needs to be examined for its full effect on the treatment process when it occurs, and be seen as a pseudodisorder.

WHAT IS MALINGERING?

Malingering is defined as the intentional production of false or grossly exaggerated physical or psychological symptoms, motivated by external incentives such as avoiding military duty, avoiding work, evading criminal prosecution, or obtaining drugs.(1)

Malingering differs from factitious disorder in that the motivation for the symptom production in malingering is an external incentive, whereas in the factitious disorder the external incentive is absent, according to the DSM. It differs from conversion disorder and other somatoform disorders through the intentionality of the behavior, as well as the external incentives.

WHAT MALINGERING IS NOT

Malingering is not a disorder. It is a set of behaviors, which can be viewed in different manners and from different arenas. The definition in the DSM, while accurate is limiting by its nature, in that it present four criteria, one of which has to do with the medical/legal arena, and another is restricted to anti-social personality. However, one need not meet either of these criteria, and still fit the definition of malingering. One could also fit those criteria and still not be a malingerer. For example, one of the other criteria, lack of cooperation during diagnostic evaluation and in complying with the prescribed treatment regimen can be explained through other clinical categories, behavioral sets, or cultural issues. These will be explored in the sections below.

MEDICAL/LEGAL VS. NONFORENSIC SETTINGS

Rogers et al. (2) found feigning of medical symptoms to play a relatively prominent role in both forensic and nonforensic cases. Sierles (3) noted malingering behavior in equal proportions in psychiatric, medical, and surgical patients at the V.A. Cunnien (4) pointed out that the traditional thoughts on malingering

Gerson, A., & Fox, D. (2006). Malingering. In J. E. Fisher, & W. T. O'Donohue (Eds.), *Practitioner's guide to evidence-based psychotherapy*. New York: Springer.

are viewed in moralistic, simplistic, or strictly behavioral manners. He indicated that malingering could not be assessed accurately because it overlaps with a great number of everyday behaviors, such as making excuses to avoid social functions.

Travin and Protter (5) view malingering as a social–psychological process in which specific goals in a social transaction are pursued in light of psychological influences. At the same time Rogers (6) criticized the criminology of the DSM model of malingering. Instead he proposed an adaptational model in which the malingerer may make choices in the context of decision theory, and not be limited to any given population.

ALTERNATIVE MODELS

Cunnien (4) offered a *threshold model*, in which the goal oriented behavior be considered when evidence is present of voluntary symptom production, environmental incentives, environmental events to be avoided, or behavior consistent with attempts at distortion. The presence of anti-social personality disorder is neither necessary nor sufficient for the consideration of malingering, which may occur in any clinical or forensic setting. Malingering should be suspected when symptom are accompanied by any of the following:

A. Suspicion of voluntary control of symptoms, as demonstrated by one or more indicators:

1. Bizarre of absurd symptoms.
2. Atypical symptoms fluctuation consistent with external incentives.
3. Unusual symptomatic response to treatment that cannot otherwise be explained, i.e., paradoxical response to medication.

B. Atypical presentation in the presence of environmental incentive, i.e., disability claims toward action obtaining drugs or shelter.
C. Atypical presentation in the presence of noxious environmental conditions such as prosecution, military duty or undesired work.
D. Complaints grossly in excess of clinical findings.
E. Substantial noncompliance with evaluation or treatment.

Dr. Cunnien also offered a *clinical decision model* in which specific findings of voluntariness in combination with clinical certainty about the pursuit of avoidance or environmental factors is required. Symptom inconsistency includes such phenomena, as bizarre or absurd symptoms not expected even in psychotic disorders, endorsement of improbable symptoms, rapidly fluctuating complaints, or physical complaints without anatomical or neurological basis. In his clinical decision model all of the following must be present:

A. Psychological and physical symptoms are clearly under voluntary controls manifested by one or more indicators.
1. Patient acknowledgment of voluntary control or deceit;
2. Gross symptom production that is inconsistent with physiological or anatomical mechanisms;
3. Direct observation of illness production;
4. Discovery of paraphernalia or substances explaining the production of physical symptoms;
5. Confirmatory lab tests, i.e., absence of EEG abnormalities during an observed "seizure".

B. Clinical certainty that symptom production occurs in response to:
   1. Pursuit of financial gain.
   2. Avoidance of work, military duty, prosecution or legal consequences.
C. Another disorder present cannot explain current symptoms.
D. Evidence of desire to assume the sick role, if present, cannot explain the totality of the current symptoms.

DAUBERT VS. FRYE

For those therapists not involved in the legal arena the presence of this portion of the chapter may be questioned as to its applicability. First, it is being brought in more for the purpose of reminding the reader to engage in critical thinking, and as a caution to be careful when dealing with data provided by the patient or collateral sources, not just as a legal standard. Furthermore, even in practices where legal aspects generally do not enter, they can slip in, for example if the issues of abuse, of child custody, or other legal entanglements find their way into the life of a patient currently in treatment.

Malingering in its present level of acceptance may pass the Frye test, but not Daubert. This is an important distinction when judging diagnoses in evidence based manner. Daubert focuses more on evidence and replicability.

The Frye test originated in a court of appeals decision [293 F. 1013 (D.C. Cir. 1923)]. It stated that the standard for admission of testimony in a court is the general acceptance in the scientific community. It was the standard in many judicial districts until Daubert. It remains the rule in many states. The issue for malingering has to do with its frequency in the legal arena. Malingering can satisfy the Frye test as put forth in the DSM, through general acceptance of the criteria in the DSM. But can it satisfy Daubert?

The Daubert decision as stated in Federal Rule 702 limits admissibility of scientific evidence by requiring that expert testimony pertain to "scientific knowledge." To qualify as scientific knowledge, an inference or assertion must be derived by the scientific method. Knowledge connotes a body of known facts or of ideas inferred from such facts, or accepted as true on good grounds. The evidence must have been tested, and have been subjected to peer review and publication, its known or potential error rate, and existence and maintenance of standards controlling its operation, and whether it has attracted widespread acceptance within a scientific community.

CULTURAL FACTORS

One of the DSM criteria for malingering deals with noncompliance, with evaluation or treatment, without taking into account cultural factors. Kirkmayer et al. found language and cultural complexity prevent adequate diagnosis, and treatment for a significant number of patients. They cite examples of patients whose apparent noncompliance was due to cultural factors, and resolved by cultural consultation services including interpreters and cultural brokers.

The National Institute on Aging in 1999–2000 study reported a high percentage (36%) of African-Americans do not take their medicine. While this would fit one of the criteria for malingering as it now exists in the DSM, they cite cultural factors including forgetting to do so, fear of possible side effects, cost, inconvenience, and disbelief in the effectiveness. The African-American patients believe, according to a Morehouse School of Medicine study from 1999, that generic medicines are not as good as name brands.

Latino patients prefer to employ spiritual and folk remedies, trusting them over western medicine, or therapeutic methods. According to Galanti (8) they are generally expressive of their pain. Their approach to "cures" may run counter to accepted medical or psychological methods. Phillips (9) noted various beliefs among Latinos patients, including the notion that cold air is a danger during a fever.

ISSUES IN MEASURING AND DETECTING MALINGERING

Typically, psychotherapists and others providing psychological diagnostic or treatment services do not consider malingering in their differential diagnoses. There are several good reasons for this. The vast majority of people seen in psychotherapy desire assistance and are more or less truthful with their therapists. It is rightly assumed that the vast majority of people wish to get better and obtain symptom relief. However, there are some circumstances in which the intentional production or severe exaggeration of symptoms should be suspected. It is difficult to estimate how frequently malingering takes place because those who engage in this form of deception rarely admit to their behavior even when confronted. Nevertheless, there are certain guidelines to assist the clinician in this area.

Among the most important distinctions to be made when symptom exaggeration occurs is the level of awareness the patient has of their behavior and the purpose of the behavior. Oftentimes, medical and occasionally psychological symptoms spring from processes out of awareness of the patient. Typically, these take the form of a somatoform disorder (for example, conversion disorder) which may involve disability from pain or imagined dysfunction. Somatoform disorders are distinguished from malingering by the level of intention typically associated with conscious awareness. Malingering requires intentional production of symptoms although unconscious motivation may also be present. In short, somatoform and malingering are not mutually exclusive. The other major disorder associated with symptom misrepresentation is Factitious Disorder. In this condition, the patient intentionally produces or grossly exaggerates symptomatology but the goals are different. In Factitious Disorder the purpose is not external reward per se (like money) but the pathological desire to adopt the "patient role." Distinguishing between Somatoform Disorder, Factitious Disorder, and malingering is difficult because they can occur together.

Further, there are some common erroneous assumptions about malingering:

- It is infrequent or rare.
- It is easily detected.
- The hallmark is inconsistency of presentation.
- It is mutually exclusive with mental illness.
- People who are habitually deceptive are always malingerers.

PREVALENCE OF MALINGERING

Research on the prevalence of malingering has focused on several identifiable subpopulations, particularly those individuals who have a clear and obvious benefit available for having symptomatology. This is typically thought to involve money but there is ample reason to believe that malingering of symptoms in order to obtain other external gain can be common as well, including avoidance of work and diminished responsibility for criminal acts.

In the past few years there has been considerable effort extended in identifying the rate of malingering in those people involved with lawsuits, disability claims and workers compensation cases involving psychological and neuropsychological symptoms. It is noted, however, that rates of malingering in individual diagnostic evaluations cannot be assumed to be identical to those from a psychotherapy practice.

One way to estimate the rate of malingering is to ask clinicians performing evaluations how often they observe such behavior. Mittenberg, Patton, & Canyock (2002) surveyed a large number of neuropsychologists who estimated the rates of malingering within their practices. The overall rate of malingering in civil cases was approximately 29%; the rate in criminal cases was 19% and in the medical or psychiatric cases not involving litigation or compensation the rate was approximately 8%. There was no difference in prevalence rates by geographic region or practice setting. The authors found that the referral source and the circumstance regarding the claim exerted powerful effects as to the prevalence of malingering. For example, malingering was much more common when the referral source was from the prosecutor in a criminal case or the defense in a civil matter.

Table 38.1 excerpted from the Mittenberg article indicates estimated rates of malingering in different diagnostic groups involved in civil litigation:

Table 38.1.

Diagnostic group	%
Mild head injury	41
Fibromyalgia or chronic fatigue	39
Pain or somatoform disorders	34
Neurotoxic disorders	29
Electrical injury	26
Depressive disorder	16
Anxiety disorder	14
Dissociative disorder	11
Seizure disorder	9
Moderate or severe head injury	9
Vascular dementia	2

Larrabee (2003a,b) has reviewed the literature and estimates of malingering neurocognitive problems in the litigated cases vary from 15% to 64%, depending upon methodology.

A survey conducted by Martelli (2001) revealed that the percentage of injured workers who fake, exaggerate or malinger as estimated by different groups (see Table 38.2).

Table 38.2.

Group estimating	% of WC claimants estimated to fake or exaggerate
Disability professionals	19
Rehabilitation/neuropsychology staff	25
Case managers	29
Health psychologists and physicians	19
Workers compensation claimants	35

The above noted studies reveal the difficulty in establishing definite rates of malingering due to the subjective nature of the diagnosis and varying perspectives of clinicians.

Another approach to estimating prevalence is to use well validated tests which measure incomplete effort that is often associated with malingering of cognitive abilities. For example, Allen, Green Richards, & Iverson (1998) found the following rates of failure on the Computerized Assessment of Response Bias (CARB), a well validated measure of poor effort/malingering, administered to a heterogeneous group of compensation seeking applicants (see Table 38.3).

Table 38.3.

Applicant group	%
Orthopedic	8.7
Distress	16.1
Chronic fatigue	20
Chronic pain	46.1
Brain injury	20.4
Neurological	15
Mixed/multisite	38

These findings suggest that the rate of CARB failure is strongly dependent on the primary complaint. Likewise, work status (working vs. disabled) strongly influences failure of such malingering tests (Gervais et. al., 2001).

Because malingering is difficult to accurately measure and many clinicians are unfamiliar with patients dramatically misrepresenting their condition, the use of objective criteria is recommended. In the neuropsychological realm specific criteria have been proposed by Slick et. al. (1999). They proposed the following criteria, many of which are applicable to nonneuropsychological cases as well.

Criteria A Presence of substantial external incentive
Criteria B Evidence from neuropsychological functioning:
1. Definite negative response bias (on symptom validity testing)
2. Probable response bias (on symptom validity testing)
3. Discrepancy between test data and known patterns of brain function
4. Discrepancy between test data and observed data
5. Discrepancy between test data and reliable collateral reports
6. Discrepancy between test data and documented background history
Criteria C Evidence from Patient Self Report:
1. Self-reported history is discrepant with documented history
2. Self-reported symptoms are discrepant with known patterns of brain functioning
3. Self-reported symptoms are discrepant with behavioral observations
4. Self-reported symptoms are discrepant with information obtained from collateral informants
5. Evidence from exaggerated or fabricated psychological (neurocognitive) dysfunction
Criteria D Behaviors meeting criteria from groups B and C are not fully accountable for by known Psychiatric, Neurological, or Developmental factors
"Definite Malingerer"
- Criterion A, Criterion B 1, and Criterion D

"ProbaFble Malingerer"
- Criterion A and two or more B Criteria (excluding B1);
- OR, met one B criterion (excluding B 1) and one or more C Criterion

"Possible Malingering"
- Criterion A and one or more C Criterion, but did not meet Criterion D;
- OR, met all criteria for Definite or Probable Malingering, but did not meet Criterion D

"Not Malingering"
  may have met criterion A, but did not meet any B, C, or D Criteria

The most important factor to be considered in suspecting malingering is the presence of any obvious relationship between psychological symptoms and an external reward. Although this may include financial compensation, such as available through a disability or workers compensation claim or personal-injury lawsuit, nonmonetary factors must be considered as well. These might include avoidance of responsibility as simple as an excuse to avoid serving on a jury or more encompassing behavior simulating psychosis to avoid criminal prosecution. At what point symptom distortion for a single, well-defined purpose becomes malingering per se is a matter of clinical judgment. The literature cited above indicates that the kind of symptoms also influences the likelihood of malingering.

The prevalence and detection techniques for malingering depend on the condition being simulated. Chronic pain, PTSD, and cognitive problems are commonly malingered psychological symptoms. However, any symptom which has the potential of producing a direct benefit from the environment can be malingered. Psychosis may be malingered, for example, if it provides a basis for avoiding criminal responsibility. On the other hand, personality disorder, sexual perversion, and substance abuse are rarely malingered because it is unusual for there to be any direct benefit for having such symptoms. Sometimes, the potential reward is interpersonal. For example, a patient may grossly exaggerate or feign psychological symptoms to avoid confronting a spouse about a conflict or to seek relief from responsibility in a relationship. Oftentimes such motivation is at an unconscious level and determining whether the simulated symptoms are intentional as compared to unconscious can be difficult.

Although the financial reward is often the motivation in malingering, another frequent but overlooked goal is access to addictive medication. Because pain is a subjective experience it is difficult for the average physician to determine the "authenticity" of pain complaints and hence potentially habituating or addictive medication is prescribed on an indefinite basis. Regardless of the initial validity of pain complaints, persisting pain may indicate goal directed behavior towards psychoactive addictive medications. Such behavior may occur at a both conscious and unconscious level.

Among the most difficult aspects of the diagnosis of malingering is the understanding that malingering is not a condition that an individual has but instead reflects situationally based behavior. Consequently, this behavior might come and go as needed and can coexist with a number of psychological conditions.

Oftentimes, clinicians make the mistake of assuming that the presence of malingering contraindicates the presence of genuine psychopathology/neuropathology. In fact, both can coexist. In addition, many clinicians think of malingering as equivalent to fraud by a person who is completely normal. While this is sometimes the case, more often, malingering behavior reflects an individual's attempt to secure a desired goal by overemphasizing the severity of their actual symptoms or exaggerating the degree of resulting disability.

HOW TO DETECT MALINGERING

In addition to clinical impression, a number of specific procedures have been developed to detect gross exaggeration of symptoms and feigned disability. Most modern measures of psychopathology such as the MMPI-2 and the Personality Assessment Inventory have built-in of validity indicators which reveal altered test taking behavior by the patient. On the MMPI there are specific scales which are sensitive to symptom exaggeration or feigning of mental disorders. This includes the original F (Infrequency) scale and the more recently developed F back (Fb) scale, the relationship between the F and K scales (F–K) and the psychiatric infrequency scale (Fp). In addition, scales particularly designed for assessing over reporting of psychological distress and physical symptoms have been developed, including the Dissimulation Scale-Revised and the Fake Bad Scale (Lees-Haley, 1994). The clinician should note that most of the scales have relevance and were designed for circumstances in which there is a high risk for malingering such as the medical legal context. Their application in purely clinical circumstances could lead to false positive identifications of exaggerated symptoms.

Another approach to the detection of malingering has been the development of a variety of tests to detect feigned cognitive disability. These include the Word Memory Test, the Computerized Assessment of Response Bias and the Test of Memory Malingering, among others (Nelson, Boone, & Dueck, 2003). Typically, these are used in neuropsychological evaluations.

Other indicators of feigning of cognitive problems include:

- poor effort on ability tests
- symptom exaggeration (extremely dramatic descriptors of distress)
- atypical test performance
- evasive behavior
- providing an unreliable history
- symptoms clearly goal directed to secure external benefit
- late onset symptoms
- resistance to treatment
- no medical findings
- bizarre complaints
- long response latencies
- vague symptoms
- over dramatized
- reluctant to accept favorable diagnosis
- self-inflicted injuries (e.g., toxic)
- recurrent injuries
- frequent requests for easily abused drugs
- also has personality disorder (particularly ASP)
- ganser-like responses
- significant resistance
- hostility
- avoidance
- inconsistencies in data
  - norms and obtained scores
  - findings and presenting problem
  - complaints and observations
  - measures of the same ability

In psychotherapy another possible indicator of malingering is unresponsiveness to appropriate treatment. Although psychological factors or unknown environmental factors can also produce interfere with effective treatment persisting complaints may be an indication of goal directed symptom over reporting.

TREATMENT

Because malingering is not a disorder, no treatment is appropriate. On the other hand, if the clinician has an ongoing relationship with the patient who shows malingering behavior it is incumbent upon the clinician to address this behavior. Simple confrontation is rarely helpful. Oftentimes, the malingering represents an attempt to secure a desired goal and the therapist might discuss with the patient the appropriate methods of securing external benefit. The most significant caution is for the therapist to not unwittingly collude with the malingering patient to deceive an insurance company or agency which not only produces social injustice but ultimately interferes with the therapeutic relationship with the patient. Of course, there is risk in falsely identifying a patient as engaging in malingering. Such a suspicion could easily undermine the therapeutic alliance and such a patient, once confronted, is not likely to trust the therapist in the future. It should also be noted that malingering can be appropriately adaptable – for example, a hostage feigning illness to escape their captor. Treatment would obviously not be needed.

There has been some research on persuading people to not malinger on psychological tests, with mixed success (Youngjohn, Lees-Haley, & Binder, 1999). However, even if malingering is no longer evident on tests, the underlying deception may be unchanged.

An individual who habitually engages in malingering may also have a diagnosable mental disorder such as a Personality Disorder that may need clinical attention. In other words, malingering behavior, like any other deception could represent a symptom of an actual disorder.

INTERNET RESOURCES

Discoveryhealth.com
    http://health.discovery.com/encyclopedias/2899.html
Emedicine.com
    http://www.emedicine.com/med/topic3355.htm
Healthopedia.com
    http://www.healthopedia.com/malingering/
Ken Pope Ph.D. Malingering Research Update
    http://kspope.com/assess/malinger.php
Psychology Today
    http://cms.psychologytoday.com/conditions/malingering.html

REFERENCES

Allen, L. M., III, Green, W. P., Richards, P. M., & Iverson, G. L. (1998). *Archives of Clinical Neuropsychology, 13(1),* 15.

American Psychiatric Association. (1994). *Diagnostic and Statistical Manual of Mental Disorders.* (4th ed). Washington, DC: American Psychiatric Association.

Gervais, R. O., Russell, A. S., Green, P., Allen, L. M., Ferrari, R., & Pieschl, S D. (2001). Effort Testing in Patients with Fibromyalgia and Disability Incentives. *Journal of Rheumatology, 28,* 1892–1899.

Larrabee, G. (2003a, October). *Advances in the assessment of malingering.* Paper presented at the National Academy of Neuropsychology, Dallas, TX.

Larrabee, G. (2003b). Exaggerated MMPI-2 symptom reporting in personal injury litigants with malingered neurocognitive deficit. *Archives of Clinical Neuropsychology, 18,* 673–686.

Martelli, M. (2001, July 9). Response Bias by Design: Table. Message posted to "*Neuropsychology*" Available from *npsych@npsych.com*

Mittenberg, W., Patton, C., & Canyock, E. M. (2002). Base rates of malingering and symptom exaggeration. *Journal of Clinical & Experimental Neuropsychology, 24(8),* 1094–1102.

Nelson, N. W., Boone, K., & Dueck, A. (2003). Relationships between eight measures of suspect effort. *The Clinical Neuropsychologist, 17(2),* 263–272.

Rogers, R. (Ed.). (1997). *Clinical Assessment of Malingering and Deception.* (2nd ed.). New York: Gilford Publications.

Slick, D. J., Sherman, E. M., & Iverson, G. L. (1999). Diagnostic criteria for malingered neurocognitive dysfunction: Proposed standards for clinical practice and research. *The Clinical Neuropsychologist, 13,* 545–561.

Youngjohn, J. R., Lees-Haley, P. R., & Binder, L. M. (1999). Comment: Warning malingerers produces more sophisticated malingering. *Archives of Clinical Neuropsychology, 14(6),* 511–515.

Marital Problems

Norman B. Epstein • Donald H. Baucom • Jaslean J. LaTaillade

CHARACTERISTICS OF MARITAL PROBLEMS

Although both social scientists and members of the public readily agree that marital problems[1] are common in today's society and are sources of great stress for couples and the people who are close to them, defining the characteristics of marital problems is complex. Most often, researchers have measured marital problems in terms of the partners' subjective evaluations; in other words, the degree to which the members of a couple report dissatisfaction with their relationship. Typically, members of a couple are asked either global questions about their overall feelings about the marriage or a set of questions that ask about the individual's level of happiness or unhappiness in a variety of specific areas such as expression of affection, finances, decision-making, sexual relations, and handling of household tasks. This approach to assessment is based on an assumption that a couple has problems if they are unhappy with their relationship. In fact, individuals' subjective reports on questionnaires such as the widely used Dyadic Adjustment Scale (Spanier, 1976) have been found to be associated with other indications of relationship problems, such as divorce, so the subjective appraisals clearly are an important aspect of marital problems. However, they do not tell us *why* the members of a couple are dissatisfied, only that something is wrong.

Bradbury and Fincham (1987) discussed the overlap between marital satisfaction and the emotions that the partners experience. Marital dissatisfaction is not only a negative cognitive evaluation of one's relationship but also an experience of unpleasant emotion. Aside from general unhappiness, members of distressed couples have been found to experience emotions such as anger, depression, anxiety, and jealousy (Beach, 2001; Epstein & Baucom, 2002; Holtzworth-Munroe, Stuart, & Hutchinson, 1997; Lazarus & Lazarus, 1994; Lundgren, Jergens, & Gibson, 1980; Noller, Beach, & Osgarby, 1997). Because the particular types of emotion experienced by members of distressed couples vary, clinicians must conduct a detailed assessment of each couple to understand the unique characteristics of their marital problems.

Another characteristic that commonly is used to determine whether a couple has marital problems is the degree to which they have taken steps toward ending the relationship; in other words, the degree of instability in the relationship. Weiss and Cerreto (1980) developed the Marital Status Inventory (MSI) to assess individuals' increasing levels of disengagement from a couple relationship, ranging from occasional thoughts of leaving to taking legal action toward divorce. Not surprisingly, individuals' scores on the MSI are significantly related to their scores on

---

[1] Although the terms "marriage" and "marital" are used throughout this chapter, the concepts and methods described are applicable for the most part to any couple, heterosexual or homosexual, in a committed relationship. There is a growing literature on the assessment and treatment of distressed gay and lesbian couples but a need for more research.

Epstein, N. B., Baucom, D. H. LaTaillade, J. L. (2006). Marital problems. In J. E. Fisher & W. T. O'Donohue (Eds.), *Practitioner's guide to evidence-based psychotherapy*. New York: Springer.

marital satisfaction questionnaires and other measures of relationship quality. However, as with level of marital dissatisfaction, the degree of instability or steps taken toward separation or divorce indicates that something is wrong in the relationship but does not identify the characteristics of the marital problems. In addition, some couples maintain stable relationships in spite of experiencing low levels of satisfaction (for example, for religious reasons, personal commitment, or a desire to provide a stable family for their children).

The existence of infidelity is commonly assumed to be an indication of marital problems even though a portion of individuals engaged in affairs report that they are happy in their marriages and have become involved in extramarital relationships for other reasons, such as a desire for variety or a very high sex drive (Glass, 2002). Nevertheless, individuals who discover a partner's affair commonly are severely distressed, often to the point of experiencing post-traumatic stress symptoms (Gordon & Baucom, 1999), and their marriages are at great risk of dissolution. As with the other indications of marital problems described earlier, the existence of infidelity often reflects dysfunction in couple relationships but does not indicate the specific factors that are interfering with the mutual fulfillment of the partners' needs. This chapter describes current knowledge about a number of those factors.

THE IMPACT OF MARITAL PROBLEMS ON THE COUPLE AND THEIR CHILDREN

Understanding the factors contributing to marital problems and what is known about effective methods for treating distressed couples is important due to the broad impact that marital dysfunction commonly has on the well being of the partners, as well as on those close to them, such as children. Studies have indicated that marital conflict is a risk factor for the spouses' development of forms of psychopathology such as depression, anxiety disorders, and alcohol abuse (Beach, 2001; Daiuto, Baucom, Epstein, & Dutton, 1998; Epstein & McCrady, 2002). Furthermore, individuals are less likely to respond well to treatments for disorders such as depression, anxiety, and substance abuse if they are involved in distressed couple relationships (Daiuto et al., 1998; Epstein & McCrady, 2002; Gollan, Friedman, & Miller, 2002). In addition, marital distress raises the probability that individuals will develop physical health problems (Sabatelli & Chadwick, 2000) and have difficulty functioning at their jobs (Forthofer, Markman, Cox, Stanley, & Kessler, 1996). Beyond the risks to the members of the couple, studies have demonstrated that parents whose marriages are conflictual provide less nurturing and effective parenting for their children (Krishnakumar & Buehler, 2000), and their children are more likely to exhibit problems such as depression, anxiety, and conduct disorders (Buehler et al., 1998; Morrison & Coiro, 1999). Thus, the costs of marital problems are far-reaching and expensive in terms of both personal well being of all family members and the economic impact of individuals with compromised interpersonal and work functioning.

PERSONAL AND INTERPERSONAL CHARACTERISTICS ASSOCIATED WITH MARITAL PROBLEMS

Theorists and researchers have attempted to understand the nature of marital problems by identifying characteristics of couple relationships that are associated with marital distress and instability, both concurrently and longitudinally. Such risk factors for marital distress then can be targets for prevention and therapeutic interventions. Among the major categories of relationship characteristics that have been examined as correlates of current distress or as predictors of the development of distress in the future are (a) the couple's demographic characteristics (e.g., age, education, socioeconomic status), (b) the individual partners' personality characteristics and psychopathology (e.g., neuroticism, depression, substance abuse), (c) the degree to which the partners have negative interactions versus engaging in positive, mutually enjoyable activities together, (d) the quality of the couple's communication, particularly when they are faced with disagreements and conflicts that need to be resolved, (e) the ways that the partners think about each other and their relationship (e.g., their personal standards concerning the characteristics of a good relationship, and the degrees to which those standards are being met), and (f) the extent to which the couple is having difficulty coping with stressors from their environment (e.g., financial problems, a child with a chronic illness). Findings regarding the role that each of these components of marital problems plays in marital distress and instability are reviewed briefly below. Marital problems commonly have multiple causes and differ from most of the other disorders described in this book in that they involve the interactions between two individuals as well as the characteristics of the two partners and the life stressors that they face together (Epstein & Baucom, 2002). Consequently, the assessment and treatment of marital problems must be multidimensional.

Demographic Characteristics

A number of demographic characteristics have been found to be associated with marital conflict and divorce, although such correlations do not necessarily indicate that these characteristics play direct causal roles in marital problems. First, the early years of marriage are a risk factor in that approximately two thirds of divorced occur during the first nine years of marriage (National Center for Health Statistics, 1995). This striking statistic most likely underestimates the frequency of distress in recent marriages, given that many unhappy couples choose to stay together rather than divorce. Furthermore, divorce statistics do not take into account those couples who are in committed relationships but are not legally married. Among the many factors that may account for early divorces are spouses' committing themselves to marriage before adequately knowing about their degree of compatibility, inadequate communication and conflict-resolution skills, and prevailing cultural beliefs emphasizing self-actualization and individualism (Glenn, 1996). In addition, although there is evidence that the presence of children reduces the risk of divorce, studies have indicated a moderate tendency for couples' marital satisfaction to be lower during the childrearing years, as demands on time, energy, financial resources, etc. affect the partners' intimacy with each other (Belsky, 1990).

Second, lower socioeconomic status and poverty are associated with marital distress. Studies have indicated that the negative impact occurs as economic strain leads to partners' greater negative interaction and less positive interaction with each other, which in turn decreases marital satisfaction (Conger et al., 1990; Falconier, 2004; Vinokur, Price, & Caplan, 1996).

Third, partners who marry younger, particularly in their teens, are more likely to experience marital problems (Feng, Giarrusso, Bengtson, & Frye, 1999), at least in part due to their limited financial resources. In addition, young marriages are more likely to be based on pregnancies, attempts to escape from conflictual or abusive homes, and other factors that may be associated with limited maturity and relationship skills. Other relationship history characteristics that have been identified as risks for marital problems are parental divorce (Amato, 1996) and the couple's cohabitation before marriage, although the results for both factors have been mixed (Gottman, 1994).

Fourth, there is a tendency for individuals to marry others who are similar to themselves in demographic characteristics and values, and similarity between partners' demographic characteristics such as education level, race, and ethnicity has been found to have a low or modest association with marital satisfaction (Watson et al., 2004; Whyte, 1990). In addition satisfaction has been found to have modest correlations with similarity in the two individuals' ideas regarding childrearing, handling money, and lifestyle, as well as in personal standards about the characteristics that their relationship should have regarding degree of boundaries between partners, the distribution of power, and the level of partners' investment in their relationship (Baucom, Epstein, Rankin, & Burnett, 1996; Benokraitis, 2002). However, Baucom et al. (1996) found that marital satisfaction depends more on whether the individuals are satisfied with the ways that the couple has developed to meet each other's standards than on degree of similarity in standards.

Personality Characteristics and Psychopathology

Although differences in partners' personality traits has not been found to have a consistent relation to marital distress (Watson et al., 2004), neuroticism and insecure attachment styles in one or both partners are associated with marital problems (Banse, 2004; Karney & Bradbury, 1995). Furthermore, forms of clinical disorders such as depression, anxiety disorders, personality disorders, and substance abuse contribute to marital distress (Beach, 2001; Daiuto et al., 1998; Epstein & Baucom, 2002; Epstein & McCrady, 2002).

Behavioral Interaction Patterns

In examining behavioral interaction patterns that are associated with marital distress, it is important to distinguish between microlevel or moment-to-moment interactions between partners and broader macrolevel patterns (Epstein & Baucom, 2002). Macrolevel patterns involve consistency across a variety of situations, along dimensions such as the distribution of power/control in decision-making, the degree of togetherness and sharing versus autonomy between partners, and the degree to which the two individuals invest time and energy into the relationship (Epstein & Baucom, 2002). In addition, marital researchers have investigated how these dimensions are enacted within gender roles in marriage. In contrast, microlevel interactions involve specific types of positive and negative behavior that affect partners' satisfaction with their relationship.

At the macrolevel, studies have indicated that couples who share power in decision-making in an equitable manner are more satisfied with their relationships (Gray-Little, Baucom, & Hamby, 1996). Regarding gender roles, women who perceive the division of responsibilities for domestic chores as inequitable are more dissatisfied with their marriages (Wilkie, Ferree, & Ratcliff, 1998). In terms of closeness and sharing, there is considerable evidence that partners who experience various forms of intimacy are more satisfied with their relationships (Prager, 1995). Finally, studies have indicated that individuals who hold standards for partners investing a high level of time and energy into their relationships report greater relationship satisfaction (Baucom et al., 1996), as do couples who provide each other with high levels of emotional support (Cutrona, 1996). Furthermore, when couples have been asked to log frequencies of positive and negative instrumental and expressive behavior exchanged on a daily basis, higher frequencies of negative acts and, to a lesser extent, lower frequencies of positive acts have been found to be associated with greater marital distress (Epstein & Baucom, 2002).

Researchers have examined specific frequencies and sequences of behavior between partners as they discuss conflictual topics in their relationships, typically by videotaping the conversation and having trained coders categorize specific types of positive and negative communication. Marital distress has fairly consistently been found to be associated with communication involving (a) more criticism, blaming, hostility, and contempt, (b) reciprocation and escalation of negative messages between partners, (c) more demand-withdrawal sequences, and (d) less validation of the other's opinions and emotions (Epstein & Baucom, 2002; Weiss & Heyman, 1997).

Relationship Cognition

The ways that members of a couple perceive and interpret the events in their relationship affect marital quality. Baucom, Epstein, Sayers, and Sher (1989) identified five types of cognition associated with marital distress: (a) *selective perceptions*, in which partners notice particular aspects of marital interaction (with distressed partners focusing on each other's negative acts) and fail to notice other aspects; (b) *negative attributions*, involving inferences that one's partner's negative behavior is due to stable, global negative traits, as well as to negative motives and a lack of love; (c) *negative expectancies*, or predictions that one's partner will behave in negative ways; (d) *inaccurate or unrealistic assumptions* about the partner and relationship, such as a belief that men and women cannot understand each other due to gender differences; and (e) *unrealistic standards* about the characteristics that one's relationship should have, such as a belief that in a close relationship partners should enjoy all of the same leisure time activities. There are research findings supporting all of these forms of cognition as risk factors for marital problems, although the majority of studies have investigated attributions and standards as predictors of marital distress and negative behavioral interactions (Epstein & Baucom, 2002).

Environmental Stressors

Marital quality can be affected by a variety of stresses that have impacts on the individual partners or on the couple's interactions and cognitions about their relationship (Epstein & Baucom, 2002; Neff & Karney, 2004). Some stressors involve the couple's physical environment (e.g., community violence, financial problems), whereas others involve interpersonal relationships (e.g., children, in-laws). Although many stressors are normative and can be predicted, such as the impact of having children, others are unexpected, such as the sudden diagnosis of a life-threatening illness. The couple's coping skills, particularly their ability to engage in joint problem solving and manage stress symptoms such as anxiety, are crucial in preventing stressors from causing deterioration in the relationship (Epstein & Baucom, 2002).

ASSESSMENT OF MARITAL PROBLEMS

Because the characteristics and potential causes of marital problems are varied, adequate assessment requires a multidimensional approach. It includes collection of information about the partners' behaviors, cognitions, and emotions, using the methods of self-report questionnaires, interviews, and direct behavioral observation (Epstein & Baucom, 2002; Snyder, Cavell, Heffer, & Mangrum, 1995). Assessment also takes into account sources of marital problems originating within the two individuals (e.g., psychopathology), the couple interaction patterns (e.g., escalating exchanges of negative behavior), and the couple's environment (e.g., conflict with in-laws). A detailed description of the procedures and instruments used in marital assessment is beyond the scope of this brief chapter, but the reader can find extensive coverage in volumes by Epstein and Baucom (2002) and Touliatos, Perlmutter, Straus, and Holden (2000). Epstein and Baucom (2002) list the overall goals of couple assessment as (a) identifying the problems that led the couple to seek help, (b) identifying factors in the couple's life (within the two individuals, the couple interactions, and the environment) contributing to the problems, (c) determining whether couple therapy is appropriate (e.g., both members want to work on the relationship; there is no danger of eliciting domestic violence), and (d) identifying existing strengths in the relationship that can be enhanced and used to solve problems.

Advantages of self-report questionnaires include the common availability of norms that assist in identifying degrees of relationship problems, efficiency in surveying areas of the relationship that can be quite time-consuming through interviews, and the opportunity for each person to report on problems privately without his or her partner's knowledge as long as the assessor sets firm limits in maintaining confidentiality. Commonly, marital therapists administer a measure of overall marital adjustment such as Spanier's (1976) Dyadic Adjustment Scale, a measure of communication such as Christensen's (1988) Communication Patterns Questionnaire (which assesses dyadic patterns of demand-withdrawal, mutual withdrawal, and mutual constructive communication), a screening instrument for partner abuse such as the revised Conflict Tactics Scale (Straus, Hamby, Boney-McCoy, & Sugarman, 1996), and a measure of individual psychopathology such as the Beck Depression Inventory (Beck, Rush, Shaw, & Emery, 1979). Although a plethora of useful scales is available to assess the various aspects of individual and relationship functioning described earlier, completion of questionnaires is time-consuming and the clinician must choose instruments judiciously.

Exclusive use of self-reports does not allow the assessor to ask follow-up questions to clarify the individual's responses, as can be done during an interview. A joint interview with the couple and a separate interview with each partner allow the assessor to tailor the inquiry to the problems and concerns that each couple presents. These interviews cover the personal histories of the two individuals (e.g., prior relationships, psychopathology, school, and job functioning) as well as the history of the couple relationship (e.g., qualities that attracted the partners to each other and how much those qualities are still present, how they decided to get married, stressors encountered over the course of the relationship, ways that the couple has coped with problems, the couple's social support network). In order to avoid placing individuals at risk for domestic abuse due to disclosures during joint interviews, inquiries about one's own and the other's prior and present psychological and physical abuse are made during the individual interviews (Epstein & Baucom, 2002). Similarly, each member of the couple is asked about his or her own and the partner's alcohol and drug use during the individual interviews.

An advantage of joint assessment sessions is the opportunity to observe the couple's behavioral interactions directly, rather than relying on their perceptions and memories of marital interactions, which are subject to distortion. The assessor can impose varying degrees of structure in conducting behavioral observations. The least structured approach involves simply focusing on the couple's interaction pattern during the interview (e.g., who responds first to questions, who interrupts or corrects whom). More structure can be imposed by asking the couple specific questions (e.g., "How do the two of you make decisions about finances?") and observing how they interact in answering. The highest degree of structure involves informing the couple that one would like to get a sample of how they discuss issues and then asking them to try to resolve an issue that they agree is a source of conflict in their relationship. The assessor can videotape the problem-solving discussion for later detailed review and can use standard communication coding systems (see Kerig and Baucom, 2004 for detailed information) as guides to identifying positive and problematic aspects of the couple's interaction. Aspects of communication that are of particular interest are each partner's skills for clearly and constructively expressing thoughts and emotions, skills for empathic listening to the other person's messages, degree of collaborative problem-solving, and forms of negative behavior such as criticism, blame, contempt messages, and withdrawal and avoidance of communication. At the dyadic level, patterns such as reciprocation of negative messages and demand-withdrawal are identified.

TREATMENT

What Treatments are Effective?

Although there currently are many theoretical orientations to couple therapy, such as structural-strategic, object relations, affective reconstruction, cognitive-behavioral, narrative, emotionally focused, and solution-focused (Gurman & Jacobson, 2002), empirical research on the effectiveness of therapy has lagged far behind the practice of most approaches. Using criteria established by Chambless and Hollon (1998), treatments are considered empirically supported if they have been shown in studies to be superior to a wait-list condition or equivalent to another efficacious treatment, there was sufficient statistical power in the studies to detect treatment effects, and they were implemented successfully by therapists other than the originators of the treatments. A treatment that has been successful in only one study or in multiple studies by the same investigator is considered "possibly efficacious." Most often, efficacy has been assessed in terms of increasing partners' self-reported relationship satisfaction, although improvements in observed communication also are used in some studies. Based on these criteria, currently three broad approaches to couple therapy have achieved empirical support: (a) traditional behavioral couple therapy and its more recent variants of cognitive-behavioral and integrative behavioral couple therapy; (b) emotionally focused couple therapy; and (c) insight-oriented couple therapy (Baucom, Shoham, Mueser, Daiuto, & Stickle, 1998).

Traditional behavior couple therapy (BCT) (e.g., Jacobson & Margolin, 1979) is based on social exchange theory (Thibaut & Kelley, 1959) and social learning theory (Bandura, 1977), with core concepts that an individual's level of relationship satisfaction depends on the ratio of positive to negative experiences he or she has with the partner, and that members of a couple shape each other's behavior through the positive or negative consequences they provide for each other's acts. The major BCT interventions are contracts in which individuals agree to enact more positive behaviors that their partners desire, communication skills training, and problem-solving skills training. Cognitive-behavioral couple therapy (CBCT) (Epstein & Baucom, 2002) adds to BCT interventions procedures for modifying partners' distorted or inappropriate cognitions such as inaccurate negative attributions, as well as procedures for modifying inappropriate emotional responses such as rage. Although BCT acknowledged that cognitions such as negative attributions contributed to individuals' upset about their partners' behavior, therapists did not intervene directly with negative cognitions, but assumed that positive behavior changes would produce more positive cognitions and greater relationship satisfaction. In contrast, the CBCT model proposes that an individual's cognitive change (e.g., a shift from attributing a partner's being late for dinner as due to disrespect to attributing it to poor time management) may be all that is needed to increase relationship satisfaction, even when the partner's behavior does not change. CBCT interventions have adapted cognitive restructuring methods from cognitive therapy (Beck et al., 1979) as well as interventions for enhancing experience and expression of emotions in inhibited partners and reducing excessive emotions in partners who experience "emotional dysregulation." Finally, Jacobson and Christensen's (1996) integrative behavioral couple therapy (IBCT) balances traditional BCT interventions for behavior *change* with interventions designed to increase partners' *acceptance* of each other's existing behaviors that are unlikely to change. IBCT is based on an assumption that a significant portion of relationship distress is due to individuals' lack of acceptance of certain partner characteristics that are for the most part unchangeable and to their attempts to coerce the partner to change, which typically results in defensiveness or counter-attacks from the partner. For example, in the acceptance-based technique of *tolerance building*, the therapist coaches the couple in thinking about the positive aspects of differences in their characteristics, to balance their awareness of the drawbacks to those differences. Published reviews (e.g., Baucom et al., 1998) of treatment outcome studies have concluded that BCT is an efficacious intervention for relationship problems, and CBCT (delivered as BCT sessions plus cognitive intervention sessions) is equally but not more efficacious as an equal number of sessions of only BCT. A recent study (Christensen et al., 2004) found that IBCT is equally efficacious as BCT, with couples receiving BCT improving more quickly initially than couples receiving IBCT but the two treatments achieving equivalent outcomes by the end of therapy.

Whereas most current approaches to couple therapy have emphasized the partners' behavioral and cognitive responses to each other, emotionally focused couple therapy (EFCT) (Johnson, 1996; Johnson & Denton, 2002) pays more attention to the emotions that individuals experience in their intimate relationships. EFCT is largely based on Bowlby's (1969) attachment theory, which proposes that humans are born with a need for emotional attachment to nurturing others. A child who experiences parents or other early caretakers as physically and psychologically available develops a secure attachment style, whereas those who experience caretakers as unavailable develop insecure attachments. Research has supported the attachment theory assumption that the attachment style that an individual develops early in life persists into adulthood, although new experiences in adult relationships can modify an individual's attachment pattern (Davila, Burge, & Hammen, 1997). Attachment theory also proposes that when an individual perceives that a significant other such as a spouse is not available physically or emotionally, the individual is likely to feel anxiety but also may experience and express negative emotions such as anger toward the spouse. These negative responses tend to backfire, increasing conflict and distance between partners rather than meeting the insecure individual's need for intimacy. In EFCT partners are guided in understanding their own and each other's negative emotional and behavioral responses that are elicited by attachment insecurity and in developing more constructive behavior toward each other that can fulfill their attachment needs. For example, the therapist "reframes" partners' negative behaviors as expressions of vulnerability and attachment needs and encourages them to express vulnerable feelings more.

Several treatment outcome studies (e.g., Denton, Burleson, Clark, Rodriguez, & Hobbs, 2000) have found EFCT to be superior to a wait list control group, and in one study couples receiving EFCT reported greater marital satisfaction than couples receiving BCT, both at post-treatment and at an 8-week follow-up (Johnson & Greenberg, 1985). Because most studies on EFCT have treated couples who ranged from nondistressed to moderately distressed, additional studies are needed to test the efficacy of EFCT with highly distressed couples. Baucom et al.'s (1998) review of outcome studies classified EFCT as an efficacious treatment for moderately distressed couples.

A variety of approaches to couple therapy emphasize increasing partners' insight into their own and each other's early relationship experiences as a means of understanding the problems in their current couple relationship. Although these approaches, typically referred to as psychodynamic, are popular among couple therapists, there has been little research on their efficacy. However, Snyder's insight-oriented couple therapy (IOCT) (Snyder & Wills, 1989) has been evaluated in studies and has shown promising impact. The theoretical model underlying IOCT proposes that members of distressed couples likely experienced emotional injuries in prior relationships that left them with vulnerabilities (e.g., fear of being controlled) and defensive strategies to protect themselves (e.g., withdrawing from significant others). In therapy, the partners are helped to see how their negative emotional and behavioral responses toward each other were shaped by the negative experiences that they had in prior relationships, thus helping them distinguish between the past and present relationships. In addition, they are guided in understanding how the coping strategies that were adaptive in earlier relationships are now inappropriate for fulfilling their personal needs within their marriage.

Snyder and Wills' (1989) study comparing the outcomes of IOCT and traditional BCT found both treatments to be efficacious in improving self-reported marital adjustment relative to a condition in which couples were on a waiting list for therapy, and IOCT and BCT couples were still comparable on marital adjustment at a six-month follow-up assessment. However, Snyder, Wills, and Grady-Fletcher (1991) found that four years after the completion of therapy significantly more of the BCT couples than the IOCT couples (38% versus 3%) had divorced, and the IOCT couples reported significantly higher levels of marital adjustment than the BCT couples. Based on the results from this one investigation, Baucom et al. (1998) classified IOCT as possibly efficacious. More such studies comparing alternative therapy approaches are needed.

The absence of research on other popular approaches to couple therapy does not mean that only the three types of therapy reviewed here are the only ones worth pursuing; rather, it seems likely that other approaches will be found to be efficacious when they are evaluated. It is important that such outcome studies be conducted so that therapists and consumers can make informed choices about treatments for marital problems.

Can Couple Interventions Prevent the Development of Marital Problems?

Given the profound negative impacts that marital problems have on the partners and the people close to them, considerable effort has been put into designing and evaluating prevention programs. In a review of research on relationship education programs, Halford & Moore (2002) concluded that only those programs that focus on improving couples' relationship skills (e.g., for communication) rather than only providing educational material have been tested for efficacy in research studies. Results of the studies have indicated that the programs do increase partners' skills and that the improvements last for at least a few years. Studies on Markman, Stanley, and Blumberg's (1994) Prevention and Relationship Enhancement

Program (PREP) have indicated that it also prevents declines in marital satisfaction, although this effect appears to occur most among couples who are more highly distressed initially (Halford & Moore, 2002). The fact that a large percentage of couples who participate in programs such as PREP report a high level of satisfaction with the programs suggests that preventive interventions appeal to couples' motivation to have successful relationships and avoid the types of marital problems described in this chapter. Despite several decades of soaring divorce rates that only recently have leveled off and begun to decrease, marriage and similar forms of committed couple relationships clearly meet a variety of basic human needs. Consequently, the continuing efforts of researchers and clinicians to develop effective preventive and therapeutic programs for relationship problems should be recognized as a high priority in the mental health field.

REFERENCES

Amato, P. R. (1996). Explaining the intergenerational transmission of divorce. *Journal of Marriage and the Family, 58*, 628–640.

Bandura, A. (1977). *Social learning theory*. Englewood Cliffs, NJ: Prentice-Hall.

Banse, R. (2004). Adult attachment and marital satisfaction: Evidence for dyadic configuration effects. *Journal of Social and Personal Relationships, 21*, 273–282.

Baucom, D. H., Epstein, N., Rankin, L. A., & Burnett, C. K. (1996). Assessing relationship standards: The Inventory of Specific Relationship Standards. *Journal of Family Psychology, 10*, 72–88.

Baucom, D. H., Epstein, N., Sayers, S. L., & Sher, T. G. (1989). The role of cognitions in marital relationships: Definitional, methodological, and conceptual issues. *Journal of Consulting and Clinical Psychology, 57*, 31–38.

Baucom, D. H., Shoham, V., Mueser, K. T., Daiuto, A. D., & Stickle, T. R. (1998). Empirically supported couple and family interventions for marital distress and adult mental health problems. *Journal of Consulting and Clinical Psychology, 66*, 53–88.

Beach, S. R. H. (Ed.) (2001). *Marital and family processes in depression: A scientific foundation for clinical practice*. Washington, DC: American Psychological Association.

Beck, A. T., Rush, A. J., Shaw, B. F., & Emery, G. (1979). *Cognitive therapy of depression*. New York: Guilford Press.

Belsky, J. (1990). Children and marriage. In F. D. Fincham & T. N. Bradbury (Eds.), *The psychology of marriage: Basic issues and applications* (pp. 172–200). New York: Guilford Press.

Benokraitis, N. J. (2002). *Marriages and families: Changes, choices, and constraints*. (4th ed.). Upper Saddle River, NJ: Prentice-Hall.

Bowlby, J. (1969). Disruption of affectional bonds and its effects on behavior. *Canada's Mental Health Supplement, 59*, 12.

Bradbury, T. N., & Fincham, F. D. (1987). Assessment of affect in marriage. In K. D. O'Leary (Ed.), *Assessment of marital discord: An integration for research and clinical practice* (pp. 59–108). Hillsdale, NJ: Erlbaum.

Buehler, C., Krishnakumar, A., Stone, G., Anthony, C., Pemberton, S., Gerard, J., et al., (1998). Interparental conflict styles and youth problem behaviors: A two-sample replication study. *Journal of Marriage and the Family, 60*, 119–132.

Chambless, D. L., & Hollon, S. D. (1998). Defining empirically supported therapies. *Journal of Consulting and Clinical Psychology, 66*, 7–18.

Christensen, A. (1988). Dysfunctional interaction patterns in couples. In P. Noller & M. A. Fitzpatrick (Eds.), *Perspectives on marital interaction. Monographs in social psychology of language* (No. 1, pp. 31–52). Clevedon, England: Multilingual Matters.

Christensen, A., Atkins, D., Berns, S., Wheeler, J., Baucom, D. H., & Simpson, L. (2004). Traditional versus integrative behavioral couple therapy for significantly and stably distressed married couples. *Journal of Consulting and Clinical Psychology, 72*, 176–191.

Conger, R. D., Elder, G. H., Lorenz, F. O., Conger, K. J., Simons, R. L., Whitbeck, L. B., et al. (1990). Linking economic hardship to marital quality and instability. *Journal of Marriage and the Family, 52*, 643–656.

Cutrona, C. E. (1996). *Social support in couples: Marriage as a resource in times of stress*. Thousand Oaks, CA: Sage.

Daiuto, A. D., Baucom, D. H., Epstein, N., & Dutton, S. S. (1998). The application of behavioral couples therapy to the assessment and treatment of agoraphobia: Implications of empirical research. *Clinical Psychology Review, 18*, 663–687.

Davila, J., Burge, D., & Hammen, C. (1997). Why does attachment style change? *Journal of Personality and Social Psychology, 73*, 826–838.

Denton, W. H., Burleson, B. R., Clark, T. E., Rodriguez, C. R., & Hobbs, B. V. (2000). A randomized trial of emotionally focused therapy for couples in a training clinic. *Journal of Marital and Family Therapy, 26,* 65–78.

Epstein, E. E., & McCrady, B. S. (2002). Couple therapy in the treatment of alcohol problems. In A. S. Gurman & N. S. Jacobson (Eds.), *Clinical handbook of couple therapy* (3rd ed., pp. 597–628). New York: Guilford Press.

Epstein, N. B., & Baucom, D. H. (2002). *Enhanced cognitive-behavioral therapy for couples: A contextual approach.* Washington, DC: American Psychological Association.

Falconier, M. K. (2004). Economic strain, friends' support, and relationship satisfaction in Argentinean couples: Paths of influence and gender differences. Unpublished doctoral dissertation, University of Maryland, College Park.

Feng, D., Giarrusso, R., Bengtson, V. L., & Frye, N. (1999). Intergenerational transmission of marital quality and marital instability. *Journal of Marriage and the Family, 61,* 451–463.

Forthofer, M. S., Markman, H. J., Cox, M., Stanley, S., & Kessler, R. C. (1996). Associations between marital distress and work loss in a national sample. *Journal of Marriage and the Family, 58,* 597–605.

Glass, S. P. (2002). Couple therapy after the trauma of infidelity. In A. S. Gurman & N. S. Jacobson (Eds.), *Clinical handbook of couple therapy* (3rd ed., pp. 488–507). New York: Guilford Press.

Glenn, N. D. (1996). Values, attitudes, and the state of American marriage. In D. Popenoe, J. B. Elshtain, & D. Blankenhorn (Eds.), *Promises to keep: Decline and renewal of marriage in America* (pp. 15–34). Lanham, MD: Rowan and Littlefield.

Gollan, J. K., Friedman, M. A., & Miller, I. W. (2002). Couple therapy in the treatment of major depression. In A. S. Gurman & N. S. Jacobson (Eds.), *Clinical handbook of couple therapy* (3rd ed., pp. 653–676). New York: Guilford Press.

Gordon, K. C., & Baucom, D. H. (1999). A multitheoretical intervention for promoting recovery from extramarital affairs. *Clinical Psychology: Science and Practice, 6,* 382–399.

Gottman, J. M. (1994). *What predicts divorce?: The relationship between marital processes and marital outcomes.* Hillsdale, NJ: Erlbaum.

Gray-Little, B., Baucom, D. H., & Hamby, S. L. (1996). Marital power, marital adjustment, and therapy outcome. *Journal of Family Psychology, 10,* 292–303.

Gurman, A. S., & Jacobson, N. S. (Eds.) (2002). *Clinical handbook of couple therapy* (3rd ed.). New York: Guilford Press.

Halford, W. K., & Moore, E. N. (2002). Relationship education and the prevention of couple relationship problems. In A. S. Gurman and N. S. Jacobson (Eds.), *Clinical handbook of couple therapy* (3rd ed., pp. 400–419). New York: Guilford Press.

Holtzworth-Munroe, A., Stuart, G. L., & Hutchinson, G. (1997). Violent versus nonviolent husbands: Differences in attachment patterns, dependency, and jealousy. *Journal of Family Psychology, 11,* 314–331.

Jacobson, N. S., & Christensen, A. (1996). *Integrative couple therapy: Promoting acceptance and change.* New York: Norton.

Jacobson, N. S., & Margolin, G. (1979). *Marital therapy: Strategies based on social learning and behavior exchange principles.* New York: Brunner/Mazel.

Johnson, S. M. (1996). *The practice of emotionally focused marital therapy: Creating connection.* New York: Brunner/Mazel.

Johnson, S. M., & Denton, W. (2002). Emotionally focused couple therapy: Creating secure connections. In A. S. Gurman & N. S. Jacobson (Eds.), *Clinical handbook of couple therapy* (3rd ed., pp. 221–250). New York: Guilford Press.

Johnson, S. M., & Greenberg, L. S. (1985). Differential effects of experiential and problem-solving interventions in resolving marital conflict. *Journal of Consulting and Clinical Psychology, 53,* 175–184.

Karney, B. R., & Bradbury, T. N. (1995). The longitudinal course of marital quality and stability: A review of theory, methods, and research. *Psychological Bulletin, 118,* 3–34.

Kerig, P. K., & Baucom, D. H. (2004). *Couple observational coding systems.* Mahwah, NJ: Erlbaum.

Krishnakumar, A., & Buehler, C. (2000). Interparental conflict and parenting behaviors: A meta-analytic review. *Family Relations, 49,* 25–44.

Lazarus, R. S., & Lazarus, B. N. (1994). *Passion and reason: Making sense of our emotions.* New York: Oxford University Press.

Lundgren, D. C., Jergens, V. H., & Gibson, J. L. (1980). Marital relationships, evaluations of spouse and self, and anxiety. *Journal of Psychology, 106,* 227–240.

Markman, H. J., Stanley, S. M., & Blumberg, S. L. (1994). *Fighting for your marriage: Positive steps for preventing divorce and preserving a lasting love.* San Francisco: Jossey-Bass.

Morrison, D. R., & Coiro, M. J. (1999). Parental conflict and marital disruption: Do children benefit when high-conflict marriages are dissolved? *Journal of Marriage and the Family, 61,* 626–637.

National Center for Health Statistics (1995). Advance report of final divorce statistics, 1989 and 1990. *Monthly Vital Statistics Reports, 43,* (9).

Neff, L. A., & Karney, B. R. (2004). How does context affect intimate relationships? Linking external stress and cognitive processes within marriage. *Personality and Social Psychology Bulletin, 30,* 134–148.

Noller, P., Beach, S., & Osgarby, S. (1997). Cognitive and affective processes in marriage. In W. K. Halford & H. J. Markman (Eds.), *Clinical handbook of marriage and couples intervention* (pp. 43–71). Chichester, UK: Wiley.

Prager, K. J. (1995). *The psychology of intimacy.* New York: Guilford Press.

Sabatelli, R. M., & Chadwick, J. J. (2000). Marital distress: From complaints to contempt. In P. C. McKenry & S. J. Price (Eds.), *Families and change: Coping with stressful events and transitions* (2nd ed., pp. 22–44). Thousand Oaks, CA: Sage.

Snyder, D. K., Cavell, T. A., Heffer, R. W., & Mangrum, L. F. (1995). Marital and family assessment: A multifaceted, multilevel approach. In R. H. Mikesell, D. D. Lusterman, & S. H. McDaniel (Eds.), *Integrating family therapy: Handbook of family psychology and systems theory* (pp. 163–182). Washington, DC: American Psychological Association.

Snyder, D. K., & Wills, R. M. (1989). Behavioral versus insight-oriented marital therapy: Effects on individual and interspousal functioning. *Journal of Consulting and Clinical Psychology, 57,* 39–46.

Snyder, D. K., Wills, R. M., & Grady-Fletcher, A. (1991). Long-term effectiveness of behavioral versus insight-oriented marital therapy: A 4-year follow-up study. *Journal of Consulting and Clinical Psychology, 59*(1), 138–141.

Spanier, G. B. (1976). Measuring dyadic adjustment: New scales for assessing the quality of marriage and similar dyads. *Journal of Marriage and the Family, 38,* 15–28.

Straus, M. A., Hamby, S. L., Boney-McCoy, S., & Sugarman, D. B. (1996). The Revised Conflict Tactics Scales (CTS2): Development and preliminary psychometric data. *Journal of Family Issues, 17,* 283–316.

Thibaut, J. W., & Kelley, H. H. (1959). *The social psychology of groups.* New York: Wiley.

Touliatos, J., Perlmutter, B. F., Straus, M. A., & Holden, G. W. (2000). *Handbook of family measurement techniques, Vols. 1–3.* Thousand Oaks, CA: Sage.

Vinokur, A. D., Price, R. H., & Caplan, R. D. (1996). Hard times and hurtful partners: How financial strain affects depression and relationship satisfaction of unemployed persons and their spouses. *Journal of Personality and Social   Psychology, 71,* 166–179.

Watson, D., Klohnen, E. C., Casillas, A., Nus Simms, E., Haig, J., & Berry, D. S. (2004). Match makers and deal breakers: Analyses of assortative mating in newlywed couples. *Journal of Personality, 72,* 1029–1068.

Weiss, R. L., & Cerreto, M. C. (1980). The Marital Status Inventory: Development of a measure of dissolution potential. *American Journal of Family Therapy, 8*(2), 80–85.

Weiss, R. L., & Heyman, R. E. (1997). A clinical-research overview of couples interactions. In W. K. Halford & H. J. Markman (Eds.), *Clinical handbook of marriage and couples interventions* (pp. 13–41). Chichester, UK: Wiley.

Whyte, M. K. (1990). Dating, mating, and marriage. New York: Aldine de Gruyter.

Wilkie, J. R., Ferree, M. M., & Ratcliff, K. S. (1998). Gender and fairness: Marital satisfaction in two-earner couples. *Journal of Marriage and the Family, 60,* 577–594.

CHAPTER 40

Mental Retardation

Frank R. Rusch • Kimberly F. Keller

WHAT IS MENTAL RETARDATION?

Definitions of mental retardation began to appear early in the 20th century and have undergone many changes, most notably by the American Association on Mental Retardation and the American Psychological Association. These definitions are more similar than they are different. For example, the 1992 AAMR definition refers to mental retardation as:

Mental retardation refers to substantial limitations in present functioning. It is characterized by significantly subaverage intellectual functioning, existing concurrently with related limitations in two or more of the following applicable adaptive skill areas: communication, self care, home living, social skills, community use, self direction, health and safety, functional academics, leisure and work. Mental retardation manifests before age 18. (AAMR, 1992, p. 1)

The American Psychological Association published a similar definition of mental retardation in the Manual of Diagnosis and Professional Practice in Mental Retardation (1996):

Mental retardation (MR) refers to (a) significant limitations in general intellectual functioning; (b) significant limitations in adaptive functioning, which exists concurrently; and (c) onset of intellectual and adaptive limitations before age 22. (p. 13).

Both definitions refer to intellectual functioning, adaptive behavior and age of onset. The AAMR and APA definitions rely upon psychometric examination of intellectual functioning to obtain a metric that can be used to assist in classifying level of mental retardation (typically referred to as mild, moderate, severe, and profound with IQ scores provided for classification purposes). Although the developmental age is different (i.e., 18 versus 22), the intent of both definitions is to identify mental retardation as an intellectual disability that occurs at some point after conception and before the individual reaches adulthood.

The reference to adaptive behavior is essential in both definitions to providing potential services across the age span. AAMR took bold steps to focus attention upon positive aspects of one's life versus long-standing references to deficits by including "systems of support" in their 1992 *Mental Retardation: Definition, Classification, and Systems of Support.* These steps included an attempt to shift attention away from the traditional classification scheme (i.e., mild, moderate, severe, and profound) toward patterns of support needed to promote positive interactions between the individual and the diverse settings that individuals learn, play, work, and live.

For the purposes of this chapter, we draw upon a definition that focuses upon the larger goals of integration and providing a voice to the consumer of services that typically is externally mediated (i.e., by teachers, trainers, and staff). The present chapter is based upon two premises. First, the person with mental retardation (and when appropriate, his/her parents/guardians) should be involved in the formation of goals associated with their education and training; secondly, these

Rusch, F. R., & Keller, K. F. (2006). Mental Retardation. In J. E. Fisher & W. T. O'Donohue (Eds.), *Practitioner's guide to evidence-based psychotherapy.* New York: Springer.

goals should focus upon the integration of individuals with mental retardation into typical communities (e.g., regular classrooms, the work environment, and the larger community that individuals without mental retardation expect to learn, work, and live in). *Typical communities* include people and resources that are linked together by common expectations and shared interests. Consequently, we refer to typical communities as integrated communities whereby "a cohesive network of people and resources are linked together by common expectations and shared interests." (Rusch, Chadsey-Rusch, White, & Gifford, 1985, p. 124). This definition is central to emerging, evidence-based practices because "integration" appears to be fueling the emergence of new, exciting research and outcomes that would eventually dispel myths and promote new thinking.

BASIC FACTS ABOUT MENTAL RETARDATION

Prevalence. The US Department of Education reported that 612,978 students between the ages of 6 and 21 were receiving special education services in 2002. This figure represents about 11% of all students with disabilities who receive education-related services as students with mental retardation. Approximately 90% of these students have been classified with mild mental retardation, or students who need limited support.

In the general population estimates vary widely as to the prevalence of mental retardation. The President's Committee on Mental Retardation (2000) estimated that between 6.2 and 7.5 million Americans have some level of mental retardation, or about 3% of the general population. The National Health Survey-Disability Supplement suggested that about 2 million people with mental retardation live in the United States (Research and Training Center on Community Services, 1999).

ASSESSMENT

Assessment Approaches

Assessments have traditionally been used to determine if a student is eligible for special education services. Unfortunately, these assessments result in labels that are difficult to rid; typically, these labels also lead to classifications that eventually result in "placements" versus the identification of education supports for children and youth to become integral members of the regular classroom. Clearly, categorizing students is limiting and more often separating and degrading. Regardless, many states still determine a student's eligibility for special services based upon one's classification. An IQ determination of 70 or below typically indicates that a student is eligible to receive special education services, for example; an IQ determination of 71 or above results in that same student not receiving special services in school.

Whether a student takes a traditional test such as the *Wechsler Preschool and Primary Scale of Intelligence-Revised (WPPSI-R)* (Wecshler, 1989) or the *Wechsler Intelligence Scale for Children-III (WISC-III)* (Wecshler 1991), there is still a number and a label associated with a level of intelligence that more often excludes versus includes these students from participating in regular education. We believe that it is more helpful to think about assessment as a process that encompasses multiple measurement options that result in identifying the supports needed for a student to remain or become an integral member of his/her classroom. Archival records, observations, and interviews define a more complete picture of an individual's educational abilities. Parents, guardians, and other significant individuals are valuable sources for providing this information when we are considering the broader goals of early childhood transition, inclusion and collaboration, and transition and self-determination, as presented above.

Fortunately, there has been a paradigm shift in assessment approaches that has gained prominence in recent years. Students are receiving services based upon the supports that are needed to participate in inclusive classrooms (Thompson et al. 2002b). The *American Association for Mental Retardation (AAMR)* efforts to identify key areas for directing assessment of needed supports was an important departure from previous assessment approaches. The AAMR manual now includes such topics as human development, teaching and education, home living, community living, employment, health and safety, behavior, social, and protection and advocacy in their assessment of metal retardation.

An assessment instrument that has been developed that addresses these diverse support needs is the *Supports Intensity Scale (SIS)* (Thompson et al., 2002a). The *SIS* is a unique approach to assessment. The *SIS* works on the premise that we should look at an individual's needs versus an individual's deficits. The *SIS* consists of 49 activities that direct the assessment. The *SIS* also measures supports needs for medical conditions, problem behaviors and protection and advocacy. The *SIS* is the first assessment to align with the AAMR definition of mental retardation. This assessment approach is important because it addresses the supports needed for a student to be become part of larger integrated communities, like regular classrooms.

EDUCATION PRACTICES

Integrated communities decidedly influence the care, education, and training of persons with mental retardation differently from communities that are defined by segregated services. As mentioned above, these typical communities include the family unit, regular classrooms, work environments, and the larger community. These are the communities where most individuals expect to play, work, and grow to assume contributing roles as adults. We defined *integrated communities* as cohesive networks of people and resources, which are linked together by common expectations and shared interests. Consequently, participation, interactions, and social roles define the quality and type of care, education and training that is received.

Throughout our lives we assume new and more demanding roles based upon our experiences while participating and interacting with our peers. For example, we learn to play games as children that result in other children around us benefiting from our participation, and ultimately, we learn to cooperate and work together toward mutual goals. When we participate with our peers in the classroom, in the workplace or while planning community activities, we draw upon our experiences (i.e., our participation in activities, interactions with our peers, and the formation of social roles) to shape the way we interact with these same peers as adults.

The goals of children, youth, and young adults with mental retardation should be no different than the goals of same-aged children, youth, and young adults without mental retardation. In fact, much of the progress we have made over the past 20 years in relation to care, education, and training has resulted from our realization that the activities that same-aged peers are enrolled/involved in typically identify the activities that define participation, interaction, and social roles that their peers with mental retardation assume. Consequently, the roles of educators, medical staff, counselors, and family are being dictated more by the regular lives of individuals without disabilities as we plan, for example, instructional activities for children with mental retardation. In the following sections we pay more attention to some of the key practices that have and continue to direct the activities of educators and professional staff across infancy and early childhood, children, youth and young adults.

Infancy and Early Childhood

The needs of infants and toddlers were recognized when the Individuals with Disabilities Education Act (PL 105-17) was reauthorized and amended in 1997. Part C of this Act recognized the role of the family in the education of infants and toddlers by including (a) multidisciplinary assessment, (b) a design to address each child's developmental needs, and (c) a written *Individual Family Service Plan* developed by a multidisciplinary team that included parents' participation.

Considerations for planning include: (a) developmentally/chronologically age-appropriate practices that highlight what the child's peers are capable of doing, the child's learning supports that will promote his/her attaining these highlights, and the identification and use of settings that are natural or typical to children without mental retardation, (b) the family as the center of planning and activities, and that the cultures and values of the family are considered, (c) the advice of multiple disciplines to address the myriad supports of each child (e.g., speech and language training, occupational therapy, physical therapy, psychological services, family training, and vision screening). Because infants and toddlers will encounter many new environments as a result of their service needs and their growth, their *transition* needs must be considered. For example, one morning they may be playing with their siblings at home and the very same day they might be playing with complete strangers in an educational environment.

Children

The fundamental provisions of the Individuals with Disabilities Education Act (PL 101-457) are well articulated and practiced throughout the United States. Consequently, these provisions are not the covered in this chapter, but can be reviewed elsewhere. Two topics deserve more attention as we consider emerging and highly charged discussions that relate to "where" children with mental retardation should receive their instruction—*inclusion and collaboration*. Historically, the educational needs of children with mental retardation have been met in one of several "least restrictive environments." These "least restrictive environments" include segregated schools and classrooms, and are considered by some educators as the "least restrictive" educational setting where the child can best benefit from instruction. The regular classroom represents the "integrated community" that we introduced above, and one where 'a cohesive network of people and resources, (can be) linked together by common expectations and shared interests." *Inclusion* is the term that is used to refer to the regular classroom placement of children with mental retardation. Inclusive classrooms appreciate student diversity and strive to promote a sense of community and social acceptance. Importantly, inclusive classrooms also strive for "cohesive networks" of educators, professionals, and families who *collaborate* to promote effective instructional practice in the classroom. *Collaboration* refers to the process of planning and providing an education that promotes learning in the classroom, typically achieved when educators from various disciplines work together to deliver an appropriate education.

Youth and Young Adults

As early as 1990, IDEA (PL 101-457) mandated that transition services be included in individualized education program (the IEP) (Rusch & Phelps, 1987). Reauthorizations of IDEA have resulted in important practices being mandated, included when and how to implement transition services. Today, transition planning must begin in the 12th year of all students with a disability and the planning must be student-focused. Including students in their planning has resulted in the emergence of several practices, including student *self-determination* and the systematic application of *self-mediation strategies*. *Self-determination* refers to the process of individuals determining their own education goals and a course of action that results in attaining those goals. A number of practices have been studied that promote self-determination, including the person-centered futures planning process (Vandercook, York, & Forest, 1989; Wehmeyer, 1998). Methods common to these practices include developing: (a) a student's vision of his future employment, living arrangement and needed training, and (b) providing supports that result in the student meeting his/her short and long term goals for participating in an education that is necessary to promote meeting the student's vision.

Self-mediation strategies refer to those strategies that students utilize to address everyday learning. These strategies differ from externally mediated strategies, which are strategies that teachers typically use to promote learning. Examples of self-mediated strategies include self-monitoring, self-instruction, and self-reinforcement (Agran, 1997; Rusch, Hughes, & Wilson, 1996). In contrast, externally mediated strategies include antecedents to (e.g., verbal prompts, gestural primes, and physical assistance) and consequences for (e.g., positive and negative reinforcement and positive and negative punishment) performance.

CONCLUSION

People with mental retardation are more like people without mental retardation than they are different. Efforts to include students in typical communities are important as the goals and methods to reach these goals in typical communities are publicly derived and also publicly monitored. Consequently, the expectations of parents, regular classroom teachers, and typical students are the goals that define our assessment approach (what we intend with our instruction), our instructional strategies (how we intend to meet these goals), and our expected and derived outcomes. Expecting students with mental retardation to participate in social interactions, for example, become the goals of our education. These expectations, often higher than those that may be formulated for only students with mental retardation, are critically important. Because these expectations are higher, the standards for our education of students with mental retardation are higher and indeed we can expect improved performance across the life span. These higher expectations, and their associated outcomes, change the expectations of students without mental retardation as well as the expectations of teachers. The resulting self-fulfilling prophecy becomes one where students with and without mental retardation are united in their common expectations for an education.

Useful Websites

American Association of Mental Retardation *www.aamr.org*
American Psychological Association *www.apa.org*
Association for Retarded Citizens *www.TheArc.org*
Internet Resources for Special Children *www.irsc.org*
National Association of Persons with Dual Diagnosis *www.thnadd.org*
National Organization on Disability *www.nod.org*
Parents helping parents website *www.php.org*
www.disabilityrights.org

State by state listing of disability resources *www.disabilityresources.org/state*
Transition Research Institute at Illinois *http://www.ed.uiuc.edu/SPED/tri/institute.htm*
Washington Alliance for Direct Support Professionals *www.wadsp.org*

RECOMMENDED READINGS

Rusch, F. R., & Chadsey-Rusch, J. (Eds.). (1998). *Beyond high school: Transition from school-to-work*. Pacific Grove, CA: Brooks/Cole Publishing.

Wehmeyer, M. L. & Patton, J. R. (Eds.). *Mental retardation in the 21ˢᵗ century*. (pp. 59–70). Austin, Tx: Pro-Ed.

REFERENCES

Agran, M. (1997). *Student-directed learning: Teaching self-determination skills*. Pacific Grove, CA: Brooks/Cole.

American Association on Mental Retardation. (1992). *Mental retardation: Definition, classification, and supports systems*. American Association for Mental Retardation: Washington, DC.

Biasini, F., Grupe, L., Huffman, L., & Bray, N. (1999). Mental Retardation: A symptom and a syndrome. In S. Netherton, D. Holmes, & C. E. Walker (Eds.), *Comprehensive textbook of child and adolescent disorders*. New York: Oxford University Press.

President's Committee on Mental Retardation. (2000). Mission [Online]. Available: http://www.acf.dhhs.gov/programs/pcmr/mission.htm

Research and Training Center on Community Services. (1999, January). 1994 National Health Interview Survey: Disability Supplement. *MR/DD Data Brief*, 1 (1), 1–7.

Rusch, F. R., Chadsey-Rusch, J. G., White, D. M., & Gifford, J. L. (1985). Programs for severely mentally retarded adults: Perspectives and methodologies. In D. Bricker & J. Filler (Eds.), *Severe mental retardation: From theory to practice* (pp. 119–140). Reston, VA: Council for Exceptional Children.

Rusch, F. R., Hughes, C., & Wilson, P. G. (1995). Utilizing cognitive strategies in the acquisition of employment skills. In W. O'Donohue & L. Krasner (Eds.). *Handbook of psychological skills training clinical techniques and applications* (pp. 363–382). New York: Pergamon Press.

Rusch, F. R., & Phelps, L. A. (1987). Secondary special education and transition from school to work: A national priority. *Exceptional Children, 53*, 487–492.

Thompson, J. R., Bryant, B., Campbell, E. M., Craig, E. M., Hughes, C., Rotholz, D. A., Schalock, R. L., Silverman, W., & Tasse, M. J. (2002a). *Supports Intensity Scale*. Unpublished assessment scale. Washington, DC: American Association on Mental Retardation.

Thompson, J. R., Hughes, C., Schalock, R. L., Silverman, W., Tasse, M. J., Bryant, B., Craig, E. M., & Campbell, E. M. (2002b). Integrating supports in assessment and planning. *Mental Retardation, 40*, 390–405.

Vandercook, T., York, J., & Forest, M. (1989). The McGill Action Planning System (MAPS): A strategy for building the vision. *Journal of the Association for Persons with Severe Handicaps, 14*, 205–215.

Wecshler, D. (1989), *Wecshler Preschool Primary Scale of Intelligence-Revised*. San Antonio: The Psychological Corporation.

Wecshler, D. (1991), *Wecshler Intelligence Scale for Children-Third Edition*. San Antonio: The Psychological Corporation.

Wehmeyer, M. L. (1998). Self-determination and individuals with significant disabilities: Examining meanings and misinterpretations. *Journal of the Association for Persons with Severe Handicaps, 23(1)*, 5–16.

Nail Biting

Wayne Fuqua • Shai Brosh

WHAT IS NAIL BITING?

Nail biting, or onychophagia involves repeated biting of the fingernails and cuticles. Typically parts of the nail, cuticle, or skin around the nail bed are removed by biting. When the frequency is high and persistent or the intensity severe, nail biting may produce acute paronychia, which involves inflammation of the tissues adjacent to the nail accompanied by infection and pus formation. The vast majority of patients requiring surgical treatment for acute paronychia reported nail biting and picking (Baran & Dawber, 1984).

Serious dental problems such as malocclusions and atypical root resorption may also occur (e.g., Wells, Haines, Williams & Brain, 1999, Woods & Miltenberger, 2001). When severe, nail biting has been associated with shorter tooth roots in 13–15 year old as a function of the severe pressure placed on the teeth (Odenrick & Brattstrom, 1985). Furthermore, fingernail biting and other oral–digital habit behaviors may lead to negative peer evaluation and avoidance of those individuals engaging in public nail biting and other digital/oral habits (Woods et al., 2001). Nail biting occurs on a continuum, with many people engaging in low frequency, low intensity nail biting that is of concern primarily for cosmetic and social reasons. At the more intense (and less prevalent) end of the severity continuum, nail biting has many similarities with self-mutilative behaviors such as body cutting and body piercing that involve repetitive, self-inflicted bodily damage (e.g., Wells et al., 1999). Unfortunately, little research has focused on this more serious end of the severity continuum.

BASIC FACTS ABOUT NAIL BITING

Comorbidity

Very little systematic research has been conducted on the behavioral and psychological correlates of nail biting. Some have speculated that nail biting might be a symptom of emotional tension and anxiety in children (e.g., Schneider & Peterson, 1982) but studies of children who bite their nails reveals little evidence of elevated anxiety levels (Deardorff, Finch, & Royall, 1974). Others have noted that nail biting in children is associated with motor restlessness and motor tics (Kanner, 1957). Data to support that claim are sketchy.

For adults, research on correlates of nail biting has yielded inconsistent results. Reports of an association between nail biting and anxiety (Klatte & Deardorff, 1981), bedwetting (Lowry, 1965) and sociopathy (Walker & Ziskind, 1977) are offset by reports of no association between nail biting and anxiety or stereotyped body movements (Clark, 1970). Observations of the similarity between nail biting and obsessive-compulsive disorder (OCD) have not been supported with empirical evidence of co morbid symptomatology. Moreover, there is evidence that nail biting, including more severe variants, may occur without any underlying psychopathology

Fuqua, W., & Brosh, S. (2006). Nail biting. In J. E. Fisher & W. T. O'Donohue (Eds.), *Practitioner's guide to evidence-based psychotherapy*. New York: Springer.

(Leonard, Lenane, Swedo, Rettew, & Rapoport, 1991). The absence of any association with psychopathology and the absence of any evidence of symptom substitution when nail biting is eliminated provide convincing evidence that nail biting is not a symptom of an underlying psychological problem, as historically claimed by psychoanalysts.

Prevalence

Nail biting is highly prevalent in children and adolescents with estimates ranging from 30% to 50% (e.g. McClanahan, 1995; Pennington, 1945). Although often considered to be a developmental problem, nail biting persists and is also common among adults. Ballinger (1970) reported a nail biting prevalence of approximately 20% among adults, a prevalence rate that approximates that reported by Pennington (1945) among naval recruits. Some variability in prevalence rates may result from different samples. Stringent versus lenient definitions of nail biting also contribute to variability in prevalence rates. For example, when a frequency criterion was added to the definition of nail biting, (five episodes or more per day), the percentage of colleges students reporting nail biting dropped from 52.7% (reporting any nail biting) to 18.2% (Brosh & Fuqua, 2004), a level that was comparable to other prevalence rates using the more stringent definition of nail biting (Woods, Miltenberger, & Flach, 1996).

Age at Onset

Nail biting behavior has been reported in children as young as four. The prevalence peaks during adolescence, between ages 10 and 18 (Ballinger, 1970). Fingernail biting is considered to be a developmental problem (Hadley, 1984). Previous studies (Malone & Masler, 1952; Wechsler, 1931) suggest that the peak period for nail biting is somewhere between the ages of 8–14. More recent research by Ballinger (1970) found that the peak period for fingernail biting was at the age range of 10–19 in a sample of nondiagnosed participants. Ballinger (1970) also found that there is a slow and gradual decrease in this behavior after it reaches its peak

Gender

Nail biting is slightly more prevalent among females than among males (Brosh & Fuqua, 2004).

Course

Nail biting typically begins in childhood or early adolescence. Many nail biters terminate the behavior or manage it at acceptable levels without special interventions, although probably motivated by social consequences. Nevertheless, nail biting is reported in approximately 20% of adults and approximately 5% of 60 year olds. This suggests that for some, the behavior pattern is highly durable. Little is known about changes in the frequency or severity over the life span

Impairment and Other Demographic Characteristics

As mentioned previously, persistent, high frequency nail biting can produce chronic infection, inflammation, bleeding and, in some cases, damage to the nail bed and loss of nails. In severe cases, the physical symptoms may be sufficiently painful to interfere with a range of daily activities involving the hands and fingers (e.g., typing, buttoning shirts). Furthermore, nail biting may also produce craniomandibular dysfunction problems and dental damage that results in orthodontic treatment.

ASSESSMENT

What Should be Ruled Out?

In severe cases, a dermatologist and/or orthodontist should be consulted to rule out other medical causes for nail bed infection, inflammation and pain and to assess dental problems and tempro mandibular joint pain. In addition to treating the behavioral causes of these physical symptoms, supplementary medical interventions (e.g., antibiotics, orthodontia, or in extreme cases, surgery) can be initiated at the same time that behavioral interventions for nail biting are implemented.

What is Involved in Effective Assessment?

Nail biting is not recognized in the DSM IV as a separate diagnostic category. Therefore, assessment efforts are not designed to yield a diagnosis but rather to characterize the severity of the nail biting problem, to monitor progress or to identify probably controlling variables for nail biting.

Clinician-administered measures There are few clinician-administered measures for the assessment of nail biting. In research studies, measures of nail length have been used to monitor progress. Using calipers to measures nail length is simple and efficient strategy for monitoring treatment progress. However, measures of nail length, if used alone, may not detect changes in the damage to soft tissue such as cuticles. Additionally, photographs, taken over the course of treatment have been used to rate skin damage and nail biting severity using a simple rating scale described by Malone and Massler (1952).

While the above assessment strategies are helpful in evaluating treatment efficacy, they provide little information about the "causes" of nail biting. Behavior assessment interviews (e.g., Miltenberger & Fuqua, 1985) may be conducted to provide a functional assessment of nail biting that is designed to clarify the response dimensions and to identify response antecedents and consequences that are plausible controlling variables for nail biting. The identification of controlling variables can often be used to develop interventions that avoid high risk situations (e.g., stressful but sedentary activities) or help to identify coping strategies, including replacement behaviors that serve the same function (e.g., manipulating an object when involved in stressful, sedentary activities). Functional assessments appear to have treatment utility in that they have been used to develop effective interventions for a number of challenging behaviors. Unfortunately, functional assessment interviews are not routinely conducted with nail biters and, as a result, there is little information about the utility of such assessment strategies for the derivation of effective and efficient interventions for nail biting.

Self-report measures Two types of self-report measures have been used in nail biting research. A number of researchers have administered a nail biting questionnaire as a screening tool. A standardized questionnaire has not been published but a number of questions are typically addressed in such questionnaires, including questions about: frequency and duration of nail biting episodes, onset, prior treatment efforts, current motivation, and, in some cases questions about self-reported causal variables.

The other type of self-report measure involves self-recording of some daily measure of nail biting. In some cases, participants record the number or duration of nail biting episodes per day or the number of "urges" to engage in this behavior. In many instances these self-report measures also include identification of the context in which nail biting occurs, such as location, time or emotional state, and on rare occasion some report on the consequences of nail biting (social reaction, changes in emotional state). There is no standard procedure or materials for such self-report measures but, in general, any procedure that is convenient and portable enough to allow recording to occur in close proximity of the nail biting occurrence is recommended to increase the accuracy of measures from self-recording. Index cards and golf wrist counters are low technology examples of such recording devices although the advent of portable electronic devices (e.g., personal data assistants) would be worthy of consideration. Of the assessment measures that are relevant to nail biting, self-reports are most clearly indicated for monitoring clinical progress.

Behavioral assessment Behavior assessment typically relies on direct observation of a target behavior, although indirect measures, such as response products (e.g., nail length or damage) are also used. Direct observation measures of nail biting have been rarely used in clinical research and treatment. The relative lack of direct observation assessments is probably a result of two factors: many direct observation assessments are reactive (the level of behavior changes when the person is aware of the observation) and direct observation may involve significant effort (personnel, arranging observation opportunities). In general, more effortful and intrusive observation procedures should be reserved for serious, disabling behavioral problems. Clinical treatment of nail biting generally does not qualify for resource intensive and potentially intrusive behavior assessment procedures such as direct observation.

Nevertheless, a small number of researchers have employed direct observation measures of nail biting. Brosh and Fuqua (2004) surreptitiously videotaped college students as they engaged in a series of activities for which participants were told that the experiment was a stuffy of physiological reactivity to the various activities. After the session, the presence of the videotape and the purpose of the experiment (a functional analysis of habit behaviors) were disclosed to participants and they were asked for permission to score the resulting videotapes for nail biting and other habit behaviors. All participants granted permission to score the videotape under the condition that their confidentiality be protected. The video tapes were subsequently scored using a 5 second partial interval scoring system (e.g., Kazdin, 1982) yielding a measure of the percentage of intervals in which at least one instance of nail biting (or other habit behavior) was recorded. A second observer independently scored half of the videotapes. Comparing the interval by interval scoring of the primary and secondary observers yielded inter observer agreement levels in excess of 95%. Such direct observation strategies are increasingly required for methodologically sound research but except in rare instances are too intrusive and resource intensive for clinical work.

Finally, a small number of studies have applied functional analysis methodology (e.g., Repp & Horner, 1999) to the identification of environmental conditions associated with elevated levels of nail biting and other habit behaviors (Brosh & Fuqua, 2004; Woods, et al., 2001; Woods & Miltenberger, 1996; Woods, Miltenberger, & Flach, 1996). This research involves the assessment of nail biting (and other habit behaviors) under test conditions designed to evaluate hypothesized causal variables. To determine if nail biting might be a variant of self-stimulatory behavior, observations have been conducted under conditions of low stimulation (designed to evoke boredom) and also while engaged in passive activities (e.g., viewing a television program). Observing nail biting under anxiety provoking conditions (having a participant prepare to give a public lecture on an unfamiliar topic) provides a test of whether nail biting is provoked by anxiety or reinforced by decreases in anxiety. Results have been somewhat inconsistent across subjects and across habit behavior topographies. Nevertheless, it appears that nail biting (and other oral habits) is more elevated under low stimulation conditions (boredom) and under passive activities with distracted attention (e.g., viewing television) than under control conditions or anxiety conditions. These observations suggest that nail biting my serve a sensory stimulation function. These results should be interpreted cautiously because of the limited number of subjects and concerns about the validity of the test conditions. Nevertheless, functional analysis methodology provides a promising strategy for the analysis of the causes of nail biting and possibly for the derivation of interventions that are tailored to the unique causal variables for nail biting.

What Assessments are Not Helpful?

Traditional psychology assessment strategies (objective and projective tests) are *not* recommended for the assessment of nail biting. There is no evidence that nail biting is related to underlying psychological or personality disorders and such testing yields no useful information for improving treatment outcomes for nail biting.

TREATMENT

What Treatments are Effective?

A behavioral intervention known as "habit reversal" appears to be the most effective intervention for habit behaviors, including nail biting. Habit reversal was initially developed as treatment package containing 10 components, which were organized into four phases, awareness training, competing response training, motivation procedures and generalization procedures (Azrin & Nunn, 1973). This multicomponent treatment package proved to be effective in the treatment of a variety of habit behaviors (see Miltenberger, Fuqua, & Woods, 1998 for a review), including nail biting (e.g., Azrin, Nunn, & Frantz, 1980).

Subsequent research has verified that a simplified version of habit reversal, consisting of three components (awareness training, response contingent competing response practice, and social support) produces decrements in habit behaviors that are comparable to the treatment effects of the original 10-component procedure (e.g., Miltenberger, Fuqua, & McKinley, 1985; Rapp, Miltenberger, Long, Elliott, & Lumley, 1998). This simplified version of habit reversal (SHR) is easier to implement in clinical settings and more efficient than the original procedure. A detailed description of the SHR treatment protocol is published elsewhere (Woods & Twohig, 2001) and will not be reproduced herein.

Furthermore, there is evidence that the topography of the competing response need not be physically incompatible with the target behavior (e.g., Sharenow, Fuqua, & Miltenberger, 1989; Woods et al., 1999). had some participants engage in a competing response (e.g., clenching the fists) that was incompatible with the habit behavior (e.g., nail biting) and other in a dissimilar competing behavior that could occur at the same time as the habit behavior (e.g., pressing the knees together). Both similar and dissimilar competing responses were associated with clinically significant reductions in the habit behaviors, although the similar competing response produced slightly larger decrements in the habit behavior. Furthermore, there is some evidence suggesting that maintenance of a contingent relationship between practice of the competing response and the habit behavior is essential to the response suppressing effect of habit reversal (Miltenberger & Fuqua, 1985). Said another way, noncontingent practice of a competing response, even one that is physically incompatible with the habit behavior, has little clinical impact. These observations are congruent with speculation that the mechanism of action for habit reversal may involve self-administered punishment.

The efficacy of a simplified habit reversal treatment package (SHR) has been replicated with nail biting with adult participants (e.g., Allen, 1996; Azrin et al., 1980; De Luca & Holborn, 1984; Horne & Wilkinson, 1980; Silber & Haynes, 1992) and with normally developing children (e.g., Woods et al., 1999). In general the results are quite impressive. Habit reversal and its simplified variants produce significant reductions in nail biting with corresponding improvements in physical damage to fingernails and cuticles. Complete and rapid elimination of nail biting and excellent maintenance of the behavior changes are commonly reported.

There is, however, an important qualifier to what is otherwise an impressive set of data that supports the efficacy of habit reversal as a treatment for nail biting. Efforts to replicate SHR with individuals diagnosed with mild to moderate mental retardation produced mixed results with three of four participants failing to show significant improvements in fingernail biting or hand to mouth behavior (Long, Miltenberger, Ellingson, & Ott, 1999). For one individual, the habit behavior was eventually eliminated after the addition of a reminder prompt to engage in the competing response after each habit behavior. For two other individuals who failed to respond favorably to the SHR, the addition of supplementary response contingencies was required to get elimination of the habit behaviors. These supplementary contingencies included monetary consequences for periods of time without engaging in the habit behavior and for engaging in the competing response contingent on a habit behavior. In addition, monetary fines for each occurrence of the habit behavior were also implemented. SHR plus these supplementary contingencies resulted in near or complete suppression of nail biting and hand to mouth oral behaviors for the remaining participants. The authors speculated that some people might require the addition of special motivational contingencies to promote adherence to the essential components of SHR. These observations underscore the importance of some minimal level of treatment adherence (including the response contingent competing response practice component of SHR) as a necessary component for producing clinically significant treatment effect.

In addition to SHR one additional punishment procedure and a positive reinforcement procedure have produced promising results with nail biting. Researchers have reported promising results from an aversive technique that involves painting the nails with a commercially available bitter substance (Allen, 1996; Silber & Haynes, 1992; Vargas & Adesso, 1976). In one study (Allen, 1996) the group treated with this form of mild aversion yielded results that were slightly better than those obtained with SHR. In the other direct comparison of the two procedures (Silber & Haynes, 1992), SHR produced better results than the bitter substance intervention. Neither study reported the collection of treatment adherence data so it is difficult to determine whether inconsistent results might be attributed to differing degrees of treatment adherence.

A small number of studies have evaluated positive reinforcement procedures for nail biting. Most of these studies have combined positive reinforcement procedures in multi component packages making it difficult to isolate the contribution of positive reinforcement along (e.g., Davidson, Denny & Elliott, 1980). Two studies have reported decrements in nail biting as function of positive reinforcement delivered contingent on either nail growth or the absence of observed nail biting (Adesso, Vargas, & Siddall, 1979; Long et al., 1999).

Finally, a small number of studies have evaluated relaxation-based interventions for nail biting. DeLuca and Holborn (1972) reported that relaxation training did not reduce nail biting. In contrast, Barrios (1977) reported that cue controlled relaxation reduced nail biting but the relaxation was implemented as a competing response, much like the response contingent competing response component of SHR. Thus it is premature to conclude that relaxation training is a promising treatment for nail biting.

What are Effective Self-Help Treatments?

Self help treatments are recommended when (1) the treatment is relatively easy to apply, even by untrained personnel; (2) when the treatment produces few, if any, adverse side effects if it is not applied effectively and (3) when failure to immediately and significantly reduce the target behavior does not pose serious health or legal problems for the person engaging in the behavior or for others in proximity of the behavior. Using these criteria, it appears that a bitter substance applied to the nails is a good candidate for self-help treatment, although some monitoring to prevent overuse of the bitter substance is recommended. In addition major components of SHR are typically implemented as a self-help treatment after some initial therapist training. In some cases (e.g., children or persons with limited instruction following capabilities), supplementary contingencies may prove helpful to insure treatment adherence (e.g., Long et al., 1999). While both interventions appear to be good candidates for self-help applications, studies evaluating the efficacy and treatment adherence of such self-contained interventions have yet to be reported.

What are Effective Therapist-Based Treatments?

SHR typically requires a qualified therapist to train the client in response detection and the application of the competing response and to train the social support person(s). Thereafter, the therapist's role shifts to focus on monitoring treatment adherence, monitoring progress and trouble-shooting treatment failures.

What is Effective Medical Treatment?

Leonard et al., (1991) report promising results from an evaluation of clomipramine hydrochloride although a high drop out rate (11 of 24 participants) and absence of replication studies limits conclusions about the efficacy of pharmacological treatment for nail biting.

Combination Treatments

Combinations of promising treatments (e.g., SHR and bitter tasting nail polish) have not been experimentally evaluated.

Other Issues in Management

Medical treatment As mentioned earlier, serious infection of the cuticles and nail beds as well as orthodontic damage should be evaluated and treated by qualified medical personnel.

Psychotherapy Psychotherapy has *not* been documented as an effective treatment for nail biting.

How Does One Select Among Treatments?

Because of its simplicity, low cost and reasonable efficacy, we recommend a trial of bitter tasting nail polish as the first line of intervention. Those fail to benefit from this intervention should seek out a behavior therapist that is qualified in the application of habit reversal techniques.

REFERENCES

Adesso, V. J., Vargas, J. M., & Siddall, J. W. (1979). The role of awareness in reducing nail biting behavior. *Behavior Therapy, 10,* 148–154.

Allen, K. W. (1996). Chronic nail biting: a controlled comparison of competing response and mild aversion treatments. *Behaviour Research and Therapy, 34,* 269–272.

Azrin, N. H., & Nunn, R. G. (1973). Habit Reversal: A method of eliminating nervous habits and tics. *Behaviour Reseaach and Therapy, 11,* 619–628.

Azrin, N. H., Nunn, R. G., & Frantz, S. E. (1980). Habit reversal versus negative practice treatment of nail biting. *Behaviour Research and Taherapy, 18,* 281–285.

Ballinger, B. R. (1970). The prevalence of nail-biting in normal and abnormal populations. *British Journal of Psychiatry, 117,* 445–446.

Baran, R., & Dawber, R. P. R. (1984). *Diseases of the nails and their management.* Oxford: Blackwell.

Barrios, B. A. (1977). Cue-controlled relaxation in reduction of chronic nervous habits. *Psychological Reports, 41,* 703–706.

Brosh, S., & Fuqua, W (May, 2004). An experimental analysis of antecedents to habit behaviors. Paper presented at the Association for Behavior Analysis, Chicago, IL.

Clark, D. F. (1970). Nail biting in subnormals. *British Journal of Medical Psychology. 43,* 69–81.

Davidson, A. M., Denny, D. R., & Elliott, C. H. (1980). Suppression and substitution in the treatment of nail biting. *Behaviour Research and Therapy, 18,* 1–9.

De Luca, R. V., & Holborn, S. W. (1984). A comparison of relaxation training and competing response training to eliminate hair pulling and nail biting. *Journal of Behaviour Therapy and Experimental Psychiatry, 15,* 67–70.

Deardorff, P. A., Finch, A. J., & Royall, L. R. (1974). Manifest anxiety and nail biting. *Journal of Clinical Psychology, 30,* 378.

Hadley, N. H. (1984). Fingernail biting: Theory, research and treatment. Jamaica, NY: Spectrum Publications.

Horne, D. J., & Wilkinson, J. (1980). Habit reversal treatment for fingernail biting. *Behaviour Research and Therapy, 18,* 287–291.

Kanner, L. (1957). *Child Psychiatry.* Springfield, IL: Charles C. Thomas Publisher.

Kazdin, A. E. (1982). *Single-case research designs.* New York: Oxford University Press.

Klatte, K., & Deardorff, P. A. (1981). Nail biting and manifest anxiety of adults. *Psychological Reports, 48,* 82.

Leonard, H. L., Lenane, M. C., Swedo, S. E., Rettew, D. C., & Rapoport, J. L. (1991). A Double-blind comparison of clomipramine and desipramine treatment of severe onychophagia (Nail biting). *Archives of General Psychiatry, 48,* 821–827.

Long, E. S., Miltenberger, R. G., Ellingson, S. A., & Ott, S. M. (1999). Augmenting simplified habit reversal in the treatment of oral-digital habits exhibited by individuals with mental retardation. *Journal of Applied Behavior Analysis, 32,* 353–365.

Lowry, D. P. (1965). Bedwetting and nail biting in military recruits. *Military Medicine, 130,* 47–54.

Malone, A. J., & Masler, M. (1952). Index of nail biting in children. *Journal of Abnormal and Social Psychology, 47,* 193–202.

McClanahan, T. M. (1995). Operant learning (R–S) principles applied to nail-biting. *Psychological Reports, 77,* 504–517.

Miltenberger, R. G., & Fuqua, R. W. (1985). Evaluation of a training manual for the acquisition of behavioral assessment interviewing skills. *Journal of Applied Behavior Analysis, 18,* 323–328.

Miltenberger, R. G., & Fuqua, R. W. (1985). A comparison of contingent versus non-contingent competing response practice in the treatment of nervous habits, 195–200.

Miltenberger, R. G., Fuqua, R. W., & McKinley, T. (1985). Habit reversal with muscle tics: Replication and component analysis. *Behavior Therapy, 16,* 39–50.

Miltenberger, R. G., Fuqua, R. W., & Woods, D. W. (1998). Applying behavior analysis to clinical problems: Review and analysis of habit reversal. *Journal of Applied Behavior Analysis, 31,* 447–469.

Odenrick, L., & Brattstrom, V. (1985). Nail biting: Frequency and association with root resportion during orthodontic treatment. *British Journal of Orthodontics, 12,* 78–81.

Pennington, L. A. (1945). The incidence of nail biting among adults. *American Journal of Psychiatry, 102,* 241–244.

Rapp, J. T., Miltenberger, R. G., Long, E. S. Elliott, A. J., & Lumley, V. A, (1998). Simplified habit reversal treatment for chronic hair pulling in three adolescents: Clinical replication with direct observation. *Journal of Applied Behavior Analysis, 31,* 299–302.

Repp, A. C., & Horner, R. H. (1999). *Functional Analysis of Problem Behaviors.* Belmont, CA: Wadsworth Publishing.

Schneider, P. E., & Peterson, J. (1982). Oral habits: Considerations in management. *Pediatric Clinics of North America.*

Sharenow, E. L., Fuqua, R. W., & Miltenberger. R. G. (1989). The treatment of muscle tics with dissimilar competing response practice. *Journal of Applied Behavior Analysis, 22,* 35–42.

Silber, K. P., & Haynes, C. E. (1992). Treating nail biting: A comparative analysis of mild aversion and competing response therapies. *Behaviour Research and Therapy, 30,* 15–32.

Vargas, J. M., & Adesso, V. J. (1976). A comparison of aversion threpies for nail biting behavior. *Behavior Therapy, 7,* 322–329.

Walker, B. A., & Ziskind, E. (1977). Relationship of nail biting to sociopathy. *Journal of Nervous and Mental Diseases, 164,* 64–67.

Wells, J. H., Haines, J., Williams, C. L., & Brain, K. L. (1999). The self-mutilative nature of severe Onychophagia: A comparison with self-cutting. *Canadian Journal of Psychiatry, 44,* 40–47.

Wechsler, D. (1931). The incidence and significance of fingernail biting in children. *Psychoanalyst, 18,* 201–209.

Woods, D. W., Fuqua, R. W., Siah, A., Murray, L. K., Welch, M., Blackman, E., et al., (2001). Understanding habits: A preliminary investigation of nail biting function in children. *Education and Treatment of Children, 24(2),* 199–216.

Woods, D. W., & Miltenberger, R. G. (1996). Are people with nervous habits nervous? A preliminary examination of habit function in a non-referred population. *Journal of Applied Behavior Analysis, 29,* 259–261.

Woods, D. W., & Miltenberger, R. G. (2001). Tic Disorders, Trichotillomania, and other repetitive behavior disorders: Behavioral approaches to analysis and treatment. Boston, MA: Kluwer Academic Publishers.

Woods, D. W., Miltenberger, R. G., & Flach, A. D. (1996). Habits, tics, and stuttering: Prevalence and relations to anxiety and somatic awareness. *Behavior Modification, 20(2),* 216–225.

Woods, D. W., Murray, L. K., Fuqua, R. W., Seif, T. A.1, Boyer, L. J., & Siah, A. (1999). Comparing the effectiveness of similar and dissimilar competing responses in evaluating the habit reversal treatment for oral–digital habits in children. *Journal of Behavior Therapy and Experimental Psychiatry, 30,* 289–300.

Woods, D. W., & Twohig, M. P. (2001). Habit reversal treatment manual for oral–digital habits. In Woods, D. W., & Miltenberger, R. G. (Eds.). Tic disorders, trichotillomania, and other repetitive behavior disorders. Norwell, MA: Kluwer Academic Publishers.

Narcissistic Personality Disorder

W. Keith Campbell • Roy F. Baumeister

AUTHOR NOTE

We thank Steven Beach, Amy Brunell, and Renee Schneider for helpful comments and suggestions regarding this manuscript.

WHAT IS NARCISSISTIC PERSONALITY DISORDER?

Narcissistic personality disorder (NPD) is one the group of cluster B disorders that also includes antisocial, histrionic, and borderline. NPD involves three elements: an inflated view of the self, a lack of warmth or empathy in relationships, and the use of a variety of strategies for maintaining the inflated self-views.

The inflated self-views of those with NPD can include the general sense of specialness, uniqueness, self-esteem, and entitlement coupled with specific inflated self-beliefs (e.g., Campbell, Bonacci, Shelton, Exline, & Bushman, 2004; Emmons, 1984). For example, there may be the belief that one is smarter, more attractive, or more creative than others. These inflated views tend to fall in the area of social dominance rather than social warmth. Narcissism is not associated with seeing one-self as more caring and kind than others (Campbell, Rudich, & Sedikides, 2002). Instead they want to be seen as beings with high status and competence.

Consistent with the view that narcissists are less concerned with warmth and intimacy than with other admirable attributes, they exhibit a relative disinterest in caring and selflessness in romantic relationships (e.g., Campbell, Foster, & Finkel, 2002). They score low on self-report measures of agreeableness (Bradlee & Emmons, 1992) and on projective measures of intimacy such as the TAT (Carroll, 1987). The lack of warmth, however, does not mean that those with NPD are not social. Quite the contrary, narcissism is associated with social extraversion (Bradlee & Emmons, 1992). Indeed, more narcissistic individuals tend to be well-liked in initial social meetings (Paulhus, 1998).

Narcissism is associated with the use of a wide range of strategies for maintaining inflated self-views. These strategies can be categorized as either intrapsychic or interpersonal. Intrapsychically, narcissism is associated with fantasies of success and power (Raskin & Novacek, 1991) as well as the self-serving bias (that is, taking credit for success but blaming the situation for failure) (e.g., Campbell, Reeder, Sedikides, & Elliot, 2000). Interpersonally, narcissism is associated with the use of social situations for enhancing status and esteem. Such strategies include bragging and boasting (Buss & Chiodo, 1991), competing (Raskin & Terry, 1988), and striving (often successfully to excel at challenging tasks when others are watching (Wallace & Baumeister, 2002). Narcissism is also associated with indirect strategies for gaining status and esteem, such as acquiring "trophy" romantic partners (Campbell, 1999) and expensive material goods (Vohs & Campbell, 2004).

When faced with the threatening information about the self, such as negative feedback, narcissism can be linked to violence or aggression against those who

Campbell, W. K., & Baumeister, R. F. (2006). Narcissistic personality disorder. In J. E. Fisher & W. T. O'Donohue (Eds.), *Practitioner's guide to evidence-based psychotherapy*. New York: Springer.

criticize the narcissist (Bushman & Baumeister, 1998) or who socially reject the narcissist (Twenge & Campbell, 2003). Narcissists will also derogate those who are critical of them (Kernis & Sun, 1994). On group tasks, narcissists are quick to blame their coworkers for any failure or poor performance, rather than risk taking blame themselves (Campbell, et al., 2000).

These interpersonal and intrapsychic patterns can be seen as self-regulatory efforts to sustain positive views of self. In that, narcissists are often successful, and narcissism in normal populations is associated with higher self-esteem, and lower depression and anxiety, as compared with other people (Rose & Campbell, in press). There is scant evidence that narcissism is associated with success in any linear way. It is more likely that narcissism is beneficial in some settings (those aided by confidence and extraversion) and harmful in others (those hampered by overconfidence) (e.g., Wallace & Baumeister, 2002; Campbell, Goodie, & Foster, in press).

This model of narcissism—inflated self-views, lack of warmth or empathy, and self-regulation strategies—can be seen in the DSM-IV criteria for NPD (American Psychiatric Association, 1994). According to the DSM-IV, NPD includes:
A pervasive pattern of grandiosity (in fantasy or behavior), need for admiration, and lack of empathy, beginning by early adulthood and present in a variety of contexts, as indicated by five (or more) of the following:

1. has a grandiose sense of self-importance (e.g., exaggerates achievements and talents, expects to be recognized as superior without commensurate achievements)
2. is preoccupied with fantasies of unlimited success, power, brilliance, beauty, or ideal love
3. believes that he or she is "special" and unique and can only be understood by, or should associate with, other special or high-status people (or institutions)
4. requires excessive admiration
5. has a sense of entitlement, i.e., unreasonable expectations of especially favorable treatment or automatic compliance with his or her expectations
6. is interpersonally exploitative, i.e., takes advantage of others to achieve his or her own ends
7. lacks empathy: is unwilling to recognize or identify with the feelings and needs of others
8. is often envious of others or believes that others are envious of him or her
9. shows arrogant, haughty behaviors or attitudes

This definition includes the positive views of self (grandiosity, specialness, entitlement), a lack of interpersonal warmth and sensitivity ("lacks empathy", exploitativeness, envy, arrogance), and several self-regulation strategies (fantasies, admiration).

Still, there is disagreement over the nature of NPD. The biggest source of disagreement in NPD involves the psychic underpinnings of the disorder. In one camp, largely psychodynamic in origin, it is argued that narcissism is a defensive response to some inner sense of abandonment, shame or hurt (e.g., Kernberg, 1975). In the other camp, based largely on research in social, cognitive, and personality psychology, narcissism is seen as an offensive rather than defensive condition, and no soft inner core of self-loathing is postulated. Narcissism in this second view is associated with overconfidence, approach orientation, and extraversion. If reality monitoring is lost, it is largely a result of excessive zeal in the quest for status and esteem. Indeed, some have argued that narcissism is in many ways like an addiction (Baumeister & Vohs, 2001), in which the positive experiences of being admired and esteeming oneself can becoming reinforcing.

The disagreement as to whether to conceptualize narcissism as offensive or defensive has not been resolved. Our opinion lies closer to the latter (offensive) view, though like many others we prefer to reserve judgment until more evidence is available. In current empirical studies, narcissism appears largely the result of a desire for status and esteem with little restraint from warm social relationships (see Morf & Rhodewalt, 2001, for review). However, there are arguments to be made on both sides, with some suggesting that there are two forms of narcissism (e.g., Millon & Davis, 1996; Rose, 2002).

A second debate involves the structure of narcissism. Is narcissism a dimensional variable, with NPD representing the top of the continuum or a subset of individuals? Or does NPD represent a discrete type? Millon and Davis (1996) and others (including ourselves) think that narcissism might be best considered a continuous variable rather than a discrete category. Although NPD would fall on the extreme end of the narcissism continuum, the clinical sample of NPD is not representative of this extreme group. Instead, so-called "failed narcissists" are overrepresented in those diagnosed with NPD (Campbell, 2000). Failed narcissists are those in whom the narcissistic self-regulatory strategies are not successful at sustaining the desired high level of self-esteem. For example, failed narcissists may be experiencing depression in the aftermath of a series of career disappointments and unmet goals. From the failed narcissist's perspective, the depression, not the NPD, is the problem. This small group of failed narcissists, then, is different from the majority of narcissists who are largely happy and nondepressed. This skewed sample of those with NPD seen by clinicians may, in part, be responsible for the view of narcissism as a defense against clandestine feelings of worthlessness (described above).

If this dimensional conceptualization of narcissism is correct, this has important implications for research. There is very little research done on individuals diagnosed with NPD. This reflects the low number of individuals with NPD seeking treatment, as well as perhaps funding priorities by the major research grant agencies. The alternative is to conduct research on nonclinical samples. This approach allows access to far more research participants and opens the door for more rapid theoretical progress. Indeed, the majority of research findings presented here are from nonclinical samples.

BASIC FACTS ABOUT NPD

Comorbidity. Comorbidity depends on the current state of the individual with NPD. Those who have experienced a series of failures may present with depression or dysthimia. In contrast, individuals with NPD who are doing well in life may present with hypomania. There also may be some link between NPD and anorexia nervosa as well as drug use. NPD is associated with the other cluster B personality disorders, and even some cluster A disorders such as paranoid personality.

Frequency. According to the DSM-IV, less than 1% of the general population suffers from NPD. Our impression is that there are far more narcissists around than that figure would suggest, but that most of those with NPD are high functioning (at least from their own perspective) and therefore do not request psychological treatment.

Age. NPD should not be diagnosed until early adulthood, because many symptoms of NPD are common (and perhaps developmentally normative) among adolescents. As a rule, the prevalence of narcissism declines with age. There is evidence for this in cross-sectional data from nonclinical samples (Foster, Campbell, & Twenge, 2003).

Gender. According to the DSM-IV, 50–75% of those with NPD are male. This same pattern is found in research on narcissism in normal samples. There is a small association between gender and narcissism, $r = .12$, with males being slightly more narcissistic (Campbell et al., 2003). This finding is similar to gender differences in self-esteem (Kling, Hyde, Showers, & Buswell, 1999).

Racial Differences. NPD is not associated with any racial differences. In normal samples, self-reported narcissism differs slightly across racial and cultural groups, with Asians being on the lower end of a continuum and African Americans on the higher end (Foster, et al., 2003). This parallels the differences found in self-esteem (Twenge & Crocker, 2002). These differences in narcissism are sufficiently small as to be regarded as without practical importance (e.g., r's < .10) and nondiagnostic.

ASSESSMENT

What Should be Ruled Out?

Narcissism can be confused with the related cluster B personality disorders, so it is important to rule those out. Antisocials are typically not as interested as narcissists in gaining admiration, although they are often hypervigilant for disrespect. Narcissism is also associated with greater extraversion than antisocial personality. Likewise, individuals with antisocial personality show greater difficulty with impulse control and are likely to have a childhood history of law breaking or other misconduct. Histrionic individuals are more emotionally buoyant and dramatic than those with NPD. NPD is associated with a "insouciant" affect—basically a detached nonchalance (Millon & Davis, 1996). Last, borderline personality disorder is relatively easy to distinguish from NPD. Borderline personality is more likely than NPD to be associated with self-destructive behavior patterns (e.g., cutting), split object relations (e.g., love or hatred for the same individual across a short period of time), and greater concern with abandonment (DSM-IV).

NPD and some cluster A personality disorders, especially paranoid, can occasionally share similarly grandiose views of the place of the self in the world (Millon & Davis, 1996). Indeed, Freud's original monograph on narcissism linked it potentially with some autistic-like, self-absorbed mental conditions. NPD is different from these other disorders in that it is usually associated with good social skills, even charm and likeability. Those with NPD typically do not appear odd or bizarre.

Grandiose states of mind similar to these in NPD can be found in states of hypomania (or the similar drug-induced states, such as cocaine use). The affective element of these manic states, as well as the nature of their onset, may help rule them out.

The DSM-IV suggests that people who are high in status such as celebrities can have NPD-like symptoms, but celebrity status should not be confused with NPD unless functioning is impaired. We would argue that NPD can be an appropriate diagnosis even when functioning is temporarily high. For example, you can have a CEO of a large company who throws lavish parties and belittles fellow employees but functions adequately in terms of the successful management of his company. If the stock market drops and people start to question the CEO's behavior, however, he or she may start engaging is potentially self-destructive behaviors (e.g., cooking the books, blaming others). We do not think that the NPD emerges when the trouble starts; more likely, it has been there the entire time, but it was not perceived as a problem as long as the profits were good. Indeed, it may be more broadly true that social circumstances dictate when NPD is seen as a pathological disorder and when it is seen as an understandable or merely annoying pattern of self-congratulation in a successful person. Nonetheless, certain circumstances, such as celebrity status, power, and fame, should be considered risk factors for NPD, because they promote and reinforce self-love to an extent that may seem appropriate during phases of worldly success but then may seem pathological when sustained through less successful periods.

What is Involved in Effective Assessment?

Assessment of NPD usually involves a structured clinical interview, such as the SCID-II (First, Spitzer, Gibbon, & Williams, 1997). This interview is based on the DSM criteria for NPD and can help a clinician make a reasonable diagnosis.

There are self-report measures that are also useful for assessing narcissism. The Millon Clinical Multiaxial Inventory-III (MCMI-III) (Million, Millon, & Davis, 1994) is consistent in large part with the DSM and can be used to diagnose NPD as well as illuminate potential subtypes (e.g., amorous, unprincipled). The narcissistic personality disorder (NPI; Raskin & Hall, 1979) is the most commonly used measure for assessing narcissism in nonclinical samples, primarily for research purposes. It is derived from the DSM-III criteria for NPD, but has no explicit "cut-off" for NPD. The Millon and NPI correlate positively in clinical samples (Prifitera & Ryan, 1984).

There are various other scales used to measure more "covert" aspects of narcissism. These have marginal reliability and tend to not correlate (or they correlate negatively) with the NPI, and we would not recommend their use (Soyer, Rovenpor, Kopelman, Mullins, & Watson, 2001).

What Assessments are Not Helpful?

Projective measures for NPD, such as the TAT or Rorschach, tend to yield mixed responses from those with NPD (Millon & Davis, 1996). This makes these measures marginally helpful. There is no known biological marker.

TREATMENT

What are Effective Therapist Based Treatments?

We know of no solid treatment outcomes studies on NPD. It is difficult to find a large sample of individuals with NPD who actually want to be treated. If you think you are better than other people, have high self-esteem, and are happy, why would you seek psychotherapy? There is certainly a small percentage of individuals with NPD who do have some insight into their problem and do want to change, but this is not the norm. Clearly, the lack of treatment outcome research for NPD is a major problem that needs to be addressed.

Despite the lack of treatment outcome research on NPD, there is a wealth of clinical treatment reports. These reports share two common similarities: (1) narcissism is difficult to treat and the treatments are not often effective, and (2) one key in treatment is to form a strong alliance with the client. This alliance is crucial to encouraging the client to remain in therapy. Beyond these basics, there are three overarching therapeutic approaches: a psychodynamic approach, an interpersonal approach, and a cognitive-behavioral approach, each broadly defined (Millon, 1999).

The historically oldest of the approaches is psychodynamic. These treatments are based largely on the work of Kernberg (1975) and Kohut (1977). The two had similar views on the appearance of narcissism, but they differed in terms of etiology, with Kernberg looking toward childhood abandonment issues as a source, and Kohut emphasizing a lack of mirroring in childhood. More recently, psychiatrists such as James Masterson have focused their practices on personality disorders. These efforts have produced well-written accounts both of therapy and of the disorder (e.g., Masterson, 1988; 1999). The commonality in these approaches is that they focus on negative childhood experience as crucial to the etiology of NPD, and they also use classic dynamic techniques in therapy (e.g., analysis of transference and countertransference, interpretation). It is also important to note that this view of the etiology of narcissism differs markedly from the learning model of narcissism proposed by Millon (e.g., Millon & Davis, 1996). Millon hypothesizes that narcissism is learned from parents who overestimate their offspring.

Interpersonal approaches are derived from the tradition of Sullivan. Interpersonal approaches focus on the structure of social relationships, both past and present, in therapy. In particular, the individual's representations of those relationships are investigated. The interpersonal approach has shown some promise in treating disorders such as NPD that have strong interpersonal components (Benjamin, 1993). (We should also note that group therapy is not generally recommended for NPD [Millon, 1999]).

More recent cognitive-behavioral approaches focus on the current manifestations of narcissism and the cognitions that accompany them. These are grandiose self-views, lack of empathy, and reactance to negative feedback. The goal of the therapy is to moderate these beliefs. Such techniques can range from the strictly cognitive (e.g., Beck & Freeman, 1990) to others that include a focus on the past more typical of psychodynamic therapies. For example, schema therapy (Young, Klosko, & Weishar, 2003) focuses on the development of early cognitive schemas or mental representation of self and other.

As noted, these different approaches to therapy have been used effectively with NPD, but there are no large scale treatment outcome studies. Given this lack of data, two other treatment approaches deserve consideration. First, there is a potential treatment for NPD that involves strengthening the narcissism rather than minimizing it. This approach, for example, may be advantageous in elderly populations (Jacobowitz & Newton, 1999). Simply reinforcing the client's narcissism should remove certain symptoms, especially those involving depression. Second, several forms of therapy based on the traditional meditation technique of "mindfulness" have been employed for a range of mental disorders (e.g., Baer, 2003; Roemer & Orsillo, 2002). Of particular note, mindfulness techniques have been used effectively as part of a broader dialectical behavior therapy (DBT) for individuals with borderline personality disorder (Linehan, 1993). Mindfulness practice has been used in the East for millennia to combat egotism, and it is plausible that these techniques might well prove useful in minimizing narcissism.

What are Effective Self-Help Treatments?

There are no known effective self-help treatments for NPD.

Useful websites There are few useful websites on NPD that we could find. Much of the information on the web is highly suspect. There are many discussion groups on NPD, but these are primarily aimed at those who have been victimized by narcissists, not at the narcissists themselves. There are also many sites on NPD that are not run by professionals. However, we could find few websites that were research based. Dr. Theodore Millon has a website on personality disorders at that is probably the best of these: http://www.millon.net.

What is Effective Medical Treatment?

Medical treatment may be effective for some of the symptoms reported by those with NPD, such as depression, but there is no known medical treatment for NPD.

How Does One Select Among Treatments?

Because treatment outcomes are so uncertain, treatment should be based on other factors, such as cost and therapist expertise. At present, our preference is for cognitive-behavioral techniques that focus on the current situation rather than those that focus on childhood etiology of the disorder. We make this recommendation because: (a) there are no good data on the etiology of narcissism, and (b) there is reason to believe that ongoing situational factors can lead to the development of narcissism (Baumeister & Vohs, 2001).

KEY READINGS

Psychodynamic approaches

Akhtar, S., & Thompson, J. A. (1982). Overview: Narcissistic personality disorder. *American Journal of Psychiatry, 139*, 12–20.

Kernberg, O. (1975). *Borderline conditions and pathological narcissism.* New York: Jason Aronson.

Kohut, H. (1977). *The restoration of the self.* New York. International Universities Press.

Masterson, J. F. (1999). *The personality disorders: A new look at the developmental self and object relations approach—Theory, diagnosis, treatment.* Connecticut: Zeig, Tucker & Theisen.

Interpersonal approaches

Benjamin, L. S. (1993). *Interpersonal diagnosis and treatment of personality disorders.* New York: Guilford Press.

Social-cognitive-personality approaches

Beck, A. T., & Freeman, A. (1990). *Cognitive therapy of personality disorders.* New York: Basic Books.

Emmons, R. A. (1987). Narcissism: Theory and measurement. *Journal of Personality and Social Psychology, 52*, 11-17.

Millon, T., & Davis, R. D. (1996). *Disorders of personality: DSM-IV and beyond.* (2nd ed.). New York: Wiley-Interscience.

Morf, C. C., & Rhodewalt, F. (2001). Unraveling the paradoxes of narcissism: A dynamic self-regulatory processing model. *Psychological Inquiry, 12*, 177–196.

Raskin, R. N., & Terry, H. (1988). A principle components analysis of the Narcissistic Personality Inventory and further evidence of its construct validity. *Journal of Personality and Social Psychology, 54*, 890–902.

REFERENCES

American Psychiatric Association (1994). *Diagnostic and statistical manual of mental disorders (4th ed., Revised).* Washington, DC: Author.

Baer, R. A (2003).Mindfulness training as a clinical intervention: A conceptual and empirical review. *Clinical Psychology: Science and Practice,* 125–143.

Baumeister, R. F., & Vohs, K. D. (2001). Narcissism as addiction to esteem. *Psychological Inquiry, 12*, 206–210.

Beck, A. T., & Freeman, A. (1990). *Cognitive therapy of personality disorders.* New York: Basic Books.

Benjamin, L. S. (1993). *Interpersonal diagnosis and treatment of personality disorders.* New York: Guilford Press.

Bradlee, P. M., & Emmons, R. A. (1992). Locating narcissism within the interpersonal circumplex and the five-factor model. *Personality and Individual Differences, 13*, 821–830.

Bushman, B. J., & Baumeister, R. F. (1998). Threatened egotism, narcissism, self-esteem, and direct and displaced aggression: Does self-love or self-hate lead to violence? *Journal of Personality and Social Psychology, 75*, 219–229.

Buss, D. M., & Chiodo, L. M. (1991). Narcissistic acts in everyday life. *Journal of Personality, 59*, 179–215.

Campbell, W. K. (1999). Narcissism and romantic attraction. *Journal of Personality and Social Psychology, 77*, 1254–1270.

Campbell, W. K., Bonacci, A. M., Shelton, J., Exline, J. J., & Bushman, B. J. (2004). Psychological entitlement: Interpersonal consequences and validation of a new self-report measure. *Journal of Personality Assessment, 83*, 29–45.

Campbell, W. K., Goodie, A. S., & Foster, J. D. (2004). Narcissism, overconfidence, and risk attitude. *Journal of Behavioral Decision Making, 17(4)*, 297–311.

Campbell, W. K., Reeder, G. D., Sedikides, C. (2000). Narcissism and comparative self-enhancement strategies. *Journal of Research in Personality, 34(3),* 329–347.

Campbell, W. K., Twenge, J. M. (2003). 'Isn't it fun to get the respect that we're going to deserve?' Narcissism, social rejection, and aggression. *Personality and Social Psychology Bulletin, 29(2),* 261–272.

Campbell, W. K., Reeder, G. D., Sedikides, C., & Elliot, A. J. (2000). Narcissism and comparative self-enhancement strategies. *Journal of Research in Personality, 34,* 329–347.

Campbell, W. K., Rudich, E., & Sedikides, C. (2002). Narcissism, self-esteem, and the positivity of self-views: Two portraits of self-love. *Personality and Social Psychology Bulletin, 28,* 358–368.

Carroll, L. (1987). A study of narcissism, affiliation, intimacy, and power motives among students in business administration. *Psychological Reports, 61,* 355–358.

Emmons, R. A. (1984). Factor analysis and construct validity of the Narcissistic Personality Inventory. *Journal of Personality Assessment, 48,* 291–300.

Foster, J. D., Campbell, W. K., & Twenge, J. M. (2003). Individual differences in narcissism: Inflated self-views across the lifespan and around the world. *Journal of Research in Personality, 37,* 469–486.

First, M. B., Spitzer, R. L., Gibbon, M., & Williams, J. B. W. (1997). Structured Clinical Interview for DSM-IV Personality Disorders, (SCID-II). Washington, DC: American Psychiatric Press, Inc.

Jacobowitz, J., & Newton, N. A. (1999). Dynamics and treatment of narcissism in later life. In M. Duffy (Ed.) *Handbook of counseling and psychotherapy with older adults,* pp. 453–469. New York: John Wiley.

Kernberg, O. (1975). *Borderline conditions and pathological narcissism.* New York: Jason Aronson.

Kernis, M. H., & Sun. C. (1994). Narcissism and reactions to interpersonal feedback. *Journal of Research in Personality, 28,* 4–13.

Kling, K. C., Hyde, J. S., Showers, C., & Buswell, B. (1999). Gender differences in self-esteem: A meta-analysis. *Psychological Bulletin, 125,* 470–500.

Kohut, H. (1977). *The restoration of the self.* New York. International Universities Press.

Linehan, M. M. (1993). *Cognitive-Behavioral Treatment of Borderline Personality Disorder.* New York: The Guilford Press.

Masterson, J. F. (1988). *The search for the real self.* New York: The Free Press.

Masterson, J. F. (1999). *The personality disorders: A new look at the developmental self and object relations approach—theory, diagnosis, treatment.* Connecticut: Zeig, Tucker & Theisen.

Millon, T. (1999). *Personality guided therapy.* New York: John Wiley.

Millon, T., Millon, C., Davis, R. (1994). *Millon Clinical Multiaxial Inventory-III (MCMI-III) Manual.* Minneapolis: National Computer Systems.

Millon, T., & Davis, R. D. (1996). *Disorders of personality: DSM-IV and beyond.(2nd ed.).* New York: Wiley-Interscience.

Morf, C. C., & Rhodewalt, F. (2001). Unraveling the paradoxes of narcissism: A dynamic self-regulatory processing model. *Psychological Inquiry, 12,* 177–196.

Paulhus, D. L. (1998). Interpersonal and intrapsychic adaptiveness of trait self-enhancement: A mixed blessing? *Journal of Personality and Social Psychology, 74,* 1197–1208.

Prifitera, A. & Ryan, J. J. (1984). Validity of the Narcissistic Personality Inventory (NPI) in a psychiatric sample. *Journal of Clinical Psychology, 40,* 140–142.

Raskin, R. N., & Hall, C. S. (1979) A narcissistic personality inventory. *Psychological Reports, 45,* 590.

Raskin, R. N., & Novacek, J. (1991). Narcissism and the use of fantasy. *Journal of Clinical Psychology, 47,* 490–499.

Raskin, R. N., & Terry, H. (1988). A principle components analysis of the Narcissistic Personality Inventory and further evidence of its construct validity. *Journal of Personality and Social Psychology, 54,* 890–902.

Roemer, L. & Orsillo, S. M. (2002). Expanding our conceptualization of and treatment for generalized anxiety disorder: Integrating mindfulness/acceptance-based approaches with existing cognitive-behavioral models. *Clinical Psychology: Science and Practice, 9,* 54–68.

Rose, P. (2002). The happy and unhappy faces of narcissism. *Personality and Individual Differences, 33,* 379–392.

Rose, P. & Campbell, W. K. (2004). Greatness feels good: A telic model of narcissism and subjective well-being. In S. P. Shohov (Ed.) *Advances in psychology research.* Hauppauge, NY: Nova Publishers, *31,* 1–25.

Soyer,. B., Rovenpor, J. L.. Kopelman, R. E., Mullins, L. S., & Watson, P. J. (2001). Further Assessment of the Construct Validity of Four Measures of Narcissism: Replication and Extension. *Journal of Psychology, 135,* 245–254.

Twenge, J., & Campbell, W. K. (2003). "Isn't it fun to get the respect that we're going to deserve?" Narcissism, social rejection, and aggression. *Personality and Social Psychology Bulletin, 29,* 261–272.

Twenge, J. M., & Crocker, J. (2002). Race and self-esteem: Meta-analyses comparing Whites, Blacks, Hispanics, Asians, and American Indians. *Psychological Bulletin, 128,* 371–408.

Vohs, K. D., & Campbell, W. K. (2004). *Narcissism and materialism.* Unpublished manuscript. University of British Columbia.

Wallace, H. M., & Baumeister, R. F. (2002). The performance of narcissists rises and falls with perceived opportunity for glory. *Journal of Personality and Social Psychology, 82,* 819–834.

Young, J. E., Klosko, J. S., & Weishaar, M. (2003). *Schema Therapy: A Practitioner's Guide.* Guilford Publications: New York.

CHAPTER 43

Nocturnal Enuresis: Evidenced-Based Perspectives in Etiology, Assessment and Treatment

Michael W. Mellon • Arthur C. Houts

WHAT IS NOCTURNAL ENURESIS?

When a child reaches the age of 5 years and is passing urine into his or her clothing or into their bedding while asleep, does so with a frequency of at least twice per week for three consecutive months, and without an organic cause for the urine accidents, this is called nocturnal enuresis (American Psychological Association, 1994). It is estimated to affect as many as 8–10% of the school age population (De Jonge, 1973; Jarvelin, Vikevainen-Tervonen, Moilanen & Huttunen, 1988; Verhulst et al., 1985), with as many as 16% of those children spontaneously remitting their symptoms each year (Forsythe & Redmond, 1974). Similar prevalence rates have been reported in other countries (Cher, Lin & Hsu, 2002). Primary enuresis describes a child who has been wetting continuously since birth, evidencing less than six consecutive months of dryness, and accounts for approximately 80% of those children who wet the bed (Rawashde, Hvistendahl, Kamperis, & Djurhuus, 2002). In the United States alone, it is estimated that as many as 4–6 million children wet their beds nearly every night.

BASIC FACTS ABOUT NOCTURNAL ENURESIS

Long gone are the days in which the common problem of nocturnal enuresis was attributed to characterological flaws in the child. For example, the neurotic triad of pyromania, sociopathy, and enuresis were thought to covary around a personality type (Baker, 1969; Glicklich, 1951). Psychodynamically conceptualized intrapsychic conflicts produced the symptom of nocturnal enuresis, and its elimination often would lead to a greater manifestation of the other legs of the triad. Fortunately for the enuretic child, emerging scientific evidence has demonstrated that a complex interaction of genetic, maturation of the urologic and neurologic systems, combined with both respondent and operant processes better accounts for the pathogenesis of bedwetting.

The exact physiological mechanisms of normal urologic functioning are quite complex and beyond the scope of this chapter. The interested reader can review the work of Krane and Siroky (1991), Holstege and Sei (2002), and Blumenfeld (2002) for a more complete discussion of those processes involved in the normal development and function of urination. Suffice it to say that urinary continence is maintained through a balance between the automatic processes of spinal cord to brainstem mediated urination and the cortical control of the pelvic floor muscles that act as an "on-off" switch for bladder emptying. Automatic bladder contractions are perceived by the child and are thought to be the relevant signal for initiation of

Mellon, M.W., Houts, & A.C. (2006). Nocturnal enuresis: Evidenced-based perspectives in etiology, assessment and treatment. In J. E. Fisher & W. T. O'Donohue (Eds.), *Practitioner's guide to evidence-based psychotherapy*. New York: Springer.

socially learned behaviors of continence (i.e., suspend current activities and visit the toilet). It is hypothesized that during sleep the signal of a full bladder is not perceived and the process of automatic bladder emptying occurs without inhibition. This also occurs within the context of a genetic predisposition for enuresis (Von Gontard, 2001; Jarvelin et al., 1991; Cohen, 1975). The possible mechanisms for this lack of inhibition are subsequently discussed.

Watanabe and Azuma (1989) developed a unique classification system based on the study of nearly 1,500 enuretic children that suggested three separate etiologic pathways. Type I enuresis is characterized by the child's incomplete arousal from sleep in response to a nearly full bladder and subsequent wetting and accounts for approximately 60% of the sample. Bladder functioning during sleep is completely normal. Type IIa enuresis shows a similar pattern of normal bladder functioning during sleep but the child never shows any level of arousal from sleep in response to a bladder contraction and subsequently has a wetting episode. Type IIa accounts for approximately 10% of the sample. Children with Type IIb enuresis demonstrate abnormal and continuous spastic bladder contractions as soon as they fall asleep and eventually have a wetting episode at much lower bladder capacities than during wakefulness. Type IIb enuresis accounts for approximately 30% of the study sample. This atypical bladder functioning is interesting as these children were medically evaluated and demonstrated normal urologic functioning during the day. Watanabe, Imada, Kawauchi, Koyama, & Shirakawa (1997) used this classification system to develop specific treatments to push Type IIa and IIb enuretic children into Type I functioning with the use of anticholinergic medications to quiet spastic bladder contractions and to possibly affect arousability from sleep. Although the reported success of these treatments are worse than basic urine alarm treatment, their work is important in that they have demonstrated ways of changing possible mechanisms of etiology for enuresis.

The Japanese research group has gone further to explain the probable neural pathways and brainstem nuclei involved in the failure to arouse from sleep for the Type I enuretic child. Watanabe et al. (1997) speculated that the "upper centrum" or cortical areas fail to perceive the signals registering in the pontine micturition center and act upon them by fully awakening to prevent wetting. This clearly suggests a problem in arousing from sleep and is echoed in the work of Wolfish (2001) who has demonstrated higher thresholds for arousal from sleep in enuretic children versus normal controls. Collectively, these findings strongly suggest neurological explanations for background noise that prevents the detection of the signal of a filling bladder.

Others have speculated that reduced bladder capacity and/or polyuria are primary etiological factors for enuresis (Djurhuus & Rittig, 2002). Simply put, children who wet the bed are thought to do so because their capacity to hold urine is less than the amount they produce during the sleeping period. There are many inconsistencies in this research in that there is evidence that enuretic children do have normal bladder capacities and can concentrate their urine just as nonbedwetters do (Kawauchi et al., 2003; Yeung et al., 2002).

However, in a unique series of investigations, Norgaard, Rittig, and Djurhuus (1989a) demonstrated that enuretic episodes are preceded by the pelvic floor relaxing, and inhibition of bladder emptying is preceded by a pelvic floor contraction that often is followed by arousal from sleep. These findings were also replicated in preliminary studies by Mellon, Scott, Haynes, Schmidt, & Houts (1997) who demonstrated increases in pelvic floor activity 30 minutes prior to a wetting episode or arousal to visit the bathroom as children progressed through urine alarm treatment. These findings may suggest the first evidence for a learning-based mechanism of action for the success of the enuresis conditioning alarm but certainly requires further investigation.

The role of the pelvic floor in the pathophysiology of and recovery from enuresis has yet to be fully investigated. With regard to bladder functioning and capacity, there is evidence that an extremely quiescent pelvic floor activates bladder instability and this leads to a diminished bladder capacity (Yeung, Chiu, & Sit, 1999). Mellon and Houts (in press) have proposed a model of enuresis that has combined these disparate findings into an explanation that accounts for the etiology and hypothesized mechanisms of action for the success of the urine alarm (Figure 43.1). The model describes the normal developmental process of achieving daytime and nighttime urinary continence, the failure to generalize urinary inhibition or the "guarding reflex" to the state of sleeping as the mechanism accounting for nocturnal enuresis, and the respondent and operant mechanisms that reestablish the guarding reflex during sleep. Other psychosocial influences affecting the optimal delivery of the urine alarm treatment are proposed.

ASSESSMENT

What Should be Ruled Out?

The conceptualization of enuresis as a "bio-behavioral" problem was perhaps most clearly articulated by Houts (1991) who contended that enuresis is clearly a physical problem but one whose optimal management is through learning based treatments that utilize the urine alarm. The "bio-behavioral" perspective for enuresis strongly mandates the importance of proper medical assessment procedures at the outset of intervention. Psychologists are particularly sensitive to the importance of our patients' overall physical health as we endeavor to care for them, and this is even more apparent for nocturnal enuresis. The medical screening should focus attention on a differential diagnosis which would rule out diseases of the urinary tract that would lead to the incomplete processing of urine resulting in excessive urination such as cystitis, pyelonephritis and diabetes. Careful history taking would review family history of diabetes or kidney problems, dramatic weight changes, and excessive eating, drinking, or urination.

The basic physical exam would include a urinalysis and urine culture as 5% of males and 10% of females will have urinary tract infections (Stansfeld, 1975) which will require antibiotic treatment prior to bed-wetting interventions. Although the chances of an active urinary tract infection or structural abnormalities are low for children with nocturnal enuresis (Jarvelin et al., 1990), these should not be overlooked as this would be a failure to meet accepted standards in care (Behrman & Kliegman, 1998; Schmitt, 1997). Most enuretic children should be considered physiologically healthy and should be reassured they are normal.

What is Involved in Effective Assessment?

The primary goal of the psychological assessment is to determine if the patient and family are able to implement a relatively demanding behavioral intervention such as the urine alarm. The basic urine alarm approach or one that is combined with other behavioral procedures requires a significant investment of time and energy from the child and parents. Factors that have been associated with poor outcome or dropout with urine alarm treatment are family history of enuresis, prior failed treatment experiences, parental attitudes and beliefs, family and home environment,

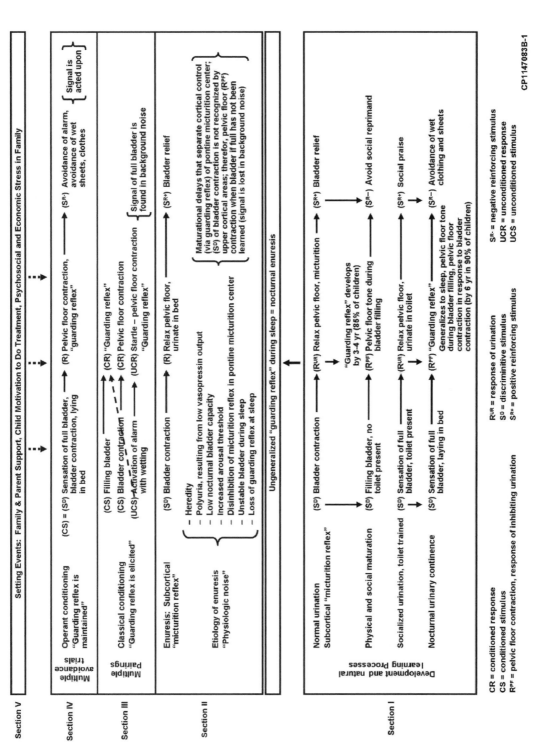

FIGURE 43.1. Bio-behavioral model on normal urinary continence, the pathophysiology of nocturnal enuresis and its remediation through conditioning treatment.

behavioral problems, and the child's current wetting pattern (Mellon & Houts, 1995; Butler & Stenberg, 2001). Psychologists should be aware that stressful situations within the family (i.e., marital problems, psychiatric problems, externalizing problems of the child, extreme parental intolerance of the wetting, or complacency) have been reported to reduce the cooperation necessary to thoroughly implement behavioral treatment long enough to be effective (Butler, Redfern, & Holland, 1994; Feilding, 1985; Morgan & Young, 1975).

Combining reliable screening questionnaires with a careful clinical interview of the child and parents helps the psychologist conduct the assessment more efficiently. Questionnaires such as the Child Behavior Checklist (CBCL) (Achenbach & Edelbrook, 1991), Behavioral Assessment System for Children (BASC) (Reynolds & Kamphaus, 1999), Parenting Stress Index (Abidin, 1995), and the Symptom Checklist (SCL-90-R) (Derogatis, 1977) are useful in identifying psychosocial problems that may need to be prioritized for intervention prior to the initiation of urine alarm treatment. Experiencing a treatment failure is likely to add to the already diminished self-esteem that is associated with a child's bed-wetting (Moffatt, 1989; also Longstaffe, Moffatt, & Whalen 2000). There has yet to be an empirically determined psychosocial profile that would allow for a clear probability statement regarding those children who would likely struggle with urine alarm treatment. The psychologist must rely on his/her clinical judgement to identify those children and parents who would have difficulty implementing this rather demanding treatment. However, it is the experience of these authors that most families are quite motivated and capable of overcoming the child's enuresis with minimal amounts of professional supervision. This has been demonstrated in the author's enuresis clinic and was recently presented at a conference for pediatric psychology (Mellon, Bannit, Whiteside, Trane, & Gutzwiller 2004).

What Assessments are Not Helpful?

Because previous research utilizing invasive medical assessment procedures (i.e., cystoscopy, voiding cystourethrogram) has led to the identification of structural abnormalities (i.e., obstructions, reflux or lesions) in only 2–5% of monosymptomatic nocturnal enuretics, these are no longer routinely recommended (American Academy of Pediatrics Committee on Radiology, 1980). Given that most children with nocturnal enuresis and their parents are highly motivated to overcome the problem and they are often described as "psychologically normal," extensive psychometric evaluations of cognitive functioning and personality characteristics have no legitimate place in assessment of nocturnal enuresis.

TREATMENT

What Treatments are Effective?

The history of treating this common childhood disorder has included interventions as bizarre as "swamp root" (patient reported treatment to authors) to medically invasive procedures such as surgically enlarging the opening of the urethra (e.g., meatotomy). However, more than 60 years of research regarding behavioral treatments for nocturnal enuresis has allowed for confident conclusions to be drawn about effective treatment. These conclusions consistently identify a primary role of the urine alarm in empirically supported treatments. As will be argued here, these conclusions are so evident that further questions regarding whether the urine alarm is effective is now irrelevant and others suggest future research should endeavor to uncover the mechanisms of action that account for its effectiveness (Mellon & McGrath, 2000; Mellon & Houts, in press).

The urine alarm consists of a urine sensor attached by wire to an alarm module. As can be discovered with an internet search with the keyword "urine alarm," it comes in numerous designs with the common versions including a rubberized pad laid on the bed or a body worn sensor, both of which attach to an alarm. The actual volume varies greatly (current author measured various models with volume ranging from 85 to 110 dB) as does the tone (i.e., electronic tone, telephone bell, fire-alarm bell). Other types of alarm feedback include vibrating devices. The prices also vary greatly from $50 to $120.

Useful Website for Purchasing Urine Alarms:
http://www.bedwettingstore.com/
The above referenced website has a variety of urine alarms, books, bedwetting treatment kits and other assessories. All of the kits include the urine alarm and this is consistent with the published literature. However, the authors are unaware of any studies directly comparing therapist supervised versus self-help treatments for bedwetting. Based on clinical experience, the authors believe that a minimal level of supervision and support from an experienced therapist is needed.

The effectiveness of the enuresis conditioning alarm has been empirically demonstrated at the level of single case methodology, in uncontrolled group studies, in randomized clinical studies with wait-list control groups or against other established treatments, and discussed in narrative and quantitative reviews of the literature. The consistent conclusion in the research literature at each level of experimental rigor is that the urine alarm treatment is proven to be effective for approximately 60–80% of monosymptomatic enuretic children regardless of age and gender. This conclusion has been argued since the first major review of the research literature by Doleys (1977), empirically supported in a meta-analytic review by Houts, Berman & Abramson (1994), and summarized in a review utilizing criteria for defining empirically established treatments (Mellon & McGrath, 2000). Further, the same findings were reported in a recent systematic review of studies that included urine alarm treatment alone, combined with other behavioral components and compared to medication treatments with inclusion criteria involving only studies with randomized or quasirandomized designs (Glazner, Evans & Peto, 2003).

Mellon and McGrath (2000) also classified the multi-component behavioral treatment called "Dry Bed Training" (DBT) by Azrin, Sneed and Foxx (1974) as another empirically supported treatment. This operant conditioning procedure, which includes the urine alarm, has an average overall success rate of 75% cured in as few as four weeks. DBT includes a method of systematically waking the child, overcorrection if a wet occurs, and cleanliness training. Mellon and McGrath (2000) reported that the singular use of the urine alarm has an average success rate of 78%, and joins "Dry Bed Training" as the only Empirically Supported Treatments. Further, treatments that combine the urine alarm with other behavioral treatments such as retention control training (i.e., Full Spectrum Home Training by Houts and Liebert, 1984) or with medications such as desmopressin have cure rates of 79% and 75%, respectively (Mellon & McGrath, 2000).

Houts et al. (1994) conducted a meta-analytic review of psychological approaches for nocturnal enuresis and included basic urine alarm treatment, urine alarm combined with other behavioral procedures, behavioral procedures without the urine alarm, and verbal psychotherapies. They also compared these behavioral treatments to medication interventions and only included studies that utilized the most rigorous experimental controls. Treatments that utilized the urine alarm were found to be clearly superior to pharmacological treatments and psychological interventions that did not include the urine alarm. However, restricted sample sizes prevented advocating approaches utilizing the urine alarm combined with behavioral procedures over basic urine alarm treatment alone.

Finally, Glazner et al. (2003) concluded the same in a recent systematic review of studies that included urine alarm treatment alone, combined with other behavioral components and compared to medication treatments with inclusion criteria involving only studies with randomized or quasi-randomized designs. This consistent pattern in the results of systematic reviews strongly indicates that further questioning of the effectiveness of the urine alarm in treating bedwetting is now irrelevant.

FUTURE RESEARCH DIRECTIONS

Mellon and Houts (in press) proposed a model accounting for the etiology of enuresis and its effective treatment via the urine alarm. This model is characterized as a "bio-behavior" model as is it accounts for physiological causes of enuresis, the learning processes involved in effective treatment, and the psychosocial influences that affect the fidelity of the urine alarm. The model also identifies specific research questions that are intended to unify various areas of current research from different disciplines to account for a complete understanding of the causes of nocturnal enuresis and the mechanisms of action through which the urine alarm works. Mellon and Houts (in press) point out that research of physiological influences on enuresis that excludes investigation of learning processes involved in urine alarm treatment and specific changes in the functioning of the pelvic floor muscles severely limits a complete understanding of bedwetting. The importance of conceptualizing bedwetting in the context of both respondent and operant processes is argued due to the fact, that regardless of different proposed etiologies for bedwetting, the urine alarm successfully cures 75–80% of enuretic children. Specific research questions are proposed which reflect the bio-behavioral nature of nocturnal enuresis in the context of learning processes and the psychosocial influences on the delivery of urine alarm treatment.

As previously mentioned, Watanabe & Azuma's (1989) work has identified three enuresis types based on simultaneous monitoring of bladder pressure and sleep activity based on polysomnography. However, these researchers have failed to study the function of the pelvic floor during sleep and the urologic and neurologic changes resulting from basic urine alarm treatment. Future research should investigate whether there is a different outcome for each of the enuresis types, whether the urine alarm changes the function of the pontine micturition center or the cortical areas involved in learned social continence, and whether bladder function and capacity changes. By randomly assigning bedwetters to urine alarm treatment or a no treatment control condition, and utilizing polysomnography, bladder and pelvic floor functioning as outcome measures, one could then specifically identify mediational variables or mechanisms through which the urine alarm works.

With regard to the respondent and operant learning processes through which conditioning treatment works, systematically manipulating the stimulus characteristics of the urine alarm is proposed. It is hypothesized that fully understanding the most potent stimulus characteristics will lead to a more effective alarm. It may also be discovered that different etiologies for enuresis will require a different combination of stimulus characteristics in the alarm to achieve an optimal outcome with conditioning treatment. For example, varying the volume of the alarm, pairing the auditory alarm with other sensory experiences such as vibration, or utilizing day-time conditioning trials may reduce the length of treatment.

Finally, better understanding the psychological characteristics of the child and parent may allow for identifying the necessary attitudes and behaviors to optimally deliver conditioning treatment. It is proposed that well validated and standardized psychological measures of child and parent behavior and attitudes will allow researchers to identify the "ideal child" for treatment that is associated with the best outcome. The use of motivational interviewing to establish the ideal behavioral and attitudinal conditions prior to treatment should also be investigated as this may increase the effectiveness of the treatment and reduce dropout. The goal of improving upon an already effective treatment is certainly a challenge not to be minimized but it is still a legitimate one.

CONCLUSIONS

Of all the childhood disorders that clinical child psychologists are called upon to treat, nocturnal enuresis is one that often leads to a sense of satisfaction in knowing that our treatment efforts are likely to lead to a good outcome. Utilizing the urine alarm, which is an empirically supported treatment, will likely lead to a cure in approximately 75–80% of those children who have been medically cleared for conditioning treatment. Exciting new research is beginning to shed light on those physiological mechanisms that appear to cause the problem of bedwetting.

It is suggested that studying those urologic and neurologic influences in the context of learning processes and other psychosocial influences that might affect the delivery of urine alarm treatment will lead to a more complete understanding of nocturnal enuresis. Even though much is already known regarding the efficacy of urine alarm treatment, further study may well push a robust psychosocial treatment closer to 100% effectiveness in nocturnally enuretic children. A brief summary of urine alarm as effective treatment for a common childhood disorder. Also mention the need for dissemination of this information to make treatment more available to those who need it.

As a final thought, barriers to the dissemination of information regarding empirically supported treatment are yet to be overcome. It is quite disappointing that today most children who present with nocturnal enuresis are likely to be treated with medications such as desmopressin, which is clearly inferior to the urine alarm in effectiveness. Clinical child psychology organizations are challenged to change this situation in light of limited medical and mental health resources. This issue was lucidly argued by Houts (2000) in a commentary regarding empirically supported treatment for nocturnal enuresis in the following quote:

"...how has it happened that the most effective treatment for a problem that affects 10% of secondary school aged children has remained so under utilized for over half a century? Something is seriously broken with our health care system and our culture of caring for children who wet the bed. What kind of health care system is it that routinely foregoes curing bedwetting and opts instead for mere palliative treatment that costs considerably more than a cure?"

Our professional responsibilities extend beyond the individual patient that we treat. We must do all that we can to make effective treatments available to all of those persons who would benefit from them.

REFERENCES

Abidin, R. (1995). *Parenting stress index, third edition. Professional manual.* Odessa, FL, Psychological Assessment Resources.

Achenbach, T. M., & Edelbrock, C. (1991). *Manual for the child behavior checklist.* Burlington, VT: Department of Psychiatry, University of Vermont.

American Academy of Pediatrics Committee on Radiology. (1980). Excretory urography for evaluation of enuresis. *Pediatrics, 65,* 644–655

American Psychiatric Association. (1994). *Diagnostic and statistical manual of mental disorders* (4th ed.). Washington, DC: American Psychiatric Association.

Baker, B. (1969). Symptom treatment and symptom substitution in enuresis. *Journal of Abnormal Psychology,* 74, 42–49.

Behrman, R., & Kliegman, R (1998). *Nelson-essentials of pediatrics, third edition.* Philadelphia: Saunders.

Blumenfeld, H. (2002). *Neuroanatomy through clinical cases.* Sunderland, MA: Sinauer Associates.

Butler, R. J., Redfern, E. J., & Holland, P. (1994). Children's notions about enuresis and the implications for treatment. *Scandinavian Journal of Nephrology, Supplement, 163,* 39–47.

Butler, R., & Stenberg, A. (2001). Treatment of childhood nocturnal enuresis: An examination of clinically relevant principles. *British Journal of Urology-International,* 88, 563–571.

Cher, T., Lin, G., & Hsu, K. (2002). Prevalence of nocturnal enuresis and associated familial factors in primary school children in Taiwan. *Journal of Urology, 168(3),* 1142–1146.

Cohen, M. (1975). Enuresis. *Pediatric Clinics of North America,* 22, 545–560.

De Jonge, G. A. (1973). Epidemiology of enuresis: A survey of the literature. In I. Kolvin, R. C. MacKeith, & S. R. Meadow (Eds.), *Bladder control and enuresis.* (pp. 39–46). London: William Heinemann.

Derogatis, L. R. (1977). *SCL-90: Administration, scoring & procedures manual for the revised version.* Baltimore: Clinical Psychometric Research.

Djurhuus, J. & Rittig, S. (2002). Nocturnal enuresis. *Current Opinion in Urology, 12,* 317–320.

Doleys, D. M. (1977). Dry-bed training and retention control training: A comparison. *Behavior Therapy, 8(4),* 541–548.

Fielding, D. (1985). Factors associated with drop-out, relapse and failure in the conditioning treatment of nocturnal enuresis. *Behavioural Psychotherapy, 13(3),* 174–185.

Forsythe, W. I., & Redmond, A. (1974). Enuresis and spontaneous cure rate: Study of 1129 enuretics. *Archives of Disease in Childhood, 49,* 259–263.

Glicklich, L. (1951). Historical account of enuresis. *Pediatrics, 8,* 859–876.

Holstege, G., & Sie, J. (2002). The central control of the pelvic floor. In J. Pemberton, M. Swash, & M. Henry (Eds.), *The pelvic floor—its function and disorders* (pp. 94–101). New York: W. B. Saunders.

Houts, A. C. (2000). Commentary: Treatments for enuresis: Criteria, mechanisms, and health care policy. *Journal of Pediatric Psychology, 25,* 219–224.

Houts, A., & Liebert, R. (1984). Bedwetting: A guide for parents and children. Springfield, IL: Charles Thomas.

Jarvelin, M. R., Moilanen, I., Kangas, P., Moring, K., Vikevainen-Tervonen, L., Huttunen, N. P., et al. (1991). Aetiological and precipitating factors for childhood enuresis. *Acta Pediatrica Scandinavia, 80,* 361–369.

Jarvelin, M. R., Vikevainen-Tervonen, L., Moilanen, I., & Huttunen, N. P. (1988). Enuresis in seven-year-old children. *Acta Paediatrica Scandinavia, 77,* 148–153.

Kawauchi, A., Tanaka, Y., Naito, Y., Yamao, Y., Ukimura, O. Yoneda, K., et al., (2003). Bladder capacity at the time of enuresis. *Urology, 61,* 1016–1018.

Krane, R., & Siroky, M. (1991). *Clinical neuro-urology.* Boston: Little, Brown and Company.

Longstaffe, S., Moffatt, M., & Whalen, J. (2000). Behavioral and self-concept changes after six months of enuresis treatment: a randomized, controlled trial. *Pediatrics, 105(4 Pt 2),* 935–940.

Mellon, M., Bannit, A., Whiteside, S., Trane, S., & Gutzwiller, E. (2004). *Outcome and Symptom Reduction for Children in Enuresis Conditioning Treatment.* Paper presented at the National Conference on Child Health Psychology, Charleston, South Carolina.

Mellon, M. W. & Houts, A. C. (1995). Psychosocial Treatments for Enuresis and Encopresis: Current Knowledge and Future Directions, *Journal of Clinical Child and Adolescent Psychology,* 341–366.

Mellon, M. W., & McGrath, M. L. (2000). Empirically supported treatments in pediatric psychology: Nocturnal enuresis. *Journal of Pediatric Psychology, 25(4),* 193–214.

Mellon, M. W., & Houts, A. C. (1995). Elimination Disorders. In R. T. Ammerman & M. Hersen (Eds.), *Handbook of child behavior therapy in the psychiatric setting* (pp. 341–366). Oxford, England: J. Wiley & Sons.

Mellon, M. W., Scott, M. A., Haynes, K. B., Schmidt, D. F. & Houts, A. C. (1997). *EMG recording of pelvic floor conditioning in nocturnal enuresis during urine alarm Treatment: A preliminary study.*

Paper presentation at the Sixth Florida Conference on Child Health Psychology, University of Florida, Gainsville, FL.

Moffatt, M. E. K. (1989). Nocturnal enuresis: Psychologic implications of treatment and non-treatment. *The Journal of Pediatrics, 114(4, Pt. 2)*, 697–704.

Morgan, R. T. T., & Young, G. C. (1975). Parental attitudes and the conditioning treatment of childhood enuresis. *Behaviour Research and Therapy, 13*, 197–199.

Norgaard, J. P., Rittig, S., & Djurhuus, J. C. (1989). Nocturnal enuresis: An approach to treatment based on pathogenesis. *Pediatrics, 14*, 705–710.

Rawashde, Y,. Hvistendahl, G., Kamperis, K., & Djurhuus, J. (2002). Demographics of enuresis patients attending a referral centre. *Scandinavian Journal of Urology & Nephrology, 36*, 348–353.

Reynolds, C., & Kamphaus, R. (1999). *Behavioral Assessment System for Children (BASC)*. American Guidance Service, Circle Pines, MN.

Schmitt, B. D. (1997). Nocturnal enuresis. *Pediatrics in Review, 18*, 183–191.

Stansfeld, J. M. (1975). Duration of Treatment for Urinary Tract Infections in Children. *British Medical Journal, 3*, 65–66.

Verhulst, F. C., van der Lee, J. H., Akkerhuis, G. W., Sanders-Woudstra, J. A. R., Timmer, F. C., & Donkhorst, I. D. (1985). The prevalence of nocturnal enuresis: Do DSM III criteria need to be changed? A brief research report. *Journal of Child Psychology and Psychiatry, 26*, 989–993.

von Gontard A., Schaumburg H., Hollmann E., Eiberg H., & Rittig S. (2001). The genetics of enuresis: A review. *Journal of Urology. 166*, 2438–2443.

Watanabe, H. & Azuma, Y. (1989). A proposal for classification system of enuresis based on overnight simultaneous monitoring of electroencephalography and cystometry. *Sleep, 12*, 257–264.

Watanabe, H., Imada, N., Kawauchi, A., Koyama, Y., & Shirakawa, S. (1997). Physiological background of enuresis type I. A preliminary report. *Scandinavian Journal of Urology & Nephrology Supplementum, 183*, 7–10.

Wolfish, N. (2001). Sleep/arousal and enuresis subtypes. *Journal of Urology, 166*, 2444–2447.

Yeung, C. K., Chiu, H. N., & Sit, F. K. Y. (1999). Sleep Disturbance and Bladder Dysfunction in Enuretic Children with Treatment Failure: Fact or Fiction? *Scandinavian Journal of Urology & Nephrology, 33(6)*, 20–23.

Yeung, C., Sit, F., To, L., Chiu, H., Sihoe, J., Lee, E., et al. (2002). Reduction in nocturnal functional bladder capacity is a common factor in the pathogenesis of refractory nocturnal enuresis. *British Journal of Urology International, 90*, 302–307.

CHAPTER 44

Nonadherence to Treatment

Eric R. Levensky

WHAT IS NON-ADHERENCE TO TREATMENT?

Although there is much variability in the definition of the term *adherence*, it generally refers to the *extent to which patients follow the instructions they are given for prescribed treatments* (Haynes, McDonald, Garg, & Montague, 2002, p. 2). In recent years, the term *adherence* has begun to be used in place of the more traditionally used term, *compliance*. This shift in terminology has occurred because many researchers and clinicians have believed that the term compliance suggests passivity and obedience on the part of patients, whereas the term adherence implies patient–provider collaboration and an active role of patients in their treatment (Rogers & Bullman, 1995). Nonadherence to treatments can take a number of forms. These include the following:

1. not initiating a recommended treatment
2. not attending or coming late to appointments
3. not completing behavioral recommendations or homework (e.g., increases in physical activity, changes in diet, self monitoring, in vivo exposure, relaxation exercises)
4. not taking medication as prescribed (e.g., taking too many or too few pills, taking medication at incorrect times, not following special dosing instructions)
5. terminating the treatment prematurely

Why Should We Care about Nonadherence to Treatments?

Although advancements in healthcare research and development have yielded effective treatments for numerous medical and behavioral health problems (e.g., Chambless, Baker, Baucum, Beutler, & Calhoun, 1998; Sackett, Straus, Richardson, Rosenberg, & Haynes, 2000), patient nonadherence is often a significant barrier to effective *delivery* of these treatments. Virtually all medical and behavioral health treatments require at least some degree of behavior change on the part of the patient (e.g., coming to appointments, agreeing to have assessments and procedures performed), and many require significant behavior change (e.g., following demanding and complex medication regimens; making dietary, activity, or other lifestyle changes; enduring sometimes aversive behavioral interventions such as self-monitoring or exposure). Unfortunately, many patients fail to make these behavior changes. In the medical treatment literature, rates of nonadherence to treatment have generally been found to be 20–40% for acute regimes, 30–60% for chronic regimes, and 50–80% for preventative regimens (Christensen, 2004). Nonadherence to treatment has also been found to be high in the psychotherapy and behavior therapy literature, with premature treatment dropout rates ranging from 30% to 60% (Garfield, 1994; Reis & Brown, 1999; Wierzbicki & Pekarik, 1993), and average rates of failing to complete assigned homework of roughly 50% (Detweiler & Whisman, 1999; Spiegler, & Guevremont, 2003).

Levensky, E. R. (2006). Nonadherence to treatment. To appear in: J. E. Fisher & W. T. O'Donohue (Eds.), *Practitioner's guide to evidence-based psychotherapy*. New York: Springer.

This nonadherence to medical and behavioral health treatments is problematic in that it often reduces the impact of potentially effective treatments, and also can lead to substantial and unnecessary health, social, and financial costs (Bryant, Simons, & Thase, 1999; Christensen, 2004; Cleemput, Kesteloot, & DeGeest, 2002; Reis & Brown, 1999; Rogers & Bullman, 1995). Health consequences can include no change or worsening of the health problem, the development of collateral health problems, the provider being unable to evaluate the effectiveness of the treatment (and potentially prematurely terminating or overprescribing the treatment), and death of the patient. Patient nonadherence can also be a source of frustration and concern for providers.

Financial consequences of patient nonadherence can include the cost of additional services and treatment (e.g., additional visits, medications, and tests; emergency room visits, hospitalizations), as well as decreases in the work productivity of the patient. Poor adherence to prescribed medications, for example, is estimated to cost over $100 billion each year in the United States through increasing healthcare utilization and decreasing patient productivity (Grahl, 1994).

HOW IS NONADHERENCE TO TREATMENT BEST ASSESSED?

As is the case with most other health problems, an important component to addressing nonadherence to treatment is identifying its occurrence in patients. With some aspects of treatment, the extent of patients' adherence can be directly observed by providers, such as with appointment attendance, in-session participation, or receiving provider-observed or administered medication or procedures. However, most often providers do not have direct access to patients' adherence to treatment (e.g., following prescribed medication regimens, completing homework assignments, making changes in diet or exercise). In these cases, other methods of assessing patient adherence must be used. There are a number of methods for measuring patients' adherence to treatment. Each has its relative strengths and weaknesses in terms of reliability, validity, utility, and practicality, and there is no clear gold standard for measuring adherence. Andrews & Friedland (2000), Miller & Hays (2000), Rand & Weeks (1998), Riekert (In press), and Vitolins, Rand, Rapp, Ribisl, & Sevick (2000) provide useful reviews of the literature on methods of assessing adherence.

Subjective-Reports

Patient-report is the most commonly used method of assessing adherence in clinical practice, due to the fact that this method is relatively quick, easy, and inexpensive. Common methods of obtaining patient-report data include questionnaires, daily self-monitoring diaries, and interviews. Although patient-report is the most practical method of adherence assessment, the accuracy of this method is often reduced by patients' hesitancy to report nonadherence, and by limitations in patients' ability to recall past adherence-related behavior, often resulting in underreporting of nonadherence (e.g., Rand & Weeks 1998).

Despite these limitations, patient-report can be a valuable clinical tool and has been found to be a predictor of adherence and clinical outcomes (Rand & Weeks, 1998; Stone, 2001). Additionally, an important advantage of the patient-report method is that it can provide information about the patterns and timing of treatment-related behavior as well as information about barriers to adherence. This can be particularly the case when patients use daily self-monitoring diaries to record the time of day of their treatment-related behaviors (e.g., medication taking, diet, behavioral activation, homework), as well as reasons for nonadherence. Methods that can increase the accuracy of patient self-report of adherence include: using brief, structured questionnaires; asking patients to report on levels of nonadherence rather than on levels of adherence; specifying a specific time-frame; assessing a recent time-frame (e.g., the last seven days); using cues to facilitate recall; having patients use a daily diary to record treatment-related behavior; and, reassuring patients that problems with adherence are normal, they will not be punished for nonadherence, and that accurate reporting of adherence problems is crucial for effective treatment (Andrews & Friedland, 2000, Dunbar-Jacob, Burke, & Puczynski, 1995; Rabkin & Chesney, 1999; Stone, 2001; Vitolins et al., 2000). Healthcare provider estimates have also been used to assess patient adherence, however, these estimates tend to be highly influenced by provider heuristics and are often no better than chance (Riekert, In press).

Indirect Measurement and Biological Indicators.

For patients who are taking medications, there are several indirect methods for assessing adherence to prescribed regimens. These include pill counts, assessing pharmacy records, and using Medication Event Monitoring System (MEMS) caps.

Pill counts and assessing pharmacy records A fairly common method for assessing patient adherence to medications is conducting pill counts. This involves determining how many pills a patient should have given the number of days since the prescription was filled (and the number of pills to be taken each day), counting all of the patient's medications to determine how many pills the patient currently has, and then calculating the difference between how many pills the patient should have and the number of pills the patient actually has. A strength of this method is that it can be more objective than patient-report in that it does not rely a patient's memory of missed doses. For clinical use, this method is limited by the requirements of patients bringing in all of their medications and of clinical staff taking the time to count the pills. The accuracy of this method is limited by patients failing to bring in all of their pills (e.g., forgetting to bring in pills not kept in bottles or intentionally leaving pills at home to appear adherent). Additionally, this method does not provide information about the patterns of adherence.

Assessing patients' pharmacy records (i.e., determining if refills were obtained on time) has also been use in research and clinical settings as an objective measure of adherence. This method suffers from many of the same problems as pill-counts, however, it also tends to be a less sensitive measure, and can be difficult to use with patients who go to more than one pharmacy to fill prescriptions.

Medication Event Monitoring System (MEMS) Caps MEMS caps are rarely used in clinical practice due to their expense, but are frequently used in research because of the relatively high accuracy of the method (e.g., Liu et al., 2001). MEMS caps are electronic devices that serve as caps to patients' medication bottles. These caps log the date and time of every opening and closing of the medication bottles. This information can then be down-loaded and examined by the clinician to assess rates and patterns of adherence and nonadherence. Strengths of this method are that it does not rely on patient report, and that it is more convenient for both the patient and the clinical staff than the pill count method. Additionally, it provides information about the timing of medication taking. Disadvantages of the method are that the caps are rather expensive, and that it cannot be determined whether or not a patient actually took pills out of the bottle when it was opened, how much was taken out, or if the patient actually consumed the medication if it was taken out. An additional disadvantage of

MEMS caps is that they are not compatible with patients using pillboxes or otherwise storing medications outside of the capped bottles.

Biological Indicators Biological markers are used in both clinical and research settings to assess patient adherence to medications. Typically this involves taking blood, saliva, or urine samples and assessing these for correlates of the presence of the medication or for traces of the medication itself. Although this method is an objective measure of adherence, its accuracy can be affected by a number of factors such as recency of ingestion, individual differences in absorption, and the presence of biological elements other than the medication that may influence readings (Miller & Hays, 2000). Additionally, this method can be expensive and impractical, and such measures are not available for many medications.

Electronic Measures

Riekert and Rand (2002) describe several electronic monitoring methods, such as blood glucose monitors, pedometers (to measure steps), heart-rate monitors, and accelerometers (to measure movement). These devices have the benefit of being more objective than self-report methods. Additional benefits of these measures are that in some cases they can identify behavioral patterns and dose-response patterns and are not affected by social desirability. Limitations of these methods are cost, malfunctions, need for ongoing calibration, and the time needed for staff to maintain devices and calculate adherence.

Health Outcomes

Although there is typically a relationship between patient adherence and treatment outcomes, there are many other factors that can also influence treatment outcomes in both positive and negative directions. Therefore, it is generally not recommended that treatment outcomes be used as a measure of adherence (DiMatteo, 2004).

Many researchers and clinicians advocate using a combination of the methods discussed here to measure patient adherence, although, it is not yet clear how this can be done most effectively (Rand & Weeks, 1998). The use of self-report in combination with a more objective measure, such as pill counts or pedometer readings would likely be useful and feasible in many clinical settings.

WHAT FACTORS CONTRIBUTE TO NONADHERENCE TO TREATMENT?

Because patient nonadherence has been found to be such a significant barrier to effective healthcare delivery, there has been much interest in understanding the causes of this problem. Over the last several decades, hundreds of studies have been conduced in this area and a wide range of factors have been found to be associated with adherence and nonadherence to treatments. Despite these efforts, however, it has been difficult to make strong conclusions from this literature. There has been wide variations across studies in definitions and measurements of examined factors as well as the definitions of adherence to treatment across. Furthermore, factors that have been identified as related to adherence have generally accounted for a relatively small proportion of the variance in adherence and are not consistently related to adherence across studies (for reviews see Burke & Ockene, 2001; Christensen, 2004, Dunbar-Jacob & Mortimer-Stephens, 2001; Fincham, 1995; Ickovics & Meisler, 1997; Meichenbaum & Turk, 1987; Morris & Schulz, 1992; Myers & Midence, 1998; Pampallona, Bollini, Tibaldi, Kupelnick, &

Munizza, 2002; Reis & Brown, 1999; Scheel, Hanson & Razzhavaikina, 2004; Shumaker, Schron, Ockene, & McBee, 1998; Vermeire, Hearnshaw, & Royen, 2001). A number of theoretical models have been developed or adapted to aid in the understanding, prediction, and control of adherence- and nonadherence-related behaviors. However, these models have been relatively unsuccessful at meeting these goals (see Christensen, 2004).

Table 44.1 summarizes clinically relevant factors that have empirical support for their association to poor adherence to treatments. In this table, these factors have been organized into those related to (1) the patient, (2) the treatment, (3) the patient–provider relationship, (4) the clinical setting, and (5) the disease, as this can be a useful way of conceptualizing barriers to treatment adherence (Ickovicks & Meisler, 1997). Several themes emerge from this literature. First, as pointed out by Meichenbaum & Turk (1987), although these factors are listed as though they are each discrete constructs, many are likely to be somewhat overlapping and should not be thought of as completely independent. Second, despite these overlaps, treatment adherence appears to be complex and multidetermined. That is, many different types of factors can impact patients' adherence to medications, including factors related the patient, disease, treatment, provider, and clinical setting. Third, patients appear to be quite heterogeneous in terms of if and how any of these factors will impact their adherence. And finally, as discussed earlier, these factors do not yet provide a reliable means for predicting whether any one patient will adhere adequately to a regimen.

Putting these themes together suggests that conducting a thorough assessment of potential barriers, and developing an individualized adherence plan with each patient is warranted. Despite the limitations of the barriers-to-adherence literature, it can serve to facilitate this process by orienting clinicians to potential barriers to patients' adherence, as well as to potentially effective interventions. Levensky (In press) presents a detailed description of how this individualized adherence barrier assessment and intervention can be done in clinical practice with HIV patients.

WHAT INTERVENTIONS ARE EFFECTIVE IN INCREASING PATIENT ADHERENCE TO TREATMENTS?

As is the case with the literature on factors related to nonadherence, the literature on the effectiveness of interventions to improve adherence is somewhat inconclusive. This is due in part to the fact that a relatively small number of studies have been conducted examining adherence interventions (see Burke & Ockene, 2001; Christensen, 2004; Dunbar-Jacob & Schlenk, 1996; Dunbar-Jacob & Mortimer-Stephens, 2001; Falvo, 2004; Fincham, 1995; Haynes, McDonald, & Garg, 2002; Ickovics & Meisler, 1997; McDonald, Garg, & Haynes, 2002; Meichenbaum & Turk, 1987; Mullen, Green, & Persinger, 1985; Myers & Midence, 1998; Roter et al., 1998; Pampallona, et al., 2002; Scheel et al., 2004; Shumaker et al., 1998; and Vermeire et al., 2001). Additionally, many of these studies have been limited by methodological and other problems that have made interpreting their results difficult, including the use of inaccurate measures of adherence; a lack random assignment or control groups; confounding variables; small sample sizes; short follow-up periods; a lack of detailed descriptions of the interventions; and differing definitions of adherence across studies. Another problem that has made it difficult to draw conclusions from this literature is that methodologically sound studies of similar interventions have produced different outcomes (e.g., Haynes, Wang, & Da Mota Gomes, 1987).

TABLE 44.1. Factors Related to Nonadherence to Treatments

Factors related to the patient:

1. Lack of knowledge of treatment requirements (e.g., what, when, how)
2. Cognitive deficits (e.g., forgetfulness)
3. Language deficits, poor literacy
4. Lack of self-management/coping skills self-management skills (e.g., self-control, problems solving)
5. Lack of tangible resources (e.g., financial, housing, transportation, time)
6. Stressful life events (e.g., death of loved one, ending of important relationship)
7. Problematic health and treatment-related beliefs (e.g., need for treatment; seriousness of the health problem; efficacy of the treatment; relative costs and benefits of adhering; self-efficacy)
8. Mental health problems (e.g., depression, substance abuse, and psychotic symptoms)
9. Inadequate social support (e.g., emotional and instrumental support; reminder and encouragement of adherence)
10. Low motivation, apathy or pessimism about health and future
11. Problematic past experiences with adherence
12. Fear of stigma for health problem
13. Treatment is an unwelcome reminder of illness
14. Problematic responses to slips in adherence

Factors related to the medication regimen:

1. High complexity and demands of the treatment (e.g., large number of pills to take, complex time-consuming homework assignments, substantial change in daily activities or diet)
2. Poor fit between treatment requirements and patient's lifestyle/daily activities (e.g., eating and sleeping patterns, work schedule, social life, other daily activities)
3. Long duration of the treatment
4. Frequent and/or severe side effects
5. High cost of treatment

Factors related to the patient–provider relationship:

1. Poor communication between patient and provider
2. Provider does not adequately assess problems with treatment and/or adherence
3. Patient has difficulty discussing problems with treatment and/or adherence
4. Patient uncertain about provider's ability to help
5. Patient lacks trust and/or comfort with provider
6. Patient and provider have differing conceptualizations or expectations of problem and/or treatment

Factors related to the clinical setting:

1. Poor accessibility of services (e.g., availability of appointments/staff, hours of operation, waits for services)
2. Lack of continuity/cohesiveness of care
3. Unfriendly/unhelpful staff
4. Poor reputation of clinic

Features of the disease:

1. Health problem not serious or threatening to health
2. Long-term duration of health problem
3. Lack of symptoms or related problems experienced by patient
4. Symptoms of health problem interfere with adherence (e.g., cognitive deficits, lack of mobility, problems with vision).

For more detailed discussions of these factors as well as their empirical support see the following sources: Bryant et al. (1999); Burke & Ockene (2001); Christensen (2004); DiMatteo (2004); Dunbar-Jacob & Mortimer-Stephens (2001); Fincham (1995); Garfield (1994); Ickovics & Meisler (1997); Meichenbaum & Turk (1987); Morris & Schulz (1992); Myers & Midence (1998); Reis & Brown (1999); Scheel, et al. (2004); Shumaker et al. (1998); Stewart (1996); Vermeire et al. (2001); Wierzbicki, & Pekarik (1993).

Finally, many adherence interventions evaluated have consisted of multiple components, as opposed to stand-alone techniques or strategies, making it difficult to identify specific strategies that may be most effective.

Despite the limitations of this research, this literature has produced some useful information regarding the effects of adherence interventions. Effective interventions have been delivered through a range of modes (e.g., face to face contact, phone, and mail), by a range of providers (e.g., physicians, nurses, adherence counselors, mental health providers, and computers), with a range of adherence targets (e.g., medication regimen adherence, appointment keeping, treatment retention, behavioral assignments), and with a range of patient populations (e.g., patients with chronic and acute medical and mental illness, patients in need of preventative health treatment). It should be noted, however, that the majority of research in this area has focused on improving adherence to medical treatments, particularly focusing on medication regimens and appointment keeping. Although no single adherence-promoting strategy appears to be clearly most effective, interventions found to significantly improve adherence generally include educational, social support, cognitive-behavioral and/or behavioral components. Additionally, multicomponent interventions are generally more effective than single-strategy interventions, and interventions that involve multiple sessions or follow-ups are more effective in sustaining adherence over time than one-time interventions. Finally, it is important to note that the impact of these interventions is generally modest with effect sizes rarely exceeding more than .34 (see Haynes et al., 2002; Haynes, McKibbon, & Kanani, 1996; Haynes, Wang, & Da Mota Gomes, 1987; Malouff & Schutte, 2004; Morris & Schulz, 1992; Pampallona, et al., 2002; Roter, Hall, Merisca, Nordstrom, Cretin, & Svarstad, 1998; Scheel, Hanson, & Razzhavaikina, 2004; and Walitzer, Dermen & Connors, 1999). These findings are consistent with the notion that adherence involves a complex and multidetermined set of behaviors that are not easily changed.

A detailed description of all the strategies included in adherence interventions that have support for their efficacy is well beyond the scope of this brief chapter. However, the primary strategies that have garnered empirical support as stand alone interventions or as part of multicomponent interventions are summarized in Table 44.2. A list of sources for more detailed discussions of these strategies as well as their empirical support is included at the bottom of Table 44.2. Again, it should be noted that strong conclusions regarding the extent and relative efficacy any one of these strategies are limited by the problems in the literature described above. It should also be noted that a number of these strategies are somewhat overlapping and, therefore, should not each be considered as a discrete and independent from one another.

WHAT ARE SOME DIRECTIONS FOR FUTURE RESEARCH?

Patient nonadherence to treatments continues to be a significant barrier to effective healthcare, and the literature on the effectiveness of nonadherence interventions is fairly inconclusive. Substantially more work is needed in better understanding and intervening on patient nonadherence to treatment. First, continued efforts are needed in the development and testing models of adherence and nonadherence that will facilitate understanding and prediction of adherence as well as guide the development of effective interventions. It is likely that researchers in will need to start thinking more "outside the box" to accomplish this. Second, further work is needed in developing and testing valid and reliable methods of assessing adherence

TABLE 44.2. Strategies for Increasing Patient Adherence to Treatments

Assessing readiness to begin treatment:

1. Assessing past adherence patterns and current beliefs/concerns about the treatment
2. Discussing pros and cons of initiating treatment
3. Asking patient to rate confidence in carrying out treatment
4. Identifying potential barriers to treatment

Increasing treatment-related knowledge:

1. Educating patient:
    −nature of health problem/action of the treatment
    −specific behavioral requirements of the treatment (what, where, when, and how)
    −importance of adherence
    −nature and management of likely aversive effects of treatment (e.g., side effects)
2. Using simple, understandable language
3. Using visual aids
4. Providing all information in written form
5. Assessing comprehension
6. Having patient demonstrate proficiency

Increasing adherence skills:

1. Providing information on treatment-related aids and training in their use:
    −using cues for engaging in treatment behaviors (e.g., alarms, notes and stickers)
    −linking treatment behaviors to daily activities such as morning/bedtime routines, meals, television shows, etc.
    −self-monitoring (e.g., tracking treatment-related behaviors)
    −using medication organizers, special medication packaging (e.g., blister packaging)
2. Teaching how to integrate treatment into routines
3. Teaching skills in anticipating, avoiding, and managing slips in adherence
4. Teaching problem-solving skills
5. Teaching skills for communicating with providers (e.g., asking questions, reporting problems)
6. Using role playing behavioral rehearsal

Increasing resources and support:

1. Referring to social services/social worker for assistance with accessing resources (e.g., financial, housing, transportation, childcare)
2. Reminder calls and letters
3. Increasing social support, including:
    −increased support and help with adherence from friends or family
    −increased contact with staff (additional appointments, telephone "check-ins," home visits)
    −support groups/individual counseling

Increasing motivation:

1. Maintaining warm, empathetic, genuine, collaborative, nonconfrontational stance
2. Having patient take an active role in treatment planning and decisions
3. Making treatment recommendations as behaviorally specific as possible
4. Simplifying treatment as much as possible to match patient capabilities
5. Tailoring treatment to fit patient's lifestyle, therapy goals, natural reinforcements
6. Helping patient reduce/manage identified barriers and aversive effects of treatment (e.g., side effects)
7. Enhancing patient's self-efficacy (e.g., pointing out past successes and successes of similar patients; affirming patient's ability to adhere)
8. Helping patient to re-frame problematic health beliefs and beliefs about the treatment

Continued

TABLE 44.2. **(Continued)**

9. Getting firm commitments from patient regarding specific treatment-related behaviors

10. Having patient self-monitor adherence and treatment progress

11. Establishing a reinforcement system for adherent behavior (e.g., self-reinforcement; praise from staff, friends or family; financial or other tangible reinforcements such as vouchers)

12. Orienting patient to benefits of adherence and costs of nonadherence (e.g., on health, treatment goals, future goals, etc.), through adherence and health-related feedback

13. Treating mental health problems (e.g., depression, substance abuse)

14. Minimizing barriers at clinic (e.g., long waits, limited appointment times)

15. Having continuity of patient care at clinic

16. Using therapy and behavior change preparatory techniques such as Treatment Contracting, Role Induction, Vicarious Therapy Retraining, and Experimental Pretraining, and Motivational Interviewing (see Lash and Burden, in press; Walitzer et al., 1999; Zweben & Zuckoff, 2004)

Maintenance:

1. Having regular follow-up visits with patient

2. Regularly assessing adherence

3. Regularly assessing barriers to adherence helping patient to reduce, manage or otherwise overcome these barriers

For more detailed discussions of these strategies as well as their empirical support see the following sources: Burke & Okene (2001); Christensen (2004); Dunbar-Jacob & Mortimer-Stephens (2001); Dunbar-Jacob & Schlenk (1996); Falvo (2004); Fincham (1995); Gray, Wykes, & Gournay (2002); Haynes, McDonald, & Garg (2002); Heiby & Lukens (in press); Helmus, Saules, Schoener & Roll (2003); Ickovics & Meisler (1997); Kirschenbaum & Flanery (1983); Lash & Burden (in press) Malouff & Schutte (2004); McDonald, et al. (2002); Meichenbaum & Turk (1987); Mullen, Green, & Persinger, (1985); Myers & Midence (1998); Newell, Bowman, & Chockburn (1999); Pampallona, et al. (2002); Roter, Hall, Merisca, Nordstrom, Cretin, & Svarstad (1998); Scheel, Hanson, & Razzhavaikina (2004); Shumaker, Schron, Ockene, & McBee (1998); Vermeire, Hearnshaw, & Royen (2001); and Zygmunt, Olfson, Boyer, & Mechanic (2002).

to treatments. This should include the development technologies for assessing adherence as well as methods for integrating these into clinical practice. Third, existing interventions, as well as new and innovative interventions, need to be tested using methodologically sound methods that will enable the determination of what interventions are effective. Specifically more outcome studies need to be conducted that the use valid and reliable measures of adherence, use random assignment to a control group, lack significant confounding variables, have adequate sample sizes (e.g., > 60 subjects per group), have longer follow-up periods (e.g., > 6 months), provide detailed descriptions of the interventions, and use standardized operational definitions of adherence (so outcomes can be compared across studies).

Fourth, although likely to be a "down the road" goal, conducting outcome research on what interventions and combinations of interventions are best for specific populations and treatments could be extremely clinically useful as well as potentially cost effective. Finally, for nonadherence assessments and interventions that are found to be effective, provider training and dissemination methods need to be developed and evaluated.

REFERENCES

Andrews, L., & Friedland, G. (2000). Progress in HIV therapeutics and the challenges of adherence to antiretroviral therapy. *Infectious Disease Clinics of North America, 14(4)*, 901–928.

Bryant, M. J., Simons, A. D., & Thase, M. E. (1999). Therapist skill and patient variables in homework compliance: Controlling an uncontrolled variable in cognitive therapy outcome research. *Cognitive Therapy and Research, 23*, 381–399.

Burke, L. E., Ockene, I. S. (Eds.). (2001). *Compliance in healthcare and research.* Armonk, NY: Futura Publishing Company.

Chambless, D. L., Baker, M., Baucum, D. H., Beutler, L. E., Calhoun, K. S. (1998). Update on empirically validated therapies, II. *The Clinical Psychologist, 51(1)*, 3–16.

Christensen, A. J. (2004). *Patient adherence to medical treatment regimens: Bridging the gap between behavioral science and biomedicine.* New Haven: Yale University Press.

Cleemput, I., Kesteloot, K., DeGeest, S. (2002). A review of the literature on the economics of noncompliance. Room for methodological improvement. *Health Policy, 59*, 65–94.

Detweiler, J. B., & Whisman, M. A. (1999). The role of homework assignments in cognitive therapy for depression: Potential methods for enhancing adherence. *Clinical Psychology: Science and Practice*, 6, 267–282.

DiMatteo, M. R. (2004). Variations in patients' adherence to medical recommendations: A quantitative review of 50 years of research. *Medical Care, 42*, 200–209.

DiMatteo, M. R., Lepper, H. S., Croghan, T. W. (2000). Depression is a risk factor for non-compliance in medical treatment. *Archives of Internal Medicine, 14*, 2101–2107.

Dunbar-Jacob, J., Burke, L. E., & Puczynski, S. (1995). Clinical assessment and management of adherence to medical regimens. In P. M. Nicassio & T. W. Smith (Eds.), *Managing chronic illness: A biopsychosocial perspective* (pp. 313–349). Washington, DC: American Psychological Association.

Dunbar-Jacob, J., & Schlenk, E. (1996). Treatment adherence and clinical outcome: Can we make a difference? In R. J. Resnick, & R. H. Rozensky (Eds.), *Health psychology through the life span: Practice and research opportunities.* (pp. 323–343). Washington DC: American Psychological Association.

Dunbar-Jacob, J., & Mortimer-Stephens, M. (2001). Treatment adherence in chronic disease. *Journal of Clinical Epidemiology, 54*, S57–S60.

Falvo, D. R. (2004). *Effective patient education: A guide to increased compliance.* Boston MA: Jones & Bartlett Publishers.

Fincham, J. (Ed.) (1995). *Advancing prescription medicine compliance: New paradigms, new practices.* Binghamton, NY: Pharmaceutical Products Press.

Garfield, S. L., (1994). Research on client variables in psychotherapy. In A. E. Bergin & S. L. Garfield (Eds.), *Handbook of Psychotherapy and Behavior Change.* (4th ed., pp. 190–228). New York: Wiley.

Grahl, C. (1994). Improving compliance: Solving a $100 billion problem. *Managed Health Care*, 11–13.

Haynes, B., McDonald, H., Garg, A. X., & Montague, P. (2002). Interventions for helping patients to follow prescriptions for medications (Chocrane Review). In: *The Chocrane Library, Issue 4.* Oxford: Update Software.

Haynes, B., Wang, E., & Da Mota Gomes, M. (1987). A critical review of interventions to improve compliance with prescribed medications. *Patient Education and Counseling, 10*, 155–166.

Helmus, T. C., Saules, K. K., Schoener, E. P., & Roll, J. M. (2003). Reinforcement of counseling attendance and alcohol abstinence in a community-based dual-diagnosis treatment program: A feasibility study. *Psychology of Addictive Behaviors, 17(3)* 249–251

Heiby, E. M., & Lukens, C. (in press). Behavioral Analysis and Modification. In W. T. O'Donohue & E. R. Levensky (Eds.), *Promoting treatment adherence: A practical handbook for healthcare providers.* New York: Sage.

Ickovics, J. R., & Meisler, A. (1997). Adherence in AIDS clinical trials: A framework clinical research and clinical care. *Journal of Clinical Epidemiology, 50*, 385–391.

Kirschenbaum, D. S., & Flanery, R. C. (1983). Behavioral contracting: Outcomes and elements. In M. Hersen, R. M. Eisler, & P. M. Miller (Eds.), *Progress in behavior modification* (Vol. 15). New York: Academic Press.

Lash, S. J., & Burden, J. L. (in press). Adherence to treatment of substance abuse disorders. In W. T. O'Donohue & E. R. Levensky (Eds.), *Promoting treatment adherence: A practical handbook for healthcare providers.* New York: Sage.

Levensky, E. L. (in press) Increasing medication adherence in chronic illnesses: Guidelines for behavioral healthcare clinicians working in primary care settings. In W. O'Donohue, M. Byrd, D. Henderson, & N. Cummings (Eds.), *Behavioral integrative care: Treatments that work in the primary care setting.* New York: Taylor & Francis.

Liu, H., Golin, C. E., Miller, L. G., Hays, R. D., Beck, C. K., Sanandaji, S., et al. (2001). A comparison study of multiple measures of adherence to HIV protease inhibitors. *Annals of Internal Medicine, 134*, 968–977.

Malouff, J. M., & Schutte, N. S. (2004). Strategies for increasing client completion of treatment assignments. *The Behavior Therapist, 27(6)*, 118–121.

McDonald, H. P., Garg, A. X., & Haynes, R. B. (2002). Interventions to enhance patient adherence to medication prescriptions. *Journal of the American Medical Association, 288*, 2868–2879.

Meichenbaum, D., & Turk, D. (1987). *Facilitating treatment adherence: A practitioner's guidebook.* New York, NY: Plenum.

Miller, L. G., & Hays, R. D. (2000). Measuring adherence to antiretroviral medications in clinical trials. *HIV Clinical Trials, 1*(1), 36–46.

Morris, L., & Schulz, R. (1992). Patient compliance—An overview. *Journal of Clinical Pharmacy and Therapeutics, 17*, 283–295.

Mullen, P., Green, L., & Persinger, G. (1985). Clinical trials of patient education for chronic conditions: A comparative meta-analysis of intervention types. *Preventative Medicine, 14,* 753–781.

Myers, L., & Midence, K. (Eds.) (1998). *Adherence to treatment in medical conditions.* United Kingdom: Harwood Academic Publishers.

Pamallona, S., Bollini, P., Tibaldi, G., Kupelnick, B., & Munizza, C. (2002). Patient adherence in the treatment of depression. *British Journal of Psychiatry, 180,* 184–189.

Rabkin, J. G., & Chesney, M. (1999). Treatment adherence to HIV medications, the achilles heal of new therapeutics. In D. G., Ostrow & S. C. Kalichman, (Eds,), *Psychosocial and public health impacts of new HIV therapies. AIDS prevention and mental health* (pp. 61–82). New York, NY: Kluwer Academic/Plenum Publishers.

Rand, C. S., & Weeks, K. (1998). Measuring adherence with medication regimens in clinical care and research. In S. Shumaker, E. Schron, J Ockene, & W. McBee (Eds.), *The handbook of health behavior change* (pp. 114–132). New York: Springer Publishing Company.

Reis, B. F., & Brown, L. G. (1999). Reducing psychotherapy dropouts: Maximizing perspective convergence in the psychotherapy dyad. *Psychotherapy, 36,* 123–136.

Riekert, K. A. (in press). How to integrate regimen adherence into clinical practice. In W. T. O'Donohue & E. R. Levensky (Eds.), *Promoting treatment adherence: A practical handbook for healthcare providers.* New York: Sage.

Riekert, K. A., & Rand, C. S. (2002). Electronic monitoring of adherence: When is high-tech best? *Journal of Clinical .Psychology in Medical Settings, 9,* 25–34.

Rogers, H., & Bullman, W. (1995). Prescription medication compliance. A review of the baseline knowledge—A report of the National Council of Patient Information and Education. *Journal of Pharmacoepidemiology, 3(2),* 3–36.

Roter, D., Hall, J., Merisca, R., Nordstrom, B., Cretin, D., & Svarstad, B. (1998). Effectiveness of Interventions to Improve Patient Compliance: A meta-analysis. *Medial Care, 36(8),* 1138–1161.

Sackett, D. L, Straus, S. E, Richardson, W. S., Rosenberg, W., & Haynes, R. B.(2000). *Evidence-based medicine: How to practice and teach EBM* (2nd ed.). New York: Churchill Livingstone.

Scheel, M. J., Hanson, W. E., & Razzhavaikina, T. L. (2004). The process of recommending homework in psychotherapy: A review of the therapist delivery methods, client acceptability, and factors that affect compliance. *Psychotherapy: Theory, Research, Practice, Training, 41(1),* 38–55.

Shumaker, S., Schron, E., Ockene, J., & McBee, W. (Eds.) (1998). *The handbook of health behavior change.* New York: Springer Publishing Company.

Spiegler, M. D, & Guevremont, D. C (2003). *Contemporary Behavior Therapy* (4th ed.). South Melbourne: Nelson Thomas.

Stewart, M. A. (1996). Effective physician–patient communication and health outcomes: A review. *Canadian Medical Association Journal, 152,* 1423–1433.

Stone, V. E. (2001). Strategies for optimizing adherence for highly active antiretroviral therapy: Lessons from research and clinical practice. *Clinical Infectious Diseases, 33,* 865–872.

Vermerie, E., Hearnshaw, H., & Van Royen, P. (2001). Patient adherence to treatment: Three decades of research. A comprehensive review. *Journal of Clinical Pharmacy and Therapeutics, 26,* 331–342.

Vitolins, M. Z., Rand, C. S., Rapp, S. R., Ribisl, P. M., & Sevick, M. A. (2000). Measuring Adherence to Behavioral and Medical Interventions. *Controlled Clinical Trials, 21,* 188S–194S.

Walitzer, K. S., Dermen, K. H., & Connors, G. J. (1999). Strategies for preparing clients for treatment. *Behavior Modification, 23,* 129–151.

Wierzbicki, M., & Pekarik, G. (1993). A meta-analysis of psychotherapy dropout. *Professional Psychology Research and Practice, 24,* 190–195.

Willey, C., Redding, C., Stafford, J., Garfield, F., Geletko, S., Flanigan, T., et al. (2000). Stages of change for adherence with medication regimens for chronic disease: Development and validation of a measure. *Clinical Therapeutics, 2, 1*

Zweben, A., & Zuckoff, A. (2004). Motivational Interviewing and treatment adherence. In W. R. Miller & S. Rollnick (Eds), *Motivational interviewing: Preparing people for change* (2nd ed.). New York: Guilford Press.

Obsessive–Compulsive Disorder

Greg Hajcak • Jonathan D. Huppert • Edna B. Foa

WHAT IS OBSESSIVE–COMPULSIVE DISORDER (OCD)?

OCD is defined by recurrent obsessions and/or compulsions that significantly impair functioning (American Psychiatric Association, 1994). Obsessions involve intrusive thoughts, images, or impulses that cause significant distress. Common obsessions include preoccupation with contamination, concerns about harming oneself or others, intrusive sexual thoughts, fear of throwing possessions away, and preoccupation with things not being "just right." Compulsions can be either mental or physical behaviors that people have a difficult time resisting; functionally, over 90% of patients with OCD report that they perform compulsions to reduce the distress associated with obsessions (Foa et al., 1995). Common compulsions include washing, checking, reviewing, hoarding, reassurance seeking, and repeating acts until they feel as if they have been performed correctly. Although DSM-IV criteria do not require the presence of both obsessions and compulsions, only 2% of patients in the DSM-IV field study reported obsessions alone (Foa et al., 1995). Covert mental actions, such as repeating a phrase mentally, or replacing an anxiety-provoking thought or image with a neutralizing thought or image, are important to identify as they can be overlooked in favor of more overt compulsive behaviors. When patients do not recognize that their obsessions and compulsions are excessive or unreasonable, they are given the diagnosis of OCD "with poor insight." From the standpoint of cognitive behavioral therapy, it is crucial to identify the functional relationship between obsessive thoughts and ritualistic behaviors, and to note the presence of poor insight.

BASIC FACTS ABOUT OCD

OCD is a relatively common disorder, estimated to occur in approximately. 5–3% of the population (Andrews, Henderson, & Hall, 2001; Rasmussen & Eisen, 1992). OCD can be observed in childhood, and has been reported as young as age 2 (Rapoport, Swedo, & Leonard, 1992), although it more commonly begins in early adolescence and young adulthood (Rasmussen & Eisen, 1992). In adult samples, approximately 50% of patients with OCD are female (Rasmussen & Tsuang, 1986). Consistent with the finding that OCD has an earlier age of onset in males (Lochner et al., 2004), reports indicate OCD in twice as many males as females in some pediatric samples (Swedo, Rapoport, Leonard, Lenane, & Cheslow, 1989).

Most patients with OCD experience a chronic course with waning and waxing symptoms (Rasmussen & Eisen, 1992). OCD has been associated with significant comorbid psychiatric illnesses, especially depression and other anxiety disorders (Denys Tenny, van Megen, de Geus, & Westenberg, 2004, LaSalle et al., 2004). In fact, these studies indicate that between one-third and two-thirds of patients with OCD meet criteria for major depressive disorder. There also appear to be high rates of comorbidity between OCD and tic disorders (Eichstedt & Arnold, 2001), as well

Hajack, G., Huppert, J. D., & Foa, E. B. (2006). Obsessive–compulsive disorder. In J. E. Fisher & W. T. O'Donohue (Eds.), *Practitioner's guide to evidence-based psychotherapy*. New York: Springer.

as potentially higher rates of comorbidity with other impulse-control disorders (cf, Foa & Franklin, 2001). In terms of impact on quality of life and functioning, OCD has been found to adversely affect employment, social functioning, physical functioning, and general quality of life (Quilty, Van Ameringen, Mancini, Oakman, & Farvolden, 2003; Bijl & Rivelli, 2000).

WHAT CAUSES OCD?

There is no single cause that currently explains why some people develop OCD. There are, however, a number of theoretical accounts regarding the development and maintenance of OCD. Dollard & Miller (1950) suggest that fear associated with obsessions begins via classical conditioning (e.g., the experience of fear is paired with a cue such as a dirty bathroom or an intrusive thought), and rituals are maintained through operant conditioning (e.g., avoiding dirty places or performing rituals reduces anxiety associated with the obsession). More cognitive theories focus on the false assumptions commonly found in patients with OCD, especially exaggerated personal responsibility (Salkovskis, 1985). Foa and Kozak (1985) proposed that patients with OCD overestimate threat because they fail to take the absence of danger as a signal of safety.

Although data indicate that there is some type of familial transmission of OCD (Nestadt et al., 2000), this also appears to be the case for most anxiety disorders (Nestadt et al., 2001). A number of genes believed to be involved in OCD have been identified; however, progress in this area seems to be hampered because of the clinical heterogeneity of OCD (Pato, Pato, & Pauls, 2002). For instance, recent studies have suggested that gender, neurobiological differences, comorbidity, and symptom types may all contribute to etiological heterogeneity in OCD. Specifically, one OCD phenotype appears to involve earlier onset, being male, a more chronic course, higher incidence of tic-related disorders, higher familial incidence of OC symptoms, and may be associated with distinct genetic susceptibility (Eichstedt & Arnold, 2001; Lochner et al., 2004).

A subset of pediatric patients develop OCD more following streptococcal infection, and these cases are referred to as Pediatric Autoimmune Neuropsychiatric Disorders Associated with Strep (PANDAS; Swedo et al., 1998). Hallmark features of PANDAS include a relatively sudden onset and symptom exacerbations and reductions that follow the course of step infections. Few data are available to date to establish the prevalence of PANDAS within patients with OCD, but our clinical experience suggests a small percentage of patients follow the hallmark features.

In terms of the neural substrates of OCD, recent neuroimaging studies have implicated hyperactivity in frontostriatal circuits, including the orbitofrontal cortex, anterior cingulate cortex, and structures of the basal ganglia (Saxena, Brody, Schwartz, & Baxter, 1998). Evidence suggests that symptom reduction following either psychotherapy or psychopharmacology is reliably related to reductions in activity in these areas of the brain. Functionally, the frontostriatal circuit has been found to be involved in action monitoring. Consistent with both OCD symptoms and OCD-related abnormalities of these areas, recent studies have reported hyperactive brain activity related to response monitoring in Obsessive–Compulsive subjects (Gehring, Himk, & Nisenson, 2000; Hajcak & Simons, 2002; Ursu, Stenger, Shear, Jones, & Carter, 2003). Although neuropsychological findings vary somewhat from study to study, patients with OCD may show deficits in some memory tasks and tasks that assess executive functions such as organization (cf, Kuelz, Hohagen, & Volderholzer, 2004).

WHAT IS INVOLVED IN EFFECTIVE ASSESSMENT?

OCD symptom severity can be assessed with either clinical interviews or self-report measures. Although structured clinical interviews can be used to determine whether or not patients meet DSM-IV criteria for OCD, the semistructured Yale-Brown Obsessive–Compulsive Scale (Y-BOCS; Goodman et al., 1989a, 1989b) is considered the gold standard in OCD assessment. The Y-BOCS is a semistructured clinician-administered interview that involves both a symptom checklist that assesses the presence of 40 obsessions and 29 compulsions, and a measure of symptom severity. Severity of obsessions and compulsions are calculated separately, where each are rated for time occupied, interference, distress, resistance, and control. The Y-BOCS total score is the sum of both the obsession and compulsion severity scales. The total scores run from 0 to 40, with the average patient in most studies ranging between a 24 and 28, and a clinical cut-score of 14.

There are several self-report instruments including the Maudsley Obsessive–Compulsive Inventory (Hodgson & Rachman, 1977), the Padua Inventory—Washington State University Revision (Burns, Keortge, Formea, & Sternberger, 1996), and the Vancouver Obsessive–Compulsive Inventory (in press). One of the most recent, and easy to administer, is the Obsessive–Compulsive Inventory—Revised (OCI-R; Foa, Huppert, et al., 2002), an 18-item self-report measure that assesses the distress associated with obsessions and compulsions. In addition to the total score, separate subscale scores can be calculated for Washing, Checking, Ordering, Obsessing, Hoarding, and Neutralizing. Foa, Huppert, et al. (2002) report excellent psychometric properties for the OCI-R in clinical patients with a range of anxiety disorders and nonanxious controls; excellent psychometric properties have also been reported in a nonclinical sample (Hajcak, Huppert, Simons, & Foa, 2004).

WHAT SHOULD BE RULED OUT?

Because of the high rates of psychiatric comorbidity in patients with OCD, it can be difficult to differentiate OCD from other disorders with related symptoms. Specifically, obsessions should be differentiated from depressive rumination and pathological worry characteristic of MDD and generalized anxiety disorder (GAD), respectively. These related symptoms can often be differentiated in the following way: the content of worry is usually verbally based, typically involves real-world concerns (e.g., the health of older parents, money in difficult financial times, etc.) and is experienced as appropriate or ego-syntonic. Ruminations generally surround negativistic thoughts about the past and the self and/or world, and depressed patients rarely struggle to suppress ruminations. On the other hand, obsessions generally involve magical or unrealistic thinking and images that are experienced as ego-dystonic; furthermore, patients with OCD continually attempt to suppress obsessions (cf, Foa & Franklin, 2001).

WHAT TREATMENTS ARE EFFECTIVE?

Behavior therapy that involves both exposure and response prevention (EX/RP) are considered the first-line treatment for OCD by experts (Greist et al., 2003). EX/RP entails exposing patients to feared stimuli in a hierarchical fashion, and having patients completely refrain from ritualizing. Exposures can be in vivo (e.g., touching contaminated objects) and/or *imaginal* (e.g., thinking about spreading contamination). Imaginal exposures should be utilized, in particular, to confront patients with their unrealistic feared catastrophes that cannot and/or should not be produced in reality (e.g., finding out that one has a brain tumor). Importantly, both imaginal and in vivo exposures must be long enough and repeated frequently enough to allow for anxiety habituation (cf, Foa & Franklin, 2001). During the course of EX/RP, patients learn that they do not need to ritualize to reduce their anxiety—that anxiety habituates on its own. Importantly, they learn that the feared disasters they anticipate do not materialize and therefore they do not need to protect themselves by ritualizing or avoiding feared situations.

A number of studies have shown EX/RP to be superior to a number of control treatments (Abramowitz, 1997). Furthermore, many studies have demonstrated that treatment gains following EX/RP are maintained over long periods of time—up to 5 years in one study (see Marks, 1997). Studies examining whether the beneficial effects of EX/RP generalize beyond therapy delivered by experts in research settings have found support for the general effectiveness of EX/RP in both nonresearch and private practice settings (Franklin, Abromawitz, Kozak, Levitt, & Foa, 2000; Warren & Thomas, 2001), as well as in ethnically diverse populations (Friedman et al., 2003). Importantly, EX/RP also appears generally effective for patients with comorbid depression (Abramowitz, Franklin, Street, Kozak, & Foa, 2000; Overbeek, Schruers, Vermetten, Griez, 2002) and personality disorders (Franklin, Harap, & Herbert, 2004), further suggesting the generalizability of EX/RP as an effective treatment.

Many studies have also found that psychopharmacological treatment with selective serotonin reuptake inhibitors (SSRIs) results in significantly greater OCD symptom reduction relative to placebo (for a review, see Dougherty, Rauch, & Jenike, 2002). However, when the medicine is discontinued, some studies have reported high rates of relapse (Koran et al., 2002), although longer-term treatment may reduce rates of relapse somewhat (Hollander et al., 2003). Relatively few studies have directly compared therapy with SSRI with EX/RP; however, the available evidence suggests that EX/RP is at least as effective if not superior to existing SSRIs (Dougherty et al., 2002). In a recent study, EX/RP was superior to clomipramine, and the combined treatment outcome was superior to medication only, but equivalent to EX/RP only (Foa et al, in press). Thus, although there is some evidence that the combination of SSRI and EX/RP produces slightly better outcome than EX/RP alone (Hohagen et al., 1998), their combination does not appear to have reliable synergistic effects (cf, Foa, Franklin, & Moser, 2002). Alternative treatments for intractable cases of OCD have also been evaluated. Notably, deep-brain stimulation (cf, Kopell, Greenberg, & Rezai, 2004) and the surgical removal of the cingulate have shown to improve some treatment-resistant cases (Dougherty et al., 2002).

WHAT PREDICTS TREATMENT OUTCOME?

Most patients that get adequate treatment with either EX/RP or pharmacotherapy will experience significant reductions in symptom severity. However, there are a number of factors that appear related to poor outcome following therapy. Some studies have found that specific patterns of pretreatment brain activity differentially predict positive treatment response to both pharmacotherapy and behavior therapy (cf, Hurley, Saxena, Rauch, Hoehn-Saric, & Taber, 2002). An early study suggested that OCD patients that have obsessions in the absence of overt rituals may fare more poorly than patients with overt rituals (Rachman & Hodgson, 1980); however, this difference may have resulted from early failures to identify and target covert mental rituals (cf, Abramowitz, Franklin, Schwartz, & Furr 2003). Subsequent studies suggest that poor insight is associated with poorer outcome with EX/RP (Abramowitz et al., 2003). Additionally, a number of studies have reported that hoarding is related to poorer outcome following both cognitive-behavioral therapy (Abramowitz et al., 2000; Mataix-Cols, Marks, Greist, Kobak, & Baer, 2002), and pharmacotherapy (Mataix-Cols, Rauch, Manzo, Jenike, & Baer, 1999). Severe depression may also be associated with a somewhat attenuated treatment response (Abramowitiz et al., 2000; Overbeek, Schruers, Vermetten, & Griez, 2002).

WHAT DO WE STILL NEED TO KNOW?

OCD is a heterogeneous disorder, and further progress may depend on research that focuses on particular symptom subtypes (cf, Calamari et al., 2003). For instance, whether hoarding represents a distinct subtype of OCD or should be considered a separate but related disorder should be a topic of future studies (see Steketee & Frost, 2003). Similarly, the OCD with childhood-onset should be investigated with respect to OCD that begins later in life. Within the latter subtype, its relationship to tic-related disorders is another area that requires further study. Identifying distinct phenotypes is a necessary step toward better understanding OCD at the level of molecular mechanisms, including the involvement of both specific genes and neurotransmitters.

   In addition to furthering our understanding of basic psychopathology and mechanisms underlying the subtypes of OCD, more research will be needed to guide practitioners in terms of how to treat treatment-resistant patients (i.e., those who do not respond to SSRIs or EX/RP), how to maintain treatment gains, and how to treat patients to full remission. Finally, how to best export the most effective treatments to the community and ensure that more patients are receiving adequate treatment also requires further examination.

WHAT ARE SOME HELPFUL RESOURCES?

- Chansky, Tamar E. (2001). *Freeing your child from obsessive-compulsive disorder: A powerful, practical program for parents of children and adolescents.* New York, NY: Three Rivers Press.
- Foa, E. B. & Wilson, R. (2001). *Stop obsessing!: How to overcome your obsessions and compulsions.* New York, NY: Bantam Doubleday Dell Publications.
- Hyman, B. M., & Pedrick, C. (1999). *The OCD workbook: Your guide to breaking free from obsessive–compulsive disorder.* Oakland, CA: New Harbinger Publications.
- March, J. S., & Mulle, K. (1998). *OCD in children and adolescents: A cognitive-behavioral treatment manual.* New York, NY: The Guilford Press.
- Rapoport, J. L. (1997). *The boy who couldn't stop washing: The experience and treatment of obsessive–compulsive disorder.* New York, NY: EP Dutton.
- Schwartz, J. M. (1997). *Brain lock: Free yourself from obsessive-compulsive behavior.* New York, NY: Regan Books, Harper Collins.
- www.adaa.org/Anxiety DisorderInfor/OCD.cfm
- www.ocfoundation.org
- www.med.upenn.edu/ctsa
- www.nimh.nih.gov/Health Information/ocdmenu.cfm
- www.nlm.nih.gov/medlineplus/obsessivecompulsivedisorder.html

REFERENCES

Abramowitz, J. S. (1997). Effectiveness of psychological and pharmacological treatments for obsessive–compulsive disorder: A quantitative review. *Journal of Consulting and Clinical Psychology, 65*, 44–52.

Abramowitz, J. S., Franklin, M. E., Schwartz, S. A., & Furr, J. M. (2003). Symptom presentation and outcome of cognitive-behavioral therapy for obsessive-compulsive disorder. *Journal of Consulting and Clinical Psychology, 71*, 1049–1057.

Abramowitz, J. S., Franklin, M. E., Street, G. P., Kozak, M. J., & Foa, E. B. (2000). The effects of pre-treatment depression on cognitive-behavioral treatment outcome in OCD clinic outpatients. *Behavior Therapy, 31*, 517–528.

American Psychiatric Association, American Psychiatric Association. (1994). *Diagnostic and statistical manual of mental disorders* (4th ed.). Washington, DC: Author.

Andrews, G., Henderson, S., & Hall, W. (2001). Prevalence, comorbidity, disability and service utilization. *British Journal of Psychiatry, 178*, 145–153.

Bijl, R. V., & Ravelli, A. (2000). Current and residual functional disability assocaited with psychopathology: findings from the Netherlands Mental Health Survey and Incidence Study (NEMESIS). *Psychological Medicine, 30*, 657–668.

Burns, G. L., Keortge, S. G., Formea, G. M., & Sternberger, L. G. (1996). Revision of the Padua Inventory of Obsessive Compulsive Disorder Symptoms: Distinctions between worry, obsessions, and compulsions. *Behavior Research & Therapy, 34(2)*, 163–173.

Calamari, J. E., Wiegartz, P. S., Riemann, B. C., et al. (2003). Obsessive–compulsive disorder subtypes: An attempted replication and extension of a symptom-based taxonomy. *Behaviour Research & Therapy.*

Denys, D., Tenney, N., van Megen, H. J. G. M., de Geus, F., & Westenberg, H. G. M. (2004). Axis I and II comorbidity in a large sample of patients with obsessive-compulsive disorder. *Journal of Affective Disorders, 80*, 155–162.

Dollard, J., & Miller, N. L. (1950). *Personality and psychotherapy: An alanysis in terms of learning, thinking and culture.* New York: McGraw-Hill.

Dougherty, D. D., Baer, L., Cosgrove, G. R., Cassem, E. H., Price, B. H., Nierenberg, A. A, et al. (2002). Prospective long-term follow-up of 44 patietns who received cingulotomy for treatment-refractory obsessive-compulsive disorder. *American Journal of Psychiatry, 159*, 269–274.

Dougherty, D. D., Rauch, S., & Jenike, M.. (2002). Pharmalogical treatments for obsessive–compulsive disorder. In P. Nathan & J. M. Gorman (Eds.), *A guide to treatments that work (2nd ed.)* (pp. 387–410). New York: Oxford University Press.

Eichstedt, J. A., & Arnold, S. L. (2001). Childhood-onset obsessive–compulsive disorder: A tic-related subtype of OCD? *Clinical Psychology Review, 21*, 137–158.

Foa, E. B., & Franklin, M. E. (2001). Obsessive–compulsive disorder. In D. H. Barlow (Ed.), *Clinical handbook of psychological disorders (3rd ed.)* (pp. 209–263). New York: Guilford Press.

Foa, E. B., Franklin, M. E., & Moser, J. S. (2002). Context in the clinic: How well do cognitive-behavioral therapies and medications work in combination? *Biological Psychiatry, 52*, 987–997.

Foa, E. B., Huppert, J. D., Leiberg, S., Langner, R., Kichic, R., Hajcak, G., & Salkovskis, P. (2002). The Obsessive–Compulsive Inventory: Development and validation of a short version. *Psychological Assessment, 14*, 485–496.

Foa, E. B., & Kozak, M. J. (1985). Treatment of anxiety disorders: Implications for psychopathology. In A. H. Tuma & J. D. Maser (Eds.), *Anxiety and the anxiety disorders* (pp. 421–452). Hillsdale, NJ: Erlbaum.

Foa, E. B., Kozak, M. J., Goodman, W. K., Hollander, E., Jenike, M., & Rasmussen, S. (1995). DSM-IV field trial: Obsessive–compulsive disorder. *American Journal of Psychiatry, 152*, 90–94.

Franklin, M. E., Abramowitz, J. S., Kozak, M. J., Levitt, J. T., & Foa, E. B. (2000). Effectiveness of exposure and ritual prevention for obsessive–compulsive disorder: Randomized compared with non-randomized samples. *Journal of Consulting and Clinical Psychology, 68*, 594–602.

Franklin, M. E., Harap, S., & Herbert, J. D. (2004). Effects of axis II personality disorders on exposure and ritual prevention treatment outcome for OCD. Manuscript in preparation.

Friedman, S., Smith, L. C., Halpern, B., Levine, C., Paradis, C., Viswanathan, R., et al. (2003). Obsessive–compulsive disorder in a multi-ethnic urban outpatient clinic: Initial presentation and treatment outcome with exposure and ritual prevention. *Behavior Therapy, 34*, 397–410.

Gehring, W. J., Himle, J., & Nisenson, L. G. (2000). Action-monitoring dysfunction in obsessive–compulsive disorder. *Psychological Science, 11(1)*, 1–6.

Goodman, W. K., Price, L. H., Rasmussen, S. A., et al. (1989a). The Yale-Brown Obsessive–Compulsive Scale: II. Validity. *Archives of General Psychiatry, 46*, 1012–1016.

Goodman, W. K., Price, L. H., Rasumssen, S. A., et al. (1989b). The Yale-Brown Obsessive–Compulsive Scale: I. Development, use, and reliability. *Archives of General Psychiatry, 46*, 1006–1011.

Greist J. H., Bandelow B., Hollander, E., Marazziti, D., Montgomery, S. A. Nutt D. J. et al. (2003). World Council of Anxiety. WCA recommendations for the long-term treatment of obsessive-compulsive disorder in adults. *CNS Spectrums, 8 Suppl 1*, 7–16.

Hajcak, G., Huppert, J. D., Simons, R. F., & Foa, E. B. (2004). Psychometric properties of the OCI-R in a college sample. *Behavior Research & Therapy, 42*, 115–123.

Hajcak, G. & Simons, R. F. (2002). Error-related brain activity in obsessive compulsive undergraduates. *Psychiatry Research, 110(1)*, 63–72.

Hodgson, R. J., & Rachman, S. (1977). Obsessional–compulsive complaints. *Behavior Research & Therapy, 15*, 389–395.

Hohagen, F., Winkelmann, G., Rasche-Rauchle, H., et al. (1998). Combination of behavior therapy with fluvoxamine in campirson with behavior therpay and placebo: Results of a multicentre study. *British Journal of Psychiatry, 173*, 71–78.

Hollander, E., Allen, A., Steiner, M., Wheadon, D. E., Oakes, R., & Burnham, D. B. (2003). Acute and long-term treatment and prevention of relapse of obsessive-compulsive disorder with paroxetine. *Journal of Clinical Psychiatry, 64*, 1113–1121.

Hurley, R. A., Saxena, S., Rauch, S. L., Hoehn-Saric, R., & Taber, K. H. (2002). Predicting treatment response in obsessive–compulsive disorder. *Journal of Neuropsychiatry and Clinical Neuroscience, 14*, 249–253.

Koran, L. M., Hackett, E., Rubin, A., et al. (2002). Efficacy of sertraline in the long term treatment of obsessive compulsive disorder. *American Journal of Psychiatry, 159*, 88–95.

Kopell, B. H., Greenberg, B., & Rezai, A. R. (2004). Deep brain stimulation for psychiatric disorders. *Journal of Clinical Neurophysiology, 21*, 51–67.

Kuelz, A. K., Hohagen, F., & Voderholzer, U. (2004). Neuropsychological functioning in obsessive-compulsive disorder: A critical review. *Biological Psychology, 65*, 185–236.

LaSalle, V. H., Cromer, K. R., Nelson, K. N., Kazuba, D., Justement, L., & Murphy, D. L. (2004). Diagnositic interview assessed neuropsychiatric disorder comorbidity in 334 individuals with obsessive–compulsive disorder. *Depression and Anxiety, 19*, 163–173.

Lochner, C., Hummings, S. M. J., Kinnear, C. J., et al. (2004). Gender in obsessive–compulsive disorder: Clinical and genetic findings. European *Neuropsychopharmacology, 14*, 105–113.

Marks, I. (1997). Behaviour therapy for obsessive-compulsive disorder: A decade of progress. *Canadian Journal of Psychiatry 42*, 1021–1027.

Mataix-Cols, D., Marks, I. M., Greist, J. H., Kobak, K. A., & Baer, L. (2002). Obsessive–compulsive symptom dimensions as predictors of compliance with and response to behavior stherapy: Results from a controlled Trial. *Psychotherapy and Psychosomatics, 71*, 255–262.

Mataix-Cols, D., Rauch, S., Manzo, P., Jenike, M., & Baer, L. (1999). Use of factor-analyzed symptom subtypes to predict outcome with serotonin reuptake inhibitors and placebo in obsessive–compulsive disorder. *American Journal of Psychiatry, 156*, 1409–1416.

Nestadt, G., Samuels, J., Riddle, M., et al. (2000). A family study of obsessive–compulsive disorder. *Archives of General Psychiatry, 57*, 358–363.

Nestadt, G., Samuels, J., Riddle, M., et al. (2001). The relationship between obsessive-compulsive disorder and anxiety and affective disorders: Results from the Johns Hopkins OCD Family Study. *Psychological Medicine, 31*, 481–487.

Overbeek, T., Schruers, K., Vermetten, E., & Griez, E. (2002). Comorbidity of obsessive-compulsive disorder and depression: Prevalence, symptom severity, and treatment effect. *Journal of Clinical Psychiatry, 63*, 1106–1112.

Pato, M. T., Pato, C. N., & Pauls, D. L. (2002). Recent findings in the genetics of OCD. *Journal of Clinical Psychiatry, 63*, 30–33.

Quilty, L. C., Van Ameringen, M., Mancini, C., Oakman, J., & Farvolden, P. (2003). Quality of life and the anxiety disorders. *Journal of Anxiety Disorders, 17*, 405–426.

Rachman, S., & Hodgson, R. (1980). *Obsessions and compulsions.* Englewood Cliffs, NJ: Prentice-Hall.

Rapoport, J. L., Swedo, S. E., & Leonard, H. L. (1992). Childhood obsessive compulsive disorder. *Journal of Clinical Psychiatry, 53*, 11–16.

Rasmussen, S. A., & Eisen, J. L. (1992). The epidemiology and clinical features of obsessive–compulsive disorder. *Psychiatric Clinics of North America, 15*, 743–758.

Rasmussen, S. A., & Tsuang, M. T. (1986). Clinical characteristics and family history in DSM-III obsessive–compulsive disorder. *American Journal of Psychiatry, 143*, 317–322.

Salkovskis, P. M. (1985). Obsessional-compulsive problems: A cognitive-behavioral analysis. *Behavior Research and Therapy, 23*, 571–583.

Saxena, S., Brody, A. L., Schwartz, J. M., & Baxter, L. R. (1998). Neuroimaging and frontal–subcortical circuitry in obsessive-compulsive disorder. *British Journal of Psychiatry, 173*, 26–37.

Simpson, H. B., Liebowitz, M. L., Foa, E. B., Kozak, M. J., Davies, S., Campeas, R., Franklin, M. E., Huppert, J. D., Kjernsted, K., Rowan, V., Schmidt, A. (2004). Clomipramine, Exposure and Response Prevention, and their combination for OCD: Long term outcomes. *Depression and Anxiety, 19*, 225–233.

Steketee, G., & Frost, R. (2003). Compulsive Hoarding: Current status of the research. *Clinical Psychology Review, b*, 905–927.

Swedo, S. E., Rapoport, J. L., Leonard, H. L., Lenane, M., & Cheslow, D. (1989). Obsessive compulsive disorder in children and adolescents: Clinical phenomenology of 70 consecutive cases. *Archives of General Psychiatry, 46*, 335–341.

Swedo, S. E., Leonard, H. L., Garvey, M., et al. (1998). Pediatric autoimmune neuropsychiatric disorders associated with streptococcal infections: Clinical description of the first 50 cases. *American Journal of Psychiatry, 155,* 264–271.

Ursu, S., Stenger, V. A., Shear, M. K., Jones, M. R., & Carter, C. S. (2003). Overactive action monitoring in obsessive-compulsive disorder: Evidence from functional magnetic resonance imaging. *Psychological Science, 14,* 347–353.

Warren, R., & Thomas, J. C. (2001). Cognitive-behavioral therapy of obsessive-compulsive disorder in private practice: An effectiveness study. *Journal of Anxiety Disorders, 15,* 277–285.

CHAPTER 46

Oppositional Defiant Disorder and Parent Training

Sheila M. Eyberg • Kelly A. O'Brien • Rhea M. Chase

WHAT IS OPPOSITIONAL DEFIANT DISORDER?

Oppositional defiant disorder (ODD) is one of two disruptive behavior disorders in the *Diagnostic and Statistical Manual of Mental Disorders* (DSM-IV; American Psychiatric Association [APA], 1994), along with Conduct Disorder (CD). In the DSM-IV, ODD is characterized by frequent disregard for adult authority, and diagnostic criteria require that four of the following eight symptoms persist for at least six months: loses temper, argues with adults, actively defies or refuses to comply with adults' requests or rules, deliberately annoys people, blames others for mistakes, is touchy or easily annoyed by others, is often angry or resentful, and is often spiteful or vindictive. In addition, these behaviors must occur more frequently than is typically seen in children of comparable age and developmental level and must cause significant impairment in social, academic, or occupational functioning.

BASIC FACTS ABOUT OPPOSITIONAL DEFIANT DISORDER

Disruptive behavior disorders are estimated to occur in 2–16% of school-age children, depending on the population sampled and the method of assessment; the rates are somewhat higher in samples of preschoolers (Loeber, Burke, Lahey, Winters, & Zera, 2000). Prevalence rates of ODD fall in late childhood and adolescence, largely due to the age-related increase in CD, which supercedes the diagnosis of ODD if characteristics of both disorders are present. If the CD behaviors are not considered, ODD tends to persist to middle adolescence and becomes more severe with age.

Among children between one and eight years of age, no gender differences are found in the prevalence of ODD, although boys with ODD demonstrate higher rates of disruptive behavior than girls (Lumley, McNeil, Herschell, & Bahl, 2002). Onset of ODD is gradual, typically beginning before age eight, and the disorder tends to be chronic without treatment. Children with ODD demonstrate substantial rates of comorbid disorders, including Attention Deficit Hyperactivity Disorder (ADHD), depression, and the anxiety disorders (Maughan, Rowe, Messer, Goodman, & Meltzer, 2004).

ETIOLOGICAL FACTORS

Genetics

Although no research suggests that the development of ODD is purely genetic, multi-rater interview data have revealed modest correlations of ODD and CD symptoms among twins, mothers, and fathers (Eaves, Rutter, Silberg, Maes, &

Eyberg, S. M., O'Brien, K. A., & Chase, R. M. (2006). Oppositional defiant disorder and parent training. In J. E. Fisher & W. T. O'Donohue (Eds.), *Practitioner's guide to evidence-based psychotherapy*. New York: Springer.

Pickles, 2000). However, it is difficult to separate genetic influences from the influences of both shared and nonshared environments, and much more work in this area is needed. It is critically important to explore genetic factors that might differentially influence the development of ODD versus CD, and particularly the genetic contributions to aggressive versus nonaggressive behaviors (Burke, Loeber, & Birmaher, 2002).

Child Temperament

Certain early temperamental characteristics, such as negative emotionality, reactive responding, inflexibility, and inhibition, are related to disruptive behaviour disorders later in childhood (Frick & Morris, 2004). The "goodness of fit" between child temperament and parenting style appears to be key. Problems are more likely to arise when child temperament and parenting style are incompatible on some dimension, such as rhythmicity. For example, if a child's sleeping and eating schedule is difficult to establish, this is more likely to cause problems if the parents are highly regimented. In general, difficult child temperament interacts with the quality of parental discipline to moderate the severity of disruptive behavior (Blackson, Tarter, & Mezzich, 1996).

Parenting Behaviors

Parenting plays a major role in the development of disruptive behavior disorders. Baumrind (1968) identified three parenting styles—permissive, authoritarian, and authoritative—and studied their effects on children's development. Authoritative parenting, which involves high parental warmth and firm control, results in the healthiest child outcomes. A low level of warmth combined with harsh disciplinary practices is linked to child disruptive behavior. Patterson (1982) described a coercive cycle of parent–child interaction in which the negative behaviors of each partner function to increase the negative behaviors of the other through the process of negative reinforcement. These fundamental principles have served as the theoretical foundation for many treatment programs designed to increase positive parent–child interactions and decrease negative disciplinary practices (Brinkmeyer & Eyberg, 2003; Kazdin, 2003).

ASSESSMENT

What Should be Ruled Out?

When diagnosing ODD in children, CD can be a difficult differential diagnosis. Although ODD and CD have been identified as distinct disorders in the DSM-IV, their symptomatology often co-occurs. CD is a more severe disorder than ODD, characterized by violation of social norms along with overt and covert aggression (Frick, Lahey, Loeber, & Tannenbaum, 1993). When ODD occurs with any other mental or physical disorders of childhood, both disorders are diagnosed.

What is Involved in Effective Assessment?

Few would argue that comprehensive initial assessment of the child with ODD is critical for determining the appropriate course of treatment. To obtain an accurate picture of the child's behavior, multiple informants and methods, including parent interviews, parent and teacher rating scales, and behavioral observation in the clinic and sometimes the school setting as well, are necessary. The integration of these assessment methods allows the clinician to evaluate the frequency, intensity, and duration of the child's behavior problems across settings and from different perspectives. Conducting a formal diagnostic interview with the child's primary caregiver, such as the NIMH Diagnostic Interview Schedule for Children Version IV (DISC IV; Shaffer, Fisher, Dulcan, & Davies, 1996) or the Child and Adolescent Psychiatric Assessment (Angold & Costello, 2000) is often a starting point for gathering thorough information on the primary symptoms of ODD and comorbid disorders, which influence the course of treatment.

Because a child's disruptive behavior affects and is affected by many environmental factors, parent and teacher questionnaires and rating scales are used to collect information on specific problematic behaviors that vary with different individuals, situations, and task demands. Common measures include the Child Behavior Checklist (CBCL; Achenbach, 1994), the Conners Ratings Scales (Conners, 1997), and the Eyberg Child Behavior Inventory (ECBI; Eyberg & Pincus, 1999). Rating scales can be particularly helpful in determining whether the severity of the child's behavior warrants an actual diagnosis, because they permit comparison of the child's behavior with a normative sample of children of the same age and gender. Measures of parenting stress and tolerance, parenting discipline practices, and parent psychopathology are also important in case conceptualization and treatment planning.

Direct observation of the child's behavior and its functional determinants provides particularly important information. Standardized behavioral observation coding systems, such as the Dyadic Parent–Child Interaction Coding System (DPICS), have been developed to assess parent–child interactions efficiently in the clinic (Eyberg, McDiarmid, Duke, & Boggs, 2004). Information gained from these observations can identify the specific parent behaviors that maintain the child's disruptive behavior and how parents can change the interactions to change the child's problem behaviors. Overall, a comprehensive assessment of ODD requires multiple methods and informants to obtain an accurate picture of the child's presenting problems and the factors that sustain them, which guides treatment planning and outcome evaluation.

TREATMENT

What Treatments are Effective for ODD?

Several effective treatments have been developed for ODD, and treatment gains have been found to generalize across settings and endure after treatment ends. Most of these treatments involve the parents, because parents are best able to identify and modify environmental factors that maintain and exacerbate their child's problem behaviors.

Parent training programs share basic behavioral principles that inform positive child management skills. Parents are taught to ignore or punish negative child behaviors and to reward positive child behaviors, particularly those that are incompatible with the negative behaviors. Parents learn to identify child behaviors they wish to change and to apply consequences (rewards or punishment) predictably and consistently. Parents also learn to recognize situations that lead to negative child behaviors and to modify these situations so as to circumvent some problem behaviors entirely.

Many parent training programs directly target parent–child relationship skills as well as disciplinary techniques. The focus on training parents must always be balanced with recognition of the transactional nature of ODD. It is the interplay of parent and child factors that creates and maintains the dysfunctional interactions characteristic of ODD. Despite bi-directional causal factors, however, the success of treatment relies almost solely on parent compliance and change. It is therefore imperative that clinicians develop a strong working alliance with the parent and remain supportive throughout treatment.

For younger children, and particularly preschoolers, behavioral parent training approaches are the treatment of choice. For older children with disruptive behavior, effective cognitive-behavioral treatments have been developed as well. It is important to note, however, that most treatment options require family involvement at some level. This reflects the importance of addressing environmental and family variables that affect the development and course of ODD.

What are Effective Therapist-based Treatments for ODD?

Parent training programs The earliest and most extensively studied program is Patterson's Parent Training model based on the operant principles of behavior change set forth in *Living with Children* (Patterson & Gullion, 1968). Parents are first introduced to basic social learning principles. They then work with the therapist to identify and monitor specific child behaviors that are most disruptive or frequent. The goal of therapy is to decrease these problem behaviors by ignoring or punishing them each time they occur and rewarding incompatible behaviors. Parents are also counseled on how to work with teachers and implement behavioral interventions in the school setting. This parent training program has evidenced significant reductions in deviant child behavior compared to a wait-list control group (Patterson, Chamberlain, & Reid, 1982).

Parent–Child interaction therapy (PCIT) is a parenting skills training program that places emphasis on improving the quality of the parent–child relationship and changing parent–child interaction patterns (Brinkmeyer & Eyberg, 2003; Eyberg, 1988). The parent and child attend treatment together, which allows monitoring and coaching of parenting skills and child behavior changes in vivo. Parents are taught relationship enhancement skill and an effective application of timeout that emphasizes parental consistency. Outcomes include statistically and clinically significant improvements in interaction quality, child disruptive behavior, parenting stress, and confidence in parenting skills when compared to a wait-list control group (Nixon, Sweeny, Erickson, Touyz, 2002; Schuhmann, Foote, Eyberg, Boggs, & Algina, 1998).

Webster-Stratton's (1994) *Incredible Years* is a group parent training program for children with disruptive behavior. Parents learn positive child management practices and stress management techniques by viewing videotaped vignettes, followed by discussion with other parents. The treatment also provides parents with strategies to enhance child social skills. This effective program has been expanded to include a teacher component with a focus on academic and social skills. The added teacher component results in greater reduction in child behavior problems both at school and at home when compared to a control condition (Webster-Stratton, Reid, & Hammond, 2001).

Multilevel programs The *Triple P-Positive Parenting Program* is a multilevel, prevention-oriented program with five levels of increasing strength and various delivery modalities designed to provide the minimally sufficient intervention required (Sanders, 1999). Level 1, the least intensive, is a "universal" approach providing parenting information and awareness of resources. The next four levels range from brief interventions targeting specific child behavior problems to family interventions targeting multiple problems (e.g., parent depression) in addition to child behavior. Depending on family need, interventions may occur in a number of settings from primary care to the home. In the Level 4 and 5 (clinician-assisted) formats of Triple-P, parents report fewer child behavior problems and greater parent competence and satisfaction after treatment than wait-list families (Sanders, Markie-Dadds, Tully & Bor, 2000).

The *Adolescent Transition Program* (ATP) is a multilevel approach that begins within the middle school setting (Dishion & Kavanagh, 2003). ATP involves three levels: (a) a "universal" level, which provides information to all parents in the school; (b) a level that identifies high-risk families; and (c) a family treatment level. Services range from parenting groups to behavioral family therapy, depending on family need. This proactive and supportive approach within the public school setting has been shown to increase engagement of high-risk families in needed interventions that improve parenting practices and reduce disruptive behavior (Dishion & Kavanagh, 2003).

Individual Child Interventions Treatment for ODD ideally involves a parent or caregiver, to address the transactional nature of the disorder and the various environmental contributions to the development and maintenance of problem behavior. Some research examining individual, child-focused interventions has supported a cognitive-behavioral approach for school age children with ODD (Southam-Gerow, 2003). Cognitive Behavioral Therapy (CBT) directly addresses the core symptoms of ODD by providing tangible problem-solving techniques such as self-monitoring, self-evaluation, and self-reinforcement.

What are Effective Self-Help Treatments?

Several self-help books are available for parents of children with oppositional behavior. Athough few studies have examined the effectiveness of self-help books as stand-alone treatments, the following books for parents are based on sound principles of behavior change and are often used by child therapists as an adjunct to parent training:

- Clark, L. & Robb, J. (1996). *SOS: Help for Parents.* Bowling Green, KY: Parents Press.
- Dishion, T. J. & Patterson, S. G. (1996). *Preventive Parenting with Love, Encouragement, and Limits: The Preschool Years.* Eugene, IL: Castalia Publishing.
- Forehand, R. & Long, N. (2002). *Parenting the Strong-Willed Child, Revised and Updated Edition: The Clinically Proven Five-Week Program for Parents of Two- to Six-Year-Olds.* Chicago, IL: Contemporary Books.
- Patterson, G.R. (1976). *Living with Children: New Methods for Parents and Teachers.* Champaign, Illinois: Research Press.

Parents and providers are also directed to the following websites for information on treatment options and links to references on ODD:

- http://www.therapyadvisor.com. (National Institute of Mental Health)
- http://www.effectivechildtherapy.com (Society of Clinical Child and Adolescent Psychology; Division 53, American Psychological Association).

What is Effective Medical Treatment?

The limited research on pharmacological treatments for disruptive behavior disorders has focused on CD, as a means of controlling the aggression and violence associated with the disorder. Stimulants decrease aggression in children with a primary diagnosis of ADHD and may have a similar effect on children with ODD alone (Waslick, Werry, & Greenhill, 1999). Clonidine may also reduce aggression in children with ADHD and comorbid ODD or CD (Connor, Barkley, & Davis, 2000). In general, findings on pharmacotherapy for aggression in children are limited and inconclusive.

Combination Treatments

Evidence suggests that even when medication is found to reduce aggression effectively, children with disruptive behavior benefit most from a combination of medication and behavioral treatment (Burke et al., 2002). Any treatment for ODD should include some level of parent/caregiver involvement to address the environmental contributions to the disorder.

How Does One Select Among Treatments?

The appropriate treatment for a particular child with ODD depends on many factors assessed in the initial evaluation, including child age, behavior problem severity, and the child's home environment. If medication is considered, it is typically used adjunctively and reserved for severe aggression and violent behavior. Parent training programs can be highly effective, but their effectiveness requires active parent involvement in treatment, and may not be possible if parents have cognitive deficits limiting their ability to learn the necessary skills. Other potential barriers to parent training programs include fees for service and needs for transportation and child care to attend therapy sessions regularly. It is necessary to consider what is feasible for the child and family in terms of cost, time, and parent willingness and ability to change.

FUTURE DIRECTIONS

Child treatment research on ODD has greatly increased our understanding of treatment options for children with ODD. For some children and families, however, effective options do not yet exist. Both advocacy and research are needed to increase treatment options for many disadvantaged children. Even with existing treatments, little is known about their efficacy for children in ethnic minority groups or for girls (Brestan & Eyberg, 1998). Establishing the efficacy of parent training approaches within diverse demographic groups is an important direction for future study.

At the same time, much more specificity in our understanding of treatments for ODD is needed. Most treatment studies of disruptive behavior combine children from different diagnostic groups (e.g., ODD, CD, ADHD) and with diverse comorbid conditions. Optimal treatments for ODD may differ from those for other disruptive behavior disorders and among children with different comorbidities. Few studies have examined the mechanisms by which a treatment reverses the course of ODD. The question originally posed by Paul in 1967 still remains: "What treatment, by whom, is most effective for this individual with that specific problem, and under what set of circumstances?" (p. 111). This is perhaps the most important of all questions as we work to find the most effective, efficient, and feasible treatment options for each child with ODD.

REFERENCES (DOES NOT INCLUDE LIST OF SELF-HELP BOOKS UNLESS OTHERWISE CITED).

Achenbach, T. M. (1994). Child Behavior Checklist and related instruments. In: M. E. Maruish (Ed.), *Use of psychological testing for treatment planning and outcome assessment.* (pp. 517–549), Hillsdale, NJ: Lawrence Erlbaum Associates, Inc.

American Psychiatric Association (1994). *Diagnostic and Statistical Manual of Mental Disorders, 4th edition* (DSM-IV), Washington, DC: Author.

Angold, A., & Costello, E. (2000). The Child and Adolescent Psychiatric Assessment (CAPA). *Journal of the American Academy of Child & Adolescent Psychiatry, 39,* 39–48.

Baumrind, D. (1968). Authoritarian vs. authoritative parental control. *Adolescence, 3,* 255–272.

Blackson, T. C. Tarter, R. E., & Mezzich, A. C. (1996). Interaction between childhood temperament and parental discipline practices on behavioral adjustment in preadolescent sons of substance abuse and normal fathers. *American Journal of Drug & Alcohol Abuse, 22,* 335–348.

Brestan, E., & Eyberg, S. M. (1998). Effective psychosocial treatments of conduct-disordered children and adolescents: 29 years, 82 studies, and 5,272 kids. *Journal of Clinical Child Psychology, 27,* 120–189.

Brinkmeyer, M. Y., & Eyberg, S. M. (2003). Parent–child interaction therapy for oppositional children. In A. E. Kazdin & J. R. Weisz (Eds.). *Evidence-based psychotherapies for children and adolescents* (pp. 204–223). New York: Guilford.

Burke, J. D., Loeber, R. & Birmaher, B. (2002). Oppositional defiant disorder and conduct disorder: A review of the past 10 years, part II. *Journal of the American Academy of Child and Adolescent Psychiatry, 41,* 1275–1293.

Conners, C. K. (1997). *Conners' Rating Scales—Revised.* Multi-Health Systems Inc.: North Tonawanda, NY.

Connor, D. F., Barkley, R. A., & Davis, H. T. (2000). A pilot study of methylphenidate, clonidine, or the combination in ADHD comorbid with aggressive oppositional defiant or conduct disorder. *Clinical Pediatrics, 30,* 19–35.

Dishion, T. J. & Kavanagh K. (2003). Intervening in adolescent problem behavior: A family-centered approach. New York: Guilford.

Eaves, L., Rutter, M., Silberg, J. L., Maes, H., & Pickles, A. (2000). Genetic and environmental causes of covariation in interview assessments of disruptive behavior in child and adolescent twins. *Behavior Genetics, 30,* 321–334.

Eyberg, S. M. (1988). Parent-child interaction therapy: Integration of traditional and behavioural concerns. *Child & Family Behaviour Therapy, 10,* 33–46.

Eyberg, S. M., McDiarmid, M. D., & Boggs, S. R. (2004). Manual for the Dyadic Parent–Child Interaction Coding System (3rd ed.) Available at www.pcit.org.

Eyberg, S. M., & Pincus, D. (1999). *Eyberg Child Behavior Inventory and Sutter-Eyberg Student Behavior Inventory: Professional manual.* Odessa, FL: Psychological Assessment Resources.

Frick, P. J. & Morris, A. S. (2004). Temperament and developmental pathways to conduct problems. *Journal of Clinical Child and Adolescent Psychology, 33,* 54–68.

Frick, P., Lahey, B., Loeber, R., & Tannenbaum, L. (1993). Oppositional defiant disorder and conduct disorder: A meta-analytic review of factor analyses and cross-validation in a clinic sample. *Clinical Psychology Review,* 13, 319–340.

Kazdin, A. E. (2003). Problem-solving skills training and parent management training for conduct disorder. In A. E. Kazdin & J. R. Weisz (Eds.), *Evidence-based psychotherapies for children and adolescents* (pp. 241–262). New York: Guilford.

Loeber, R., Burke, J. D., Lahey, B. B., Winters, A., & Zera, M. (2000). Oppositional defiant disorder and conduct disorder: A review of the past 10 years, part I. *Journal of the American Academy of Child and Adolescent Psychiatry, 39,* 1468–1484.

Lumley, V. A., McNeil, C. B., Herschell, A. D., & Bahl, A. B. (2002). An examination of gender differences among young children with disruptive behavior disorders. *Child Study Journal, 32,* 89–100.

Maughn, B., Rowe, R., Messer, J., Goodman, R., & Meltzer, H. (2004). Conduct disorder and oppositional defiant disorder in a national sample: Developmental epidemiology. *Journal of Child Psychology and Psychiatry, 45,* 609–621.

Nixon, R. D. V., Sweeny, L., Erickson, D. B., & Touyz, S. W. (2003). Parent-child interaction therapy: A comparison of standard and abbreviated treatments for oppositional defiant preschoolers. *Journal of Consulting and Clinical Psychology, 71,* 257–260.

Patterson, G. R., (1982), Coercive Family Process, Eugen, OR: Castalia.

Patterson, G. R., & Guillion, M. E. (1968). *Living with children: New methods for parents and children.* Research Press: Champaign, IL.

Patterson, G., Chamberlain, P., & Reid, J. B. (1982). A comparative evaluation of a parent-training program. *Behavior Therapy, 13,* 638–650.

Paul, G. (1967). Outcome research in psychotherapy. *Journal of Consulting Psychology, 31,* 109–118.

Sanders, M. R. (1999). Triple P -positive parenting program: Towards an empirically validated multilevel parenting and family support strategy for the prevention of behavior and emotional problems in children. *Clinical Child & Family Psychology Review, 2,* 71–90.

Sanders, M. R., Markie-Dadds, C., Tully, L. A., & Bor, W. (2000). The Triple-P—positive parenting program: A comparison of enhanced, standard, and self-directed behavioral family intervention for parents of children with early onset conduct problems. *Journal of Consulting & Clinical Psychology, 68,* 624–640.

Shaffer, D., Fisher, P., Dulcan, M., & Davies, M. (1996). The NIMH Diagnostic Interview Schedule for Children Version 2.3 (DISC-2.3): Description, acceptability, prevalence rates, and performance in the MECA study. *Journal of the American Academy of Child & Adolescent Psychiatry,* 35, 865–877.

Schuhmann, E. M., Foote, R. C., Eyberg, S. M., Boggs, S. R., & Algina, J. (1998). Efficacy of parent-child interaction therapy: Interim report of a randomized trial with short-term maintenance. *Journal of Clinical Child Psychology, 27,* 34–45.

Southam-Gerow, M. A. (2003). Child-focused cognitive-behavioral therapies. In C. A. Essau (Ed.), *Conduct and oppositional defiant disorders: Epidemiology, risk factors, and treatment* (pp. 257–277). Mahwah, NJ: Lawrence Erlbaum Associates.

Waslick, B, Werry, J. S., & Greenhill, L. L. (1999). Pharmacotherapy and toxicology of oppositional defiant disorder and conduct disorder. In H. C. Quay & A. E. Hogan (Eds.). *Handbook of Disruptive Behavior Disorders* (pp. 455–474). New York: Kluwer Academic/Plenum.

Webster-Stratton, C. (1994). Advancing videotape parent training: A comparison study. *Journal of Consulting and Clinical Psychology, 66,* 715–730.

Webster-Stratton, C., Reid, M. J., & Hammond, M. (2001). Preventing conduct problems, promoting social competence: A parent and teacher training partnership in head start. *Journal of Clinical Child Psychology, 30,* 283–302.

Orgasmic Disorders

Lisa G. Regev • Antonette Zeiss • Robert Zeiss

WHAT ARE THE ORGASMIC DISORDERS?

Orgasm follows the excitement and plateau phases of the sexual response cycle and is considered to be the sexual "peak" that results in the release of sexual tension (Masters and Johnson, 1966). Heart rate, breathing, and blood pressure reach their physiological peak, followed by a loss of muscle control. Women experience rhythmic contractions in the uterus, vagina, anus, and pelvic floor muscles, and men experience contractions in the urethra, anus, and pelvic floor muscles, which is usually accompanied by the emission of semen. With orgasm, endorphins are released and produce a general sense of well-being. An orgasmic disorder constitutes a disruption in the orgasm phase of the sexual response cycle.

DSM-IV-TR (APA, 2000) identified three orgasmic disorders, including Female Orgasmic Disorder, Male Orgasmic Disorder, and Premature Ejaculation. This chapter will discuss male and female orgasmic disorder. Premature ejaculation is discussed in chapter 28 of this volume.

Female orgasmic disorder (formerly labeled "inhibited female orgasm") is defined as a "persistent or recurrent delay in, or absence of, orgasm following a normal sexual excitement phase" that causes "marked distress or interpersonal difficulty." Clinicians are asked to take into account contextual factors prior to making a diagnosis, such as the woman's sexual experience and adequacy of the sexual stimulation.

Male orgasmic disorder (a.k.a. retarded ejaculation; formerly labeled "inhibited male orgasm") is defined as a "persistent or recurrent delay in, or absence of, orgasm following a normal sexual excitement phase during sexual activity that the clinician judges to be adequate in focus, intensity, and duration" that causes "marked distress or interpersonal difficulty."

Masters and Johnson (1970) distinguish between "masturbatory dysfunction," "coital dysfunction," and "random dysfunction." They also distinguish between primary and secondary anorgasmia. Primary anorgasmia refers to the inability to reach orgasm by any means of sexual stimulation (e.g., manual, oral, vibrator, intercourse, alone or with a partner). If the individual has experienced at least one orgasm, the current problem is classified as secondary anorgasmia.

BASIC FACTS ABOUT THE ORGASMIC DISORDERS

Prevalence. According to a national study of the prevalence of sexual dysfunction, male orgasmic disorder is a relatively rare condition, affecting up to 8% of the population. Female orgasmic disorder is more prevalent, affecting up to 26% of women for at least 12 months (Laumann, Paik, & Rosen, 1999). A national sample in the UK found lower estimates, with 5% of men and 14% of women reporting inability to reach orgasm for at least 1 month within a year and 1% of men and 4% of women reporting inability to reach orgasm for six months within a year (Mercer et al. 2003).

Regev, L. G., Zeiss, A., & Zeiss, R. (2006). Organic disorders. In J. E. Fisher & W. T. O'Donohue (Eds.), *Practitioner's guide to evidence-based psychotherapy.* New York: Springer.

Age. Among men aged 18–59, men in their 40s may be more likely to experience difficulties related to orgasm (Laumann et al. 1999).

Marital status. Nonmarried women are significantly more likely to experience orgasm difficulties than their married counterparts (Laumann et al. 1999).

Education level. Women with less than a high school education were significantly more likely to experience an inability to reach orgasm than women who were college educated (Laumann et al. 1999).

Etiology. A variety of neurophysiological and psychosocial factors may influence a person's orgasmic capacity.

Neurophysiological factors. Intact genital (i.e., clitoris, vagina, penis, anus) sensitivity and vasocongestive capacity positively impact orgasmic capacity. Vascular disease can inhibit vasocongestion and therefore inhibit orgasmic capacity. Diabetic neuropathy can reduce sensation in the genital area, inhibiting orgasmic capacity. Increased availability of serotonin and decreased dopamine (i.e., the effects of antidepressant medications such as SSRIs) can inhibit orgasm in either sex. The brain is another important source of sexual arousal and can result in "phantom orgasms" through hypnosis, fantasy, or direct stimulation of the brain (Money, 1960). Despite popular beliefs, it remains unclear whether stimulation of the "G-spot" (an area on the anterior vaginal wall, a few centimeters from the vaginal opening) helps women reach orgasm.

Physiological components of orgasm (e.g., heart rate, respiration rate, and pelvic contractions) do not appear to be correlated with reported subjective intensity or satisfaction of orgasm (Bohlen, Held, & Sanderson, 1983).

Women's orgasmic capacity was thought to be influenced by the strength and tone of the pubococcygeal (PC) muscle located in the vagina. Women with orgasmic difficulties were encouraged to engage in Kegel exercises to strengthen the PC muscles. More recently, it appears that the correlations between PC muscle tone and orgasmic capacity are low (Heiman, 2000).

Psychological factors that affect orgasmic capacity:

- Poor sexual skills (i.e., lacking information as to what kind of stimulation and contextual factors will produce orgasm)
- Depression can be associated with low desire and thus indirectly with orgasmic difficulties
- Sexual abuse
- Anxiety (e.g., fear of losing control, fears of high levels of arousal)
- Relationship factors
  - Inadequate level of comfort with partner
  - Inadequately sexually aroused by partner
  - Poor communication regarding sex
- *Sexual myths.* There are also numerous sexual myths related to orgasm that may interfere with sexual pleasure, particularly when orgasm is viewed as the pinnacle sexual experience and as a necessary endpoint (see Zilbergeld, 1999). Sample myths:
  - If I can't have an orgasm, what's the point of engaging in sexual activity with my partner?
  - Our relationship would be perfect if she could only have an orgasm.
  - If I can't have an orgasm, why bother getting into a relationship?
  - A good lover is able to give his partner an orgasm each time they have intercourse
  - Simultaneous orgasm is the most fulfilling sexual experience for a couple
  - I shouldn't start something I can't finish
  - A woman should be most able to experience orgasm through vaginal intercourse

ASSESSMENT

What is involved in effective assessment (see Wincze & Carey, 2001; Zeiss, Zeiss, & Davies, 1999)

- Assess both partners' sexual functioning where relevant and possible (as delineated below)
- Build rapport—sexuality is a sensitive and private issue and can be embarrassing for people to talk about. Some techniques for enhancing rapport/openness to discuss sexual issues include:
  - Asking permission to talk explicitly about sex
  - Discussing confidentiality
  - Asking more general questions first to help establish rapport and to give the patient time to become comfortable in the session
  - Keeping a nonjudgmental tone
  - Using precise, clear terms
  - Not leaping to conclusions too quickly; be sure you check out precise meanings, especially when the patient is using slang terms

When assessing orgasmic dysfunction it is important to keep in mind that some patients have difficulty identifying the presence or absence of orgasm. For example:

- Men may confuse ejaculation with orgasm and say that they are not experiencing orgasm when, in fact, they are reaching orgasm but are not ejaculating. This happens commonly, for instance, with certain medical conditions.
  - Help patients distinguish between ejaculation and orgasm by asking them to describe their subjective experience during sexual activity despite their inability to ejaculate
  - Normal age-related changes result in reduced ejaculatory volume, but do not directly affect orgasmic experience
  - Men who experience retrograde ejaculation (where ejaculate travels to the bladder rather than out the urethra) are especially likely to think that they are not experiencing orgasm
    - For men who say they are not ejaculating, ask if they have cloudy urine the next time they empty the bladder
- Men with erectile dysfunction may lose their erection prior to orgasm and mistake an orgasmic difficulty with an arousal problem
  - Ask couples if they continue engaging in sexual stimulation even when the male partner loses his erection
  - Case studies suggest that almost all men can experience orgasm despite losing an erection if they continue to engage in sexual stimulation
- Women may confuse high levels of arousal with the experience of orgasm, such that they report experiencing orgasm when they, in fact, are not
  - This can be difficult to assess, because we do not have an objective measure or agreed-upon subjective definition of orgasm
  - Thoroughly assess the patient's physiological and subjective experience of orgasm
- Women may experience orgasm but say that they do not because of unrealistic expectations regarding the orgasmic experience

A step-by-step assessment of sexual functioning and contextual factors.
- Medical evaluation
  - Genital functioning
  - Health problems/conditions, including menopausal status
  - Medications

- Psychological factors to assess
  - Life situation—people's level of stress and whether or not they have time to engage in sexual activity in a relaxed atmosphere will be an important aspect to consider when assessing orgasmic capacity. Assess the following areas:
    - Relationship status
    - Children
    - Living situation
    - Work
    - Current stressors
  - Comorbid mental disorders, such as:
    - Depression—especially anhedonia/loss of interest in sexual activity that predates the orgasmic dysfunction
    - Anxiety—especially performance anxiety or PTSD resulting from sexual assault
  - Substance use
    - Alcohol
    - Tobacco
    - Caffeine
    - Illicit drugs
  - Sexual functioning in the past month
    - *Desire.* Frequency of sexual interest, thoughts, urges, feelings; frequency of engaging in sexual activity (including masturbation); contextual factors that enhance or inhibit desire.
    - *Arousal.* % erection/lubrication–swelling response, typically and maximally, with partner and in masturbation (for male patients, also assess morning erections).
    - Orgasm
      - Does the patient experience orgasm? Ask to describe the experience and ask about the specific physiological changes
      - How often?
      - During which sexual activity(s) (intercourse, oral sex, masturbation, etc.)?
      - With what kind(s) of stimulation (manual, vibrator, visual, auditory, etc.)?
      - How much time is spent in foreplay?
      - *Genital pain.* presence, intensity, during which type of sexual activity, response of partner.
  - Baseline sexual functioning (prior to time sexual difficulties began):
    - *Desire.* Frequency of sexual interest, thoughts, urges, feelings; frequency of engaging in sexual activity (including masturbation)
    - *Arousal.* % erection/lubrication–swelling response typically and maximally, with partner and in masturbation (for male patients, assess morning erections).
    - *Orgasm.* presence, timing, amount of foreplay, with a partner and during masturbation.
    - Genital pain. presence, intensity, during which type of sexual activity, response of partner.
  - Onset—when did the sexual problem begin?
    - Did the problem develop gradually or abruptly?
    - Did the problem start around the same time as any of the psychological factors assessed above (e.g., life stressors, mental disorders)?
    - Did the problem start around the time of beginning a new medication, giving birth, or other event that could have led to biological changes?

- Context—global versus situational
  - Does the person experience low desire with all partners and during all sexual activities (e.g., intercourse, masturbation) or does it only occur in certain situations (e.g., with a specific partner or a specific sexual activity)?
- Are there thoughts/fears related to sexual activity that might be affecting orgasmic capacity?
  - E.g., fears of STDs, pregnancy, loss of control, failure, closeness, feeling of vulnerability, disgust or that sex is morally wrong
- Relationship issues
  - Quality of emotional intimacy/communication
  - Do the sexual difficulties adversely affect the overall relationship?
  - Communication patterns regarding sex in general and sexual difficulties
- Causal beliefs
  - What does the patient think is causing the problem?
- Goals for treatment
  - Are the stated goals realistic?

What should be ruled out?

- Another Axis I disorder (except another sexual dysfunction) that better accounts for the problem, such as depression or PTSD resulting from sexual assault
- Physiological effects of a substance that exclusively accounts for the problem, including prescription and street drugs
- Physiological effects of a medical disorder that reduces genital sensation to a degree incompatible with building arousal
- Unrealistic expectations regarding how often or during which sexual activity a person "should" reach orgasm

According to DSM-IV-TR (APA, 2000), specify:
- Onset
  - Whether the person never experienced an orgasm ("lifelong") or the disorder was "acquired" at some point
- Context
  - Whether the orgasmic difficulty is true in all situations ("generalized") or only some situations ("situational")
    - E.g., experiences orgasmic difficulties with all sexual activities or only intercourse; experiences orgasmic difficulties with all potential sexual partners or only with a specific partner
- Etiological factors
  - Whether the orgasmic difficulty is due to "psychological factors" (e.g., relationship distress, anxiety, depression), "physiological factors," or "combined factors" (including both psychological and physiological factors)
  - According to DSM-IV-TR (APA, 2000), when the orgasmic difficulty is due exclusively to the physiological effects of a general medical condition, the appropriate diagnosis is "Sexual dysfunction due to a general medical condition"

TREATMENTS

What treatments are effective?

Historically, Masters and Johnson's (1970) two-week intensive therapy was considered the standard of care. More recently, research has found that one therapist is as effective as two therapists (LoPiccolo, Heiman, Hogan, & Roberts, 1985), longer-term therapy is as effective as intensive therapy (about 12 weeks; Ulrich-Clement &

Schmidt, 1983), and group and bibliotherapy (with minimal therapist contact) formats are as effective as full-therapist contact conditions (Libman, Fichten, & Brender, 1985; van Lankveld, 1998).

The vast majority of the research on orgasmic dysfunction has focused on the treatment of female orgasmic dysfunction. Directed masturbation, which primarily consists of education and self-exploration of the woman's body, has been shown to be most effective with primary anorgasmic women in that over 80% experienced masturbatory orgasm and 20–60% experienced orgasm with a partner. This treatment also positively influences women's attitudes towards sex, their bodies, and sexual satisfaction (Ersner-Hershfield & Kopel, 1979; Nairne & Hemsley, 1983). Directed masturbation can also be effective in treating secondary anorgasmia, particularly with younger, emotionally healthier, and more happily married women (LoPiccolo & Stock, 1986; Schneidman & McGuire, 1976). Zeiss, Rosen and Zeiss (1977) offer a six-step treatment program for women who are orgasmic only in masturbation seeking to increase their coital orgasmic capacity using conditioning principles to pair orgasm with intercourse.

Male orgasmic dysfunction is a relatively rare condition and therefore has not been sufficiently studied. Most clinical accounts of male orgasmic disorder consist of secondary dysfunction, where the male can reach orgasm and ejaculate on his own but experiences greater difficulty with a partner. Apfelbaum (2000) suggests that treatment that focuses on the male's emotional experience and lack of arousal, while trying to reduce performance pressures, is likely to produce favorable outcomes.

For both males and females who experience orgasmic dysfunction, selecting the appropriate treatment will be informed by a thorough assessment of the etiological and maintaining factors (as delineated above). Consider the following treatment components (see Barbach, 2000; Heiman & LoPiccolo, 1988; Leiblum & Rosen, 2000):

Use the PLISSIT Model—a stepped-care approach (see Annon, 1976):

- Permission
  - Help patients give themselves permission to engage in sexual activity, to experience orgasm, or not to experience orgasm
- Limited information
  - Provide psychoeducation regarding their sexual concerns
- Specific suggestions
  - Provide specific suggestions on how they can improve their sexual functioning (as delineated above)
- Intensive treatment
  - when necessary, provide or refer for more intensive treatment

More specifically, steps that can be taken linked to the PLISSIT conceptual model include:

- Provide psychoeducation (as appropriate):
  - Debunk myths—many people experiencing orgasmic difficulties may have unrealistic ideas about the ways in which treatment will impact their lives
  - Discuss or provide reading/viewing materials helping the individual or couple learn about their bodies, including areas and types of stimulation that produce pleasure
  - Normalize and validate their experiences
  - Discuss possible etiological factors (as delineated above)
- Encourage self-exploration of beliefs about sex

- Teach relaxation exercises
- Encourage physical self-exploration—exploring areas of pleasure
- Discuss fears about orgasm and encourage the patient to role-play orgasm on own
- Ask patients to self-monitor arousal and orgasm triggers
- Explore the use of vibrators to maximize stimulation
- Encourage communication and sharing of self-discoveries with the partner
- Encourage physical affection, without the performance demands of sexual intercourse
- Treat the sexual dysfunction causing the orgasmic dysfunction
  - Desire, arousal, and pain disorders may contribute or cause the orgasmic dysfunction (see Leiblum & Rosen, 2000; Wincze & Carey, 2001)
- Treat the relationship issues causing the orgasmic dysfunction
  - Teach assertiveness, communication and problem-solving skills (see Gottman & Silver, 2000)
- Treat the psychological condition causing low desire
- E.g., depression, anxiety, PTSD, substance abuse, negative body image.

What treatments are not effective?

Medical treatments such as bupropion hydrochloride, testosterone and sildenafil (Viagra) have not been shown to be effective (Carney, Bancroft, & Matthews, 1978; Crenshaw, Goldberg, & Stern, 1987; Kaplan et al., 1999; Matthews, Whitehead, & Kellet, 1983).

Therapist Manuals

There are a variety of therapist manuals that address sexual dysfunction in general and orgasmic dysfunction more specifically. Recommended manuals include:

Annon, J. (1976). *Behavioral treatment of sexual problems* (vols. 1 & 2). Harper Collins.

Leiblum, S., & Rosen, R. (Eds.) (2000). *Principles and practice of sex therapy.* (3rd ed.). New York: Guildford Press.

Levine, S., Althof, S., & Risen, C. (Eds.) (2003). *Handbook of clinical sexuality for mental health professionals.* Brunner-Routeledge.

O'Donohue, W., & Geer, J. (Eds.) (1993). *Handbook of assessment and treatment of sexual dysfunctions.* Boston: Allyn & Bacon.

Wincze, J., & Carey, M. (2001). *Sexual dysfunction: A guide for assessment and treatment.* (2nd ed.). New York: Guilford Press.

Zeiss, A, & Zeiss, R. (1999). Sexual dysfunction: Using an interdisciplinary team to combine cognitive-behavioral and medical approaches. In M. Duffy's (Ed.) *Handbook of counseling and psychotherapy with older adults.* (pp. 294–313). New York: Wiley.

Zeiss, A., Zeiss, R., & Davies, H. (1999). Assessment of sexual function and dysfunction in older adults. In P. Lichtenberg's (Ed) *Handbook of assessment in clinical gerontology.* (pp. 270–296). New York: Wiley.

Self-Help Alternatives

Self-help has been shown to be effective in treating female orgasmic disorder, especially with periodic follow-up to maintain motivation to follow-through with readings and homework exercises. Recommended self-help books include:

Barbach, L. G. (2000). *For yourself: The fulfillment of female sexuality.* New York: Bantam Doubleday Dell Publishing Group Inc. (to treat female orgasmic dysfunction), $7.50.

Barbach, L. (1984). *Pleasures: Women write erotica.* New York: Doubleday & Co. (a sexual fantasy guide) $13.95.

Friday, N. (1991). *Women on top.* New York: Pocket Books (a sexual fantasy guide) $7.99.

Gottman, J. & Silver, N. (2000). *The seven principles for making marriage work.* Three Rivers Press (to treat relationship distress), $13.95.

Heiman, J., & LoPiccolo, J. (1988). Becoming orgasmic: *A sexual and personal growth program for women* (revised and expanded edition). New York: Simon & Schuster (to treat female orgasmic dysfunction) $13.

Zilbergeld, B. (1999) *The new male sexuality* (2nd ed.). New York: Bantam Books. $14.95.

Websites

Websites related to sexual health are plentiful. Here are a few that are particularly useful.

To purchase sexual materials, such as videos, books and intimacy aids:

The Sinclair Intimacy Institute's professional library at www.intimacyinstitute. com/library/professional/index.html includes a variety of instructive videos developed by human sexuality professionals for clinical and educational purposes.

Good Vibrations at www.goodvibes.com also provides a selection of videos and books that may appeal to a wide variety of viewers, including lesbian, gay, and bisexual individuals.

For General sexual information: www.sexualhealth.com, www.siecus.org, and www.sexuality.org.

For medical information: www.gettingwell.com and www.webmd.com

People can get their sexual health questions answered at www.goaskalice. columbia.edu

Additional Research

The empirical evidence suggests that cognitive-behavioral treatment is effective in treating female orgasmic disorder, particularly lifelong anorgasmia. These cases appear particularly straightforward in that many women who have never reached orgasm lack the necessary sexual skills. Therefore, treatments that emphasize psychoeducation and directed masturbation are particularly effective.

Secondary anorgasmia is understandably more challenging to treat, given that people in this category tend to be more heterogeneous. Some may have infrequently experienced orgasm, while others enjoyed frequent orgasms in the past. The etiology of the disorder in these cases is more likely to vary from person to person, thereby making treatment packages more diffuse and less potent. It may be beneficial to categorize the orgasmic disorders on a continuous, rather than dichotomous scale. Additionally, categorizing based on etiological and maintaining variables may be more efficient in developing effective treatments.

Given the low prevalence of male orgasmic disorder, studying this disorder is difficult. We currently rely on clinical case studies for information on this topic. Continuing to collect these case studies in a more systematic fashion may be particularly helpful in furthering our knowledge base.

REFERENCES

American Psychiatric Association (2000). *Diagnostic and statistical manual of mental disorders, fourth edition, text revision.* Washington, DC: Author.

Annon, J. (1976). *Behavioral treatment of sexual problems* (vols. 1&2). Harper Collins.

Apfelbaum, B. (2000). Retarded ejaculation. In S. Leiblum & R. Rosen (Eds.) *Principles and practice of sex therapy* (3rd ed.). New York: Guilford Press.

Barbach, L. G. (2000). *For yourself: The fulfillment of female sexuality.* New York: Bantam Doubleday Dell Publishing Group Inc.

Bohlen, J. G., Held, J. P., & Sanderson, M. O. (1983). Update on sexual physiology research. *Marriage and Family Review, 6,* 21–33.

Carney, A., Bancroft, J., & Matthews, A. (1978). Combination of hormonal and psychological treatment for female sexual unresponsiveness: A comparative study. *British Journal of Psychiatry, 132,* 339–346.

Crenshaw, T. L., Goldberg, J. P., & Stern, W. C. (1987). Pharmacologic modification of psychosexual dysfunction. *Journal of Sex and Marital Therapy, 13,* 239–253.

Ersner-Herschfield, R. & Kopel, S. (1979). Group treatment of preorgasmic women: Evaluation of partner involvement and spacing of sessions. *Journal of Consulting and Clinical Psychology, 47,* 750–759.

Gottman, J. & Silver, N. (2000). *The seven principles for making marriage work.* Three Rivers Press.

Heiman, J. (2000). Orgasmic disorders in women. In S. Leiblum & R. Rosens's (Eds.) *Principles and practice of sex therapy* (3rd ed.). New York: Guilford Press.

Heiman, J., & LoPiccolo, J. (1988). Becoming orgasmic: *A sexual and personal growth program for women* (revised and expanded edition). New York: Simon & Schuster.

Kaplan, S. A., Reis, R. B., Kohn, I. J., Ikeguchi, E. F., Laor, E., Te, A. E., et al., (1999). Safety and efficacy of sildenafil in postmenopausal women with sexual dysfunction. *Urology, 53*, 481–486.

Laumann, E. O., Paik, A., & Rosen, R. C. (1999). Sexual dysfunction in the United States: Prevalence and predictors. *Journal of the American Medical Association, 281*, 537–544.

Leiblum, S., & Rosen, R. (Eds.) (2000). *Principles and practice of sex therapy.* (3rd ed.). New York: Guildford Press.

Libman, E., Fichten, C. S., & Brender, W. (1985). The role of therapeutic format in the treatment of sexual dysfunction: A review. *Clinical Psychology Review, 5*, 103–117.

LoPiccolo, J., Heiman, J., Hogan, D., & Roberts, C. (1985). Effectiveness of single therapists versus cotherapy teams in sex therapy. *Journal of Consulting and Clinical Psychology, 53*, 287–294.

LoPiccolo, J., & Stock, W. E. (1986). Treatment of sexual dysfunction. *Journal of Consulting and Clinical Psychology, 54*, 158–167.

Masters, W., & Johnson, V. (1966). *Human sexual response.* Boston: Little, Brown.

Masters, W., & Johnson, V. (1970). *Human sexual inadequacy.* Boston: Little, Brown.

Matthews, A., Whitehead, A., & Kellett, J. (1983). Psychological and hormonal factors in the treatment of female sexual dysfunction. *Psychological Medicine, 13*, 83–92.

Mercer, C. H., Fenton, K. A., Johnson, A. M., Wellings, K., Macdowall, W., McMannus, et al., (2003). Sexual function problems and help seeking behaviour in Britain: National probability sample survey. *British Medical Journal, 327*, 426–427.

Money, J. (1960). Phantom orgasm in the dreams of paraplegic men and women. *Archives of General Psychiatry, 3*, 373–382.

Nairne, K. D., & Hemsley, D. R. (1983). The use of directed masturbation training in the treatment of primary anorgasmia. *British Journal of Clinical Psychology, 22*, 283–294.

Schneidman, B., & McGuire, L. (1976). Group therapy for nonorgasmic women: Two age levels. *Archives of Sexual Behavior, 5*, 239–247.

Ulrich-Clement, D., & Schmidt, G. (1983). The outcome of couple therapy for sexual dysfunctions using three different formats. *Journal of Sex and Marital Therapy, 9*(1), 67–78.

van Lankveld, J. J. D. M. (1998). Bibliotherapy in the treatment of sexual dysfunctions: A meta-analysis. *Journal of Consulting and Clinical Psychology, 66*, 702–708.

Wincze, J., & Carey, M. (2001). *Sexual dysfunction: A guide for assessment and treatment.* (2nd ed.). New York: Guilford Press.

Zeiss, A. M., Rosen, G. M., & Zeiss, R. A. (1977). Orgasm during intercourse: A treatment strategy for women. *Journal of Consulting and Clinical Psychology, 45*(3), 891–895.

Zeiss, A. M., Zeiss, R. A., & Davies, H. (1999). Assessment of sexual function and dysfunction in older adults. In P. Lichtenberg's (Ed.) *Handbook of assessment in clinical gerontology* (pp. 270–296). New York: John Wiley and Sons.

Zilbergeld, B. (1999). *The new male sexuality* (2nd ed.). New York: Bantam Books.

CHAPTER 48

Other Paraphilias

Tamara Penix • Lezlie Pickett

WHAT IS A PARAPHILIA?

Paraphilia is a term whose root word and prefix combined mean "to one side of love." The implication is that paraphilia is love gone astray, an abnormal or defective kind of attraction. The Greek was appropriately commandeered by the Diagnostic and Statistical Manual of the American Psychiatric Association (DSM-TR; APA, 2000) to refer to a general category of recurrent, intense sexually arousing sexual fantasies, urges and behaviors lasting at least six months that involve nonhuman objects, the suffering or humiliation of oneself or one's sexual partner, or nonconsenting persons (Criterion A). They range from private behaviors that garner attention only when they cause distress or a loss of social functioning in an individual, to those that may be unwanted and/or harmful to the object of the sexual behavior. The unusual object of sexual desire is necessary for sexual arousal in some cases, and in others, is sometimes included in sexual behavior, particularly during times of stress. These paraphilias are the varieties of sexually deviant behavior recognized by the medical and psychological communities, formally through the DSM and more informally through real, unusual case presentation, in North America.

Nine paraphilias garner DSM-TR diagnoses. In addition to Criterion A above, a diagnosis of Pedophilia, Voyeurism, Exhibitionism, or Frotteurism is given if the person has acted on the sexual thoughts or they have caused significant distress or interpersonal difficulty. For Sexual Sadism, the diagnosis is made if the person has acted on the sexual urges with a nonconsenting person or the urges have caused significant distress or interpersonal difficulty. For the remaining four paraphilias, the diagnosis is given if the sexual thoughts or behaviors cause clinically significant distress or impairment in social, occupational, or other important areas of functioning. Each paraphilia is further defined by the form of the sexual behavior.

Exhibitionism is exposing the genitals to an unsuspecting person.
Fetishism is using nonliving objects to achieve sexual gratification.
Frotteurism is touching and rubbing against a nonconsenting person.
Pedophilia is sexual activity with a prepubescent child or children (generally age 13 or younger). The person must be at least 16 years old and five years senior to the child or children involved. This is the best-researched paraphilia. As such, it is addressed separately in Chapter 53 this volume.
Sexual Masochism is receiving sexual pleasure from humiliation or suffering.
Sexual Sadism is receiving sexual pleasure from inflicting humiliation or suffering.
Transvestic Fetishism is receiving sexual pleasure from cross-dressing.
Voyeurism is observing an unsuspecting person who is naked in the process of disrobing or engaging in sexual activity.

Penix, T. M., & Pickett, L. (2006). Other paraphilias. In J. E. Fisher & W. T. O'Donohue (Eds.), *Practitioner's guide to evidence-based psychotherapy*. New York: Springer.

Paraphilia NOS is a general diagnosis for sexual behavior that may be considered aberrant, but which does not fit into one of the other categories, such as necrophilia (sexual arousal to corpses).

Adult sexual assault is not explicitly diagnosed as a paraphilia in the DSM-TR. Assessors may diagnose Sexual Sadism or Paraphilia NOS depending on the details surrounding the crime.

It should be noted that the paraphilias fail to engender distress in some people who experience the symptoms. For them, it is the reaction of others and the ensuing social difficulties that become problematic. For others, there is tremendous guilt and shame associated with the paraphilia. They may be embarrassed by the behavior, afraid of being discovered, or depressed by being involved in activities they view as immoral. Attention to the object of the sexual behavior may preclude reciprocal affectionate sexual activity. It is a loss in the range of sexual behavior that appears related to other diagnoses including sexual dysfunctions, personality disorders, and various types of depression.

BASIC FACTS

Studies of the paraphilias are rare. Thus, much of the most basic information about these problems is unknown. A review of the literature from the last 15 years revealed only 200 articles covering all of the paraphilias except pedophilia. The content of these papers is largely descriptive in nature. Less than a handful address assessment and the treatment outcome studies are overwhelmingly limited to single case studies without the application of formal single case design methodology, and pharmacological interventions. The dearth of research seems a byproduct of the fact that these issues are rarely diagnosed in general medical settings (APA, 2000). People do not pursue traditional avenues of treatment for the paraphilias, first, because many are not distressed by their behaviors, and secondly, due to the sexual, and therefore, private and to some, embarrassing nature of the problem. People with sexual problems in general do not present for treatment en mass. Of course there is even greater stigmatism associated with the paraphilias, the "sexual deviance" disorders. As a result, some of the best epidemiological studies have focused on incidence and prevalence across a range of paraphilias in community, college, and incarcerated samples. Few studies have investigated the characteristics and theories surrounding particular paraphilias. As a result the following information is limited.

Basic facts about exhibitionism In limited college and community samples 40–60% of women reported having been victims of exhibitionism (Murphy, 1997). A non-incarcerated sample of 142 exhibitionists conceded 72,974 victims (Abel & Rouleau, 1990). In two studies of college males, results indicated that 2–4% had engaged in exhibitionism while 7% indicated the desire to do so (Person, Terestman, Myers, Goldberg, & Salvadori, 1989; Templeman & Stinnett, 1991). In general sex offender populations, rates of exhibitionism were higher, from 14% to 23% (Abel, Osborn, & Twigg, 1993; Barnard, Hankins, & Robbins, 1992). There appear to be two periods of onset for exhibitionism, in the middle teen years and in the mid-20s' (Berah & Myers, 1983; Mohr, Turner, & Jerry, 1964). It is not known if adolescent exhibitionism continues into adulthood or if there are any important differences between exhibitionists who begin in adolescence and those who begin later in life. It is not known if victim characteristic preferences exist. Exhibitionists may expose themselves to victims of any age (Maletzky, 1998). Exhibitionism is considered a male disorder, although there have been a few reports of females engaging in the behavior (Murphy, 1997).

The course of exhibitionism is unknown. No prospective studies of exhibitionists have been published. Frisbie and Dondis (1965) followed untreated exhibitionists for six years. They found that 41% had reoffended after one year. This increased to 57% for those with a history of multiple arrests. Reported recidivism rates for treated exhibitionists vary significantly. Maletzky (1987) and Wolfe (1989) reported similar reoffense rates of 14–15% for treated outpatient offenders who were followed for 1–14 years. Treated incarcerated samples have demonstrated weaker treatment outcomes at 41% (Langevin et al., 1979) and 48% (Marshall & Barbaree, 1990). No specific psychological impairment is associated with exhibitionism, although lifetime comorbidity with Axis I disorders and substance abuse disorders is common (Kafka & Prentky, 1994). Exhibitionism is highly comorbid with the other paraphilias. Abel & Rouleau (1990) found that 93% of their sample of exhibitionists met criteria for another paraphilia and 73% met criteria for more than one additional paraphilia.

Basic Facts about Fetishism

The prevalence and incidence of fetishism are unknown. Chalkley & Powell (1983) found only 48 cases of reported fetishism in a large London hospital in a 20-year period. In the Abel et al. (1993) sample 8% of adolescents and 5% of adults were diagnosed with a fetish. In a clinical sample, the rate was 25% (Barnard et al., 1992). Fetishism is believed to be significantly more common in males (Mason, 1997); however, there are reports of female fetishists in the literature (Greenacre, 1979; Zavitzianos, 1971). It has been theorized that this is due to the fact that female sexual arousal is not easily conditioned (Kinsey, Pomeroy, Martin, & Gebhard, 1953), supported by Letourneau & O'Donohue (1997). Gamman & Makinen (1995) have argued that there is a concerted effort to ignore fetishism in women because it is a "taboo" practice. Studies of the cultural determinants of fetishistic behavior are lacking; however, there is evidence that culture shapes the form of the behavior. For example, Money (1977) noted the sexual appeal of a foot that had been bound to make it smaller than its natural size in China, a fetish that is not apparent in other cultures. The course of fetishism is unknown. Bancroft (1989) identified three major categories of fetishistic stimuli: a part of the body, an inanimate extension of the body (clothes or accessories), or a source of specific tactile stimulation (certain types of material). The comorbidity of fetishism with other clinical problems is unknown.

Basic Facts about Frotteurism

Few prevalence and incidence studies have been conducted with people who engage in frotteurism. In the Templeman and Stinnett (1991) sample of college men, they found that 35% had engaged in this behavior. This figure is slightly elevated in the Barnard et al. (1992) sample of sex offenders at 39%. The frequency of the behavior is significant. A 1987 study by Abel et al. with nonincarcerated participants found that the mean number of acts of frottage per person was 849.5. A later study by Abel et al. (1993) found that adolescents who had engaged in the behavior offended 31 times on average, with a range of 1–180 times. The age of onset is unknown. There are no published accounts of female frotteurs.

The course of frottage is unknown. Abel, Becker, Cunningham-Rather, Mittelman, & Rouleau (1988) found that only 21% of frotteurs exclusively engaged in frottage. On average, frotteurs in this sex offender sample were diagnosed with five paraphilias. Bradford, Boulet, & Pawlak (1992), in an inpatient sample of court-involved males, found similar results. Thus, there appears to be a high co-occurrence of frotteurism with the other paraphilias. However, frotteurs are not usually arrested, therefore these samples may not be representative of the typical frotteur. Exclusive studies of frotteurs aside from case studies have not been published.

Basic Facts about Sexual Masochism

It has been estimated that 5-10% of the general population has engaged in masochistic sex play, twice as many masochistic fantasy, and that fewer than 1% engages in masochistic behavior with any frequency (Baumeister, 1989). In the Abel et al. (1993), Barnard et al. (1992) and Person et al. (1989) community, sex offender, and college student samples, the prevalence ranged from 1% to 3%. Females appear to engage in masochistic sexual behavior at a slightly lower rate than males (Baumeister, 1989; Moser & Levitt, 1987). It has been suggested that females practice masochism differently than do males. Females appear to emphasize less severe pain than do males and they seek out that pain more in the context of an ongoing relationship (Baumeister, 1988). Baumeister also noted that for males, the humiliation aspect of masochism is more related to loss of status and infidelity of the partner whereas for females having to make oral sexual displays and being displayed naked were more arousing activities (Baumeister 1988, 1989).

Culturally, sexual masochism appears to be a modern Western phenomenon, with no evidence of the practice until the 1500s (Baumeister, 1988, 1989). Socioeconomic influences on the practice are marked. Masochism is strongly correlated with wealth and high social status (Baumeister & Butler, 1997). Clubs that cater to sadists and masochists report upper-middle class, well-educated clientele (Moser & Levitt, 1987; Scott, 1983). Baumeister and Butler (1997) also reported that prostitutes with upper class clientele are more often asked for sexual domination than are those who cater to the lower classes (Diana, 1985; Janus, Bess, & Saltus, 1977; Smith & Cox, 1983). The course of masochism is unknown. Masochism appears to be practiced by relatively healthy, successful individuals who engage in the practice safely (Scott, 1983). Cowan (1982) reported that masochists are above average in terms of adjustment and mental healthfulness. However, there are people who engage in dangerous masochistic behavior and accidental suicide does occur (O'Halloran & Dietz, 1993).

Basic Facts about Sexual Sadism

Sexual sadism includes practices ranging from tying up a sexual partner to causing that partner injury or even death. Hunt (1974) found that 5% of men and 2% of women achieved sexual gratification from inflicting pain on another person whereas Arndt, Foehl, & Good found in 1985 that one-third of women and half of males fantasized about binding a sexual partner. There appears to be a 4:1 ratio of masochists to sadists in terms of fantasy and practice (Friday, 1980; Scott, 1983). Both Baumeister (1988, 1989) and Scott (1983) reported that the majority of sadists became sadists only after practicing masochism for some time. Most sadistic males (75%) report having been aware of their sadistic interests prior to age 18 (Breslow, Evans, & Langley, 1985) while female sadism more often has its onset in adulthood in the context of adult sexual relationships with masochistic men (Scott, 1983).

The typical course of sexual sadism is unknown. A distinction is made between consensual sadomasochistic encounters and predatory sadism. Consensual sadomasochism is generally established as a mutually satisfying sexual encounter between someone who likes to be submissive and one who prefers to dominate. It typically involves humiliating verbalizations and actions that are arousing to both partners. Predatory sadism involves an unwilling victim and often significant harm or death. Forms include piquerism, in which the sadist stabs an unsuspecting victim in an erogenous zone (De River, 1958), vampirism (Jaffe & DiCataldo, 1994), sadistic rape (Dietz, Hazelwood, & Warren, 1990), and sadistic (lust) murder (Arndt, 1991; Dietz et al., 1990). Sexual sadism is highly comorbid with the other paraphilias. Abel et al. (1988) found that 18% of sadistic participants were masochistic, 46% had raped another person, 21% were exhibitionists, 25% were voyeurs, 25% were frotteurs, and 33% were pedophiliacs. Only one recent study of sexual sadists alone was found in the literature. In a six-year follow-up of 60 untreated sexual sadists, a third relapsed with a sexual offense (Berner, Berger, & Hill, 2003).

Basic Facts about Transvestic Fetishism

The prevalence and incidence of transvestic fetishism are unknown. In the Person et al. (1989) study, 1% of a college male sample acknowledged cross-dressing in the previous month. The Abel et al. (1993) study found that 9% of adolescents and 5% of adults in the sample met criteria for this diagnosis. The 1992 Barnard et al. sex offender sample yielded a 21% rate of transvestism. While the incidence of this type of fetishism appears to be on the rise, Zucker and Blanchard (1997) note that there may simply be greater visibility of individuals with the disorder due to an increase in organized activities such as support groups. Contrary to popular belief, men with transvestic fetishism do not typically exhibit effeminate behaviors (Doorn, Poortinga, & Verschoor, 1994; Zucker & Bradley, 1995). They are "unremarkably masculine in their adult hobbies and in their career choices (Zucker & Blanchard, 1997)." There is a subgroup of men with transvestic fetishism who experience gender dysphoria, a desire to be regarded as a member of the opposite gender (Blanchard, 1994; Levine, 1993). Zucker and Bradley (1995) found the age of onset to be in childhood or puberty and rarely later than midadolescence. Dressing in women's clothes comes to elicit sexual arousal. While some males and females may enjoy cross-dressing and exhibit the behavior in nonerotic environments, the paraphilia diagnosis is explicitly linked to sexual arousal to traditionally opposite sex clothing.

The diagnosis is limited to heterosexual men only, despite the fact that nearly half of men who meet criteria for the disorder have had one or more homosexual experiences (Brown et al., 1996). According to Adshead (1997), while the behavior may be restricted to looking at and touching the clothing, increased arousal and orgasm usually require the wearing of the articles. The course and recidivism rates for the disorder are unknown. Comorbidity data are also lacking, although in one study of people involved in cross-dressing at all levels, participants showed elevations on the Brief Symptom Inventory compared with a group of noncross-dressing heterosexual males (Fagin, Wise, & Derogatis, 1988). In a nonclinical sample, personality disorders were not found (Bentler & Prince, 1970).

Basic Facts about Voyeurism

The rates of voyeurism are highly variable from sample to sample. Fourteen percent of the adolescents and 13% of adults in the Abel et al. (1993) sample could be diagnosed as voyeurs. The two college samples differed significantly, with 4% in the Person et al. sample (1989) and 42% of the Templeman and Stinnett (1991) sample. The Barnard et al. sex offender sample also revealed a prevalence of 42%. In a study by Abel, Mittelman and Becker (1985) 62 men (13% of the sample) admitted more than 52,000 voyeuristic acts and victims. A later study by Abel (1989) found the median number of voyeuristic acts to be 17. The onset of these activities appears to be prior to age 15 according to the DSM (APA, 2000). Voyeuristic behavior appears to continue untreated and it is sometimes a precursive behavior to contact sexual offenses. However, voyeurs are not typically arrested for peeping because they are mistaken for trespassers or loiterers (Kaplan & Krueger, 1997). No studies that examined female voyeuristic activity were found. Other than case studies, few studies have looked at voyeurs alone. Beyond the difficulty in finding a population of voyeurs, exclusive voyeurs are rare in the literature. Abel and Rouleau (1990) found that of 62 voyeurs in their sample, only 1 was exclusively voyeuristic. The remainder of the sample could be diagnosed with two or more paraphilias and 47% could be diagnosed with four or more of them. In similar findings, Freund and Watson (1990) reported that of 125 voyeurs 50 were exhibitionists, 50 were frotteurs, and 73 had another paraphilia. The comorbidity with psychological disorders is unknown.

Basic Facts about Paraphilia NOS

Paraphilia NOS is a catch-all category for the many remaining forms of paraphilias ranging from zoophilia (bestiality) to necrophilia and every variation in between. These are behaviors that infrequently come to the attention of the legal and medical systems. As a result, the prevalence and incidence rates are unknown. Women are involved in these behaviors as well as men, but it is impossible to say at what rate. It is impossible to review the literature for all of these behaviors in this space. Two excellent review chapters may assist the reader, one by Milner and Dopke (1997) and another by Schewe (1997).

WHAT CAUSES PARAPHILIC BEHAVIOR?

The etiology of paraphilic behavior is unknown. Theories of the causal and maintaining factors surrounding these behaviors abound; however, large-scale investigations of these theories are notably absent from the literature. Models of paraphilic behavior that are spurring research and treatment development include the courtship disorder theory, social learning theories including cognitive-behavioral theory, and biological models.

Courtship Disorder

Albert Ellis proposed that the paraphilias are the reflection of arrested sexual development, of not moving through the normal phases of courtship (Ellis & Brancala, 1956). Freund and his colleagues elaborated on and have tested the theory (Freund 1990; Freund, Seto, & Kuban, 1997). Paraphilias are, from this perspective, a failure to pass through the phases of sexual behavior that precede sexual intercourse. The theory posits that human courtship is sequential, that the paraphilia appears when an intensification or distortion occurs in the sequence, and that the behavior reflects the desire for instant conversion of sexual arousal to orgasm. Frotteurism, exhibitionism, voyeurism, and preferential rape are viewed as forms of this disorder.

Social Learning and Cognitive-Behavioral Theory

Social learning theory offers that human behavior is related to causal factors including reciprocal determinism, observational learning, attentional and motivational processes, self-regulatory and self-reflective capacities, self-efficacy, and social interaction (Bandura, 1992). Cognitive-behavioral theory suggests that sexually deviant behavior is caused by an interplay among thoughts, feelings, and behaviors (Marshall & Fernandez, 1998). Included in the behavioral component is the idea that paraphilias develop as a result of conditioning and the reinforcing quality of the orgasm specific to deviant activities (Tollison & Adams, 1979). Ward and Beech (2004) have examined these affective, cognitive, and behavioral factors with an eye toward risk of sexual offending, suggesting that it is the interaction of significant learning events, psychological vulnerabilities, and contextual or proximal variables that produces an acute, dynamic risk of offending.

Biological Theory

Biological theories of the paraphilias suggest that these behaviors may be correlated with physical (mainly brain) abnormalities (Grubin & Mason, 1997; Saleh & Guidry, 2003). Many studies are investigating a wide variety of hypothesized abnormalities with promising, but inconclusive results thus far. Proposed loci of dysfunction include orbitofrontal brain tumors (Burns & Swedlow, 2003), traumatic brain injuries (Simpson, Blaszczynski, & Hodgkinson, 1999), temporal lobe abnormalities (Mendez, Chow, Ringman, Twitchell, & Hinkin, 2000), lesions of the central nervous system (Frohman, Frohman, & Moreault, 2002), abnormally high levels of testosterone (Aromaki, Lindman, & Eriksson, 2002), hyperarousal of the hypothalamus (Galski, Thornton, & Shumsky, 1990), malfunctions in serotonin production (Kafka & Prentky, 1992), and high androgen levels (Gijs & Gooren, 1996).

ASSESSMENT

What is Involved in Effective Assessment?

Assessment of the paraphilias is naturally dependent on the referral question, that is, whether the purpose of the assessment is clinical and/or forensic in nature. Clinical assessments must begin with a thorough clinical interview in which a functional analysis of behavior is conducted to determine the antecedents that may be setting the stage and consequences that may be maintaining the paraphilic behavior(s) for the individual. This information should be supplemented by and compared with additional data from relevant collateral sources, a thorough records review if the client has had prior institutional contact related to the problem, and objective assessment with psychometrically sound measures. Data should be gathered in the following areas. Useful objective measurement instruments are suggested.

Self-report measures

Sexual history

The Clarke Sexual History Questionnaire (SHQ; Langevin, Paitich, Russon, Handy, & Langevin, 1990). This is a self-report measure that is used to assess the variety of expressions of sexual behavior.

Multidimensional Assessment of Sex and Aggression (MASA; Knight, Prentky, & Cerce, 1994). This is a self-report measure used to assess the full range of sexual and aggressive behaviors. An adolescent form is available.

The Multiphasic Sex Inventory (MSI; Nichols & Molinder, 1984). This is a self-report measure used to assess the full range of sexual behaviors. A juvenile form is available.

The Sexual Fantasy Questionnaire (SFQ; O'Donohue, Letourneau, & Dowling, 1997). This is a self-report measure that assesses the full range of sexual fantasy content.

Deviant sexual arousal

Attraction to Sexual Aggression Scale (ASA; Malamuth, 1989). This self-report measure was designed to measure the appeal of sexually aggressive behavior.

Erotic Preferences Examination Scheme (EPES; Freund, Watson, & Rienzo, 1988). This is a self-report measure of a variety of paraphilic interests. It has been shown to discriminate between paraphiliacs and nonparaphiliacs on a number of indices.

Phallometry. Measuring physiological arousal genitally may be useful in the assessment of sexual sadism. A distinctive arousal profile has been identified for sexual sadists (Fedora et al., 1992). No distinctive physiological profiles have emerged relative to the other paraphilias. A useful review of the promise and perils of phallometry is found in O'Donohue and Letourneau (1992). Additional less intrusive physiological measures of sexual arousal are in development, but have not been validated for use in assessing or treating the "other" paraphilias.

Social cognitive needs

Poor thinking, alternatively referred to as cognitive distortion or irrational belief has been implicated as a maintaining factor in paraphilic behavior. These thoughts are usually assessed in the context of a clinical interview. Social skills deficits are believed to impair the paraphilic's ability to engage in more normative sexual behavior. McFall (1990) describes how to assess for these social skills deficits using an information-processing model.

Psychological distress

Emotional and psychological vulnerabilities have been implicated as precursive factors in losses of sexual self-control, although there is no one-to-one correspondence between having an emotional problem or psychological disorder and displaying paraphilic behavior. General psychological distress should be evaluated using psychometrically sound measures. Description of these measures reaches beyond the scope of this chapter. There is no particular Minnesota Multiphasic Personality Inventory-2 profile associated with any of the paraphilias; therefore, it is not useful in their diagnosis; however, it may be useful in detecting comorbid symptoms or syndromes.

Clinician-administered measures

Risk

If a sexual offense has been committed the following instruments may be useful in the actuarial prediction of risk of sexual offense recidivism.

Juvenile Sexual Offense Assessment Protocol II (J-SOAP-II; Prentky, Harris, Frizell, & Righthand, 2000). This is a clinician-generated measure of both static and dynamic risk factors for reoffense in juveniles. It produces a percentage of likelihood of reoffending.

Minnesota Sex Offender Screening Tool-Revised (MnSOST-R; Epperson, Kaul, & Hesselton, 1998). This clinician completed measure uses 16 items to assess the risk of reoffense for child molesters and rapists (who may meet criteria for sexual sadism or another paraphilia).

Psychopathy Checklist-Revised (PCL-R; Hare, 1990). This is a clinician completed measure that uses a lengthy clinical interviews and records review to assess for psychopathic characteristics. These characteristics have been correlated with less successful treatment outcomes for sex offenders (Firestone, et al., 1999; Harris & Rice, 1997).

Rapid Risk Assessment for Sexual Offense Recidivism (RRASOR; Hanson, 1997). The RRASOR is a four-item measure of the proclivity of sex offender to reoffend.

Sex Offense Reassessment Guide (SORAG; Quinsey, Harris, Rice, & Cormier, 1998) The SORAG is a clinician completed measure that employs 14 static and dynamic risk factors to predict risk.

Static-99 (Hanson & Thornton, 1999). The STATIC-99 is comprised of 10 items. It was created out of the RRASOR and another sexual offense risk assessment instrument (the SACJ) and has been found to be superior to both of them in its prediction prowess.

Assessment data should be integrated into a reasonable analysis of the causal and maintaining factors and viable treatment and/or risk containment recommendations.

TREATMENT

What Treatments are Effective?

Treatment of these paraphilias has either been developed on a case-by-case basis or has been the extrapolation of pedophilia treatment techniques to new, but conceptually related problems. There have been no concerted, large-scale treatment development efforts for any of these paraphilias. Logical reasons for the scarcity of larger treatment development and outcome study efforts abound. First, paraphilic behaviors are somewhat rare and often do not result in efforts to access treatment. Unearthing populations of fetishists or masochists for study would require ingenuity targeting pocket populations or large-scale community surveys, both of which require significant drive and financial support. The financial support for human sexuality research is on the wane in recent years, particularly deviant sexuality. It seems important to state that for many of these behaviors, fetishism, sexual masochism, and transvestic fetishism in particular, the presence of the behaviors is not sufficient to make a diagnosis and initiate treatment. There may be no distress, harm, or impairment in functioning accompanying these behaviors, thus many people who engage in these behaviors will not present for treatment. When treatment is requested or mandated as a result of a sexual offense, it is experimental due to the impediments to more broad ranging treatment development noted above. These conditions not do appear conducive to paraphiliacs knocking down the door for an effective treatment. What follows then, is a description of the best available treatments for the paraphilias thus far, with the recognition that there is a long way to go in terms of fully understanding and efficiently treating these problems.

The aims of treatment for the paraphilias are fourfold: decrease deviant sexual arousal, increase adaptive sexual arousal, improve overall well being, and maintain treatment gains. Biological interventions attempt to alter the physiological substrates believed to produce deviant sexual arousal, psychological disorder, and lifestyle imbalances. The major focus of these efforts has been altering neurotransmitters or hormones in order to produce changes in cognition, affect and external behavior.

What are Effective Therapist Based Treatments?

Decreasing paraphilic arousal Sexual arousal to nonnormative objects or persons has been altered by a number of different means. Most of these interventions fall into the realm of behavior therapy. They include such techniques as aversion therapy, covert sensitization, and various satiation interventions. Aversion therapy is a counterconditioning approach that involves pairing paraphilic sexual arousal with an aversive experience, such as smelling ammonia. Sexual arousal to the paraphilic stimulus, for example, a silk scarf, is punished by forcing oneself to smell the noxious substance in the presence of the arousal. Covert sensitization is a more cognitive approach that is based on behavioral principles. It involves thinking of a paraphilic sexual fantasy with awareness. At the height of sexual arousal in the fantasy, the person must alter the fantasy to include a horribly aversive event that will sharply diminish the arousal, for example, being publicly humiliated, smelling a disgusting smell, or being hurt during the sexual activity. The person imagines what it would be like to avoid such events in the future.

Sexual satiation is accomplished therapeutically in a number of different ways. Satiation is a behavioral term meaning satisfied, or full. One has had enough of something when one is sated. Laws (1991) reviews the following masturbatory satiation techniques. Directed masturbation involves masturbating to ejaculation using only nonparaphilic fantasies. Following orgasm, this is often paired with another approach, masturbatory satiation, which involves masturbating to paraphilic fantasies during the refractory period, thus pairing them with minimal sexual arousal and presumably producing boredom. Verbal satiation involves saying the paraphilic sexual fantasy aloud, often into a tape recorder repeatedly until it is no longer arousing. There is evidence that verbal satiation produces similar results to its masturbation counterpart (Laws, 1995) and is easier to prescribe in a professional psychological setting. An additional intervention aimed at managing deviant sexual arousal is stimulus control. The paraphilic stimulus, whether an object, preferred person or scenario is avoided, escaped, or controlled by someone other than the paraphiliac. Thus, the frotteur who offends in subway cars might buy an automobile. The transvestic fetishist might donate all of his women's clothes to the Goodwill organization. The sexual sadist might relinquish membership in an S&M club if that is where she finds sexual partners.

Increasing normative sexual behavior The more challenging aspect of treating the paraphilias is increasing normative sexual behavior. Many of the aforementioned approaches succeed in decreasing paraphilic sexual behavior. Unfortunately, they often wipe out sexual behavior entirely, thereby producing a gap in life that needs crossing. The clinician and client must wrestle with the fact that most clients do not wish to be asexual. Therefore, additional interventions are necessitated for normal functioning. Approaches that have some evidential support for use in accomplishing these goals in addition to the orgasmic reconditioning procedures noted above include systematic desensitization, cognitive restructuring, and social-sexual skills training.

Systematic desensitization involves gradually and repeatedly pairing the experience of fear (anxiety) with relaxation moving from less feared stimuli to those that are most feared. For a person with a paraphilia, the anxiety-provoking stimulus might be engaging in more normative sexual activities. For example, an exhibitionist might be afraid of being rejected in a consensual sexual interaction. Desensitization would focus on cooperatively generating a fear hierarchy which might range from searching for a potential sexual partner to talking casually to that person, to asking for a date, and finally, after a number of intervening steps, arriving at having sex with that person. Exposure to these feared scenarios is done in the psychotherapy session along with diaphragmatic breathing and relaxation. The client rates his or her anxiety throughout the process on a scale from 0 to 100 (subjective units of distress: SUDS). When the anxiety for the scenario dips below 20, the therapeutic dyad tackles the next most feared item.

Cognitive restructuring involves challenging irrational, distorted, or ineffective beliefs about deviant and nondeviant sexual behavior that are linked to engaging in paraphilic behavior and not engaging in more normative activities. Clients are first taught to become aware of their thoughts surrounding their sexual behavior and that of others. They may be given homework assignments to track those thoughts for days or weeks at a time, perhaps writing them for use in therapy.

They then learn how to challenge the veracity of those thoughts and to generate viable and pragmatic alternatives. If, for example, the client has a recurrent thought such as, "I can only enjoy sex if I am humiliated by my partner," the goal would be to help the client contact memories of times when he experienced pleasure without being humiliated, perhaps while masturbating alone. Thus, the thought would be countered. Vigilance on the part of the client is required for cognitive restructuring to be effective. The client must challenge the thoughts repeatedly, perhaps many times a day and maintain an awareness of new problematic thoughts in need of challenging.

Social and/or sexual skills training is another approach that has been used to increase positive sexual behaviors. It may be conceived of as a positive conditioning approach. This intervention assumes that paraphiliacs have a deficiency in interpersonal skills including those related to communicating with others and intimacy. McFall (1990) has outlined an approach for assessing and intervening when skills deficits appear related to enacting paraphilic behavior. There have been no studies of the impact of social skills training on any of the paraphilias apart from the multiple intervention programs of which they are a part.

Improving overall well-being Finally, relapse prevention (RP) for sexual offenders (Laws, 1989) has been utilized with people with paraphilias. Relapse prevention is a general intervention intended to follow a successful program of treatment that has as its focus the maintenance of treatment gains. Relapse prevention aids individuals in anticipating the high-risk situations including feelings, thoughts, and external events that would probabilistically produce the desire to engage in the paraphilic behavior. A relapse prevention plan with proven strategies for escaping, avoiding or coping directly with high risk situations is generated and revised over time for relevance. The RP plan implies that the individual has reasoned through a variety of ways to effectively manage these situations and that she only needs to be able to access one option in a threatening situation in order to not engage in the paraphilia. RP has been the treatment of choice for sexual offenders for the past 15 years; however, its faults have been the focus of many papers and presentations in the recent years (Marques, Nelson, Alarcon, & Day, 2000; Marshall & Anderson, 1996; Thornton, 1997). It is best viewed as an adjunctive intervention to the more focused CBT interventions. It has been used with sexual offenders who exhibit multiple paraphilias, with some reported success in conjunction with mainly cognitive-behavioral treatment interventions such as those noted above. Relapse prevention has not been investigated as a stand-alone treatment for any of these paraphilias.

The paraphilias may be comorbid with a variety of psychological problems including most commonly mood and substance abuse disorders. Clients should be referred and/or treated for these problems with techniques with the strongest empirical support and ideally a therapist with expertise in treating sexual behavior problems.

What are Effective Medical Treatments?

Biological interventions aimed at decreasing sexual drive have included surgical and chemical castration, neurosurgery, and pharmacotherapy. Of these approaches, surgical castration is the most effective because it permanently eradicates the secretion of testosterone; however, it is highly controversial because it may be used in a punitive fashion and is irreversible (Rosler & Witztum, 2000). Ethical objections have rendered surgical castration impotent for now. Neurosurgery involved damaging parts of the brain thought to drive deviant sexual behavior. It is no longer in use due to its imprecise and destructive nature (Gijs & Gooren, 1996).

Pharmacological interventions fall into two realms: hormone-focused and psychotropic medications. Treatment with antiandrogens, most commonly cyproterone acetate (CPA) and medroxyprogesterone acetate (MPA) has produced mixed results with apparently limited use for these paraphilias. These interventions appear to inhibit the sexual reaction, that is, they decrease sexual responding; however, they do not selectively decrease deviant sexual arousal and are accompanied by numerous aversive side effects (Rosler & Witztum, 2000). Therefore, people taking these hormonal agents have the same urges taking them as they did previously. They simply cannot fully act on those urges. While this approach may prove useful for people who are willing to lose sexual responding, it is unlikely to be a palatable long-term solution for people for whom sexuality has been so central in life. Antiandrogens do not offer any hope of having a normal sex life.

Long-acting gonadotropin-releasing hormone (GnRH) agonists have been the focus of more recent antiandrogen development for the paraphilias (Briken, Nika, & Berner, 2001; Rosler & Witztum, 2000). They demonstrate fewer side effects, are completely reversible, and may be administered by injection every one to three months according to Rosler and Witztum. It has been suggested that the GnRH agonists in conjunction with psychotherapy offer promise for the paraphilias including exhibitionism and voyeurism (Rosler & Witztum, 2000). Psychotropic medications such as fluoxetine (Greenburg, Bradford, Curry, & O'Rourke, 1996; Masand, 1993), sertraline (Greenburg et al., 1996; Kafka, 1994), fluvoxamine (Greenburg et al., 1996), clomipramine (Clayton, 1993) and paroxetine have also been tested as interventions for the paraphilias due to their sexual side effects and assumption that these sexual manifestations could be obsessive-compulsive spectrum behaviors (Abouesh & Clayton, 1999). Greenburg et al. (1996) found no differences in effects between fluoxetine, fluvoxamine and sertraline. Nefazadone produced the fewest sexual desire and arousal side effects while reducing sexual obsessions and compulsions in a study by Coleman, Gratzer, Nesvacil and Raymond (2000). The effectiveness of the selective serotonin reuptake inhibitors SSRIs in reducing sexual fantasy, sexual desire, masturbation, and other sexual behavior in patients with paraphilias has been demonstrated (see Bradford, 2000 for a review). These interventions target only those sexual behaviors that appear to have compulsive or affective substrates. Despite the apparent successes of the SSRIs in treating the paraphilias, it should be cautioned that these findings are not well-established. Studies have typically used small samples, follow-up periods of less than three months, and have not employed either placebo controls or a double-blind methodology (Hill, Briken, Kraus, Strohm, & Berner, 2003).

What are Effective Self-help Treatments?

There is only one self help intervention that is applicable to the paraphilias that teaches the interventions noted above. The Sexual Addiction Workbook: Proven Strategies to Regain Control of Your Life (Sbraga & O'Donohue, 2004) introduces people with sexual self-control problems to treatment in lay language using a colloquial style and empirically supported techniques in a workbook format. This workbook emphasizes lifestyle balance. Readers learn how to create a vital life that has sexuality as one part of a whole instead of being all-encompassing. Ward and Stewart (2003) similarly advocate for lifestyle balance in the treatment of problems of sexual self-control. While this manual refers to the paraphilias as "sexual addictions," using the lay lingo, it does not conceptualize them as such. In contrast, apparently all of the remaining self-help resources focused specifically on these paraphilias (as opposed to sexual offending behaviors) are based on a 12-step addiction model of causality and recovery. There is no persuasive empirical evidence supporting the use of these approaches in treating the paraphilias. Links to many 12-step resources for sexual self-control problems may be found through the National Council on Sexual Addiction and Compulsivity, found at *www.ncsac.org*. Many on-line and in-person support groups are available for people who view their problem as a sexual addiction or compulsion. These include Sexaholics Anonymous, Sexual Compulsives Anonymous, Sex and Love Addicts Anonymous, and Sex Addicts Anonymous. For those whose paraphilic behaviors have become sexually abusive, the following organizations offer the cognitive-behavioral and pharmacological treatments noted above in addition to useful information: the Association for the Treatment of Sexual Abusers, Correctional Service of Canada, National Organisation for the Treatment of Sexual Abusers, The Safer Society Foundation, and Stop It Now!. These organizations offer reading materials and referral sources for institutions and therapists with expertise in treating out-of-control sexual behavior.

REFERENCES

Abel, G. (1989). Paraphilias. In H. I. Kaplan & B. J. Sadock (Eds.), *Comprehensive textbook of Psychiatry* (5th ed., pp. 1069–1085). Baltimore: Williams & Wilkins.

Abel, G., Becker, J., Cunningham-Rather, J., Mittelman, M., & Rouleau, J. L. (1988). Multiple paraphilic diagnoses among sex offenders. *Bulletin of the American Academy of Psychiatry and the Law, 16*, 153–168.

Abel, G., Becker, J., Cunningham-Rather, J., Mittelman, M., Rouleau, J., & Murphy, W. (1987). Self-reported sex crimes of nonincarcerated paraphiliacs. *Journal of Interpersonal Violence, 2*, 3–25.

Abel, G., Mittelman, M. S., & Becker, J. V. (1985). Sexual offenders: Results of assessments and recommendations for treatment. In M. H. Ben-Aron, S. J. Hucker, & C. D. Webster (Eds.), *Clinical criminology: Current concepts* (pp. 191–205). Toronto: M & M Graphics.

Abel, G., Osborn, C., & Twigg, D. (1993). Sexual assault through the life span: Adult offenders with juvenile histories. In H. E. Barbaree, W. L. Marshall, & S. M. Hudson (Eds.), *The juvenile sex offender* (pp. 104–117). New York: Guilford Press.

Abel G., & Rouleau, J. (1990). The nature and extent of sexual assault. In W. L. Marshall, D. R. Laws & H. E. Barbaree (Eds.), Handbook of sexual assault: Issues, theories, and treatment of the offender (pp. 9–21) New York: Plenum Press.

Abouesh, A., & Clayton, A. (1999). Compulsive voyeurism and exhibitionism: A clinical response to paroxetine. *Archives of Sexual Behavior, 28*, 23–30.

Adshead, G. (1997). Trasvestic fetishism: Assessment and treatment. In. D. R. Laws & W. O'Donohue (Eds.), *Sexual deviance: Theory, assessment and treatment* (pp. 280–296). New York: Guilford Press.

American Psychiatric Association. (2000). *Diagnostic and statistical manual of mental disorders* (4th ed., text revision). Washington, DC: Author.

Arndt, W. (1991). *Gender disorders and the paraphilias*. Madison, CT: International Universities Press.

Arndt, W., Foehl, J., & Good, F. (1985). Specific fantasy themes: A multidimensional study. *Journal of Personality and Social Psychology, 48*, 472–480.

Aromaki, A. S., Lindman, R. E., & Eriksson, C. J. P. (2002). Testosterone, sexuality, and antisocial personality traits in rapists and child molesters: A pilot study. *Psychiatry Research, 110*, 239–247.

Bancroft, J. (1989). *Human sexuality and its problems* (2nd ed.). Edinburgh: Churchill Livingstone.

Bandura, A. (1992). Social cognitive theory. In L. A. Perrin, J. Ed, & P. Oliver (Eds.), Handbook of personality: Theory and research (2nd ed., pp. 154–196). New York: Guilford Press.

Barnard, G., Hankins, G., & Robbins, L. (1992). Prior life trauma, posttraumatic stress symptoms and character traits in sex offenders: An exploratory study. *Journal of Traumatic Stress, 5*, 393–420.

Baumeister, R. (1989). *Masochism and the self*. Hillsdale, NJ: Erlbaum.

Baumeister, R., & Butler, J. (1997). *Sexual masochism: Deviance without pathology*.

Baumeister, Ri., (1988), Masochism as an escape from self. *Journal of Sex Research, 25*, 28–59.

Bentler, P. M., & Prince, C. (1970). Personality characteristics of male transvestites. *Journal of Clinical Psychology, 26*, 287–291. In. D. R. Laws and W. O'Donohue (Eds.), *Sexual deviance: Theory, assessment and treatment* (pp. 225–239). New York: Guilford.

Berah, E. F., & Myers, R. G. (1983). The offense records of a sample of convicted exhibitionists. *Bulletin of the American Academy of Psychiatry and Law, 11*, 365–369.

Berner, W., Berger, P., & Hill, A. (2003). Sexual sadism. *International Journal of Offender Therapy and Comparative Criminology, 47,* 383–395.

Blanchard, R. (1994). A structural equation model for age at clinical presentation in nonhomosexual male gender dysphorics. *Archives of Sexual Behavior, 23,* 311–320.

Bradford, J. M. W. (2000). The treatment of sexual deviation using a pharmacological approach. *Journal of Sex Research, 37,* 248–257.

Bradford, J. M., Boulet, J., & Pawlak, A. (1992). The paraphilias: A multiplicity of deviant behaviors. *Canadian Journal of Psychiatry, 37,* 104–108.

Briken, P., Nika, E., & Berner, W. (2001). Treatment of paraphilia with lutenizing hormone-releasing hormone (LHRH)—a systematic review. *Journal of Clinical Psychiatry, 27,* 45–55.

Breslow, N., Evans, N., & Langley, J. (1985). On the prevalence and roles of females in sadomasochistic sub-culture: Report of an empirical study. *Archives of Sexual Medicine, 14,* 303–317.

Brown, G. R., Wise, T. N., Costa, P. T., Herbst, J. H., Fagan, P. J., & Schmidt, C. (1996). Personality characteristics and sexual functioning of 188 cross-dressing men. *Journal of Nervous and Mental Disease, 184,* 265–273.

Burns, J. M., Swedlow, R. H. (2003). Right orbitofrontal tumore with pedophilia symptoms and constructional apraxia sign. *Archives of Neurology, 60,* 437–440.

Chalkley, A. J., & Powell, G. E. (1983). The clinical description of forty-eight cases of sexual fetishism. *British Journal of Psychiatry, 143,* 292–295.

Clayton, A. H. (1993). Fetishism and clomipramine. *American Journal of Psychiatry, 48,* 730–738.

Coleman, E., Gratzer, T., Nesvacil, L., & Raymond, N. C. (2000). Nefazodone and the treatment of nonparaphilic compulsive sexual behavior: A retrospective study. *Journal of Clinical Psychiatry, 61,* 282–284.

Cowan, L. (1982), Masochism'. A Jungian view, Dallas, TX: Spring.

De River, P. (1958). *Crime and the criminal psychopath.* Springfield, IL: Charles C. Thomas.

Diana, L. (1985). *The prostitute and her clients.* Springfield, IL: Charles C. Thomas.

Dietz, P., Hazelwood, R., & Warren, J. (1990). The sexually sadistic criminal and his offenses. *Bulletin of the American Academy of Psychiatry and Law, 18,* 163–178.

Doorn, C. D., Poortinga, J., & Verschoor, A. M. (1994). Cross-gender identity in trans-vestites and male transsexuals. *Archives of Sexual Behavior, 23,* 185–201.

Ellis, A., & Brancala, R. (1956). The psychology of sex offenders. Springfield, IL: Charles C. Thomas.

Epperson, D. L., Kaul, J. D., & Hesselton, D. (1998, October). Final report of the development of the Minnesota Sex Offender Screening Tool-Revised (MnSOST-R). Presentation at the 17th annual research and treatment conference of the Association for the Treatment of Sexual Abusers, Arlington, VA.

Fagan, P., Wise, T., & Derogatis, L. (1988). Distressed transvestites: Psychometric characteristics. *Journal of Nervous and Mental Disease, 176,* 626–632.

Fedora, O., Reddon, J., Morrison, J., Fedora, S., Pascoe, H., & Yeudall, C. (1992). Sadism and other paraphilias in normal controls and aggressive and nonaggressive sex offenders. *Archives of Sexual Behavior, 21,* 1–15.

Firestone, P., Bradford, J. M., McCoy, M., Greenberg, D. M., Larose, M. R., & Curry, S. (1999). Prediction of recidivism in incest offenders. *Journal of Interpersonal Violence, 14,* 511–531.

Freund, K. (1990). Courtship disorder. In W. L. Marshall, D. R. Laws, & H. E. Barbaree (Eds.), *Handbook of sexual assault: Issues, theories, and treatment of the offender* (pp. 195–207). New York: Plenum Press.

Freund, K., Seto, M., & Kuban, M. (1997). The theory of courtship disorder. In. D. R. Laws & W. O'Donohue (Eds.), Sexual deviance: Theory, assessment and treatment (pp. 111–130). New York: Guilford Press.

Freund, K., & Watson, R. (1990). Mapping the boundaries of courtship disorder. *Journal of Sex Research, 27,* 589-606.

Freund, K., Watson, R., & Rienzo, D. (1988). The value of self-reports in the study of voyeurism and exhibitionism. *Annals of Sex Research, 1,* 243–262.

Friday, N. (1980). Men in love. New York: Dell.

Frisbie, L. U., & Dondis, E. H. (1965). Recidivism among treated sex offenders (California Mental Health Research Monograph No. 5), Sacramento, CA: Department of Mental Hygiene.

Frohman, E. M., Frohman, T. C., & Moreault, A. M. (2002). Acquired sexual paraphilia in patients with multiple sclerosis. *Archives of Neurology, 59,* 1006–1010.

Galski, T., Thornton, K. E., Y Shumsky, D. (1990). Brain dysfunction in sex offenders. *Journal of Offender Rehabilitation, 16,* 65–80.

Gamman, L., & Makinnen, M. (1995). *Female fetishism.* New York: NYU Press.

Gijs, L., & Gooren, L. (1996). Hormonal and psychopharmacological interventions in the treatment of paraphilias: An update. *Journal of Sex Research, 33,* 273–290.

Greenacre, P. (1979). Fetishism. In I. Rosen (Ed.), Sexual deviation. Oxford: Oxford University Press.

Greenburg, D. M., Bradford, J. M. W., Curry, S., & O'Rourke, A. B. (1996). A comparison of treatment of the paraphilias with three serotonin reuptake inhibitors. A retrospective study. *Bulletin of the American Academy of Psychiatry and Law, 24,* 525–532.

Grubin, D., & Mason, D. (1997). Medical models of sexual deviance. In. D. R. Laws & W. O'Donohue (Eds.), *Sexual deviance: Theory, assessment and treatment* (pp. 434–448). New York: Guilford Press.

Hanson, R. K., & Thornton, D. (1999). *STATIC-99: Improving actuarial risk assessments for sex offenders. Report No. 1999-02.* Ottawa: Office of the Solicitor General of Canada.

Hare, R. (1991). The hare psychopathy checklist-revised. Toronto, Ontario, Canada: Multi-Health Systems.

Harris, G. T., & Rice, M. E. (1997). Risk appraisal and management of violent behavior. *Psychiatric Services, 48,* 1168–1176.

Hill, A., Briken, P., Kraus, C., Strohm, K., & Berner, W. (2003). Differential pharmacological treatment of paraphilias and sex offenders. *International Journal of Offender Therapy and Comparative Criminiology, 47,* 407–421.

Hunt. M., (1974), Sexual behavior in the 1970s, New York: Playboy Press.

Jaffe, P. D., & DiCataldo, F. (1994). Clinical vampirism: Blending myth and reality. *Bulletin of the American Academy of Psychiatry and Law, 22,* 533–544.

Janus, S., Bess, B., & Saltus, C. (1977). *A sexual profile of men in power.* Englewood Cliffs, NJ: Prentice-Hall.

Kafka, M. P. (1994). Sertraline pharmacotherapy for paraphilias and paraphilia-related disorders. An open trial. *Annals of Clinical Psychiatry, 6,* 189–195.

Kafka, M. P., & Prentky, R. (1992). Fluoxetine treatment of nonparaphilic sexual addictions and paraphilias in men. *Journal of Clinical Psychiatry, 53,* 351–358.

Kaplan, M., & Krueger, R. (1997). Voyeurism: Psychopathology and theory. In. D. R. Laws & W. O'Donohue (Eds.), Sexual deviance: Theory, assessment and treatment (pp. 297–310). New York: Guilford Press.

Kinsey, A. C., Pomeroy, W. B., Martin, C. E., & Gebhard, P. H. (1953). Sexual behavior in the human female. New York: Simon & Schuster.

Knight, R., Prentky, R., & Cerce, D. (1994). The development, reliability, and validity of an inventory for the multidimensional assessment of sex and aggression. *Criminal Justice and Behavior, 21,* 72–94.

Langevin, R., Paitich, D., Hucker, S., Newman, S., Ramsay, G., Pope, S., et al. (1979). The effect of assertiveness training, Provera, and sex of therapist in the treatment of genital exhibitionism. *Journal of Behavior Therapy and Experimental Psychiatry, 10,* 275–282.

Langevin, R., Paitich, D., Russon, A., Handy, L., & Langevin, R. (1990). *The Clarke Sexual History Questionnaire for Males: Manual.* Toronto: Juniper Press.

Laws, D. R. (1989). Relapse prevention with sex offenders. New York: Guilford Press.

Laws, D. R. (1995). Verbal satiation: Notes on procedure with speculation on its mechanism of effect. *Sexual Abuse: A Journal of Research and Treatment, 7,* 155–166.

Laws, D. R., & Marshal, W. L. (1991). Masturbatory reconditioning with sexual deviates: An evaluative review. *Advances in Behavior Research and Therapy, 13,* 13–25.

Letourneau, E., & O'Donohue, W. (1997). Classical conditioning of female sexual arousal. *Archives of Sexual Behavior, 26,* 63–78.

Levine, S. B. (1993). Gender-disturbed males. *Journal of Sex and Marital Therapy, 19,* 131–141.

Malamuth, N. M. (1989). The Attraction to Sexual Aggression: Part One. *Journal of Sex Research, 26,* 26–49.

Marshall, W. L., & Anderson, D. (1996). An evaluation of the benefits of relapse prevention programs with sexual offenders. *Sexual Abuse: A Journal of Research and Treatment, 8,* 209–221.

Masand, P. S. (1993). Successful treatment of sexual masochism and transvestic fetishism associated with depression with fluoxetine hydrochloride. *Depression, 1,* 50–52.

Maletzky, B. (1987). Data generated by an outpatient sexual abuse clinic. Paper presented at the 1st annual Conference on the Assessment and Treatment of Sexual Abusers, Newport, Oregon.

Maletzky, B. (1998). The paraphilias: Research and treatment. In P. E. Nathan & J. M. Gorman (Eds.), *A guide to treatments that work* (pp. 474–500). New York: Oxford University Press.

Marques, M. J. K., Nelson, C., Alarcon, J. M., Day, D. M. (2000). Preventing relapse in sexual offenders: What we learned from SOTEP's experimental program. In D. R. Laws, S. M. Hudson, & T. Ward (Eds.), *Remaking relapse prevention for sexual offenders* (pp. 321–340). Thousand Oaks, CA: Sage.

Marshall, W. L., & Barbaree, H. E. (1990). An integrated theory of the etiology of sexual offending. In W. L. Marshall, D. R. Laws, & H. E. Barbaree (Eds.), *Handbook of sexual assault: Issues, theories, and treatment of the offender* (pp. 257–275). New York: Plenum Press.

Marshall, W. L., & Fernandez, Y. (1998). Cognitive-behavioral approaches to the treatment of the paraphilias: Sex offenders. In V. E. Caballo (Ed.), *International handbook of cognitive and behavioral treatments for psychological disorders.* Oxford: Englander Science Limited.

Mason, F. (1997). Fetishism: Psychopathology and theory. In D. R. Laws and W. O'Donohue (Eds.), *Sexual deviance: Theory, assessment and treatment* (pp. 75–91). New York: Guilford Press.

McFall, R. M. (1990). The enhancement of social skills. In W. L. Marshall, D. R. Laws, & H. E. Barbaree (Eds.), *Handbook of sexual assault: Issues, theories and treatment of the Offender* (pp. 311–330). New York: Plenum Press.

Mendez, M., Chow, T., Ringman, J., Twitchell, G., & Hinkin, C. (2000). Pedophilia and temporal lobe disturbances. *Journal of Neuropsychiatry and Clinical Neurosciences, 12,* 71–76.

Milner, J., & Dopke, C. (1997). *Paraphilia not otherwise specified: Psychopathology and theory.* In D. R. Laws & W. O'Donohue (Eds.), *Sexual deviance: Theory, assessment and treatment* (pp. 394–423). New York: Guilford Press.

Mohr, J. W., Turner, R. E., & Jerry, M. B. (1964). *Pedophilia and exhibitionism.* Toronto: University of Toronto Press.

Money, J. (1977). Peking: The sexual revolution. In J. Money & H. Mustaph (Eds.), *Handbook of sexology.* Amsterdam: Excerpta Medica.

Moser, C., & Levitt, E. E. (1987). An exploratory-descriptive study of a sadomaso-chistically oriented sample. *Journal of Sex Research, 23,* 273–275.

Murphy, W. (1997). Exhibitionism: Psychopathology and theory. In D. R. Laws & W. O'Donohue (Eds.), *Sexual deviance: Theory, assessment and treatment* (pp. 22–39). New York: Guilford Press.

Nichols, H., & Molinder, I. (1984). Manual for the Multiphasic Sex Inventory. (Available from the authors at 437 Bowes Dr., Tacoma, WA 98466).

O'Donohue, W., & Letourneau, E. (1992). The psychometric properties of the penile tumescence assessment of child molesters. *Journal of Psychopathology and Behavioral Assessment, 14,* 123–174.

O'Donohue, W., Letourneau, E., & Dowling, H. (1997). The measurement of sexual fantasy. *Sexual Abuse: A Journal of Research and Treatment, 9,* 167–178.

O'Halloran, R. L., & Dietz, P. E. (1993). Autoerotic fatalities with power hydraulics. *Journal of Forensic Sciences, 38,* 359–364.

Person, E. S., Terestman, N., Myers, W. A., Goldberg, E. L., & Salvadori, C. (1989). Gender differences in sexual behaviors and fantasies in a college population. *Journal of Sex and Marital Therapy, 15,* 187–198.

Prentky, R., Harris, B., Frizell, K., & Righthand, S. (2000). An actuarial procedure for assessing risk with juvenile sex offenders. *Sexual Abuse: A Journal of Research and Treatment, 12,* 71–93.

Quinsey, V. L., Harris, G. T., Rice, M. E., & Cormier, C. A. (1998). *Violent offenders: Appraising and managing risk.* Washington, DC: American Psychological Association.

Rosler, A., & Witztum, E. (2000). Pharmacotherapy of the paraphilias in the next millennium. *Behavioral Sciences and the Law, 18,* 43–56.

Saleh, F. M., & Guidry, L. L. (2003). Psychosocial and biological treatment considerations for the paraphilic and nonparaphilic sex offender. *The Journal of the American Academy of Psychiatry and the Law, 31,* 486–493.

Sbraga, T. P., & O'Donohue, W. T. (2004). The sex addiction workbook: Proven strategies to help you regain control of your life. Oakland, CA: New Harbinger Press.

Schewe, P. (1997). Paraphilia not otherwise specified: Assessment and treatment. In D. R. Laws & W. O'Donohue (Eds.), Sexual deviance: Theory, assessment and treatment (pp. 424–433). New York: Guilford Press.

Scott, G. G. (1983). Erotic power: An exploration of dominance and submission. Secaucus, NJ: Oxford University Press.

Simpson, G., Blaszczynski, A., & Hodgkinson, A. (1999). Sexual offending as a psychosocial sequela of traumatic brain injury. *Journal of Head Trauma Rehabilitation, 14,* 569–580.

Smith, H., & Cox, C. (1983). Dialogue with a dominatrix. In T. Weinberg & G. Kamel (Eds.), S and M: Studies in sadomasochism (pp. 80–86). Buffalo, NY: Prometheus.

Templeman, T. L., & Stinnett, R. D. (1991). Patterns of sexual arousal and history in a "normal" sample of young men. *Archives of Sexual Behavior, 20,* 137–150.

Thornton, D. (1997, October). Is relapse prevention really necessary? Paper presented at the 17th annual research and treatment conference of the Association for the Treatment of Sexual Abusers, Arlington, VA.

Tollison, C. D., & Adams, H. E. (1979). Sexual disorders: Theory, treatment, and research. New York: Gardner Press.

Ward, T., & Beech, A. R. (2004). The etiology of risk: A preliminary model. *Sexual Abuse: A Journal of Research and Treatment, 16,* 271–284.

Ward, T., & Stewart, C. A. (2003). Good lives and the rehabilitation of sexual offenders. In T. Ward, D. R. Laws, & S. M. Hudson (Eds.), Sexual deviance: Issues and controversies (pp. 21–44). Thousand Oaks, Sage.

Wolfe, R. (1989). Novel techniques in treating the sexual offender. Workshop presented at the 3rd annual Conference on the Assessment and Treatment of Sexual Abusers, Seattle, Washington.

Zavitzianos, G. (1971). Fetishism and exhibitionism in the female and their relationship to psychopathology and kleptomania. *International Journal of Psycho-Analysis, 52,* 297–305.

Zucker, K., & Blanchard, R. (1997). Transvestic fetishism: Psychopathology and theory. In D. R. Laws & W. O'Donohue (Eds.), Sexual deviance: Theory, assessment and treatment (pp. 253–279). New York: Guilford Press.

Zucker, K., & Bradley, S. J. (1995). Gender identity disorder and psychosexual problems in children and adolescents. New York: Guilford Press.

Panic Disorder

Kristin Vickers • Richard J. McNally

PANIC DISORDER

What is Panic Disorder?

Panic disorder is characterized by repeated, unexpected panic attacks, and by persistent concern about subsequent attacks. The *Diagnostic and Statistical Manual of Mental Disorders* (DSM-IV; American Psychiatric Association [APA], 1994) defines panic attack and panic disorder separately. DSM-IV states that panic is:

A discrete period of intense fear or discomfort, in which four (or more) of the following symptoms developed abruptly and reached a peak within 10 minutes:

1. palpitations, pounding heart, or accelerated heart rate
2. sweating
3. trembling or shaking
4. sensations of shortness of breath or smothering
5. feeling of choking
6. chest pain or discomfort
7. nausea or abdominal distress
8. feeling dizzy, unsteady, lightheaded, or faint
9. derealization (feelings of unreality) or depersonalization (being detached from oneself)
10. fear of losing control or going crazy
11. fear of dying
12. paresthesias (numbness or tingling sensations)
13. chills or hot flushes (p. 395)

The occurrence of repeated, unexpected panic attacks (at least two) is necessary, but insufficient, for a diagnosis of panic disorder, which requires that:
at least one of the [panic] attacks has been followed by 1 month (or more) of one (or more) of the following:

a. persistent concern about having additional attacks
b. worry about the implications of the attack or its consequences (e.g., losing control, having a heart attack, "going crazy")
c. a significant change in behavior related to the attacks (APA, 1994, p. 402)

Because panic attacks occur in patients with other disorders (e.g., specific phobia; see this volume), DSM-IV requires that the attacks are not better explained by another mental condition. Additionally, the attacks must not result directly from substance use or general medical conditions (e.g., hyperthyroidism). Many patients who meet these criteria for panic disorder also have agoraphobia (see this volume), an avoidance of situations from which escape might be difficult or help unavailable should a panic attack occur. The remainder receive a diagnosis of panic disorder without agoraphobia.

Vickers, K., & McNally, R. J. (2006). Evidence-based therapy for panic disorder. In J. E. Fisher & W. T. O'Donohue (Eds.), *Practitioner's guide to evidence-based psychotherapy*. New York: New York.

Because panic is characterized by a sudden onset of terror accompanied by intense cardiorespiratory and other physiologic symptoms, most theorists distinguish it from anxiety—a state of heightened worry. Whether panic arises from a distinct abnormality, such as misfiring of a suffocation alarm system (e.g., Klein, 1993), or whether it merely reflects intense fear (e.g., Barlow, 2002, pp. 106–107), remains a topic of debate (e.g., Vickers & McNally, in press-a).

Basic Facts About Panic Disorder

According to the National Comorbidity Survey (Kessler et al., 1994), the current and lifetime prevalences of panic disorder among American adults is 2.3% and 3.5%, respectively. Twice as many women as men develop panic disorder, and syndrome can be chronic if left untreated.

Panic disorder usually erupts in late adolescence or early adulthood; it rarely begins before puberty or late in life (McNally, 1994, pp. 167–169). Panic attacks often begin during periods of life stress such as losing a job, marital conflict, or in anticipation of major life events (e.g., getting married). Isolated panic attacks are not uncommon in the general population (McNally, 1994, pp. 14–16). Only when people develop dread of subsequent attacks or alter their life in response to fear of panic is the disorder diagnosed.

People with panic disorder often meet criteria for other anxiety disorders, mood disorders, or both (e.g., Kessler et al., 1998). Alcohol abuse is not uncommon. Although pure panic disorder does not appear to increase risk for suicide attempt (e.g., Vickers & McNally, in press-b), panic sufferers are at heightened risk when they have comorbid depression and substance abuse.

ASSESSMENT

What Should be Ruled Out?

Several medical conditions can produce heightened physiological arousal that can mimic panic symptoms. For example, inner ear problems can produce dizziness, mitral valve prolapse can produce heart palpitations, and excessive caffeine intake can produce jitteriness. These conditions should be ruled out prior to psychological treatment.

What is Involved in Effective Assessment?

Many panic patients have already received general medical assessments prior to contacting a mental health professional, but if not, then such assessment may be needed. The presence of depression, suicidal ideation, and substance abuse are also assessed (APA, 1998).

After clinicians have confirmed the diagnosis of panic disorder, often via semi-structured interview, most administer a battery of questionnaires to gauge the severity of the disorder. These often include measures of the fear of anxiety symptoms, such as the Anxiety Sensitivity Index (ASI; McNally, 2002; Reiss, Peterson, Gursky, & McNally, 1986), the Agoraphobic Cognitions Questionnaire (Chambless, Caputo, Bright, & Gallagher, 1984), or the Body Sensations Questionnaire (Chambless et al., 1984), and self-report measures of avoidance behavior, such as the Fear Questionnaire (Marks & Mathews, 1979) and the Mobility Inventory for Agoraphobia (Chambless, Caputo, Jasin, Gracel, & Williams, 1985). A measure of depressive symptoms is often included (e.g., Beck Depression Inventory; Beck, Steer, & Brown, 1996).

In addition to establishing the diagnosis via semi-structured interview, assessment entails having patients use a structured diary to record their panic attacks prospectively (e.g., Antony & Swinson, 2000, pp. 169–170). Self-monitoring forms often contain a checklist of panic symptoms, and require patients to rate their intensity. Forms ask about the circumstances surrounding the onset of panic attack, thereby enabling identification of any antecedent triggers. They also ask about any catastrophic thoughts that occurred to the patient, such as fear of dying, losing control, fainting, and so forth. Clinicians also ask patients why their feared disasters have yet to materialize so far. Answers to such questions usually uncover safety behaviors—actions taken by patients in response to feared sensations that they believe prevent feared disasters. Engaging in safety behaviors prevents patients from learning that their feared catastrophes do not occur.

The key goals of the assessment are to identify panic triggers, feared symptoms (e.g., dizziness), catastrophic thoughts (e.g., "I'm going to collapse!"), and extent of agoraphobic avoidance.

What Assessments are Not Helpful?

Traditional psychological tests (e.g., the Rorschach, MMPI) are seldom useful in panic assessment. No laboratory test can establish a diagnosis of panic disorder (APA, 1994).

TREATMENT

What Treatments are Effective?

Both certain pharmacologic agents and a specific form of psychological treatment called cognitive behavioral therapy (CBT) are empirically supported treatments for panic (Barlow, 2002, pp. 364–375).

What are Effective Self-Help Treatments?

Researchers have increasingly turned their attention to examining the effectiveness of self-help approaches to panic. For example, Clark et al. (1999) found that five CBT sessions, plus self-study modules, were just as effective as the standard 12-session CBT protocol. Furthermore, some panic patients respond well to a bibliotherapy, self-help protocol (Lidren et al., 1994). Reviewing this literature, Hofmann and Spiegel (1999, p. 7) commented that self-help approaches to panic seem "viable." It is, however, essential that self-help material provide accurate information about panic (Graham, 2003). Moreover, further research is warranted to determine whether patients who are severely impaired benefit from self-help treatment (Hofmann & Spiegel, 1999).

Useful Websites:

For patients, the National Institute of Mental Health provides information about panic, as well as a link to locate mental health services in a particular area, at: http://www.nimh.nih.gov/HealthInformation/panicmenu.cfm

For practitioners, the APA's (1998) treatment guidelines for panic disorder are online at:

http://www.psych.org/psych_pract /treatg/pg/pg_panic.cfm

What are Effective Therapist-Based Treatments?

The psychological approach to panic holds that the core feature maintaining the disorder is elevated fears of anxiety symptoms. Accordingly, the major treatment derived from this approach, CBT, focuses on reducing these fears. Recent research confirms that reduction in the "fear of fear" mediates clinical improvement in response to CBT (Smits, Powers, Cho, & Telch, 2004). To accomplish this aim, CBT therapists rely on both cognitive techniques (psychoeducation about panic and cognitive restructuring) and behavioral methods (interoceptive exposure; e.g., Taylor, 2000, pp. 340–351).

CBT therapists first provide patients with information about panic disorder. This psychoeducation provides the basis for subsequent interventions and facilitates patients' active collaboration. Most panic patients harbor many misconceptions about the bodily sensations associated with panic attacks, and these call for correction. For example, many patients mistake intercostal muscle tension in the chest as indicative of a heart attack, not realizing that cardiac arrest entails a crushing pain in the chest, usually accompanied by pains that shoot downward through the arm. Many patients mistake hyperventilation-related dizziness as indicative of impending faint, not realizing that fainting results from a sudden *drop* in heart rate and blood pressure. Hence, elevated heart rate during panic protects against faint, dizziness notwithstanding. Patients often fail to realize that panic—or the "fight–flight" fear reaction—defends against threat; it is not itself dangerous. Finally, unfamiliar with the symptoms of psychosis, patients sometimes fear that their panic symptoms may evolve into serious mental illness. These mistaken beliefs about bodily sensations provide the basis for their fearful response to dizziness, heart palpitations, and so forth, and these catastrophic misinterpretations can aggravate symptoms, leading to a full-blown panic attack (Clark, 1986).

Many patients continue to hold catastrophic beliefs and misconceptions about bodily sensations because their safety behaviors have prevented testing (and refutation) of these beliefs. Accordingly, clinicians will ask the patients what has prevented them from falling victim to their feared catastrophes. Patients will typically indicate that they have taken certain actions when symptoms strike that they believe have prevented the disaster from materializing. Consider a patient who believes that she will collapse if dizzy. When asked, "Why have you not collapsed so far?", the patient is likely to mention safety behaviors that have prevented the feared event from occurring (e.g., leaning against a wall, sitting down).

Cognitive restructuring of catastrophic beliefs entails conducting behavioral experiments (Clark, in press) in addition to providing psychoeducation about symptoms. Behavioral experiments are designed to provide direct, experiential evidence to refute these beliefs. Consider the patient who fears fainting when dizzy, and who always sits down (safety behavior) when this sensation occurs. A behavioral experiment might entail having the patient hyperventilate while sitting down, thereby producing sensations of dizzy lightheadedness. The patient's catastrophic prediction is that he or she will faint upon standing, whereas the alternative prediction is that only slight unsteadiness will result. Having the patient confront the feared bodily sensations without engaging in the accustomed safety behavior is among the most powerful methods of changing catastrophic beliefs that maintain panic disorder. The therapist's goal is to design convincing behavioral experiments that will permit refutation of beliefs associated with the different feared bodily sensations. Cognitive restructuring is thereby accomplished by psychoeducation plus behavioral experiments.

Panic patients fear bodily sensations in the same sense that a height phobic fears high places or a dog phobic fears dogs. Prolonged, systematic exposure to feared, but nondangerous, stimuli is a core feature of behavioral treatment of anxiety disorders. Applied to panic disorder, the exposure principle requires patients to practice exposure to bodily sensations until these sensations lose their capacity to incite fear. Exposure to internal sensations—interoceptive exposure—is integral to the treatment of panic disorder. This can entail brisk running up and down stairs to produce increases in heart rate, breathing through straws to simulate dyspnea, hyperventilation to produce dizziness, and tensing chest muscles to simulate intercostal tension.

Some clinicians continue to provide patients with anxiety management skills, such as applied muscle relaxation and breathing retraining, designed to counteract hyperventilation. Although the rationale for these procedures was originally to help patients attenuate the intensity of feared bodily sensations, some therapists now question the wisdom of these methods. That is, teaching patients methods for attenuating sensations seems to imply that experiencing these sensations is bad, undesirable, or harmful, and this implication runs counter to psychoeducational procedures that teach the harmlessness of the feared sensations. Indeed, one study showed that panic patients whose treatment omitted breathing retraining responded better to CBT than those who had received this anxiety management technique (Schmidt et al., 2000). Alternatively, teaching anxiety management techniques as a means of imparting to patients a sense of control over their bodies may prove useful. Framed in this manner, anxiety management techniques need not imply that the sensations thereby controlled are harmful and must be suppressed.

Fear of panic attacks motivates many patients to avoid certain places and activities. Residual agoraphobic avoidance can linger, even after the aforementioned CBT antipanic methods have worked. Accordingly, therapists customarily design in vivo ("real life") exposure assignments whereby patients practice entering feared situations (e.g., subways, shopping malls) and engaging in feared activities (e.g., driving on the expressway, flying in planes) until their discomfort subsides (see Agoraphobia, this volume).

Numerous randomized, controlled studies attest to the efficacy of this multicomponent approach against panic. CBT, delivered in either individual sessions (e.g., Barlow, Gorman, Shear, & Woods, 2000) or in group format (e.g., Telch et al., 1993), significantly reduces panic. About 74% of CBT-treated patients are panic-free posttreatment (Gould, Otto, & Pollack, 1995). Comparable outcomes occur when CBT is transported to community mental health settings (Stuart, Trent, & Wade, 2000; Wade, Treat, & Stuart, 1998). CBT has outperformed other efficacious interventions, such as applied relaxation and imipramine (Clark et al., 1994) and emotion-focused therapy (Shear, Houck, Greeno, & Masters, 2001).

What is Effective Medical Treatment?

Controlled trials show that three classes of drugs—high-potency benzodiazepines, tricyclic antidepressants (TCAs), and selective serotonin reuptake inhibitors (SSRIs)—are efficacious against panic disorder (Barlow, 2002, pp. 364–368; Cross-National Collaborative Panic Study, 1992; Lecruiber et al., 1997). Because benzodiazepines carry the risk of physical dependence after long-term use (Kasper & Resinger, 2001), some researchers restrict use of these drugs to obtain short-term, rapid control over symptoms (APA, 1998). TCAs and SSRIs are both effective pharmacologic options for longer treatment. The side effect burden of TCAs, however, is greater than that of SSRIs. Accordingly, some researchers currently consider SSRIs to have a better balance of efficacy and adverse effects for many panic patients (e.g., APA, 1998).

Researchers know more about the short-term efficacy of these agents than about the long-term outcome of pharmacotherapy. Evidence to date suggests that some patients relapse or suffer symptom exacerbation when medication is discontinued (e.g., Doyle & Pollack, 2004; Rapaport et al., 2001). Researchers have also reported that some patients who are maintained on adequate pharmacotherapy after remission relapse (Simon et al., 2002). Accordingly, researchers continue to investigate how to minimize chance of relapse in patients treated with pharmacotherapy.

Because both CBT and certain pharmacologic agents have demonstrated efficacy against panic, researchers have investigated whether their simultaneous combination enhances long-term outcome. Findings to date suggest are inconsistent with this hypothesis (Foa, Franklin, & Moser, 2002). For example, patients treated with both CBT and imipramine (a TCA) were more likely to relapse six months after treatment discontinuation than were patients who received CBT alone (Barlow et al., 2000). Similarly, five months posttreatment, fewer patients treated with the combination of alprazolam (a benzodiazepine) and exposure therapy remained well than patients treated with the combination of pill placebo and exposure therapy (Marks et al., 1993).

Other Issues in Management

Researchers are currently examining other issues in management of panic symptoms, such as the appropriate length of treatment. CBT usually extends over 12 weeks, although some improvement occurs as soon as after the second session (Penava, Otto, Maki, & Pollock, 1998), and encouraging results have occurred from abbreviated forms of CBT (Clark et al., 1999). Researchers continue to investigate the optimal duration of pharmacologic treatment with TCAs or SSRIs. Although earlier research suggested that extending the length of this treatment decreased relapse risk upon discontinuation (Mavissakalian & Perel, 1992), this finding has not replicated. Specifically, approximately 37% of panic patients treated with imipramine for either six months or for 12–30 months relapsed after discontinuation (Mavissakalian & Perel, 2002). Similarly, Dannon et al. (in press) found that extending paroxetine (an SSRI) treatment from one year to two years did not reduce relapse rate.

Another important management issue concerns strategies that enhance the chances of successful medication discontinuation. Along these lines, researchers have found that adding CBT during benzodiazepine taper significantly reduces relapse risk. Indeed, patients who underwent benzodiazepine taper alone were 13.5 times more likely to have relapsed and resumed medication at six-month follow-up than were those who received 12 individual weekly sessions of CBT during taper (Spiegel et al., 1994). Building on the success of CBT during benzodiazepine taper, researchers have recently added CBT to antidepressant discontinuation, with encouraging results (Schmidt, Woolaway-Bickel, Trakowski, Santiago, & Vasey, 2002; Whittal, Otto, & Hong, 2001).

How Does One Select Among Treatments?

Efficacy studies have revealed that CBT performs as well as pharmacotherapy in the short-term and may be more durable over the long-term (Barlow et al., 2000). Thus, the success of these two monotherapies —CBT and certain pharmacologic interventions —in ameliorating panic symptoms presents practitioners and patients with a choice. Unfortunately, researchers have yet to establish the factors that predict which treatment modality will be most effective for an individual patient (Otto, Pollack, & Maki, 2000). Further complicating matters, predictors of better response to a particular type of medication than another type (e.g., SSRIs or TCAs), or to a particular drug within a medication class (e.g., sertraline or fluoxetine within the SSRI class), are largely lacking.

In the absence of this information, researchers have turned to other factors, such as tolerability, cost, and patient preference, to inform their choice of treatment strategy. For example, the balance of the evidence suggests that CBT is more tolerable than pharmacotherapy (e.g., Gould et al., 1995). Although individual CBT costs more over four months than does pharmacotherapy, individual CBT is more affordable over one year (Otto et al., 2000). Examining patient preference, researchers have found that pretreatment refusal occurs less commonly with CBT than with pharmacotherapy. Only one of 305 panic patients gave the reason of refusal to undergo psychotherapy as the basis for not entering a treatment trial; in contrast, over 33% refused because they were unwilling to take the medication (Hofmann et al., 1998).

Clearly, many factors must guide the choice of treatment. For example, medications have varied side effect profiles (e.g., Barlow, 2002, pp. 364–368); therapists require suitable training to administer CBT (e.g., Clark et al., 1999). Patients' physical health, suicide risk, and previous response to treatment must always be carefully considered. It is beyond the scope of this brief chapter to review such material; practitioners are urged to consult the treatment guidelines set forth by the APA (1998).

In summary, the aforementioned considerations suggest that CBT alone should be the first treatment option. If access to a CBT therapist is unavailable, then an SSRI or a TCA should be prescribed.

KEY READINGS

American Psychiatric Association. (1998). Practice guidelines for the treatment of patients with panic disorder. *American Journal of Psychiatry, 155(Suppl. 5)*.

Antony, M. M., & Swinson, R. P. (2000). *Phobic disorders and panic in adults: A guide to assessment and treatment*. Washington, DC: American Psychological Association.

Barlow, D. H. (2002). *Anxiety and its disorders: The nature and treatment of anxiety and panic* (2nd ed.). New York: Guilford Press.

McNally, R. J. (1994). *Panic disorder: A critical analysis*. New York: Guilford Press.

McNally, R. J. (2002). Anxiety sensitivity and panic disorder. *Biological Psychiatry, 52*, 938–946.

Taylor, S. (2000). *Understanding and treating panic disorder: Cognitive-behavioural approaches*. Chichester, UK: Wiley.

REFERENCES

American Psychiatric Association. (1994). *Diagnostic and statistical manual of mental disorders* (4th ed.). Washington, DC: Author.

American Psychiatric Association. (1998). Practice guidelines for the treatment of patients with panic disorder. *American Journal of Psychiatry, 155(Suppl. 5)*.

Antony, M. M., & Swinson, R. P. (2000). *Phobic disorders and panic in adults: A guide to assessment and treatment*. Washington, DC: American Psychological Association.

Barlow, D. H. (2002). *Anxiety and its disorders: The nature and treatment of anxiety and panic* (2nd ed.). New York: Guilford Press.

Barlow, D. H., Gorman, J. M., Shear, K., & Woods, S. W. (2000). Cognitive-behavioral therapy, imipramine, or their combination for panic disorder. *Journal of the American Medical Association, 283*, 2529–2536.

Beck, A. T., Steer, R. A., & Brown, G. K. (1996). *Beck Depression Inventory manual* (2nd ed.). San Antonio, TX: Psychological Corporation.

Chambless, D. L., Caputo, G. C., Bright, P., & Gallagher, R. (1984). Assessment of fear of fear in agoraphobics: The body sensations questionnaire and the agoraphobic cognitions questionnaire. *Journal of Consulting and Clinical Psychology, 52*, 1090–1097.

Chambless, D. L., Caputo, G. C., Jasin, S. E., Gracel, E. J., & Williams, C. (1985). The Mobility Inventory for Agoraphobia. *Behaviour Research and Therapy, 23*, 35–44.

Clark, D. M. (1986). A cognitive approach to panic. *Behaviour Research and Therapy, 24*, 461–470.

Clark, D. M. (in press). Developing new treatments: On the interplay between theories, experimental science and clinical innovation. *Behaviour Research and Therapy*.

Clark, D. M., Salkovskis, P., Hackmann, A., Middleton, H., Anastasiades, P., & Gelder, M. (1994). A comparison of imipramine, applied relaxation, and imipramine in the treatment of panic disorder. *British Journal of Psychiatry, 164,* 759–779.

Clark, D. M., Salkovskis, P., Hackmann, A., Wells, A., Ludgate, J., & Gelder, M. (1999). Brief cognitive therapy for panic disorder: A randomized controlled trial. *Journal of Consulting and Clinical Psychology, 67,* 583–589.

Cross-National Collaborative Panic Study, Second Phase Investigators. (1992). Drug treatment of panic disorder. Comparative efficacy of alprazolam, imipramine, and placebo. *British Journal of Psychiatry, 160,* 191–202.

Dannon, P. N., Iancu, I., Lowengraub, K., Cohen, A., Grunhaus, L. J., & Kotler, M. (in press). Three year naturalistic outcome study of panic disorder patients treated with paroxetine. *BMC Psychiatry.*

Doyle, A., & Pollack, M. H. (2004). Long-term management of panic disorder. *Journal of Clinical Psychiatry, 65(Suppl. 5),* 24–28.

Foa, E. B., Franklin, M. E., & Moser, J. (2002). Context in the clinic: How well do cognitive-behavioral therapies and medications work in combination? *Biological Psychiatry, 52,* 987–997.

Graham, C. (2003). Reading about self-help books on obsessive–compulsive and anxiety disorders: A review. *Psychiatric Bulletin, 27,* 235–237.

Gould, R. A., Otto, M. W., & Pollack, M. H. (1995). A meta-analysis of treatment outcome for panic disorder. *Clinical Psychology Review, 15,* 819–844.

Hofmann, S. G., Barlow, D. H., Papp, L. A., Detweiler, M. F., Ray, S. E., Shear, M. K., Woods, S. W., & Gorman, J. M. (1998). Pretreatment attrition in a comparative treatment outcome study on panic disorder. *American Journal of Psychiatry, 155,* 43–47.

Hofmann, S. G., & Spiegel, S. G. (1999). Panic control treatment and its applications. *Journal of Psychotherapy Practice and Research, 8,* 3–11.

Kasper, S., & Resinger, E. (2001). Panic disorder: The place of benzodiazepines and selective serotonin reuptake inhibitors. *European Neuropsychopharmacology, 11,* 307–321.

Kessler, R. C., McGonagle, K. A., Zhao, S., Nelson, C. B., Hughes, M., Eshleman, S., Wittchen, H.-U., & Kendler, K. S. (1994). Lifetime and 12-month prevalence of DSM-III-R psychiatric disorders in the United States: Results from the National Comorbidity Survey. *Archives of General Psychiatry, 51,* 8–19.

Kessler, R. C., Stang, P. E., Wittchen, H.-U., Ustun, T. B., Roy-Byrne, P. P., & Walters, E. E. (1998). Lifetime panic-depression comorbidity in the National Comorbidity Survey. *Archives of General Psychiatry, 55,* 801–808.

Klein, D. F. (1993). False suffocation alarms, spontaneous panics, and related conditions: An integrative hypothesis. *Archives of General Psychiatry, 50,* 306–317.

Lecruiber, Y., Bakker, A., Dunbar, G. Judge, R., & the Collaborative Paroxetine Panic Study Investigators. (1997). A comparison of paroxetine, clomipramine, and placebo in the treatment of panic disorder. *Acta Psychiatrica Scandinavica, 95,* 145–152.

Lidren, D. M., Watkins, P. L., Gould, R. A., Clum, G. A., Asterino, M., & Tulloch, H. L. (1994). A comparison of bibliotherapy and group therapy in the treatment of panic disorder. *Journal of Consulting and Clinical Psychology, 62,* 865–869.

Mavissakalian, M. R., & Perel, J. M. (1992). Protective effects of imipramine maintenance treatment in panic disorder with agoraphobia. *American Journal of Psychiatry, 149,* 1053–1057.

Mavissakalian, M. R., & Perel, J. M. (2002). Duration of imipramine therapy and relapse in panic disorder with agoraphobia. *Journal of Clinical Psychopharmacology, 22,* 294–299.

Marks, I. M., & Mathews, A. M. (1979). Brief standard self-rating for phobic patients. *Behaviour Research and Therapy, 17,* 263–267.

Marks, I. M., Swinson, R. P., Basoglu, M., Kuch, K., Noshirvani, H., O'Sullivan, G., et al. (1993). Alprazolam and exposure alone and combined in panic disorder with agoraphobia: A controlled study in London and Toronto. *British Journal of Psychiatry, 162,* 776–787.

McNally, R. J. (1994). *Panic disorder: A critical analysis.* New York: Guilford Press.

McNally, R. J. (2002). Anxiety sensitivity and panic disorder. *Biological Psychiatry, 52,* 938–946.

Otto, M. W., Pollack, M. H., & Maki, K. M. (2000). Empirically supported treatments for panic disorder: Costs, benefits, and stepped care. *Journal of Consulting and Clinical Psychology, 68,* 556–563.

Penava, S. J., Otto, M. W., Maki, K. M., & Pollack, M. H. (1998). Rate of improvement during cognitive-behavioral group treatment for panic disorder. *Behaviour Research and Therapy, 36,* 665–673.

Rapaport, M. H., Wolkow, R., Rubin, A., Hackett, E., Pollack, M., & Otoa, K. Y. (2001). Sertraline treatment of panic disorder: Results of a long-term study. *Acta Psychiatrica Scandinavica, 104,* 289–298.

Reiss, S., Peterson, R. A., Gursky, D. M., & McNally, R. J. (1986). Anxiety sensitivity, anxiety frequency and the prediction of fearfulness. *Behaviour Research and Therapy, 24,* 1–8.

Schmidt, N. B., Woolaway-Bickel, K., Trakowski, J., Santiago, H., Storey, J., Koselka, M. et al. (2000). Dismantling cognitive-behavioral treatment for panic disorder: Questioning the utility of breathing retraining. *Journal of Consulting and Clinical Psychology, 68,* 417–424.

Schmidt, N. B., Woolaway-Bickel, K., Trakowski, J. H., Santiago, H. T., & Vasey, M. (2002). Antidepressant discontinuation in the context of cognitive behavioral treatment for panic disorder. *Behaviour Research and Therapy, 40,* 67–73.

Shear, M. K., Houck, P., Greeno, C., & Masters, S. (2001). Emotion-focused psychotherapy for patients with panic disorder. *American Journal of Psychiatry, 158,* 1993–1998.

Simon, N. M., Safren, S. A., Otto, M. W., Sharma, S. G., Lanka, G. D., & Pollack, M. H. (2002). Longitudinal outcome with pharmacotherapy in a naturalistic study of panic disorder. *Journal of Affective Disorders, 69,* 201–208.

Smits, J. A. J., Powers, M. B., Cho, Y., & Telch, M. J. (2004). Mechanism of change in cognitive-behavioral treatment of panic disorder: Evidence for the fear of fear mediational hypothesis. *Journal of Consulting and Clinical Psychology, 72,* 646–652.

Spiegel, D. A., Bruce, T. J., Gregg, S. F., & Nuzzarello, A. (1994). Does cognitive behavior therapy assist slow-taper alprazolam discontinuation in panic disorder? *American Journal of Psychiatry, 151,* 876–881.

Stuart, G. L., Treat, T. A., & Wade, W. A. (2000). Effectiveness of an empirically based treatment for panic disorder delivered in a service clinic setting: 1-year follow-up. *Journal of Consulting and Clinical Psychology, 68,* 506–512.

Taylor, S. (2000). *Understanding and treating panic disorder: Cognitive-behavioural approaches.* Chichester, UK: Wiley.

Telch, M. J., Lucas, J. A., Schmidt, N. B., Hanna, H. H., Jaimez, T. L., & Lucas, R. A. (1993). Group cognitive-behavioral treatment of panic disorder. *Behaviour Research and Therapy, 31,* 279–287.

Vickers, K., & McNally, R. J. (in press-a). Respiratory symptoms and panic in the National Comorbidity Survey: A test of Klein's suffocation false alarm theory. *Behaviour Research and Therapy.*

Vickers, K., & McNally, R. J. (in press-b). Panic disorder and suicide attempt in the National Comorbidity Survey. *Journal of Abnormal Psychology.*

Wade, W. A., Treat, T. A., & Stuart, G. L. (1998). Transporting an empirically supported treatment for panic disorder to a service clinic setting: A benchmarking strategy. *Journal of Consulting and Clinical Psychology, 66,* 231–239.

Whittal, M. L., Otto, M. W., & Hong, J. J. (2001). Cognitive-behavior therapy for discontinuation of SSRI treatment of panic disorder: A case series. *Behaviour Research and Therapy, 39,* 939–945.

Paranoia

Thomas F. Oltmanns • Mayumi Okada

WHAT IS PARANOIA?

The principal defining features of paranoia are pervasive and unwarranted mistrust and suspiciousness of others. People who are paranoid are locked into a rigid and maladaptive pattern of thought, feeling, and behavior based on the conviction that others are "out to get them." Their perception of the world as a threatening place drives them to be highly alert to any evidence suggesting that they are being victimized. A constant search for proof of their victimization often leads them to misinterpret others' comments and behaviors. Hypersensitivity to slights, both imagined and real, combined with the tendency to have excessive confidence in their own knowledge and abilities, create tension in interpersonal relationships and leave social networks depleted. This description is a summary of the definition for paranoid personality disorder (PD) found in the *Diagnostic and Statistical Manual of Mental Disorders* (DSM-IV; American Psychiatric Association).

The DSM-IV criteria for paranoid PD are quite similar to those presented in the most recent edition of the *International Classification of Diseases* (ICD-10). Both manuals agree that paranoid people are suspicious and prone to jealousy. They construe other's actions as hostile and hold grudges. There are also some interesting differences between the APA and WHO diagnostic systems. The following ICD criteria are not included in the DSM-IV-TR: excessive sensitivity to setbacks and rebuffs, tendency toward excessive self-importance that is manifested in persistent self-referential attitude, and a combative sense of personal rights. This comparison suggests that the characteristic features of paranoia remain open to further consideration.

Factor analytic results suggest that one of the DSM-IV criteria for paranoid personality disorder— "Is suspicious that his/her sexual partner might be cheating"— may be less useful than the others. In a data set obtained using a nonclinical sample of military recruits, factor analysis found that this item was not significantly related to the other criteria used to diagnose paranoid PD (Thomas, Turkheimer, & Oltmanns, 2003). The other diagnostic features for paranoid PD all loaded together on one factor that included items related primarily to mistrust and aggression. This result raises the possibility that jealousy involving one's sexual partner is not necessarily a core feature of paranoia. In fact, research grounded in an evolutionary approach to personality suggests that jealousy may be a specialized emotion that is specifically related to the issue of mate retention (Buss, 1999).

The rigid and maladaptive patterns of thought that are characteristic of paranoid personality disorder are clearly pathological. On the other hand, suspiciousness and vigilance are not unique to paranoia. For example, popular books on leadership styles in the business world proclaim that "only the paranoid survive" (Grove, 1996). This argument hinges on the notion that it pays to anticipate negative events. Rigid patterns of thought are also common. Most people adhere to a preconceived notion, even when they are confronted with evidence that ought to persuade them otherwise (Nisbett & Ross, 1980). We all notice the relevance of

Oltmanns, T. F., & Okada, M. (2006). Paranoia. In J. E. Fisher & W. T. O'Donohue (Eds.), *Practitioner's guide to evidence-based psychotherapy*. New York: Springer.

confirming cases more readily than that of disconfirming ones. Therefore, the sustained vigilance and suspicion of being harmed are not sufficient to justify a diagnosis.

When does a cautious approach to the motives of other people cross the line into pathological paranoia? The distinction depends, in part, on the consideration of associated features—characteristics that are not considered primary diagnostic signs but are nevertheless often associated with paranoia (Frances, First, & Pincus, 1995). One issue involves irritability and hostility. Because they believe that other people are causing problems for them, paranoid people are often extremely angry. Another consideration involves fear. Paranoid people can also become anxious and withdrawn. Again, this fear is based largely on the conviction that others intend to cause them harm. In an effort to avoid the threats that seem to be all around them, paranoid people try to protect themselves by avoiding other people. When a chronically suspicious person begins to experience problems with exaggerated interpersonal anger and aggression, or if that person is markedly fearful and withdrawn, it seems reasonable to conclude that the suspicions are no longer adaptive or normal.

Another way to distinguish between normal and abnormal suspicions involves the amount of time that the person spends thinking about threats posed by other people. While most people become suspicious from time to time, paranoid people are *preoccupied* with the notion that others are out to get them. They are unable to think otherwise. As Shapiro (1965) put it, "These people are not merely capable of remarkably active, intense, and searching attention; they seem essentially incapable of anything else (p. 59)." Paranoid people are also impaired in their ability to consider information from another person's point of view. Most of us are able to seek and consider another person's perception or interpretation of uncertain events; paranoid people cannot do so. Another way of looking at the rigidity in thought patterns that mark this disorder is to examine how a paranoid individual's behavior and, or perception differs from those around him or her. In this regard, criterion six of paranoid PD "perceives attack on his or her reputation that are not apparent to others . . ." (APA, 2000) represents an important consideration.

There is considerable overlap between paranoia and features of related personality disorders. Clues to these associated features can be found in previous versions of the official diagnostic manual (e.g., DSM-III). For example, people who are paranoid tend to be tense, stubborn, and argumentative. They can be aggressive and counterattack when they feel they are being attacked. They find it difficult to accept criticism of themselves. They can appear to be serious, cold, and lacking in emotional response. These diagnostic features overlap with the formal descriptions of Narcissistic PD and Antisocial PD in DSM-IV. Criteria related to restricted affect and absence of tender or sentimental feelings were dropped from the diagnostic manual, perhaps to reduce overlap with the descriptive features of Schizoid PD (Bernstein, Useda, & Siever, 1995). The criterion related to being easily slighted and quick to take offense was also dropped, primarily in an effort to reduce overlap with Narcissistic PD.

Distinctions between paranoia and other forms of personality pathology can be clarified using descriptions based on the Five-Factor Model of personality. Individuals with paranoid PD are characterized primarily by low Agreeableness, particularly on the specific facets (lower level traits) of trust, straightforwardness, and compliance. They are also high on Neuroticism, and more specifically on the facet of angry-hostility. Other personality disorders that share similar profiles of low Agreeableness include narcissistic and antisocial personality disorders. Not surprisingly, there is a fairly high rate of cooccurrence among these categories. While low scores on the Agreeableness scale characterize paranoid, narcissistic, and antisocial PDs, they can be distinguished in terms of the specific components of agreeableness. Prototypic cases of Narcissistic PD produce low scores on the facets of modesty, altruism, and tendermindedness. In contrast, paranoid people produce high scores on mistrust. Unlike Paranoid PD that emphasizes low trust, prototypic cases of Antisocial PD are characterized by low scores on altruism (Costa, Widiger, & Costa, 2002).

BASIC FACTS ABOUT PARANOIA

Prevalence. Approximately 10–14% of adults in the general population (i.e., those not seeking treatment for a mental disorder) would meet diagnostic criteria for at least one type of personality disorder (Torgersen, Kringlen, & Cramer, 2001). Rates for specific personality disorders vary from one study to the next, depending on the assessment procedures employed and the way in which participants were identified. Studies that have used semi-structured diagnostic interviews with community residents have reported a lifetime prevalence of approximately 1% for paranoid personality disorder (Mattie & Zimmerman, 2001).

Comorbidity. Many people would qualify for a diagnosis of more than one type of personality disorder. Among people who meet the criteria for paranoid personality disorder, the most frequent cooccurring conditions are schizotypal, narcissistic, borderline, and avoidant personality disorders (Bernstein, et al., 1995).

Gender. Epidemiological evidence regarding gender differences for personality disorders (other than antisocial PD) is ambiguous. Very few community-based studies have been done using standardized interviews as a basis for diagnosis. There has been some speculation that paranoid personality disorder may be somewhat more common among men than women (Bernstein, et al., 1995).

Age at onset. According to DSM-IV, paranoia may be evident in childhood and adolescents. Early manifestations may take the form of social isolation, poor peer relationships, social anxiety, and hypersensitivity. Some people who are later recognized as being frankly paranoid may have appeared to be odd or eccentric during childhood and adolescence.

Temporal stability is one of the most important assumptions about personality disorders. Evidence for the assumption that personality disorders appear during adolescence and persist into adulthood has, until recently, been limited primarily to antisocial personality disorder. One longitudinal study has collected information regarding the prevalence and stability of personality disorders among adolescents (Bernstein et al., 1993). This investigation is particularly important because it did not depend solely on subjects who had been referred for psychological treatment and because it was concerned with the full range of personality disorders. The rate of personality disorders was relatively high in this sample: 17% of the adolescents received a diagnosis of at least one personality disorder. While many of these people continued to exhibit the same problems over time, fewer than half of the adolescents who were originally considered to have a personality disorder qualified for that same diagnosis two years later. This evidence suggests that maladaptive personality traits are frequently transient phenomena among adolescents.

Course. Follow-up studies indicate that paranoid personality characteristics are typically long-term problems that change relatively little over time (Seivewright, Tyrer, & Johnson, 2002; Stephens, Richard, & McHugh, 2000). For many patients, their paranoid beliefs become more pronounced over time.

ETIOLOGY

Most attempts to explain the development of paranoia share an interest in two underlying themes. One involves a strategy for protecting the self. For example, some therapists have suggested that paranoid people are trying to protect themselves from a tumultuous family background characterized by parental dominance and mistreatment. There is no strong empirical support for this hypothesis.

The second common feature is the idea that the central mechanism that drives paranoid thinking is low self-esteem. Some theorists trace this deeply ingrained feeling of personal failure to early family interactions, which are presumably characterized by parental dominance, mistreatment, and lack of consistent affection (Benjamin, 1996). A somewhat different perspective on the role of low self-esteem begins with a focus on rejection and ridicule, which may be the consequence of the paranoid person's personality style. The person behaves in a rigid, self-important, and suspicious manner and is therefore rejected by others. Rejection leads to a further reduction in self-esteem (Fenigstein, 1996).

Colby's (1977, 1981) information-processing view of paranoid thinking incorporated both factors, i.e., self-protection and low self-esteem. According to this view, paranoid people scan the verbal content of conversations with other people for evidence suggesting that the self is inadequate or defective. Upon finding the "evidence," the person searches for ways to deal with it. Acknowledging their inadequacy will result in humiliation and shame, which would in turn lend support to their inner belief that they are somehow inadequate or unworthy. Therefore, they turn to alternative methods of coping that allow them to deflect this sense of shame. Rather than accepting responsibility, they blame others and assert that they are being victimized. This defensive reaction sets in motion a pernicious cycle: by viewing others as hostile, the paranoid person maintains his or her self-esteem, but he or she then behaves in a defensive and perhaps offensive manner. This in turn elicits anger from others, and these reactions lend further support to the paranoid person's belief that others are hostile.

In addition to the self-protective function of deflecting shame and fault away from the self, Maher (1988) suggested that blaming others also allows the paranoid person to make sense of (or impose order and meaning on) seemingly random events and vaguely threatening experiences. It may be less frightening to find an enemy to blame than to accept the fact that some events happen randomly and accidentally. The paranoid person may choose to blame others because the identification of a specific, tangible threat reduces anxiety and enables the person to organize efforts to combat the threat, even if they are in fact misconceived and inappropriate (Fenigstein, 1996).

In the paranoid style of thinking, all events are seen as bearing reference to the self, even when they do not (Magaro, 1980; Shapiro, 1981). Their self-focused style of thinking in which all events, including behaviors of others, are rigidly perceived to be relevant to the self, leads them to believe that they are being watched, targeted, or even plotted against. Self-focused attention contributes to the maintenance of paranoia. Attention that is directed to the self, especially to aspects of the self that are observable by others, can induce an exaggerated feeling of visibility and conspicuousness. The person is inclined to believe that others are similarly preoccupied by his or her appearance or behavior and that they act with him or her in mind. Insignificant and irrelevant events are perceived as being personally relevant, and the person continues to believe that he or she is the target of others' malevolent acts.

ASSESSMENT

What Should be Ruled Out?

The principal issue regarding differential diagnosis and paranoid PD concerns the distinction between this category and delusional disorder, in which the patients exhibit persistent persecutory delusions or delusional jealousy. The paranoid ideas in paranoid personality disorders are presumably not of sufficient severity to be considered delusional, but the criteria to be used in making this distinction are not entirely clear. When does pervasive suspicion and mistrust become a paranoid belief? The two categories may be etiologically distinct, but it has not been demonstrated that they carry different treatment implications. *DSM-IV-TR* lists the categories separately, but the reliability and validity of the two categories remain open questions (Bernstein, et al., 1995).

Cultural factors also raise difficult issues regarding the differential diagnosis of paranoia. Within a particular society, the experiences of people from cultural and ethnic minorities should be considered carefully before diagnostic decisions are made. Strong feelings of suspicion, alienation, and distrust, illustrate this issue. People who belong to minority groups (and those who are recent immigrants from a different culture) are more likely than members of the majority or dominant culture to hold realistic concerns about potential victimization and exploitation. For example, black Americans may develop and express mild paranoid tendencies as a way of adapting to ongoing experiences of oppression (Whaley, 1998). Clinicians may erroneously diagnose these conditions as paranoid personality disorder if they do not recognize or understand the cultural experiences in which they are formed. In this particular case, it is obviously important for the clinician to consider the person's attitudes and beliefs regarding members of his or her own family or peer group, as well as the person's feelings about the community as a whole.

What is Involved in Effective Assessment?

Disordered views of the self and others prevent most paranoid people from seeking help. When they do enter treatment, they may not describe their problems in a way that allows the therapist to recognize the true nature of their problems. Because they believe that all faults lie with others and not with the self, most paranoid individuals do not complain about being suspicious, lacking in trust, or hypervigilant. Instead, they typically present with problems that reflect hostile and or adversarial relationships with others.

The assessment process requires openness to scrutiny that many paranoid individuals cannot tolerate. Given their hypersensitivity to threat, direct confrontation may cause the paranoid person to become more guarded and less trusting of the therapist or to terminate therapy prematurely. Exaggerated empathy can also be counterproductive. If the therapist appears to be too open and understanding, the client may become increasingly guarded and wary. Therefore, the therapist must walk a fine line, balancing acceptance with objectivity.

The most widely recognized approach to the assessment of personality disorders, in both research and clinical practice, involves the use of interviews. Many different semistructured interviews have been developed for the diagnosis of personality disorders (Zimmerman, 1994). Examples include the Structured Interview for DSM-IV Personality (SIDP-IV; Pfohl, Blum, & Zimmerman, 1997) and the Personality Disorders Interview (PDI-IV; Widiger et al., 1995). Each of the interview schedules provides a list of opening questions on topics related to the diagnostic features as well as suggested follow-up probes to be used whenever the person admits problems in a particular area. Clark and Harrison (2001) have described in detail

the advantages and potential weaknesses of these instruments. Most efforts to evaluate empirically the utility of semistructured interviews have focused on the issue
of reliability. Interrater reliability estimates in a joint interview format are higher
(average κ above .60) than either short-interval test–retest or the long interval
test–retest. Reliability increases when personality disorders are computed using
dimensional scores rather than categorical scores (Zimmerman & Coryell, 1989;
Pilkonis et.al., 1995). Less attention has been paid to the validity of diagnostic interviews in the assessment of personality disorders. Convergent reliability (different
interviews compared to each other or an interview compared to a self-report questionnaire) has been shown to be relatively poor (Clark, Livesley, & Morey, 1997).
Clinicians should therefore consider the results of diagnostic interviews with some
caution. These instruments are considered to be the "gold standard" with regard to
the diagnosis of personality disorders, but they depend largely on the ability or willingness of the person to recognize the nature of his or her problems.

Another popular approach to the assessment of paranoid PD involves the
administration of self-report questionnaires. Several different instruments are available. Some focus on symptoms of paranoid PD, others focus on personality traits
that are related to paranoia, and a final option would be to collect information
regarding interpersonal difficulties that follow as a consequence of paranoia.

The Minnesota Multiphasic Personality Inventory (MMPI-II) is the most widely
used self-report inventory in clinical practice and research. The test includes ten clinical scales, one of which is Paranoia (Pa). This scale was originally developed to identify
patients with paranoid symptoms, such as ideas of reference, feelings of persecution,
grandiose self-concepts, suspiciousness, excessive sensitivity, and rigid opinions and
attitudes (Graham, 2000). Elevated scores on this scale signify suspiciousness, sensitivity, delusions of persecution, ideas of reference, rigidity, and externalizing defenses,
correspond reasonably well with both DSM-IV and ICD-10 criteria for paranoid PD.

Rather than focusing on diagnostic scales, with an emphasis on somewhat arbitrary thresholds and a categorical view regarding the presence or absence of paranoia, some self-report instruments place greater emphasis on personality dimensions.
Some of these focus exclusively on normal personality traits. One popular alternative
of this type is the NEO-PI-R, a questionnaire that provides scores based on the Five
Factor Model of personality (Costa & McCrea, 1989). Using this measure for the
assessment of traits that are related to paranoia, one might expect low scores on
Agreeableness, especially the more specific facets of trust, straightforwardness, and
compliance. A person who is paranoid would also be expected to produce a high
score on Neuroticism, and more specifically on the facet of angry-hostility.

The Schedule for Nonadaptive and Adaptive Personality (SNAP) is a factor ana-
lytically derived, self-report instrument that is designed to measure trait dimensions
that are important in the domain of personality disorders (Clark, 1990; 1993). The
instrument includes both obvious and more subtle items which are intended to tap
the high and low ends of all of the trait dimensions. The core of the SNAP is composed of 15 scales, including 12 trait scales associated with relatively specific forms
of personality pathology and three more general "temperament" scales (negative
temperament, positive temperament, and disinhibition). The specific trait scales
most related to paranoia include mistrust, aggression, and detachment. The SNAP
also includes five validity scales that can be used to identify subjects who have
responded carelessly or defensively. They are also sensitive to various other response
sets that might contribute to an invalid profile. In addition to the 15 trait scales, the
SNAP can also be used to derive scores on 13 diagnostic scales, which correspond to
each of the specific PD categories included in DSM-IV. The combination of validity

scales, trait scales, and diagnostic scales makes the SNAP an especially useful instrument to be used in an assessment aimed at the identification of personality problems related to paranoia.

Another approach to the assessment of paranoia would be to focus on interpersonal problems that follow as a consequence of rigid, unwarranted suspicions. An example of such an instrument is the Inventory of Interpersonal Problems (IIP). The IIP was originally designed as a way to measure and track interpersonal problems commonly seen in patients presenting for therapy. The items comprising the original IIP were derived from complaints reported by clinical patients. These items were structured as either "It is hard to…" statements (e.g., "It is hard for me to feel close to other people") or "These are things I do too much" statements (e.g., "I am too suspicious of other people") (Horowitz, Rosenberg, Baer, Ureño, & Villaseñor, 1988). The analytic model used to score the IIP has focused on a combination of two orthogonal bipolar dimensions: a vertical dimension representing dominance, status, or control, and a horizontal dimension representing love, warmth, or affiliation. These dimensions have been expanded to include a set of eight scales following a circumplex model, in which traits are arrayed around these two dimensions in a circular space. The closer two traits are on the circle, the more highly they are correlated. Scales most relative to the assessment of paranoia are: vindictive/self-centered (characterized by distrust and suspicion of others and an inability to care about others) and cold/distant (characterized by an inability to express affection).

The fact that semistructured interviews and self-report questionnaires have traditionally been used in the assessment of PDs should not imply that they are the best sources of information. Like everyone else, people with personality disorders are frequently unable to view themselves realistically and are unaware of the effects of their behavior on others (Oltmanns, Turkheimer, & Strauss, 1998; Westen & Schedler, 1999). Because realistic, accurate information about a client's behavior may not be obtained from the clients themselves, it is often useful to collect information from other sources. Family members, friends, and other acquaintances may provide an important perspective. Studies that have examined the relation between self-report data and informant report data regarding personality pathology have found that the two sources often disagree (Klonsky, Oltmanns & Turkheimer, 2002; Thomas et al., 2003).

Comparisons between self and peer reports reveal an interesting paradox regarding paranoia. People who are viewed by their peers as being paranoid do not see themselves as being suspicious or lacking in trust. Rather, they described themselves as being angry and hostile (Clifton, Turkheimer, & Oltmanns, 2004). Research has shown that those who had thought of themselves as being paranoid were often regarded by others as cold and unfeeling. While it has not yet been determined how the two very different types of information should be used, it is fair to state that patient and informant evaluation represent two different assessment approaches to personality that produce two different portrayals of a client's personality disorder. Perhaps utilizing information from both sources may help a clinician gain a more comprehensive picture of a client's personality disorder than if the clinician were to rely solely on one source of information.

TREATMENT

What Treatments are Effective?

Psychotherapy can be beneficial for patients with various kinds of personality disorder (Perry, Banon, & Ianni, 1999; Sanislow & McGlashan, 1998). Unfortunately, relatively little evidence is available specifically with regard to the effects of treatment for paranoid PD. Clinical experience suggests that therapy is often of limited value with paranoid patients because it is so difficult to establish a trusting therapeutic relationship with them (Bernstein, 2001).

Although several treatment techniques have been proposed, some of which have appeared to be successful based on case reports and uncontrolled clinical reports, to date, there have not been controlled treatment studies on patients with paranoid PD (Sperry, 2003). It is interesting, however, that despite the differences in vocabulary and theoretical orientations, the limited number of treatment approaches that have been developed for paranoid PD are quite similar. Almost all techniques prescribe a series of phases beginning with developing a trusting therapeutic relationship with the client, improving the client's sense of self-efficacy, followed by modifying their belief system, and concluding with an adoption of a more flexible and adaptive style of thinking and interpersonal behavior.

The first phase of treatment involves the development of a trusting therapeutic relationship with the client. Without this base, treatment cannot succeed. Numerous strategies have been developed to encourage the development of such a relationship; examples include explicitly acknowledging and accepting the person's difficulty in trusting the therapist, giving clients control over scheduling appointments and content of sessions, and establishing your role as a professional person whose interest in the client is solely professional (Lipkin & Cohen, 1998). The cognitive therapy approach recommends beginning the treatment process by helping the client specify and prioritize goals for therapy, and working toward a goal that appears manageable; this serves several purposes. First, having the clients specify and prioritize goals demonstrates that the client is in control of the treatment process. Second, the process of jointly agreeing on a goal lays the foundation for the client and the therapist to work together collaboratively. Third, if the client is able to make demonstrable progress toward the goal, not only would this encourage the client to proceed with the therapy, but it will also increase the client's self-esteem.

Increasing the individual's self-esteem and sense of self-efficacy is the next focal point. Many theorists assume that while paranoid individuals are often resistant and contentious, behind their defensiveness and arrogance may be strong feelings of inferiority, shame, humiliation, personal rejection and longing for dependence (Sperry, 1995; Lipkin & Cohen, 1998). Paranoia can be viewed as a defense mechanism that is used to protect the self from further exposure to these strong negative feeling. Therefore, in the hopes of helping the clients reach a point in which they can begin to let go of their defensive strategy, their self-esteem must be bolstered.

Cognitive therapy also has interesting applications for the treatment of paranoid patients. The central assumption of this approach is that personality disorders are associated with deeply ingrained, maladaptive beliefs (Beck et al., 2001). In the case of paranoid personality, these include thoughts such as "people cannot be trusted" and "if I get close to people, they will find out my weaknesses and hurt me." The therapist works with the client to identify and recognize these cognitive distortions and their influence on the person's behavior. The paranoid person is encouraged to test the validity of these maladaptive thoughts. Over time, the goal is to help the person learn to replace them with more adaptive thoughts are more accurate attributions (Bentall & Kinderman, 1998; Kinderman, 2001).

As treatment progresses, emphasis should shift to modifying their belief system regarding the self and others. Many of the techniques that are used during this phase of treatment are borrowed from cognitive therapy (CT) and schema therapy, a type of cognitive therapy that was developed specifically for treating PDs. The central assumption of cognitive therapy is that personality disorders are associated with deeply ingrained, maladaptive beliefs that are often inaccurate (Beck et al., 2001). Therefore, the goal of CT is to replace their maladaptive beliefs with those that are more "adaptive" and "accurate." As these thoughts are intrinsic to the personality-disordered individual, it is hard, if not impossible, for them to recognize and acknowledge that their core beliefs need to be changed. With the help of the therapist, clients are encouraged to identify and recognize cognitive distortions and their influence on behavior.

Once the maladaptive schemas have been identified, the client is encouraged to test the validity of these maladaptive thoughts. Examining evidence for and against the schemas of mistrust and abuse that are predominantly found in those with paranoid PD, may be achieved by having a series of structured dialogues between the client and the therapist in which both parties try to constructively argue for and against the schema (Young, 1999). Such a method allows the patient to systematically confront and challenge his or her maladaptive schemas.

In the process of challenging and changing their maladaptive schemas, clinicians should encourage patients to think about how their behavior may have elicited certain reactions from others. Paranoid individuals have learned to be hypersensitive to the judgments of others, and as a result, they behave in ways that invite the type of reaction they anticipate and fear. As they react in hostile manners that drive people away, paranoid individuals become convinced that their suspicions were correct. In order to break the cycle, clients should be taught how to be less sensitive to criticism and how to act in ways that will not invite attack or avoidance (Turkat & Maisto, 1985). The latter is achieved by utilizing social skills training techniques such as instructional role-playing, behavior rehearsal, and videotaped feedback, through which they are taught to attend to more appropriate social stimuli, to interpret information more accurately and to receive feedback from others in a non-defensive way.

What are Effective Self-Help Treatments?

The literature on self-help methods for paranoid personality disorder is quite limited. Paranoid people are unlikely to seek treatment of any kind (therapist-based or otherwise) because they seldom view the origins of their emotional and interpersonal difficulties in terms of their own behavior. Recognize the nature of the problem is, in many respects, the most important step in setting the stage for positive change. One book that might be helpful is Martin Kantor's "Understanding Paranoia: A Guide for Professionals, Families, and Sufferers." Kantor describes a number of self-help techniques that may be useful for people who are able to acknowledge the possibility that their difficulties with other people can be traced, at least partially, to themselves. Included in this list are strategies to increase and enhance self-acceptance, improve relationships with others, manage anger, learn to trust and love one's self and others, and learn to identify and correct cognitive errors that may lead to distortions of oneself and/or others. Journaling is one example. It is recommended as a procedure that can increase self-awareness and encourage alternative ways of reacting to specific situations. These techniques may also help the person to consider alternative perspectives, that is, ways that others may view and react to their suspicious behaviors. Taken together, the program may help some people to create a social network that seems less dangerous and threatening.

What is Effective Medical Treatment?

With the growing number of research and clinical trials that suggest a link between personality disorders and neurochemical abnormalities, there has been an increased interest in finding biological treatments for personality disorders (Crits-Christoph &

Barber, 2004). Unfortunately, due to the lack of controlled pharmacological trials that have been conducted for paranoid PD, there is a great deal of disagreement regarding both the type of medication that should be used and the effectiveness of such medication. Some have argued that because the symptoms that are character-istic of paranoid PD are similar to the delusional beliefs often evident in schizo-phrenia, these patients should be treated with atypical antipsychotic medication such as risperidone (Grossman, 2004). Others have argued that fluoxetine hydrochloride (Prozac) is effective in reducing suspiciousness and irritability, symp-toms that are characteristic of both depression and paranoid personality disorder (Fieve, 1994). Finally, since the publication of an open-clinical trial of pimozide for treating paranoia (Munro, 1992), numerous researchers have cited its effectiveness in reducing symptoms associated with Cluster A personality disorders. However, contrary to this view, the original article by Munro did not include any empirically supported evidence to suggest that pimozide would be effective for treating para-noid PD. Furthermore, the original article clearly stated that paranoid personality disorder is one of the few "principle disorders to be excluded" (p. 337) from what was then referred to as delusional (paranoid) disorder (DSM-III-R) which did seem to benefit from the use of pimozide [see Friedman, next chapter].

REFERENCES

American Psychiatric Association. (2000). *Diagnostic and statistical manual of mental disorders, fourth edition text revision (DSM-IV-TR)*. Washington, DC: Author.

Beck, A. T., Butler, A. C., Brown, G. K., Dahlsgaard, K. K., Newman, C. F., & Beck, J. S. (2001). Dysfunctional beliefs discriminate personality disorders. *Behaviour Research & Therapy, 39*(10), 1213–1225.

Benjamin, L. S. (1996). *Interpersonal diagnosis and treatment of personality disorders* (2nd ed.). New York, NY, US: Guilford Press.

Bernstein, D. P., Useda, D., & Siever, L. J. (1995). Paranoid personality disorder. In W. J. Livesley (Ed.), *The DSM-IV Personality Disorders* (Vol. 7, pp. 45–57). New York: Guilford Press.

Clark, L. A., & Harrison, J. A. (2001). Assessment instruments. In W. J. Livesley (Ed.), *Handbook of personality disorders: Theory, research, and treatment.* New York: Guilford. (pp. 277–306).

Clifton, A., Turkheimer, E., & Oltmanns, T. F. (2004). Contrasting perspectives on personal-ity problems: Descriptions from the self and others. *Personality and Individual Differences, 36*, 1499–1514.

Colby, K. M. (1977). Appraisal of four psychological theories of paranoid phenomena. *Journal of Abnormal Psychology, 86*(1), 54–59.

Colby, K. M. (1981). Modeling a paranoid mind. *Behavioral & Brain Sciences, 4*(4), 515–560.

Costa, P.T., & McCrae, R.R. (1989). Normal personality assessment in clinical practice: The NEO Personality Inventory. *Psychological Assessment, 4*, 5–13.

Costa, P. T., & McCrae, R. R. (1992). The five-factor model of personality and its relevance to personality disorders. *Journal of Personality Disorders, 6*(4), 343–359.

Costa, P. T., Widiger, T. A., & Costa, P. T., Jr. (2002). *Personality Disorders and the Five-Factor Model of Personality* (2nd edition ed.). Washington DC: American Psychological Association (APA).

Crits-Christoph, P., & Barber, J. P. (2004). Empirical Research on the Treatment of Personality Disorders. In J. J. Magnavita (Ed.), Handbook of Personality Disorders: Theory and Practice (pp. 513–527). Hoboken, NJ: John Wiley & Sons, Inc.

Fenigstein, A. (1995). Paranoia and self-focused attention. In A. Oosterwegel & R. A. Wicklund (Eds.), *The self in European and North American culture.* Amsterdam: Kluwer Academic Publishers.

Fenigstein, A. (1996). Paranoia. In C. G. Costello (Ed.), *Personality Characteristics of the Personality Disordered* (pp. 242–275). New York: Wiley Interscience Pub.

Fieve, R. (1994). *Prozac.* New York: Avon Books.

Frances, A., First, M. B., & Pincus, H. A. (1995). *DSM-IV guidebook.* Washington, DC: American Psychiatric Press.

Graham, J. R. (2000). *MMPI-2: Assessing personality and psychopathology* (3rd ed.). New York: Oxford University Press.

Grossman, R. (2004). Pharmacotherapy of Personality Disorders. In J. J. Magnavita (Ed.), *Handbook of Personality Disorders: Theory and Practice* (pp. 331–355). Hoboken, NJ: John Wiley & Sons.

Grove, A. S. (1996). *Only the paranoid survive: How to exploit the crisis points that challenge every company.* New York: Doubleday.

Kantor, M. (2004). *Understanding paranoia: A guide for professionals, families, and sufferers.* Westport, CT: Praeger.

Klonsky, E. D., Oltmanns, T. F., & Turkheimer, E. (2002). Informant-reports of personality Disorder: Relation to self-reports and future research directions. *Clinical Psychology: Science and Practice, 9,* 300–311.

Lipkin, G. B., & Cohen, R. G. (1998). *Effective approaches to patients' behavior* (5th ed.): *A guide book for health care professionals, patients, and their caregivers.* New York, NY: Springer Publishing Co.

Magaro, P. A. (1980). *Cognition in schizophrenia and paranoia: The interpretation of cognitive processes.* Hillsdale, NJ: Erlbaum.

Maher, B. (1974). Delusional thinking and perceptual disorder. *Journal of Individual Psychology, 30,* 98–113.

Maher, B. (1988). Anomalous experience and delusional thinking: The logic of explanation. In T. F. Oltmanns & B. Maher (Eds.), *Delusional beliefs* (pp. 15–33). New York: Wiley.

Munro, A. (1992). Psychiatric disorders characterized by delusions: Treatment in relation to specific types. *Psychiatric Annals, 22,* 232–240.

Nisbett, R. E., & Ross, L. (1980). *Human inferences: Strategies and shortcomings of social judgement.* Englewood Cliffs, NJ: Prentice Hall.

Oltmanns, T. F., Turkheimer, E., & Strauss, M. E. (1998). Peer assessment of personality traits and pathology in female college students. *Assessment, 51*(1), 53–66.

Pilkonis, P. A., Heape, C. L., Proietti, J. M., Clark, S. W., McDavid, J. D., & Pitts, T. E. (1995). The reliability and validity of two structured diagnostic interviews for personality disorders. *Archives of General Psychiatry, 52,* 1025–1033.

Pretzer, J. (2004). Cognitive therapy for Personality Disorders. In J. J. Magnavita (Ed.), *Handbook of Personality Disorders: Theory and Practice* (pp. 169–193). Hoboken, NJ: John Wiley & Sons, Inc.

Raczek, S. W. (1992). Childhood abuse and personality disorders. *Journal of Personality Disorders, 6*(2), 109–116.

Shapiro, D. (1965). *Neurotic styles.* New York: Basic Books.

Shapiro, D. (1981). *Autonomy and rigid character.* New York: Basic Books.

Sperry, L. (2003). *Handbook of the diagnosis and treatment of DSM-IV-TR personality disorders* (2nd ed.). New York: Brunner-Routledge.

Tarter, R. E., & Perley, R. N. (1975). Clinical and perceptual characteristics of paranoids and paranoid schizophrenics. *Journal of Clinical Psychology, 31*(1), 42–44.

Thomas, C., Turkheimer, E., & Oltmanns, T. F. (2003). Factorial structure of pathological personality as evaluated by peers. *Journal of Abnormal Psychology, 112*(1), 81–91.

Turkat, I. D., & Banks, D. S. (1987). Paranoid personality and its disorder. *Journal of Psychopathology & Behavioral Assessment, 9*(3), 295–304.

Westen, D., & Shedler, J. (1999). Revising and assessing axis II, Part II: Toward an empirically based and clinically useful classification of personality disorders. *American Journal of*

Widiger, T. A. (1993). The DSM-III—R categorical personality disorder diagnoses: A critique and an alternative. *Psychological Inquiry, 4*(2), 75–90.

World Health Organization. (1992). *International statistical classification of diseases and related health* problems (10th ed.). New York: Author.

Young, J. (1999). *Cognitive therapy for personality disorders: A schema-focused approach* (3rd ed.). Sarasota, FL: Professional Resource Press.

Zimmerman, M. (1994). Diagnosing personality disorders: A review of issues and research methods. *Archives of General Psychiatry, 51,* 225–245.

Zimmerman, M. & Coryell, W. (1989). The Reliability of personality disorder diagnoses in a non-patient sample. *Journal of Personality Disorders, 3,* 53–57.

Zimmerman, M., & Coryell, W. H. (1990). Diagnosing personality disorders in the community: A comparison of self-report and interview measures. *Archives of General Psychiatry, 47*(6), 527–531.

CHAPTER 51

Pediatric Feeding Disorders

Kyong-Mee Chung • SungWoo Kahng

WHAT IS PEDIATRIC FEEDING DISORDER?

Eating is one of the most important skills children acquire in the first few years of life. However, feeding difficulties are some of the most common behavioral disturbances in young children, particularly in children with developmental disabilities (Jenkins, Owens, Bax, & Hart, 1984; Sanders, Patel, Le Grice, & Shepherd, 1993). Studies have reported that between 6% and 40% of typically developing preschool children have feeding problems (Archer, Rosenbaum, & Streiner, 1991; Rozin, 1990). The prevalence of feeding problems for children with developmental disabilities was reported to be much higher, ranging from 19% to 80% (Palmer, Thompson, & Linscheid, 1978; Perske, Clifton, McLean, & Stein, 1977).

Some children with pediatric feeding disorders manifest their problems in the form of refusal (i.e., refusing to consume any food by mouth). Alternatively, they may exhibit selectivity, which results in the acceptance of a limited number of select foods (e.g., soft textures or preferred foods). If left untreated, feeding problems may lead to malnourishment; dehydration; weight loss; electrolyte imbalance; impaired intellectual, emotional, and academic development; growth retardation; conditions secondary to artificial feeding (e.g., infections at tube sites); and, in severe and protracted cases, a life-threatening condition (Budd et al., 1992; Linscheid, Oliver, Blyler, & Palmer, 1978). Consequently, pediatric feeding disorders may be a potential burden to society mainly due to the cost of hospitalization; resultant treatment of chronic physical, developmental, and behavioral disorders; and the possible expense of institutionalization and foster care placement for severe cases (Linscheid & Murphy, 1999). The purpose of this chapter is to review the most common pediatric feeding problems in children with developmental disabilities, chronic food refusal and selectivity, and provide empirically based assessment and treatment strategies for children with these problems and their families.

DIAGNOSIS AND CLASSIFICATION

Historically, several different terms have been used to describe children with disturbances or difficulties in feeding. They include failure to thrive (Kessler, 1966), infantile anorexia nervosa (Chatoor & Ganiban, 2003), food phobia (Pliner & Lowen, 1997), and posttraumatic feeding disorder (Benoit, Green, & Arts-Rodas, 1997). The confusion and inconsistency surrounding the diagnosis of pediatric feeding problems can be attributed to many factors. These include the variety of topographies of feeding problems; the existence of heterogeneous theoretical perspectives; the various and diverse training backgrounds of professionals involved in assessing and treating feeding difficulties; and the coexistence of feeding problems with multiple diagnostic, intervention, and treatment issues (Kedesdy & Budd, 1998).

Chung, K-M., & Kahng, S. W. (2006). Pediatric feeding disorders. In J. E. Fisher & W. T. O'Donohue (Eds.), *Practitioner's guide to evidence-based psychotherapy*. New York: Springer.

The Diagnostic and Statistical Manual, Fourth Edition (DSM-IV; American Psychiatric Association, 1994) includes three categories of disorders likely to first manifest in infancy and early childhood: pica, rumination disorder, and feeding disorders of infancy (FDI) and early childhood. FDI is a new diagnosis in the DSM-IV and defined as feeding disturbances not associated with gastrointestinal or other general medical conditions but resulting in significant failure to gain weight or weight loss for at least a month with onset prior to the age of 6 (APA, 1994). The addition of FDI in the DSM-IV increased awareness among mental health professionals of the severity of pediatric feeding problems. However, the new diagnostic criteria have not been widely adopted, primarily because they are not specific enough to enable mental health specialists to differentiate children with various feeding disorders manifested by similar symptoms (Linscheid & Murphy, 1999). The definition also excludes feeding disorders without general growth failure but with specific nutritional deficiencies (i.e., vitamin, iron, zinc, or protein deficiencies) and with various medical conditions.[1]

Three alternative approaches for classifying pediatric feeding problems are descriptive, causal, and multidimensional classification (Kedesdy & Budd, 1998). Descriptive classification is used when pediatric feeding problems are classified on the basis of some descriptive characteristics of the feeding problem. Several descriptive classifications are available, but they are different from each other because different aspects of feeding are being described and classified. Kedesky and Budd (1998) listed 11 descriptive categories based on different descriptive characteristics including the amount and type of food ingested, the properties of the meal, and associated behavior problems. A descriptive classification system is preferred by clinicians due to its practical utility given that it provides useful information for developing a behavioral treatment plan (Budd et al., 1992; Luiselli, 2000).

Causal classification organizes pediatric feeding disorders by their suspected etiologies. Several theoretical models of feeding problems are summarized by Linscheid and Murphy (1999). Though a few different systems have been developed, pediatric feeding disorders are frequently classified as having organic, nonorganic, or mixed etiologies (Budd et al., 1992; Kedesdy & Budd, 1998). When the physical examination and medical tests identify related organic factors for feeding difficulties, the problem is classified as organic. Organic factors include structural physiological defects, metabolic disorders, and food intolerance due to allergies (Kedesdy & Budd, 1998).

When these medical tests results fall within the normal range, the feeding problem is categorized as being of nonorganic etiology. Behavior mismanagement—including, but not limited to, not being able to introduce solid foods at the appropriate age, forced feeding, excessive attention through coaxing, or removal from the feeding situation after problem behaviors—is considered the primary nonorganic factor (Luiselli, 2000).

The third category, mixed etiologies, evolved from recognition that most feeding and growth disorders may result from interactions between organic and nonorganic factors. That is, environmental factors may play a significant role in the development, maintenance, or exacerbation of existing feeding problems due to organic factors (Iwata, Riordan, Wohl, & Finney, 1982; Linscheid et al., 1978). Theories of the etiology of feeding disorders increasingly reflect the complex

---

[1] Some specialists have reported that the new diagnosis may actually perpetuate confusion amongst clinicians and researchers about the nature and appearance of feeding disorders (Chatoor & Ganiban, 2003).

interplay of biological, behavioral, and social factors. This biopsychosocial approach is in fact the most widely accepted one because it allows various practical factors related to feeding problems to be considered and provides a framework for evaluating feeding problems and for guiding intervention planning (Luiselli, 2000).

ASSESSMENT

What Should be Ruled Out?

If a child's feeding problem is purely due to organic factors, medical treatments should be the first treatment of choice. Comprehensive and extensive medical and physiological examination should be conducted during assessment periods to determine if the problem is solely caused and maintained by medical reasons (Kedesky & Budd, 1998).

What is Involved in Effective Assessment?

The purpose of feeding assessments are to collect information about presenting problems and the history of behaviors; identify factors affecting feeding, feeding skills, and caregiver behaviors during meals; and establish realistic treatment goals. In a clinical setting, it is very common for coordination within an interdisciplinary team to address the multiple interacting characteristics of pediatric feeding disorders. This approach allows diagnostic conclusions and the subsequent plan for treatment to reflect the input and collaboration of the multiple disciplines required to address complex problems, especially for those present in individuals with developmental disabilities and complex medical problems (Babbitt, Hoch, & Coe, 1994; Miller, Burklow, & Santoro, 2001). The specific roles of various specialists including pediatricians, gastroenterologists, psychologists, occupational therapists, nutritionists, social workers, and speech pathologists are summarized elsewhere (Kedesdy & Budd, 1998; Wren & Tarbell, 1998).

A typical comprehensive clinical assessment includes a parental report (parents' perceptions of mealtime behaviors and nutrient intake); a review of the child's health, developmental, medical, nutritional, motor, feeding, and growth history; and observation of a meal. These are done through interviews and rating scales, such as the Screening Tool of Feeding Problems (Matson & Kuhn, 2001) or Behavioral Pediatrics Feeding Assessment Scale (BPFAS; Crist, McDonnell, & Beck, 1994), and direct observation with or without structured observation systems, such as an ABC checklist (Miltenberger, 2001; O'Neill, Horner, Albin, Storey, & Sprague, 1997), Global Rating Scale for Feeding Situations (GRSFS; Stark, Bowen, Tyc, Evans, & Passero, 1990), or Mealtime Observation Schedule (MOS; Sanders et al., 1993).[2]

Behavioral Assessments

Assuming that feeding problems are partly maintained by environmental influences, a functional assessment may be conducted as part of a feeding assessment. A functional assessment involves the identification of functional relationships between a specified set of target behaviors and various environmental factors. The functional assessment has been adapted to the evaluation of pediatric feeding disorders with the assumption that regardless of the original etiology of a feeding disorder, environmental factors such as interactions with parents, will affect

---

[2] Some of these scales (e.g., BPFAS, GRSFS, & MOS) have also been used to examine treatment outcomes.

children's behaviors during mealtimes because parents use a variety of consequences to motivate their children to eat (Piazza, Fisher et al., 2003). Identification of these environmental determinants ultimately guides the selection and development of treatment.

The most direct and systematic method of identifying the function is through experimental functional analysis (Iwata, Dorsey, Slifer, Bauman, & Richman, 1994). Functional analyses were originally developed to identify environmental factors that affect self-injurious behaviors; however, this method has been widely adopted for a variety of other behaviors, including aggression, stereotypy, pica, and elopement, not only with persons with developmental disabilities but also typically developing children. Although a limited number of studies have used functional analyses to assess pediatric feeding disorders (Levin & Carr, 2001; Piazza, Fisher et al., 2003), researchers have shown that many children exhibiting food refusal have shown behaviors consistent with an escape or avoidance function, such as a physical resistance to feeding, expulsion of food, or other incompatible behaviors such as aggression and attempts to leave the table (Kitfield & Masalsky, 2000; Levin & Carr, 2001; Piazza, Patel, Gulotta, Sevin, & Layer, 2003). These functional analysis results explain why procedures used to eliminate avoidance or escape (e.g., extinction) are the major treatment components for these populations.

What Assessments are Not Helpful?

Focusing on only one aspect of feeding (e.g., mother–child relationship, medical problems, nutritional aspects) will not provide necessary information for effective treatment. Also, traditional psychological tests projective tests, cognitive assessment, and neuropsychological tests are not useful.

TREATMENT

What is Effective Medical Treatment?

Typical medical treatment include medication, hyperalimentation (e.g., supplementation, forced feeding), intravenous feeding, and the use of oral-gastric, nasogastric, or gastrostomy tubes. Diverse medications frequently used for or impacting feeding problems are well summarized elsewhere (Kedesky & Budd, 1992). These procedures are essential to deal with cases of immediate risk from dehydration or severe malnutrition. However, medical treatments alone are not recommended as long-term strategies because they do not only actively promote appropriate feeding behavior and are associated with additional health risks (Farell, Hagopian, & Kurtz, 2001).

What Methods are Not Helpful?

Mere exposure to food or food deprivation is typically recommended by pediatricians and nutritionists (Skuse, 1993) when parents bring up the issues of feeding difficulties. Some research supports that mere exposure to foods could increase food preference among typically developing children (Birch & Marlin, 1982). However, no studies have supported the effectiveness of mere exposure for treating children with pediatric feeding problems. In addition, Levin and Carr (2001) indicated that deprivation alone, in the absence of other intervention methods, was not sufficient to facilitate consumption of the target food item. Nutritional consultation is a necessary component for developing an effective treatment, but it is not sufficient to reduce feeding problems (Stark et al., 1990).

What Treatments are Effective?

Research has demonstrated that, in many cases, interventions using applied behavior analysis (Baer, Wolf, & Risley, 1968) are effective for treating pediatric feeding disorders (Kerwin, 1999). These behavioral interventions have included one or more of the following components: reinforcement, escape extinction, and stimulus fading.

Many treatments included reinforcement alone or in combination with other treatment components for appropriate eating. Typically, these reinforcement contingencies have included the presentation of tangible items (e.g., toys) or preferred foods contingent on food consumption (Johnson & Babbitt, 1993; Linscheid et al., 1978; Riordan, Iwata, Wohl, & Finney, 1980; Siegel, 1982). For example, Riordan et al. (1980) evaluated positive reinforcement as a treatment for food selectivity. Their participants were two children and their treatment consisted of providing social praise and preferred foods contingent on acceptance of nonpreferred foods. This treatment resulted in a significant increase in food consumption and decrease in problem behaviors during mealtimes.

Although positive reinforcement-based interventions are more common, interventions based on negative reinforcement (e.g., escape) may also prove effective in increasing food acceptance. This is particularly likely given that in most instances, food refusal and selectivity may be maintained by escape from the meal. Kahng, Boscoe, and Byrne (2003) evaluated the use of meal termination as a reinforcer for food acceptance. They initially terminated the meal on the acceptance of a small amount of food. They gradually increased the termination criterion so that the child had to consume larger amounts of food before being permitted to leave the meal. They were able to successfully increase food acceptance through the termination of meals.

Although reinforcement-based interventions are successful in increasing food acceptance, it is oftentimes necessary to incorporate escape extinction in order to eliminate attempts to escape or avoid food (Ahearn, Kerwin, Eicher, Shantz, & Swearingin, 1996; Babbitt et al., 1994; Hoch, Babbitt, Coe, Krell, & Hackbert, 1994; Kerwin, Ahearn, Eicher, & Burd, 1995). This is particularly true if a child has a limited history of oral intake given that the child would have minimal opportunities to obtain reinforcement for appropriate eating. The two most effective and widely used escape extinction procedures for pediatric feeding disorders are nonremoval of spoon (Ahearn et al., 1996; Babbitt et al., 1994; Hoch et al., 1994; Riordan, Iwata, Finney, Wohl, & Stanley, 1984) and physical guidance (Ahearn et al., 1996; Babbitt et al., 1994; Kerwin et al., 1995). Nonremoval of the spoon involves keeping the spoon in front of the child's lips until the bite of food has been accepted. Physical guidance consists of applying gentle pressure to the child's jaw in order to open the child's mouth. The bite of food is then inserted into the mouth.

Ahearn et al. (1996) conducted a direct comparison of both escape–extinction procedures, nonremoval of the spoon and physical guidance. They used an alternating treatments design to compare the efficacy of the two escape–extinction procedures. Their results showed that both were equally effective in increasing food acceptance. However, physical guidance was associated with fewer corollary behaviors, shorter meal durations, and parental preference.

In most cases, behavioral treatments for pediatric feeding disorders include a stimulus fading procedure to increase the amount or type of food consumed. The most common example of stimulus fading involves increasing the number of bites (Luiselli, 2000; Najdowski, Wallace, Doney, & Ghezzi, 2003; Riordan et al., 1980) that a child must be consumed before a reinforcer is delivered. Another stimulus fading procedures consists of increasing the amount of food presented on the spoon. Kerwin, et al. (1995) initially presented a spoon without food on it. They initially increased it to a "dipped" spoon (i.e., the spoon was coated with food), then to a quarter-full, half-full, and finally full spoon. A similar procedure consists of having the child gradually move from touching the food to the lip to swallowing it. Siegel (1982) gradually introduced a six-year old boy to family meals by initially having the child smell the food. This was eventually faded to touching the food with the tongue, then to holding the food in the mouth for few seconds, then to chewing the food, and finally to swallowing the food.

If the child is food selective, stimulus fading can be done by combining nonpreferred foods with preferred foods and increasing the ratio of nonpreferred to preferred foods (e.g., Piazza, et al. 2002). examined the use of blending nonpreferred foods with preferred foods to increase consumption of the nonpreferred foods. The food initially presented to their participants consisted of 10% nonpreferred foods and 90% preferred foods, which their participants consistently consumed. They gradually increased the ratio of nonpreferred foods to preferred foods so that their participants ate up to 16 different foods. Finally, some children may have difficulty consuming certain textures of food. In these cases, it may be possible to change the texture from an easier texture (e.g., pureed) to a more difficult texture (e.g., diced) (Freeman & Piazza, 1998; Shore Babbit, Williams, Coe, & Snyder 1998). Shore, et al., (1998) introduced pureed food to 3 children with severe food selectivity. They gradually increased the texture to junior, ground, and chopped fine using different combinations of textures (e.g., 75% previously successful texture/25% new texture, 50% previously successful texture/50% new texture, etc.) depending upon acceptance and swallowing. They were able to successfully increase food texture using this stimulus fading procedure with their participants.

How do Behavioral Treatments Impact Feeding?

Hoch et al. (1994) and Kerwin et al. (1995) provided an explanation of how these behavioral treatment components might work for treating feeding problems. First, the stimulus fading may have a prompt function, bringing an infrequent behavior (food acceptance) into frequent contact with a positive reinforcement contingency, thereby accelerating the reinforcement effect, hence the term "contingency contacting." Second, continued food presentation despite refusal may extinguish refusal if that refusal was maintained by a meal or presentation termination in a naturally occurring negative reinforcement contingency. Finally, if food presentation is an aversive event, accepting the food would be negatively reinforced by terminating the food presentation following acceptance.

Other Considerations

In addition to these treatment components, other environmental variables are important in the behavioral treatment of pediatric feeding disorders. These variables include rearranging the environment to optimize eating such as manipulating the conditions of mealtime. This can include altering where the meal occurs, who is presenting the food during meals, and where the child and parent are seated. Furthermore, the frequency of meals and snacks in a given day can influence treatment success as can the duration of the meals (Werle, Murphy, & Budd, 1998).

For the majority of studies, the treatment agents were trained therapists, mainly due to an assumption that behavior mismanagement by caregivers plays a major role in pediatric feeding disorders. Identified effective treatment methods are generalized to caregivers after demonstrated success with therapists. Recently, some researchers have successfully examined the use of trained parents to serve as treatment agents (Najdowski et al., 2003; Werle et al., 1998) to facilitate generalization. In addition, a few studies have demonstrated the effectiveness of behavioral group parent training in increasing oral food intake for children with feeding problems associated with cystic fibrosis (Stark et al., 1990). More research should be conducted to establish the effectiveness of these programs and issues involved with successful caregiver training.

What are Effective Self-Help Treatments?

Unfortunately, there are no self-help or parent-governed treatment materials/manual available. In fact, implementation of a treatment program without professional supervision is not recommended because it may worsen the existing problems, especially for severe cases (Luiselli, 2000). The following is the list of feeding clinics across the nation providing intensive behavioral treatment. Some of them include basic information about various feeding disorders.

Useful Websites

http://www.chw.org/display/PPF/DocID/8100/router.asp (Children's Hospital of Wisconsin)

http://www.hmc.psu.edu/childrens/feeding/clinic.htm (Penn State Children's Hospital Feeding Disorder Clinic)

http://www.kennedykrieger.org/kki_cp.jsp?pid=1408 (Kennedy Krieger Feeding Disorders Clinic)

http://www.marcus.org/kki_cp.jsp?pid=2446 (Marcus Institute Feeding Disorders Clinic)

http://www.nlm.nih.gov/medlineplus/print/ency/article/00 (Basic information about pediatric feeding disorders by NIH)

http://www.uihealthcare.com/depts/uibehavioralhealth/pat (University of Iowa Health Care Feeding Clinic)

How Does One Select Among Treatments?

As indicated above, feeding is a relatively complex procedure, which requires simultaneous motor, developmental, and social–emotional maturation. Any interruption in these areas significantly impact typical development in feeding. In addition, significant individual differences exist across different children in these domains. Hence, a treatment should be individualized based on each child's need considering levels of maturation across these domains. Although research has demonstrated the effectiveness of behavioral interventions, due to complex nature of pediatric feeding disorders, it is recommended that a multidisciplinary team select/design an appropriate treatment program for each child. In fact, this approach is the most widely adopted for most of feeding disorder clinics in the nation.

SUMMARY

Eating is one of the most important and complex skills acquired during early childhood. In this chapter, diagnosis, assessment, and treatment for food refusal/selectivity in children were reviewed. Prevalence data indicate that many children, especially those with developmental disabilities, have problems in feeding, and these problems are increasing mainly due to increased mortality because of medical and technical advances. Pediatric feeding disorders may represent a potentially significant cost to society, which might lead to serious problems such as malnutrition. Although the inclusion of pediatric feeding disorders of infancy and early childhood in the DSM-IV was a significant advance, this diagnosis has not been used widely due to its limited coverage. Additional efforts to classify food problems (e.g., descriptive and causal classification) do have merit for developing appropriate assessment and treatment programs; however, more effort should be made to improve the diagnostic system. Considering the complex nature of feeding, a multi-disciplinary approach to assessing and treating the feeding problems is highly suggested.

The literature on pediatric feeding problems consistently indicates that behavioral treatments are effective for increasing oral food intake and decreasing refusal behaviors during feeding, although specific treatment components vary across different types of feeding problems. A combination of positive reinforcement for appropriate food consumption, escape extinction, and stimulus fading appears to be the most effective and widely used behavioral treatment program for pediatric feeding disorders. Consideration of factors affecting feeding including hunger manipulation and contextual variables are necessary for successful treatment. Methodologically sound treatment outcome studies, especially comparing behavioral treatment to other alternative treatment methods; component analysis identifying responsible treatment components for change; and continuous efforts to develop treatment manuals are needed to establish empirically supported treatments for pediatric feeding disorders.

Current efforts to identify empirically supported treatment methods increase the need for more treatment outcome research with solid research design. Continuous attention should be given to comparative treatment outcome studies as well as to the identification of individual contributions of treatment components to increase food consumption. The development of a treatment manual and the dissemination of the manual to frontline clinicians are other important goals to pursue.

REFERENCES

Ahearn, W. H., Kerwin, M. E., Eicher, P. S., Shantz, J., & Swearingin, W. (1996). An alternating treatments comparison of two intensive interventions for food refusal. *Journal of Applied Behavior Analysis, 29*, 321–332.

Archer, L. A., Rosenbaum, P. L., & Streiner, D. L. (1991). The children's eating behavior inventory: Reliability and validity results. *Journal of Pediatric Psychology, 16*, 629–642.

American Psychiatric Association (1994). *Diagnostic and statistical manual of mental disorders* (4th ed.). Washington, DC: Author.

Babbitt, R. L., Hoch, T. A., & Coe, D. A. (1994). Behavioral feeding disorders. In D. N. Tuchman & R. S. Walter (Eds.), *Disorders of feeding and swallowing in infants and children* (pp. 77–95). San Diego, CA: Singular Publishing Group, Inc.

Baer, D. M., Wolf, M. M., & Risley, T. R. (1968). Some current dimensions of applied behavior analysis. *Journal of Applied Behavior Analysis, 1*, 91–97.

Benoit, D., Green, G., & Arts-Rodas, D. (1997). Posttraumatic feeding disorders. *Journal of the American Academy of Child and Adolescent Psychiatry, 36*, 577–578.

Birch, L. L., & Marlin, D. W. (1982). I don't like it; I never tried it: Effects of exposure on two-year-old children's food preferences. *Appetite, 3*, 353–360.

Budd, K. S., McGraw, T. E., Farbisz, R., Murphy, T. B., Hawkins, D., Heilman, N., et al. (1992). Psychosocial concomitants of children's feeding disorders. *Journal of Pediatric Psychology, 17*, 81–94.

Chatoor, I., & Ganiban, J. (2003). Food refusal by infants and young children: Diagnosis and treatment. *Cognitive and behavioral practice, 10*, 138–146.

Crist, W., McDonnell, P., & Beck, M. (1994). Behavior at mealtimes and the young child with cystic fibrosis. *Journal of Developmental & Behavioral Pediatrics, 15*, 157–161.

Farell, D. A., Hagopian, L. P., & Kurtz, P. F. (2001). A hospital- and home-based behavioral intervention for a child with chronic food refusal and gastrostomy tube dependence. *Journal of Developmental and Physical Disabilities, 13*(4), 407–418.

Freeman, K. A., & Piazza, C. C. (1998). Combining stimulus fading, reinforcement, and extinction to treat food refusal. *Journal of Applied Behavior Analysis, 31*, 691–694.

Hoch, T. A., Babbitt, R. L., Coe, D. A., Krell, D. M., & Hackbert, L. (1994). Contingency contracting: Combining positive reinforcement and escape extinction procedures to treat persistent food refusal. *Behavior Modification, 18*, 106–128.

Iwata, B. A., Dorsey, M. F., Slifer, K. J., Bauman, K. E., & Richman, G. S. (1994). Toward a functional analysis of self-injury. *Journal of Applied Behavior Analysis, 27*, 197–209.

Iwata, B. A., Riordan, M. M., Wohl, M. K., & Finney, J. W. (1982). Pediatric feeding disorders: Behavioral analysis and treatment. In P. J. Accardo (Ed.), *Failure to thrive in infancy and early childhood* (pp. 297–329). Baltimore, MD: University Park Press.

Jenkins, S., Owens, J. C., Bax, M., & Hart, H. (1984). Continuities of common behaviour problems in preschool children. *Journal of Child Psychology & Psychiatry, 27*, 75–89.

Johnson, C. R., & Babbitt, R. L. (1993). Antecedent manipulation in the treatment of primary solid food refusal. *Behavior Modification, 17*, 510–521.

Kahng, S., Boscoe, J. H., & Byrne, S. (2003). The use of an escape contingency and a token economy to increase food acceptance. *Journal of Applied Behavior Analysis, 36*, 349–353.

Kedesdy, J. H., & Budd, K. S. (1998). *Childhood feeding disorders: Behavioral assessment and intervention*. Baltimore, MD: Paul. H. Brookes Publishing.

Kerwin, M. E. (1999). Empirically supported treatments in pediatric psychology: Severe feeding problems. *Journal of Pediatric Psychology, 24*, 193–214.

Kerwin, M. E., Ahearn, W. H., Eicher, P. S., & Burd, D. M. (1995). The costs of eating: A behavioral economic analysis of food refusal. *Journal of Applied Behavior Analysis, 28*, 245–260.

Kessler, J. W. (1966). *Psychopathology of children*. Englewood Cliffs, NJ: Prentice Hall.

Kitfield, E. B., & Masalsky, C. J. (2000). Negative reinforcement-based treatment to increase food intake. *Behavior Modification, 24*(4), 600–608.

Levin, L., & Carr, E. G. (2001). Food selectivity and problem behavior in children with developmental disabilities. *Behavior Modification, 25*(3), 443–470.

Linscheid, T. R., & Murphy, L. B. (1999). Feeding disorders of infancy and early childhood. In S. D. Letherton & D. Holmes (Eds.), *Child & Adolescent Psychological Disorders: A comprehensive textbook* (pp. 139–155). London: Oxford University Press.

Linscheid, T. R., Oliver, J., Blyler, E., & Palmer, S. (1978). Brief hospitalization for the behavioral treatment of feeding problems in the developmentally disabled. *Journal of Pediatric Psychology, 3*, 72–76.

Luiselli, J. K. (2000). Cueing, demand fading, and positive reinforcement to establish self-feeding and oral consumption in a child with chronic food refusal. *Behavior Modification, 24*(3), 348–358.

Matson, J. L., & Kuhn, D. E. (2001). Identifying feeding problems in mentally retarded persons: Development and reliability of the screening tool of feeding problems. *Research in Developmental Disabilities, 21*, 165–172.

Miller, C. K., Burklow, K. A., & Santoro, K. (2001). An interdisciplinary team approach to the management of pediatric feeding and swallowing disorders. *Children's Health Care, 30*(3), 201–218.

Miltenberger, R. G. (2001). *Behavior modification: Principles and procedures*. Pacific Grove, CA: Wadsworth.

Mueller, M. M., Michael, M., Piazza, C. C., Patel, M. R., Kelley, M. E., & Pruett, A. E. (2004). Increasing vareity of foods consumed by blending nonpreferred foods into preferred foods. *Journal of Applied Behavioral Analysis, 37*, 159–170.

Najdowski, A. C., Wallace, M. D., Doney, J. K., & Ghezzi, P. M. (2003). Parental assessment and treatment of food selectivity in natural settings. *Journal of Applied Behavior Analysis, 36*, 383–386.

O'Neill, R. E., Horner, R. H., Albin, R. W., Storey, K., & Sprague, J. R. (1997). *Functional assessment and program development for problem behavior: A practical handbook* (2nd ed.). Pacific Grove, CA: Brooks/Cole.

Palmer, S., Thompson, R. J., & Linscheid, T. R. (1978). Applied behavior analysis in the treatment of childhood feeding problems. *Developmental Medicine and Child Neurology, 17*, 333–339.

Perske, R., Clifton, A., McLean, B. M., & Stein, J. I. (1977). *Mealtimes for severely and profoundly handicapped persons: New concepts and attitudes*. Baltimore, MD.: University Park Press.

Piazza, C. C., Fisher, W. W., Brown, K. A., Shore, B. A., Patel, M. R., Katz, R. M., et al. (2003). Functional analysis of inappropriate mealtime behaviors. *Journal of Applied Behavior Analysis, 36*, 187–204.

Piazza, C. C., Patel, M. R., Santana, C. M., Goh, H., Delia, M. D., & Lancaster, B. M. (2002). An evaluation of simultaneous and sequential presentation of preferred and nonpreferred food to treat food selectivity. *Journal of Applied Behavior Analysis, 35*, 259–269.

Piazza, C. C., Patel, M. R., Gulotta, C. S., Sevin, B. M., & Layer, S. A. (2003). On the relative contributions of positive reinforcement and escape extinction in the treatment of food refusal. *Journal of Applied Behavior Analysis, 36*, 309–324.

Pliner, P., & Lowen, E. R. (1997). Temperament and food neophobia in children and their mothers. *Appetite, 28*, 239–254.

Riordan, M. M., Iwata, B. A., Finney, J. W., Wohl, M. K., & Stanley, A. E. (1984). Behavioral assessment and treatment of chronic food refusal in handicapped children. *Journal of Applied Behavior Analysis, 17*, 327–341.

Riordan, M. M., Iwata, B. A., Wohl, M. K., & Finney, J. W. (1980). Behavioral treatment of food refusal and selectivity in developmentally disabled children. *Applied Research in Mental Retardation, 1,* 95–112.

Rozin, P. (1990). Development in the food domain. *Developmental Psychology, 26,* 555–562.

Sanders, M. R., Patel, R. K., Le Grice, B., & Shepherd, R. W. (1993). Children with persistent feeding difficulties: An observational analysis of the feeding interactions of problem and non-problem eaters. *Health Psychology, 12*(1), 64–73.

Shore, B. A., Babbitt, R. L., Williams, K. E., Coe, D. A., & Snyder, A. (1998). Use of texture fading in the treatment of food selectivity. *Journal of Applied Behavior Analysis, 31,* 621–633.

Skuse, D. (1993). Identification and management of problem eaters. *Archives of Disease of Childhood, 69,* 604–608.

Siegel, L. J. (1982). Classical and operant procedures in the treatment of a case of food aversion in a young child. *Journal of Clinical Child Psychology, 27,* 105–110.

Stark, L. J., Bowen, A. M., Tyc, V. L., Evans, S., & Passero, M. A. (1990). A behavioral approach to increasing calorie consumption in children with cystic fibrosis. *Journal of Pediatric Psychology, 15,* 309–326.

Werle, M. A., Murphy, L. B., & Budd, K. S. (1998). Broadening the parameters of investigation in treating young children's chronic food refusal. *Behavior Therapy, 29*(1), 87–105.

Wren, F. J., & Tarbell, S. E. (1998). Feeding and growth disorders. In R. T. Ammerman & J. V. Campo (Eds.), *Handbook of pediatric psychology and psychiatry: Disease, injury, and illness* (Vol. 2, pp. 133–165). Needham Heights, MA: Allyn & Bacon.

Practice Guidelines: Pediatric Sleep Disturbance

Brie A. Moore

WHAT IS PEDIATRIC SLEEP DISTURBANCE?

Sleep disturbance in infants, children and adolescents is defined as significant and persistent difficulty initiating and/or maintaining sleep. (Lozoff, Wolf & Davis, 1985) The most common manifestations include resisting bedtime at least three times per week, delays in sleep onset of at least 30 minutes to 1 hour, prolonging and resisting morning wake-up, daytime fatigue, and night awakenings at least four times per week. Sleep problems are most common during the toddler period and may often persist into early childhood.

Differences between normal and abnormal sleep onset and duration are often defined more so by age than by sleep pattern. For example, whereas newborns may sleep in excess of 16 hours, by school age, children require significantly less sleep (Ferber, 1996; see Figure 52.1). Guidelines for typical sleep requirements can provide appropriate expectations for parents and health professionals.

The presentation of pediatric insomnia also differs with age. Whereas infants are more likely to experience difficulties settling and awaken frequently throughout the night, preschoolers often resist bedtime, delay the onset of sleep, and engage in disruptive night awakenings. School-aged children are most likely to resist bedtime while adolescents with sleep difficulties report insomnia and difficulty initiating sleep (Thiedke, 2001).

It is not uncommon for child sleep behaviors that are considered "typical," such as delaying bedtime and frequent night awakenings, to be difficult for parents to accept, understand and respond to in effective ways.

Basic Facts About Pediatric Insomnias

Pediatric insomnias represent one type of Dyssomnia or secondary sleep disturbance. Primary Hypersomnia, or excessive sleepiness, is also a Dyssomnia. However, Hypersomnia in young children is often related to poor sleep habits or inadequate nighttime sleep. Dyssomnias are distinct from Parasomnias (e.g., Sleep Terrors (see this volume), Nightmares, Nocturnal Enuresis (see this volume), and Sleep Walking) or primary sleep disturbances that involve abnormal variations in sleep physiology and are related to central nervous system immaturity.

Sleep disturbances tend to persist, especially from infancy to later childhood. Some studies indicate that as high as 84% of children's sleep problems persist after three years (Kataria, Swanson & Trevathan, 1987).

The persistence of sleep problems often results in clinically significant distress for children and their families, including distressing parent–child interactions during the evening hours, complications in the marital relationship, delays in the development of independent practice of bedtime skills and disruptions in daytime

Moore, B. A. (2006). Practice Guidelines: Pediatric Sleep Disturbance. In Fisher, J. E., & O'Donohue, W. T. (Eds.), *Practitioner's guide to evidence-based psychotherapy*. New York: Springer.

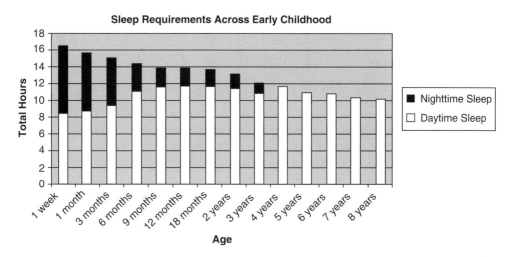

FIGURE 52.1. Sleep Requirements Across Early Childhood (Adapted from Ferber, 1996).

functioning for parents and children. A growing body of literature suggests that pediatric sleep disturbances have a widespread impact on children's health, behavior, mood, attention, cognition, memory, and school performance (Gelman & King, 2001; Kataria et al., 1987; Paavonen et al., 2002; Pollock, 1994).

Comorbidities in young children may include:

Externalizing Behavior Problems

ADHD

Emotional Lability

In adolescents may include:

Anxiety　　　　　　　Depression　　　　　　　Inattentiveness　　　　　　Conduct Disorder

Parent presence and involvement in the sleep process has been associated with sleep problems. Children who fall asleep in a parent's presence or are put to bed asleep awaken more often during the night than infants who are put to bed awake and are left to fall asleep independently. Given this history, children with sleep onset and maintenance problems may have difficulty quieting (day or night) or falling asleep independently at bedtime or after night awakenings because they have come to rely on adult assistance in this process (Kuhn & Weidinger, 2000).

Sleep behaviors are among the most common concerns that parents of young children bring to their physicians. After oppositional behavior (60% occurrence rate), sleep and bedtime problems (42% occurrence rate) are the second most frequently encountered behavioral problem presenting in primary care (Lozoff, Wolf & Davis, 1985).

Between 20% and 30% of children under the age of four-years-old, especially those under the age of 2-years-old, are regarded by their parents as having a sleep problem. Approximately 27% of parents of school aged children report bedtime resistance, while 11% report sleep-onset delays (Blader et al., 1997; Richman, 1981).

According to the National Sleep Foundation's 2006 poll, only 20 percent of adolescents get the recommended nine hours of sleep on school nights.

Age. Occurs in all ages. During the toddler period, sleep disturbance rates may increase with the common onset of fears, such as fear of parental separation or fear of the dark.

Gender. No significant differences in prevalence exist between the sexes.
Racial differences. Investigations of racial differences have not been conducted.

ASSESSMENT

What Should be Ruled Out?

Caveat. Although a thorough assessment considers possible rule-outs, common sleep problems typically result from poor sleep habits and are seldom caused by an underlying medical condition. Unless there is evidence to support a thorough medical evaluation, practitioners should consider behavioral interventions as the first line of treatment.

Sleep disturbance due to the direct physiological effects of a substance (e.g., abuse of a drug, a medication) or general medical condition.
Sleep disturbance due to other sleep disorders including Narcolepsy, Breathing-Related Sleep Disorder, Circadian Rhythm Disorder, a Parasomnia.
Sleep disturbance due to another mental disorder such as Major Depressive Disorder, Generalized Anxiety Disorder or delirium.

What is Involved in Effective Assessment?

Because pediatric insomnias are related to parent–child interactions at bedtime, effective assessment should result in information regarding typical bedtime routines, child behavior at bedtime, and parental responses. Asking questions about sleep assists in identification of treatable sleep problems. Discussing sleep routines and patterns provides an opportunity to evaluate family interactions, learn about parents' current strategies for handling sleep problems, educate parents about good sleep hygiene, and increases the likelihood of preventing more chronic sleep-related problems.

- Assessment
  - Questions about general sleep behavior
    - About how many hours each night does the child sleep?
    - Does the child take naps?
    - How many, how often and for how long?
  - Questions about bedtime
    - Is their a bedtime routine?
    - When is the child's bedtime?
    - Is this bedtime consistent throughout the week?
    - What time does the child actually go to bed?
    - Does the child delay bedtime (e.g., make multiple requests)?
    - Are the child's requests granted?
    - In the parent's opinion, is bedtime a struggle?
  - Questions about sleep onset
    - Is the child put to bed awake or asleep?
    - How long does it take for the child to fall asleep?
    - Is a parent present when the child falls asleep?
    - Is the child held or rocked to sleep?
  - Questions about night awakenings
    - Does the child wake during the night?
    - How often do night awakenings occur?
    - Does (s)he require parental assistance to fall back asleep?
    - How does the parent typically respond?
    - How often do these interactions last?

- Questions about diurnal behavior
  - Does the child require assistance to wake in the morning?
  - Does the child wake fatigued, irritable or in a bad mood?
  - Does the parent have concerns about the child's daytime behavior in general (noncompliance, attention difficulties, aggression, etc.)?
- Questions about parents' current strategies
  - In general, how does the parent typically respond to the child's sleep problems?
- Questions about parents' distress
  - How much of a problem is this for the parents, siblings, and/or family?

If additional information is desired, the practitioner may utilize:

- Sleep Diary (National Sleep Foundation, 2006)
- Child Behavior Check List: Sleep Problems Scale (Achenbach, & Edelbrock, 1983)

What Assessments are Not Helpful?

Traditional developmental assessments such as the Bayley Scales of Infant Development or extensive medical and neurological examinations. Common behavioral sleep problems, such as bedtime resistance and recurrent night awakening, are rarely caused by an underlying medical condition.

TREATMENT

What Treatments are Effective?

1. Education as prevention: prevention of sleep problems in children may be facilitated by simply providing parents with written instructions about sleep (Adair et al., 1992;.
2. Establishment of bedtime routines including 4-7 quiet activities lasting no longer than a total of 20 minutes (Adams & Rickert, 1989; Rickert & Johnson, 1988)
3. Day correction of bedtime problems: development of self-quieting skills during the day encourage the development of sleep-onset skills (Christopherson & Mortweet, 2001)
4. Scheduled awakenings: parents instructed to awaken their child at scheduled times during the evening and to do things like soothe the child or change a diaper (Rickert & Johnson, 1988).

What are Effective Self-Help Treatments?

There are several good books that can have all elements of effective treatments. These include:

American Academy of Pediatrics. Ferber, R. *Solve your Child's Sleep Problems.* New York, NY: Fireside Books; 1985.

Christophersen, E.R. *Little People: Guidelines for Common Sense Child Rearing.* (4th ed.). Kansas City, MO: Westport; 1988.

Christophersen, E.R. *Beyond Discipline: Parenting That Lasts a Lifetime.* (2nd ed.). Shawnee Mission, KS: Overland Press; 1998b.

Finally, Useful Websites are.

1. The University of Michigan Health Systems' guide to development and behavior resources provides information to help promote better sleep hygiene for both parents and children from birth to adolescence. *http://www.med.umich.edu/1libr/yourchild/sleep.htm*

2. About.com's children's sleep problems site provides links to related books, quizzes, and links to information regarding treating sleep problems. *http://pediatrics.about.com/cs/sleep.*

3. The American Academy of Pediatrics simple and efficient guide to establishing good sleep habits in infants and young children. *http://pediatrics.about.com/gi/dynamic/offsite.htm?site=http%3A%2F%2Fwww.medem.com%2Fsearch%2Farticle_display.cfm%3Fpath%3Dn%3A%3A%26mstr%3D%2FZZZYCAGNH4C.html%26soc%3DAAP%26srch_typ%3DNAV_SERCH*

4. Women's Health child sleep site provides information on the causes, types, and signs of sleep disturbances in young children, tips for helping children fall asleep and guidelines for typical sleep requirements from 1 week to 16 years old. *www.mplan.com/womens%20health/childs_sleep.htm*

5. Web MD's Your Child and Sleep site provides guidelines for typical amounts of sleep required from 1-week to 18-years-old, links to articles explaining why sleep is important and instructions how to facilitate healthy sleep behaviors in children. *http://my.webmd.com/content/article/65/79514.htm*

What are Effective Therapist-Based Treatments?

Treatment is generally most effective when employed in the home by parents and can be guided by a therapist if parents need additional support in applying these procedures. Therapists knowledgeable about general parent training can provide individualized consultation. In the case of comorbidity with externalizing behavior problems, Parent–Child Interaction Therapy (PCIT; Eyberg, 1988) is one of the most commonly evaluated and promising treatments. PCIT is a manualized, empirically supported, psychosocial treatment that can be applied in an individual or group format to reduce child behavior problems and promote positive parent–child relationships. The group format can be more cost-effective and parents can gain support from one another.

What is Effective Medical Treatment?

Few empirical studies demonstrate the effectiveness of medication in helping children fall asleep. In most cases, the possible side effects of medications that help children fall asleep outweigh the usefulness of the drugs. Depending on medications pharmacological approaches could result in delays in learning how to fall asleep independently or in dependency (Edwards & Christophersen, 1994). On the basis of many successful reports with reliable measures, behavioral procedures have shown that children's sleep difficulties are often related to how their parents interact with them at bedtime (Blum & Carey, 1996; Edwards & Christophersen, 1994; Ferber, 1985). Behavioral interventions are the most effective and efficient means of treating child behavior problems.

Other Issues in Management

When prescribing behavioral interventions, the practitioner should provide empathic support and discuss parents' views and worries about extended child crying. Providing a thorough rationale in a compassionate manner can help persuade parents to consistently respond in a new way. Additional phone support from the practitioner or office staff may assist in promoting treatment adherence.

Bedtime problems can be due to inconsistent parenting, with the parents intermittently reinforcing problematic behavior such as allowing the child to sleep with them after repeated pleas. Research has established that intermittently reinforced behavior is the most difficult to extinguish (Skinner, 1938; 1991). Thus, it is particularly important to teach the parents to be consistent. The children are escalating aversive behavior in order to try to find a parent "breaking point" in which they will comply with the child's wishes. Also, parents may have some secondary gain, such as gaining pleasant time with their child. Thus, the amount of child-centered time and physical contact experienced throughout the day also needs to be examined.

When implementing bedtime routines, improvements should occur in four weeks time.

Scheduled awakenings, although much more socially valid than ignoring-based procedures, may result in a less rapid behavior change (Rickert & Johnson, 1988).

When day correction of bedtime problems is employed, after the day component is completed, children may settle themselves at bedtime or upon night awakening within three nights (Christophersen & Mortweet, 2001).

HOW DOES ONE SELECT AMONG TREATMENTS?

Cost—self-help protocols are more cost effective than therapist-based treatments and may provide sufficient guidance for families not requesting high levels of support. Developmental level—treatments for infant sleep disturbance will require solely parent involvement, whereas toddlers and older children can be integrated more actively into treatment.

Parent motivation—how motivated and agreeable are parents to treatment procedures? Although highly effective, behavioral interventions require active parental involvement, high levels of motivation and consistent parent compliance.

Differential compliance to different modalities—how much support do parents need to successfully implement the intervention? Highly motivated families with many resources may benefit from low-cost, minimally intensive interventions.

Child preference and temperament—how may this child's typical response style influence his or her parents' ability to follow through with treatment and the level of support parents' may require?

KEY READINGS

Achenbach, T. M., & Edelbrock, T. (1983). *Manual for the Child Behavior Check List and Revised Child Behavior Profile*. Burlington, VT: University of Vermont.

Adair, R., Zuckerman, B., Bauchner, H., Philipp, B., & Levenson, S. (1992). Reducing night waking in infancy: A primary care intervention. *Pediatrics, 89*, 585–588.

Adams, L. A., & Rickert, V. I. (1989). Reducing bedtime tantrums: Comparison between positive routines and graduated extinction. *Pediatrics, 84*, 756–761.

Blader, J. C., Koplewicz, H. S., Abikoff, H., & Foley, C. (1997). Sleep problems of elementary school children: A community survey. *Archives of Pediatric and Adolescent Medicine, 151*, 473–380.

Blum N.J., & Carey, W.B. (1996). Sleep problems among infants and young children. *Pediatric Review, 17*, 88–93.

Christophersen, E. & Mortweet, S. L. (2001). *Treatments that work with children: Empirically supported strategies for managing childhood problems*. Washington, DC: American Psychological Association.

Edwards, K. J., & E. R. Christophersen. (1994). Treating common sleep problems in young children. *Developmental Behavioral Pediatrics, 15*, 207–213.

Eyberg, S. (1988). Parent-child interaction therapy: Integration of traditional behavioral concerns. *Child and Family Behavior Therapy, 10*, 33–46.

Ferber, R. (1985). *Solve your child's sleep problems*. New York: NY: Fireside Books.

Ferber, R. (1996). Childhood sleep disorders. *Neurologic Clinics, 14*(3), 493–511.

Gelman, V. S., & King, N. J. (2001). Wellbeing of mothers with children exhibiting sleep disturbance. *Australian Journal of Psychology, 53*, 18–22.

Kataria, S., Swanson, M. S., & Trevathon, G. E. (1987). Persistence of sleep disturbances in preschool children. *Behavioral Pediatrics, 110*, 642–646.

Kuhn B. R. & Weidinger, D. (2000). Interventions for infant and toddler sleep disturbance: A review. *Child & Family Behavior Therapy* 22(2):33–50.

Lozoff, B., Wolf, A. W. & N. S. Davis. (1985). Sleep problems in pediatric practice. *Pediatrics, 75,* 477–483.

National Sleep Foundation. (2006). Sleep in America Poll. Accessed on April 6, 2006 from: http://www.sleepfoundation.org/hottopics/index.php?secid=16&id=392.

National Sleep Foundation. (2006). Sleep diary for kids. Accessed on April 8, 2006 from: http://www.sleepfoundation.org/content/hottopics/FinalDiary.pdf

Paavonen, E. J., Almqvist, F., Tamminen, T., Moilanen, I., Piha, J., Räsänen, E., & Aronen, E. T. (2002). Poor sleep and psychiatric symptoms at school: An epidemiological study. *European Child & Adolescent Psychiatry, 17,* 10–17.

Pollock, J. L. (1992). Night waking at 5 years of age: Predictor and prognosis. *Journal of Child Psychology and Child Psychiatry and Allied Disciplines, 35,* 699–708.

Richman, N. (1981). Sleep problems in young children. *Archives of Diseases of Children, 56,* 491–493.

Rickert, V. I., & Johnson, C. M. (1988). Reducing nocturnal awakening and crying episodes in infants and young children: A comparison between scheduled awakenings and systematic ignoring. *Pediatrics, 81,* 203–212.

Skinner, B. F. (1938). *The Behavior of Organisms: An Experimental Analysis.* Copley Publishing group: 1991.

Thiedke, C. (2001). Sleep disorders and sleep problems in childhood. *American Family Physician, 63,* 277–284.

CHAPTER 53

Pedophilia

Dawn Fisher • Tony Ward • Anthony R. Beech

WHAT IS PEDOPHILIA?

The term pedophile has come to be used variously in the scientific and journalistic literature, ranging from being used loosely to describe all individuals who sexually molest children through to a more restrictive subset of child molesters who are only sexually attracted to children. Not surprisingly this has led to confusion as to what the term actually means and what type of person is being included in this category.

Groth, Hobson, and Gary (1982) and Howells (1981) have proposed typologies that distinguish between those offenders who have a long-standing exclusive preference for children both as sexual partners and social companions (i.e., preferential), from those who turn to children as surrogates when adult partners are unavailable in times of stress (i.e., situational). Beech (1998) notes that such a dichotomy is often used to divide sex offenders into either "fixated pedophiles," (i.e., those who commit extrafamilial offenses) or regressed (incestuous) perpetrators. However, it would be wrong to view all incest offenders as "regressed" or "situational" and to assume that they only turn to children sexually when an adult partner is unavailable. This is because a number of studies have found that incestuous offenders frequently offend against several victims within and outside their family (e.g., Bagley & Thurston, 1996).

Attempts have also been made to define pedophilia in a precise manner by using the American Psychiatric Association's Diagnostic and Statistical Manual of Mental Disorders (DSM-IV, 1994; DSM-IV-TR, 2000). In this manual, pedophilia is defined in the following way: the offender has experienced, for at least six months, recurrent and intense sexually arousing fantasies, sexual urges, or behaviors involving sexual activity with a prepubescent child or children (aged 13 years or younger; and these fantasies, sexual urges, or behaviors cause clinically significant distress or impairment in social, occupational, or other important areas of functioning to the offender. Another caveat to this description is that the person being assessed should be at least age 16 years and is at least five years older than his/her victim/s. Marshall (1997) observes that the DSM-IV (1994) classification of pedophilia probably only applies to about 25–40% of those who commit contact offenses against children and, therefore, excludes the majority of those who commit this type of sexual offense.

For the purposes of this chapter, we will use the term pedophilia in its widest sense to describe all contact sexual offenses against children, whether they are inside or outside of the family, while retaining the use of the term "fixated pedophile" to describe those who appear to have a primary sexual interest in children.

BASIC FACTS

Comorbidity

Marshall (1997) concludes that, "very few child molesters suffer from either any form of psychopathology or disturbances in personality functioning" (p. 162). Marshall

Fisher, D., Ward, T., & Beech, A. R. (2006). Pedophilia. In J. E. Fisher & W. T. O'Donohue (Eds.), *Practitioner's guide to evidence-based psychotherapy*. New York: Springer.

also notes that fewer than 5% of sexual offenders are psychotic, and antisocial personality disorder is the only diagnosis that has been applied to sex offenders with any consistency. Although not a formal psychiatric diagnosis, some researchers have suggested there is a significant relationship between psychopathy and sexual offending. However, those rated as high on psychopathic traits tend not be specialized sexual offenders (Hare, 1995) in that they are criminally "versatile" rather than "specialist" offenders. Therefore, if such individuals offend sexually this is more likely to reflect their general criminal predispositions rather than deviant sexual interests. Despite these caveats, if an individual is both psychopathic and has deviant sexual interests this is the profile of the most dangerous recidivist sexual offender (Hildebrand, de Ruiter & de Vogel, 2002).

Prevalence

There are problems in ascertaining the actual level of sexual offending against children. The primary difficulty being that only a small fraction of sexual offenses are ever reported. In addition to under-reporting of sexual offenses, there is also the problem of sexual offenses being difficult to prosecute satisfactorily and result in a conviction. Figures generally suggest of child abuse offenses reported, only 10% end in prosecution (e.g., Prior, Glaser, & Lynch, 1997). Thus, relying on conviction figures and the number of men in prison or on probation for sexual offenses at a given time, is likely to result in a gross underestimation of the true level of sexual offending against children.

Despite the limitations outlined above, our best data suggests that the prevalence of sexual offences against children is alarming. A recent study in the UK (Cawson, Wattam, Brooker, & Kelly, 2000) found that 16% of girls and 7% of boys have been sexually assaulted before the age of 13. More than twice the number reported that they had been abused by somebody they knew (parents or carers, other relatives, or by other known people) than had been abused by a stranger or by someone that they had just met, indicating that it is much more likely that a child will be abused by somebody they know.

Gender

Most known child molestation offenses would appear to be committed by males. However, the reported rate of female offending may be a severe underestimation of the number of offenses actually committed by women/adolescent females. Current criminal statistics in the UK indicate that around 99% of convicted sexual offenders are male and 1% offenders are female. However, the latest figures from Childline (a telephone helpline in the UK for those who are being abused or know about individuals who are being abused) for April 2002—March 2003, suggest that the female perpetrator figures are actually far higher than the official conviction data reveal. According to Childline, the overall percentage of those calling about being abused by a female perpetrator was 12%. When this figure is broken down by gender of victim it was found that 4% of girls calling reported being abused by a female and 37% of boys calling about being abused by a female (Ford, in press).

Age of onset

Hanson (2001) notes that sexual offenders are generally older than other offenders, with child abusers being older than rapists. There would appear to be two peaks in the onset of child sexual offending with the largest peak being at the age of 13 (here it should be noted that a third of all sexual offenses are committed by adolescents—

e.g., Snyder & Sickmund, 1999) and a second peak in the mid to late 30s (Canadian Center for Justice Statistics, 1999).

Course

The early peak of offending at 13 may be due to the fact that some individuals who have a primary interest in children have started offending at this time as well as the more generally antisocial aggressive individuals. However, life histories of those who may be regarded as fixated pedophiles reveal that typically they begin offending around the age of 12–14 and have committed numerous further sexual offenses through adulthood (Beech, Fisher, & Beckett, 1999; Sullivan & Beech, 2004). Therefore, the more fixated juvenile offenders are likely to represent a high level of risk across their lifespan unless interventions are undertaken to reduce their level of risk. While, the more generalist juvenile offender who has targeted children of a similar age may desist from sexual offending against children as adults. Indeed, there is no strong evidence to suggest that the majority of sexually abusive adolescents will become adult sexual offenders (Beech, Tudway, Parrish, Print, & Thornton, in preparation).

For adult offenders, Hanson (2001) states that recidivism rates differ for extrafamilial and intrafamilial (incestuous) offenders. Generally, extrafamilial child molesters recidivate at twice the level of incestuous offenders e.g., 19.5% compared to 8.4% reported by Hanson, 2001). In terms of life course the highest risk age period for extrafamilial offenders occurs between the ages of 25 and 35 with relatively little decline in risk until the age of 50. For those offenders who have committed incestuous offenses, Hanson reports that recidivism is generally low (less than 10%). However, incestuous offenders who originally were convicted between the age of 18–24 age range recidivated at a much higher level (30.7%), indicating that young age at assessment is a particular risk factor for incestuous offenders.

Impairment

Child sexual abuse has been described as being related to impairment in socioaffective functioning, although some would argue that intimacy deficits and poor attachment actually play a causative role in sexual offending, specifically child sexual abuse (Marshall, 1989; Marshall & Marshall, 2000).

ASSESSMENT

Beech, Fisher and Thornton (2003) recommend that the following steps be followed in order to assess the level of risk a sexual offender individual poses and to identify his/her treatment needs:

- functional analysis of the offense process in order to determine how the offender's problems contributed to their offending and the motivation for offending;
- the application of a suitable actuarial risk predictor to assess the offender's global level of risk;
- the identification of psychological problems that make potential treatment targets;
- the monitoring of acute dynamic factors that indicate offending is imminent.

Functional Analysis

Beech, Fisher and Thornton (2003) suggest that any assessment of a sex offender should include a detailed functional analysis to determine the underlying motives and functions for the offending behavior. Functional analysis typically involves obtaining detailed information about, the *antecedents*, the *behaviors*, and *consequences* of offending (the ABC model). This should include the actual behaviors carried out along with the accompanying thoughts and emotions. Unfortunately this is not always a straightforward task with sex offenders due to their tendency to deny aspects of the offence and therefore being unwilling to be completely truthful about the areas that the assessor needs to obtain information about. Indeed, even in those offenders who are open about the level of their offending behaviors, there is often a reluctance to disclose their thoughts and feelings around their offending. In order to assist in gaining the information for the functional analysis it can be helpful to provide the offender with a framework to understand the process of offending.

Currently the most useful framework is probably what is called a "Decision Chain" or individualized model of the offence process (Ward, Louden, Hudson, & Marshall, 1995). A decision chain is a sequence of choices leading to an offense. Each choice is characterized in terms of the situation it took place in, the thoughts that made sense of and responded to the situation, and the emotions and actions that arose from these thoughts. Thus, in any analysis of offence behaviors it is important to take account of the diversity in offending, and to accommodate individuals whose firmly entrenched beliefs about the legitimacy of sexual contact with children lead them to experience positive emotions during the offence process. When constructing a decision chain or offence process model it is important to collect as much collateral information as possible, for example, police reports, victim statements, and so on. Relying solely on self-report data is a real problem and may result in a distorted account of what happened and result in a decision chain that will prove insufficient (and misleading!) for treatment planning purposes.

Actuarial Risk Assessment

In recent years there has been an increasing interest in the development of actuarial risk predictors for sexual offenders (e.g., Static-99, Hanson & Thornton, 2000; the Sex Offence Risk Appraisal Guide, Quinsey et al., 1998; the Minnesota Sex Offender Screening Tool-Revised, Epperson, Kaul, & Hesselton, 1998). These predictors use risk factors identified in research studies and then devise ways of coding the presence of these factors to arrive at a score for an individual, which gives a probability of reconviction for a sexual offense over some specified follow-up period. Most actuarial risk predictors designed for sexual offenders rely almost exclusively on static factors (those factors that cannot change), such as in Static-99: *persistence*, (i.e., having committed a number of previous sexual offenses); *wide range of potential victims* (i.e., whether the individual being assessed has previously offended against unrelated or stranger victims which widens his/her scope of potential victims compared to those who only offend against those who they know/ are within their family circle); *sexual deviance* (i.e., whether the individual has offended against male victims, and has committed nonsexual offenses); and *general level of antisocial acts* (i.e., has committed other nonsexual violent offenses.). It can be seen that those individuals scoring highly on such measures of risk (i.e., have committed numerous sexual offenses against stranger victims who are male children) are more likely to fit the pedophilic fixated description than incestuous offenders who would typically have a low score on static measures of risk.

Psychological Problems as Potential Treatment Targets

Recently, in an attempt to overcome the limitations of purely static actuarial instruments, some researchers have developed classification schemes that additionally incorporate factors that are amenable to change. One form of this is what are called risk-needs instruments (Bonta, 1996). Here, static risk factors are used to characterize risk whereas potentially changeable risk factors are used to characterize need.

The most comprehensive description of dynamic risk factors has been described by Thornton (2002), here he describes four dynamic risk domains: (1) deviant sexual interests, (2) distorted attitudes, (3) problems in socioaffective functioning, and (4) self-management problems. For child sexual abusers, problems across these four domains would mean that the individual would have: a sexual preference for children (Domain 1 problems); distorted attitudes about children and children's sexuality which would mean that individual saw children as being happy to engage in sexual activity with adults (Domain 2 problems); socioaffective problems, such as low self esteem, emotional loneliness, and chronic under-assertiveness (Domain 3 problems); and self management problems, i.e., lifestyle impulsiveness, poor problem solving, poor emotional control (Domain 4 problems).

Hence any thorough assessment of a sexual offender should measure problems in these domains. We will now briefly describe what is available in terms of psychological assessment of these domains.

Assessing deviant sexual interest The three assessments most commonly used for the assessment of sexual interests are the Penile Plethysmograph (PPG), response-time-based measures, and the Polygraph. The PPG measures changes in penile circumference or volume in response to audio or visual stimuli. PPG seeks to assess the direction of sexual interests. There have also been attempts to develop alternative measures of sexual interest using response time. For example, the Abel Assessment™ measures the length of time an individual looks at a particular image in order to ascertain his sexual interests. It is marketed in North America and is reported in some research studies (e.g., Abel, Huffman, Warberg, & Holland, 1998). It is less intrusive than the PPG and seems to be associated with past offending as strongly as the PPG does but has not yet been related to sexual recidivism.

The Polygraph, an instrument for the simultaneous recording of several involuntary physiological activities, including pulse rate and perspiration, is also used widely in North America to facilitate judgments about whether someone is being truthful. Combined with a sexual history questionnaire, it seems to facilitate fuller disclosure of past offending and so may indirectly indicate the direction of sexual interests (Ahlmeyer, Heil, McKee, & English, 2000). However, its usefulness is dependent upon the employment of highly trained polygraphers, which limits it availability. Some psychometric tests might also be considered helpful in the measurement of sexual interests such as the Multiphasic Sex Inventory (Nichols & Molinder, 1984). However, the problems with such self-report measures are that they are dependent upon the offender being honest about his sexual interests.

Assessing attitudes supportive of sexual assault The second area that needs to be assessed is attitudes supportive of sexual assault. These refer to sets of generalized beliefs about offenses, sexuality or potential victims that can be used to justify or give permission for sexual offenses (Thornton, 2002). Distorted beliefs of various kinds seem to be more common among child molesters than they are in comparison groups (e.g., Beech et al., 1999; Hanson, Gizzarrelli & Scott, 1994; Hanson & Scott, 1995).

Assessing socioaffective problems The third domain refers to ways of relating to other people and to the motivating emotions felt in the context of these interpersonal interactions (Thornton, 2002). Thornton's review suggests that at least four aspects of socioaffective functioning are relevant to child molestation: *inadequacy* (external locus of control, low self-esteem), *emotional congruence with children* (being more emotionally open to children than to adults), *lack of emotionally intimate relationships with adults* (marked by shallow relationships or the absence of relationships, and *emotional loneliness*. These factors have been found to typically be more marked in analyses comparing the more repetitive sexual offenders to less repetitive sexual offenders (e.g. Thornton, 2002) or in analyses comparing convicted sexual offenders to nonoffenders (e.g., Fisher, Beech, & Browne, 1999). Similar socioaffective factors have been identified as acute offense-precursors. For example, Pithers, Kashima, Cumming and Beal (1988) found various kinds of negative affect (anger, anxiety, depression, and low self-esteem) to play this role, as did Hanson and Harris (2000). Hence some of these factors seem to be both stable and acute dynamic factors. Again a number of measures have been developed to assess problems in this and the other risk domains, see Table 53.1.

Assessing self-management—general self-regulation problems Ward and Hudson (1998) have identified problems in self-management in the type of offender who uses passive strategies in his offending. Bickley and Beech (2002) found that those child molesters who have used passive strategies in their offending were found to be somewhat more impulsive, under-assertive and externally controlled than those that used active strategies in their offending. Lifestyle impulsivity is measured partly by Factor 2 in the Hare Psychopathy Checklist (Hare, 1991), which has been found to predict sexual recidivism in child abusers (Rice & Harris, 1997) and in incest offenders (Firestone et al., 1999). Hence it is important to measure this lifestyle impulsivity component of dynamic risk. Sections of the PCL-R (Hare, 1991) that measure lifestyle impulsivity can also be used to measure this problem domain. There are also self-report instruments that have been constructed to measure impulsivity such as the Barratt Impulsivity Scale (BIS-II, Barratt, 1994), as well as performance tasks such as the Porteus mazes (Porteus, 1955).

Table 53.1. Instruments to Consider When Assessing Stable Dynamic Domains

Domains	*Instruments*
Assessing deviant sexual interest	• The Penile Plethysmograph
	• The Polygraph
	• The Sexual Obsessions Scale of the Multiphasic Sex Inventory (MSI, Nichols & Molinder, 1984)
	• Rating of sexual interest from file information
Assessing attitudes supportive of sexual assault/pro-offending/ distorted attitudes	• The Justifications Scale of the MSI
	• The Bumby RAPE and MOLEST scales (Bumby, 1996)
	• The Children and Sex: Cognitive Distortions Scale (Beckett, 1987)
	• Burt Rape Scales (including rape myths. adversarial sexual attitudes, acceptance of interpersonal violence against women, sex role stereotyping, Burt, 1980)
	• Hostility towards women scale (Check 1984)
Assessing intimacy deficits/ socio-affective problems/ socio-affective thinking	• The Children and Sex: Emotional Congruence Scale (Beckett, 1987)
	• The UCLA Loneliness scale (Russell, Peplau, & Cutrona 1980)
	• The Novaco Anger Scale (Novaco, 1975)
	• The Dissipation-Rumination Scale (Caprara, 1986)
Assessing self management/ General self-regulation problems	• The PCL-R (Hare, 1991) Factor 2 - which measures lifestyle impulsivity
	• The Barratt Impulsivity Scale (BIS-II, Barratt, 1994)
	• Emotion Control Questionnaire (Roger & Najarian, 1989)
	• The Porteus Mazes (Porteus, 1955)

The Monitoring of Factors that Indicate Offending is Imminent

In terms of identifying acute risk factors, Hanson and Harris (2000) identified the types of behavior that indicated increased risk in a group of sex offenders under supervision. The best acute predictors were found to be victim access behaviors, noncooperation with supervision and shifts in mood. Hanson and Harris suggest that these behaviors act as warning signs for increased risk and should be monitored by supervisors.

From this research, and work reported by Hanson & Bussière (1998), Hanson and Harris (2001) have identified the following dynamic risk factors: victim access; emotional collapse, i.e., evidence of severe emotional disturbance/emotional crisis, collapse of social supports; hostility; substance abuse; sexual preoccupations and rejection of supervision. The final factor in this system is what Hanson and Harris term a "unique factor" in that some offenders have unique characteristics that represent a real risk factor for that offender. The type of factors that could be important for an offender could be such events as: a specific date or event (i.e., anniversary) that causes an emotional response, pain or discomfort-possibly triggering alcohol or drug abuse; homelessness, contact with a specified family member, health problems of a cyclical nature that may enter and leave the offender's situation with little warning, and being bothered by intrusive thoughts regarding their own victimization.

TREATMENT

We will briefly outline the major approaches to treatment that have been shown to have some impact upon sexual offending: behavioral therapy and cognitive behavioral therapy. Drug therapy is also a useful adjunct in some cases but we do not have space to review this option in any detail (see Adi et al. 2002; Kafka (2003). We would also note that other therapies are available, such psychodynamic therapy and counseling. However, these types of therapy have not been associated with any reductions in the level of offending in pedophiles (Marshall, Anderson, & Fernandez 1999).

Behavioral Therapy

Clinicians and researchers have commonly used a number of techniques using learning principles in order to change deviant sexual interest in children and create new, more appropriate ones. The following is not an inclusive list but gives an idea of the techniques that have been developed to alter deviant sexual interest and fantasy. These include: (1) *Olfactory aversion therapy* (Marshall et al., 1999; (2) *Covert sensitization* (Marshall et al., 1999); (3) *Masturbatory reconditioning* (Marquis, 1970); (4) *Directed masturbation* (Laws & O'Neil, 1981); (5) *Verbal satiation* (Laws, 1995)

Cognitive–Behavioral Treatment

The method of treatment primarily used in the UK and North America is best described as cognitive–behavioral therapy (CBT). This approach has developed through the combination of both cognitive and behavioral approaches to therapy. (For a systematic overview of the CBT approach see Marshall et al., 1999.) To give a brief synopsis, the behavioral component addresses the overt and covert behavior of an individual using the principles of learning theory. Originally this was confined to the use of procedures to alter behavior, i.e., rewarding desired behaviors and punishing unwanted behaviors, see above, but has since broadened out to include modeling (demonstrating a desired behavior) and skills training (teaching specific skills through behavioral rehearsal). The cognitive component of the

CBT approach addresses the thoughts or cognitions that individuals' experience, which are known to affect mood state and hence have an influence upon subsequent behavior. Cognitive therapy therefore aims to encourage an individual to think differently about events, thus giving rise to different affect and behavior. The use of self-instruction and self-monitoring, and the development of an awareness of how one thinks affects how one feels and behaves, are vital components in cognitive therapy. By combining these two approaches, CBT provides a comprehensive approach to treating sex offenders, which now has research evidence to support its efficacy (Alexander, 1999; Friendship, Mann, & Beech, 2003; Hanson, et al., 2002).

Group, rather than individual work is the usual method of delivery of CBT for sexual offenders. The group work approach is seen as being suitable for all types of sexual offender. Beech and Fordham (1997) outlined the benefits of being in a group and group work as the following: groups provide an environment that can offer both support and challenge to the individual; group work provides the opportunity for discussion with peers; and provides opportunities for increasing self-esteem and empathic responding; groups also offer a forum for support and sharing of problems which may be a completely new experience for many child sex abusers who are generally isolated individuals, often with interpersonal deficits and feelings of inadequacy. Having the experience of being valued, being able to help others, practicing social skills and getting to know others in detail can greatly improve an individual's self-esteem and interpersonal functioning. Given that feelings of inadequacy and lack of appropriate relationships may be an important vulnerability factor for many child sex abusers (Thornton, Beech, & Marshall, 2004), improvement in these areas is an important element in reducing re-offending.

Web Addresses

We have found the following websites to contain excellent resources related to the treatment of sexual offenders:

1. Stop It Now!
www.stopitnow.com
2. National Organisation for the Treatment of Abusers
www.nota.co.uk
3. Association for the Treatment of Sexual Abusers
www.atsa.com
4. Pacific Psychological Assessment Corporation
www.pacific-psych.com
5. Correctional Service Canada
www.csc-scc.gc.ca
6. HM Prison Service
www.hmprisonservice.gov.uk
7. The Safer Society Foundation Inc
www.safersociety.org

Self-Help Resources

A particularly useful self-help book is *The sex addiction workbook* by Tamara Penix Sbraga and William O'Donohue (2003). It speaks directly to individuals with sexual disorders in a down-to-earth and respectful manner. The quality of the research is impeccable and the book should prove to be a valuable adjunct resource for sexual offenders and therapists alike. In addition, The Safer Society Foundation (see above) has a number of good self-help books on their publication list.

CONCLUSIONS

We are currently in the situation where we know a lot more about the basic facts of child molestation and the best ways to assess and treat this serious problem. Careful research has enabled the development of risk assessment schedules by looking at the relationship of historical information/demographic variables to future offending (e.g., Hanson & Bussière, 1998) in order to inform risk and treatment need. It is also becoming increasingly evident that cognitive–behavioral treatment represents the most effective way to reduce recidivism and help offenders turn their lives around.

REFERENCES

Abel, G. G., Huffman, J., Warberg, B. W., & Holland, R. (1998). Visual reaction time and plethysmography as measures of sexual interest in child molesters. *Sexual Abuse: A Journal of Research and Treatment, 10*, 317–335.

Adi, Y, Ashcroft, D., Browne, K., Beech, A., Fry-Smith, A., & Hyde, C. (2002). Clinical effectiveness and cost-consequences of selective serotonin reuptake inhibitors in the treatment of sex offenders. *Health Technology Assessment, 6*, 1–66. Available from *www.hta.nhsweb.nhs.uk/fullmono/mon628.pdf.*

Ahlmeyer, S., Heil, P, & English, K. (2000). The impact of polygraphy on admissions of victims and offenses in adult sexual offenders. *Sexual Abuse: A Journal of Research and Treatment, 12*, 123–138.

Alexander, M. A. (1999). Sexual Offender Treatment Efficacy Revisited. *Sexual Abuse: A Journal of Research and Treatment, 19*, 101–116.

American Psychiatric Association (1994). *Diagnostic and statistical manual of mental disorders: Fourth edition.* Washington: American Psychiatric Association.

American Psychiatric Association (2000). *Diagnostic and statistical manual of mental disorders: Fourth edition, text revision.* Washington: American Psychiatric Association.

Bagley, C., & Thurston, W. (1996). *Understanding and preventing child sexual abuse: Critical summaries of 500 key studies* (Vol. 2). Aldershot: Arena.

Barratt, E. S. (1994). Impulsiveness and aggression. In J. Monahan & H. J. Steadman (Eds.), *Violence and mental disorder: Developments in risk assessment* (pp. 21–79). Chicago, IL: University of Chicago.

Beckett, R. C. (1987). The children and sex questionnaire. Available from Richard Beckett, Room FF39, The Oxford Clinic, Littlemore Health Centre, Sandford Rd., Littlemore, Oxford, England.

Beech, A. R. (1998). A psychometric typology of child abusers. International *Journal of Offender Therapy and Comparative Criminology, 42*, 319–339.

Beech, A. R., Fisher, D., & Beckett, R. C. (1999). *An evaluation of the Prison Sex Offender Treatment Programme.* UK Home Office Occasional Report. Available from Home Office Publications Unit, 50, Queen Anne's Gate, London, SW1 9AT, England. Available electronically from: www.homeoffice.gov.uk/rds/pdfs/occ-step3.pdf.

Beech, A. R., Fisher, D. D., & Thornton, D. (2003). Risk assessment of sex offenders. *Professional Psychology: Research and Practice, 34*, 339–352.

Beech, A. R., & Fordham, A. S. (1997). Therapeutic climate of sex offender treatment programmes. *Sexual Abuse: A Journal of Research and Treatment, 9*, 219–237.

Beech, A. R., Tudway, J., Parrish, R, Print, R., & Thornton, D. (in revision), *The effectiveness of actuarial risk assessment with adolescent sex offenders.*

Bickley, J., & Beech, A. R. (2002). An empirical investigation of the Ward & Hudson self-regulation model of the sexual offence process with child abusers. *Journal of Interpersonal Violence, 17*, 371–393.

Bonta, J. (1996). Risk-needs assessment. In A. T. Harland (Ed.), *Choosing correctional options that work: Defining the demand and evaluating the supply* (pp. 18–32). London: Sage.

Bumby, K. (1996). Assessing the cognitive distortions of child molesters and rapists. Development and validation of the RAPE and MOLEST scales. *Sexual Abuse: A Journal of Research and Treatment, 8*, 37–54.

Burt, M. (1980). Cultural myths and support for rape. *Journal of Personality and Social Psychology, 39*, 217–230.

Canadian Center for Justice Statistics (1999). Sex offenders. Juristat Catalogue no. 85-002-XIE, Vol. 19. Ottawa: Statistics Canada.

Caprara, G. V. (1986). Indications of aggregation: The dissipation-rumination scale. *Personality and Individual Differences, 7,* 763–769.

Cawson, P., Wattam, C. Brooker, S., & Keely, G. (2000). *Child maltreatment in the United Kingdom. A study of the prevalence of child abuse and neglect.* London: NSPCC.

Epperson, D. L., Kaul, J. D., & Hesslton, D. (1998). *Final report on the development of the Minnesota Sex Offending Screening Tool-Revised (MnSOST-R).* St. Paul: Minnesota Department of Corrections.

Firestone, P., Bradford, J. M., McCoy, M., Greenberg, D. M., Larose, M. R., & Curry, S. (1999). Prediction of recodivism in incest offenders. *Journal of Interpersonal Violence, 14,* 511–531.

Fisher, D., Beech, A. R., & Browne, K. D. (1999). Comparison of sex offenders to non-sex offenders on selected psychological measures. *International Journal of Offender Therapy and Comparative Criminology. 43,* 473–491.

Ford, H. (in press). *Women who sexually abuse children.* Chichester: Wiley.

Friendship, C., Mann R., & Beech, A. (2003). Evaluation of a national prison-based treatment program for sexual offenders in England and Wales. *Journal of Interpersonal Violence, 18,* 744–759.

Groth, A. N., Hobson, W. F., & Gary, T. S. (1982). The child molester: Clinical observations. In J. Conte & D. Shore (Eds.), *Social work and child sexual abuse* (pp. 129–142). New York: Haworth Press.

Hanson, R. K. (2001). Age and sexual recidivism: A comparison of rapists and child molesters. Public Works and Government Services, Catalogue no. JS42-96/ 2001.

Hanson, R. K., & Bussière, M. T. (1998). Predicting relapse: A meta-analysis of sexual offender recidivisim studies. *Journal of Consulting and Clinical Psychology, 66,* 348–362.

Hanson, R. K., Gizzarelli, R., & Scott, H. (1994). The attitudes of incest offenders: Sexual entitlement and acceptance of sex with children. *Criminal Justice and Behavior, 21,* 187–202.

Hanson, R. K., Gordon, A., Harris, A. J. R., Marques, J. K., Murphy, W., Quinsey, V. L., et al., (2002). First report of the collaborative outcome data project on the effectiveness of psychological treatment for sex offenders. *Sexual Abuse: A Journal of Research and Treatment, 14,* 169–194.

Hanson, R. K., & Harris, A. J. R. (2000). Where should we intervene? Dynamic predictors of sexual offense recidivism. *Criminal Justice and Behavior, 27,* 6–35.

Hanson, R. K., & Harris, A. (2001). The sex offender need assessment rating (SONAR): a method for measuring change in risk levels. Available electronically from *www.sgc.gc.ca/epub/corr/e200001a/* e200001b/e200001b.htm. The authors note that this is an older version of SONAR and should not be used for assessment.

Hanson, R. K., & Scott, H. (1995). Assessing perspective-taking among sexual offenders, non-sexual criminals, and non-offenders. *Sexual Abuse: A Journal of Research and Treatment, 7,* 259–277.

Hanson, R. K., & Thornton, D. (2000). Improving risk assessments for sex offenders: A comparison of three actuarial scales. *Law and Human Behavior, 24,* 119–136.

Hare, R. D. (1991). *Manual for the Revised Psychopathy Checklist.* Toronto: Multi-Health Systems.

Hare, R. D. (1995). Psychopaths: New trends in research. *Harvard Mental Health Letter, 12,* 4–5.

Hildebrand, M., de Ruiter, C., & de Vogel, V. (2004). Psychopathy and sexual deviance in treated rapists: Association with sexual and non-sexual recidivism. *Sexual Abuse: A Journal of Research and Treatment, 16,* 1–24.

Howells, K. (1981). Adult sexual interest in children: Considerations relevant to theories of aetiology. In M. Cook & K. Howells (Eds.), *Adult sexual interest in children.* London: Academic Press.

Kafka, M. P. (2003). The monoamine hypothesis for the pathophysiology of paraphilic disorders. In R. Prentky, E. Janus, M. Seto, & A. W. Burgess (Eds.), *Understanding and managing sexually coercive behavior. Annals of the New York Academy of Sciences, 989,* 86–94.

Laws, D. R. (1995). Verbal satiation: Notes on procedure, with speculation on its mechanism of effect. *Sexual Abuse: A Journal of Research and Treatment, 7,* 155–166.

Laws, D. R., & O'Neil, J. A. (1981). Variations on masturbatory reconditioning. *Behavioral Psychotherapy, 9,* 111–136.

Marquis, J. N. (1970). Orgasmic reconditioning: changing sexual object choice through controlling masturbation fantasies. *Journal of Behavioral Therapy and Experimental Psychiatry, 1,* 263–271.

Marshall, W. L. (1989). Invited essay: Intimacy, loneliness and sexual offenders. *Behaviour Research and Therapy, 27,* 491–503.

Marshall, W. L. (1997). Pedophilia: Psychopathology and theory. In D. R. Laws & W. O'Donahue (Eds.), *Sexual deviance: Theory, assessment, and treatment* (pp. 152–174). New York: Guildford Press.

Marshall, W. L., Anderson, D., & Fernandez, Y. (1999). *Cognitive–behavioural treatment of sexual offenders.* New York: Wiley.

Marshall, W. L., & Marshall, L. E. (2000). The origins of sexual offending. *Trauma, Violence, & Abuse, 1,* 250–263.

Nichols, H. R., & Molinder, I. (1984). Multiphasic Sex Inventory manual. Available from the authors, 437 Bowes Drive, Tacoma, WA, 98466, USA.

Novaco, R. (1975). *Anger control: the development and evaluation of an experimental treatment.* Lexington: MA: D. C. Heath.

Pithers, W. D., Kashima, K. M., Cumming, G. F., & Beal, L. S. (1988). Relapse prevention: A method of enhancing maintenance of change in sex offenders. In A. C. Salter, *Treating child sex offenders and victims* (pp. 131–170). London: Sage.

Porteus, S. D. (1955). *The maze test: Recent advances.* Palo Alto, CA: Pacific Books.

Prior, V., Glaser, D., & Lynch, M. A. (1997). Responding to child sexual abuse: The criminal justice system. *Child Abuse Review, 6,* 128–140.

Quinsey, V. L., Harris, G. T., Rice, M. E., & Cormier, C. A. (1988). *Violent offenders: Appraising and managing risk.* Washington, DC: American Psychological Association.

Rice M. E., & Harris, G. T. (1997). Cross-validation and extension of the Violence Risk Appraisal Guide for child molesters and rapists. *Law and Human Behavior, 21,* 231–241.

Roger, D., & Najarian, B. (1989). The construction and validation of a new scale for measuring emotion control. *Personality and Individual Differences, 10,* 845–853.

Russell, D., Peplau, L. A., & Cutrona, C. A. (1980). The revised UCLA loneliness scale: concurrent and discriminant validity evidence. *Journal of Personality and Social Psychology, 39,* 472–480.

Sbraga, T. P, & O'Donohue. W. T. (2003). *The sex addiction workbook.* Oakland, CA: New Harbinger Publications, Inc.

Snyder, H., & Sickmund, M. (1999). *Juvenile sexual offenders and victims: 1999 national report.* Washington, DC: Office of Juvenile Justice and Delinquency Prevention.

Sullivan, J., & Beech, A. (2004). A comparative study of demographic data relating to intra- and extra-familial child sexual abusers and professional perpetrators. *Journal of Sexual Aggression, 10,* 39–50.

Thornton (2002) Constructing and testing a framework for dynamic risk assessment. *Sexual Abuse. A Journal of Research and Treatment, 14,* 139–154.

Thornton, D., Beech, A., & Marshall, W. L. (2004). Pre-treatment self-esteem and post-treatment sexual recidivism. *International Journal of Offender Therapy and Comparative Criminology, 48,* 587–599.

Ward, T., & Hudson, S. M. (1998). A model of the relapse process in sexual offenders. *Journal of Interpersonal Violence, 13,* 700–725.

Ward, T., Louden, K., Hudson, S. M, & Marshall, W. L. (1995). A descriptive model of the offence chain for child molesters. *Journal of Interpersonal Violence, 10,* 452–472.

CHAPTER 54

Pica

Linda A. LeBlanc • Brian J. Feeney • Christine M. Bennett

WHAT IS PICA?

Pica is defined as persistent ingestion of nonnutritive substances for a period of at least one month other than as part of a culturally sanctioned practice (APA, 2000). This behavior occurs in many typically developing infants and toddlers as a result of failure to discriminate appropriate things to put in their mouth. The prevalence of pica for children under 6 in the general population is between 10% and 32% with the highest rates among children aged 12–24 months (MedlinePlus, 2002). Mouthing and accidentally ingesting objects is considered a normal aspect of development for young children; however, pica may persist beyond infancy in individuals with pervasive developmental disorders, mental retardation, and is sometimes seen in typically developing individuals, particularly those who have nutritional or mental health conditions. Typical ingested objects include paint, string, hair, cloth, leaves, pebbles, cigarette butts, and feces (i.e., coprophagia).

Pica can be a life threatening disorder and is often considered a form of self-injurious behavior due to the potential severe consequences. Pica can result in choking, suffocation, parasites (associated with feces ingestion), poisoning (e.g., lead toxicity), esophageal or intestinal tears, and intestinal blockage (Matson & Bamburg, 1999; Ricciardi, Luiselli, Terrill, & Reardon, 2003). Individuals with persistent pica often have to undergo surgical intervention to remove objects and mend torn internal tissue. Cigarette butts, the most commonly ingested item, present additional health hazards such as nicotine addiction and withdrawal, dental problems (e.g., periodontal disease, gingival recession), elevated blood pressure, exposure to communicable diseases, and oral cancer (Goh, Iwata, & Kahng, 1999; Matson & Bamburg, 1999; Piazza, Hanley & Fisher, 1996). In addition to health risks, pica can negatively impact an individual's social well-being by creating social stigma and resulting in avoidance by care providers (Matson & Bamburg, 1999).

FACTS ABOUT PICA

In general, the most severe and life threatening cases of pica occur in individuals with mental retardation and autism (Ali, 2001) who live in institutional settings. Pica can occur in individuals with normal intellect such as pregnant and nursing women, individuals with dementia, schizophrenia, bipolar disorder, and eating disorders such as anorexia and bulimia (Ali, 2001). Rare cases of pica have also been documented in typically developing individuals with no known mental health condition but the majority of published studies on assessment and treatment of pica focus on individuals with developmental disabilities and this will be the primary focus of the rest of this chapter.

Most prevalence studies on pica examine individuals with developmental disabilities such as mental retardation and autism within an institutional setting and their results suggest a strong link between type of pica, severity of intellectual deficits, and

LeBlanc, L. A., Feeney, B. J., & Bennett, C. M. (2006). Pica. In J. E. Fisher & W. T. O'Donohue (Eds.), *Practitioner's guide to evidence-based psychotherapy.* New York: Springer.

institutionalization (Ali, 2001; Danford & Huber, 1982; Ellis et al., 1997; Lofts, Schroeder, & Maier, 1990; McAlpine & Singh, 1986; Tewari, Krishnan, Valsalan, & Roy, 1995). Rates of pica in institutional settings range between 9.2% and 25% with variability in estimates due differences in operational definitions. Following early childhood, the incidence of pica decreases with age and then increases again after the age of 70 (Danford & Huber, 1982; McAlpine & Singh, 1986).

Matson and Bamburg (1999) conducted a survey of 45 individuals in an institutional setting who engaged in pica. The most frequently consumed pica items were cigarette butts and pieces of paper, perhaps because these items were more frequently available for consumption. Their results indicate that most cases of pica were not maintained by social variables and this finding has been supported by several other experimental functional analysis studies (Hagopian & Adelinis, 2001; Piazza et al., 1996, 1998; Piazza, Roane, Keeney, Boney, & Abt, 2002).

ASSESSMENT

Ruling Out Conditions

Individuals presenting with pica should be evaluated by medical professionals to identify or rule out vitamin, mineral, and other nutritional deficiencies (Ali, 2001). For example, if a zinc or iron deficiency is present, individuals may crave and ingest nonfood substances like clay to satisfy their body's natural urge to supplement the deficiency (Pace & Toyer, 2000; Ali, 2001). The clinician should also consider whether the behavior is common to the individual's culture as indicated in the DSM IV-TR (APA, 2000). Behaviors accepted by the individual's culture, such as chewing ice and clay, are not appropriately considered pica (Ali 2001; Reid, 1992). The clinician should also attempt to determine if another psychological disorder is more appropriate in accounting for pica (e.g., borderline personality disorder, bulimia). Finally, medical consultation is crucial in order to determine if the pica is at a life-threatening stage and/or if an invasive medical procedure is warranted and to determine if any parasites or orally transmitted diseases have been contracted as a result of pica (Marcus & Stambler, 1979).

Effective Assessment Procedures

Two categories of assessment information are critical for guiding intervention planning. The first category is functional assessment of the environmental determinants that may be maintaining pica (Mace & Knight, 1986). Several studies support the finding that pica is typically maintained independent of social consequences (Matson & Bamburg, 1999; Piazza et al, 1996); however, specific cases have been identified where pica was at least partially maintained by social consequences such as attention from others (Piazza et al., 1998). In cases where social variables are identified, these variables can be directly manipulated in the context of a function-based intervention such as noncontingent reinforcement. Functional assessment typically begins with a descriptive informant assessment in the form of an interview or checklist (Carr & LeBlanc, 2003). The most commonly used interview tool is the Functional Assessment Interview (O'Neill, Horner, Albin, Storey, & Sprague, 1990), which samples both environmental and biological factors that may impact pica. The Motivational Assessment Scale (Durand & Crimmins, 1988) is a commonly used checklist and the Questions About Behavioral Function scale (Matson & Vollmer, 1995) has support for use specifically with pica (Matson & Bamburg, 1999).

Preference assessments also yield extremely important information for treatment planning, particularly when pica is maintained by automatic or sensory reinforcers that cannot be easily withheld (LeBlanc, Carr, & Patel, 2000). Several studies demonstrate a model for conducting multiple preference assessments designed to identify the critical sensory properties of the ingested items (Goh et al., 1999; Piazza et al., 1996; Piazza et al., 1998). Piazza, Hanley, et al used a forced choice preference assessment procedure in which they presented the potentially relevant components of a cigarette in a series of pairings until all components had been presented with all other components. The most highly preferred component was the tobacco which was confirmed in an analysis where pica of tobacco butts occurred at much higher frequency that herbal butts. Piazza et al. (1998) used a single item preference assessment procedure to determine which food items and items that could be safely mouthed would effectively compete with pica during brief presentations of commonly ingested materials. A follow up analysis examined the critical aspects of the items that competed most effectively with pica and revealed that the texture or hardness of the items was a critical factor. Information obtained from these assessments can directly guide the selection of items used in developing interventions and studies support that use of items that are matched to the relevant stimulus features increases the effectiveness of environmental enrichment interventions.

When conducting either functional analyses or preference assessments that include the opportunity to engage in pica, the clinician should carefully consider safety issues and dependent measures. Recent studies have incorporated latency to the first attempt at pica rather than frequency as a measure to minimize actual object ingestion (Goh et al., 1999). When frequency measures are used, an environment can be cleaned and then baited with items that are safe when ingested in small amounts (e.g., small bits of paper) or that mimic typically ingested items (e.g., uncooked beans for rocks).

Traditional psychological assessment procedures such as personality measures and projective tests do not provide particularly useful information for treating pica. However, neuropsychological assessments including intellectual assessments have been used with children who have suffered lead poisoning (Banks, Ferretti, & Shucard, 1997) which can be an effect of pica. These tools are not used to predict development of pica or to select interventions for pica but may be helpful in planning academic interventions for children who have a history of pica and may have sustained cognitive impairments.

TREATMENT

Effective Treatments

Unlike many psychological problems, pica is generally not treated by traditional psychotherapy either at the individual or group level. Instead, structured behavioral interventions using basic operant strategies have proven most effective. Effective intervention for pica typically requires the skills of a professional with expertise working with individuals with severe behavior problems and developmental disabilities. All interventions discussed in this section have some level of empirical support for use in treating pica and are all based on operant theory. However, each intervention has also failed to work for certain individuals and the practitioner may need to combine several of the interventions in a package or conduct sequential trials of different interventions to achieve the best effect for a client. The interventions are arranged in order of suggested progression from those interventions that are perceived as least intrusive to interventions that may be more intrusive.

Antecedent interventions The most common antecedent intervention has been referred to by several terms including enriched environment (EE) and alternate sensory activities (Ellis et al., 1997). This intervention involves providing access to enjoyable alternative activities or items, usually on a continuous basis. Several studies have supported the utility of this type of intervention particularly when preference assessments are used to identify highly preferred items that are matched to the hypothesized sensory properties of the ingested items (Piazza et al., 1998). Delivery of social attention on a dense schedule independent of the occurrence of pica (often referred to as noncontingent reinforcement) has also been used to decrease pica when pica was sensitive to attention as a functional reinforcer (Piazza et al., 1998). The effectiveness of EE interventions are variable and dependent upon the degree to which the alternative items compete with or substitute for the sensory reinforcers inherent in the act of pica at any given moment. EE is often used as a component in multicomponent interventions and is generally considered beneficial to quality of life of the client even if pica is not completely suppressed by the procedure.

Reinforcement-based procedures Several reinforcement-based procedures have shown promise for individuals with pica. Differential reinforcement has been used in the form of differential reinforcement of other behavior (DRO) and differential reinforcement of alternative behavior (DRA) or incompatible behavior (DRI) (Donnelly & Olczak, 1990; Ellis et al., 1997). DRO involves providing a preferred stimulus contingent upon the passage of the period of time without an occurrence of pica while DRA involves directly reinforcing the occurrence of an alternative behavior that may or may not be incompatible with pica. Reasonable alternative behaviors might be putting trash in a receptacle, delivering pica items to a care provider or engaging with a leisure item. One particular use of DRA is discrimination training, which involves teaching an individual to only eat items directly off of a plate. This intervention has been demonstrated effective with young typically developing children with lead poisoning (Madden, Russo, & Cataldo, 1980). Either of these interventions requires vigilance on the part of the care provider and may be difficult to sustain over time resulting in lessening of the effectiveness of the procedure.

Response blocking Response blocking involves preventing the engagement of pica by removing the stimulus from the client's possession prior to the stimulus crossing the threshold of the lips. Blocking is typically accomplished by manually providing a physical removal of the inedible item just prior to ingestion, brief restraint of the hand delivering the item to the mouth, or restraining the person from approaching a suspected preferred item. This intervention also requires constant proximity of a care provider and can often prove effortful especially when physical management involved in attempts to block pica result in aggression.

Response blocking is typically included as one component in a multicomponent intervention (e.g., EE with response blocking). A recent study compared the effects of a condition in which pica was ignored, a condition in which pica was physically blocked, and a condition in which response blocking was enhanced with the redirection of behavior and access to an alternative edible item (Hagopian & Adelinis, 2001). The response blocking condition alone was ineffective in reducing pica and resulted in an increase in client aggressive behaviors compared to the enhanced condition. In another study, Piazza et al. (1998) enhanced an EE intervention with stimuli matched to the sensory properties associated with preferred pica items by including response blocking and redirection to produce an acceptable decrease in pica. These studies suggest that blocking can be most effective when used in conjunction with redirection to a competing stimulus. Blocking may interrupt the response–reinforcer contingency or may increase the response effort associated with pica in comparison to the response effort for accessing alternative reinforcers. In each of the studies after the behavior was blocked the client was redirected away from the inedible stimuli and/or prompted to engage or move toward an area where more appropriate stimuli were placed.

Simplified habit reversal One study has illustrated the utility of simplified habit reversal with a typically developing six-year old boy who constantly mouthed items such as his shirt and remote controls (Woods, Miltenberger, & Lumley, 1996). The protocol includes awareness training, competing response training, and social support. The awareness training component involves having the child identify instances of their own target behavior (i.e., chewing his shirt) either live or from video. The competing response component involves having the child engage in an alternative response (i.e. removing the object and pursing lips for 1 minute) contingent upon occurrence of the target behavior. Social support involves prompting and social praise from loved ones for engaging in the target behavior. The intervention proved effective and socially acceptable for this one child and may be a useful intervention option for typically developing children. The clinician should note that the competing response component may operate via a punishment process.

Punishment procedures Although the trend in intervention with individuals with developmental disabilities is toward less intrusive interventions, several punishment procedures have been successfully used to decrease pica. In cases where pica is dangerous and other interventions have proven ineffective, the clinician might implement a punishment procedure in conjunction with an antecedent or reinforcement procedure. Piazza et al. (1996) used a verbal reprimand to decrease cigarette pica following a functional analysis that demonstrated that pica was not sensitive to the effects of attention as a consequence. The clinician should be extremely cautious in using verbal reprimands because of the potential for reprimands to directly reinforce problem behavior such as pica.

Various overcorrection procedures have been used to successfully decrease pica (Ellis et al., 1997; Singh & Winton, 1985). In a recent investigation, Ricciardi et al., (2003) successfully reduced pica in a school setting by requiring a child with automatically reinforced pica to practice an alternative response of discarding multiple objects contingent upon pica attempts. Contingent presentation of aversive odors, tastes, and water mists have also been successfully used to decrease pica (Ellis et al.) although no recent studies have investigated these procedures, perhaps because of recent trends in intervention toward less intrusive procedures.

Punishment procedures have their effect because the aversive properties of the programmed consequence overcome the reinforcing properties of engaging in pica and the effects are typically robust. However, there is great individual variability with regard to which stimulus will function effectively as an aversive consequence and how well any event will function at any given moment. If prior enrichment and reinforcement based intervention attempts have failed and the clinician must resort to a punishment based procedure, it is recommended that assessment be conducted prior to implementation of the procedure using a model such as the empirically derived consequences (EDC) model described by Fisher et al (1994) to determine which stimulus is most likely to be effective as a punisher. In this procedure, several potential consequences are tried in brief sessions prior to large-scale implementation. Measures are obtained to determine which procedures are most likely to produce the largest and most rapid decreases in the behavior and which interventions can be implemented with the highest procedural integrity.

Effective Medical Treatments

When medical screening confirms a metabolic or nutritional problem such as a vitamin or mineral deficiency (e.g., iron, zinc, calcium), vitamin therapy is an appropriate intervention. The addition of a daily multivitamin has been shown to decrease pica in individuals with anemia or other vitamin deficits (Pace & Toyer, 2000). A serum zinc supplement has also been shown to significantly impact pica in a typically developing young girl (Lofts, et al., 1990) and a daily oral elemental diet supplement called Vivonex® has proven beneficial for individuals with mental retardation (Bugle & Rubin, 1993) who exhibited coprophagia. This supplement comes in powder form and is readily mixed with water. Note that these nutritional interventions have typically resulted in a decrease rather than elimination of pica and it is recommended that vitamin therapies be implemented in conjunction with behavioral interventions as described above.

There are no well-controlled treatment outcome studies evaluating the effects of pharmacological interventions for pica. Many individuals included in studies of behavioral interventions have previously been unresponsive to pharmacological interventions suggesting that medications may often prove ineffective at decreasing pica. However, recent case studies have documented some beneficial effects of selective serotonin reuptake inhibitors on pica (Bashir, Loschen, Baluga, & Kirchner, 2002; Gundogar, Demir, & Eren, 2003). However, these studies are preliminary in nature and further studies are needed to determine if pharmacological interventions will reliably prove effective in decreasing pica.

Selecting Among Treatments

The clinician should consider several factors when selecting an intervention for pica. First, consider the level of monitoring and supervision that can be provided by caregivers and the amount of effort required to implement the procedure. Most interventions for pica have to be in place for all waking hours and fatigue will lead to poor procedural integrity and decreased intervention effectiveness. Second, always proceed using a least restrictive intervention approach beginning with less intrusive interventions that add preferred stimuli or experiences to the life of the client before moving to more intrusive interventions that involve adding aversive stimuli or increasing sedation or restrictions. However, pica is often a life-threatening condition that requires almost complete suppression in order to maintain health status for the client. If other interventions are not effective, the clinician should consider punishment procedures that are carefully selected based on an assessment of empirically derived consequences.

Recommended Websites and Online Resource Articles

There are few useful websites on pica that are professional rather than oriented for general parent information. One useful website for parent information is available at KidsHealth at *http://kidshealth.org/parent/emotions/behavior/pica.html*.

KEY READINGS

Ali, Z. (2001). Pica in people with intellectual disability: A literature review of aetiology, epidemiology and complications. *Journal of Intellectual & Developmental Disability, 26,* 205–215.

Ellis, C. R., Singh, N. N., Crews, W. D., Bonaventura, S. H., Gehin, J. M., & Ricketts, R. W. (1997). Pica. In N. N. Singh (Ed.), *Prevention and treatment of severe behavior problems: Models and methods in developmental disabilities* (pp. 253–269). Belmont, CA: Brooks/Cole Publishing Co.

Goh, H. L., Iwata, B. A., & Kahng, S. W. (1999). Multicomponent assessment and treatment of cigarette pica. *Journal of Applied Behavior Analysis, 32,* 297–316.

Matson, J. L., & Bamburg, J. W. (1999). A descriptive study of pica behavior in persons with mental retardation. *Journal of Developmental and Physical Disabilities, 11,* 353–361.

McAdam, D. B., Sherman, J. A., Sheldon, J. B., & Napoliano, D. A. (2004). Behavioral interventions to reduce the pica of persons with developmental disabilities. *Behavior Modification, 28,* 45–72.

Myles, B. S., Simpson, R. L., & Hirsch, N. C. (1997). A review of literature on interventions to reduce pica in individuals with developmental disabilities. *Autism, 1,* 77–95.

Piazza, C. C., Fisher, W. W., Hanley, G. P., LeBlanc, L. A., Worsdell, A. S., Lindauer, S. E., (1998). Treatment of pica through multiple analyses of its reinforcing functions. *Journal of Applied Behavior Analysis, 31,* 165–189.

REFERENCES

Ali, Z. (2001). Pica in people with intellectual disability: A literature review of aetiology, epidemiology and complications. *Journal of Intellectual & Developmental Disability, 26,* 205–215.

American Psychiatric Association. (2000). *Diagnostic and statistical manual of mental disorders: DSM-IV-TR.* Washington, DC: Author.

Banks, E. C., Ferretti, L. E., & Shucard, D. W. (1997). Effects of low level lead exposure on cognitive functioning in children: A review of behavioral, neuropsychological, and biological evidence. *Neurotoxicology, 18,* 237–281.

Bashir, A., Loschen, E., Baluga, J., & Kirchner, L. (2002). A case of pica in a patient with mental retardation treated with venlafaxine extended release. *Mental Health Aspects of Developmental Disabilities, 5,* 87–89.

Bugle, C., & Rubin, H. B. (1993). Effects of a nutritional supplement on coprophagia: A study of three cases. *Research in Developmental Disabilities, 14,* 445–456.

Carr, J. E., & LeBlanc, L. A. (2003). Functional Analysis. In W. O'Donohue, J. E. Fisher, & S. C. Hayes (Eds.), *Empirically Supported Techniques of Cognitive Behavior Therapy: A Step by Step Guide for Clinicians* (pp. 167–175). Hoboken, NJ: Wiley.

Danford, D. E., & Huber, A. M. (1982). Pica among mentally retarded adults. *American Journal of Mental Deficiency, 87,* 141–146.

Donnelly, D. R., & Olczak, P. V. (1990). The effect of differential reinforcement of incompatible behaviors DRI on pica for cigarettes in persons with intellectual disability. *Behavior Modification, 14,* 81–96.

Dumaguing, N. I., Singh, I., Sethi, M., & Devanand, D. P. (2003). Pica in the geriatric mentally ill: Unrelenting and potentially fatal. *Journal of Geriatric Psychiatry & Neurology, 16,* 189–191.

Durand, V. M., & Crimmins, D. B. (1988). Identifying the variables maintaining self-injurious behavior. *Journal of Autism and Developmental Disorders, 18,* 99–117.

Ellis, C. R., Singh, N. N., Crews, W. D., Bonaventura, S. H., Gehin, J. M., & Ricketts, R. W. (1997). Pica. In N. N. Singh (Ed.), *Prevention and treatment of severe behavior problems: Models and methods in developmental disabilities* (pp. 253–269). Belmont, CA: Brooks/Cole Publishing Co.

Fisher, W. W., Piazza, C. C., Bowman, L. G., Kurtz, P. F., Sherer, M. R., & Lachman, S. R. (1994). A preliminary evaluation of empirically derived consequences for the treatment of pica. *Journal of Applied Behavior Analysis, 27,* 447–457.

Goh, H. L., Iwata, B. A., & Kahng, S. W. (1999). Multicomponent assessment and treatment of cigarette pica. *Journal of Applied Behavior Analysis, 32,* 297–316.

Gundogar, D., Demir, S. B., & Eren, I. (2003). Is pica in the spectrum of obsessive-compulsive disorders? *General Hospital Psychiatry, 25,* 293–294.

Hagopian, L. P., & Adelinis, J. D. (2001). Response blocking with and without redirection for the treatment of pica. *Journal of Applied Behavior Analysis, 34,* 527–530.

LeBlanc, L. A., Patel, M. R., & Carr, J. E. (2000). Recent advances in the assessment of aberrant behavior maintained by automatic reinforcement in individuals with developmental disabilities. *Journal of Behavior Therapy & Experimental Psychiatry, 31,* 137–154.

Lofts, R. H., Schroeder, S. R., & Maier, R. H. (1990). Effects of serum zinc supplementation on pica behavior of persons with mental retardation. *American Journal on Mental Retardation, 95,* 103–109.

Mace, F. C., & Knight, D. (1986). Functional analysis and treatment of severe pica. *Journal of Applied Behavior Analysis, 19,* 411–416.

Madden, N. A., Russo, D. C., & Cataldo, M. F. (1980). Behavioral treatment of pica in children with lead poisoning. *Child Behavior Therapy, 2,* 67–81.

Marcus, L. C., & Stambler, M. (1979). Visceral larva migrans and eosinophilia in an emotionally disturbed child. *Journal of Clinical Psychiatry, 40,* 139–140.

Matson, J. L., & Bamburg, J. W. (1999). A descriptive study of pica behavior in persons with mental retardation. *Journal of Developmental and Physical Disabilities, 11,* 353–361.

Matson, J. L., & Vollmer, T. R. (1995). The Questions About Behavioral Function (QABF). Scientific Publishers: Baton Rouge, LA.

McAlpine, C., & Singh, N. N. (1986). Pica in institutionalized mentally retarded persons. *Journal of Mental Deficiency Research, 30,* 171–178.

MedlinePlus (2002). Pica. *Online Medical Encyclopedia.* US National Library of Medicine and National Institutes of Health. Available: www.nlm.nih.gov/encyclopedia.html

O'Neill, R. E., Horner, R. H., Albin, R. W., Storey, K., & Sprague, J. R. (1990). *Functional analysis of problem behavior: A practical assessment guide.* Sycamore, IL: Sycamore Publishing Company.

Pace, G. M., & Toyer, E. A. (2000). The effects of a vitamin supplement on the pica of a child with severe mental retardation. *Journal of Applied Behavior Analysis, 33,* 619–622.

Piazza, C. C., Fisher, W. W., Hanley, G. P., LeBlanc, L. A., Worsdell, A. S., Lindauer, S. E., et al. (1998). Treatment of pica through multiple analyses of its reinforcing functions. *Journal of Applied Behavior Analysis, 31,* 165–189.

Piazza, C. C., Hanley, G. P., & Fisher, W. W. (1996). Functional analysis and treatment of cigarette pica. *Journal of Applied Behavior Analysis, 29,* 437–450.

Piazza, C. C., Roane, H. S., Keeney, K. M., Boney, B. R., & Abt, K. A. (2002). Varying response effort in the treatment of pica maintained by automatic reinforcement. *Journal of Applied Behavior Analysis, 35,* 233–246.

Reid, R. M. (1992). Cultural and medical perspectives on geophagia. *Medical Anthropology, 13,* 337–351.

Ricciardi, J. N., Luiselli, J. K., Terrill, S., & Reardon, K. (2003). Alternative response training with contingent practice as intervention for pica in a school setting. *Behavioral Interventions, 18,* 219–226.

Singh, N. N., & Winton, A. S. (1985). Controlling pica by components of an overcorrection procedure. *American Journal of Mental Deficiency, 90,* 40–45.

Tewari, S., Krishnan, V. H. R., Valsalan, V. C., & Roy, A. (1995). Pica in a learning disability hospital: A clinical survey. *British Journal of Developmental Disabilities, 41,* 13–22.

Woods, D. W., Miltenberger, R. G., & Lumley, V. A. (1996). A simplified habit reversal treatment for pica related chewing. *Journal of Behavior Therapy and Experimental Psychiatry, 27,* 257–262.

Premenstrual Syndromes: Guidelines for Assessment and Treatment

Mary Macdougall • Leslie Born • Catherine E. Krasnik • Meir Steiner

PREMENSTRUAL SYNDROMES

What are Premenstrual Syndromes?

Up to 75% of women of reproductive age experience some physical or psychological symptoms attributed to the premenstrual phase of the menstrual cycle. This phenomenon is often classified by the generic term premenstrual syndrome or PMS, and refers to a combination of symptoms that appear during the week before menstruation and resolve within a week of onset of menses. For most women the symptoms are mild and manageable. However, 3–8% of women report premenstrual irritability, tension, dysphoria and mood lability that seriously interfere with daily living and relationships. These women meet diagnostic criteria for Premenstrual Dysphoric Disorder or PMDD, the most severe form of PMS.

This chapter will provide guidelines for assessment and treatment of premenstrual syndromes.

ASSESSMENT

What is the Etiology of PMS?

The etiology of PMS and PMDD is not fully known. Premenstrual syndromes are heritable. Research suggests that normal ovarian function, not hormone imbalance, is the cyclical trigger for biochemical events in the central nervous system and other organs. The current consensus is that women with severe PMS or PMDD may have an altered serotonergic sensitivity to gonadal steroid fluctuations.

What are Risk Factors for PMS?

Risk factors for the development of PMDD include a past history of affective disorders and family loading for premenstrual symptoms.

How do we Diagnose PMS?

A diagnosis of PMS requires the presence of one or more negative mood, physical or behavioural symptoms attributed to the premenstrual phase of the menstrual cycle. Women will vary in the type and severity of symptoms. A series of diagnostic criteria for PMDD are found in The Diagnostic and Statistical Manual of Mental Disorders, 4th edition (American Psychiatric Association, 1994, p 715):

A. Symptoms must occur during the week before menses and remit a few days after onset of menses. Five of the following symptoms must be present and at least one must be (1), (2), (3), or (4).

Macdougall, M., Born, L., Krasnik, C. E., Steiner, M. (2006). Premenstrual syndromes: Guidelines for assessment and treatment. In J. E. Fisher & W. O'Donohue (Eds.), *Practitioner's guide to evidenced-based psychotherapy.* New York: Springer.

1. Depressed mood or dysphoria
2. Anxiety or tension
3. Affective lability
4. Irritability
5. Decreased interest in usual activities
6. Concentration difficulties
7. Marked lack of energy
8. Marked change in appetite, overeating, or food cravings
9. Hypersomnia or insomnia
10. Feeling overwhelmed
B. Symptoms must interfere with work, school, usual activities or relationships
C. Symptoms must not merely be an exacerbation of another disorder
D. Criteria A, B, and C must be confirmed by prospective daily ratings for at least two consecutive symptomatic menstrual cycles

(*Modified DSM-IV criteria for PMDD)

There are no objective diagnostic tests for PMS and PMDD. However, the Premenstrual Symptoms Screening Tool (PSST) is a simple, effective tool which is based on DSM-IV PMDD criteria and which measures the severity and impact of premenstrual symptoms. It can quickly establish if a woman is likely to qualify for PMDD (see Table 55.1).

TABLE 55.1. The Premenstrual Symptoms Screening Tool

Symptom	Not at all	Mild	Moderate	Severe
1. Anger/irritability				
2. Anxiety/tension				
3. Tearful/Increased sensitivity to rejection				
4. Depressed mood/hopelessness				
5. Decreased interest in work activities				
6. Decreased interest in home activities				
7. Decreased interest in social activities				
8. Difficulty concentrating				
9. Fatigue/lack of energy				
10. Overeating/food cravings				
11. Insomnia				
12. Hypersomnia (needing more sleep)				
13. Feeling overwhelmed or out of control				
14. Physical symptoms: breast tenderness, headaches, joint/muscle pain, bloating weight gain				

Have your symptoms, as listed above, interfered with:

	Not at all	Mild	Moderate	Severe
A. Your work efficiency or productivity				
B. Your relationships with coworkers				
C. Your relationships with your family				
D. Your social life activities				
E. Your home responsibilities				

TABLE 55.1. (Continued)

Scoring

The following criteria must be present for a diagnosis of PMDD

1) at least one of #1, #2, #3, #4 is **severe**

2) in addition at least four of #1 – #14 are **moderate to severe**

3) at least one of A, B, C, D, E is **severe**

The following criteria must be present for a diagnosis of **moderate to severe PMS**

1) at least one of #1, #2, #3, #4 is **moderate to severe**

2) in addition at least four of #1 – #14 are **moderate to severe**

3) at least one of A, B, C, D, E is **moderate to severe**

Do you experience some or any of the following premenstural symptoms that *start before* your period and *stop* within a few days of bleeding? (please mark an "X" in the appropriate box)

What Should be Ruled Out?

If a diagnosis of PMDD or severe PMS is probable, the clinician can then begin to rule out other psychiatric and/or medical conditions. All psychological and physical symptoms should be charted on a daily basis for at least *two* consecutive symptomatic cycles. Daily prospective symptoms ratings will confirm if a woman's symptoms are found largely during the premenstrual phase and are relatively absent during the follicular phase. If the symptoms occur across the cycle, it may indicate that a concurrent depression or anxiety disorder with premenstrual magnification is present. Also, medical conditions such as endometriosis, polycystic ovary disease, thyroid disorders, anemia, hyperprolactinemia and other endocrine disorders may mimic symptoms of PMS.

TREATMENTS

What Treatments are Effective?

A wide range of treatments has been tested in the management of PMS.

Conservative Treatments

These treatments are appropriate and recommended for women with mild to moderate symptoms.

Daily charting of symptoms to identify vulnerable times in the cycle
Reduce or eliminate (especially in the premenstrual phase) salt, chocolate, caffeine, alcohol and tobacco.
Small, frequent meals with complex carbohydrates (whole grain foods and cereal products, fruits, vegetables)
10,000 lux light therapy for 30 minutes in the evening
Moderate, regular, aerobic exercise
Stress management or relaxation courses/audio tapes
Relationship or self counselling
Self-help groups if available

Evidence-Based, Low-risk, Pharmacologic Treatments for Mild to Moderate PMS

Some of these interventions are effective for more than one symptom, while others are symptom-specific.

Calcium 1,200 g daily has shown significant benefit in reduction of negative affect, water retention, food cravings, and physical symptoms

Vitamin B6 50–100 mg daily may decrease nervous tension, mood swings, irritability, or anxiety

Magnesium Ion 50–200 mg daily may reduce weight gain, swelling of extremities, breast tenderness and abdominal bloating

Chasteberry extract 20 mg daily may decrease severity of symptoms including mood alteration, irritability/anger, headache and breast fullness

Psychological Interventions for Moderate to Severe PMS

Women seeking treatment for moderate to severe PMS with strong preferences for nonpharmacological interventions may consider a psychological intervention. Behavior Therapy and Relaxation Therapy have demonstrated effectiveness in reducing intensity of symptoms associated with PMS. Cognitive Behavior Therapy (a minimum of 10 sessions) can be particularly effective for PMS or PMDD with predominant symptoms of anxiety and depression.

Cognitive Behavioral Therapy* has shown significant improvement in symptoms of anxiety and depression although no significant effect on physical symptoms

Relaxation Therapy, Behavior Therapy may help reduce intensity of affective and physical symptoms.

Self-monitoring of symptoms has shown significant improvement for most symptoms, not including depression

*Most effective of all psychological interventions

Prescribed Pharmacologic Interventions for Severe PMS or PMDD

The first line pharmacologic treatment for severe PMS and PMDD is psychotropic medication. Overall, selective serotonin reuptake inhibitors (SSRIs) demonstrate a 60–70% efficacy rate, compared with an approximate 30% efficacy rate with placebo. In general the SSRI dose that is effective for PMDD is similar to the effective dosage ranges for major depression. However, a more rapid response to SSRIs has been observed in women with PMDD compared to women with major depression, suggesting a different mechanism of action. This allows for intermittent dosing, i.e., a SSRI can be administered on symptomatic days only and discontinued on the first or second full day of bleeding (daily charting will show the symptomatic days).

Antidepressants: Fluoxetine 20 mg/d*; Sertraline 50–150 mg/d*; Paroxetine 10–30 mg/d*; Citalopram 5–20 mg/d*; Clomipramine 25–75 mg/d*; Venlafaxine 50–200 mg/d; L-tryptophan 6 g/d (14 days before menses)

*Continuous (daily) or intermittent (daily during symptomatic days in the premenstrual [luteal] phase only)

Efficacy has been shown with anxiolytics although the magnitude of the therapeutic response is less than that of SSRIs and the side effect profile and potential for dependence are of concern.

Anxiolytics: Alprazolam 0.25–1.0 mg/tid (6–14 days before menses); Buspirone 25 mg/d (12 days before menses)

Hormonal agents are a second line of pharmacologic treatment for severe PMS/PMDD. The induction of "medical menopause" with gonadotrophin-releasing hormone agonists tends to successfully relieve many premenstrual symptoms. However, the occurrence of side effects that mimic menopause and the potential for hypoestrogenism and osteoporosis limits their use. Similar concerns are present with surgical oophorectomy. Oral contraceptives, while suppressing ovulation, have not been shown to be an effective treatment for severe PMS/PMDD.

Ovulation suppression (GnRH agonists): Buserelin 100–900 mug/d (intranasal); Leuprolide 3.75–7.5 mg/mo (intramuscular injection); Danazol 200–400 mg/d (intermittent)

Issues to Consider When Selecting a Treatment

The average age of onset of severe PMS or PMDD is about 26 years, although in many women the onset can be much earlier. There is evidence that premenstrual symptoms tend to worsen over time, especially after childbirth, and recur when treatment is halted. Treatment should always begin with conservative and low-risk interventions prior to the initiation of pharmacologic therapy, given that otherwise healthy women may need to be on the medication for the duration of their reproductive lifecycle. Further research on the long-term use of SSRI agents is necessary.

Websites and Self-Help Resources

The American College of Obstetricians and Gynecologists
ACOG Education Pamphlet AP057—Premenstrual Syndrome
http://www.acog.org/from_home/pubqry.cfm
Medline Plus
http://www.nlm.nih.gov/medlineplus/ premenstrualsyndrome.html
The North American Society for Psychosocial Obstetrics and Gynecology
http://www.naspog.org/
Journal of Women's Health
www.liebertpub.com/jwh/
National Association for Premenstrual Syndrome
http://www.pms.org.uk/
The National Women's Health Information Center
http://www.4woman.gov/faq/pms.htm

KEY READINGS

American Psychiatric Association. (1994). Diagnostic and statistical manual of mental disorders, (4th ed.) Washington DC: American Psychiatric Association, p. 715.

Busse J. W., Montori, V., Krasnik, C. E., & Guyatt, G. (in press). The effect of psychological intervention on premenstrual syndrome: A systematic review and meta-analysis of randomized controlled trials. *British Medical Journal.*

Dimmock, P. W., Wyatt, K. M., Jones P. W., et al. Efficacy of selective serotonin reuptake-inhibitors in premenstrual syndrome: a systematic review. *Lancet 2000, 356,* 1131–1136.

Kahn, L. S., & Halbreich, U. (2001). Oral contraceptives and mood. *Expert Opinions in Pharmacotherapy, 2,* 1367–1382.

Macdougall, M., & Steiner, M. (2003). Treatment of premenstrual dysphoria with selective serotonin reuptake inhibitors: Focus on safety. *Expert Opinions in Drug Safety 2,* 161–166.

Steiner, M., Macdougall, M., & Brown, E. (2003). The premenstrual symptoms screening tool (PSST) for clinicians. *Archieves in Womens Mental Health,* 6, 203–209.

Stevinson, C., Ernst, E. (2001). Complementary/alternative therapies for premenstrual syndrome: A systematic review of randomized controlled trials. *American Journal of Obstetrics Gynecology, 185,* 227–235.

CHAPTER 56

Posttraumatic Stress Disorder

James D. Herbert • Evan M. Forman

WHAT IS POSTTRAUMATIC STRESS DISORDER?

Posttraumatic Stress Disorder (PTSD) is a syndrome characterized by persistent anxiety-related symptoms provoked by a traumatic event. These symptoms are comprised of three clusters: Re-experiencing symptoms such as recurrent intrusive thoughts about the trauma, nightmares, and flashbacks, numbing symptoms such as detachment from others and loss of interest in usual activities, and a third cluster of miscellaneous symptoms including an exaggerated startle response, sleep disturbance, and memory impairment. Estimates of the prevalence of PTSD vary widely; the National Comorbidity Survey found rates of 8.2% among men and 20.4% among women (Kessler et al., 1995). The National Vietnam Veterans Readjustment Study (NVVRS, Kulka et al., 1990) reported that 30.9% of American soldiers who served in Vietnam developed PTSD; this figure rose to 50% if subsyndromal PTSD was counted. Although these figures continue to be widely cited, the NVVRS has been widely criticized on several grounds, including reliance on undocumented, retrospective self-reports of trauma, lack of measurement of impairment, and most importantly the simple fact that only 15% of those serving in Vietnam were actually in combat units.

BASIC FACTS ABOUT POSTTRAUMATIC STRESS DISORDER

The Origin of the PTSD Diagnosis

Both military and civilian psychologists and psychiatrists have long recognized the potentially debilitating effects of extreme trauma, including those related to war and industrial accidents. However, a specific diagnostic syndrome related to post-traumatic symptoms did not emerge until publication of the third edition of the *Diagnostic and Statistical Manual of Mental Disorders* (DSM-III) in 1980 (APA, 1980). Antiwar psychiatrists argued that many veterans returning from Vietnam experienced debilitating effects resulting from war experiences, and proposed a diagnosis of post-Vietnam syndrome. The DSM-III task force was understandably reluctant to create a diagnostic entity related to a specific and highly politically charged event. The proponents of the diagnosis then argued that the posttraumatic symptoms experienced by combatants in Vietnam were similar to those induced by other forms of severe trauma such as rape and natural disasters. They also argued that posttraumatic reactions were characterized by a unique symptom profile that was not adequately captured by existing diagnostic entities such as mood or anxiety disorders. Post-Vietnam syndrome therefore became PTSD, which was included in the DSM-III. In the two-and-a-half decades since, PTSD has attracted a great deal of attention from both researchers and clinicians. This attention has highlighted several contentious issues related to the disorder. In fact, PTSD has likely become the most controversial contemporary diagnostic syndrome, with virtually every aspect of the disorder and its treatment currently debated.

Herbert, J. D., Forman, E. M. (2006). Posttraumatic stress disorder. In J. E. Fisher, & W. T. O'Donohue (Eds.), *Practitioner's guide to evidence based psychotherapy*. New York: Springer.

Consideration of the scientific status of the extant issues related to PTSD holds important implications for treatment. Thus, while debate continues and many issues remained unresolved, we discuss in the sections below several of the major issues surrounding PTSD, followed by a discussion of the more efficacious treatments for posttraumatic reactions.

The Problem of Defining Trauma

As a diagnosis of PTSD presupposes exposure to a traumatic event, a great deal rides on what counts as trauma (McNally, 2004). The original architects of PTSD conceptualized the precipitating traumatic experiences as life-threatening event such as war combat, violent assault, or natural disasters. Indeed, the DSM-III defined traumatic stressors as falling "outside the range of usual human experience" (APA, 1980, p. 236). This definition was expanded in the revision of the DSM-III to include learning about or witnessing a friend or family member's exposure to a life-threatening event. The DSM-IV further expanded the concept to trauma as "the person experienced, witnessed, or was confronted with an event or events that involved actual or threatened death or serious injury, or a threat to the physical integrity of self or others," as long as the event resulted in "intense fear, helplessness, or horror" (APA, 1994, pp. 427–428). There are several noteworthy aspects of this evolution. First, not only does one no longer need to have direct experience with a life-threatening event, but the vicarious experience no longer needs to involve a family member or friend. Second, the event need not be unusual or outside the range of normal experience. Third, the trauma is no longer defined solely by objective external standards, but now considers the individual's psychological reaction to the event. And finally, trauma can now include "developmentally inappropriate sexual experiences" (p. 424), even if these involved no actual or threatened violence or injury.

McNally (2003a, 2004) argues that these changes have led to a "bracket creep" in the definition of trauma, noting that they permit events such as hearing off-color jokes in the workplace (Avina & O'Donohue, 2002), extramarital affairs (Dattilio, 2004), or witnessing the terrorist attacks of September 11, 2001 on the television to count as traumatic stressors capable of producing PTSD. In fact, the majority of Americans have experienced at least one traumatic event according to the DSM-IV definition (Breslau & Kessler, 2001). This expansion of the concept of trauma complicates the search for psychobiological correlates of and treatments for PTSD, as it is highly unlikely that the typical reaction to events such as hearing off-color jokes is comparable to that of war combat or brutal rape.

The Causal Role of Trauma

PTSD and its cousin, Acute Stress Disorder, are the only disorders in the DSM-IV (other than the Adjustment Disorders) that refer to a specific external etiological event. The traumatic event is presumed to be the proximal cause of the resulting symptoms. However, one cannot necessarily conclude that an event caused symptoms merely because it preceded the onset of those symptoms, especially when the symptoms include such common symptoms as depressed mood, difficulty concentrating, or sleep disturbances (cf. the logical fallacy known as post hoc ergo propter hoc, "after this therefore because of this").

Furthermore, not everyone exposed to a traumatic event develops PTSD. In fact, epidemiological data reveal that only a minority of those who experience trauma develop the disorder (Kessler et al., 1995). This raises the possibility that the severity of the traumatic event may determine the outcome. Although some studies support such a dose–response effect, many others do not (Bowman, 1999). Moreover, interpretation of those studies that do support a connection between trauma and symptom severity are complicated by the fact that trauma severity is typically assessed through a subjective self-report of severity which is likely to be highly influenced by one's current clinical state.

Whereas evidence is mixed on the role of severity of trauma in the development of PTSD, research has found that the development of the disorder is highly related to a number of individual (pretrauma) risk factors, including intelligence, neuroticism, and preexisting mood or anxiety disorder. Despite these findings, most clinical descriptions of PTSD, including the DSM-IV, focus primarily or exclusively on the trauma event itself as the cause of the disorder.

Problems with Symptoms

As previously observed, PTSD is thought to reflect a unique symptom profile. Yet there exists surprisingly little prospective data on the actual frequency of the cardinal PTSD symptoms following trauma (McNally, 2004). Rather, patients are typically asked to report their symptoms retrospectively. Most of the symptoms of PTSD overlap substantially with other diagnostic entities, especially mood and anxiety disorders. Moreover, Neal et al. (2004) recently found that disability was more strongly predicted by depression than by symptoms of posttraumatic stress.

Perhaps the most contentious issue surrounding PTSD concerns the symptom of psychogenic amnesia, especially in the context of childhood sexual abuse. The original DSM-III noted that memory impairments in the form of everyday forgetfulness associated with difficulties concentrating could occur. During the 1980s some psychotherapists built on the Freudian notion of repression to suggest that traumatic memories, especially of childhood sexual abuse, were "repressed" from consciousness, yet leaked out to produce intrusive thoughts, images, and other re-experiencing symptoms (Brown et al., 1998; Herman & Schatzow, 1987). As this perspective gained popularity, the forgetfulness symptom in DSM-III was replaced in DSM-III-R and DSM-IV with the "inability to recall an important aspect of the trauma (psychogenic amnesia)" (p. 250). Such amnesia assumes that the information was accurately encoded and subsequently blocked from awareness by an active psychological mechanism.

At current, the debate rages on. Some (e.g., Gleaves et al., 2004) argue that clinical and empirical evidence support the phenomenon of recovered memories. Many others (e.g. McNally, 2003b; Kihlstrom, 2004) take the position that the evidence for psychogenic amnesia is unreliable and/or misconstrued, and that the construct of "motivated forgetting" is inconsistent with a scientific understanding of memory. A failure to report a past trauma might best be explained not by forgetting, but by either a failure to *encode* the event at the time or a simple unwillingness to report. Moreover, research demonstrates that even the most traumatic of memories, far from being forgotten, are highly memorable and particularly vivid. Additionally, "recovered" memories are not necessarily descriptions of events that actually took place. Memory does not operate like a video camera, accurately recording external events then filing them away for later retrieval, but instead is a reconstructive process in which information is influenced by historical and contextual factors (Schacter, 1996).

Is PTSD a Social Construction?

Given the various problems on both the trauma and the symptom sides of PTSD noted above, it is not surprising that some scholars have raised the possibility that the disorder may in some sense represent a social construction. This argument takes two closely related forms. First, some suggest that PTSD pathologizes normal reactions to timeless human experiences (Summerfield, 2004). These scholars note the political origins of PTSD, and question equating normative human suffering with mental illness. Other scholars acknowledge the considerable suffering associated with PTSD, but suggest that the specific symptoms that define the disorder are largely a product of prevailing cultural theories of psychopathology (Herbert & Sageman, 2002).

Most traumatologists reject this view, and insist that PTSD is a "natural kind" phenomenon like heart disease or AIDS, existing independently of our theories about it. In support of this view, they adduce evidence from biological studies, crosscultural studies, and historical analyses, which purport to demonstrate the universal nature of PTSD across time and social contexts. Careful examination of each of these literatures, however, raises serious questions about evidence supporting the universality of the disorder. Regarding biological studies, although PTSD is associated with psychophysiologic reactivity to autobiographical accounts of trauma, between one-third and one-half of those with PTSD do not show heightened reactivity. In addition, similar reactivity is shown by individuals who claim traumatic memories of events that are highly unlikely to have occurred, such as abduction by space aliens (Clancy et al., 2002), suggesting that heightened reactivity reflects the emotional intensity of memory rather than its accuracy. Another line of biological inquiry suggests that traumatic stress, especially chronic and/or extreme trauma, may result in hippocampal atrophy through the effects of chronically elevated levels of stress hormones. Although some neuroimaging studies have in fact found smaller hippocampi in individuals with PTSD relative to controls (Bremner, 2001), most assessments of cortisol levels in persons with PTSD have found that they are not elevated. Moreover, Gilbertson et al. (2002) found that monozygotic twins in which one pair had served in Vietnam and developed PTSD while the other had not been in the war both had comparably small hippocampi, strongly suggesting that reduced hippocampus volume may be a preexisting risk factor for PTSD rather than a result of traumatic stress.

Crosscultural studies and transhistorical analyses are frequently cited in support of the legitimacy of the PTSD concept. The "natural kind" perspective would be supported by findings that the specific symptoms comprising the PTSD syndrome occur in other (and especially non-Western) cultures, and that the syndrome can be documented more-or-less in its present form across historical contexts. The limited crosscultural research to date has yielded mixed results. Some studies have found moderate to high rates of PTSD symptoms in indigent non-Western peoples (e.g., Carey, Stein, Zungu-Dirwayi, & Seedat, 2003; Howard et al., 1999; McCall & Resick, 2003). However, such studies simply asked individuals known to have experienced negative reactions to trauma to endorse symptoms of PTSD as defined by the DSM-IV. Setting aside the issues of translation and possible interviewer demand characteristics, such methods do not permit an assessment of normative responses to trauma, since base rate data on traumatized individuals are not collected and since only symptoms associated with PTSD are assessed. Indeed, other studies using more ethnosemantic interview methods in which open-ended interviews assess a wider range of experiences reveal considerable variability across cultures both in the nature of what is considered traumatic, and in the normative responses to trauma (Marsella, Friedman, Gerrity, & Scurfield, 1996). It is often argued that history reveals case examples of PTSD symptoms strikingly similar to contemporary conceptualizations of the disorder.

However, recent scholarly historical analyses have tended to support the opposite view, i.e., that both the frequency of pathological reactions to trauma, as well as the specific nature of those reactions, vary considerably across historical contexts (Herbert & Sageman, 2002).

In summary, the issue of the essential nature of PTSD remains unresolved. There is no question that some individuals who experience extreme traumatic stressors develop longstanding and debilitating symptoms that impact their psychosocial functioning. Nevertheless, the current conceptualization of the disorder is complicated by problems with the definition of trauma, questions about the etiological significance of traumatic events, and questions about the uniqueness of the symptom profile. Moreover, psychobiological, crosscultural, and historical studies cast doubt on the notion that PTSD exists independently of prevailing cultural conceptualizations of psychopathology. In fact, as discussed below, some scholars now suggest that some modern intervention technologies may actually contribute to the development of the disorder.

ASSESSMENT

PTSD-related assessment requires the identification of qualifying traumas in a patient's life history and a determination of the presence, quality, and intensity of trauma-related symptoms. In both types of assessments the interviewer is challenged by the possibility of having to work to extract information that may be difficult for a patient to acknowledge, while not creating a climate of suggestion or expectation. For a variety of reasons, including shame, the wish to avoid unpleasant and overwhelming affect, and a sense that the trauma is irrelevant to their psychological difficulties, many individuals do not at first report their trauma histories. The clinician must therefore be prepared to ask directly about such events. However, given the concerns raised earlier about the creation of false memories, it is essential that the assessor avoid leading questions or comments that overtly or covertly suggest that a particular experience occurred.

In addition to the clinical interview, a number of tools are available to assist in the assessment of PTSD. Structured interviews include instruments such as the Structured Clinical Interview for DSM-IV (SCID; First, Spitzer, Gibbon, & Williams, 1995), the Diagnostic Interview Schedule (DIS; Robins, Helzer, Croughan, & Ratcliffe, 1981), and more targeted interviews such as the PTSD Symptom Scale—Interview (Foa, Riggs, Dancu & Rothbaum, 1993) and the Clinician-Administered PTSD Scale (CAPS; Blake, Weathers, Nagy, & Kaloupek, 1995). Self-report scales include the PTSD Symptom Scale—Self-Report (Falsetti, Resnick, Resick & Kirkpatrick, 1993) and the Postraumatic Stress Diagnostic Scale (PDS; Foa, 1995). Of note is the Trauma Symptom Inventory (TSI; Briere, 1995), as it includes a number of validity indices such as tendencies to endorse unusual items and to respond in an inconsistent manner.

What Assessments are Not Helpful?

Traditional psychological tests (e.g., MMPI, projective tests like figure drawings and the Rorschach inkblot test) are not useful in assessing PTSD. Likewise, no medical tests are available. Given the concerns discussed above about suggestibility following the experience of trauma, questioning under hypnosis should be avoided given its tendency to produce confabulation. Similarly, questions regarding PTSD symptoms should avoid creating the expectation that such symptoms are inevitable and, if present, will be long-lasting.

TREATMENT

What Treatments are Effective?

As PTSD is not diagnosed until at least one month following a traumatic event, most of the treatment research on the disorder has focused on patients with persistent symptoms. However, some studies have begun to examine interventions in the immediate aftermath of trauma. Findings from these studies are supplemented by the considerable military experience over the past several decades in treating acutely traumatized soldiers. There is mounting evidence that the most effective approach to intervention depends upon the phase at which the patient presents for treatment in relation to the experience of trauma.

The Acute Posttraumatic Phase Many traumatologists paint a highly pessimistic picture of the typical sequelae of trauma, suggesting that most individuals will go on to experience chronic, debilitating symptoms if not treated. In fact, the evidence suggests the opposite is true. Although subjective distress is common in the immediate hours and days following a traumatic event, such effects are transient for the vast majority of individuals, who demonstrate surprising resilience (Bryant, 2004). Also discussed earlier was the possibility that the development of posttraumatic symptoms is partly a product of cultural context. These observations have direct therapeutic implications. First, well-intentioned messages suggesting trauma creates pathology could be predicted to *increase* the likelihood of persistent symptoms, whereas messages emphasizing the transient nature of symptoms and the high likelihood of recovery should foster resiliency. In fact, some theorists have suggested that the time immediately following a traumatic event is critical as victims are especially prone to morbid suggestion during this time (Herbert & Sageman, 2002).

Evidence in support of this perspective comes from two sources. First, the accumulated experience of military psychiatry and clinical psychology has demonstrated the value of treating psychiatric casualties close to the front with rest (including temporary sedation if necessary), while avoiding any hint of pathology and with the expectation of a quick return to the front (Shephard, 1999, 2000; Solomon & Benbenishty, 1986). The second source of evidence comes from the effects of interventions that, ironically, are designed to prevent the development of PTSD among recently traumatized persons. "Psychological debriefing" programs bring acutely traumatized individuals together into groups in which information is presented about the typical psychological effects of trauma, and emotional discussion of details of the traumatic experience is encouraged. Most research on such programs has failed to demonstrate beneficial effects relative to untreated controls, although several studies have found that debriefing actually *increases* the likelihood of the development of chronic symptoms, including PTSD (Devilly & Cotton, 2003; Gist & Devilly, 2002). It is possible that these well-intentioned interventions encourage morbid, pessimistic expectancies, thereby impeding the natural recovery process. Thus, the available evidence suggests that interventions in the immediate aftermath of trauma should be limited to immediate restorative and recuperative measures (e.g., adequate sleep using short-term tranquillizers if necessary) in the context of supportive, optimistic messages about recovery (National Institute of Mental Health, 2002). Meaningful activities should be encouraged to prevent morbid preoccupation with the trauma.

The subacute phase Even if morbid suggestions are carefully avoided, some individuals will develop persistent symptoms. Several recent studies suggest that short-term cognitive–behavior therapy (CBT), delivered between two and four weeks posttrauma, is effective in reducing symptoms and arresting the development of a chronic course (Bryant, Harvey, Dang, Sackville, & Basten 1998; Bryant, Sackville, Dang, Moulds, & Guthrie, 1999; Foa, Hearst-Ikeda, & Perry, 1995), even at four-year follow-up (Bryant, Moulds, & Nixon, 2003). Unlike debriefing programs, which target everyone who experiences a trauma, these CBT programs target only individuals who are experiencing clinically significant symptoms at least two weeks following the traumatic event. Although promising, these studies are limited to victims of assault or accident; no studies have yet evaluated such programs for combat, natural disasters, or terrorism.

Chronic symptoms A growing literature supports the effectiveness of exposure-based psychotherapies for chronic PTSD. These treatments are designed to confront the tendency to avoid distressing reminders of the trauma, including distressing memories. Exposure is conducted both in imagery (thoughts, feelings, images), as well as in vivo (relevant environmental stimuli). The therapist and patient typically work together to construct a hierarchy of distressing stimuli, which are then systematically presented. Exposure is typically conducted under the general rubric of CBT, in which other techniques such as cognitive restructuring or relaxation training may be incorporated. Exposure-based therapies have been shown to be effective for various traumatized populations, including victims of combat, accidents, rape, physical assault, and natural disasters (e.g., Devilly & Spence, 1999; Foa et al., 1999; Keane et al., 1989; Marks, Lovell, Noshirvani, Livanou, & Thrasher, 1998). Although the precise mechanism through which systematic exposure operates remains controversial, the central theme of all exposure-based interventions is confronting the natural tendency to avoid distressing material. Prolonged (imaginal) exposure (PE) represents a particularly well-validated form of exposure treatment in which patients are asked to remember and describe traumatic events during an extended therapy session (e.g., 90 minutes). The therapy apparently depends on the patient reliving the experience as vividly as possible through the use of present tense narratives and highly detailed sensory cues such as sounds and smells (Foa et al., 1999).

Cognitive restructuring is another well established treatment for posttraumatic symptoms. Foa and Rothbaum (1998) proposed that two dysfunctional cognitions are implicated in the development of PTSD: (1) The world is highly dangerous, and (2) I am incompetent. Based on Beck's paradigm of cognitive therapy (Beck & Emery, 1985), cognitive restructuring for PTSD involves helping patients identify and revise PTSD-related negative automatic thoughts (e.g., "If I get in a car again I'll surely be in another accident and then I'll never recover") stemming from these dysfunctional beliefs. Although cognitive restructuring appears to be an effective treatment (Foa, Keane, & Friedman, 2000; Marks et al., 1998), the addition of cognitive restructuring to exposure treatments has been found to be no more effective than exposure treatment alone (Foa & Rauch, 1999; Marks et al., 1998).

Closely related to cognitive restructuring is Stress Inoculation Training (SIT; Kilpatrick et al. 1982), a multicomponent intervention involving relaxation, guided self-dialogue, covert modeling (visualizing the successful confrontation of an anxiety-provoking situation), role-playing, and thought stopping (e.g. subvocally saying the word "stop!" to interrupt ruminative or disturbing thoughts). Although SIT appears to be effective, some evidence suggests it is not as powerful as PE and that it does not add anything above and beyond PE-only (Foa, Rothbaum, Riggs, & Murdock, 1991; Foa et al., 1999). Moreover, there is now support for the notion that attempting to suppress trauma-related cognitions may, in fact, paradoxically increase the frequency and intensity of the thoughts (Harvey & Bryant, 1998).

The paradoxical effects of thought stopping point to the more general role of experiential avoidance (i.e. the avoidance of aversive thoughts, memories and emotions) in the development and maintenance of PTSD. Acceptance-based therapies, especially Acceptance and Commitment Therapy (ACT; Hayes, Strosahl, & Wilson, 1999), directly address experiential avoidance and have been increasingly used in the treatment of PTSD (Orsillo & Batten, in press; Walser & Hayes, 1998). Although promising, little research has investigated ACT for trauma-related disorders.

What are Effective Self-Help Treatments?

Little is known about self-directed treatment of PTSD, although at least one study (Ehlers et al., 2003) found that self-treatment through any self-help booklet was no better than no treatment. A number of self-help books have been published, but most are inconsistent with scientifically based treatment guidelines such as those outlined here. For example, almost without exception the available books emphasize pathological responses to trauma as the norm, and many endorse the idea of repressed memories and encourage various techniques to "recover" such memories. Many also highlight dubious techniques (e.g., massage therapy, rapid eye movements) as keys to "unlocking" traumatic experiences. Nevertheless, potentially useful self-help guides include:

- Williams, M. B., & Poijula, S. (2002). *The PTSD workbook: Simple, effective techniques for overcoming traumatic stress symptoms.* Oakland, CA: New Harbinger.
- Greist, J. H., Jefferson, J. W., & Katzelnick, D. J. (2000). *Posttraumatic stress disorder: A guide.* Madison, WI: Information Centers, Madison Institute of Medicine. (Downloadable online at: *http://ptsd.factsforhealth.org/PTSDGuide.pdf*)
- Rothbaum, B. O., & Foa, E. B. (1999). *Reclaiming your life after rape.* San Antonio: Psych. Corp.
- Bourne, E. J. (2000). *The anxiety and phobia workbook.* Oakland, CA: New Harbinger.

In addition, a number of useful informational websites about PTSD are available, including:

- *http://www.ncptsd.org*
- *http://www.ptsdalliance.com*
- *http://www.mhsanctuary.com/ptsd*
- *http://www.apa.org/practice/ptsd.html*
- *http://ptsd.factsforhealth.org/whatisit.html*

What is Effective Medical Treatment?

A variety of medications have been shown to be helpful in uncontrolled, open-label studies, including the selective serontonin reuptake inhibitors and other antidepressants, mood stabilizers, and benzodiazepines. The general finding is that all of these classes of agents are helpful. There have been only a few randomized controlled trials of medications, and only two antidepressants (Sertraline and Paroxetine) are currently FDA approved for the treatment of PTSD. Given the high rates of comorbidity between PTSD and other conditions, especially mood and anxiety disorders, it is not clear if drug therapy addresses symptoms specific to PTSD, or if the observed improvements are a function of amelioration of comorbid conditions. Either way, as with other anxiety disorders, a major limitation of drug therapy for PTSD is the high risk of relapse following discontinuation of medication.

Therapies without Empirical Support There are several forms of psychotherapy that, despite being widely practiced, either have minimal or no data to support their effectiveness, involve dramatic techniques that are devoid of therapeutic powers, or may even be harmful. There is no controlled research supportive of psychoanalytic/psychodynamic psychotherapy or of supportive psychotherapy for PTSD. "Recovered memory" therapy involves a number of techniques such as hypnosis, age regression, and guided imagery that are designed to uncover "repressed" traumatic memories, often of childhood sexual abuse. In addition to the problems with the notion of traumatic repression reviewed above, these therapies involve highly suggestive techniques that can actually create memories, which are then experienced as veridical.

The past decade has witnessed the ascendance of the so-called "power" therapies, which promise quick relief from distressing symptoms in as little as a single treatment session. Foremost among these is Eye Movement Desensitization and Reprocessing (EMDR; Shapiro, 2001), which entails therapist-guided back-and-forth eye movements in the context of imaginal exposure. Although proponents of EMDR highlight the powers of eye movements, controlled research has shown this component is utterly devoid of therapeutic effects (Davidson & Parker, 2001; Devilly, 2002; Herbert et al., 2000). Some studies even suggest that eye movements may interfere with effective treatment relative to imaginal exposure without eye movements, especially in the long-term. Although EMDR appears to be more effective than no treatment at all, its proposed mechanism of action is highly suspect, and it appears to be less effective than CBT (Devilly & Spence, 1999).

How Does One Select Among Treatments?

Given the high rates of relapse following medication discontinuation, drug therapy is generally not considered the initial treatment of choice for PTSD per se. However, medications can be very useful in three circumstances. First, short-term use of minor tranquilizers (e.g., benzodiazepines) or related sleep-inducing medications can often be helpful in the immediate aftermath of trauma to promote adequate sleep and recuperation. Second, antidepressant medications can be useful in treating clinically significant comorbid mood or anxiety symptoms. Finally, medications are sometimes useful in treatment refractory cases in which psychotherapy has failed. In all cases, a risk-benefit calculus based on a consideration of possible side effects and likely benefits should be discussed with the patient. As discussed above, several psychotherapies have been shown to be effective in treating traumatic stress, including exposure-based therapies, cognitive restructuring, and relaxation-based interventions. Such treatments should generally be considered first-line interventions.

Useful resources for the professional that discuss specific treatment considerations include:

- Foa, E. B., Keane, T. M., & Friedman, M. J. (Eds.) (2000). *Effective treatments for PTSD: Practice guidelines from the International Society for Traumatic Stress Studies.* New York: Guilford.
- Wilson, J. P., Friedman, M. J., & Lindy, J. D. (Eds.) (2001). *Treating psychological trauma and PTSD.* New York: Guilford.
- Bryant, R. A., & Harvey, A. G. (2000). *Acute stress disorder: A handbook of theory, assessment, and treatment.* Washington, DC: American Psychological Association.
- Nutt, D. J., Davidson, J. R. T., & Zohar, J. (Eds) (2000). *Posttraumatic stress disorder: Diagnosis, management and treatment.* London: Martin Dunitz.
- Rosen, G. M. (Ed.) (2004), *Posttraumatic stress disorder: Issues and controversies.* Chichester, England: John Wiley & Sons.

CONCLUSION

PTSD has become a lightening rod for the storms currently raging in the field of clinical psychology and related disciplines between scientifically minded researchers and practitioners and those whose theories and interventions are less rooted in science. Recent research has cast in sharp relief many of the issues surrounding PTSD. Although many questions remain unanswered, emerging data point to the potential importance of avoiding suggestion of permanent pathology in the critical period immediately following the experience of trauma, and support the efficacy of various CBT treatments for those who develop persistent posttraumatic symptoms.

REFERENCES

American Psychiatric Association (1980). Diagnostic and statistical manual of mental disorders (3rd ed.). Washington, DC: Author.

American Psychiatric Association (1994). Diagnostic and statistical manual of mental disorders (4th ed.). Washington, DC: Author.

Avina, C., & O'Donohue, W. (2002). Sexual harassment and PTSD: Is sexual harassment diagnosable trauma? *Journal of Traumatic Stress, 15*, 69–75.

Beck, A. T., & Emery, G. (1985). *Anxiety disorders and phobias.* New York: Basic Books.

Blake, D. D., Weathers, F. W., Nagy, L. M., & Kaloupek, D. G. (1995). The development of a clinician-administered PTSD scale. *Journal of Traumatic Stress, 8*, 75–90.

Bowman, M. (1999). Individual differences in posttraumatic stress: Problems with the DSM-IV model. *Canadian Journal of Psychiatry, 44*, 21–33.

Bremner, J. D. (2001). Hypotheses and controversies related to effects of stress on the hippocampus: An argument for stress-induced damage to the hippocampus in patients with posttraumatic stress disorder. *Hippocampus, 11*, 75–81.

Breslau, N., & Kessler, R. C. (2001). The stressor criterion in DSM-IV posttraumatic stress disorder: An empirical investigation. *Biological Psychiatry, 50*, 699–704.

Briere, J. (1995). *Trauma Symptom Inventory professional manual.* Lutz, FL: Psychological Assessment Resources.

Brown, D., Scheflin, A. W., & Hammond, D. C. (1998). *Memory, trauma treatment, and the law.* New York: Norton.

Bryant, R. A., Harvey, A. G., Dang, S. T., Sackville, T., & Basten, C. (1998). Treatment of acute stress disorder: A comparison of cognitive-behavioral therapy and supportive counseling. *Journal of Consulting and Clinical Psychology, 66*, 862–866.

Bryant, R. A., Moulds, M. L., & Nixon, R. V. D. (2003). Cognitive-behaviour therapy of acute stress disorder: A four-year follow-up. *Behaviour Research & Therapy, 41*, 489–494.

Bryant, R. A., Sackville, T., Dang, S. T., Moulds, M., & Guthrie, R. (1999). Treating acute stress disorder: An evaluation of cognitive behavior therapy and supportive counseling techniques. *American Journal of Psychiatry, 156*, 1780–1786.

Carey, P. D., Stein, D. J., Zungu-Dirwayi, N., & Seedat, S. (2003). Trauma and PTSD in an Urban Xhosa Primary Care Population: Prevalence, Comorbidity, and Service Use Patterns. *Journal of Nervous and Mental Disease, 191*, 230–236.

Clancy, S. A., McNally, R. J., Schacter, D. L., Lenzenweger, M. F., & Pitman, R. K. (2002). Memory distortion in people reporting abduction by aliens. *Journal of Abnormal Psychology, 111*, 455–461.

Dattilio, F. M. (2004). Extramarital affairs: The much-overlooked PTSD. *The Behavior Therapist, xx*, 76–78.

Davidson, P. R., & Parker, K. C. H. (2001). Eye movement desensitization and reprocessing (EMDR): A meta-analysis. *Journal of Consulting and Clinical Psychology, 69*, 305–316.

Devilly, G. J. (2002). Eye movement desensitization and reprocessing: A chronology of its development and scientific standing. The Scientific Review of Mental Health Practice, 1, 113–138.

Devilly, G. J., & Cotton, P. (2003). Psychological debriefing and the workplace: Defining a concept, controversies and guildelines for intervention. *Australian Psychologist, 38*, 144–150.

Devilly, G. J., & Spence, S. H. (1999). The relative efficacy and treatment distress of EMDR and a cognitive behavioral trauma treatent protocol in the amelioration of posttraumatic stress disorder. *Journal of Anxiety Disorders, 13*, 131–157.

Ehlers, A., Clark, D. M., Hackmann, A., McManus, F., Fennell, M., Herbert, C., et al. (2003). A randomized controlled trial of cognitive therapy, a self-help booklet, and repeated assessments as early interventions for posttraumatic stress disorder. *Archives of General Psychiatry, 60*, 1024–1032.

Falsetti, S. A., Resnick, H. S., Resick, P. A., & Kilpatrick, D. G. (1993). The modified PTSD Symptom Scale: A brief self-report measure of posttraumatic stress disorder. *Behavior Therapist, 16,* 161–162.

First, M. B., Spitzer, R. L., Gibbon, M., & Williams, J. B. W. (1995). *Structured Clinical Interview for* DSM-IV *Axis I disorders—Patient edition* (SCID-I/P, Version 2.0). New York: Biometrics Research Department.

Foa, E. B. (1995). *PDS (Posttraumatic Stress Diagnostic Scale) manual.* Minneapolis, MN: National Computer Systems

Foa, E. B., Dancu, C. V., Hembree, E. A, Jaycox, L. H., Meadows, E. A., & Street, G. P. (1999). A comparison of exposure therapy, stress inoculation training, and their combination for reducing posttraumatic stress disorder in female assault victims. *Journal of Consulting & Clinical Psychology. 67,* 194–200.

Foa, E. B., Hearst-Ikeda, D., & Perry, K. J. (1995). Evaluation of a brief cognitive-behavioral program for the prevention of chronic PTSD in recent assault victims. *Journal of Consulting and Clinical Psychology, 63,* 948–955.

Foa, E. B., Keane, T. M., & Friedman, M. J. (2000). Effective treatments for PTSD: Practice guidelines from the International Society for Traumatic Stress Studies. *New York: Guilford Press.*

Foa, E. B., & Rauch, S. A. M. (2004). Cognitive changes during prolonged exposure versus prolonged exposure plus cognitive restructuring in female assault survivors with posttraumatic stress disorder. *Journal of Consulting & Clinical Psychology, 72,* 879–884.

Foa, E. B., Rothbaum, B. O., Riggs, D. S., & Murdock, T. B. (1991). Treatment of posttraumatic stress disorder in rape victims: A comparison between cognitive–behavioral procedures and counseling. *Journal of Consulting and Clinical Psychology, 59,* 715–723.

Foa, E. B., & Rothbaum, B. O. (1998). *Treating the trauma of rape: Cognitive-behavioral therapy for PTSD.* New York: Guilford Press.

Gilbertson, M. W., Shenton, M. E., Ciszewski, A., Kasai, K., Lasko, N. B., Orr, S. P. et al. (2002). Smaller hippocampal volume predicts pathologic vulnerability to psychological trauma. *Nature Neuroscience, 5,* 1242–1247.

Gist, R., & Devilly, G. J. (2002). Post-trauma debriefing: The road too frequently traveled. *The Lancet, 360,* 741–742.

Gleaves, D. H., Smith, S. M., Butler, L. D., & Spiegal, D. (2004). False and recovered memories in the laboratory and clinic: A review of experimental and clinical evidence. *Clinical Psychology: Science & Practice, 11,* 3–28.

Harvey, A. G., & Bryant, R. A. (1998). The role of valence in attempted thought suppression. *Behaviour Research & Therapy. 36,* 757–763.

Hayes, S. C., Strosahl, K., & Wilson, K. G. (1999). *Acceptance and commitment therapy: An experiential approach to behavior change.* New York: Guilford Press.

Herbert, J. D., Lilienfeld, S. O., Lohr, J. M., Montgomery, R. W., O'Donohue, W. T., & Rosen, G. M. (2000). Science and pseudoscience in the development of eye movement desensitization and reprocessing: Implications for clinical psychology. *Clinical Psychology Review, 20,* 945–971.

Herbert, J. D., & Sageman, M. (2002). *"First do no harm": Emerging guidelines in the treatment of posttraumatic reactions.* In G. M. Rosen (Ed.), *Posttraumatic stress disorder: Issues and controversies.* Chichester, England: John Wiley & Sons.

Herman, J. L., & Schatzow, E. (1987). Recovery and verification of memories of childhood sexual trauma. *Psychoanalytic Psychology, 4,* 1–14.

Howard, W., Loberiza, F., Pfohl, B., Thorne, P., Magpantay, R., & Woolson, R. (1999). Initial results, reliability, and validity of a mental health survey of Mount Pinatubo disaster victims. *The Journal of Nervous and Mental Disease, 187,* 661–672.

Keane, T. M., Fairbank, J. A., Caddell, J. M., & Zimering, R. T. (1989). Implosive (flooding) therapy reduces symptoms of PTSD in Vietnam combat veterans. *Behavior Therapy, 20,* 245–260.

Kessler, R. C., Sonnega, A., Bromet, E., Hughes, M., & Nelson, C. B. (1995). Posttraumatic stress disorder in the National Comorbidity Survey. *Archives of General Psychiatry, 52,* 1048–1060.

Kihlstrom, J. F. (2004). An unbalanced balancing act: Blocked, recovered, and false memories in the laboratory and clinic. *Clinical Psychology: Science & Practice, 11,* 34–41.

Kulka, R. A., Schlenger, W. E., Fairbank, J. A., Hough, R. L., Jordan, B. K., Marmar, C. R., et al. (1990). *Trauma and the Vietnam war generation: Report of findings from the National Vietnam Veterans Readjustment Study.* New York: Brunner/Mazel.

Marks, I., Lovell, K., Noshirvani, H., Livanou, M., & Thrasher, S. (1998). Treatment of posttraumatic stress disorder by exposure and/or cognitive restructuring. *Archives of General Psychiatry, 55,* 317–325.

Marsella, A. J., Friedman, M. J., Gerrity, E. T., & Scurfield, R. M. (Eds.). (1996). *Ethnocultural aspects of posttraumatic stress disorder: Issues, research, and clinical applications.* Washington, DC: American Psychological Association.

McCall, G., & Resick, P. (2003). A pilot study of PTSD symptoms among Kalahari Bushmen. *Journal of Traumatic Stress, 16,* 445–450.

McNally, R. J. (2003a). Progress and controversy in the study of posttraumatic stress disorder. *Annual Review of Psychology, 54,* 229–252.

McNally, R. J. (2003b). *Remembering Trauma.* Cambridge, MA: Harvard University Press.

McNally, R. J. (2004). Conceptual problems with the DSM-IV criteria for posttraumatic stress disorder. In G. M. Rosen (Ed.), *Posttraumatic stress disorder: Issues and controversies.* Chichester, England: John Wiley & Sons.

National Institute of Mental Health (2002). *Mental health and mass violence: Evidenced-based early psychological interventions for victims/survivors of mass violence. A workshop to reach consensus on best practices.* NIH Publication No. 02-5138, Washington, DC: US Government Printing Office.

Neal, L. A., Green, G., & Turner, M. A. (2004). Post-traumatic stress and disability. *British Journal of Psychiatry, 184,* 247–250.

Orsillo, S. M., & Batten, S. V. (in press). Acceptance and Commitment Therapy for PTSD. *Behavior Modification.*

Robins, L., Helzer, H., Croughan, J., & Ratcliff, K. (1981). National Institute of Mental Health Diagnostic Interview Schedule: Its history, characteristics, and validity. *Archives of General Psychiatry, 38,* 381–389.

Schacter, D. L. (1996). *Searching for memory: The brain, the mind, and the past.* New York: Basic Books.

Shapiro, F. (2001). *Eye movement desensitization and reprocessing: Basic principles, protocols, and procedures* (2nd ed.). New York: Guilford Press.

Shephard, B. (1999). "Pitiless psychology": The role of prevention in British military psychiatry in the second world war. *History of Psychiatry, 10,* 491–510.

Shephard, B. (2000). *A war of nerves: Soldiers and psychiatrists 1914–1994.* London: Jonathan Cape.

Solomon, Z., & Benbenishty, R. (1986). The role of proximity, immediacy, and expectancy in frontline treatment of combat stress reaction among Israelis in the Lebanon War. *American Journal of Psychiatry, 143,* 613–617.

Summerfield, D. (2004). Cross-cultural perspectives on the medicalization of human suffering. In G. M. Rosen (Ed.), *Posttraumatic stress disorder: Issues and controversies.* Chichester, England: John Wiley & Sons.

Veronen, L. J., & Kilpatrick, D. G. (1983). Stress management for rape victims. In D. Meichenbaum & M. E. Jaremko (Eds.), *Stress reduction and prevention* (pp. 341–374). New York: Plenum.

Walser, R. D., & Hayes, S. C. (1998). Acceptance and trauma survivors: Applied issues and problems. In V. M. Follette, Victoria M & J. I. Ruzek (Eds.), Cognitive-behavioral therapies for trauma (pp. 256–277). New York: Guilford Press.

Recurrent Headache Disorders

Victoria E. Mercer • Melanie P. Duckworth

WHAT IS RECURRENT HEADACHE DISORDER?

For most people headaches are relieved with rest, re-hydration, or use of over-the-counter analgesics. Unfortunately, a significant proportion of the population is not able to relieve their headache through these common means. These people experience recurrent headaches most commonly in the form of migraine or tension-type headaches. Migraine and tension headaches are significant in terms of the number of persons suffering from such headaches, the level of distress and impairment associated with the often chronic course of such headaches, and the economic burden born by the individual headache sufferer and society.

In 2004, the International Headache Society (IHS) published the most current version of The *International Classification of Headache Disorders, 2nd edition* (ICHD-II; International Headache Society, 2004). This classification includes precisely operationalized diagnoses and reliable headache categories that can be used for research and clinical purposes. The ICHD-II headache categories are listed in Table 57.1, the diagnostic criteria provided by the ICHD-II for certain types of primary headaches are listed in Table 57.2. A clinical description of the more common migraine and tension-type headaches are provided below. The reader is encouraged to review the full listing and criteria provided in the ICHD-II supplement (classification available online at http://*www.cephalalgia.org*).

The IHCD-II differentiates between six subtypes of migraines; the two primary subtypes are migraine with and without aura. Migraine without aura is the most frequent and disabling type of migraine. The general description of migraine without aura (International Headache Society, 2004) is:

Recurrent headache disorder manifesting in attacks lasting 4–72 hours. Typical characteristics are unilateral location, pulsating quality, moderate or severe intensity, aggravation by routine physical activity and association with nausea and/or photophobia and phonophobia (p. 24).

The description of migraine with aura is as follows (International Headache Society, 2004):

Recurrent disorder manifesting in attacks of reversible focal neurological symptoms that usually develop over 5–20 minutes and last for less than 60 minutes. Headache with the features of migraine without aura usually follows the aura symptoms. Less commonly, headache lacks migrainous features or is completely absent (p. 25–26).

The ICHD-II term "tension-type" headache replaces terms like muscle-contraction headache, psychogenic headache, and idiopathic headache (International Headache Society, 2004). This ICHD-II classification includes four subtypes of tension-type headache: infrequent episodic, frequent episodic, chronic episodic, and probable tension-type. Each of these first three is again separated by the presence or absence of pericranial tenderness, as evidenced by manual palpation.

Mercer, V. E. & Duckworth, M. P. (2006). Recurrent headache disorders. In J. E. Fisher & W. T. O'Donohue (Eds.), *Practitioner's guide to evidence-based psychotherapy*. New York: Springer.

TABLE 57.1 The International Headache Society's Classification of Headache Disorders, 2nd Ed.

Primary headache

1. Migraine
    1.1. Migraine without aura
    1.2. Migraine with aura
        1.2.1. Typical aura with migraine headache
        1.2.2. Typical aura with non-migraine headache
        1.2.3. Typical aura without headache
        1.2.4. Familial hemiplegic migraine (FHM)
        1.2.5. Sporadic hemiplegic migraine
        1.2.6. Basilar-type migraine
    1.3. Childhood periodic syndromes that are commonly precursors of migraine
    1.4. Retinal migraine
    1.5. Complications of migraine
    1.6. Probable migraine
2. Tension-type headache (TTH)
    2.1. Infrequent episodic tension-type headache
        2.1.1. Infrequent episodic tension-type headache associated with pericranial tenderness
        2.1.2. Infrequent episodic tension-type headache not associated with pericranial tenderness
    2.2. Frequent episodic tension-type headache
        2.2.1. Frequent episodic tension-type headache associated with pericranial tenderness
        2.2.2. Frequent episodic tension-type headache not associated with pericranial tenderness
    2.3. Chronic tension-type headache
        2.3.1. Chronic tension-type headache associated with pericranial tenderness
        2.3.2. Chronic tension-type headache not associated with pericranial tenderness
    2.4. Probable tension-type headache
        2.4.1. Probable infrequent episodic tension-type headache
        2.4.2. Probable frequent episodic tension-type headache
        2.4.3. Probable chronic tension-type headache
3. Cluster headache and other trigeminal autonomic cephalalgias
4. Other primary headache

Secondary headache

5. Headache attributed to head and/or neck trauma
6. Headache attributed to cranial or cervical vascular disorder
7. Headache attributed to nonvascular intracranial disorder
8. Headache attributed to a substance or its withdrawal
9. Headache attributed to infection
10. Headache attributed to disorder of homeostasis
11. Headache of facial pain attributed to disorder of cranium, neck, eyes, ears, nose, sinuses, teeth, mouth or other facial or cranial structures
12. Headache attributed to psychiatric disorder
13. Cranial neuralgias and central causes of facial pain
14. Other headache, cranial neuralgia, central or primary facial pain

Source: The International Classification of Headache Disorders, 2nd edition; International Headache Society, 2004

TABLE 57.2 Diagnostic Criteria of The International Classification of Headache Disorders, 2nd edition

1.1. Migraine without aura:

  A. At least five attacks fulfilling criteria B–D

  B. Headache attacks lasting 4–72 hours (untreated or unsuccessfully treated)

  C. Headache has at least two of the following characteristics:

    1. Unilateral location

    2. Pulsating quality

    3. Moderate or severe pain intensity

    4. Aggravation by or causing avoidance of routine physical activity (eg, walking or climbing stairs)

  D. During headache at least one of the following:

    1. nausea and/or vomiting

    2. photophobia and phonophobia

  E. Not attributed to another disorder (p. 24–25)

1.2. Migraine with aura:

  A. At least two attacks fulfilling criterion B

  B. Migraine aura fulfilling criteria B and C for one of the subforms 1.2.1–1.2.6

  C. Not attributed to another disorder (p. 26)

2.1. Infrequent episodic tension-type headache:

  A. At least 10 episodes occurring on <1 day per month on average (<12 days per year) and fulfilling criteria B–D

  B. Headache lasting from 30 minutes to 7 days

  C. Headache has at least two of the following characteristics:

    1. bilateral location

    2. pressing/tightening (nonpulsating) quality

    3. mild or moderate intensity

    4. not aggravated by routine physical activity such as walking or climbing stairs

  D. Both of the following:

    1. no nausea or vomiting (anorexia may occur)

    2. no more than one of photophobia or phonophobia

  E. Not attributed to another disorder (p. 38)

2.2. Frequent episodic tension-type headache:

  A. At least 10 episodes occurring on ≥1 but <15 days per month for at least 3 months (≥12 and <180 days per year) and fulfilling criteria B-D

  B. Headache lasting from 30 minutes to 7 days

  C. Headache has at least two of the following characteristics:

    1. bilateral location

    2. pressing/tightening (nonpulsating) quality

    3. mild or moderate intensity

    4. not aggravated by routine physical activity such as walking or climbing stairs

  D. Both of the following:

    1. no nausea or vomiting (anorexia may occur)

    2. no more than one of photophobia or phonophobia

  E. Not attributed to another disorder (p. 39)

2.3. Chronic tension-type headache:

  A. Headache occurring on ≥15 days per month on average for >3 months (≥180 days per year) and fulfilling criteria B–D

  B. Headache lasts hours or may be continuous

TABLE 57.2 (Continued)

   C. Headache has at least two of the following characteristics:
      1. bilateral location
      2. pressing/tightening (nonpulsating) quality
      3. mild or moderate intensity
      4. not aggravated by routine physical activity such as walking or climbing stairs
   D. Both of the following:
      1. no more than one of photophobia, phonophobia, or mild nausea
      2. neither moderate or sever nausea nor vomiting
   E. Not attributed to another disorder (p. 39)

Source: The International Classification of Headache Disorders, 2nd edition; International Headache Society, 2004

All subtypes of tension-type headache involve pain that is typically bilateral, pressing or tightening in quality, of mild to moderate intensity, and that does not worsen with routine physical activity (International Headache Society, 2004). Infrequent and frequent tension-type headaches do not involve nausea but may involve photophobia or phonophobia. The diagnosis of infrequent tension-type headache requires that at least 10 episodes occur in total, but episodes occur less than one day per month; frequent type diagnosis requires that at least 10 episodes in total, and that the episodes occur at least one day, but less than 15 days per month for at least three months. Chronic tension-type headache may involve mild nausea, photophobia, or phonophobia, and requires that a headache occur at least 15 days per month for more than three months.

BASIC FACTS ABOUT RECURRENT HEADACHE DISORDERS

Comobidity

The relation between migraine headache and mood and anxiety disorders has been documented in two large community based samples (Breslau, & Davis, 1993; Breslau, Davis, Schultz, & Peterson, 1994; Breslau, Merikangas, & Bowden, 1994; Merikangas, Angst, & Isler, 1990; Merikangas, Merikangas, & Angst, 1993). The data from Breslau and colleagues (Breslau et al., 1994; Breslau, Lipton, Stewart, Schultz & Welch 2003) found that migraine history predicted the first-onset of depression and a depression history predicted the first-onset of migraine. In contrast, Merikangas and colleagues (1990; Low, & Merikangas, 2003) found a stronger relation of migraine to the combined presentation of anxious and depressive symptoms, rather than to purely anxious or purely depressive presentations. The data from the Zurich Cohort Study of Young Adults found that anxiety preceded the onset of migraine in about 80% of individuals whereas the onset of depression followed the onset of migraine in about 74% of individuals (Merikangas et al., 1990; 1993).

There are fewer epidemiological studies of tension-type headache and psychopathology. The data suggests that the prevalence of anxiety or mood disorders is not increased in episodic tension-type headache (Merikangas, 1994; Merikangas, Stevens, & Angst, 1993). However, in a survey of nonspecific tension-type headache patients, it was found that at least one psychosocial stressor or psychiatric disorder was detected in 84.8% of all patients. Moreover, 52.5% of patients experienced anxiety and within this group of patients 83.3% were diagnosed with generalized anxiety disorder. A little more than 36.4% of all nonspecific tension-type headache patients experienced depression, with 45.6% of this group being diagnosed with dysthymia (Puca, Genco, Prudenzo, et al., 1999).

Prevalence

Data gathered from the American Migraine Study II suggest that migraine prevalence is not changing over time (Lipton, Stewart, Diamond, Diamond, & Reed, 2001). In 1999, it was estimated that 27.9 million Americans experienced migraine headaches; this figure reflects an increase of 4.3 million migraine sufferers over a 10-year period. Despite this absolute increase in the number of migraine sufferers, the increase in the number of people with migraine reflects the increase in US population over the same 10-year period (Holroyd, & Penzien, 1994; Hagen, Zwart, Stovner, & Bovim, 2000; Rasmussen, 2001; Russell, Rasmussen, Throvaldsen, & Olesen, 1995).

While it is difficult to pool prevalence rates reported for tension-type headache due to variability in reported severity, frequency, duration, and extent of disability, it has been estimated that the 1-year prevalence rate for regular tension-type headache (more than once a month) is 20–30% of the general US population, with 10-15% of these people suffering from chronic tension-type headache (more than 180 days per year) (Breslau, Davis, & Andreski, 1991; Holroyd, & Penzien, 1994; Rasmussen, 2001; Schwartz, Stewart, Simon, & Lipton, 1998). Some studies have estimated the prevalence of tension-type headache to be as high as 78% (International Headache Society, 2004).

Age at onset

Early cases of migraine headache have been reported in infancy and early childhood (Barlow, 1994). The prevalence of migraine headache among children under the age of 7 years ranges from 1.4% to 3.2%, the prevalence among school-age children ranges from 4% to 11% (Lipton, 1997; Sillanpaa, & Anttila, 1996). Tension-type headache in children between the ages of 5–15 years accounts for about 10% of recurrent headache disorders, early cases of tension-type headache have been reported with an overall prevalence rate of 0.9% (Abu-Arefeh, & Russell, 1994).

Gender

Within adult migraine sufferers the 1-year prevalence rate is higher among females (15–18%) than among males (6–8%) (Hagen et al., 2000; Rasmussen, 2001). The lifetime prevalence rate of migraine headache has been estimated to be as high as 33% in women, and 13.3% in men (Launer, Terwindt, & Ferrari, 1999). Like migraine headaches, tension-type headaches are also more prevalent in females (8%) than in males (2%) (Hagen, et al., 2000; Pryse-Phillips et al., 1992; Schwartz, Stewart, Simon, & Lipton, 1998).

Course

Prevalence of migraine increases from age 12 to 45 then decreases steadily in both females and males (Hagen et al., 2000; Rasmussen, 2001). Like migraine headache, tension-type headache prevalence increases into the fourth decade of life and then decreases, peaking between the ages of 30 and 39 (Hagen et al., 2000; Rasmussen, 2001).

Impairment and other demographic characteristics

One-year prevalence rates are reported to be higher in Caucasians than African Americans in both males (40.1% vs. 22.8%) and females (46.8% vs. 30.9%), and prevalence is inversely related to household income, at least in the United States (Schwartz et al., 1998).

The American Migraine Study II estimates that 14.8 million Americans suffer from headaches severe enough to cause impairment of normal daily activities or to cause bed-rest; however, it is difficult to estimate the socio-economic burden of headaches because nearly half of all adult migraine sufferers and four-fifths of persons with tension-type headache have never contacted their general practitioner concerning their headache experience (Rasmussen, 2001; Rasmussen, Jensen, & Olesen, 1992),. Approximately 31% of migraine sufferers report missing at least one day of work or school in the previous three months; 51% report being only 50% effective while at work or school due to presence of migraine symptoms (Gerth, Carides, Dasbach, Visser, & Santanello, 2001; Lipton, Stewart, Diamond, Diamond, & Reed, 2001). One in four households contains an adult migraine sufferer, with nearly 15 million of these people found to be functionally impaired. In the United States, the annual cost of migraine-related work loss to the employer is $3309 per employee with migraine, with the total cost of lost productivity due to adult migraine sufferers estimated to be nearly $13 billion dollars (Gerth, et al., 2001).

Chronic tension-type headaches also have a large impact on work and social functioning. Two thirds of sampled chronic tension-type headache sufferers report impairments in sleep, energy level, and emotional wellbeing; 74% of the same sample report taking a mean of seven headache-related disability days in the last six months (Holroyd et al., 2000). Because most patients continue to carry out daily life responsibilities, even though they are in pain and may have diminished role performance, an accurate estimate of the socioeconomic burden of such headaches is more difficult to calculate (Holroyd, et al., 2000). Looking across types, headache can be considered a significant public health problem, requiring evaluation and intervention aimed at decreasing pain and suffering and improving functioning across the various life domains.

ASSESSMENT

What Should be Ruled Out?

While some headaches are benign, others are not. It is essential that a physician perform a neurological evaluation of a person's symptoms before psychological intervention begins. If the patient describes symptoms that are not typical of a benign headache, or the patient reports sudden changes in their headache, the clinician should ensure a physician or specialist evaluates the patient. Diagnosis of migraine or tension-type headache should not be given unless the disorders associated with the other specific types of headache have been ruled out and the headaches did not begin at the same time as the onset of any other disorder. These diagnoses include headaches attributed to head and/or neck trauma, cranial or cervical vascular disorder, nonvascular intracranial disorder, substance use or its withdrawal, infection, disorder of homeostasis, disorders of the cranium, neck, eyes, ears, nose, sinuses, teeth, mouth or other facial or cranial structures, psychiatric disorder, or cranial neuralgias (International Headache Society, 2004).

What is Involved in Effective Assessment?

A comprehensive assessment of headache typically requires that the patient self-monitor their headache, complete a battery of headache specific and more global measures of function and undergo a diagnostic interview. While the ordering of assessment is left up to the clinician it is often efficient and cost-effective to have self monitoring and self-report measures completed in the week prior to the diagnostic interview.

Clinician-administered measures Depending on the level of breadth and specificity of information gathered from self-report instruments, the information gathered from the interview can duplicate that obtained from self-report instruments to a considerable extent. Such duplication allows for a measure of the consistency of patient report of headache, the clarification of discrepancies and omissions in reporting due to confusion or misreading, and identifying individual and environmental variables that may account for some precipitous change in the patient's headache between assessment points.

Self-report measures When completing a self-report headache diary, the patient may be asked to include information about the quality of a headache, pain experienced, treatment employed, and antecedent circumstances. The quality of a headache includes duration (e.g., minutes, days) and warning signs (e.g., nausea, photophobia); headache pain includes the type (e.g., piercing, throbbing), intensity (usually a 6–9 point rating scale), and location of the pain (e.g., between eyes, back of head); treatment includes the treatment employed (e.g., medication, behavioral techniques, rest) and treatment effectiveness (e.g., did it work, how well); and assessment of the common antecedent triggers such as sleep (e.g., time, quality), diet (e.g., chocolate, aged cheese, monosodium glutamate), and stressful events (e.g., work, life stress).

Headache specific measures generally assess the parameters of the headache experience, and the impact of the headache experience on the individual's functioning across various life domains. The most commonly used headache-specific measures include: the Migraine Disability Assessment (MIDAS; Stewart, Lipton, Simon, Von Korff, & Liberman, 1998; Stewart, Lipton, Kolodner, Liberman, & Sawyer, 1999); the Migraine-Specific Quality of Life Questionnaire (MSQ; Jhingran, Osterhaus, Miller, Lee, & Kirchdoerfer, 1998); the Headache Disability Inventory (HDI; Jacobsen, Ramadan, Aggarwal, & Newman, 1994); the Migraine Work and Productivity Loss Questionnaire (MWPLQ; Davies, Santanello, Gerth, Lerner, & Block, 1999); and the Headache Impact Test (HIT; Bjorner, Kosinski, & Ware, 2003). The MIDAS is particularly useful in the context of health care provision and clinical research as it assesses information about headache-related disability that only about one-third of patients commonly volunteer; and this information, when provided, is described by physicians as being primary in assessing a patient's treatment needs (Lipton, Stewart, Sawyer, & Edmeads, 2001). The HIT is noteworthy because of its accessibility to and use by patients. The HIT is a reliable and valid computerized adaptive tool designed to assess impact of headache on patient functional health and well-being (Holroyd, 2002; Lipton, Bigal, Amatniek, & Stewart, 2004).

Behavioral assessment Because recurrent headache disorder is characterized by the frequency of occurrence of headache pain, the clinician is often in the position of engaging with the patient while headache pain is active. Such occasions serve as an opportunity to observe both verbal and nonverbal pain behaviors and to obtain real time data related to the impact of headache pain on the patient's engagement in routine activities.

What assessments are Not Helpful?

Although traditional measures of psychological dysfunction such as the MMPI are useful in evaluating response styles that may exacerbate and maintain headache pain, such instruments should not be used as stand alone instruments in the evaluation of characteristic headache pain and the associated life disruptions.

TREATMENT

What Treatments are Effective?

Behavioral management of headache includes three empirically supported methods of intervention: relaxation training, biofeedback (frequently administered with relaxation training), and cognitive-behavioral therapy (or stress-management) (Campbell, Penzien, & Wall, 2000; Goslin, Gray, & McCrory, 1999; Holroyd, 2002). Although all of these strategies may be implemented across migraine and tension-type headaches, the application of these strategies and their primacy in clinical management of these two headache disorders will be reviewed separately. The four empirically supported treatments for migraine headache are, (1) relaxation training (PRT), (2) thermal biofeedback combined with relaxation training (TBF), (3) electromyographic biofeedback (EMG-BF), and 4) cognitive-behavioral therapy (CBT) (Campbell et al., 2000). The four empirically supported treatments for tension-type headache are, (1) PRT, (2) EMG-BF, (3) EMG-BF plus PRT, and (4) CBT (Campbell, et al., 2000; McCrory, Penzien, Hasselblad, & Gray, 2001). In a number of more inclusive meta-analyses of the headache treatment literature, EMG-BF, relaxation therapy, and a combination of the two are found to be most effective of all behavioral techniques reviewed (Blanchard, Andrasik, Ahles, Teders, & O'Keefe, 1980; Bogaards, & ter Kuile, 1994; Holroyd, & Penzien, 1986). An evidence report of behavioral and physical treatments for migraines was prepared by the Agency for Health Care Policy and Research (AHCPR) and is available for download from their web site (http://www.clinpl.mc. duke.edu; Goslin, Gray, & McCrory, 1999). An evidence report of behavioral treatments for tension-type headache was prepared by the Agency for Health Care Research and Quality (McCrory et al., 2001) and is available for review. Readers who are interested in a more detailed explication of the strategies used in establishing the evidence for the effectiveness of the psychological treatments for both migraine and tension-type headache are referred to the sources above, as well as Holroyd's (2002) review of the assessment and management of recurrent headache disorders.

What are Effective Self-Help Treatments?

Patients usually report the use of rest and over-the-counter medications to relieve headache pain. Activity scheduling and a balance between stressful and leisure activities, sufficient sleep, and decreased caffeine consumption are all self-help treatments that can assist in reducing a person's headache related pain. Listed below are several self-help books and Internet sites that may be helpful to clients who are seeking psychoeducation about the triggers and course of their recurrent headache, who would like to establish a relationship with other members of the community who suffer from recurrent headache disorders, and who are looking for strategies that may assist them in coping and managing their recurrent headache. These self-help resources have not been empirically evaluated for effectiveness. The client's should use author credentials (e.g., doctoral or medical degrees and citation of empirical studies) and website host credentials (e.g., university or federal affiliation) as guidelines in their selection of self-help material.

Self-Help Books

- Swanson, J. W. (2004). *Mayo clinic on headaches: Manage headache pain and reduce its impact on your daily life.* New York: Kensington Publishing.

- Kandel, J., & Sudderth, D. B. (2000). *Migraine what works! A complete guide to overcoming and preventing pain.* Roseville, CA: Prima Publishing.
- Constantine, L. M., & Scott, S. (1994). Migraine: *The complete comprehensive resource book for people with migraine, their families, and physicians.* New York: Bantam Doubleday Dell Publishing Group.
- Stafford, D., & Shoquist, J. (2003). *Migraine for dummies.* Indianapolis, IN: Wiley Publishing.
- Fox, B., & Mauskop, A. (2001). *What your doctor may not tell you about migraines: The breakthrough program that can help end your pain.* New York: Warner Books.
- Buchholz, D., & Reich, S. (2002). *Heal your headache: The 1–2–3 program for taking charge of you pain.* New York: Workman Press.
- Bic, Z., & Bic L. (1999). *No more headaches no more migraines.* New York: Avery Publishing Group.

Self-Help Websites
- *http://www.headache-help.org* (Help for Headaches)
- *http://www.achenet.org* (The American Council for Headache Education)
- *http://www.headaches.org* (National Headache Foundation)
- *http://www.ahsnet.org* (American Headache Society)
- *http://www.migrainetrust.org* (The Migraine Trust)
- *http://www.ninds.nih.gov* (The National Institute of Neurological Disorders and Stroke)
- *http://www.painandhealth.org* (The Mayday Pain Project)
- *http://www.headachecentral.net* (Michigan Headache Treatment Network)
- *http://www.healingwell.com* (Healing Well Online Support and Information)
- *http://www.headachecare.com* (Headache Care Center)

What are Effective Therapist Based Treatments?

Both migraine and tension-type headaches are responsive to behavioral treatments. When treating recurrent headache disorders, the techniques employed differ more in their primacy of application than the specifics of the procedures used. Therefore, with the exception of TBF, the treatments described below will be assumed to apply to the management of both migraine and tension-type headache.

Relaxation training Today there are many clinical and nonclinical relaxation techniques employed to relieve the tension and stress experienced in people's lives. The most frequently employed relaxation technique is progressive muscle relaxation training (PRT; Jacobsen, 1938). Since the origin of PRT there have been a number of adaptations to its execution (Wolpe, 1990; Poppen, 1988; and Bernstein, & Borkovec, 1973). These adaptations overlap to a considerable extent, differing in subtle specifics of execution more than anything else. Bernstein and Borkovec (1973) present PRT as including a comprehensive rationale, a specific training procedure, and explicit requirements for practice of tension and release of muscle groups. The rationale for PRT includes: 1) an introduction to the concept of the stress response, with emphasis placed on the physiological component of the stress response ; 2) an identification of the skeletomuscular system as a physiological response system that is particularly amenable to voluntary control; and 3) an explication of the synergy that exists among response channels, that synergy allowing total system changes in stress level to occur as a function of targeting and exerting voluntary control over the skeletomuscular response channel. Patients are taught to increase and release muscle tension in various muscle groups and to attend to and contrast feelings of tension and relaxation in the various muscle groups. Patients are then assigned the task of monitoring and measuring their basal level of muscle tension and using this index of excessive basal arousal

TABLE 57.3 Tension-Release Cycles for 16 PRT Muscle Groups

The tension-release cycle in the order conducted for a right hand dominant person are as follows:

1. (Dominant hand and forearm) Right lower arm and hand: make a tight fist with your right hand; tense the right hand and lower arm. Relax the muscles you have tensed.

2. (Dominant bicep) Right upper arm: push your elbow down and back against the chair; tense your upper arm. Relax these muscles.

3. (Nondominant hand and forearm) Lower left arm and hand: make a tight fist with your left hand; tense the left hand and lower arm. Relax the muscles you have tensed.

4. (Nondominant bicep) Left upper arm: push your elbow down and back against the chair; tense your upper arm. Relax these muscles.

5. Forehead: lift your eyebrows as high as possible; tense the muscles in your forehead. Relax.

6. Cheeks and upper face: squint your eyes and wrinkle your nose; tense the muscles in your upper cheeks and jaw. Relax.

7. Lower face and jaws: clench your teeth and pull the corners of your mouth backward in an exaggerated grin; tense the muscles in your lower face and jaw. Relax.

8. Neck: pull your chin toward your chest while keeping it from touching your chest; tense the muscles in your neck. Relax.

9. Chest, shoulders, and upper back: pull your shoulder blades together; tense the muscles in your chest, shoulders, and upper back. Relax.

10. Stomach: take a deep breath and hold it. While making your stomach hard; tense your stomach muscles. Then breathe out and relax.

11. (Dominant thigh) Right upper leg: lifting your right leg slightly off the chair, tense the muscles of your right upper leg. Relax.

12. (Dominant calf) Right calf: extend your right leg and pull your toes toward your head; tense the muscles in your right calf. Relax these muscles.

13. (Dominant foot) Right foot: straighten your right leg, turn your foot down and inward, and curling your toes, tense your right foot. Relax.

14. (Nondominant thigh) Left upper leg: lift your left leg slightly off the chair, tense the muscles of your left upper leg. Relax these muscles.

15. (Nondominant calf) Left calf: extend your left leg and pull your toes toward your head; tense the muscles in your left calf. Relax.

16. (Nondominant foot) Left foot: straighten your left leg, turning your foot down and inward, and curling your toes, tense your left foot. Relax.

Source: Berstein and Borkovec (1973) adapted by Penzien and Holroyd (1994).

as a cue for practice of PRT. Finally, patients are provided information regarding the proper context for employing PRT. The patient should not use PRT to manage situations involving extreme anxiety or extreme stress. PRT should be practiced as a strategy for reducing baseline levels of tension and arousal and to manage mild to moderate increases in anxiety or tension.

The initial PRT training procedure for all 16-muscle groups is provided in Table 57.3. With practice, these muscle groups can be condensed to 7 or 4 muscle groups and these groups cue full relaxation. Bernstein and Borkovec (1973) emphasize the necessity of home practice. It is critical that the patient understands the nature of PRT and makes a commitment to participate in their self-management; this is all the more necessary if they have a therapeutic history of passive therapies (pharmaceuticals and bed-rest).

PRT can be delivered using a variety of protocols including a group or individual format, and training occurring in 6–12 sessions over a 6-week to 3-month period, or in a minimal contact treatment format. The minimal contact procedure includes an introduction to the PRT skills in the clinic and the greater part of the skill acquisition is done by the patient at home using instruction manuals and audiotapes (Blanchard et al., 1990; Penzien, & Holroyd, 1994).

Biofeedback When training a headache patient to use biofeedback strategies in the prevention or management of recurrent headache, the techniques allow a patient to manage their physiology through control of peripheral temperature in thermal biofeedback (TBF) and muscle tension of the head and neck in electromyographic biofeedback (EMG-BF). The actual physiological response channel being targeting for observation and manipulation is determined by headache type with biofeedback for migraine headache targeting thermal and skeleto-muscular responses, and biofeedback for tension-type headache targeting the skeleto-muscular responses.

There are a number of distinct types of biofeedback used to treat migraine headaches: TBF, EMG-BF, autogenic feedback, blood volume pulse biofeedback, and transcranial doppler biofeedback. Research shows TBF and EMG-BF to be empirically supported (Campbell et al., 2000). TBF employs measurement of peripheral temperature as an indirect measure of peripheral vasoconstriction (Peek, 1995). Vasoconstriction has been implicated in the onset and severity of migraine headache disorders. Consequently, management of temperature through TBF correlates with management of vasoconstriction and a decrease in the severity and or duration of a patient's migraine headache. EMB-BF is typically used to treat tension-type headaches; however, it has also been endorsed as an empirically supported treatment for migraine (Campbell, et al., 2000; Goslin et al., 1999). Similar to the role of peripheral temperature in migraine, recordings of muscle contraction are used to provide observable evidence of muscle activity, and act as a component of migraine headache that can be manipulated. Although the exact mechanism acting in TBF and EMG-BF is unclear, most research shows that biofeedback training helps patients gain increased awareness and voluntary control of their autonomic functioning (Rokicki et al., 1997; French, Gauthier, Roberge, Bouchard, et al., 1997). This awareness and control has been found to reliably decrease headache frequency and duration. There are a number of physiological and cognitive changes that occur when a patient undergoes biofeedback. These changes include such things as enhanced confidence and self-efficacy, which promotes more varied and active attempts to cope (Rokicki et al., 1997).

Thermal biofeedback combined with relaxation training People with migraine headaches can learn hand-warming or thermal biofeedback (TBF) skills in a group or individual format. Generally, the trained biofeedback therapists offer 6–12 treatment sessions over a 6-week to 3-month period of time. A training session in the clinic generally lasts from 30 minutes to 1 hour. Research also shows that TBF can be successfully and cost-effectively delivered in a minimal contact format (Blanchard et al., 1985). Research also shows that while TBF alone produces a reduction in the frequency of migraine headache; it is most effective when combined with a relaxation component (Blanchard et al., 1982). TBF may be combined with autogenic therapy to form what is often termed "autogenic feedback." Autogenic training involves the repetition of phrases such as "I feel quiet . . . I am beginning to feel quite relaxed . . . My hands and arms are heavy and warm . . . I feel quite peaceful and calm . . ." that seem to help a person to raise the temperature of their peripheral limbs (Penzien, & Holroyd, 1994).

Patients should be reminded that these skills are learned and must be practiced at home to become effective at managing their headache. Use of a biofeedback practice log may be useful in getting a patient to practice at home and monitor their progress. Thermal biofeedback works best if employed in the early stages of a headache, when the headache-related physiology is still increasing (Schwartz, 1995). The hand-warming skills should be used whenever a patient notices that their hands are cool, or they are beginning to get a headache. If used preventatively, the person may stave-off a migraine episode.

EMG biofeedback In current EMG-BF approaches, it is common to create an individualized assessment of muscle tension and place the electrodes at the appropriate muscle locations; the patient is then given information (in the form of an auditory tone that is directionally proportional to the tension level of the muscles) about the ongoing level of muscle activity in this area. The patient is then coached in strategies facilitating relaxation and reduction in muscle tension level, and a resultant decrease in headache activity (Andrasik, 1992).

Cognitive-behavioral therapy Many chronic pain patients feel hopeless, helpless, and demoralized. Patients who are severely impeded by their negative thoughts and beliefs about their headache, disability, and quality of life due to their headache may benefit from CBT. In a headache context, CBT is used to teach patients skills for identifying and controlling stress and the effects of stress on their body. These patients are encouraged to develop a positive expectation about their headache and to adopt a sense of self-control. An underlying assumption of CBT as it applies to headache treatment is that the way a patient copes with stress (both environmental and headache-related stress) influences the production and the course of headache and headache-related disability (Holroyd et al., 2001; Mosley, Grotheus, & Meeks, 1995). CBT has been shown to be effective as a primary and adjunct therapy in the behavioral management of migraine (Goslin et al., 1999). Appelbaum et al. (1990) propose that a patient's perception and experience of stressful situations accounts for the worsening and/or maintenance of headaches. Automatic thoughts that accompany perceptions may mediate stress reactivity and headache onset. In tension-type headaches, one of two factors may be mediating the headache experience: (1) the individual's perception of a lack of control when facing these stressful situations; and (2) the chronic muscle tension and arousal that occurs in response to these situations.

CBT in the treatment of headache can be conceptualized as a stress-management therapy aimed at teaching a patient the skills necessary to manage the pain and disability associated with their headache. Stress management includes four components: (1) a psychoeducational overview of the biopsychosocial model of stress; (2) creation of a behavioral plan that lists concrete cognitive and behavioral strategies to be employed to reduce their stress and tension (if a patient can eliminate the stressor then they should do so, if the stressor cannot be eliminated then the patient should avoid contact or interaction with the stressor, if the stressor cannot be eliminated or avoided then attempts should be made to reduce the impact of the stressor); (3) implementation of lifestyle changes around health promoting behavior (more leisure time, reduce time spent in proximity to the stressor, or increase time for relaxation or exercise); and (4) education around lifestyle trends contributing to headache initiation and maintenance (problem solving techniques, practice cognitive restructuring strategies, or practice mindfulness).

What is Effective Medical Treatment?

Preventative drugs are used to reduce migraine severity, frequency, and duration (Silbertein, & Goadsby, 2002). Indications for the use of preventative drugs (β-adrenergic blockers, antidepressants, calcium-channel antagonists, serotonin antagonists, anticonvulsants, and nonsteroidal antiinflammatory drugs) includes migraine headaches that interfere with patient's daily life, a migraine that is recurrent despite routine acute treatment, problems with or overuse of acute drugs, or very frequent headaches (more than two per week) (Silberstein, 2003).

If a migraine headache occurs it is treated with acute or abortive drugs (ergots and triptans), or nonspecific drugs (analgesics and opioids) (Silberstein, 2003). Nonspecific drugs are used to control pain disorders and therefore the pain of migraine. Specific drugs are effective for migraine headache attacks, but not effective for nonheadache disorders. Triptans, the most frequently used abortive drugs, are effective in the treatment of a range of mild to severe migraine attacks (Lipton, Stewart, Cady, et al., 2000). Using a stepped care approach to migraine treatment, analgesics can be used for the treatment of mild to moderate headaches; and triptans are first-line drugs for severe attacks or less-severe attacks that are not responding to analgesics (Lipton, Stewart, Stone, Lainez, & Sawyer, 2000). If these treatments fail then rescue drugs (opioids, neuroleptics, and corticosteroids) are needed (Silbertein, 2003). Although these drugs do provide pain relief because of their sedating effects, they often cause severe restrictions in functioning, as well as unpleasant side effects.

There are a dearth of studies that investigate specific pharmacotherapies for tension-type headache (Stillman, 2002; Zhao, & Stillman, 2003). Most of the pharmacotherapy drugs used to treat tension-type headache are available in over-the-counter generic forms, and are unprofitable. The few studies that exist to evaluate the effectiveness of traditional drug therapies find that the standard drug classes, tricyclic antidepressants, and nonsteroidal antiinflammatory drugs are most effective. Currently, research is pointing to the potential usefulness of botulinum toxin type A, magnesium, and nitric synthase inhibitors (Sycha, Kranz, Auff, & Schnider, 2004).

Combination Treatments

Research trials have found the addition of drug therapy to one of the psychological forms of migraine treatment (PRT, TBF, or CBT) to be beneficial (Holroyd, 2002). Within these trials, drug treatment alone and combined drug and psychological treatments were comparable in their effectiveness for migraine symptom reduction. Initially, it appears that the combination of drug and psychological treatment for tension-type headache is more successful than either of the treatments alone; however, over time the advantage of the combined therapy seems to diminish. The effectiveness of combined treatment is equal to biofeedback alone. Overall the combined treatment appears to be better for tension-headache.

Other Issues in Management

Medical treatment If a client has a history of pharmacological management of headache pain and if the client is on a cocktail of pain medications at the point of assessment by the clinician, support from a medical professional may be needed in determining a schedule of titration for getting the patient off of certain medications, many of which are associated with headache rebound, sleep disturbances, impaired cognitive, and motor functioning.

Psychological treatment. For recurrent headache sufferers, the experience of headache pain can sometimes be interpreted as a signal of lifestyle imbalance, in attempting to continue functioning without addressing this imbalance, the patient may continue to engage in headache sustaining activities such as caffeine use and smoking.

How Does One Select Among Treatments?

Characteristics of headache and history of previous treatments direct initial treatment approach, with modifications to the treatment package being based on ongoing evaluation of changes in headache pain and functional status over the course of treatment.

In spite of advances in medicine most individuals with recurrent headache disorder still do not have the means to effectively manage their headaches. Furthermore, up to a third of patients who receive medical care for headaches discontinue treatment because they are unsatisfied with their care (Edmeads et al., 1993). Effective management of recurrent headache disorder lies in the integration of biological and psychosocial approaches aimed at increasing management of headache related pain and impairment and decreasing health reducing behaviors such as smoking and drinking.

REFERENCES

Self help books listed in text are not listed here.

Abu-Arefeh, I., & Russell, G. (1994). Prevalence of headache and migraine in schoolchildren. *British Medical Journal, 309,* 765–769.

Appelbaum, K. A., Blanchard, E. B., Nicholson, N. L., Radnitz, C., Michultka, D., Attanasio, V., et al. (1990). Controlled evaluation of the addition of cognitive strategies to a home-based relaxation protocol for tension headache. *Behavior Therapy, 21,* 293–303.

Andrasik, F. (1992). Assessment of patients with headaches. In D. C. Turk & R. Melzack (Eds.), *Handbook of pain assessment* (pp. 213–239). New York: Springer.

Barlow, C. F. (1994). Migraine in the infant and toddler. *Journal of Child Neurology, 9,* 92–94.

Berstein, D. A., & Borkovec, T. D. (1973). *Progressive relaxation training: A manual for the helping professions.* Champaign, IL: Research Press.

Bjorner, J. B., Kosinski, M., & Ware, J. E. (2003). Calibration of an item pool for assessing the burden of headaches: An application of item response theory to the Headache Impact Test (HIT™). *Quality of Life Research, 12,* 913–933.

Blanchard, E. B., Andrasik, F., Ahles, T. A., Teders, S. J., & O'Keefe, D. M. (1980). Migraine and tension headache: A meta-analytic review. *Behavior Therapy, 11,* 613–631.

Blanchard, E. B., Andrasik, F., Appelbaum, K. A., Evans, D. D., Jurish, S. E., Teders, S. J., et al. (1985). The efficacy and cost-effectiveness of minimal-therapist-contact, non-drug treatments of chronic migraine and tension-headache. *Headache, 25,* 214–220.

Blanchard, E. B., Andrasik, F., Neff, D. F., Arena, J. G., Ahles, T. A., Jurish, S. E., et al. (1982). Biofeedback and relaxation training with three kinds of headache: Treatment effects and their prediction. *Journal of Consulting and Clinical Psychology, 50,* 562–575.

Blanchard, E. B., Appelbaum, K. A., Radnitz, C. L., Michultka, D., Morrill, B., Kirsch, C. et al. (1990). Placebo-controlled evaluation of abbreviated progressive muscle relaxation and of relaxation combined with cognitive therapy in the treatment of tension headache. *Journal of Consulting and Clinical Psychology, 58(2),* 210–215.

Bogaards, M. C., & ter Kuile, M. M. (1994). Treatment of recurrent tension headache: A meta-analytic review. *Clinical Journal of Pain, 10,* 174–190.

Breslau, N., & Davis, G. C. (1993). Migraine, major depression and panic disorder: A prospective epidemiologic study of young adults. *Cephalalgia, 12,* 85–90.

Breslau, N., Davis, G. C., Schultz, L. R., & Peterson, E. L. (1994). Migraine and major depression: A longitudinal study. *Headache, 34,* 387–393.

Breslau, N., Davis, G. C., & Andreski, P. (1991). Migraine, psychiatric disorders, and suicide attempts: An epidemiologic study of young adults. *Psychiatry Research, 37(1),* 11–23.

Breslau, N., Lipton, R. B., Stewart, W. F., Schultz, L. R., & Welch, K. M. A. (2003). Comorbidity of migraine and depression. *Neurology, 60,* 1308–1312.

Breslau, N., Merikangas, K., & Bowden, C. L. (1994). Comorbidity of migraine and major affective disorders. *Neurology, 44(Suppl 7),* S17–S22.

Campbell, J. K., Penzien, D. B., & Wall, E. M. (2000). *Evidence-based guidelines for migraine headache: Behavioral and physical treatments.* US Headache Consortium. Retrieved April 7, 2004, from *http://www.aan.com/public/practiceguidelines/headache_gl.htm*

Davies, G. M., Santanello, N., Gerth, W., Lerner, D., & Block, G. A. (1999). Validation of a migraine work and productivity loss questionnaire for use in migraine studies. *Cephalalgia, 19,* 497–502.

Edmeads, J., Findlay, H., Tugwell, P., Pryse-Phillips, W., Nelson, R. F., & Murray, T. J. (1993). Impact of migraine and tension-type headache on life-style, consulting behavior, and medication use: A Canadian population survey. *Canadian Journal of Neurological Science, 19(3)*, 333–339.

French, D. J., Gauthier, J. G., Roberge, C., Bouchard, S., et al., (1997). Self-efficacy in the thermal biofeedback treatment of migraine sufferers. *Behavior Therapy, 28(1)*, 109–125.

Gerth, W. C., Carides, G. W., Dasbach, E. J., Visser, W. H., & Santanello, N. C. (2001). The multinational impact of migraine symptoms on healthcare utilisation and work loss. *Pharmacoeconomics, 19(2)*, 197–206.

Goslin, R., Gray, R., & McCrory, D. (1999) *Behavioral and physical treatments for migraine headache* (Technical Review 2.2). Retrieved April 7, 2004, Available: http://www.clinpol.mc.duke.edu

Hagen, K., Zwart, J-A., Vatten, L., Stovner, L. J., & Bovim, G. (2000). Prevalence of migraine and non-migrainous headache—head-HUNT, a large population-based study. *Cephalalgia, 20*, 900–906.

Holroyd, K. A. (2002). Assessment and psychological management of recurrent headache disorders. *Journal of Consulting and Clinical Psychology, 70(3)*, 656–677.

Holroyd, K. A., O'Donnell, F. J., Stensland, M., Lipchik, G. L., Cordingley, G. E., & Carlson, B. (2001). Management of chronic tension-type headache with tricyclic antidepressant medication, stress-management therapy, and their combination: A randomized controlled trial. *JAMA, 285*, 2208–2215.

Holroyd, K. A., & Penzien, D. (1986). Client variables in the behavioral treatment of recurrent tension headache: A meta-analytic review. *Journal of Behavioral Medicine, 9*, 515–536.

Holroyd, K. A, & Penzien, D. B. (1994). Psychosocial interventions in the management of recurrent headache disorders. 1: Overview and effectiveness. *Behavioral Medicine, 20(2)*, 53–63.

Holroyd, K. A., Stensland, M., Lipchik, G. L., Hill, K. R., O'Donnell, F. S., & Cordingley, G. (2000). Psychosocial correlates and impact of chronic-tension-type headaches. *Headache, 40*, 3–16.

International Headache Society. (2004). The international classification of headache disorders, (2nd ed). *Cephalalgia, 24(Suppl 1)*.

Jacobsen, E. (1938). *Progressive Relaxation*. Chicago: University of Chicago.

Jacobsen, G. P., & Ramadan, N. M., Aggarwal, S. K., & Newman, C. W. (1994). The Henry Ford Hospital Headache Disability Inventory (HDI). *Neurology, 44*, 837–842.

Jhingran, P., Osterhaus, J. T., Miller, D. W., Lee, J. T., Kirchdoerfer, L. (1998). Development and validation of the Migraine-Specific Quality of Life Questionnaire. *Headache, 38*, 295–302.

Launer, L. J., Terwindt, G. M., & Ferrari, M. D. (1999). The prevalence and characteristics of migraine in a population-based cohort: The GEM Study. *Neurology, 53(3)*, 537–542.

Lipton, R. B. (1997). Diagnosis and epidemiology of pediatric migraine. *Current Opinion in Neurology, 10*, 231–236.

Lipton, R. B., Bigal, M. E., Amatniek, J. C., & Stewart, W. F. (2004). Tools for diagnosing migraine and measuring its severity. *Headache, 44*, 387–398.

Lipton, R. B., Stewart, W. F., Cady, R., Hall, C., O'Quinn, S., Kuhn, T., et al. (2000). Sumatriptan for the range of headaches in migraine sufferers: Results of the spectrum study. *Headache, 40*, 783–791.

Lipton, R. B., Stewart, W. F., Diamond, S., Diamond, M. L., & Reed, M. (2001). Prevalence and burden of migraine in the United States: Data from the American Migraine Study II. *Headache, 41*, 646–657.

Lipton, R. B., Stewart, W. F., Sawer, J., & Edmeads, J. G. (2001). Clinical utility of an instrument assessing migraine disability: The Migraine Disability Assessment (MIDAS) Questionnaire. *Headache, 41*, 854–861.

Lipton, R. B., Stewart, W. F., Stone, A. M., Lainez, M. J. A., & Sawyer, J. P. C. (2000). Stratified care vs step care strategies for migraine: The disability in strategies of care (DISC) study: A randomized trial. *JAMA, 284*(20), 2599–2605.

Low, N. C. P., & Merikangas, K. R. (2003). The comorbidity of migraine. *CNS Spectrums, 8*(6), 433–444.

McCrory, D., Penzien, D., Hasselblad, V., & Gray, R. (2001). *Behavioral and physical treatments for tension-type and cervicogenic headache* (No. 2085). Des Moines, IA: Foundation for Chiropractic Education and Research.

Merikangas, K. R. (1994). Psychopathology and headache syndromes in the community. *Headache, 34*, S17–S26.

Merikangas, K. R., Angst, J., & Isler, H. (1990). Migraine and psychopathology: Results of the Zurich Cohort Study of Young Adults. *Archives of General Psychiatry, 47*, 849–853.

Merikangas, K. R., Merikangas, J. R., & Angst, J. (1993). Headache syndromes and psychiatric disorders: Association and familial transmission. *Journal of Psychiatric Research, 27(2)*, 197–210.

Merikangas, K. R., Stevens, D. E., & Angst, J. (1993). Headache and personality; Results of a community sample of young adults. *Journal of Psychiatric Research, 27(2)*, 187–196.

Mosley, T. H., Grothues, C. A., & Meeks, W. M. (1995). Treatment of tension headache in the elderly: A controlled evaluation of relaxation training and relaxation combined with cognitive–behavior therapy. *Journal of Clinical Geropsychology, 1*, 175–188.

Peek, C. J. (1995). A Primer of Biofeedback Instrumentation. In M. S. Schwartz (Ed.), *Biofeedback: A Practitioner's Guide, (2nd ed.*, pp. 47–48). New York: The Guilford Press.

Penzien, D. B., & Holroyd, K. A. (1994). Psychosocial interventions in the management of recurrent headache disorders 2: Descriptions of treatment techniques. *Behavioral Medicine, 20,* 64–73.

Poppen, R. (1988). Behavioral relaxation training and assessment. *Psychology practitioner guidebooks.* (p. 139). Elsmford, NY: Pergamon Press, Inc.

Pryse-Phillips, W., Findlay, H., Tugwell, P., Edmeads, J., Murray, T. J., & Nelson, R. F. (1992). A Canadian population survey on the clinical, epidemiologic and societal impact of migraine and tension-type headache. *The Canadian Journal of Neurological Sciences, 19,* 333–339.

Puca, F., Genco, S., Prudenzano, M. P., Savarese, M., Bussone, G., D'Amico, D., et al. (1999). Psychiatric comorbidity and psychosocial stress in patients with tension-type headache from headache centers in Italy. *Cephalalgia, 19,* 159–164.

Rasmussen, B. K. (2001). Epidemiology of headache. *Cephalalgia, 21,* 774–777.

Rasmussen, B. K., Jensen, R., & Olesen, J. (1992). Impact of headache on sickness absence and utilization of medical services: A Danish population study. *Journal of Epidemiological Community Health, 46(4),* 443–446.

Rokicki, L. A., Holroyd, K. A., France, C. R., Lipchik, G. L., France, J. L., & Kvaal, S. A. (1997). Change mechanisms associated with combined relaxation/EMG biofeedback training for chronic tension headache. *Applied Psychophysiology and Biofeedback, 22(1),* 21–41.

Russell, M. B., Rasmussen, B. K., Throvaldsen, P., & Olesen, J. (1995). Prevalence and sex-ratio of the stubtypes of migraine. *International Journal of Epidemiology, 24(3),* 612–618.

Schwartz, M. S. (1995). Headache: Selected issues and considerations in the evaluation and treatment. Part B: Treatment. *Biofeedback: A Practitioner's Guide, (2nd ed.* pp. 354–410). New York: The Guilford Press.

Schwartz, B. S., Stewart, W. F., Simon, D., & Lipton, R. B. (1998). Epidemiology of tension-type headache. *JAMA, 279(5),* 381–383.

Silberstein, S. D. (2003). Migraine. *Lancet, 363,* 381–391.

Silberstein, S. D., & Goadsby, P. J. (2002). Migraine: Preventive treatment. *Cephalalgia, 22,* 491–512.

Sillanpaa, M., & Anttila, P. (1996). Increasing prevalence of headache in 7-year old school-children. *Headache, 36,* 466–470.

Stewart, W. F., Lipton, R. B., Kolodner, K., Liberman, J., & Sawyer, J. (1999). Reliability of the migraine disability assessment score in a population-based sample of headache sufferers. *Cephalalgia, 19,* 107–114.

Stewart, W. F., Lipton, R. B., Simon, D., Von Korff, M., & Liberman, J. (1998). Reliability of an illness severity measure for headache in a population sample of migraine sufferers. *Cephalalgia, 18,* 44–51.

Stillman, M. J. (2002). Pharmacotherapy of tension-type headaches. *Current Pain and Headache Reports, 6(5),* 408–413.

Sycha, T., Kranz, G., Auff, E., & Schnider, P. (2004). Botulinum toxin in the treatment of rare head and neck pain syndromes: A systematic review of the literature. *Journal of Neurology, 251(Suppl. 1),* 1/19–1/30.

Wolpe, J. (1990). *The practice of behavior therapy, (4th ed.)* Elmsford, NY: Pergamon Press, Inc.

Zhao, C., & Stillman, M. J. (2003). New developments in the pharmacotherapy of tension-type headaches. *Expert Opinion in Pharmacotherapy, 4(12),* 2229–2237.

CHAPTER 58

Schizophrenia

Thea L. Rothmann • Srividya N. Iyer • Jason E. Peer • William D. Spaulding

WHAT IS SCHIZOPHRENIA?

Increasingly, research efforts in schizophrenia seek to understand schizophrenia not as a disorder with a single causal deficit but as a biosystemic disorder in which component processes are in a state of dysregulation (Spaulding, 1997). These components include processes related to neurophysiology (i.e., neurotransmitter systems), neurocognition (i.e., basic cognitive functions such as attention and memory), social cognition (i.e., higher order cognitive functions such as the formation of beliefs and abstract reasoning), and sociobehavioral functioning (i.e., performing behavioral activities in a socially meaningful context) (Spaulding, 1997; Spaulding, Sullivan, & Poland, 2003). By identifying the relative contribution of these multiple levels of functioning to the clinical impairments in schizophrenia, researchers can approach the investigation of schizophrenia with far greater precision (Spaulding et al., 2003).

The biosystemic conceptualization is directly informed by general systems theory which suggests that the pathology of schizophrenia is a result of biosystemic dysregulation (Ciompi, 1989; Spaulding, 1997; Strauss, 1989). Specifically, the nature of the course, the observed deficits, and recovery in schizophrenia are all reflections of varying degrees of dysregulation within the person (Ciompi, 1989; Spaulding, 1997; Spaulding et al., 2003) and between the person and their environment (Strauss, 1989). In biosystemic models of schizophrenia, dysregulation not only occurs within a given domain but *between* domains. Impairment does not proceed in a linear cascade from molecular to molar, but instead is a result of reciprocal interactions (Spaulding, 1997; Spaulding et al., 2003). Thus, dysregulation at any domain of functioning may affect performance in other domains and interventions targeting multiple domains are needed to reregulate the system.

BASIC FACTS ABOUT SCHIZOPHRENIA

Prevalence, Gender, Age of Onset, and Cost

Approximately 1% of the population develops schizophrenia in the course of a lifetime. The disorder affects men and women with equal frequency, but onset typically occurs earlier for men than women. Age of onset typically occurs in late adolescence or early adulthood, however, premorbid characteristics (e.g., impaired social functioning) are apparent in some, but not all, individuals during childhood. The Global Burden of Disease Study identified mental illness as one of the leading burdens of disease, second only to cardiovascular conditions (Murray & Lopez, 1996). The cost of mental illness in the United States is estimated at $79 billion each year, and there is no mental illness more costly to treat than schizophrenia (Hall & Graf, 2004).

Diagnosis and Symptomatology

Schizophrenia is now widely understood as a heterogeneous group of disorders rather than a specific disorder with clear, identifiable symptoms and etiological

Rothmann, T. L., Iyer, S. N., Peer, J. E., & Spaulding (2006). Schizophrenia. In J. E. Fisher & W. T. O'Donahue (Eds). *Practitioner's guide to evidenced-based psychotherapy*. New York: Springer.

patterns. Schizophrenia represents a profound disruption of the most fundamental human attributes: emotion, language, thought, and perception. The symptoms vary widely for each individual and no single symptom is definitive for diagnosis. Various combinations of persisting psychotic symptoms, along with impairments in daily functioning, make up the criteria typically used for diagnosis (American Psychiatric Association DSM-IV-TR, 2000). Symptoms have often been dichotomized into *positive* (features which are *added* to an individual's typical presentation) and negative symptoms (features which are *taken away*). Positive symptoms include delusions, hallucinations, and bizarre behaviors (e.g., posturing). Negative symptoms include alogia, avolition, psychomotor retardation, and flat affect. Positive symptoms are often considered more responsive to treatment, especially psychopharmacological treatment, but more variable over time. On the other hand, negative symptoms tend to be treatment-resistant and follow a more chronic and stable course.

There is discussion within the field regarding the need to include "disorganization" as a third category of symptoms. These symptoms include thought disorder, disorientation, and memory difficulties. Some argue that symptoms of disorganization are connected with another hallmark feature of schizophrenia, cognitive impairment. This includes difficulties with concept formation, abstract thinking, attention, and memory. Impairments in cognition, in conjunction with all the symptoms of schizophrenia, result in a gross disruption across most major areas of functioning, such as occupational, interpersonal, neurocognitive, and self-care. As described in the treatment section below, these functional impairments cannot be overlooked in the treatment of schizophrenia. In fact, these functional impairments represent the bulk of the treatment action particularly in a psychiatric rehabilitation framework.

In addition, people with schizophrenia also have significant mood symptoms, including anxiety and depression. Depression in schizophrenia is associated with its high suicide rate, one out of every ten individuals. Symptoms of anxiety are often related to paranoid delusions or hallucinations, but are also a result of impaired social skills. Substance abuse is the most common comorbid diagnosis with schizophrenia. However, treatments designed to address substance abuse problems have not demonstrated efficacy within this population (Drake & Mueser, 1996).

Etiology

It was generally accepted early in the twentieth century that schizophrenia had biological origins (Kraepelin, 1919/1971). In the 1950s and 1960s, many investigators hypothesized that schizophrenia resulted from disturbed family relationships (Bateson, Jackson, Haley, & Weakland, 1956). No data supports this hypothesis, although family interactions may influence the course of schizophrenia. Most current theories include interacting biological and environmental causes in *diathesis stress* models. Many studies of people with schizophrenia have found structural anatomic abnormalities (e.g., enlargement of cerebral ventricles and decrease of other brain regions) or brain function abnormalities (e.g., decreased metabolic activity in certain brain regions and abnormality of neurotransmitter activity across synapses). The most widely researched brain function abnormality in schizophrenia is dysregulation of dopaminergic activity (activity in neurons using dopamine as a neurotransmitter). The D2 dopamine receptor is especially implicated in this dysregulation, although there are probably numerous other mechanisms involved (Kapur & Mamo, 2003). Dysregulation of the mesolimbic dopamine subsystem is thought to be associated with positive psychotic symptoms, while negative symptoms and cognitive impairment appear more attributable to dysregulation of the mesocortical subsystem

(Stahl & Wets, 1988). Dopamine systems also play a key role in responding to stress in the normal brain, suggesting a link to the diathesis-stress nature of schizophrenia. There are numerous other hypotheses about neurophysiological dysregulation in schizophrenia, not necessarily incompatible with the dopamine hypothesis.

Neurodevelopmental theories identify neurobiological abnormalities present early in life which interact in the course of development to produce the actual illness (Green, 1998; de Haan & Bakker, 2004). Problems may not manifest until puberty or early adulthood, when environmental demands increase and as normal maturational brain changes interact adversely with developmental abnormalities. The origins of the early abnormalities may include genetic, viral, toxic, physical trauma, or stress factors. Neurodevelopmental models incorporate a diathesis-stress hypothesis, including such environmental factors as family interactions, negative or traumatic life events (Zubin & Steinhauer, 1981) and sociocultural factors such as ethnicity, and cultural background (Sartorius, et al., 1986).

Course and prognosis

Generally schizophrenia is understood to be an *episodic* disorder, meaning there are periods of acute exacerbations or *psychotic episodes* interspersed with relative stability. However, most individuals experience residual symptoms or cognitive impairments between episodes, sometimes so severe that the episodic course is obscured. A deteriorating course is classically considered a key feature in the diagnosis of schizophrenia (see McGlashan, 1998). However, research suggests a great deal of heterogeneity in the course patterns of schizophrenia. Several studies have found only a small portion of individuals with schizophrenia show a deteriorating course with most showing a stable or fluctuating course and some actually improving (Carpenter & Strauss, 1991; Harding, 1988; Mason et al., 1996; Quinlan, Schuldberg, Morgenstern & Glazer, 1995). The "Law of 1/3's" is often applied, meaning that about one third of people who develop schizophrenia have nearly complete remission with only mild relapses and little disruption to their daily lives, one third have a variable pattern of symptom exacerbation with more interruption to daily functioning, and one third have chronic symptoms that impair most aspects of daily life.

ASSESSMENT

What Should be Ruled Out?

Thorough assessment of schizophrenia must rule out other possible causes of the psychotic symptomatology of delusions, hallucinations, and bizarre behavior. These symptoms may manifest as a result of various conditions including, but not limited to, neurological conditions, delirium, dementia, drug intoxication, severe depression and bipolar disorder. One must also consider psychotic behavior which results from extreme situational factors such as stress and depression. Sometimes cultural factors contribute to the presence of behaviors perceived by others as psychotic (e.g., religious practices or beliefs). Finally, one must rule out malingering and/or the presence and contribution of personality disorders when assessing for schizophrenia.

What is Involved in Effective Assessment?

Diagnosis of schizophrenia does little to determine the treatment strategy that should be employed. Functional assessments that identify specific areas of vulnerability, impairment and relative strength are generally more informative. Since current conceptualizations of schizophrenia recognize that impairment occurs at multiple levels, assessment should likewise address multiple levels of functioning.

This includes assessing current symptoms, neurocognitive functioning, medication response, and side-effects, occupational functioning, social functioning, and history of treatment compliance. Family interaction and level of involvement is also an important area to be aware of in planning treatment. Finally, issues related to competency for the purpose of treatment decisions and possibly more general decision making should be considered. By identifying the relative contribution of these multiple levels of functioning to the clinical impairments in schizophrenia, researchers can approach the investigation and treatment of schizophrenia with far greater precision (Spaulding et al., 2003). To fully assess and treat each level of functioning, a multidisciplinary approach is necessary. Psychologists, social workers, occupational and recreational therapists, psychiatrists, nurses and others all contribute knowledge and expertise to a full assessment of schizophrenia. Algorithms for stepwise assessment and treatment application have been proposed (see Spaulding et al., 2003; Spaulding, Johnson, Coursey, 2001).

What Assessments are not Helpful?

Assessment which considers only current symptomatology usefully guides selection of pharmacological treatment, especially in an acute episode, but it does not effectively guide treatment or rehabilitation. Similarly psychiatric diagnosis, generally based on identification of the same symptoms as pharmacological treatment, provides too little information about functional assets and liabilities to guide a comprehensive treatment and rehabilitation approach

TREATMENT

The last three decades have been marked by significant advances in specific psychopharmacological and psychosocial treatments for schizophrenia (see American Psychological Association [APA], n.d.; Hofman & Thompson, 2002; Kendall, 1998; Lehman, Thompson, Dixon, & Scott, 1995; McEvoy, Scheifler, & Frances, 1999; Spaulding et al., 2003). Currently, treatments in schizophrenia are not viewed as a "cure" for the illness, but rather as strategies which help manage the illness and minimize disruption in life. Any specific treatment addresses only a subset of an individual's problems. As a group, people with schizophrenia have much in common, but at the same time each individual represents a unique set of impairments, requiring multiple approaches in varying combinations. *Psychiatric rehabilitation* (Wallace, Liberman, Kopelowicz & Yeager, 2001) has emerged as an approach to organizing a diversity of treatments for the purpose of overcoming disabilities, rather than "curing" the condition.

What Treatments are Effective?

From its beginnings four decades ago (e.g. Anthony, Buell, Sharratt, & Althoff, 1972; Paul & Lentz, 1977) psychiatric rehabilitation has evolved along with the specific technologies it incorporates (e.g. Liberman, 1972; Spaulding et al., 2003) toward an increasingly complex, but integrated approach. Psychiatric rehabilitation efforts, in general, target multiple levels of functioning to optimize treatment outcome and prevent relapse. Although state-of-the-art psychiatric rehabilitation is not universally available, for over 20 years now it has been practiced in many scattered venues, usually associated with academic research programs and/or academic/public sector collaborations (e.g. Bachrach, 1980; Talbott, 1981; Bond, Dincin, Setze, & Witheridge, 1984; Paul, 1984; Bellack & Mueser, 1986; Perris, 1992; Sullivan, Richardson, & Spaulding, 1991). While the treatment approaches below are discussed under the familiar headings of the chapters of this text, they are better understood as components of psychiatric rehabilitation. In this sense, one rarely chooses a single treatment from the list below, but rather chooses the most effective combination. This constitutes effective treatment of schizophrenia.

What are Effective Self-Help Treatments?

Individuals with severe mental illnesses such as schizophrenia are increasingly recognized as active participants in, rather than recipients of, mental health services. The last 25 years has seen a significant increase in the number of self-help programs for individuals with schizophrenia. The programs are increasingly recognized as beneficial for dispelling stigma surrounding schizophrenia, empowering individuals to decrease dependence and helplessness, and maintaining greater accountability within the mental health system and individual treatment programs. The services provided by consumer-run programs vary greatly. They may include case management, homeless services, crisis response, housing programs, benefits acquisition, peer support groups, employment, advocacy, and research. Because these programs vary greatly and also because they are a recent development within in the mental health system, the known efficacy is not well-established. The Substance Abuse and Mental Health Service Administration has recently issued a report reviewing a series of federally-funded demonstration self-help programs over the last two decades (Van Tosh & del Vecchio, 2000). The report also outlines the future direction of self-help programs. Self-help groups and client empowerment programs are currently advocated by organizations such as the National Alliance for the Mentally Ill (NAMI).

In addition to the overall movement of client empowerment and more active roles in treatment, there are isolated self-help strategies available to address specific symptoms. For example, self-help strategies for the management of auditory hallucinations have been proposed, especially by practitioners in England and Australia (for more information, see http://www.pwer2u.org/articles/selfhelp/voices.html).

Useful informational websites about schizophrenia and related resources include:

- http://www.nami.org/ (National Alliance for the Mentally Ill)
- http://www.narsad.org/ (National Alliance for Research on Schizophrenia and Depression)
- http://www.aabt.org/ (Association for the Advancement of Behavioral Therapy)
- http://www.power2u.org/index.html (National Empowerment Center)
- http://www.nimh.nih.gov/health information/schizophreniamenu.cfm (National Institute of Mental Health)
- http://www.brmh.org (Behavioral Health Recovery Management)

What are Effective Therapist Based Treatments?

Cognitive–behavioral therapy (CBT). The development of cognitive–behavioral strategies for schizophrenia has primarily occurred in Great Britain (for reviews, see Haddock, Tarrier, Spaulding, Yusupoff, Kinney, & McCarthy, 1998; Drury, Birchwood, Cochrane, & MacMillan, 1996) and is only recently gaining momentum in the United States. These strategies focus on key cognitions (e.g., voices or delusional beliefs) and behaviors (e.g., ways of coping with voices) similar to other cognitive–behavioral interventions (Kingdon, 2000). One of the primary differences between the strategies being employed in the United States and those in Great Britain is that the former include problem-solving strategies as a key component while the latter do not. Targeting problem-solving was found to be effective in improving social functioning and the strategy was rapidly assimilated into Social Skills Training (SST) and now in CBT interventions. Reviews of CBT interventions have found that they tend to be primarily effective at reducing psychotic symptoms (Bustillo, Lauriello, Horan, & Keith, 2001; Huxley, Rendall, & Sederer, 2000; Penn & Mueser, 1996).

Family intervention strategies. The original application of social learning principles to develop cognitive–behavioral family strategies for major mental disorders is typically credited to Liberman (1970). Since then, many researchers have developed interventions aimed towards treating families (for a review, see Lam, 1991). This is an important consideration since many adults with schizophrenia live with their families and the burden, stress, and guilt can be considerable. The development of empirically supported intervention strategies is largely credited to Ian R.H. Falloon, Gerard Hogarty, and their colleagues (Falloon, et al., 1985; Hogarty, et al., 1986). Family intervention strategies include a diverse array of components including psychoeducation about the disorder, social support, and development of coping, communication, and problem-solving skills.

Social skills training. Poor social functioning has been identified as a negative prognostic factor for schizophrenia (Strauss & Carpenter, 1974) and subtle premorbid signs of social dysfunction often precede onset of the disorder (Cornblatt et al., 2003). This understanding has made SST a primary treatment and rehabilitative strategy for people with schizophrenia. SST modalities have typically been found to be an effective intervention for social skills deficits associated with schizophrenia (Bustillo, et al., 2001; Heinssen, Liberman, & Kopelowicz, 2000; Penn & Mueser, 1996). SST interventions have been used to teach skills necessary for a range of functional behaviors, such as medication management or having a conversation (Heinssen, et al., 2000; Bellack, Mueser, Gingerich, & Agresta, 1997). Theoretically, SST interventions, often using techniques like role-play, improve social functioning by gradually and incrementally training patients in necessary molecular social skills until more complex social behavior can consistently be performed (Liberman et al., 1986).

Occupational skills training. Supported employment has found to be an effective intervention in schizophrenia (Drake, 1996). In addition, training in specific occupational skills (e.g., following directions, staying on task) has been found to improve work functioning and overall quality of life. Often, occupational skills training incorporates training in other instrumental role areas such as leisure and recreation.

Neurocognitive therapy. Neurocognitive impairments have been closely linked to functional impairments and can act as rate limiting factors for other forms of psychosocial interventions (Green, 1998). As such, these deficits have become the targets of a class of psychosocial interventions that produce improvement in both neurocognition and social functioning (Spaulding, Reed, Sullivan, Richardson, & Weiler, 1999). Strategies such as these are collectively referred to as neurocognitive therapy, cognitive training, cognitive remediation, or neurocognitive training. Specific strategies target verbal and visual memory, attention, cognitive flexibility, and mental state. A review of 17 studies found that cognitive training interventions can improve neurocognitive functioning and in turn improve functional behavior, and even reduce symptoms (Twamley, Jeste, & Bellack, 2004). Cognitive training also has been demonstrated to improve gains made in work rehabilitation (Bell, Bryson, Greig, Corcoran, & Wexler, 2001).

What is Effective Medical Treatment?

Psychopharmacological interventions. Antipsychotic drugs are almost always used to suppress psychotic symptoms and prevent relapses. It is not within the scope of this chapter to review these interventions, but interested readers are referred to the American Psychiatric Association guidelines (1997) regarding prescription of antipsychotic medications for schizophrenia. However, antipsychotic medications are rarely sufficient in and of themselves to treat all levels of functional impairment associated with this disorder. Researchers estimate that 25–50% of patients with schizophrenia experience residual medication resistant symptoms, which highlights the importance of psychosocial interventions (Garety, Fowler, & Kuipers, 2000; Spaulding, Johnson, & Coursey, 2001).

Other Issues in Management

Contingency management. Contingency management constitutes of group of techniques designed to increase adaptive behaviors and suppress maladaptive behaviors. These techniques, as well as social skills training, family intervention strategies, and other techniques described below were borne out of the social-learning theories of the 1960s and later informed by theories of operational learning. Contingency management for schizophrenia was first applied in the form of token economies (Ayllon & Azrin, 1968; Liberman, 1972). These techniques continue to be important in inpatient settings and have been effective for a variety of behaviors such as reducing aggression (Beck, Menditto, Baldwin, Angelone, & Maddox, 1991) and increasing participation in treatment (Paul & Menditto, 1992). Despite their utility, these techniques tend to be underused due to difficulties with implementation, mostly because of the amount of staff training and supervision required for ethical and effective application.

Case management and related services. Despite advances in treatment and rehabilitation strategies, outcomes remain modest, especially for the most severe psychiatric disorders, like schizophrenia (reviewed by Wallace et al, 2001). Ample data on the response of specific problems to various treatments, and common sense, have produced broad agreement that in practice a diverse armamentarium of credible treatments is better than any specific treatment alone. However, having a wide diversity of approaches makes it difficult to choose and apply them at appropriate and key points in an intervention plan. *Case management* services coordinate the efforts of interdisciplinary treatment teams to provide the most cost-effective treatment (Holloway, Oliver, Collins, & Carson, 1995: Mueser, Bond, Drake, & Resnick, 1998). Assertive Community Treatment (ACT) is a program closely linked to case management. ACT is designed to provide comprehensive rehabilitation services including case management and psychiatric services in an outpatient setting. There have been inconsistent results about the effectiveness of this approach (see Mueser et al., 1998 for a review).

How Does One Select Among Treatments?

Treatment must target the impaired domains of functioning for each individual. Current conceptualizations of schizophrenia, as previously described, require interventions targeting multiple domains to re-regulate the system. As such, the process of recovery in schizophrenia reflects varying degrees and timing of reorganization across these domains. Recovery in one domain can impact other domains and recovery can occur at different rates depending on the phase of disorder (acute or postacute). With this conceptualization of schizophrenia, it is necessary to use multiple treatments systematically to address multiple problems. Often these multiple treatments must delivered flexibly over a sustained duration of time to ensure reorganization and recovery as well as to prevent psychotic relapse.

REFERENCES

American Psychiatric Association (1997). Practice guidelines for the treatment of patients with schizophrenia. *American Journal of Psychiatry, 154(Suppl. 4)*, 1–63.

American Psychiatric Association (2000). *Diagnostic and statistical manual of mental disorders* (4th ed., text revision). Washington, DC: Author.

American Psychological Association, Division 12 (n.d.). *Empirically supported treatments*. Retrieved June 6, 2004, from http://www.apa.org/divisions/div12/rev_est/index.html.

Anthony, W., Buell, G., Sharratt, S., & Althoff, M. (1972). Efficacy of psychiatric rehabilitation. *Psychological Bulletin, 78*, 447–456.

Ayllon, T., & Azrin, N. (1968). *The token economy: A motivational system for therapy and rehabilitation*. New York: Appleton-Century-Crofts.

Bachrach, L. (1980). Model programs for chronic mental patients. *American Journal of Psychiatry, 137*, 1023–1031.

Bateson, G., Jackson, D., Haley, J., & Weakland, J. H. (1956). Toward a theory of schizophrenia. *Behavioral Science, 1*, 251–264.

Beck, N., Menditto, A., Baldwin, L., Angelone, E., & Maddox, M. (1991). Reduced frequency of aggressive behavior in forensic patients in a social learning program. *Hospital and Community Psychiatry, 42*, 750–752.

Bell, M., Bryson, G., Greig, T., Corcoran, C., & Wexler, B. (2001). Neurocognitive enhancement therapy with work therapy: Effects on neurocognitive test performance. *Archives of General Psychiatry, 58*, 763–768.

Bellack, A., & Mueser, K. (1986). A comprehensive treatment program for schizophrenia and chronic mental illness. *Community Mental Health Journal, 22*, 175–189.

Bellack, A. S., Mueser, K. T., Gingerich, S., & Agresta, J. (1997). *Social skills training for schizophrenia: A step-by-step guide*. New York: Guilford Press.

Bond, G., Dincin, J., Setze, P., & Witheridge, T. (1984). The effectiveness of psychiatric rehabilitation: A summary of research at thresholds. *Psychosocial Rehabilitation Journal, 7*, 6–22.

Bustillo, J. R., Lauriello, J., Horan, W. P., & Keith, S. J. (2001). The psychosocial treatment of schizophrenia: An update. *American Journal of Psychiatry, 158*, 163–175.

Carpenter, W. T., & Strauss, J. S. (1991). The prediction of outcome in schizophrenia: IV. Eleven year follow-up of the Washington IPSS cohort. *Journal of Nervous and Mental Disease, 179*, 517–525.

Ciompi, L. (1989). The dynamics of complex biological–psychosocial systems: four fundamental psycho-biological mediators in the long-term evolution of schizophrenia. *British Journal of Psychiatry, 155(Suppl. 5)*, 15–21.

Cornblatt, B. A., Lencz, T., Smith, C. W., Correll, C. U., Auther, A. M., & Nakayama, E. (2003). The schizophrenia prodrome revisited: A neurodevelopmental perspective. *Schizophrenia Bulletin, 29*(4), 633–651.

de Haan, L., & Bakker, J. M. (2004). Overview of neuropathological theories of schizophrenia: From degeneration to progressive developmental disorder. *Psychopathology, 37*, 1–7.

Drake, R. E. (1996). Day treatment versus supported employment for persons with severe mental illness: A replication study. *Psychiatric Services, 47*(10), 1125–1127.

Drake, R., & Mueser, K. (1996). *Dual diagnosis of major mental illness and substance abuse disorder. II: Recent research and clinical implications. New directions in mental health services*. San Francisco: Jossey-Bass.

Drury, V., Birchwood, M., Cochrane, R., & MacMillan, F. (1996). Cognitive therapy and recovery from psychosis: A controlled trial. I: Impact on schizophrenic symptoms. *British Journal of Psychiatry, 169*, 593–601.

Falloon, R. H., Boyd, J. L., McGill, C. W, Williamson, M., Razani, A., Moss, H. B. et al. (1985). Family management in the prevention of morbidity of schizophrenia: Clinical outcome of a two-year longitudinal study. *Archives of General Psychiatry, 42*, 887–896.

Garety, P. A., Fowler, D., & Kuipers, E. (2000). Cognitive-behavioral therapy for medication resistant symptoms. *Schizophrenia Bulletin, 26*, 73–86.

Green, M. (1998). *Schizophenia as a neurocognitive disorder*. Boston: Ayllon & Bacon.

Haddock, G., Tarrier, N., Spaulding, W., Yusupoff, L., Kinney, S., & McCarthy, E. (1998). Individual cognitive–behavioral therapy in the treatment of hallucinations and delusions: A review. *Clinical Psychology Review, 18*(7), 821–838.

Hall, L., & Graf, A. (2004, February). *Roadmap to recovery and cure: Final report of the NAMI policy research institute task force on serious mental illness research*. Arlington, VA: National Alliance for the Mentally IL.

Harding, C. M. (1988). Course types in schizophrenia: An analysis of European and American studies. *Schizophrenia Bulletin, 14*, 633–642.

Heinssen, R. K., Liberman, R. P., & Kopelowicz, A. (2000). Psychosocial skills training for schizophrenia: Lessons from the laboratory. *Schizophrenia Bulletin, 26,* 21–46.

Hofman, S. G., & Tompson, M. C. (2002). *Treating chronic and severe mental disorders: A handbook of empirically supported interventions.* New York: Guilford Press.

Hogarty, G., Anderson, C., Reiss, D., Kornblith, S., Greenwald, D., Javna, C., et al. (1986). Family psychoeducation, social skills training, and maintenance chemotherapy in the aftercare treatment of schizophrenia: One-year effects of a controlled study on relapse and expressed emotion. *Archives of General Psychiatry, 43,* 633–642.

Holloway, F., Oliver, N., Collins, E., & Carson, J. (1995). Case management: A critical review of the outcome literature. *European Psychiatry, 10,* 113–128.

Huxley, N., Rendall, M., & Sederer, L. (2000). Psychosocial treatments in schizophrenia: A review of the past 20 years. *Journal of Nervous and Mental Disease, 188,* 187–201.

Kapur, S., & Mamo, D. (2003). Half a century of antipsychotics and still a central role for dopamine D2 receptors. *Progress in Neuropsychopharmacology & Biological Psychiatry, 27*(7), 1081–1090.

Kendall, P. C. (1998). Empirically supported psychological therapies. *Journal of Consulting and Clinical Psychology.*

Kingdon, D. (2000). Cognitive–behavior therapy of schizophrenia. *Directions in Psychiatry, 20,* 265–273.

Kraepelin, E. (1919/1971). *Dementia praecox and paraphrenia* (R. M. Barclay, Trans.). New York: Kreiger.

Lam, D. (1991). Psychosocial family intervention in schizophrenia: A review of empirical studies. *Psychological Medicine, 211,* 423–441.

Lehman, A. F., Thompson, J. W., Dixon, L. B., & Scott, J. E. (1995). Introduction. Schizophrenia: Treatment outcomes research. *Schizophrenia Bulletin, 21,* 561–566.

Liberman, R. P. (1970). Behavioral approaches to family and couple therapy. *American Journal of Orthopsychiatry, 40,* 106–118.

Liberman, R. P. (1972). Behavioral modification of schizophrenia: A review. *Schizophrenia Bulletin, 1*(6), 37–48.

Liberman, R. P., Mueser, K. T., Wallace, C. J., Jacobs, H. E., Eckman, T., & Massel, H. K. (1986). Training skills in the psychiatrically disabled: Learning coping and competence. *Schizophrenia Bulletin, 12,* 631–647.

Mason, P., Harrison, G., Glazebrook, C., Medley, I., et al. (1996). The course of schizophrenia over 13 years: A report from the international study on schizophrenia (ISOS) coordinated by the world health organization. *British Journal of Psychiatry, 169,* 580–586.

McEvoy, J., Scheifler, P., & Frances, A. (Eds.). (1999). Treatment of schizophrenia. *Journal of Clinical Psychiatry, 60(Suppl. 11),* 4–80.

McGlashan, T. (1998). The profiles of clinical deterioration in schizophrenia. *Journal of Psychiatric Research, 32,* 133–141.

Mueser, K., Bond, G., Drake, R., & Resnick, S. (1998). Models of community care for severe mental illness: A review of research on case management. *Schizophrenia Bulletin, 24,* 37–73.

Murray, C. J. L., & Lopez, A. D. (Eds.). (1996). *The global burden of disease and injury series, volume 1: A comprehensive assessment of mortality and disability from diseases, injuries, and risk factors in 1990 and projected to 2020.* Cambridge, MA: Published by the Harvard School of Public Health on behalf of the World Health Organization and the World Bank, Harvard University Press.

Paul, G. L. (1984). Residential treatment programs and after care for the chronically institutionalized. In M. Mirabi (Ed.), *The chronically mentally ill: Research and services.* New York: S. P. Medical & Scientific Books.

Paul, G., & Menditto, A. (1992). Effectiveness of inpatient treatment programs for mentally ill adults in public psychiatry facilities. *Applied and Preventive Psychology, 1,* 41–63.

Paul, G. L., & Lentz, R. J. (1977). *Psychosocial treatment of chronic mental patients: Milieu vs. social learning programs.* Cambridge, MA: Harvard University Press.

Penn, D. L., & Mueser, K. T. (1996). Research update on the psychosocial treatment of schizophrenia. *American Journal of Psychiatry, 153,* 607–617.

Perris, C. (1992). A cognitive–behavioral treatment program for patients with a schizophrenic disorder. In R. P. Liberman (Ed.), *Effective psychiatric rehabilitation* (Vol. 53, pp. 7–20). San Francisco: Jossey-Bass.

Poland, J., Von Eckardy, B., & Spaulding, W. (1994). Problems with the DSM approach to classifying psychopathology. In G. Graham & G. L. Stephens (Eds.). *Philosophical psychopathology.* Cambridge, MA: The MIT Press.

Quinlan, D., Schuldberg, D., Morgenstern, H., & Glazer, W. (1995). Positive and negative symptom course in chronic community based patients: A two-year prospective study. *British Journal of Psychiatry, 166,* 634–641.

Sartorius, N., Jablensky, A., Korten, A., Ernberg, G., Anker, M., Cooper, J. E., et al. (1986). Early manifestations and first-contact incidence of schizophrenia in different cultures. *Psychological Medicine, 16,* 909–928.

Spaulding, W., Johnson, D., & Coursey, R. (2001). Treatment and rehabilitation of schizophrenia. In M. Sammons & N. Schmidt (Eds.), *Combined treatments for mental disorders: A guide to psychological and pharmacological interventions*. Washington, DC: American Psychological Association.

Spaulding, W. D. (1997). Cognitive models in a fuller understanding of schizophrenia. *Psychiatry, 60*, 341–346.

Spaulding, W. D., Reed, D., Sullivan, M., Richardson, C., & Weiler, M. (1999). Effects of cognitive treatment in psychiatric rehabilitation. *Schizophrenia Bulletin, 25*(4), 657–676.

Spaulding, W. D., Sullivan, M. E., & Poland, J. S. (2003). *Treatment and rehabilitation of severe mental illness*. New York: Guildford Press.

Stahl, S. M., & Wets, K. M. (1988). Clinical pharmacology of schizophrenia. In P. Bebbington & P. McGuffin (Eds.), *Schizophrenia: The major issues* (pp. 135–136). Oxford, England: Heinemann Professional Publishing.

Strauss, J. S., & Carpenter, W. T. (1974). The prediction of outcome in schizophrenia II: Relationships between predictors and outcome variables. *Archives of General Psychiatry, 31*, 37–42.

Strauss, J. S. (1989). Mediating processes in schizophrenia toward a new dynamic psychiatry. *British Journal of Psychiatry, 155 (Suppl. 5)*, 22–28.

Sullivan, M., Richardson, C., & Spaulding, W. (1991). University-state hospital collaboration in an inpatient psychiatric rehabilitation program. *Community Mental Health Journal, 27*(6), 441–453.

Talbott, J. E. (1981). *Chronic mental patients: Treatment, programs, systems*. New York: Human Services Press.

Twamley, E. W., Jeste, D. V., & Bellack, A. S. (2003). A review of cognitive training in schizophrenia. *Schizophrenia Bulletin, 29*, 359–382.

Van Tosh, L., & del Vecchio, P. (2000). *Consumer-operated self-help programs: A technical report*. US Center for Mental Health Services. Rockville, MD.

Wallace, C. J., Liberman, R. P., Kopelowicz, A., & Yaeger, D. (2001). Psychiatric rehabilitation. In G. O. Gabbard (Ed.), *Treatment of psychiatric disorders* (3rd ed., pp.1093–1112). Washington, DC, American Psychiatric Publishing.

Zubin, J., & Steinhauer, S. (1981). How to break the logjam in schizophrenia. *Journal of Nervous and Mental Disease, 169*, 477–492.

Schizotypal Personality Disorder

Irwin S. Rosenfarb • Michael A. Juan

WHAT IS SCHIZOTYPAL PERSONALITY DISORDER?

Schizotypal personality disorder (SPD) is characterized by a pervasive pattern of cognitive or perceptual distortions, eccentricities of behavior, and discomfort in close relationships. This persistent style must begin by early adulthood and be present across a wide variety of contexts (APA, 2000). Cognitive or perceptual distortions may include ideas of reference (e.g., "That person on the TV was talking directly to me."), odd beliefs (e.g., "I feel an evil presence in this room."), and magical thinking (e.g., the individual believes that he or she is clairvoyant or has telepathic abilities). Eccentricities of behavior include odd dress (e.g., wearing a heavy coat in the middle of the summer) or odd speech (using words in a unusual context or having loose or tangential associations among ideas). Social discomfort may include having few or no close friends, excessive anxiety around other people, and paranoid fears about others.

Research suggests that first-degree relatives of individuals with schizophrenia are at increased risk of developing SPD (Asarnow et al., 2001; Kendler, Gruenberg, & Strauss, 1981; Onstad, Skre, Lowing, Mirsky, & Kringlen, 1991). In addition, first-degree biological relatives of those with SPD are at increased risk of developing schizophrenia (Battaglia et al., 1991; Siever et al., 1990; Thaker, Adami, Moran, Lahti, & Cassady, 1993). Thus, there is a clear genetic link between SPD and schizophrenia and SPD is often referred to as a "schizophrenia-spectrum disorder" or a "schizophrenia-related personality disorder." In addition, research also suggests that those with SPD are at an increased risk of developing schizophrenia in the future (Fenton & McGlashan, 1989; Mason et al., 2004; Weiser et al., 2001). The number of individuals with SPD, however, who will go on to develop schizophrenia is unclear.

Research suggests three dominant factors or dimensions define SPD: positive symptoms (e.g., hallucinations, delusions, odd beliefs), negative symptoms (e.g., restricted affect, social avoidance, avolition) and conceptual disorganization (odd speech and behavior) (Chen, Hsiao, & Lin, 1997; Fossati, Raine, Carretta, Leonardi, & Maffei, 2003; Raine, 1991). Research also suggests that these three dimensions are present in schizophrenia (e.g., Andreasen, Arnott, Alliger, Miller, & Flaum, 1995; Ratakonda, Gorman, Yale, & Amador, 1998). Thus, symptoms are organized similarly in SPD and schizophrenia which suggests that SPD may represent an attenuated or mild form of schizophrenia (Lenzenweger, 1999).

BASIC FACTS ABOUT STPD

- There is approximately a 1% prevalence rate of schizotypal personality disorder in the general population (Torgersen, Kringlen, & Cramer, 2001).
- Schizotypal personality disorder has been associated with increased rates of substance abuse and dependence, childhood trauma, and cooccurring mood disorders (McGlashan et al., 2000; Bornstein, Klein, Mallon, & Slater, 1988; Berenbaum, Valera, & Kerns, 2003).

Rosenfarb, I. S., & Juan, M. A. (2006). Schizotypal personality disorder. In J. E. Fisher & W. T. O'Donohue (Eds.), *Practitioner's guide to evidence-based psychotherapy*. New York: Springer.

- Positive symptoms, such as ideas of reference, tend to be more common in women while negative symptoms, such as isolation and lack of close friendships, tend to be more common in men (Raine, 1992).
- The large Collaborative Longitudinal Personality Disorders study (McGlashan et al., 2000; n=668) found that those diagnosed with SPD could also be diagnosed with an average of 2.4 additional Personality Disorders. The most common additional diagnoses were Avoidant PD (49%) and Paranoid PD (36%). In addition, 66% of those with SPD were also diagnosed with Major Depressive Disorder and 41% with Panic Disorder.
- African Americans tend to be diagnosed with SPD more frequently than Whites (Chavira et al., 2003). The reasons for this are unclear.

ASSESSMENT

What Should be Ruled Out?

Schizophrenia. The primary distinction between SPD and Schizophrenia is in the severity of symptoms and the period of symptom expression. SPD symptoms tend to be less severe than symptoms of schizophrenia. In schizophrenia, for example, delusions tend to be well-formed and pervasive. Paranoid delusions in schizophrenia, for example, may dominate a person's life and affect all of their interactions with others. In SPD, however, the paranoi may occur only in certain contexts. Moreover, the onset of schizophrenia must be preceded by a clear deterioration in the level of one's social or occupational functioning. In SPD, however, symptoms are usually present for many years and there is no clear deterioration in functioning.

Major depressive disorder (MDD) with psychotic features. In MDD with psychotic features, the depressed mood tends to dominate and the psychotic features (hallucinations and/or delusions) are secondary to the depression. The psychotic features occur only when the individual is depressed and the hallucinations and/or delusions typically have a depressive theme (e.g., "God is punishing me for my sins"). Moreover, as with schizophrenia, in MDD, there is a clear deterioration of functioning prior to or concordant with the onset of symptoms.

Schizoid personality disorder. As with SPD, schizoid PD is characterized by the absence of a desire to develop close interpersonal relationships. Individuals with schizoid PD, however, lack the cognitive or perceptual distortions and the marked peculiarity or oddness of SPD. One characteristic that distinguishes the two disorders is "eccentricity." Eccentric or odd traits are associated only with SPD. These eccentricities may be manifested behaviorally, perceptually, and/or interpersonally.

Borderline personality disorder (BPD). Individuals with BPD may have psychotic symptoms that may look similar to the symptoms of SPD. In BPD, however, psychotic symptoms tend to be transient while in SPD, subclinical psychotic features are a core part of the disorder. In addition, in BPD, hallucinations and/or delusions are often secondary to affective mood changes and are usually associated with changes in mood (e.g., paranoid symptoms and/or hearing voices to harm others after interpersonal rejection). Moreover, individuals with SPD often have little desire to develop and tend to avoid close interpersonal relationships while those with BPD typically have a strong desire for intimacy and closeness.

WHAT IS INVOLVED IN EFFECTIVE ASSESSMENT?

The Structured Clinical Interview for DSM-IV Personality Disorders (Pfohl, Blum, & Zimmerman, 1995) is the most effective way to assess SPD. Individuals with SPD, however, may deny or minimize symptoms because of their level of discomfort in social situations. Thus, it is important to develop adequate rapport with clients before attempting to obtain an accurate diagnosis. It is also important to take one's subculture into account when diagnosing SPD. Odd or unusual beliefs that seem abnormal may be prevalent in one's subculture.

The schizotypal personality questionnaire (Raine, 1991). The SPQ is a 74-item, self report questionnaire developed to assess an individual on the nine domains of the DSM-IV criteria for SPD. The scale has been shown to have good internal and test–retest reliability and to correlate well with interview measures of SPD (Raine, 1991). The test has also been translated into Italian (Fossati, Raine, Carretta, Leonardi, & Maffei, 2003), German (Klein, Andresen, & Jahn, 1997), French (Dumas, Bouifia, Gutknecht, Sauod, & Damato 2000), Chinese (Chen et al., 1997), and Greek (Stefanis et al., 2004). A 22-item brief version of the test has also been developed (Raine & Benishey, 1995) which has been shown to have good reliability and validity with an adolescent inpatient population (Axelrod, Grilo, Sanislow, & McGlashan, 2001).

WHAT ASSESSMENTS ARE NOT HELPFUL?

Although neuropsychological assessments may be helpful in assessing neurocognitive functions central to the schizophrenia-spectrum disorders (Barch et al., in press), no guidelines has been established for their use in assessing SPD. Similarly, projective testing may be helpful as the open-ended nature of these instruments may allow individuals with SPD to demonstrate odd perceptual experiences or unusual thinking. Moreover, these tests provide little information with which to "fake good" (Perry, Minassian, Cadenhead, Sprock, & Braff, 2003). As with neuropsychological assessments, however, no empirical research has demonstrated the usefulness of projective testing in assessing SPD.

TREATMENT

What Treatments are Effective?

Most individuals with SPD never come to treatment because of their high anxiety in social situations. There are several empirical studies, however, which suggest that the combination of antipsychotic medication and cognitive–behavior therapy may be most effective with this population. In addition, since family psychoeducation has the greatest research base of any psychosocial treatment for schizophrenia (McFarlane, Dixon, Lukens, & Lucksted, 2003), this treatment may also be effective in treating SPD.

Cognitive–Behavior Therapy McGorry et al. (2002) have developed a specially designed clinic, known as the PACE (Personal Assessment and Crisis Evaluation) clinic to treat individuals at "ultra-high-risk" of developing schizophrenia. Although the clinic does not specifically target individuals with SPD, those with a family history of schizophrenia as well as individuals with attenuated or subclinical positive psychotic symptoms are included. Thus, many of the patients in their clinic may be diagnosed with SPD. Treatment consisted of respiridone (see below) and cognitive–behavior therapy. The specific cognitive–behavioral treatment was tailored to each individual patient, but included stress management, coping with positive symptoms, and cognitive–behavioral strategies for dealing with depression, substance abuse, and social anxiety. Results of a randomly controlled trial indicated that, compared with supportive treatment alone, this combination treatment significantly reduced the risk of transition to psychosis over a one-year period.

Morrison et al. (2004) attempted to determine whether cognitive therapy alone (with no medication) could prevent the onset of psychotic symptoms in individuals at "ultra-high risk" of developing schizophrenia. As with the McGorry et al. (2002) study, the treatment did not specifically target individuals with SPD. Yet, since their inclusion criteria were identical to those used in the previous study, many individuals with SPD were most likely included in their sample. Treatment consisted of up to 26 individual sessions over a six month period and followed the guidelines developed by Beck (see Beck, Freeman, & Davis, 2004). The central features of the treatment included normalizing the interpretations patients make for psychotic symptoms, helping patients develop alternative explanations for events and then test out those alternative explanations, and decatastrophizing fears about "being crazy." Results of a randomly controlled trial indicated that this treatment significantly improved positive symptoms, significantly reduced the likelihood of clients being prescribed antipsychotic medication, and significantly decreased the likelihood of clients developing a DSM-IV psychotic disorder over a 12 month period. Thus, cognitive therapy alone, without antipsychotic medication, appears to be an efficacious treatment for this population.

Pharmacotherapy–Antipsychotics Second generation antipsychotics have been implicated as effective forms of intervention for this population. Koenigsberg, Reynolds, & Goodman. (2003) randomly assigned 25 patients with SPD to receive either low-dose respiridone or a placebo in a double-blind manner. Results of the study indicated that respiridone was significantly more effective than a placebo in reducing both positive and negative symptoms over a 9-week period. Keshavan, Shad, Soloff, and Schooler (2004) conducted a 26-week open-label study of olanzapine with 11 patients with SPD. Results indicated that patients showed significant reductions in psychotic symptoms and depression as well as a significant improvement in overall level of functioning. Finally, as mentioned previously, McGorry et al. (2002), in a randomly controlled trial, found open-label respiridone, in combination with cognitive-behavior therapy, significantly reduced the onset of psychotic symptoms in patients at ultra-high risk of developing schizophrenia over a 12 month period.

It should be noted, however, that the use of antipsychotics with this population has been controversial, especially with patients who have had stable psychotic symptoms for long periods of time (Bentall & Morrison, 2002). There are multiple side effects to these medications including sexual dysfunction, significant weight gain, and an increased risk of developing diabetes. Moreover, the long-term effect of these medications on brain development, especially in adolescents or young adults, is unknown. These risks, however, must be balanced against the pernicious effects of developing schizophrenia on both psychosocial functioning and brain development.

Family psychoeducational treatment As mentioned previously, family psychoeducational treatments have the greatest research support of any psychosocial intervention in schizophrenia (McFarlane et al., 2003). There have now been more than 30 randomized controlled trials showing that family psychoeducation can significantly reduce relapse risk in schizophrenia. Although the specific components of treatment that are most effective are unclear at this time, most treatments include psychoeducation on the symptoms of the disorder, and help families improve their communication and problem-solving skills.

What are Effective Self-Help Treatments?

To our knowledge, there are no self-help treatments designed specifically for individuals with SPD. Several books, however, that may be helpful to individuals with schizophrenia and their families may also be helpful to this population. *Surviving schizophrenia: A manual for families, consumers, and providers* (Torrey, 2001) is now in its fourth edition and is considered the "Bible" of self-help books on schizophrenia. Although heavily focused on biological aspects of the disorder, the book contains much useful information on the causes, symptoms, and treatments of the disorder, as well as useful information for families of patients. *Diagnosis Schizophrenia* (Miller & Mason, 2002) includes 35 first-person accounts by individuals with schizophrenia as well as good information on medications, ways to cope with the disorder, and how to obtain adequate social services. Finally, *I am Not Sick I Don't Need Help!* by Amador and Johanson (2000) may be useful in helping those with SPD accept their disorder and consent to needed treatments.

Conclusion

The relatively small body of research in schizotypal personality disorder has left many questions unanswered. In recent years, however, interest has increased greatly as researchers continue to examine the close link between SPD and schizophrenia. Much important recent research has attempted to identify individuals with SPD who may develop schizophrenia in the future and intervene early to prevent the onset of florid psychotic symptoms. Although this research is still in its infancy, this is a an exciting and productive time for clinicians and researchers working in this area.

Useful Websites

http://www-rcf.usc.edu/%7Eraine/spq.htm. A sample version of the Schizotypal Personality Questionnaire.

http://www.schizophrenia.com. Excellent information, support, and education for those affected by the disorder and their family members.

http://www.toad.net/~arcturus/dd/schtypal.htm. A very good informational Web site that also addresses substance use issues with this population.

http://council.nami.org/programs.html. A very influential national organization providing information to consumers. NAMI also offers support groups for consumers and their families.

http://www.narsad.org/. The National Alliance for Research on Schizophrenia and Depression. A good overview of current research in this area.

REFERENCES

Amador, X., & Johanson, A. (2000). *I am not sick, I don't need help! Helping the seriously mentally ill accept treatment.* Peconic, NY: Vida Press.

American Psychiatric Association. (2000). *Diagnostic and Statistical Manual of Mental Disorders* (4th ed. text rev.). Washington, DC: Author.

Andreasen, N. C., Arndt, S., Alliger, R., Miller, D., & Flaum, M. (1995). Symptoms of schizophrenia: Methods, meanings, and mechanisms. *Archives of General Psychiatry, 52,* 341–351.

Asarnow, R. F., Nuechterlein, K. H., Fogelson, D., Subotnik, K. L., Payne, D. A., Russell, A. T., et al. (2001). Schizophrenia and schizophrenia-spectrum personality disorders in the first-degree relatives of children with schizophrenia: The UCLA family study. *Archives of General Psychiatry, 58,* 581–588.

Axelrod, S. R., Grilo, C. M., Sanislow, C., & McGlashan, T. H. (2001). Schizotypal Personality Questionnaire-Brief: Factor structure and convergent validity in inpatient adolescents. *Journal of Personality Disorders, 15,* 168–179.

Barch, D. M., Mitropoulou, V., Harvey, P. D., New, A. S., Silverman, J. M., & Siever, L. J. (in press). Context processing deficits in schizotypal personality disorder. *Journal of Abnormal Psychology.*

Battaglia, M., Gasperini, M., Sciuto, G., Scherillo, P., Diaferia, G., & Bellodim L. (1991). Psychiatric disorders in the families of schizotypal subjects. *Schizophrenia Bulletin, 17,* 659–668.

Beck, A. T., Freeman, A., & Davis, D. D. (2004). *Cognitive Therapy of Personality Disorders* (3rd ed.). New York: Guilford Press

Bentall, R. P, & Morrison, A. (2002). More harm than good: The case against using antipsychotic drugs to prevent severe mental illness. *Journal of Mental Health, 11,* 351–356.

Berenbaum, H., Valera, E. M., & Kerns, J. G. (2003). Psychological trauma and schizotypal symptoms. *Schizophrenia Bulletin, (29),* 143–152.

Bornstein, R. F., Klein, D. N., Mallon, J. C., & Slater, J. F. (1988). Schizotypal personality disorder in an outpatient population: Incidence and clinical characteristics. *Journal of Clinical Psychology, 4,* 322–325.

Chavira, D. A., Grilo, C. M., Shea, M. T., Yen, S., Gunderson, J. G., Morey, L., et al. (2003). Ethnicity and four personality disorders. *Comprehensive Psychiatry, 44,* 483–491.

Chen, W. J., Hsiao, C. K., & Lin, C. H. (1997). Schizotypy in community samples: The three-factor structure and correlation with sustained attention. *Journal of Abnormal Psychology, 106,* 649–654.

Dumas, P., Bouafia, S., Gutknecht, C., Sauod, M., & Damato, T. (2000). Schizotypal Personality Questionnaire (SPQ): Validation and factorial structure of its French translation in a sample of 232 students. *Encephale, 26),* 23–29.

Fenton, W., & McGlashan, T. (1989). Risk of schizophrenia in character disordered patients. *American Journal of Psychiatry, 146,* 1280–1284.

Fossati, A., Raine, A., Carretta, I., Leonardi, B., & Maffei, C. (2003). The three-factor model of schizotypal personality: Invariance across age and gender. *Personality & Individual Differences, 35,* 1007–1019.

Kendler, K. S., Gruenberg, A. M., & Strauss, J. S. (1981). An independent analysis of the Copenhagen sample of the Danish adoption study of schizophrenia. II. The relationship between schizotypal personality disorder and schizophrenia. *Archives of General Psychiatry, 38,* 982–984.

Keshavan, M., Shad, M., Soloff, P., & Schooler, N. (2004). Efficacy and tolerability of olanzapine in the treatment of schizotypal personality disorder. *Schizophrenia Research, 71,* 97–101.

Klein, C., Andresen, B., & Jahn, T. (1997). Psychometric assessment of the schizotypal personality according to DSM-III-R criteria: Psychometric properties of an authorized German translation of Raine's "Schizotypal Personality Questionnaire" (SPQ). *Diagnostica, 43,* 347–369.

Koenigsberg, H. W., Reynolds, D., & Goodman, M. (2003). Risperidone in the treatment of schizotypal personality disorder. *Journal of Clinical Psychiatry, 64(6),* 628–634.

Lenzenweger, M. F. (1999). Schizotypic psychopathology: Theory, evidence, and future directions. In T. Millon, P. H. & Blaney, P. H. (Eds), *Oxford textbook of psychopathology,* (pp. 605–627). London: Oxford University Press.

Mason, O., Startup, M., Halpin, S., Schall, U., Conrad, A., & Carr, V. (2004). Risk factors for transition to first episode psychosis among individuals with 'at-risk mental states'. *Schizophrenia Research, 71,* 227–237.

McFarlane, W. R., Dixon, L., Lukens E., & Lucksted, A. (2003). Family psychoeducation and schizophrenia: A review of the literature. *Journal of Marital and Family Therapy, 29,* 223–245.

McGlashan, T. H., Grilo, C. M., Skodol, A. E., Gunderson, J. G., Shea, M. T., Morey, L. C., et al. (2000). The collaborative longitudinal personality disorders study: Baseline axis I/II and II/II diagnostic co-occurrence. *Acta Psychiatrica Scandinavica, 102,* 256–264.

McGorry, P. D., Yung, A. R., Phillips, L. J., Yuen, H. P., Francey, S., Cosgrave, E. M., et al. (2002). Randomized controlled trial of interventions designed to reduce the risk of progression to first-episode psychosis in a clinical sample with subthreshold symptoms. *Archives of General Psychiatry, 59,* 921–928.

Miller, R., & Mason, S. E. (2002). *Diagnosis Schizophrenia.* New York: Columbia University Press.

Morrison A. P., French, P., Walford, L., Lewis, S. W., Kilcommons, A., Green, J., et al. (2004). Cognitive therapy for the prevention of psychosis in people at ultra-high risk: Randomised controlled trial. *British Journal of Psychiatry, 185,* 291–297.

Onstad, S., Skre, I., Edvardsen, J., Torgersen, S., & Kringlen, E. (1991). Mental disorders in first-degree relatives of schizophrenics. *Acta Psychiatrica Scandinavia, 83,* 463–467.

Perry, W., Minassian, A., Cadenhead, K., Sprock, J., & Braff, D. (2003). The use of the ego impairment index across the schizophrenia spectrum. *Journal of Personality Assessment, 80(1),* 50–57.

Pfohl, B., Blum, N., & Zimmerman, M. (1995). *Structured interview for DSM-IV personality disorders.* Iowa City: University of Iowa.

Raine, A. (1991). The SPQ: A scale for the assessment of schizotypal personality based on DSM-III-R Criteria. *Schizophrenia Bulletin, 17(4),* 555–564

Raine, A. (1992). Sex differences in schizotypal personality in a nonclinical population. *Journal of Abnormal Psychology, 101,* 361–364.

Raine, A., & Benishay, D. (1995), The SPQ-B: A brief screening instrument for schizotypal personality disorder. *Journal of Personality Disorders, 9,* 346–355.

Ratakonda S, Gorman, J. M., Yale, S. A., & Amador X. F. (1998). Characterization of psychotic conditions. Use of the domains of psychopathology model. *Archives of General Psychiatry, 55,* 75–81.

Reynolds, C. A., Raine, A., Mellingen, K., Venables, P. H., & Mednick, S. A. (2000). Three-factor model of schizotypal personality: Invariance across culture, gender, religious affiliation, family adversity, and psychopathology. *Schizophrenia Bulletin, 26,* 603–618.

Siever, L. J., Silverman, J. M., Horvath, T. B., Klarm H., Coccaro, E., Keefe, R. S., et al. (1990). Increased morbid risk for schizophrenia-related disorders in relatives of schizotypal personality disordered patients. *Archives of General Psychiatry, 47,* 634–640.

Thaker, G., Adami, H., Moran, M., Lahti, A., & Cassady, S. (1993). Psychiatric illnesses in families of subjects with schizophrenia-spectrum personality disorders: high morbidity risks for unspecified functional psychoses and schizophrenia. *American Journal of Psychiatry, 150,* 66–71.

Stefanis, N. C., Delespaul, P., Lembesi, A., Avramopoulos, D. A., Evdokimidis, I. K., et al. (2004). Is the excess risk of psychosis-like experiences in urban areas attributable to altered cognitive development? *Social Psychiatry & Psychiatric Epidemiology, 39,* 364–368.

Torgersen, S., Kringlen, E., & Cramer, V. (2001). The prevalence of personality disorders in a community sample. *Archives of General Psychiatry, 58,* 590–596.

Torrey, E. F. (2001). *Surviving schizophrenia: A manual for families, consumers, and providers* (4th ed.). New York: Harper Perennial.

Weiser, M., Reichenberg, A., Rabinowitz, J., Kaplan, Z., Mark, M., Bodner, E., et al. (2001). Association between nonpsychotic psychiatric diagnoses in adolescent males and subsequent onset of schizophrenia. *Archives of General Psychiatry, 58,* 959–964.

CHAPTER 60

School Refusal

David Heyne

INTRODUCTION

While most children and adolescents attend school regularly and without difficulty, there is a sizable group of young people who experience what can be regarded as a school attendance problem. Kearney (2003) proposed a distinction between non-problematic and problematic absenteeism, whereby young people with problematic absenteeism were defined as those who: "(a) have missed most (i.e., >50%) school time for at least 2 weeks and/or (b) experience difficulty attending school for at least 2 weeks such that significant interference occurs in the child's or the family's daily life routine" (p. 59). Further, with respect to point (a), the absences are not due to factors which parents and school officials regard as legitimate, such as illness or arrangements for home schooling. Even though the definition includes a non-specific criteria (i.e., significant interference in daily life), it goes a long way towards helping to bring much needed consensus to the important field of school attendance problems.

Terms and Definitions

An inordinate number of terms has been used in association with school attendance problems, including "disallowed absence," "truancy," "psychoneurotic truancy," "school phobia," "school refusal," "separation anxiety," "anxiety-based school refusal," "school refusal behavior," "school withdrawal," "parent withholding," "early school-leaving," and "school drop-out," to name just some of them. Sometimes authors use the same term to refer to different types of school attendance problems. For example, while the term "truancy" is often used in relation to the school attendance problem characterized by a young person's absence from school without parental knowledge or consent (e.g., Galloway, 1982; Huffington & Sevitt, 1989), some have used the term "truancy" to refer more generally to all types of school attendance problems (e.g., Bimler & Kirkland, 2001). Adding further confusion, the term 'school refusal' has been used as an umbrella term for both anxiety-based school attendance problems and truancy-related school attendance problems (e.g., Egger et al., 2003). Terminological ambiguity and indeed, inconsistencies in conceptualizing different types of school attendance problems pose a considerable roadblock in efforts to advance both scientific knowledge and effective practice in the management of these problems (Kearney, 2003).

The specific attendance problem focused upon in this chapter is "school refusal" as defined by Berg and colleagues (Berg, 1997; 2002; Berg, Nichols, & Pritchard, 1969; Bools, Foster, Brown, & Berg, 1990). This is a type of school attendance problem characterized by: (1) a young person's reluctance or refusal to attend school, often (but not necessarily) leading to prolonged absence; (2) the young person usually remaining at home during school hours, rather than concealing the problem from parents; (3) the young person displaying emotional upset at the prospect of attending school, which may be reflected in excessive fearfulness,

Heyne, D. (2006). School refusal. In J. E. Fisher & W. T. O'Donohue (Eds.), *Practitioner's guide to evidence-based psychotherapy*. New York: Springer.

temper tantrums, unhappiness, or possibly in the form of unexplained physical symptoms; (4) an absence of severe antisocial tendencies, beyond the young person's resistance to parental attempts to get them to school; and (5) reasonable parental efforts to secure the young person's attendance at school, at some stage in the history of the problem. These criteria are often drawn upon to differentiate between 'school refusal' and other types of attendance problems, including 'truancy' (which frequently occurs as part of a constellation of antisocial behaviors; e.g., Egger et al., 2003), and 'school withdrawal' (whereby nonattendance is related to parental ambivalence or opposition toward the child attending school regularly; e.g., Kahn & Nursten, 1962). Differentiation of this kind can help focus due attention upon the different factors likely to be important in tailoring intervention plans to varying types of school attendance problems.

Prevalence

Heyne and King (2004) described earlier studies from the USA, UK, and Venezuela which suggested that between 1% and 2% of all school-age young people will exhibit school refusal at some point. This range is in keeping with Egger, Costello, & Angold' (2003) recent community study of 1,422 young people (aged 9–16 years) in North Carolina, USA. Two percent of the young people met criteria for "pure anxious school refusal," defined according to "school nonattendance (of at least a half-day's duration) due to worry/anxiety; staying home mornings from school because of anxiety; failing to reach school or leaving school and going home; and/or having to be taken to school because of worry and anxiety about attending school," at least once in a three-month period (p. 799). While the community prevalence of school refusal is low compared to some other child and adolescent problems, persistent school refusal poses a significant threat to the young person's social, emotional, and academic development and it has been associated with mental health problems in adult life (e.g., Flakierska-Praquin, Lindstrom, & Gillberg, 1997). It can also have a negative impact upon the parents of the school-refusing child or adolescent, and upon school staff (McAnanly, 1986).

Early estimates of the incidence of school refusal among clinic-referred young people were around 5% (Burke & Silverman, 1987; Hersov, 1985), with the suggestion that this figure may be higher among secondary school students (Hersov, 1985). Last and Strauss' (1990) study of 63 school refusers with anxiety disorders lends some support to this age-related contention. That is, referrals were accepted for young people from 5 years of age, but most (92%) of the school refusers were at least 10 years old, and the peak age for referral was 13–15 years. In a more recent Australian study, McShane, Walter, & Rey (2001) reported that school refusal cases in adolescence (10–17 years) constituted 7% of a clinic population. The majority (78%) of the 192 school refusers initially exhibited school refusal in the first two years of high school, with a mean age of onset of 12.3 years. Adolescence might be regarded as an important developmental period from the point of view of school refusal onset and referral.

Presentation

School refusal is marked by substantial heterogeneity, with respect to refusal-related characteristics and associated symptoms. Onset of the refusal to attend school may be sudden or gradual, and attendance may be full, partial, or nonexistent. Behaviorally, when pressured to attend school, there may be complaints about school, temper tantrums, and even threats to run away or to harm oneself (Berg, 2002; Coulter, 1995). Some school refusers begin to head towards school but rush home in a state of anxiety before they arrive there, while others appear to behave normally after arriving at school, and then their fearfulness returns the next day when it is time to get ready for school again (Berg, 2002). Somatic complaints such as headache and stomachache are commonly expressed by school refusers, and many other symptoms such as sweating, dizziness, and frequent urination have also been reported. In a Japanese study (Honjo et al., 2001), almost 80% of 34 children and adolescents refusing to attend school expressed somatic complaints, significantly higher than the 30% of depressed children and adolescents in a small comparison group (n=10) who expressed such complaints. The cognitive component of school refusal involves irrational or dysfunctional thoughts associated with school attendance. School refusers may, for example, overestimate the likelihood of anxiety-provoking situations occurring at school, underestimate their own ability to cope with anxiety-provoking situations, magnify or selectively attend to the unpleasant aspects of school attendance, or misinterpret the thoughts and actions of others at school (e.g., Kearney, 2001; King, Ollendick, et al., 1998).

School refusal is not a formal diagnosis in DSM-IV (American Psychiatric Association, 1994), but young people presenting with school refusal are often diagnosed with one or even a number of disorders (e.g., Bernstein & Garfinkel, 1986; Last, Strauss, & Francis, 1987). Many meet criteria for anxiety disorders and to a lesser extent depressive disorders, the latter often overlapping with anxiety disorders (e.g., Bernstein, 1991; Last & Strauss, 1990; Martin et al., 1999; McShane et al., 2001). Even when full diagnostic criteria are not met for a specific anxiety disorder, the presence of prominent anxious or phobic symptoms may contribute to a diagnosis of Anxiety Disorder Not Otherwise Specified (e.g., Heyne et al., 2002). School refusal, while defined by an absence of severe antisocial behavior such as stealing and destructiveness, is sometimes associated with other externalising behavior such as the young person's argumentativeness and aggression when parents attempt to get him or her to go to school (e.g., Berg, 2002; Hoshino et al., 1987). Some school refusers consistently display multiple externalizing behaviors over time, and a diagnosis of oppositional defiant disorder might be made (e.g., McShane et al., 2001).

There are suggestions that the development, clinical presentation, and severity of school refusal vary according to age. Hersov (1985) suggested that sudden onset is more typical of younger school refusers, whereas older refusers are more likely to display an insidious onset. Age-related trends in diagnoses and symptoms are also observed. For example, separation anxiety disorder is more common among younger school refusers (e.g., Last & Strauss, 1990), and adolescent school refusers are more likely to experience social phobia and possibly panic disorder (e.g., Bernstein & Borchardt, 1991; Last & Strauss, 1990) as well as depressive symptoms (e.g., Baker & Wills, 1978). Regarding severity of the problem, Eisenberg (1959) observed that the adolescent school refuser is far more disturbed than the younger school refuser, and this impression has received empirical support (see review by Atkinson, Quarrington, Cyr, 1985). Hansen, Sanders, Massaro, and Last (1998) found that age was the strongest predictor of school absenteeism (a measure of school refusal severity) among a sample of clinic-referred anxious school refusers (aged 6–17 years); increased age was predictive of greater levels of absenteeism, whereas no relationship was found between absenteeism and the length of the problem or the occurrence of a prior school refusal episode. Heyne's (1999) unpublished data from a treatment outcome study of 61 school refusers also indicated that at pretreatment, school refusers from the secondary school level attended school significantly less regularly (12% mean attendance) than school refusers from the primary school level (31% mean attendance). As possible explanations for the greater absenteeism among adolescent school refusers, Hansen et al. (1998) proposed that the complexity of the adolescent developmental period presents a heightened challenge for adolescents in coping with school-based fears, and that in adolescence young people are more likely to resist (and are more capable of resisting) parents' and teachers' efforts to return them to school. These and other developmental factors are likely to account, in some part, for the suggestion that treatment outcome is inferior for adolescents relative to children (e.g., Last, Hansen, & Franco, 1998).

Etiology and Course

The etiology of school refusal is incompletely understood (King & Ollendick, 1989). What is most apparent is that school refusal is often complexly determined. A helpful way to conceptualize the range of potentially relevant etiological factors is to consider the domains of predisposing, precipitating, and perpetuating influences. Within (and indeed across) each domain there is likely to be a confluence of individual, family, school, and community factors.

At the individual level, young people prone to anxiety, depression, and associated social difficulties may be particularly susceptible to school refusal (Elliott, 1999). However, questions about whether school refusal precedes other problems such as anxiety or depression or is an outcome of these other problems are often unanswered (Kearney, 2001). Much discussion and research highlights the potential role of parent and family factors in predisposing young people to the development of school refusal. Early reports suggested that the child's dependency is fostered or condoned by the mother (e.g., Berg & McGuire, 1974; Eisenberg, 1958), and some recent reports similarly emphasise the over-protection and over-involvement of mothers in the families of some school refusers (e.g., Kameguchi & Murphy-Shigematsu, 2001; Kearney & Silverman, 1995). Detached family relationships have also been associated with school refusal (Bernstein, Warren, Massie, & Thuras, 1999; Kearney & Silverman, 1995). Regarding family constellation, Bernstein and Borchardt (1996) speculated that the characteristics of single parent family situations may predispose the young person to school refusal. Conversely, in dual parent families characterized by marital conflict, the child may come to fear that, in his or her absence during school-time, the family structure will disintegrate (Valles & Oddy, 1984). The frustration and impairment in academic performance as a result of language disorders and learning difficulties may contribute to the development of school refusal for some young people (Naylor, Staskowski, Kenney, & King, 1994). At the community level, increasing social pressure for students to achieve academically and the associated competitiveness of school environments are held to contribute to nonattendance problems in Japan (Iwamoto & Yoshida, 1997; Kameguchi & Murphy-Shigematsu, 2001).

Many different precipitants have been associated with the onset of school refusal. Among a referred sample of 192 adolescent school refusers, McShane et al. (2001) identified conflict with family or peers, academic difficulties, family separation, change of home or school, and physical illness as key stressors associated with onset. Bullying at school is commonly reported by young people with school refusal (e.g., Place, Hulsmeier, Davis, & Taylor, 2000). Other school-based situations which might be avoided by some young people include tests, oral presentations, athletic performance, undressing for showers, having to complete homework, and the reactions of teachers (Kearney & Beasley, 1994; Leung, 1989; Ollendick & Mayer, 1984). High risk times for onset also include the times following major holidays (King, Heyne, Tonge, Gullone, & Ollendick, 2001), mother's commencing work (Ollendick & Mayer, 1984), and the death of someone in the close or extended social network of the young person (Davidson, 1960). In many cases a combination of precipitating events is reported (e.g., Silove & Manicavasagar, 1993), and in some cases precipitating events are not identifiable (e.g., Baker & Wills, 1978; Smith, 1970), especially if the onset is not so recent (cf. Baker & Wills, 1978).

Regarding the perpetuation of school refusal, the secondary gain associated with not being at school is a common factor in school refusers' ongoing avoidance of school (Burke & Silverman, 1987; Kearney, 2001). The secondary gain might be in the form of parental attention and tangible reinforcement such as access to the television, the computer, pets, toys, and certain foods. Negative reinforcement of school refusal may be another significant factor in its continuation, in that the young person's nonattendance is reinforced by the avoidance of negative affect associated with being at school (Kearney, 2001). The cognitions of the young person are also linked to the perpetuation of school refusal; the more time that is spent away from school, the more likely it is that some young people will think that they cannot cope with the social and academic aspects of school (Okuyama, Okada, Kuribayashi, & Kaneko, 1999). In particular, they may expect difficulty in answering peers' or teacher's questions about their absence (Heyne et al., 1998). At the family-level, Bernstein & Garfinkel (1990) suggested that the parents of school refusers may be ineffective in their role to facilitate a return to school, and that the child may assume a hostile, defiant and controlling role within the family. Similarly, King, Ollendick, and Tonge (1995) suggested that overly dependent mothers and uninvolved fathers lack effective parenting strategies important to the management of school refusal. The psychopathology that is frequently evidenced in the parents of school refusers (e.g., Bernstein & Garfinkel, 1988; Bools et al., 1990; Last, Francis, Hersen, Kazdin, & Strauss, 1987; Martin et al., 1999) may perpetuate the problem, inasmuch as the parents' own anxiety or depression may make it difficult for them to appropriately support their child. At a community level, inconsistent professional advice (e.g., Coulter, 1995) and inadequate support services may serve to perpetuate the problem.

From a developmental point of view it can be argued that, as the child grows older, school attendance problems are increasingly under the influence of school-based factors (Galloway, 1985). The increasing academic demands placed upon the young person during the years of secondary schooling may contribute to the development or exacerbation of a young person's feeling uncomfortable in the school setting. Further, secondary schools generally constitute more complex environments with larger student populations. With the increasing importance of peer influences during adolescence and the increased complexity of the secondary school environment, some vulnerable youth may become overwhelmed in this context, escaping to the security of the home environment. Parents' perspectives on the role of school-related experiences in the development of their children's school attendance problems have indeed suggested that problems at school more often played a role in secondary school absenteeism than in primary school absenteeism (Galloway, 1985). Unpublished data from the treatment outcome study of Heyne et al. (2002) indicated that the diagnosis of Adjustment Disorder with Anxiety was commonly applied to adolescents who had difficulty making the transition to secondary school. Further attention needs to be paid to the relationship between the developmental challenges associated with adolescence, and the development and maintenance of school refusal.

The course of school refusal is also insufficiently researched. Clinical observations suggest that, over time, the school-refusing young person may become progressively withdrawn, disengaging from usual activities and refusing to have any contact with peers. Mood problems may intensify, and anxiety may generalize across situations (Berg, 2002; Torma & Halsti, 1975). The young person's self-worth can deteriorate as he or she labels himself/herself as different to peers and falls further behind academically. Through all of this, family tension and parental distress are prone to mount. Despite the obvious importance of longitudinal data, few follow-up studies of young people with school refusal have been reported. Relying mainly on register data, Flakierska and her colleagues (Flakierska, Lindstorm, & Gillberg, 1988; Flakierska-Praquin et al. 1997) conducted two controlled follow-up investigations of a sample of school refusers who received inpatient or outpatient treatment in Sweden. In the second follow-up study, the follow-up interval was 20- to 29 years, with all individuals being older than 30 years at the time of follow-up. The original sample was confined to school refusers seen at ages 7–12 years, and whose chart histories met DSM-III criteria for separation anxiety disorder (n=35). At 20- to 29-year follow-up this group was compared with age- and sex-matched subjects who had been non school refusal child psychiatric patients (n=35) and a sample who were children from the general population (n=35). The investigation revealed that the original school refusal group received more psychiatric consultations and continued to live with their parents more often than the general population group, and they had fewer children than both comparison groups. These findings suggest that many separation anxious school refusers may continue to have problems with independence into adulthood.

ASSESSMENT

The best understanding of the factors associated with a young person's refusal to attend school is achieved using a multisource, multimethod approach to assessment (Ollendick & King, 1998). This approach yields the breadth of information required to develop and test hypotheses about the development and maintenance of school refusal (i.e., the predisposing, precipitating, and perpetuating factors), and thus to inform treatment planning. Accordingly, assessment typically involves clinical-behavioral interviews with the young person and their parents (e.g., Blagg, 1987; Heyne & Rollings, 2002); diagnostic interviews with both parties (e.g., Anxiety Disorders Interview Schedule for Children; Silverman & Albano, 1996); the young person's reports of emotional, social, behavioral, and family functioning, via questionnaires and self-monitoring procedures; parent- and teacher-completed reports of the young person's functioning; parent reports of their own functioning and of family functioning; a review of the young person's school attendance record; consultation with school staff and with any other involved professionals; and arrangements for a physical examination in order to determine whether biological etiologies are linked to the young person's difficulty in attending school. For a detailed review of self-report and other-report measures used in the assessment of school refusal see Ollendick and King (1998) and Kearney (2001). As outlined below, contemporary developments in the field include the systematic functional analysis of behaviors associated with school refusal, and the assessment of cognitions which may play a role in the maintenance of a young person's refusal to attend school and the maintenance of parents' suboptimal management of the problem.

The need to develop a sound system for determining treatment-relevant differences among school refusers was underscored in a review article in which Burke and Silverman (1987) evaluated existing models for the classification of school refusal subtypes. In turn, a functional analytic model was proposed and tested (Kearney & Silverman, 1990), and the School Refusal Assessment Scale (SRAS; Kearney & Silverman, 1993) was developed so as to provide a standardized functional analysis of the behaviors of school refusers. A revised version of the scale has since been published (SRAS-R; Kearney, 2002). The SRAS-R comprises a youth-report questionnaire and a parent-report questionnaire, each containing 24 items rated on a 0–6 scale (from "never" to "always"). The items were intended to measure the relative strength of four hypothesized functions of (i.e., reasons for the maintenance of) a young person's school refusal behavior.[1] The hypothesized functions are represented in the following functional categories: (1) avoidance of school-related stimuli that provoke a sense of general negative affectivity; (2) escape from aversive social and/or evaluative situations at school; (3) pursuit of attention from significant others; and (4) pursuit of tangible reinforcement outside the school setting. Exemplary items include, respectively: (1) "How often to you have bad feelings about going to school because you are afraid of something related to school (e.g., tests, school bus, teacher, fire alarm)?"; (2) "How often do you stay away from school because it is hard to speak with the other kids at school?"; (3) "How often do you feel you would rather be with your parents than go to school?"; and (4) "When you are not in school during the week (Monday- to Friday) how often do you leave the house and do something fun?" Psychometric evaluation of the SRAS and SRAS-R (Higa, Daleiden, & Chorpita, 2002; Kearney, 2002; Kearney & Silverman, 1990, 1993) supports the presence of three, and not four separate factors: negative reinforcement (made up of a combination of the first two hypothesized functional categories), attention-seeking, and tangible reinforcement.

Importantly, the SRAS and its revision were intended to aid the development of treatment plans which best account for the specific factors maintaining a young person's refusal to attend school. Kearney and Albano (2000a,b) published a therapist guide and parent workbook which include treatment recommendations corresponding with each of the four hypothesized functional categories. While there is some support for the clinical utility of this systematic functional analytic approach to the assessment of school refusal behavior (e.g., Chorpita, Albano, Heimberg, & Barlow, 1996; Kearney & Silverman, 1990, 1999), further research on the benefits of assigning prescriptive treatments is required. Based on the fore-mentioned finding regarding the presence of three and not four functional categories, further research needs to also address the question of whether differentiation between the first and second hypothesized functional categories is possible and even desirable (Kearney, 2002). Perhaps it is a reflection of the perceived utility of the systematic functional approach that the original SRAS has been translated into German (Overmyer, Schmidt, & Blanz, 1994) and French (Brandibas, Jeunier, Gaspard, & Fouraste, 2001), and evaluation of the Dutch translation of the SRAS-R is underway (Heyne, Vreeke, & Maric, in preparation).

Attention to assessment of the cognitions of school refusers and their parents was stimulated by Mansdorf and Lukens' (1987) pioneering report in which "cognitive analysis" was used to help guide treatment with school refusers and their parents. Based on the notion that attitudes and beliefs interfere with the effectiveness of behavioral interventions, Mansdorf and Lukens used self-instruction techniques to help two children (10 and 12 years old) employ coping self-statements to guide

---

[1] Kearney (2003) uses the umbrella term "school refusal behavior" to refer to the behaviors of the group of young people often regarded as truants, as well as the behaviors of the group of young people often regarded as school refusers.

positive behavior. A cognitive restructuring process was used with parents to challenge distorted beliefs about their child's problem and about management of the problem. Recognizing the potential clinical and research value of a standard assessment of young people's cognitions associated with school attendance, Heyne et al. (1998) developed the Self-Efficacy Questionnaire for School Situations (SEQ-SS). The SEQ-SS is a 12-item self-report measure in which young people indicate, on a 1–5 scale (from "really sure I couldn't" to "really sure I could") the strength of their belief that they could cope with potential stressful or anxiety-provoking situations like being separated from parents during school-time, doing school work, and handling peers' questions about absence from school. Evaluation of the instrument's properties indicated that it comprises two logically cohesive factors (academic/social stress and separation/discipline stress) and that it is a stable measure over time.

More extensive information about a young person's cognitive content and to some extent their cognitive processes may be achieved by targeting private speech via the use of a self-statement assessment procedure (Kendall & Korgeski, 1979). With the aim of bringing to light cognitive data overlooked by highly standardized measures such as pencil-and-paper questionnaires, the young person can be engaged in a think-aloud task that encourages a continuous monologue via a variation on the free association method (Genest & Turk, 1981). Heyne and Rollings (2002) described a Self-Statement Assessment-Child Form which aims to elicit school refusers' cognitions in relation to seven aspects of school attendance (e.g., separation from parents; school work; teachers; peers at school). The self-statement assessment is introduced in the context of a word game, with initial practice items focused on words and then on situations not related to school (e.g., "Tell me the first things that come into your head about going to the beach"). During the practice phase the clinician also models thinking aloud in response to items suggested by the young person. Once the practice phase has indicated that the young person is able to think aloud, the practitioner begins the assessment of self-statements about the school-related items. The young person's self-statements are recorded verbatim by audio/video recording or in-session transcription. In order to identify targets for cognitively orientated interventions, subsequent analysis of the recorded cognitions focuses on the identification of specific thoughts and ways of thinking that may be associated with the development or maintenance of school refusal (e.g., overestimation of the likelihood of a parent falling ill while the young person is at school; young person's belief that the teacher will growl at him if he gives a wrong answer in class). Coding of the self-statements (e.g., positive, neutral, and negative) permits an evaluation of cognitive change during intervention.

Heyne and Rollings (2002) also recommended the use of a Self-Statement Assessment—Parent Form aimed at eliciting parents' cognitions in response to issues concerning school attendance problems (e.g., cognitions associated with why their child does not attend school regularly and voluntarily, who ought to be most responsible for the young person's attendance at school, what things parents can do to help manage the problem, and how quickly a young person should return to school after an absence due to school refusal). By presenting the self-statement assessment as a routine part of assessment with the parents of school-refusing children, parents may be less defensive in their responses, increasing the likelihood that the assessment procedure leads to the identification of pivotal attitudes and beliefs warranting cognitive intervention (e.g., "My child has a serious mental problem and I shouldn't push her to go to school"; "The school has the answers and there is nothing that I can do"). Whilst the fore-mentioned child and parent self-statement assessment procedures are not evaluated with respect to their reliability, validity, and clinical utility, they have strong clinical appeal in that they permit identification of cognitive data not addressed in questionnaires.

INTERVENTION

Many types of intervention have been employed in cases of school refusal, including psychodynamic psychotherapy (e.g., Malmquist, 1965), family therapy (e.g., Bryce & Baird, 1986), behavioral therapy (e.g., Blagg & Yule, 1984), cognitive–behavioral therapy (CBT; e.g., King, Tonge et al., 1998), and pharmacotherapy (e.g., Bernstein et al., 2000). King and Bernstein's (2001) review of school refusal research indicated that, during the decade prior to their review, most treatment efficacy research was confined to CBT and pharmacotherapy. This has continued to be the case during the six years since then. Following is a brief summary of the evidence base for cognitive–behavior therapy. An outline of the major components of CBT for school refusal is then presented, followed by an account of the ways in which components might be selected for inclusion in an intervention plan. (Readers interested in a review of studies on pharmacological interventions are directed to Heyne, King, & Tonge [2004]).

Scientific Evidence

Of the psychosocial treatment approaches used with school refusal, only CBT has been subjected to rigorous evaluation in randomized controlled clinical trials. In a comparison with a wait-list control condition (n=17), King, Tonge, Heyne et al. (1998) reported that a 4-week CBT condition (n=17) consisting of six sessions with the young person (aged 5–15 years), five parent sessions, and one school visit lead to superior outcomes with respect to increased school attendance and self-efficacy, and reduced emotional distress. Thirteen of the sixteen treated young people who were able to be located at long-term follow-up (between three to five years after treatment) demonstrated maintenance of improvements in school attendance, and an absence of new psychological problems (King, Tonge, Heyne et al., 2001). Given that the follow-up data was acquired via telephone interviews, claims for the long-term efficacy of CBT still need to be supported by more rigorous follow-up studies incorporating standardized measures and diagnostic interviews.

In another controlled study of school-refusing young people (aged 6–17 years), Last et al. (1998) compared the outcome of a CBT condition (n=20) consisting of 12 weekly sessions with the young person, and the outcome of a control condition (n=21) also consisting of 12 weekly sessions with the young person and comprising education and support therapy (EST). The two major components of CBT consisted of graduated in vivo exposure and coping self-statement training. The EST condition controlled for the non-specific effects of treatment, incorporating educational presentations, encouragement for young people to talk about their fears, and a daily diary for recording feared situations and associated thoughts and feelings. Unlike CBT, the EST condition did not include any skills training (i.e., no training in the use of coping self-statements) nor any therapist-prescribed in-session or out-of-session exposure tasks. The young people in both conditions displayed improvements in attendance and reductions in emotional distress.

Last et al. (1998) concluded that the structured CBT approach may not be superior to the less structured EST approach. This conclusion is perhaps mitigated by the disparate nonresponse rates at 4-week follow-up: the attendance of 40% of the EST group had not improved, whereas the attendance of just 14% of the CBT group had not improved. Further, the functioning of the two groups at longer-term follow-up periods is unclear. Telephone interviews were conducted in the new school year, but no data on attendance levels or on the young person's emotional functioning were reported, and the length of time since the end of treatment was not specified. Well conducted long-term follow-ups (e.g., at least one year after treatment) are regarded as the ultimate test of the utility of an intervention (Blanchard et al., 2004), and currently there are no such data on CBT for school refusal relative to a psychological placebo control condition such as EST. It is conceivable that the skills training component of CBT may yield increased longevity of gains relative to the EST placebo condition. Silverman and Berman's (2001) review of research on psychosocial interventions for anxiety in young people suggested that Last and colleagues' study warrants replication before conclusions about the clinical significance of their results are drawn. Given that the Last et al. (1998) treatment conditions focused solely on work with the young people, future comparisons between CBT and EST may include parent sessions in both conditions as an additional test of the benefits of behavior management skills training with the parents of school refusers.

King, Tonge, Heyne, & Ollendick (2000) evaluated the two controlled studies of CBT (i.e., King et al., 1998; Last et al., 1998) in the light of Lonigan, Elbert, & Johnson's (1998) stringent criteria for determining evidentiary support for psychosocial interventions. On the basis of this evaluation it was suggested that CBT could not yet be described as a "well-established" treatment for school refusal. At best, it has been regarded as having sparse but encouraging empirical support. Adding to this encouraging support is Heyne et al.'s (2002) more recent randomized trial which, while not including a control group, indicated that (i) child/adolescent-focused CBT (n = 21), (ii) parent-focused CBT (n = 20), and (iii) the combination of child/adolescent-focused CBT and parent-focused CBT (n = 20) were all associated with school refusers' increased school attendance and self-efficacy and reduced emotional distress at 4.5 month follow-up. The usefulness of CBT is further bolstered by uncontrolled case studies and open clinical trials (see review by King et al., 2000). However, King et al. (2000) remind us of a number of considerations that should temper enthusiasm regarding the empirical support for CBT for school refusal. With respect to the two randomized controlled trials for example, samples were based upon American and Australian subjects only, and few of the young people in the studies were diagnosed with depression despite the fact that some studies have found depression to be common among young people refusing to attend school (e.g., Martin et al., 1999). Further, the broader benefits of CBT (i.e., benefits beyond increased school attendance and reduced emotional distress, such as enhanced school, social, and family functioning) are generally not reported.

CBT for School Refusal

The cognitive–behavioral approach to therapy is not a unitary approach, and as such it does not lend itself to any simple definition (Herbert, 2001). CBT is, rather, an umbrella term for a broad range of cognitive and behavioral techniques which are employed in different permutations (Drinkwater, 2004). While CBT might thus be regarded by some as a "ragbag eclecticism," Herbert (2001) observed that the present ethos of CBT as an "informed eclecticism" stems from its deep roots in empirical psychology and its growing track record of successful outcomes for many of the problems encountered by young people. Below is an overview of the cognitive–behavioral strategies which commonly constitute the various components of a

CBT approach to treating school refusal. Thereafter, consideration is given to the issues in determining how components can be selected for inclusion in a comprehensive CBT intervention.

Intervention components with the young person

(a) *Psychoeducation.* To promote readiness for active collaboration in CBT, the young person is provided with information and engaged in discussion about the nature of his or her difficulties and the way in which CBT can help him or her alleviate the difficulties. The notion of "normalizing + forecasting + linking" may help prompt the clinician to consider addressing: the common occurrence of school attendance difficulties and associated problems such as anxiety; factors leading to the development and maintenance of these problems, including the relationships between thoughts, feelings, and behaviors; shorter- and longer-term outcomes in the absence of, but especially in the presence of intervention, including improved quality of life; the components of CBT, how they relate to specific goals for the young person and how they will be sequenced during intervention, with an initial skills-building phase preceding school return mid-way through intervention; and the process of CBT, whereby the clinician serves as "coach" as the young person learns new ways of handling things, the involved parties (clinician, young person, parents, and school staff) figuratively form a team in a collaboration to make a positive difference, and between-session practice tasks help the young person to develop strengths and to change things for themselves.

(b) *Relaxation training.* Training in relaxation aims to provide the young person with an efficient means of managing physiological discomfort in situations associated with school attendance (e.g., preparing for school on the morning of school return; approaching the school grounds; giving class talks). In learning to identify and manage discomforting feelings, young people are better placed to confront challenging situations and to employ other skills and strategies in the process of coping with school attendance. The young person's relaxation skills are also drawn upon in more structured exposure procedures such as systematic desensitization. The clinician must be creative in engaging young people in relaxation training. Two useful training scripts are those by Koeppen (1974) for younger children and Ollendick and Cerny (1981) for older children and adolescents. Alternative forms of relaxation training which may be used include guided imagery, autogenic relaxation training, and breathing retraining.

(c) *Social skills training.* Interventions aimed at enhancing the young person's social competence are indicated in two main situations. First, underdeveloped social skills (e.g., lacking strategies for developing friendships or for dealing with teasing) may have contributed to the development and maintenance of the refusal to attend school. Training the young person in skills for joining in with peers and dealing assertively with harassment can be most beneficial. Typically, training makes use of educational handouts and involves the clinician modeling desired social behaviors, having the young person rehearse these behaviors during role-plays, and providing reinforcing and corrective feedback. Second, social skills training can be important for young people who are socially anxious with respect to answering peers' or teachers' questions about their absence from school, especially when the young person has been absent for a long time. A social problem-solving approach is employed wherein options for responding to questions are brainstormed, evaluated, and selected, following which the young person is engaged in rehearsal of the selected response(s). Supplementary strategies such as social perspective skills training may further enhance social competence (Spence, 2003).

(d) *Cognitive therapy.* In the field of school refusal, the importance of cognitive interventions relative to behavioral interventions is yet to be subjected to systematic investigation. From a clinical point of view cognitive interventions are suggested to be a vital aspect of school refusal treatment (Heyne & Rollings, 2002). The aim of cognitive therapy is to effect a change in the young person's emotions and behavior, mobilising them towards school attendance, by helping them modify maladaptive cognitions. School refusers may, for example, misinterpret situations (e.g., "John didn't ask me to his party—he hates me!"; "I know the teacher doesn't like me because she raises her voice"), overestimate the probability of negative events occurring (e.g., "Other kids will make fun of me"; "Mum will fall ill while I'm at school"), underestimate coping resources (e.g., "I won't know what to do if the teacher asks me a question"; "It's all too much"), and engage in negative self-evaluations (e.g., "Why would anybody want to be my friend?"; "I'm hopeless at sport"). The "Seven D's" is a clinician aid in the process of conducting cognitive therapy, emphasising key components involved in *Describing* the cognitive therapy model, *Detecting* cognitions, *Determining* which cognitions to address, *Disputing* (or *Dealing with*) maladaptive cognitions, *Discovering* more adaptive cognitions, *Doing* a between-session practice task, and *Discussing* the outcome of the task (Heyne & Rollings, 2002).

(e) *Exposure.* Logically, exposure to school attendance constitutes a key component of CBT for school refusal. In conjunction with the above preparatory strategies, school-return arrangements must be negotiated with the young person, parents, and school staff. For school refusers exhibiting high levels of anxiety, a graduated return to school is usually planned, constituting in vivo desensitisation. This involves a step-by-step approach to conquering the anxiety elicited by school return (e.g., attending for one class on the first day, two classes the next day, etc.). The young person draws on his or her relaxation skills and cognitive coping strategies to manage the anxiety associated with the successive steps. When the young person's anxiety is very high, imaginal desensitisation may need to occur prior to planned school return, perhaps incorporating emotive imagery with younger children (see King, Heyne, Gullone, et al. 2001). Some young people and their families prefer that the resumption of attendance occur on a full-time basis from the first day of school return. This is usually more stressful than a graduated return, but it is intended to prevent or minimise the embarrassment for young people of having to explain why they are leaving school part way through the day. Kennedy's (1965) open clinical trial suggests that rapid return to full-time attendance may be appropriate for children of primary school age whose refusal to attend school has a recent onset. To date there has been no comparative study of the relative effectiveness of graduated versus full-time return to school. The question of their relative efficacy should include consideration of the moderating influences of severity, chronicity, and developmental level.

Intervention components with the caregivers (parents and school staff)

(a) *Psychoeducation.* As for intervention with the young person, parents' readiness for active collaboration in CBT is facilitated through information and discussion around the nature of school refusal, anxiety, and CBT. The "normalizing + forecasting + linking" model is once again helpful. A key objective during this initial stage is for parents to appreciate the important role they can play in addressing school refusal, whilst not feeling blamed for the situation. Information about the known efficacy of CBT for school refusal may also be helpful during the psychoeducation process.

(b) *Attending to setting events.* Problem-solving discussions take place with the parents in relation to their child's class, level, and school placement, with a view to determining the extent to which current and alternative placements might exacerbate or reduce difficulties associated with school return. Parents are helped to manage the young person's access to reinforcing events and experiences when at home during school hours, in order to reduce the secondary gain that may otherwise strengthen their child's resolve not to attend school. A problem-solving discussion also takes place in relation to the specific day for school return, aiming for it to be a day which, for example, involves more of the young person's favourite subjects or teachers. The clinician helps parents to plan and institute smooth routines in the lead-up to school return (e.g., bed-time and wake-up routines; showering and dressing routines). Further, parents learn how to remain calm and to model confidence in the young person's ability to cope with a school return, lest the parents' own anxiety heighten that of their child.

(c) *Training in instruction giving.* Following the work of Forehand and McMahon (1981), parents receive training in instruction giving via educational handouts, modeling, rehearsal, and feedback. Emphasis is placed upon gaining the young person's attention and using clear and specific instructions. This is particularly important for those parents who give vague and imprecise instructions about school-related issues such as getting out of bed in the morning, getting ready for school, and leaving home to go to school. If, following parents' clear expectations and instructions regarding attendance, the young person does not come to the point of attending school voluntarily, parents may need to escort their child to school. This process of "professionally informed parental pressure" (cf. Gittelman-Klein & Klein, 1971), which requires good planning and support (Kearney & Roblek, 1998; Kennedy, 1965), can be an important aspect of treatment as it allows parents to block the young person's entrenched avoidance of school.

(d) *Contingency management training.* Consistent with operant principles, parents are instructed in the recognition and reinforcement of the young person's appropriate coping behaviors and school attendance, and the planned ignoring of inappropriate behaviors such as tantrums, arguments, excessive seeking of reassurance, and somatic complaints without known organic cause (Blagg, 1987; Kearney & Roblek, 1998). Contingency contracting can be used by parents to limit their child's access to certain privileges contingent upon agreed-to arrangements regarding such things as school attendance and homework. Again, the training process draws upon instructional handouts and especially in the case of planned ignoring, performance-based methods. To balance the parents' firmness in managing their child's school attendance behavior, parents are also encouraged to schedule regular non-contingent positive interactions with their child.

(e) *Cognitive therapy.* Clinical experience suggests that, in some instances, cognitive therapy needs to be employed with parents before (and during) their involvement in the aforementioned components of CBT, in order for them to be more invested in acquiring and using the various behavior management strategies, and so that they may avoid modeling unhelpful attitudes and beliefs for their children, and may instead model confidence in their child's capacity to cope with school attendance. Unhelpful parental attitudes and beliefs to be addressed during cognitive therapy may include: "my child is incapable of coping with school attendance" (e.g., Coulter, 1995); "I shouldn't push" (e.g., Mansdorf & Lukens, 1987); and "something has to change in my child's mind in order for him to be able to attend school" (e.g., Anderson et al., 1998). Coping self-statements (as well as behavioral strategies) may also help parents remain calm and committed during difficult times in managing their child's nonattendance (Kearney & Roblek, 1998).

(f) *School-based interventions.* Consultation with school staff is aimed at ensuring that the young person's re-integration into full-time schooling is successful. There is much scope for attention to setting events, including: advising the young person's class-mates and teachers of the timing of his/her return to school, and the need to be supportive and to refrain from probing about nonattendance; identifying one or two peers to act as "buddies" who will provide support during the early stages of school re-entry; identifying a supportive teacher or counsellor who can help the young person settle in on arrival at school and familiarize him/her with the routine for the day; making arrangements to temporarily or permanently accommodate the young person's special needs, such as reduced homework requirements, academic remediation, or a change of classroom; and engineering positive experiences for the young person such as special classroom responsibilities or lunch-time privileges, so as to help make the school environment a more reinforcing place to be. Planned positive reinforcement of appropriate behaviors, and ignoring of inappropriate behaviors such as tantrums and pleading to go home, are also applicable in the school situation.

Developing a Treatment Plan

Various methods exist for determining which components of a multicomponent approach to intervention are best applied in a particular case. Two methods at respective ends of a "flexibility–inflexibility" continuum include, on the one hand, the idiographic approach based upon individual case formulations, and on the other hand the standardized approach based upon strict adherence to manualized treatment protocols. When treatments are evaluated in outcome research, external validity is enhanced via use of the flexible method in determining treatment (i.e., the findings are readily generalizable to day-to-day clinical practice), and internal validity is enhanced via the use of the standardized method (i.e., the findings related to outcome may be more readily attributed to the treatment applied). Somewhere along the "flexibility–inflexibility" continuum is the treatment-match-ing method. This involves the use of a set of criteria to match characteristics of the client (or more systemically, characteristics of the case) with those components of a multicomponent intervention which are theoretically (and preferably, empiri-cally) indicated by the characteristics of the case. In treatment outcome studies, treatment-matching may thus help to achieve what is regarded as an important balance between external and internal validity (Chorpital, Barlow, Albano, & Daleiden, 1998).

Kearney's (2002) functional analytic approach to treatment planning constitutes a treatment-matching method. Data arising from administration of the SRAS-R are used to guide the selection of cognitive and behavioral treatment compo-nents or "techniques." (See Kearney [2003] for a summary of the recommended matching between SRAS-R functional categories and treatment techniques.) Among initial support for this approach to treatment planning is a noncon-trolled clinical trial involving seven young people who were prescribed treatment on the basis of scores on a preliminary version of the SRAS (Kearney & Silverman, 1990), and a small randomized trial in which four young people were offered the treatment components indicated by the data arising from administration of the SRAS and another four young people were offered an alternative to the indi-cated treatment (Kearney & Silverman, 1999). Daleiden, Chorpita, Kollins, & Drabman (1999) expressed concerns about relying upon the SRAS as the sole means for prescribing treatments, on account of its suboptimal psychometric properties. A revised scale, the SRAS-R, was developed by Kearney (2002) in an effort to improve the psychometric properties of the original scale. However, as noted above, factor analysis of responses to the SRAS-R yielded three functional conditions instead of the hypothesized four. Because of its significant potential in guiding decisions about treatment planning, further research is warranted, including: (a) additional exploration of the psychometric properties of the SRAS-R; (b) redressing the current (mis)match between the empirically derived model suggesting that there are three main functions served by the refusal to attend school, and the treatment guidelines in which four different treatments are recommended; (c) clarification of the role of clinical judgement in determining which functional category is most applicable (cf. Daleiden, et al., 1999); and (d) evaluation of the relative merits of permitting clinical judgement in treatment planning vis-à-vis relying solely on the results of the SRAS-R to plan treatment.

Heyne and Rollings' (2002) account of the assessment and treatment of school refusal also constitutes a treatment-matching method. Drawing on information derived from the multisource, multimethod assessment, the form of the associated psychopathology is described diagnostically and a case formulation is developed. The case formulation summarizes the central problems for the young person, the family, and the school, as well as the respective strengths of each; it identifies those factors at the individual level (e.g., anxiety symptoms; problems with social skills; academic difficulties; comorbid mood problems), the family level (e.g., parental anxiety/depression; incidental reinforcement of nonattendance), and the school level (e.g., conflict with the teacher; isolation in the playground) which are associated with the development and maintenance of the young person's refusal to attend school; and related, the case formulation specifies the targets for intervention, with the ultimate goal being the reduction of emotional distress and the resumption of regular and voluntary school attendance. Specific components of the CBT intervention (outlined above in "CBT for School Refusal") are then selected on the basis of the case formulation. This flexibility in matching treatment components to characteristics of the case is held to be necessary in view of the complex array of factors associated with the refusal to attend school. As well as advocating flexibility in the selection of treatment components, Heyne and Rollings (2002) suggested that flexibility in the delivery of the treatment components is warranted, accounting in particular for the developmental level of the young person. Flexibility in the delivery of treatment components with parents (e.g., variation in the amount of time spent discussing and practicing planned ignoring during the training in contingency management) is guided by factors such as the parents' current competencies in the use of certain behavior management strategies. Support for the efficacy of the treatment-matching method in Heyne and Rollings' (2002) practitioner guide comes from the studies of King et al. (1998) and Heyne et al. (2002).

There are several key issues pertaining to treatment-matching which warrant attention in outcome research. At the broadest level, the question remains as to whether a treatment-matching approach yields superior, readily disseminable outcomes relative to the standard implementation of a manualized treatment, and relative to the highly individualized case formulation approach. Within the realm of treatment matching, Wilson (1996) noted that the process of matching components from within multicomponent treatment manuals to clients' situations is only of value when there are reliable and valid systems for determining which components best fit the clients' difficulties. While progress is being made in this area, especially in relation to Kearney's (2002) functional analytic model, further specification and evaluation of treatment-matching processes need to occur.

CONCLUSION

The field of school refusal has long been the subject of much discussion and research, and new developments are still occurring. In particular, the functional analysis of school refusers' behaviors and the systematic assessment of their cognitions and the cognitions of their parents are important advances for the cognitive–behavioral approach to intervention. There is mounting evidence for the utility of CBT in helping to reduce the emotional distress experienced by school refusers, and for helping them to resume regular school attendance. At the same time there has been an insufficient number of controlled evaluations which can uphold CBT as a well-established treatment for school refusal. Adolescence appears to be an important developmental period with respect to the onset, referral, severity, and treatment of school refusal, and current treatments may need to be tailored so as to better respond to the confluence of developmental issues arising during this period (cf. Holmbeck et al., 2000). The development and evaluation of reliable and valid methods for determining the most appropriate intervention for each school-refusing young person and his or her family remain key research priorities.

REFERENCES

American Psychiatric Association (1994). *Diagnostic and statistical manual of mental disorders* (4th ed.). Washington, DC: Author.

Anderson, J., King, N., Tonge, B., Rollings, S., Young, D., & Heyne, D. (1998). Cognitive-behavioral intervention for an adolescent school refuser: A comprehensive approach. *Behavior Change, 15*, 67–73.

Atkinson, L., Quarrington, B., & Cyr, J. J. (1985). School refusal: The heterogeneity of a concept. *American Journal of Orthopsychiatry, 55*, 83–101.

Baker, H., & Wills, U. (1978). School phobia: Classification and treatment. *British Journal of Psychiatry, 132*, 492–499.

Berg, I. (1976). School phobia in the children of agoraphobic women. *British Journal of Psychiatry, 128*, 86–89.

Berg, I. (1997). School refusal and truancy. *Archives of Disease in Childhood, 76*, 90–91.

Berg, I. (2002). School avoidance, school phobia, and truancy. In M. Lewis (Ed.), *Child and adolescent psychiatry: A comprehensive textbook* (pp. 1260–1266). Sydney: Lippincott Williams & Wilkins.

Berg, I., & McGuire, R. (1974). Are mothers of school-phobic adolescents overprotective? *British Journal of Psychiatry, 124*, 10–13.

Berg, I., Nichols, K., & Pritchard, C. (1969). School phobia: Its classification and relationship to dependency. *Journal of Child Psychology and Psychiatry, 10*, 123–141.

Bernstein, G. A. (1991). Comorbidity and severity of anxiety and depressive disorders in a clinic sample. *Journal of the American Academy of Child and Adolescent Psychiatry, 30*, 43–50.

Bernstein, G. A., & Borchardt, C. M. (1991). Anxiety disorders of childhood and adolescence: A critical review. *Journal of the American Academy of Child and Adolescent Psychiatry, 30*, 519–532.

Bernstein, G. A., & Borchardt, C. M. (1996). School refusal: Family constellation and family functioning. *Journal of Anxiety Disorders, 10*, 1–19.

Bernstein, G. A., Borchardt, C. M., Perwien, A. R., Crosby, R. D., Kushner, M. G., Thuras, P. D., et al. (2000). Imipramine plus cognitive–behavioral therapy in the treatment of school refusal. *Journal of the American Academy of Child and Adolescent Psychiatry, 39*, 276–283.

Bernstein, G., & Garfinkel, B. D. (1986). School phobia: The overlap of affective and anxiety disorders. *Journal of the American Academy of Child Psychiatry, 25*, 235–241.

Bernstein, G. A., & Garfinkel, B. D. (1988). Pedigrees, functioning, and psychopathology in families of school phobic children. *American Journal of Psychiatry, 145*, 70–74.

Bernstein, G. A., Svingen, P. H., & Garfinkel, B. D. (1990). School phobia: Patterns of family functioning. *Journal of the American Academy of Child and Adolescent Psychiatry, 29*, 24–30.

Bernstein, G. A., Warren, S. L., Massie, E. D., & Thuras, P. D. (1999). Family dimensions in anxious-depressed school refusers. *Journal of Anxiety Disorders, 13*, 513–528.

Bimler, D., & Kirkland, J. (2001). School truants and truancy motivation sorted out with multidimensional scaling. *Journal of Adolescent Research, 16*, 75–102.

Blagg, N. (1987). *School phobia and its treatment.* New York: Croom Helm.

Blagg, N. R., & Yule, W. (1984). The behavioral treatment of school refusal: A comparative study. *Behavior Research and Therapy, 22*, 119–127.

Blanchard, E. B., Hickling, E. J., Malta, L. S., Freidenberg, B. M., Canna, M. A., Kuhn, E., et al. (2004). One- and two-year prospective follow-up of cognitive behavior therapy or supportive psychotherapy. *Behavior Research and Therapy, 42*, 745–759.

Bools, C., Foster, J., Brown, I., & Berg, I. (1990). The identification of psychiatric disorders in children who fail to attend school: A cluster analysis of a non-clinical population. *Psychological Medicine, 20*, 171–181.

Brandibas, G., Jeunier, B., Gaspard, J.-L., & Fouraste, R. (2001). Evaluation des modes de refus de l'ecole: Validation francaise de la SRAS (School Refusal Assessment Scale). *Psychologie et Psychometrie, 22*, 45–58.

Bryce, G., & Baird, D. (1986). Precipitating a crisis: Family therapy and adolescent school refusers. *Journal of Adolescence, 9*, 199–213.

Burke, A. E., & Silverman, W. K. (1987). The prescriptive treatment of school refusal. *Clinical Psychology Review, 7*, 353–362.

Chorpita, B. F., Albano, A. M., Heimberg, R. G., & Barlow, D. H. (1996). A systematic replication of the prescriptive treatment of school refusal behavior in a single subject. *Journal of Behavior Therapy and Experimental Psychiatry, 27*, 281–290.

Chorpita, B. F., Barlow, D. H., Albano, A. M., & Daleiden, E. L. (1998). Methodological strategies in child clinical trials: Advancing the efficacy and effectiveness of psychosocial treatments. *Journal of Abnormal Child Psychology, 26*, 7–16.

Coulter, S. (1995). School refusal, parental control and wider systems: Lessons from the management of two cases. *Irish Journal of Psychological Medicine, 12*, 146–149.

Daleiden, E. L., Chorpita, B. F., Kollins, S. H., & Drabman, R. S. (1999). Factors affecting the reliability of clinical judgements about the function of children's school-refusal behavior. *Journal of Clinical Child Psychology, 28*, 396–406.

Davidson, S. (1960). School phobia as a manifestation of family disturbance: Its structure and treatment. *Journal of Child Psychology and Psychiatry, 1*, 270–287.

Drinkwater, J. (2004). Cognitive case formulation. In P. J. Graham (Ed.), *Cognitive behavior therapy for children and families* (pp. 84–99). Cambridge: Cambridge University Press.

Egger, H. L., Costello, E. J., & Angold, A. (2003). School refusal and psychiatric disorders: A community study. *Journal of the American Academy of Child and Adolescent Psychiatry, 42*, 797–807.

Eisenberg, L. (1958). School phobia: Diagnosis, genesis and clinical management. *Pediatric Clinics of North America, 5*, 645–666.

Eisenberg, L. (1959). The pediatric management of school phobia. *Journal of Pediatrics, 55*, 758–766.

Elliott, J. G. (1999). Practitioner review: School refusal: Issues of conceptualisation, assessment, and treatment. *Journal of Child Psychology and Psychiatry, 40*, 1001–1012.

Flakierska, N., Lindstrom, N., & Gillberg, C. (1988). School refusal: A 15–20-year follow-up study of 35 Swedish urban children. *British Journal of Psychiatry, 152*, 834–837.

Flakierska-Praquin, N., Lindstrom, M., & Gillberg, C. (1997). School phobia with separation anxiety disorder: A comparative 20- to 29-year follow-up study of 35 school refusers. *Comprehensive Psychiatry, 38*, 17–22.

Forehand, R. L., & McMahon, R. J. (1981). *Helping the noncompliant child: A clinician's guide to parent training.* New York: The Guilford Press.

Galloway, D. (1982). A study of persistent absentees and their families. *British Journal of Educational Psychology, 52*, 317–330.

Galloway, D. (1985). *Schools and persistent absentees.* Oxford: Pergamon Press.

Genest, M., & Turk, D. C. (1981) Think-aloud approaches to cognitive assessment. In T. V. Merluzzi, C. R. Glass, & M. Genest (Eds.), *Cognitive assessment* (pp. 233–269). New York: The Guilford Press.

Gittelman-Klein, R., & Klein, D. F. (1971). Controlled imipramine treatment of school phobia. *Archives of General Psychiatry, 25*, 204–207.

Hansen, C., Sanders, S. L., Massaro, S., & Last, C. G. (1998). Predictors of severity of absenteeism in children with anxiety-based school refusal. *Journal of Clinical Child Psychology, 27*, 246–254.

Herbert, M. (2001). Clinical formulation. In T. Ollendick (Ed.), *Children and adolescents: Clinical formulation and treatment* (pp. 25–55). Amsterdam: Elsevier.

Hersov, L. (1985). School refusal. In M. Rutter, & L. Hersov (Ed.), *Child and adolescent psychiatry: Modern approaches* (pp. 382–399). Oxford: Blackwell.

Heyne, D. (1999). Evaluation of child therapy and caregiver training in the treatment of school refusal. Unpublished doctoral dissertation, Monash University, Melbourne, Australia.

Heyne, D., & King, N. J. (2004). Treatment of school refusal. In P. M. Barrett and T. H. Ollendick (Ed.), *Handbook of interventions that work with children and adolescents: Prevention and treatment* (pp. 243–272). West Sussex: John Wiley & Sons.

Heyne, D., King, N. J., & Tonge, B. (2004). School refusal. In T. H. Ollendick, & J. S. March (Ed.), *Phobic and anxiety disorders in children and adolescents: A clinician's guide to effective psychosocial and pharmacological interventions* (pp. 236–271). Oxford: Oxford University Press.

Heyne, D., King, N., Tonge, B., Rollings, S., Pritchard, M., Young, D. et al. (1998). The self-efficacy questionnaire for school situations: Development and psychometric evaluation. *Behavior Change, 15*, 31–40.

Heyne, D., King, N. J., Tonge, B., Rollings, S., Young, D., Pritchard, M., et al. (2002). Evaluation of child therapy and caregiver training in the treatment of school refusal. *Journal of the American Academy of Child and Adolescent Psychiatry, 41*, 687–695.

Heyne, D., & Rollings, S. (2002). *School refusal.* Oxford: Blackwell Scientific Publications.

Heyne, D., Vreeke, L., & Maric, M. (in preparation). Development and psychometric evaluation of the Dutch version of the School Refusal Assessment Scale—Revised.

Holmbeck, G. N., Colder, C., Shapera, W., Westhoven, V., Kenealy, L. & Updegrove, A. (2000). Working with adolescents: Guides from developmental psychology. In P. C. Kendall (Ed.), *Child and adolescent therapy: Cognitive-behavioral procedures* (pp. 334–385). New York: The Guilford Press.

Honjo, S., Nishide, T., Niwa, S., Sasaki, Y., Kaneko, H., Inoko, K., et al. (2001). School refusal and depression with school inattendance in children and adolescents: Comparative assessment between the children's depression inventory and somatic complaints. *Psychiatry and Clinical Neurosciences, 55*, 629–634.

Hoshino, Y., Nikkuni, S., Kaneko, M., Endo, M., Yashima, Y., & Kumashiro, H. (1987). The application of DSM-III diagnostic criteria to school refusal. *The Japanese Journal of Psychiatry and Neurology, 41*, 1–7.

Huffington, C. M., & Sevitt, M. A. (1989). Family interaction in adolescent school phobia. *Journal of Family Therapy, 11*, 353–375.

Iwamoto, S., & Yoshida, K. (1997). School refusal in japan: The recent dramatic increase in incidence is a cause for concern. *Social Behavior and Personality, 25*, 315–320.

Kahn, J. H., & Nursten, J. P. (1962). School refusal: A comprehensive view of school phobia and other failures of school attendance. *American Journal of Orthopsychiatry, 32*, 707–718.

Kameguchi, K & Murphy-Shigematsu, S. (2001). Family psychology and family therapy in Japan. *American Psychologist, 56*, 65–70.

Kearney, C. A. (2001). *School refusal behavior in youth: A functional approach to assessment and treatment.* Washington, DC: American Psychological Association.

Kearney, C. A. (2002). Identifying the function of school refusal behavior: A revision of the school refusal assessment scale. *Journal of Psychopathology and Behavioral Assessment, 24*, 235–245.

Kearney, C. A. (2003). Bridging the gap among professionals who address youths with school absenteeism: Overview and suggestions for consensus. *Professional Psychology: Research and Practice, 34*, 57–65.

Kearney, C. A., & Albano, A. M. (2000a). *When children refuse school: A cognitive-behavioral therapy approach—Parent workbook.* The Psychological Corporation United States of America: Graywind Publications Incorporated.

Kearney, C.A., & Albano, A.M. (2000b). *When children refuse school: A cognitive-behavioral therapy approach—Therapist guide.* The Psychological Corporation United States of America: Graywind Publications Incorporated.

Kearney, C. A., & Beasley, J. F. (1994). The clinical treatment of school refusal behavior: A survey of referral and practice characteristics. *Psychology in the Schools, 31*, 128–132.

Kearney, C. A., & Roblek, T. L. (1998). Parent training in the treatment of school refusal behavior. In J. M. Briesmeister, & C. E. Schaefer (Ed.), *Handbook of parent training: Parents as co-therapists for children's behavior problems* (pp. 225–256). New York: John Wiley & Sons, Inc.

Kearney, C. A., & Silverman, W. K. (1990). A preliminary analysis of a functional model of assessment and treatment for school refusal behavior. *Behavior Modification, 14*, 340–366.

Kearney, C. A., & Silverman, W. K. (1993). Measuring the function of school refusal behavior: The school refusal assessment scale. *Journal of Clinical Child Psychology, 22*, 85–96.

Kearney, C. A., & Silverman, W. K. (1995). Family environment of youngsters with school refusal behavior: A synopsis with implications for assessment and treatment. *The American Journal of Family Therapy, 23*, 59–72.

Kearney, C., & Silverman, W. (1999). Functionally based prescriptive and nonprescriptive treatment for children and adolescents with school refusal behavior. *Behavior Therapy, 30*, 673–695.

Kendall, P. C., & Korgeski, G. P. (1979). Assessment and cognitive-behavioral interventions. *Cognitive Therapy and Research, 3*, 1–21.

Kennedy, W. A. (1965). School phobia: Rapid treatment of fifty cases. *Journal of Abnormal Psychology, 70*, 285–289.

King, N., & Bernstein, G. A. (2001). School refusal in children and adolescents: A review of the past 10 years. *Journal of the American Academy of Child and Adolescent Psychiatry, 40*, 197–205.

King, N. J., Heyne, D., Gullone, E., & Molloy, G. N. (2001). Usefulness of emotive imagery in the treatment of childhood phobias: Clinical guidelines, case examples and issues. *Counselling Psychology Quarterly, 14*, 95–101.

King, N. J., Heyne, D., Tonge, B., Gullone, E., & Ollendick, T. H. (2001). School refusal: Categorical diagnoses, functional analysis and treatment planning. *Clinical Psychology and Psychotherapy, 8*, 352–360.

King, N. J., & Ollendick, T. H. (1989). School refusal: Graduated and rapid behavioural treatment strategies. *Australlian and New Zealand Journal of Psychiatry, 23*, 213–223.

King, N. J., Ollendick, T. H., & Tonge, B. J. (1995). *School refusal: Assessment and treatment.* Boston: Allyn & Bacon.

King, N., Ollendick, T. H., Tonge, B. J., Heyne, D., Pritchard, M. Rollings, S., et al. (1998). School refusal: An overview. *Behavior Change, 15*, 5–15.

King, N., Tonge, B., Heyne, D., & Ollendick, T. (2000). Research on the cognitive-behavioral treatment of school refusal: A review and recommendations. *Clinical Psychology Review, 20*, 495–507.

King, N. J., Tonge, B. J., Heyne, D., Pritchard, M., Rollings, S., Young, D., et al. (1998). Cognitive-behavioral treatment of school-refusing children: A controlled evaluation. *American Academy of Child and Adolescent Psychiatry, 37*, 395–403.

King, N., Tonge, B., Heyne, D., Turner, S., Pritchard, M., Young, D., et al. (2001). Cognitive-behavioral treatment of school-refusing children: Maintenance of improvement at 3- to 5-year follow-up. *Scandinavian Journal of Behavior Therapy, 30*, 85–89.

Koeppen, A. S. (1974). Relaxation training for children. *Elementary School Guidance and Counseling*, 14–21.

Last, C. G., Francis, G., Hersen, M., Kazdin, A. E., & Strauss, C. C. (1987). Separation anxiety and school phobia: A comparison using DSM-III criteria. *American Journal of Psychiatry, 144*, 653–657.

Last, C. G., Hansen, C., & Franco, N. (1998). Cognitive-behavioral treatment of school phobia. *Journal of the American Academy of Child and Adolescent Psychiatry, 37*, 404–411.

Last, C. G. & Strauss, C. C. (1990). School refusal in anxiety-disordered children and adolescents. *Journal of the American Academy of Child and Adolescent Psychiatry, 29*, 31–35.

Last, C. G., Strauss, C. C., & Francis, G. (1987). Comorbidity among childhood anxiety disorders. *The Journal of Nervous and Mental Disease, 175*, 726–730.

Leung, A. K. C. (1989). School phobia: Sometimes a child or teenager has a good reason. *Postgraduate Medicine, 85*, 281–282, 287–289.

Lonigan, C. J., Elbert, J. C. & Johnson, S. B. (1998). Empirically supported psychosocial interventions for children: An overview. *Journal of Clinical Child Psychology, 27*, 138–145.

Malmquist, C. P. (1965). School phobia: A problem in family neurosis. *Journal of the American Academy of Child Psychiatry, 4*, 293–319.

Mansdorf, I. J., & Lukens, E. (1987). Cognitive-behavioral psychotherapy for separation anxious children exhibiting school phobia. *Journal of the American Academy of Child and Adolescent Psychiatry, 26*, 222–225.

Martin, C., Cabrol, S., Bouvard, M. P., Lepine, J. P., & Mouren-Simeoni, M. C. (1999). Anxiety and depressive disorders in fathers and mothers of anxious school-refusing children. *Journal of the American Academy of Child and Adolescent Psychiatry, 38*, 916–922.

McAnanly, E. (1986). School phobia: The importance of prompt intervention. *Journal of School Health, 56*, 433–436.

McShane, G., Walter, G. & Rey, J. M. (2001). Characteristics of adolescents with school refusal. *Australian and New Zealand Journal of Psychiatry, 35*, 822–826.

Naylor, M. W., Staskowski, M., Kenney, M. C., & King, C. A. (1994). Language disorders and learning disabilities in school-refusing adolescents. *Journal of the American Academy of Child and Adolescent Psychiatry, 33*, 1331–1337.

Okuyama, M., Okada, M., Kuribayashi, M., & Kaneko, S. (1999). Factors responsible for the prolongation of school refusal. *Psychiatry and Clinical Neurosciences, 53*, 461–469.

Ollendick, T. H., & Cerny, J. A. (1981). *Clinical behavior therapy with children.* New York: Plenum Press.

Ollendick, T. H., & King, N. J. (1998). Assessment practices and issues with school-refusing children. *Behavior Change, 15*, 16–30.

Ollendick, T. H. & Mayer, J. A. (1984). School phobia. In S. M. Turner (Ed.), *Behavioral treatment of anxiety disorders* (pp. 367–411). New York: Plenum Press.

Overmeyer, S., Schmidt, M. H. & Blanz, B. (1994). Die einschätzungsskala der schulverweigerung (esv)—modifizierte deutsche fassang der school refusal assessment scale (sras) nach c.A. Kearney und w.K. Silverman (1993). *Kindheit und Entwicklung, 3*, 238–243.

Place, M., Hulsmeier, J., Davis, S., & Taylor, E. (2000). School refusal: A changing problem which requires a change of approach? *Clinical Child Psychology and Psychiatry, 5*, 345–355.

Silove, D., & Manicavasagar, V. (1993). Adults who feared school: Is early separation anxiety specific to the pathogenesis of panic disorder? *Acta Psychiatrica Scandinavia, 88*, 385–390.

Silverman, W. K., & Albano, A. M. (1996). *Anxiety disorders interview schedule for DSM-IV, child and parent versions.* San Antonia, TX: Psychological Corporation.

Silverman, W. K., & Berman, S. L. (2001). Psychosocial interventions for anxiety disorders in children: Status and future directions. In W. K. Silverman & P. D. A. Treffers (Ed.), *Anxiety disorders in children and adolescents: Research, assessment and intervention* (pp. 313–334). Cambridge: Cambridge University Press.

Smith, S. L. (1970). School refusal with anxiety: A review of sixty-three cases. *Canadian Psychiatric Association Journal, 15,* 257–264.

Spence, S. H. (2003). Social skills training with children and young people: Theory, evidence and practice. *Child and Adolescent Mental Health, 8,* 84–96.

Torma, S. & Halsti, A. (1975). Factors contributing to school phobia and truancy. *Psychiatria Fennica, 76,* 209–220.

Valles, E., & Oddy, M. (1984). The influence of a return to school on the long-term adjustment of school refusers. *Journal of Adolescence, 7,* 35–44.

Wilson, G. T. (1996). Manual-based treatments: The clinical application of research findings. *Behavior Research and Therapy, 34,* 295–314.

CHAPTER 61

Self-Injurious Behavior

W. Larry Williams • Michele Wallace

WHAT IS SIB?

Self-injurious behavior (SIB) viewed as a general area of pathology (e.g., McAllister, 2003) has been associated with obvious significant danger and persistence (Emerson et al. 2001), uncertain etiology (Pooley, Houston, Hawton & Harrison, 2003), and controversy in its treatments (Boyce, Carter, Penrose-Wall, Wilhelm, & Goldney, 2003; Linscheid & Reichenbach, 2002). At the broadest level, SIB could be considered to include all forms of human behavior that produce or lead to physical or psychological harm such as in its most extreme, suicide, (e.g., Tyrer et al. 2003) or as related to eating disorders (Favaro & Santonastaso, 2002), drug addictions (e.g., alcoholism), participation in dangerous activities (e.g., unusual rituals or extreme sports) or even participation in unhealthy relationships (e.g., codependency). These topics are covered elsewhere in this volume. The present chapter will discuss SIB more narrowly as it pertains to acts deliberately performed to inflict immediate physical damage to one's body. Specifically, we will discuss SIB as it is known to occur in the population of persons with diagnosed psychopathologies and to greater extent as it occurs in persons with developmental disabilities (DD) or both DD and psychopathology.

BASIC FACTS ABOUT SIB

Etiology of SIB

SIB is currently thought to be multiply controlled by genetic/structural features interacting with changing physiological and environmental conditions. Whereas research is beginning to isolate genetic factors associated with SIB (Pooley et al. 2003; Robey, Reck, Giacomini, Barabas, & Eddey, 2003) there has been ample demonstration of environmental (learned) variables controlling SIB (Iwata, Dorsey, Slifer, Bauman, & Richard 1982/1994; Kahng, Iwata, & Lewin, 2002) and recently investigation into sequential effects of SIB on itself (Marion, Touchette, & Sandman, 2003). For a recent comprehensive discussion of gene, brain and behavior relationships associated with SIB the reader is referred to Schroeder, Oster-Granite, and Thompson (2002).

SIB-Related to Known Psychopathology

SIB has been associated with several traditional psychopathologies such as borderline personality disorder (Verheul et al. 2003), dissociative disorders (Saxe, Chawla, & Van Der Kolk, 2002) and has often been observed in cases involving post traumatic stress syndrome (Gratz, 2003). Indeed a recent study by Klonsky, Oltmanns, and Turkheimer (2003) involving 1,986 nonclinical military recruits reported that 4% of participants who engaged in self-harm behaviors when compared with participants without a history of deliberate self-harm, scored higher on self and peer report measures of borderline, schizotypal, dependent, and avoidant personality

Williams, W. L., & Wallace, M. (2006). Self-injurious behavior. In J. E. Fisher & W. T. O'Donohue (Eds.), *Practitioner's guide to evidence-based psychotherapy.* New York: Springer.

disorder symptoms and reported more symptoms of anxiety and depression. Gratz (2003) has indicated that risk factors for development of later SIB include childhood sexual and physical abuse, neglect, childhood separation and loss, security of attachment to caregivers, and emotional reactivity and intensity.

SIB in Persons with Developmental Disabilities

SIB has been observed more prominently in persons with a variety of developmental disabilities and functioning at the severe and profound levels of mental retardation. SIB has been observed to occur at significant rates in persons diagnosed with Chri-du-chat syndrome (Collins & Cornish, 2002), Cornelia de Lange syndrome (Hyman, Oliver, & Hall, 2002) and most dramatically as a major feature of Lesch-Nyhan syndrome (Robey et al., 2003).

One of the most significant improvements in the assessment and treatment of SIB that has occurred over the last two decades is the prescription of interventions based on the findings from functional behavioral assessments. Prior to the development of this model of assessment, the only treatments that had been demonstrated to be routinely effective in treating self-injury were those based on punishment (Birnbrauer, 1968; Corte, Wolfe & Locke., 1971; Dorsey, Iwata, Ong, & McSween, 1980; Sajwaj, Libet, & Agras, 1974; Tanner & Zeiler, 1975). The functional behavioral assessment model focuses on the identification of the underlying cause and effect relationship responsible for the occurrence of a particular response. Current approaches to functional behavioral assessment include three general categories: indirect assessments, descriptive assessments, and functional analyses (see Iwata, Kahng, Wallace, & Lindberg, 2000 for a review).

WHAT IS INVOLVED IN EFFECTIVE ASSESSMENT?

Indirect Assessment

With this method of assessment, the clinician attempts to identify environmental correlates of behavior by soliciting verbal reports from significant others. Rather than by direct observation of behavior, typically, caregivers are asked to rate the likelihood that SIB will occur under various situations or environmental circumstances, answer interview questions designed to assess the relative influence of several variables on the occurrence of self-injury, or a combination of both. Some of the most common indirect assessment utilized in the assessment of SIB include: the Motivation Analysis Rating Scale (MARS; Wieseler, Hanson, Chamberlain, & Thompson, 1985); the Motivation Assessment Scale (MAS; Durand & Crimmins, 1988); the Stimulus Control Checklist (SCC; Rolider & Van Houten, 1993); and the Functional Analysis Interview Form (FAIF; O'Neil, Horner, Albin, Storey, & Sprague, 1990). The main advantage of this type of assessment is its ease of use; however, the major disadvantage of such assessments is that the verbal reports on which conclusion on function are based tend to be highly subjective, unreliable, and insufficient for treatment development. Thus, it should be noted that indirect assessments are more appropriately characterized as a preliminary guide to structure descriptive assessments and functional analyses rather than as an assessment tool to direct intervention development.

Descriptive Assessments

These methods of assessment are based on direct observation of the behavior and the circumstances under which the behavior occurs. Typically these assessments are conducted under naturalistic conditions during which an observer passively observes and records the occurrence of events as they happen. A number of methodologies have been utilized to assess SIB; however, the most common form of descriptive analysis is continuous observation. Continuous observation consists of observing and recording the events that occur prior to the self-injury, the typographical form of the self-injury, and the events that immediately occur after the self-injury. These data are then either summarized with respect to the most common cause and effect relationship recorded (see Groden, 1989) or conditional probabilities are calculated for given event–behavior occurrences (see Lerman & Iwata, 1993). The main advantage of utilizing a descriptive assessment is that the hypotheses regarding the maintaining causes of the self-injury are based on direct observation versus verbal reports. Despite this advantage, it should be noted that the information obtained may be only correlational in nature and may itself be subjective. For example, observers may record subjective descriptions of antecedent or consequence events (e.g., "mad" for antecedent and "upset" for consequence). In addition, due to the passivity of descriptive assessments (i.e., the observer must wait for the self-injury to occur naturally), the analysis may be time consuming and ineffectual. One accommodation with respect to this disadvantage that has been developed is the structured descriptive assessment (Freeman, Anderson, & Scotti, 2000; Anderson & Long, 2002). In this assessment, antecedent events are manipulated to occasion the self-injury, while naturally occurring consequences are maintained (see Wallace, Kenzer, & Penrod, 2004 for a review).

Functional Analysis

Iwata et al. (1982/1994) proposed a general model for conducting a functional analysis in order to identify the environmental contingencies responsible for the maintenance of self-injury. This assessment relies on direct observation as well as the direct manipulation of antecedent and consequent events that are suspected to be influencing the self-injury. Specifically, three test conditions (alone: test for automatic reinforcement; attention: test for social positive reinforcement, and demand: test for social negative reinforcement) are implemented whereby a specific antecedent designed to establish the motivation to engage in the self-injury and a consequence that may serve as reinforcement are arranged. Results of these conditions are compared to a control condition to determine the function of the self-injury. For example, to test for attention, a therapist ignores the individual throughout the session unless the individual engages in self-injury at which time the therapist delivers attention in the form of reprimand. In this condition, the ignoring establishes the motivation to engage in the behavior if attention is a reinforcer. If the individual's self-injury is maintained by attention, responding in this condition should be higher when compared to the control condition (see O'Neill, et al. 1990 for how to conduct a functional analysis).

TREATMENT

Treatment of SIB in persons without a diagnosis of mental retardation has consisted of a variety of formats of Cognitive–Behavior Therapy (CBT, Tyrer et al. 2003). Boyce et al., (2003) report that dialectical behavior therapy (DBT, Verheul et al., 2003) appears to show most benefit. They also report that although there is no one who recommended pharmacological treatment, lithium may be effective for those with bipolar disorder, and there is evidence for the benefit of clozapine for patients with schizophrenia and schizo-affective disorder.

What Treatments are Effective?

The successful identification of behavioral function improves the development of effective treatments by allowing for the specification of antecedent conditions under which self-injury occurs such that their alteration will make self-injury less likely and the identification of the source of reinforcement that can then be eliminated in order to produce extinction as well as be used to establish and strengthen alternative behaviors. Moreover, results of a functional behavioral assessment can identify reinforcers and treatment components that are irrelevant as well as lessen the need for the inclusion of punishment procedures (see Kahng, Iwata, & Lewin, 2002 for a review).

Antecedent manipulations Interventions focusing on antecedent manipulations either manipulate antecedent events to evoke desirable behaviors (e.g., present cues that evoke the desired behavior, arrange a motivational state that makes the consequence for engaging in the desirable behavior more reinforcing, decreasing the effort involved in engaging in the desirable behavior) or manipulate antecedent events to decrease undesirable behavior (e.g., remove cues for the undesirable behavior, eliminate the motivation for engaging in the undesirable behavior, increase the effort involved in engaging in the undesirable behavior; Miltenberger, 2003). However, it should be noted that these are categories of antecedent manipulations and the specific procedures one would implement to decrease SIB would depend on the identified function. For example, if the function of the SIB was determined to be negative reinforcement, in the form of escape from demands, a common antecedent manipulation involving the presentation of cues to evoke the desired behavior (i.e., compliance) is the high-p low-p procedure (e.g., Mace & Belfiore, 1990). Noncontingent reinforcement (NCR) is a common antecedent manipulation implemented to decrease SIB maintained by social positive reinforcement (e.g., Vollmer, Iwata, Zarcone, Smith, & Mazaleski, 1993) as well as automatic reinforcement (e.g., Lindberg, Iwata, Roscoe, Worsdell, & Hanley, 2003). One of the ways NCR decreases SIB is by eliminating the motivation for engaging in the SIB by providing the functional reinforcer in abundance irrespective of behavior.

Extinction If SIB is occurring, then there must be a reinforcing consequence maintaining it. Therefore, to decrease the behavior, an important component of any intervention is to eliminate the maintaining reinforcer (whenever possible). Thus, if the SIB is maintained by social positive reinforcement, extinction would be implemented by not delivering the social positive reinforcer contingent on the occurrence of the SIB. If, on the other hand, the SIB is maintained by social negative reinforcement, extinction would be implemented by not allowing the individual to escape the demand contingent on the occurrence of the SIB and would actually involve making the individual comply with the demand. Implementing extinction to decrease SIB maintained by automatic reinforcer is, however, more difficult. Extinction of automatic reinforced behavior would mean eliminating the sensory stimulation produced by the SIB. Thus, an additional assessment is necessary to implement extinction for SIB that is maintained by automatic reinforcement to identify the actual source of sensory stimulation (Goh et al., 1995). When implementing extinction, it is necessary to have identified the function of the SIB or by definition extinction of the behavior will not occur and the procedure will not be effective (see Iwata, Pace, Cowdery, & Mildtenberger, 1994).

Differential reinforcement procedures. Besides eliminating the reinforcer contingency, one can utilize the functional reinforcer to decrease SIB (Differential Reinforcement of

Other Behavior; DRO) and/or to increase an alternative behavior (Differential Reinforcement of an Alternative Behavior; DRA). In DRO procedures, SIB is reduced by delivering a reinforcer in the absence of self-injury. In DRA procedures, SIB is reduced by increasing an alternative behavior that either serves the same function as the self-injury (i.e., a communicative response) or is incompatible with the self-injury (i.e., cannot physically occur simultaneously). Both DRO and DRA procedures have been extremely effective in eliminating SIB (see Vollmer & Iwata, 1992, for a review). As with the other interventions, treatment procedures will vary depending on the identified function.

Punishment Although the current philosophy in the treatment of self-injury is based on the Least Restrictive Alternative (LRA; Carr, Coriaty, & Dozier, 2000), when function-based interventions fail it is then necessary to include punishment procedures within the intervention. The most common punishment based interventions utilized to decrease SIB are: restraint fading (Fisher, Piazza, Bowman, Hanley, & Adelinis, 1997), response blocking (Lerman, Kelley, Vorndran, & Van Camp, 2003), and The Self-Injurious Behavior Inhibiting System (SIBIS; Linschied, Iwata, Ricketts, Williams, & Griffin, 1990). It should be noted, however, that when utilizing a punishment based procedure to decrease SIB, a positive reinforcement component should always be included to increase the interventions overall effectiveness and to avoid potential negative side effects.

Medical Treatments

Pharmacological treatment of SIB in this population has been more specific. One line of research has postulated that SIB increases the release of natural endorphins and that opiate antagonists such as naltrexone should be effective in reducing SIB (Sandman, 1990/1991; Sandman et al. 1998; Sandman, Touchette, Lenjavi, Marion, & Chicz-DeMet, 2003). Another line of research (Valdovinos, et al., 2002; Zarcone et al., 2001; Zarcone et al., 2004) have provided evidence of the effectiveness of resperidone in reducing SIB. This latter work importantly also combines functional analysis methodology with traditional drug trials to parcel out the relative effects of medication versus sociobehavior interactions.

FINAL CONSIDERATIONS

SIB by definition is a very serious and immediate problem. Indeed, the very significance of SIB places the clinician at risk for immediate solutions that may be counter-indicated. Clinicians are well advised to assure that assessment and treatment are guided by those with ample experience and knowledge of SIB relevant to the presenting situation. There are two primary errors that the clinician must avoid with SIB. The first is to underestimate the obvious immediate danger it presents and to not simultaneously eliminate any medical cause. This is especially true when SIB is present in persons with intellectual disabilities. The second, also of primary importance in persons with intellectual disabilities, is to not accurately assess possible environmental causes such as those involved through attention or escape functions, by conducting an appropriate functional assessment, including if necessary, a complete functional analysis.

Resources

The Association for Behavior Analysis: *www.abainternational.org*
The Cambridge Center for Behavioral Studies: *www.behavior.org*
The Journal of Applied Behavior Analysis: *http://seab.envmed.rochester.edu/jaba*

REFERENCES

Anderson, C. M., & Long, E. S. (2002). Use of structure descriptive assessment methodology to identify variables affecting problem behavior. *Journal of Applied Behavior Analysis, 35,* 137–154.

Birnbrauer, J. (1968). Generalization of punishment effects—A case study. *Journal of Applied Behavior Analysis, 1,* 201–211.

Boyce, P., Carter, G., Penrose-Wall, J., Wilhelm, K., & Goldney, R. (2003). Summary Australian and New Zealand clinical practice guideline for the management of adult deliberate self-harm. *Australasian Psychiatry, 11(2),* 150–155.

Carr, J. E., Coriaty, S., & Dozier, C. L. (2000). Current issues in the function-based treatment of aberrant behavior in individuals with developmental disabilities. In J. Austin & J. E. Carr (Eds.), *Handbook of applied behavior analysis.* Reno, NV: Context Press.

Collins, M., & Cornish, K.(2002). A survey of the prevalence of stereotypy, self-injury and aggression in children and young adults with Cri du Chat syndrome. *Journal of Intellectual Disability Research, 46(2),* 133–140.

Coret, H. E., Wolf, M. M., & Locke, B. J. (1971). A comparison of procedures for eliminating self-injurious behavior of retarded adolescents. *Journal of Applied Behavior Analysis, 4,* 201–213.

Dorsey, M. F., Iwata, B. A., Ong, P., & McSween, T. E. (1980). Treatment of self-injurious behavior using a water mist: Initial response suppression and generalization. *Journal of Applied Behavior Analysis, 13,* 343–353.

Durand, V. M., & Crimmins, D. B. (1988). Identifying the variables maintaining self-injurious behavior. *Journal of Autism and Developmental Disorders, 18,* 99–117.

Emerson, E., Kiernan, C., Alborz, A., Reeves, D., Mason, H., Swarbrick, R., et al. (2001). Predicting the persistence of severe self injurious behavior. *Research in Developmental Disabilities. 22,* 67–75

Favaro, A., & Santonastaso, P. (2002). The spectrum of self-injurious behavior in eating disorders. *Eating Disorders: The Journal of Treatment & Prevention, 10(3),* 215–225.

Fisher, W. W., Piazza, C. C., Bowman, L. G., Hanley, G. P., & Adelinis, J. D. (1997). Direct and collateral effects of restraints and restraint fading. *Journal of Applied Behavior Analysis, 33,* 105–120.

Freeman, K. A., Anderson, C. M., & Scotti, J. R. (2000). A structured descriptive methodology: Increasing agreement between descriptive and experimental analyses. *Education and Training in Mental Retardation and Developmental Disabilties, 35,* 406–414.

Goh, H., Iwata, B. A., Shore, B. A. (1995). An analysis of the reinforcing properties of hand mouthing. *Journal of Applied Behavior Analysis, 28(3),* 269–283.

Gratz, K. L. (2003). Risk factors for and functions of deliberate self-harm: An empirical and conceptual review. *Clinical Psychology: Science & Practice, 10(2),* 192–205.

Groden, G. (1989). A guide for conducting a comprehensive behavioral analysis of a target behavior. *Journal of Behavior Therapy and Experimental Psychiatry, 20,* 163–169.

Hyman, P., Oliver, C., & Hall, S. (2002). Self-injurious behavior, self-restraint, and compulsive behaviors in Cornelia de Lange syndrome. *American Journal on Mental Retardation,107(2),* 146–154.

Iwata, B. A., Dorsey, M. F., Slifer, K. J., Bauman, K. E., & Richman, G. S. (1994). Toward a functional analysis of self-injury. *Journal of Applied Behavior Analysis, 27,* 197–209.

Iwata, B. A., Kahng, S., Wallace, M. D., & Lindberg, J. S. (2000). The Functional Analysis Model of Behavioral Assessment. In J. Austin & J. E. Carr (Eds.), *Handbook of applied behavior analysis.* Reno, NV: Context Press.

Iwata, B. A., Pace, G. M., Cowdery, G. E., & Miltenberger, R. G. (1994). What makes extinction work: An analysis of procedural form and function. *Journal of Applied Behavior Analysis, 27,* 131–144.

Kahng, S., Iwata, B. A., & Lewin, A. B. (2002). Behavioral treatment of self-injury, 1964 to 2000. *American Journal on Mental Retardation, 107,* 212–221.

Klonsky, E. D., Oltmanns, T. F., & Turkheimer, E. (2003). Deliberate self-harm in a nonclinical population: Prevalence and psychological correlates. *American Journal of Psychiatry, 160(8),* 1501–1508.

Lerman, D. C., & Iwata, B. A. (1993). Descriptive and experimental analyses of variables maintaining self-injurious behavior. *Journal of Applied Behavior Analysis, 26,* 293–319.

Lerman, D. C., Kelley, M. E., Vorndran, C. M., & Van Camp, C. M. (2003). Collateral effects of response blocking during the treatment of stereotypic behavior. *Journal of Applied Behavior Analysis, 36,* 119–123.

Lindberg, J. S., Iwata, B. A., Roscoe, E. M., Worsdell, A. S., & Hanley, G. P. (2003). Treatment efficacy of noncontingent reinforcement during brief and extended application. *Journal of Applied Behavior Analysis, 36,* 1–19.

Linscheid, T. R., & Reichenbach, H. (2002). Multiple factors in the long-term effectiveness of contingent electric shock treatment for self-injurious behavior: A case example. *Research in Developmental Disabilities, 23(2),* 161–177.

Linschied, T. R., Iwata, B. A., Ricketts, R. W., Williams, D. E., & Griffin, J. C. (1990). Clincial evaluation of SIBIS: The Self-Injurious Behavior Inhibiting System. *Journal of Applied Behavior Analysis, 23,* 53–78.

Mace, F. C., & Belfiore, P. J. (1990). Behavioral momentum in the treatment of escape-motivated stereotypy. *Journal of Applied Behavior Analysis, 23,* 507–514.

Marion, S., Touchette, P., & Sandman, C. (2003) . Sequential analysis reveals a unique structure for self-injurious behavior. *American Journal on Mental Retardation,108(5),* 301–313.

McAllister, M. (2003) Multiple meanings of self harm: A critical review. International *Journal of Mental Health Nursing, 12(3),* 177–185.

Miltenberger, R. G. (2003). *Behavior Modification: Principles and Procedures.* Belmont, CA: Wadsworth/Thomson Learning.

O'Niel, R. E., Horner, R. H., Albin, R. W., Storey, K., & Sprague, J. R. (1990). *Functional analysis: A practical assessment guide.* Sycamore, IL: Sycamore, Publishing Co.

Pooley, E. C., Houston, K., Hawton, K., Harrison, P. J. (2003). Deliberate self-harm is associated with allelic variation in the tryptophan hydroxylase gene (TPH A779C), but not with polymorphisms in five other sertonergic genes. *Psychological Medicine, 33(5),* 775–783.

Robey, K., Reck, J., Giacomini, K., Barabas, G., & Eddey, G. (2003). Modes and patterns of self-mutilation in persons with Lesch–Nyhan disease. *Developmental Medicine & Child Neurology, 45(3),* 167–171.

Rolider, A., & Van Houten, R. (1993). The interpersonal treatment model. In R. Van Houten & S. Axelrod (Eds.), *Behavior analysis and treatment* (pp. 127–168) New York: Plenum

Sajwaj, T., Libet, J., & Agras, S. (1974). Lemon-juice therapy: The control of life-threatening rumination in a six-month-old infant. *Journal of Applied Behavior Analysis, 7,* 557–563.

Sandman, C. A. (1990/1991). The opiate hypothesis in autism and self-injury. *Journal of Child and Adolescent Psychopharmacology, 1,* 237–248.

Sandman, C. A., Thompson, T., Barret, R. P., Verhoeven, W. M. A., McCubbin, J. A., Schroeder, S. R., & Hetrick, W. P. (1998). Opiate blockers. In S. Reiss & M. G. Aman (Eds.), *The international consensus handbook on psychopharmacology* (pp. 291–302). Columbus: The Ohio State University, Nisonger Center.

Sandman, C. Touchette, P. Lenjavi, M., Marion, S., & Chicz-DeMet, A. (2003). beta-endorphin and ACTH are dissociated after self-injury in adults with developmental disabilities. *American Journal on Mental Retardation, 108(6),* 414–424.

Saxe, G. Chawla, N., & Van Der Kolk, B. (2002). Self-destructive behavior in patients with dissociative disorders. *Suicide & Life-Threatening Behavior, 32(3),* 313–320.

Schroeder, S. R, Oster-Granite, M., & Thompson, T. (2002). *Self-injurious behavior: Gene, brain, behavior relationships.*

Tyrer, P. Thompson, S. Schmidt, U., Jones, V., Knapp, M., et al. (2003) Randomized controlled trial of brief cognitive behaviour therapy versus treatment as usual in recurrent deliberate self-harm: the POPMACT study. *Psychological Medicine, 33(6),* 969–976.

Valdovinos, M., Napolitano, D., Zarcone, J., Hellings, J., Williams, D., & Schroeder, S. R. (2002). Multimodal evaluation of Risperidone for destructive behavior: Functional analysis, direct observations, rating scales, and psychiatric impressions. *Experimental & Clinical Psychopharmacology, 10(3),* 268–275.

Verheul, R., van den Bosch, L., Koeter, M. de Ridder, M., Stijnen, T., & van den Brink, W. (2003). Dialectical behaviour therapy for women with borderline personality disorder: 12-month, randomized clinical trial in The Netherlands. *British Journal of Psychiatry, 182(2),* 135–140.

Vollmer, T. R., & Iwata, B. A. (1992). Differential reinforcement as treatment for behavior disorders: Procedural and functional variations. *Research in Developmental Disabilties, 13,* 393–417.

Vollmer, T. R., Iwata, B. A., Zarcone, J. R., Smith, R. G., & Mazaleski, J. L. (1993). The role of attention in the treatment of attention-maintained self-injurious behavior: Noncontingent reinforcement and differential reinforcement of other behavior. *Journal of Applied Behavior Analysis, 26,* 9–21.

Wallace, M. D., Kenzer, A., & Penrod, B. (2004). Innovation in functional behavioral assessment. In W. L. Williams (Ed.), *Developmental disabilities: Etiology, assessment, intervention, and integration.* Reno, NV: Context Press.

Wieseler, N.A., Hanson, R. H., Chamberlain, T. P., & Thompson, T. (1985). Functional taxonomy of stereotypic and self-injurious behavior. *Mental Retardation, 23,* 230–243.

Zarcone, J. R., Hellings, J. A., Crandall, K., Reese, R. M., Marquis, J., Fleming, K., et al. (2001). Effects of risperidone on aberrant behavior of persons with developmental disabilities: I. A double-blind crossover study using multiple measures. *American Journal on Mental Retardation, 106,* 525–538.

Zarcone, J.R., Lindauer, S.E., Morse, P.S.,Crosland, K.A., Valdovinos, M.G.,McKerchar, T. L., et al. (2004). Effects of risperidone on destructive behavior of persons with developmental disabilities: III. Functional Analysis. *American Journal on Mental Retardation, 109 4,* 310–321.

Separation Anxiety Disorder

Andreas Dick-Niederhauser • Wendy K. Silverman

WHAT IS SEPARATION ANXIETY DISORDER?

Separation anxiety disorder (SAD) is a common psychiatric disorder of childhood and early adolescence and is characterized by an unrealistic and excessive fear of separation from an attachment figure, usually the mother. Separation anxiety can be a characteristic of normal development or a symptom of an anxiety disorder. Anxieties about separation are regarded as clinically significant if they are excessive, lead to age-inappropriate behaviors, or interfere with social, family, or academic functioning.

It has been suggested that SAD can be prevalent throughout the entire life course and may be less recognizable in adults than in children and adolescents (Silove & Manicavasagar, 2001). However, SAD is currently defined by the *Diagnostic and Statistical Manual of Mental Disorders* (DSM-IV; American Psychiatric Association, 1994) as a disorder that occurs prior to age 18. A diagnosis may be made in adults who have a history of onset before age 18. The symptoms of SAD (which must be present for a minimum of 4 weeks) include distress prior to and during times of separation, anxiety about being separated from attachment figures, school refusal, clinging to attachment figures, difficulty sleeping alone, nightmares, and somatic complaints.

Prevalence

SAD is likely to occur in 3–4% of children and is slightly less frequent in adolescents. About 15% of schoolchildren report subclinical symptoms of SAD. Approximately one third of children referred to anxiety disorders specialty clinics receive a diagnosis of SAD. Most studies have found an overrepresentation of SAD in girls (see Perwien & Bernstein, 2004; Silverman & Dick-Niederhauser, 2004, for review).

ETIOLOGY

Research on the etiology of SAD is relatively sparse. Risk factors that have been investigated with SAD samples include biological/genetic factors, temperament, family processes and attachment, parental anxiety and depression, and presence of certain stressors in the family environment (e.g., marital conflicts, absence of the father).

Possible genetic links with SAD have been investigated on the basis of four different twin pair samples (see Cronk, Slutske, Madden, Bucholz, & Heath, 2004; Eley & Gregory, 2004). The majority of investigators found that both genetic and environmental influences play a role in SAD. The relevance of the shared environment has been less consistently demonstrated than the influence of the nonshared environment and of genetic hereditability. All studies found higher hereditability for girls than for boys. There are large discrepancies between children's and parents' reports, indicating that the findings are highly dependent on the definition and assessment of SAD.

Niederhauser, A., & Silverman, W. K. (2006). Separation anxiety disorder. In J. E. Fisher & W. T. O'Donohue (Eds.), *Practitioner's guide to evidence-based psychotherapy*. New York: Springer.

Behavioral inhibition as a stable trait across childhood is the central construct in studies linking SAD with child temperament. Behavioral inhibition represents the tendency to exhibit fear, restraint, and withdrawal in new and unfamiliar situations. Behaviorally inhibited children have been found to show higher rates of SAD than uninhibited children (Biederman et al., 1993).

Case illustrations with a psychodynamic or systemic background often portray SAD children as being in competition with their father for the mother's interest and attention. Mother and child are viewed to be enmeshed in their alliance with each other with the mother displaying heightened anxiety about being separated from the child as well as heightened dependence on her own mother (e.g., Gardner, 1992; Hamilton, 1994). Controlled empirical studies investigating these mechanisms among SAD children and their parents are, however, nonexistent at this point as far as we are aware.

In contrast, links between an insecure mother–child attachment, controlling and rejecting parental rearing styles, and general anxiety in children have been established (see Rapee, 1997; Manassis, 2001, for review). The highest risk for developing an anxiety disorder comes from anxious-ambivalent attachment with the mother being only intermittently available for the child and from insecure-disorganized attachment associated with unresolved trauma and loss. In addition, parents of anxious children are less likely to grant autonomy to their children and are more likely to influence their children to avoid taking risks than parents of healthy children.

The strongest evidence for a particular risk-factor for SAD comes from studies investigating parental anxiety and depression. Mothers of SAD children show a heightened risk of a lifetime diagnosis or a current diagnosis of an anxiety disorder or major depression (Last, Hersen, Kazdin, Finkelstein, & Strauss, 1987). Offspring of parents with panic disorder have been shown to have a threefold greater risk of SAD, and offspring of parents with panic disorder plus major depression have more than a tenfold greater risk (Leckman, et al. 1985). In a sample of 4- to 10-year old children of mothers with a lifetime diagnosis of panic disorder, mothers' display of emotional overinvolvement was highly related to SAD in their children (Hirshfeld, Biederman, Brody, Faraone, & Rosenbaum, 1997).

Several other stressful factors related to the family environment have been found to be related to a heightened risk of SAD in youths. Parents with few social supports, no spouse, and high levels of stress have an increased risk of developing insecure attachments with their infants, thus increasing the risk of a later development of SAD in their children (e.g., Last, Perrin, Hersen, & Kazdin, 1992). Moreover, conditions of chronic stress affecting the child that may lead to SAD include physical and mental illness of family members and family violence (Turner, Beidel, & Costello, 1987). SAD was found to be associated with mother-reported marital conflict and dissatisfaction and with father-reported oppositional defiant disorder in the child, suggesting difficulties in the father–child relationship and tensions in the parents' marital relationship for families of SAD children (Foley, et al. 2004).

In a sample of 1,887 female twin pairs born in Missouri between 1975 and 1987, Cronk et al. (2004) examined the influences of paternal absence (in addition to genetic influences and socioeconomic disadvantage) on the development of mother-reported SAD at the time when the twins ranged from 13 to 23 years of age. Genetic hereditability and parental absence were both found to have a significant influence on vulnerability for SAD, whereas the effects of socioeconomic disadvantage were washed out in the presence of paternal absence.

In summary, existing findings suggest that the influences on the development of SAD may be the result of different types of reciprocal relations between the primary caregiver (usually the mother) and characteristics of the child: in one type of reciprocal relation, anxious and behaviorally inhibited children elicit more emotional ambivalence or even rejection in their mothers than assertive and temperamentally easy children. Attachment ambivalence in mothers in turn encourages children to use clingy behavior in order to receive emotional support. In another type of reciprocal relation, anxious and withdrawn children elicit overprotection in their mothers, who directly or indirectly prevent children from making positive coping experiences with temporary separation. Maternal overprotection may be related to the mother's own fears about separation, possibly due to unresolved loss or trauma in the past, separation from the spouse (i.e., absence of a father for the child), and/or current psychopathology. In a third type of reciprocal relation, maternal anxious and depressive symptoms and different family stressors (such as divorce or violence) may serve as a source of threat to the child, thus reinforcing his or her fears about the welfare of the mother (see also Manassis, 2001).

Reciprocal relations between genetic vulnerability and family-related influences may predispose a child to develop selective attention mechanisms with a bias towards interpreting separation situations as more dangerous than they are and towards interpreting their own coping mechanisms as insufficient (see Boegels & Zigterman, 2000). Due to this cognitive distortion, these children try to avoid being separated from their parents and thus maintain their anxiety symptoms.

What is involved in Effective Assessment?

It is important to assess all forms of interference of SAD on children's and adolescents' lives including internal distress such as high physiological arousal, somatic symptoms, or nightmares, as well as more overt behavior such as refusing to go to school, to sleep alone, or to stay at home alone. In the case of school refusal behavior, it is important to distinguish children who refuse to go to school because of separation anxiety concerns from cases involving social anxiety or truancy.

There are several methods available to diagnose separation anxiety symptoms and SAD in youths, including (1) clinical interviews, (2) clinician rating scales, (3) child and parent self-report measures, and (4) observational measures. These methods are briefly discussed in this section. For a more extensive review of assessment methods for SAD see Perwien & Bernstein (2004) and the January 2000 issue of the *Journal of the American Academy of Child and Adolescent Psychiatry*.

Several reliable structured and semi-structured interviews to assess childhood anxiety disorders have been developed, most of which are based on DSM-IV criteria. Structured diagnostic interviews are highly specific in their wording, criteria for assessing responses, and instructions for conducting them (e.g., *Diagnostic Interview Schedule for Children*, DISC-IV: Shaffer, Fisher, Lucas, Dulcan, & Schwab-Stone, 2000). Semistructured interviews, on the other hand, do not require that questions be asked exactly as they are written (e.g., *Anxiety Disorders Interview Schedule for Children*, ADIS: Silverman & Albano, 1996). The ADIS with separate child and parent versions is the only interview schedule specifically designed to diagnose anxiety-related disorders in children and adolescents.

Clinician rating scales assess overall levels of anxiety severity. The *Anxiety Rating Scale for Children-Revised* (Bernstein, Crosby, Perwien, & Borchardt, 1996) includes an anxiety subscale with five items (anxious mood, cognitive, tension, fears, and separation anxiety) and a physiological subscale with six items (muscular, sensory, cardiovascular, respiratory, gastrointestinal, and autonomic).

Self-report measures assessing symptoms of anxiety in children and adolescents include either general questions about anxiety (e.g., *Revised Children's Manifest Anxiety Scale*, RCMAS; Reynolds & Richmond, 1978) or scales related to specific anxiety disorders. Three widely used self-report measures specifically assessing separation anxiety are the *Multidimensional Anxiety Scale for Children* (MASC; March, Parker, Sullivan, Stallings, & Conners, 1997) with 39 items (age range 8–19 years), the *Screen for Anxiety Related Emotional Disorders* (SCARED; Birmaher, et al. 1997) with 41 items (age range 8–18 years), and the *Spence Children's Anxiety Scale* (SCAS; Spence, 1997) with 44 items (age range 8–12 years). For the SCARED, a parent-report form is also available.

Because of weaknesses of questionnaire and interview strategies (e.g., children's potential cognitive limitations, response bias and social desirability, low correspondence between child and parent reports), clinicians and researchers may attempt to assess separation anxiety in youths by means of behavioral observation. Attachment researchers have used different types of laboratory procedures that allow for the observation of child behaviors during separation and reunion situations with the parent (e.g., Main & Cassidy, 1987). In the *Separation Anxiety Test* (SAT; Hansburg, 1972), children are asked to respond to drawings of separation situations. Emotional openness as an indicator of separation anxiety is coded according to verbal and nonverbal reactions of the children.

The different methods of assessing separation anxiety and SAD in youths have their specific advantages and disadvantages (see Perwien & Bernstein, 2004). Ideally, clinicians will base a diagnosis of SAD on a structured or semistructured clinical interview (e.g., the ADIS, with the mother and the child being interviewed separately), on at least one self-report measure specifically assessing separation anxiety symptoms (e.g., the SCARED with separate child and parent versions) and—in younger children—on the clinical impression of the observed behavior of the child during separation from the mother (i.e., while the mother is being interviewed).

TREATMENT

What Treatments are Effective?

Research from randomized clinical trials has produced consistent evidence showing that cognitive–behavioral therapy (CBT) can play an important role in reducing SAD in children and adolescents (see Silverman & Berman, 2001, for review). We will briefly present the main therapeutic procedures and strategies used in CBT for treating SAD in youths. To ease presentation, we discuss the therapy along three phases: Education, Application, and Relapse Prevention. In practice, however, there is overlap among the procedures and strategies used across the phases.

In the *Education Phase*, children first receive general information that anxiety may manifest itself in three ways: (1) bodily reactions; (2) behavior/avoidance; (3) thoughts/worries. It is explained that children will learn to reduce these reactions in therapy. For children who experience bodily reactions when feeling anxious, the Education Phase might involve teaching relaxation strategies. Primary emphasis, however, is placed on informing children about the importance of "facing their fears."

It is explained that when children avoid what makes them feel anxious (i.e., a temporary separation from the parents), the anxiety is maintained because they do not have the opportunity to learn that the events are not that "bad" after all. It is further explained that exposures to separation situations will be done in a gradual fashion, not "all at once." As much information as possible is elicited about the situations avoided. This information will be included on the "ladder" or fear/anxiety hierarchy.

Therapy will involve asking the child to complete each rung on the ladder or do each exposure. Three important dimensions need to be taken into account when developing the hierarchy: (1) duration of time spent in the situation; (2) distance from home or parental figure; (3) presence or absence of other individuals.

For children with SAD who also manifest school refusal behavior, two separate hierarchies should be constructed: one will contain items associated with school attendance, the other one will include items relating to separation from home and significant others. The number of items on each hierarchy may be reduced if two separate hierarchies are being constructed. School refusal behavior should be addressed prior to other situations related to separation, since school refusal usually interferes most in children's and their parents' lives. Telephone contact with the school counselor should be made prior to the initiation of gradual exposure to ensure the school's cooperation.

Although parental involvement is not essential for positive treatment response, therapists may decide that in some cases, parental involvement may be helpful. This may be particularly true for parents who seem to encourage child avoidance behavior, or when working with young children. If parents are involved, they are taught behavioral strategies to help increase child exposure and decrease child avoidance.

Because exposure can be scary and difficult, it is important to teach children skills they can use while "facing their fears." This involves teaching children cognitive or self control strategies. Children learn the mnemonic *STOP*: Scared, Thoughts, Other thoughts or Other things I can do to handle my fear, and Praise myself for successful handling of my fear and exposure.

In the *Application Phase*, children (and parents, if they are involved), practice the principles and procedures taught in the beginning sessions. This application occurs in the therapy session and out-of-session as "homework" assignments. The therapist's role is similar to a coach in terms of providing feedback, support, and encouragement, as the child engages in increasingly difficult anxiety provoking exposure tasks.

If parents are involved, contingency management may be applied. The therapist helps generate a contingency contract, which is a detailed written agreement about the specific exposure task that the child will try, the specific reward the parent will provide to the child for the child's successful attempt and/or completion of the task, and when the reward will be provided.

Although in vivo exposures are encouraged during the Application Phase, in some circumstances it may be difficult to devise an in vivo exposure. Imaginal exposures involve having children imagine anxiety provoking situations on their hierarchy. The details of the scene should be elicited prior to having the child imagine it to help ensure a vivid image on the part of the child. The child should imagine the scene for as long as possible, but definitely until the anxiety decreases. STOP can be used to help decrease the anxiety response, upon its evocation.

As the child meets with continued success, the therapist should begin discussing with the child issues relating to termination in the *Relapse Prevention Phase*. Specifically, the importance of continued exposures is emphasized. However, children also should understand that like any accomplishment, "if you don't use it, you lose it," and the possibility for "slips."

This treatment has empirical evidence for producing positive treatment response in youths with SAD. Therefore, the main therapeutic procedures, particularly exposure exercises, should be included in any treatment plan for children and adolescents presenting with this disorder. The other strategies, such as the contingency contracting and self-control procedures, may be used to help facilitate the likelihood that children will engage in successful exposures (see Silverman & Kurtines, 1996 for further details).

What is Effective Medical Treatment?

The pharmacological literature for the treatment of childhood anxiety disorders, including SAD, is in its infancy when compared to the treatment literature on exposure-based CBT. Although some research shows that benzodiazapines, selective serotonin reuptake inhibitors, and trycyclic antidepressants may be effective in treating children and adolescents with SAD, firm inferences cannot be drawn from the findings in light of methodological constraints. Overall, pharmacological intervention has been recommended with more difficult or "resistant" cases rather than the frontline approach to be used with all cases (see Stock, Werry, & McClelland, 2001).

FUTURE ISSUES

Many issues related to SAD require further investigation. With regards to the next revision of the DSM, the question of whether SAD is a disorder first manifesting itself in childhood and adolescence or whether SAD can emerge at any point in people's lives should be further explored. With regards to etiological models of SAD, it is important to understand more clearly which risk factors lead to the development of SAD, directly or indirectly, and which factors are merely byproducts of SAD risk factors. For example, it may be possible that socioeconomic disadvantage is but a byproduct of parental absence; absence of the father may be a risk factor mediating the influence of the mother's own separation anxiety on the child's fears.

When investigating family processes and their influence on SAD, it is important to include the father–child relationship, the relationship between the parents, and even relationships to siblings in the research design. Family processes should be studied from a more systemic perspective rather than to rely on simple linear relations between mother variables or general family variables (e.g., parenting) and symptoms of SAD in children.

Despite the evidence for benefits of CBT in treating children and adolescents with SAD, future research should be conducted on examining the essential components of psychosocial interventions for use with SAD children in terms of identifying and evaluating the main mediators of change. In addition, there remains the question of whether more specialized or focused interventions might be needed for certain subtypes of SAD cases. It also would be important that future research focus on comparing CBT with other treatments, including other psychosocial interventions as well as psychopharmacological, alone or in combination.

REFERENCES

American Psychiatric Association (1994). *Diagnostic and statistical manual of mental disorders. 4th edition.* Washington, DC: American Psychiatric Association.

Bernstein, G. A., Crosby, R. D., Perwien, A. R., & Borchardt, C. M. (1996). Anxiety rating for children-revised: Reliability and validity. *Journal of Anxiety Disorders, 10,* 97–114.

Biederman, J., Rosenbaum, J. F., Bolduc-Murphy, E. A., Faraone, S. V., Charloff, J., Hirshfeld, D. R., et al. (1993). A 3-year follow-up of children with and without behavioral inhibition. *Journal of the American Academy of Child and Adolescent Psychiatry, 32,* 814–821.

Birmaher, B., Khetarpal, S., Brendt, D., Cully, M., Balach, L., Kaufman, J., et al. (1997). The screen for child anxiety-related emotional disorders (SCARED): Scale construction and psychometric characteristics. *Journal of the American Academy of Child and Adolescent Psychiatry, 36,* 545–553.

Boegels, S. M., & Zigterman, D. (2000). Dysfunctional cognitions in children with social phobia, separation anxiety disorder, and generalized anxiety disorder. *Journal of Abnormal Child Psychology, 28,* 205–211.

Cronk, N. J., Slutske, W. S., Madden, P. A. F., Bucholz, K. K., & Heath, A. C. (2004). Risk for separation anxiety disorder among girls: Paternal absence, socioeconomic disadvantage, and genetic vulnerability. *Journal of Abnormal Psychology, 113*, 237–247.

Eley, T. C., & Gregory, A. M. (2004). Behavioral genetics. In T. L. Morris & J. S. March (Eds.), *Anxiety disorders in children and adolescents* (pp. 71–97). New York: Guilford.

Foley, D., Rutter, M., Pickles, A., Angold, A., Maes, H., Silberg, J., et al. (2004). Informant disagreement for separation anxiety disorder. *Journal of the American Academy of Child and Adolescent Psychiatry, 43*, 452–460.

Gardner, R. A. (1992). Children with separation anxiety disorder. In J. D. O'Brien, D. J. Pilowsky, & O. W. Lewis (Eds.), *Psychotherapies with children and adolescents: Adapting the psychodynamic process* (pp. 3–25). Washington, DC: American Psychiatric Press.

Hamilton, B. (1994). A systematic approach to a family and school problem: A case study in separation anxiety disorder. *Family Therapy, 21*, 149–152.

Hansburg, H. G. (1972). *Adolescent separation anxiety: A method for the study of adolescent separation problems.* Springfield, IL: Charles C. Thomas.

Hirshfeld, D. R., Biederman, J., Brody, L., Faraone, S. V., & Rosenbaum, J. F. (1997). Associations between expressed emotion and child behavioral inhibition and psychopathology: A pilot study. *Journal of the American Academy of Child and Adolescent Psychiatry, 36*, 205–214.

Last, C. G., Hersen, M., Kazdin, A. E., Finkelstein, R., & Strauss, C. (1987). Comparison of DSM-III separation anxiety and overanxious disorders: Demographic characteristics and patterns of comorbidity. *Journal of the American Academy of Child and Adolescent Psychiatry, 26*, 527–531.

Last, C. G., Perrin, S., Hersen, M., & Kazdin, A. E. (1992). DSM-III-R anxiety disorders in children: Sociodemographic and clinical characteristics. *Journal of the American Academy of Child and Adolescent Psychiatry, 31*, 1070–1076.

Leckman, J. F., Weissman, M. M., Merikangas, K. R., Pauls, D. L., Prusoff, B. A., & Kidd, K. K. (1985). Major depression and panic disorder: A family study perspective. *Psychopharmacology Bulletin, 21*, 543–545.

Main, M., & Cassidy, J. (1987). *Reunion based classifications of child-parent attachment organization at 6 years of age.* Unpublished scoring manual, University of California at Berkeley.

Manassis, K. (2001). Child–parent relations: Attachment and anxiety disorders. In W. K. Silverman & P. D. A. Treffers (Eds.), *Anxiety disorders in children and adolescents: Research, assessment, and intervention* (pp. 255–272). Cambridge, UK: Cambridge University Press.

March, J. S., Parker, J. D., Sullivan, K., Stallings, P., & Conners, C. K. (1997). The Multidimensional Anxiety Scale for Children (MASC): Factor structure, reliability, and validity. *Journal of the American Academy of Child and Adolescent Psychiatry, 36*, 554–565.

Perwien, A. R., & Bernstein, G. A. (2004). Separation anxiety disorder. In T. H. Ollendick & J. S. March (Eds.), *Phobic and anxiety disorders in children and adolescents: A clinician's guide to effective psychosocial and pharmacological interventions* (pp. 272–305). New York: Oxford University Press.

Rapee, R. M. (1997). Potential role of childrearing practices in the development of anxiety and depression. *Clinical Psychology Review, 17*, 47–67.

Reynolds, C. R., & Richmond, B. O. (1978). What I think and feel: A revised measure of children's manifest anxiety. *Journal of Abnormal Child Psychology, 6*, 271–280.

Shaffer, D., Fisher, P., Lucas, C. P., Dulcan, M. K., & Schwab-Stone, M. E. (2000). NIMH Diagnostic Interview Schedule for Children Version IV (NIMH DISC-IV): Description, differences from previous versions, and reliability of some common diagnoses. *Journal of the American Academy of Child and Adolescent Psychiatry, 39*, 28–38.

Silove, D., & Manicavasagar, V. (2001). Early separation anxiety and its relationship to adult anxiety disorders. In M. W. Vasey & M. R. Dadds, (Eds.), *The developmental psychopathology of anxiety* (pp. 459–480). New York: Oxford University Press.

Silverman, W. K., & Albano, A. M. (1996). *Anxiety Disorders Interview Schedule for DSM-IV, Child and Parent Versions.* San Antonio, TX: Psychological Corporation.

Silverman, W. K., & Berman, S. L. (2001). Psychosocial interventions for anxiety disorders in children: Status and future directions. In Silverman, W. K. & Treffers, P. D. A. (Eds.), (2001). *Anxiety disorders in children and adolescents: Research, assessment and intervention* (pp. 313–334). Cambridge, UK: Cambridge University Press.

Silverman, W. K., & Dick-Niederhauser, A. (2004). Separation anxiety disorder. In T. L. Morris & J. S. March (Eds.), *Anxiety disorders in children and adolescents* (pp. 164–188). New York: Guilford.

Silverman, W. K., & Kurtines, W. M. (1996). *Anxiety and phobic disorders: A pragmatic approach.* New York: Plenum Press.

Spence, S. H. (1997). Structure of anxiety symptoms among children: A confirmatory factor-analytic study. *Journal of Abnormal Psychology, 106*, 280–297.

Stock, S. L., Werry, J. S., & McClellan, J. M. (2001). Pharmacological treatment of paediatric anxiety. In W. K. Silverman & P. D. A. Treffers (Eds.), *Anxiety disorders in children and adolescents: Research, assessment, and intervention* (pp. 335–367). Cambridge, UK: Cambridge University Press.

Turner, S. M., Beidel, D. C., & Costello, A. (1987). Psychopathology in the offspring of anxiety disordered parents. *Journal of Consulting and Clinical Psychology, 55*, 229–235.

Sexual Pain Disorders

Alina Kao • Marie-Andrée Lahaie • Samir Khalifé • Irv Binik

WHAT ARE SEXUAL PAIN DISORDERS?

The DSM-IV-TR uses the term "Sexual Pain Disorders" to categorize and describe the diagnoses of dyspareunia and vaginismus (APA, 2000). Although these diagnoses have traditionally been used to denote distinct disorders, a growing body of evidence suggests that dyspareunia and vaginismus are not easily differentiable (Reissing, Binik, Khalifé, Cohen, & Amsel, 2004). Furthermore, there is some controversy concerning whether or not these disorders should be classified as sexual dysfunctions (Binik, in press a; in press b). Nonetheless, for the purpose of the present chapter, we will adhere to the DSM definition and classification.

WHAT IS DYSPAREUNIA?

Dyspareunia is defined in the DSM-IV-TR (APA, 2000) as "Recurrent or persistent genital pain associated with sexual intercourse in either a male or female" (p. 556). The pain may be characterized as lifelong or acquired, as generalized or situational, and as due to psychological or combined factors. A separate category of "Dyspareunia Due to a General Medical Condition" is also listed; however, no criteria are provided to distinguish between exclusively medical and combined etiologies. Although they are commonly used, our view is that such causation-based categories should be avoided.

Dyspareunia in males is often associated with medical conditions such as STDs and Peyronie's disease, and prostatitis, but may also occur in the absence of physical pathology (Luzzi, 2003). The prevalence of male dyspareunia is far less than that in women and is rarely a presenting complaint seen by mental health professionals.

BASIC FACTS ABOUT DYSPAREUNIA

Currently, there is no clear consensus concerning the best way to categorize potentially different types of chronic dyspareunia. Nevertheless, they can be tentatively classified into two groups based on the anatomical location of pain, superficial or deep. However, pain can occur simultaneously in both locations (Meana, Binik, Khalifé, & Cohen, 1997). Only chronic dyspareunia will be discussed below because mental health professionals seldom treat acute forms.

Superficial Dyspareunia

This encompasses pain in the external genitalia (most commonly in the vulva) and vagina. There are numerous overlapping terms used to describe these problems and it is not clear to what extent they are separate syndromes.

Kao, A., Lahaie, M.-A., Khalifé, & Binik, I. (2006). Sexual pain disorders. In J. E. Fisher W. T. O'Donohue (Eds.), *Practitioner's guide to evidence-based psychotherapy*. New York: Springer.

- *Vulvodynia* is constant or intermittent vulval discomfort or pain for which no explanatory pathology is found. Patients most often describe burning sensations but also report stinging or raw pain.
- *Vulvar Vestibulitis Syndrome* (VVS), also called vestibulodynia, is the most common form of dyspareunia in premenopausal women (Meana et al., 1997). VVS is characterized by localized burning or sharp pain at the vulvar vestibule (i.e., vaginal entry) in response to touch or pressure.
- *Clitorodynia* is pain in the clitoris and surrounding area.

Deep Dyspareunia

Pain experienced internally, in the pelvic and abdominal areas, falls under this classification. It is often described as a diffuse or localized tenderness felt during or after penetration (Bachmann & Phillips,1998).

Prevalence Dyspareunia is reported to affect approximately 10–15% of women (Laumann, Gagnon, Michaci, & Micheals, 1994), and is the most common complaint in gynecological settings (Steege, 1984). Specifically, about 6–7% of women experience superficial dyspareunia (Harlow, 2003). The prevalence of deep dyspareunia is unknown.

Etiology Pukall, Lahaie, and Binik (in press) provide a comprehensive review which suggests that our knowledge of etiological information is limited. Superficial dyspareunia has been associated with medical factors such as yeast infections, vulvar abnormalities, dermatological conditions, early contraceptive use, menopause, a genetic susceptibility to inflammation, and surgical and chemical treatments. It has also been linked to psychosocial factors such as anxiety, hypervigilance, and pain catastrophization. Deep dyspareunia has been associated with a variety of medical conditions such as ovarian cysts, endometriosis, fibroids, ectopic pregnancy, pelvic adhesions, and bowel disease (Bachmann & Phillips, 1998). Childhood physical and sexual abuse have been frequently mentioned as specific psychosocial etiological factor for deep dyspareunia (Jacob & DeNardis, 1998). Inadequate sexual arousal has been associated with both superficial and deep dyspareunia (Bachmann et al., 1998).

Comorbidity Women suffering from superficial dyspareunia have higher rates of other somatic pain-related complaints (Danielsson, Eisemann, Sjöberg, & Wikman, 2001). Regardless of whether the pain is superficial or deep, dyspareunia can adversely affect desire, arousal, and orgasm (Meana et al., 1997).

ASSESSMENT OF DYSPAREUNIA

What Should be Ruled Out?

The possibility of a general medical condition that can cause genital or pelvic pain needs to be eliminated. However, even if one is found, it is unlikely to fully account for the pain. Often, the original causes of chronic dyspareunia may no longer be the effective maintaining ones. By the time that dyspareunia sufferers reach mental health professionals, they are frequently caught in a vicious cycle of pain, sexual dysfunction, negative affect, and relationship problems. Assessing the psychological and interpersonal effects of dyspareunic pain is important so that prevention of further sexual dysfunction and relationship difficulties can be incorporated into treatment.

What is Involved in Effective Assessment?

A psychosexual history Maurice (1999) provides guidelines for taking an in depth sexual history which involves both partners whenever possible. Assessment should include inquiry about parental attitudes towards sexuality, early sexual experiences, sexual abuse or trauma experiences, past and present sexual functioning, and couple dynamics. Also, discussing the reasons for consultation and assessing for the presence of other significant psychological problems can provide valuable information and help in the choice of a treatment plan.

A pain history Binik, Bergeron, and Khalifé (2000) describe a systematic dyspareunia pain assessment that includes asking about:

- *Location.* Questions such as "Where exactly does it hurt?", "Is the pain superficial or deep?", and "Does the pain travel?" are important. A diagram may help patients point to the site of pain.
- *Quality.* Descriptors of painful sensations such as "burning," "sharp," or "tender" facilitate differential diagnosis. The descriptor list of the McGill–Melzack Pain Questionnaire (Melzack & Katz, 1992) can help patients to describe their pain.
- *Intensity.* Have the patient rate their pain and the associated distress on scales of 0–10 (no pain—worst pain ever, and no distress—extremely distressing).
- Time course and elicitors. How long has the client had dyspareunia? Is it chronic or remitting? What activities cause pain or make it worse? How long does it last when it occurs?
- Interference. What activities does the patient's pain interfere with?
- Meaning. Patients' "personal theories" and attributions about the causes of their pain can significantly impact their levels of distress, influence interpersonal relationships and hinder treatment adherence (Meana, Binik, Khalifé, & Cohen, 1999).

TREATMENT OF DYSPAREUNIA

What Treatments are Effective?

There have been few controlled treatment outcome studies for either superficial or deep dyspareunia. Psychotherapeutic interventions are typically aimed at alleviating pain and improving sexual functioning. A multidisciplinary approach combining the efforts of medical, physical, and psychological specialists is preferred (Bergeron et al., 2001).

What are Effective Self-Help Treatments?

There are no empirically supported self-help treatments for dyspareunia. However, helpful recommendations may include:

- Stopping the use of soaps, creams, fragrances or deodorants, douches, etc. in or around the genital area.
- Reducing activities that cause irritation such as bicycling and wearing tight fitting pants.
- Cool or lukewarm sitz baths may offer temporary relief.
- Lists of helpful websites and readings are provided in the Informational Resources section at the end of this chapter.

What are Effective Therapist Based Treatments?

Only two randomized controlled trials have studied the efficacy of therapist-based interventions for VVS (Bergeron et al., 2001; Weijmar Schultz et al., 1996); these investigations found that cognitive-behavioral approaches were effective. No randomized controlled studies examining psychotherapeutic treatment for other forms of superficial or deep dyspareunia exist. However, cognitive–behavioral therapies are often used to address pain coping strategies, sexual dysfunction, as well as couple and interpersonal issues. Treatment should incorporate both sex therapy and pain management interventions because pain reduction does not necessarily bring about increased intercourse frequency or improvement in overall sexual functioning (Bergeron et al., 2001).

Cognitive–Behavioral Therapy

Cognitive–behavioral sex therapy techniques are used to educate the patient about anatomy, the sexual response cycle, sexual skills, and to counter myths and dysfunctional beliefs about sexuality. Also, the clients learn to increase behaviors that reduce pain (e.g., nonpenetrative sex) and facilitate arousal and desire (e.g., sensate focus). Realistic therapy goals such as mutual sexual comfort for couples, increased satisfaction, and reasonable decreases in pain should be discussed because complete pain removal is sometimes unlikely.

- Cognitive–behavioral pain management techniques for the treatment of dyspareunia include educating the client about how cognitive, emotional, and physiological factors influence and are affected by the dyspareunic pain. Exercises such as keeping a pain diary are aimed at increasing the client's knowledge about their pain and how it may change with their emotional and psychological states. Therapists also help them to identify maladaptive responses to pain and facilitate positive coping procedures. Relaxation training is taught to reduce anxiety associated with pain. In vivo desensitization procedures include mapping the location of the pain using a mirror, and finger or graduated dilator insertions.

Couples therapy It is often useful to treat dyspareunia sufferers with their partners. This helps the couple cope together with the interference in their sex life and the associated effects on their relationship. Since the experience of dyspareunia is relatively uncommon in males, it also provides the partner with necessary information and may facilitate his participation in couple homework exercises.

WHAT ARE EFFECTIVE MEDICAL TREATMENTS?

There is promising evidence that these are efficacious treatments for VVS:

- Vestibulectomy, the surgical removal of a thin sliver of skin on the vulvar vestibule, is the only medical treatment that has been proven effective by randomized controlled clinical trials (Bergeron et al., 2001; Weijmar Schultz et al., 1996).
- Pelvic floor physical therapy is shown to improve pain and sexual functioning in women with VVS (Bergeron et al., 2002). Physiotherapists provide a combination of hands-on techniques, exercises, and behavioral approaches such as biofeedback, progressive vaginal dilatation, and Kegel's exercises (Rosenbaum, in press; Bergeron, 2002). Some of the goals of physical therapy are to gain greater awareness and control of the musculature, improve muscle discrimination and relaxation, increase elasticity of the vaginal opening, and relieve pain (Rosenbaum, in press). Moreover, pelvic floor physical therapy can be very helpful in the process of desensitizing the client to vaginal penetration (Bergeron et al., 2002).

There is a paucity of evidence concerning medical treatments for other forms of superficial dyspareunia. Treatments commonly prescribed despite limited evidence of effectiveness include:

- Topical analgesic agents and corticosteroid creams may offer temporary pain relief, but can irritate the vulvar area.
- Low dose tricyclic antidepressants have been recommended as an adjunctive treatment, but no double-blind placebo controlled studies have been performed (Fischer, 2004).
- Topical or systemic hormone replacement is prescribed for secondary dyspareunia associated with lack of lubrication due to inadequate hormone levels (Graziottin, 2003).

Medical treatments offered for deep dyspareunia are typically aimed at treating the identified organicity such as endometriosis, adhesions, and pathology of the uterus, bladder, and internal reproductive organs.

Other Issues in Management

The following issues should be kept in mind when treating patients with dyspareunia:

- Comorbid sexual dysfunctions are common in the patient and her partner.
- Women with dyspareunia have increased anxiety (Meana et al., 1997).

How does One Select Among Treatments?

Where possible, medical, cognitive–behavioral, and physical therapeutic treatments should be administered concurrently (Bergeron & Lord, 2003; Weijmar Schultz, 1996). Vestibulectomy is often considered the last resort treatment for chronic VVS that has not responded to less invasive treatments (Stewart & Spencer, 2002).

What is Vaginismus?

The DSM-IV-TR (APA, 2000) defines vaginismus as a "recurrent or persistent involuntary spasm of the musculature of the outer third of the vagina that interferes with intercourse" (p. 558). This spasm-based definition has recently been challenged (Reissing, Binik, Khalifé, Cohen, & Amsel, 2004) and there is currently no consensus about which vaginal/pelvic are muscles involved. While vaginal spasm does not appear to be a reliable diagnostic criterion for vaginismus, recent studies have suggested that avoidance of intercourse and level of fear displayed during gynecological examinations are useful in differentially diagnosing vaginismus from dyspareunia (Reissing et al., 2004; Binik et al., 2002). Although vaginismus is classified as a sexual pain disorder in the DSM, the experience of pain is not required for its diagnosis and no information is provided on the location, intensity, duration, or quality of the pain typically experienced by women with vaginismus. Reissing et al. (2004) have proposed a new conceptualization of vaginismus as a specific phobia of vaginal penetration. Most authors agree with the related idea that women suffering from vaginismus fear vaginal penetration and therefore avoid sexual intercourse.

Basic Facts about Vaginismus

Prevalence Although 12–17% of patients who attend clinics for sexual dysfunction are reported to suffer from vaginismus (Spector & Carey 1990; Hirst, Baggaley, & Watson 1996), the general population prevalence remains unknown.

Etiology Numerous biological, psychological, and social factors have been implicated in the development of vaginismus. However, a recent comprehensive and critical review of the vaginismus literature suggests that most of the etiological studies are seriously methodologically flawed (Reissing, Binik, Khalifé, Cohen, & Amsel, 2003).

- The condition of the pelvic floor musculature has often been suggested as playing a role in the development and maintenance of vaginismus (e.g., Fordney, 1978; Barnes, Bowman, & Cullen, 1984). However, the principal diagnostic criterion for vaginismus, involuntary vaginal spasm, has not been found to be reliable or valid (Reissing et al., 2004; Van der Velde & Everaerd, 1999, 2001). Rather, women with vaginismus show elevated vaginal/pelvic muscle tone and lower muscle strength (Reissing et al., 2004). The pelvic floor muscle activity that women with vaginismus experience might be part of a general learned bodily defense mechanism that can be induced in both sexual and nonsexual situations that are threatening (Buytendijk, 1957; Van der Velde et al., 2001).
- Fear of pain, of vaginal penetration, or of sexual intimacy have been suggested causes of vaginismus (e.g., Walthard, 1909; Kaplan, 1974; Ward & Ogden, 1994). Women with vaginismus share important features with individuals with specific phobias such as behavioral and affective fear/panic reactions to attempted vaginal penetration, avoidance of vaginal penetration activities, and physiological arousal responses (Reissing et al., 2004).

Several commonly believed causes of vaginismus are not empirically supported:

- Lack of sexual education and knowledge; although women with vaginismus hold less positive sexual self-views, they do not differ from unaffected women on level of sexual knowledge and education (Duddle, 1977; Reissing et al., 2003).
- Higher prevalence of sexual abuse in women with vaginismus has not been found in the vast majority of studies (e.g., Hawton & Catalan, 1990; van Lankveld Brewaeys, Ter Kuile, & Weijenborg, 1995). However, one recent controlled study found that women with vaginismus were twice as likely to report a history of sexual abuse experiences in childhood (Reissing et al., 2003).
- Limited investigations of couple factors in the etiology of vaginismus have not shown significant differences in marital adjustment between women with vaginismus and controls (Reissing et al., 2003; Rust, Golombok, & Collier, 1988).

Comorbidity Dyspareunia and vaginismus tend to co-occur and may be very difficult, if not impossible, to differentially diagnose reliably (e.g., van Lankveld et al., 1995), even if information from clinical interviews, gynecological examination, and characteristics of the pain experienced during vaginal penetration are included in the assessment (de Kruiff, ter Kuile, Weijenborg & van Lankveld, 2000; Reissing et al., 2004). However, women with vaginismus display avoidance of intercourse and greater fear during gynaecological examinations (Reissing et al., 2004). Also, according to one well-controlled study, women with vaginismus are more likely to report lower levels of desire, pleasure, arousal, and masturbation compared to controls (Reissing et al., 2004). It still remains unknown whether these problems occur prior to or as a consequence of vaginismus.

ASSESSMENT OF VAGINISMUS

What Should be Ruled Out?

It is important to rule out any gynecological and medical conditions which may cause or exacerbate difficulties with vaginal penetration such as hymeneal abnormalities, endometriosis, vaginitis, herpes, pelvic inflammatory disorder, and birth and surgical injuries of the genitals.

What is Involved in an Effective Assessment?

A comprehensive biopsychosocial assessment which includes a careful gynecological examination, an assessment of the pelvic floor musculature, and a thorough psychosexual history is essential.

A gynecological examination This should be performed by a professional who is familiar with vaginismus, since it will often require great patience and sensitivity. The internal and external genitalia and reproductive organs should be examined and information concerning the quality, intensity, location, and duration of the pain (see Assessment of Dyspareunic Pain) should be obtained at this time. Affective and behavioral responses to the gynecological examination should be carefully observed since they are good indicators of how distressed the woman is during vaginal penetration. In certain cases, undergoing a gynaecological examination before treatment may be impossible and even traumatic and should be postponed until the women is psychologically and physically ready. Although highly anxious or fearful patients might be capable undergoing a gynecological examination, they may become traumatized by the experience. In such cases, the examination should be postponed until the woman is psychologically and physically ready.

An assessment of the pelvic floor musculature A trained pelvic floor physiotherapist should evaluate pelvic floor muscle tone, contractility, reactivity, and stability. The assessment should include an external and internal exam focusing on the mobility and integrity of the muscular, fascial, and connective tissue components (Rosenbaum, in press).

A psychosexual history The assessment outline previously discussed for dyspareunia is recommended for vaginismus. It is also critical to assess and deal with the women's motivation for treatment. For instance, it is not uncommon to see women with vaginismus coming to treatment with the goal of becoming pregnant or of pleasing their partners rather than experiencing pleasurable intercourse.

What Assessments are Not Effective?

Assessments focusing exclusively on the confirmation of vaginal muscle spasm are not effective since there are no specific guidelines to measure involuntary muscle spasm, no generally accepted definition of the term spasm and no consensus on which vaginal/pelvic muscles are involved in vaginismus (Reissing, Binik, & Khalife, 1999). Moreover, when vaginismus is situational and limited to attempts at sexual intercourse, the vaginal spasm may not be present during the gynecological examination.

TREATMENT OF VAGINISMUS

What Treatments are Effective?

The most popular treatment for vaginismus has focused primarily on the main diagnostic criteria, involuntary muscle spasms which interfere with intercourse. However, Reissing et al.'s (1999) review of the literature found that treatment outcome is highly variable. Given that vaginismus and sexual functioning involves an intricate interaction between biological, social, psychological, and relational factors, an effective treatment plan should not focus exclusively on vaginal containment; indeed, a more holistic and multidisciplinary approach is needed (e.g., Reissing, Binik, & Khalifé 2003; Kleinplatz, 1998). Essential elements which should be addressed in the treatment of vaginismus are: fear and avoidance of vaginal penetration, genital pain, sexual functioning, and pelvic floor tonicity.

What are Effective Self-Help Treatments?

There are presently no empirically validated self-help treatments. However, there are a number of websites and self-help books which can be helpful (see Informational Resources).

What are Effective Therapist-Based Treatments?

Cognitive–Behavioral Therapy. Cognitive–behavioral sex therapy programs focus on helping the woman overcome her fears and anxieties about vaginal penetration as well as improving sexual functioning and enjoyment. They typically include:

- Education and basic information on sexuality in general (e.g., sexual anatomy and physiology, the sexual response cycle).
- Cognitive restructuring aimed at reducing negative thoughts and feelings toward sexuality and addressing specific fears such as fear of pain, penetration, or sexual intimacy. The therapist should also address any sexually inhibiting thoughts and challenge sexual myths which may have a negative impact on sexual functioning.
- Systematic desensitization to increase tolerance to anxiety surrounding vaginal penetration. The rationale behind this technique is that the feared situation (vaginal penetration) will gradually be associated with positive feelings (relaxation and arousal) rather than with negative feelings (anxiety and fear) by exposing repeatedly the woman to increasingly fear inducing stimuli (i.e., at first imagined and then actual vaginal penetration) while she is in a relaxed state.

What are Effective Medical Treatments?

There are currently no empirically validated medical treatments for vaginismus. However, the following treatments should be used in conjunction with the standard cognitive–behavioral sex therapy approach:

- Pelvic floor physical therapy (see Effective Medical Treatments for Dyspareunia).
- Anxiolytics have been recommended for severe cases of vaginismus or fear of penetration (Plaut & Rach Beisel, 1997).
- Botulinum toxin injections have been proposed to be an effective and safe way of relieving muscle spasms in vaginismus (Brin & Vapnek, 1997; Jankovic & Brin, 1991).

Other Issues in Management

- Since women with vaginismus commonly experience dyspareunia, pain management (see Effective Treatments of Dyspareunia) should be incorporated into the standard treatment approach.
- When problems within the sexual response cycle (e.g., low sexual desire and arousal) or when other important psychological disorders which can impact sexual functioning coexist with vaginismus, they should be addressed and incorporated into the treatment plan.

How Does One Select Among Treatments?

Given that vaginismus appears to be a complex disorder with possibly multiple different paths leading to its development, the treatment of choice should be multidisciplinary and involve the cooperation of different health professionals such as a gynecologist, a pelvic floor physical therapist, and a psychotherapist skilled in sex therapy.

KEY READINGS

Informational and Self-Help and Books

Goodwin, A.J. & Agronin, M.E. (1997). *A woman's guide to overcoming sexual fear and pain.* Oakland, CA: New Harbinger Publications Inc.

Katz, D. & Tabisel, R.L. (2002). *Private pain. It's about life, not just sex. Understanding vaginismus and dyspareunia.* Plainview, NY: Katz-Tabi Publications.

Stewart, E. G., & Spencer, P. (2002). *The V book: A doctor's guide to complete vulvovaginal health.* New York, NY: Bantam Books, Random House Inc.

Useful Websites

http://www.nva.org (National Vulvodynia Association)
http://www.vulvodynia.com (Vulvar Pain Foundation)
http://www.sstarnet.org (Society for Sex Therapy and Research)
http://www.endometriosisassn.org (Endometriosis Association)
http://www.issvd.org (International Society for the Study of Vulvovaginal Disease)
http://www.acog.org (American College of Obstetricians and Gynecologists)
http://www.pelvicpain.org (International Pelvic Pain Society)
http://www.theacpa.org (American Chronic Pain Association)

REFERENCES

American Psychiatric Association (2000). *Diagnostic and statistical manual of mental disorders* (4th ed., Text Rev.) Washington, DC: Author, 2000.

Bachmann, G.A. & Phillips, N.A. (1998). Sexual Dysfunction. In J. F. Steege, D.A. Metzger, & B. S. Levy (Eds.). *Chronic pelvic pain: An integrated approach.* Philadelphia, PA: W.B. Saunders Company.

Barnes, J., Bowman, E. P., & Cullen, J. (1984). Biofeedback as an adjunct to psychotherapy in the treatment of vaginismus. *Biofeedback and Self-Regulation, 9,* 281–289.

Basson, R., Berman, J., Burnett, A., Derogatis, L., Ferguson, D., Fourcroy, J., et al. (2000). Report of the international consensus development conference on female sexual dysfunction: Definitions and Classifications. *The Journal of Urology, 163,* 888–893.

Bergeron, S., Binik, Y. M., Khalifé, S., Pagidas, K., Glazer, H. I., Meana, M. et al. (2001). A randomized comparison of group cognitive–behavioral therapy, surface electromyographic biofeedback, and vestibulectomy in the treatment of dyspareunia resulting from vulvar vestibulitis. *Pain, 91(3),* 297–306.

Bergeron, S., Brown, C., Lord, M.-J., Oala, M., Binik, Y.M., & Khalifé, S. (2002). Physical therapy for vulvar vestibulitis syndrome: a retrospective study. *Journal of Sex and Marital Therapy, 28,* 183–192.

Bergeron, S., & Lord, M. (2003). The integration of pelvi-perineal re-education and cognitive-behavioral therapy in the multidisciplinary treatment of the sexual pain disorders. *Sexual & Relationship Therapy, 18(2),* 135–141.

Binik, Y. M. (in press, a). Should dyspareunia be retained as a sexual dysfunction in DSM-V? A painful classification decision. *Archives of Sexual Behavior.*

Binik, Y. M. (in press, b). Dyspareunia looks sexy on first but how much pain will it take for it to score? *Archives of Sexual Behavior.*

Binik, Y. M., Bergeron, S., & Khalifé, S. (2000). Dyspareunia. In S. R. Leiblum & R. C. Rosen (Eds.). *Principles and Practice of Sex Therapy* (3rd ed.). New York, NY, US: Guilford Press.

Binik, Y. M., Reissing, E. D., Pukall, C. F., Flory, N., Payne, K. A., & Khalifé, S. (2002). The female sexual pain disorders: Genital pain or sexual dysfunction? *Archives of Sexual Behavior, 31,* 425–429.

Brin, M. F. & Vapnek, J. M. (1997). Treatment of vaginismus with botulinum toxin injections. *The Lancet, 349,* 252–253.

Buytendijk, F. J. J. (1957). *Algemene theorie der menselijke houding en beweging.* [General theory of human posture and movement] Utrecht: Spectrum.

Danielsson, I., Eisemann, M., Sjöberg, I., & Wikman, M. (2001). Vulvar vesitbulitis: A multifactorial condition. *British Journal of Obstetrics and Gynaecology, 108,* 456–461.

de Kruiff, M. E., ter Kuile, M. M., Weijenborg, P. Th. M., & van Lankveld, J. J. D. M. (2000). Vaginismus and dyspareunia: Is there difference in clinical presentation? *Journal of Psychosomatic Obstetrics & Gynaecology, 21,* 149–155.

Duddle, M. (1977). Etiological factors in the unconsummated marriage. *Journal of Psychosomatic Research, 21,* 157–60.

Fischer, G. (2004). Management of vulvar pain. *Dermatological Therapy, 17,* 134–149.

Fordney, D. (1978). Dyspareunia and Vaginismus. *Clinical Obstetrics and Gynecology,* 21, 205–221.

Grazziottin, A. (2003). Etiology and diagnosis of coital pain. *Journal of Endocrinological Investigation, 26(Suppl. no. 3),* 115–121.

Harlow, B. L. & Stewart, E. G. (2003). A population based assessment of chronic unexplained vulvar pain: Have we underestimated the pain? *JAMWA, 58,* 82–88.

Hawton, K. & Catalan, J. (1990). Sex therapy for vaginismus: Characteristics of couples and treatment outcome. *Sex & Marital Therapy, 5,* 39–48.

Hirst, J. F., Baggaley, M. R., & Watson. J. P. (1996). A four-year survey of an inner-city psychosexual problems clinic. *Sexual and Marital Therapy, 11,* 19–36.

Jacob, M. C., & DeNardis, M. C. (1998). Sexual and physical abuse and chronic pelvic pain. In J. F. Steege, D. A. Metzger, & B. S. Levy (Eds.). *Chronic pelvic pain: An integrated approach.* Philadelphia, PA: W.B. Saunders Company.

Jankovic, J., & Brin, M. (1991). Therapeutic uses of botulinum toxin. *New England Journal of Medicine, 324,* 1186–1194.

Kaplan, H. S. (1974). *The New Sex Therapy.* New York: Brunner/Mazel.

Kleinplatz, P. (1998). Sex therapy for vaginismus: A review, critique, and humanistic alternative. *Journal of Sex and Marital Therapy, 27,* 153–55.

Laumann, E. O., Gagnon, J. H., Michaci, R. T., & Micheals, S. (1994). *The social organization of sexuality.* University of Chicago Press, Chicago.

Luzzi, G. (2003). Male genital pain disorders. *Sexual & Relationship Therapy, 18,* 225–235.

Masters, W. H. & Johnson, V. E. (1970). *Human sexual inadequacy.* Boston: Little, Brown.

Maurice, W. L. (1999). *Sexual Medicine in Primary Care.* St. Louis, MO: Mosby Inc.

Meana, M., Binik, Y. M., Khalifé, S., & Cohen, D. (1997). Dyspareunia: Sexual dysfunction or pain syndrome? *The Journal of Nervous and Mental Disease, 185(9),* 561–569.

Meana, M., Binik, Y. M., Khalifé, S., & Cohen, D. (1999). Psychosocial correlates of pain attributions in women with dyspareunia. *Psychosomatics, 40(6),* 497–502.

Melzack, R. & Katz, J. (1992). The McGill Pain Questionnaire: Appraisal and current status. In D. C. Turk & R. Melzack (Eds.). *Handbook of pain assessment.* New York, NY: Guilford Press.

Plaut, S. M. & Rach Beisel, J. (1997). Use of anxiolytic medication in the treatment of vaginismus and severe aversion to penetration: Case report. *Journal of Sex Education and Therapy, 22,* 43–45.

Pukall C. F., Lahaie M.-A., & Binik Y. M. (in press). Sexual pain disorders: Etiologic factors. In I. Goldstein, C. M. Meston, S. Davis, & A. Traish (Eds.) *Female sexual dysfunction.* London: Taylor & Francis.

Reissing, E. D., Binik, Y. M. & Khalifé, S. (1999). Does vaginismus exist?: A critical review of the literature. *Journal of Nervous & Mental Disease, 187(5),* 26–274.

Reissing, E. D., Binik, Y. M., Khalifé, S., Cohen, D., & Amsel, R. (2003). Etiological correlates of vaginismus: Sexual and physical abuse, sexual knowledge, sexual self-schema, and relationship adjustment. *Journal of Sex and Marital Therapy, 29,* 47–59.

Reissing, E. D., Binik, Y. M., Khalifé, S. Cohen, D., & Amsel, R. (2004). Vaginal spasm, pain, and behavior: An empirical investigation of the diagnosis of vaginismus. *Archives of Sexual Behavior. 33(1),* 5–17.

Rosenbaum, T. H. (in press). Physiotherapy treatment of sexual pain disorders. *Journal of Sex and Marital Therapy.*

Rust, J., Golombok, S., & Collier, J. (1988). Marital problems and sexual dysfunction: How are they related? *British Journal of Psychiatry,* 152, 629–631.

Spector, I. P. & Carey, M. P. (1990). Incidence and prevalence of the sexual dysfunctions: A critical review of the empirical literature. *Archives of Sexual Behavior, 19,* 389–408.

Steege, J. F. (1984). Dyspareunia and vaginismus. *Clinical Obstetrics & Gynecology. 27(3),* 750–759.

Stewart, E. G., & Spencer, P. (2002). *The V book: A doctor's guide to complete vulvovaginal health.* New York, NY: Bantam Books, Random House Inc.

Van der Velde, J., & Everaerd, W. (1999). Voluntary control over pelvic floor muscles in women with and without vaginistic reactions. *International Urogynecology Journal and Pelvic Floor Dysfunction, 10,* 230–236.

Van der Velde, J., & Everaerd, W. (2001). The relationship between involuntary pelvic floor muscle activity, muscle awareness and experienced threat in women with and without vaginismus. *Behavior Research & Therapy, 39,* 395–408.

van Lankveld, J. J. D. M., Brewaeys, A. M. A., Ter Kuile, M. M., & Weijenborg, P. Th. M. (1995). Difficulties in the differential diagnosis of vaginismus, dyspareunia and mixed sexual pain disorder. *Journal of Psychosomatic Obstetrics & Gynaecology, 16,* 201–209.

Walthard, M. (1909). Die Psychogene Aetiologie und die Psychotherape des Vaginismus. *Muencheher Medizinische Wochenzeitscrift, 56,* 1997–2000.

Ward, E., & Ogden, J. (1994). Experiencing vaginismus: Sufferers' beliefs about causes and effects. *Sexual & Marital Therapy, 9(1),* 33–45.

Weijmar Schultz W. C. M., Gianotten, W. L., van der Meijden, W. I., van de Wiel, H. B. M., Blindeman, L., Chadha, S. et al. (1996). Behavioral approach with or without surgical intervention to the vulvar vestibulitis syndrome: a prospective randomized and non-randomized study. *Journal of Psychosomomatic Obstetrics and Gynecology, 17,* 143–148.

Wincze, J. P. & Carey, M. P. (2001). *Sexual dysfunction: A guide for assessment and treatment,* 2nd ed. New York, NY: Guilford Press.

Specific Phobias

Raphael D. Rose • Michelle A. Blackmore • Michelle G. Craske

WHAT IS SPECIFIC PHOBIA?

Specific phobias (also known as simple phobias) refer to excessive fears and avoidance of a wide range of circumscribed situations or objects (American Psychiatric Association, 1994). In contrast to more commonly occurring fears, phobias are severe enough to cause significant interference in life functioning and/or cause significant distress (Craske, 2003). Individuals who meet DSM-IV criteria for specific phobia recognize that their fear is excessive or more than what would be expected. Unlike adults, children are not required to acknowledge that their fears are unreasonable or excessive, and in order to prevent the overdiagnosis of transitory developmental fears, persistence of symptoms is required for at least six months. Historically, the various specific phobias (e.g., animals, heights, blood, flying) were grouped together, but recent research suggests marked differences across the various phobias (Himle, McPhee, Cameron, & Curtis, 1989; Öst, 1987), including age of onset (Curtis, Hill, & Lewis, 1998; Öst, 1987), rates of cooccurring disorders (Himle et al., 1989), response profiles (Craske, Zarate, Burton, & Barlow, 1993), familial aggregations data (Himle et al., 1989), and genetic variance data (Kendler, Neale, Kessler, Heath, & Eaves, 1993). Hence, while phobias vary greatly in terms of the particular feared stimulus and other factors mentioned above, typically individuals with specific phobias fall into the following four subtypes: animal fears (e.g., snakes, insects), natural environment fears (e.g., storms, heights), blood injection–injury fears (e.g., receiving or observing needle injections or blood injuries), and situational fears (e.g., flying or enclosed spaces).

When individuals with specific phobias are *not* exposed to their feared object or situation, they experience the *least* severe and impairing anxiety disorder (Barlow et al., 1985). However, when encountering feared objects or situations, individuals with phobias tend to experience severe discomfort and may attempt to escape the situation or else endure it with great distress. This distress is often accompanied by physical symptoms such as palpitations, sweating, blushing, and trembling, which may take the form of a situationally bound panic attack. Individuals may also experience similar distress in advance or anticipation of exposure to a feared situation or object (e.g., before a scheduled flight, prior to a medical appointment). As a result, feared situations are often avoided. Such fear and avoidance may significantly interfere with the individual's functioning, often resulting in a change in normal routines, a decline in occupational opportunities, negative impact on social relationships, or changes in regular health maintenance behaviors (e.g., medical checkups).

BASIC FACTS ABOUT SPECIFIC PHOBIAS

Prevalence

Mild fears of specific situations and objects are quite common in the general population (King et al., 1989); however, specific phobias (that cause clinically significant interference and/or distress) are among the most common of the anxiety

Rose, R. D., Blackmore, A., & Craske, M. G. (2006). Specific phobias In J. E. Fisher & W. T. O'Donohue (Eds.), *Practitioner's guide to evidence-based psychotherapy*. New York: Springer.

disorders. The National Comorbidity Survey found lifetime prevalence rates for specific phobias, using DSM-IV criteria, to be 12.5% (Kessler, Berglund, Demler, Jin, & Walters, 2005). Fredrikson, Annas, Fischer, and Wik (1966) found slightly higher prevalence rates (16.3%) among their Swedish sample of 704 adults.

Gender

Women (15.7%) are more likely than men (6.7%) to receive a specific phobia diagnosis (Kessler et al., 1994). Overall, 75–90% of individuals with animal, natural environment, or situational specific phobia are female, with slightly lower rates (55–70%) for individuals with phobias of heights or blood-injection (Himle et al., 1989).

Age of onset, course, and demographic characteristics

The majority of individuals with animal and blood-injection specific phobia report an onset of difficulties by childhood (ages 7–9), whereas situational and natural environment subtypes exhibit a bimodal distribution of onset, in early childhood and early adulthood (Himle et al., 1989), with situational subtypes more commonly developing in young adulthood (Öst & Treffers, 2001). Additionally, for those phobias occurring during childhood, elevations are often seen between 10 and 13 years of age (Strauss & Last, 1993).

Untreated specific phobias tend to be chronic or recurrent (Yonkers, Dyck, &, Keller, 2001), with a remission rate over a seven-year period as low as 16% (Wittchen, 1988). Interestingly, despite the relatively high prevalence and chronicity of specific phobias, individuals rarely seek treatment, perhaps because most people with specific phobias are able to function despite strong fears and phobias. Individuals with higher levels of functional impairment, multiple phobias, panic symptoms in the phobic situation, and surprisingly, *absence* of blood phobias, injury or medical procedures were all related to higher help-seeking (Chapman, Fyer, Mannuzza, & Klein, 1993). As a result of the generally circumscribed nature of specific phobias, they are associated with less distress overall in comparison to other anxiety disorders (Craske, 2003).

Comorbidity The cooccurrence of a specific phobia with other disorders, such as panic disorder and agoraphobia, depression, or additional specific phobias is very common. With respect to cooccurring depressed mood, research suggests this may be the result of anxiety and mood disorders sharing a vulnerability of negative affectivity (Brown, Chopita, & Barlow, 1998; Craske, 2003; Zinbarg & Barlow, 1996). Although specific phobias yield the lowest rates of cooccurring anxiety disorders when compared to other anxiety disorders (Brown & Barlow, 1992), panic disorder and agoraphobia are commonly found to cooccur. Ehlers (1993) found that individuals with specific phobia who occasionally panic are more likely to develop panic disorder when compared to those that do not panic. Situational phobias most often overlap with panic disorder and agoraphobia as individuals with these disorders are often more sensitive to bodily sensations and believe them to be dangerous (Craske, Lang, Aikins, & Mystkowski, 2003). Therefore, the feared stimuli in situational phobias, such as claustrophobia (Febbraro & Clum, 1995) and driving phobias (Ehlers, Hofmann, Herda, & Roth, 1994), may render bodily sensations more salient and threatening, often triggering panic attacks. Individuals with natural environment phobias also demonstrate a stronger propensity toward panic attacks when compared to those with other specific phobias such as the animal-subtype diagnosis (Verburg, Griez, & Meijer, 1994).

ASSESSMENT

What Should be Ruled Out?

Specific phobia is only diagnosed when the presenting symptoms are not better accounted for by another mental disorder. Some individuals with specific phobias (e.g., driving, flying, heights, enclosed places) may experience panic attacks in their feared situations. For these individuals, a diagnosis of panic disorder should be ruled out, as they may also experience non-circumscribed attacks and apprehension about future panic attacks. For individuals who experience situationally bound or circumscribed panic attacks and do *not* have panic attacks in other situations or do *not* worry about future attacks, then a diagnosis of specific phobia would remain appropriate. Additionally, multiple specific phobia diagnoses would be appropriate when an individual has significant fear and avoidance of one or more distinct situations or objects (e.g., situational—driving, and animal—dogs). Lastly, it is possible to have multiple specific phobia diagnoses *within* a specific phobia specifier when the focus of the fear is distinctly different (e.g., phobia of dogs and a phobia of insects within the animal-subtype diagnosis).

What is Involved in Effective Assessment?

A thorough psychological assessment of specific phobia should include examination of:

- DSM-IV criteria for specific phobia
- Severity of specific fear
- Range of feared situations or objects (multiple phobias)
- Severity of distress when encountering feared situation
- Frequency and severity of avoidance behavior
- Functional impairment
- Severity of anticipatory anxiety
- Substance use to self-medicate anxiety (e.g., while flying)

Clinician-administered measures Structured clinical interviews, such as the Anxiety Disorders Interview Schedule for DSM-IV, Lifetime version (DiNardo, Brown, & Barlow, 1994), provide substantial information about the presence of diagnostic features and fear and avoidance of specific phobias. The Structured Clinical Interview for DSM-IV-*Patient Version* (SCID-I/P) is another commonly used interview for the assessment and diagnosis of specific phobias (First, Spitzer, Gibbon, & Williams, 1996).

Self-report measures The Fear Survey Schedule-II (FS-II) (Geer, 1965) and FSS-III (Wolpe & Lang, 1969) measure specific objects and situations that an individual fears. The FS-II is a research-based 51-item measure while the FS-III is a 72-item scale designed for use in clinical settings. In addition to specific phobias (e.g., flying, blood-injection), the scales include items related to social phobia (e.g., public speaking) and agoraphobia (e.g., crowds), as well as items for situations that people fear (e.g., fear of sirens, noise from vacuum) that are *not* typically reported by individuals with specific phobias. Therefore, the FSS may not be ideal for assessing specific phobias. There are several other self-report measures that focus solely on certain specific phobias (e.g., animals, insects, medical procedures, flying, dental visits) some examples include: The Spider Questionnaire (SPQ) is a 31-item measure with each item being a fearful on nonfearful statement about spiders (Klorman, Hastings, Weerts, Melamed, & Lang, 1974). The Medical Fear Survey

(MFS) is a 50-item measure that assesses the severity of medical fears (Kleinknecht, Thorndike, & Walls, 1996). The Acrophobia Questionnaire (AQ) is a 40-item scale in which individuals rate their fear and avoidance in relation to 20 different height situations (Cohen, 1977). The Fear of Flying Scale (FSS) is a 21-item measure for assessing fears of flying (see Haug et al., 1987, for more information).

Behavioral assessment Observation of behavior in anxiety-provoking situations may be helpful in understanding the severity of anxiety and behavior in specific situations. A standardized behavioral assessment task (BAT) can involve approach–avoidance exercises where the proximity to and duration spent with a phobic stimulus (e.g., spider) is measured and can be utilized pre- and posttreatment to gauge treatment response (e.g. Rachman & Hodgson, 1974). Behavioral assessment for specific phobias is critical because the data one collects is often discordant with self-report and physiological measures (Lang, 1971; Rachman & Hodgson, 1974), and one can also obtain information that is critical for treatment development, as would be the case if clients were unaware of aspects of the their behavioral responses.

What Assessments are Not Helpful?

Psychological tests such as the Minnesota Multiphasic Personality Inventory (MMPI), projective tests (e.g., Rorschach Inkblot test), neuropsychological tests, or medical tests are not particularly useful in assessing specific phobias.

TREATMENT

What Treatments are Effective?

Mastery of your Specific Phobia (Antony, Craske, & Barlow, 1995) is a manualized CBT treatment approach for specific phobias that was influenced by the ground-breaking efforts of Wolpe (1958) who described the therapeutic technique of systematic desensitization. Wolpe's approach of systematic desensitization involved repeated pairings of progressively more anxiety-provoking images of phobic stimuli with a contrary response of relaxation. Such repeated pairings lead to the relaxation response eventually inhibiting the anxiety response such that the individual can imagine the phobic stimulus without experiencing anxiety. Mastery of your Specific Phobia divides treatment into three areas; psychoeducation, cognitive restructuring, and systematic exposure exercises (see Craske, Antony, & Barlow, 1997). Treatment strategies are applicable to all specific phobias, but there are also phobia specific chapters (e.g., flying, blood injection, animals, and insects).

Cognitive–behavioral therapy (CBT) for specific phobias has demonstrated efficacy and empirical support stemming from randomized controlled trials (e.g., Chambless et al., 1996). CBT interventions for specific phobias share several common characteristics: treatments are generally short and time-limited lasting anywhere from one to eight sessions, they are present-focused, and through a collaborative working relationship between therapist and patient, treatments attempt to broaden the range of patients' cognitive and behavioral skills. Specific phobia treatments are similar in that they involve many of the following educational, cognitive, and behavioral strategies; they differ in that they would target the patient's specific feared stimuli (e.g., flying, spiders). The key component of specific phobia treatment is in vivo exposure to the feared stimulus (see Antony, et al., 1995 for a detailed description of these specific phobia management strategies in manualized format):

1. Psychoeducation teaches clients about common features of specific phobias including etiology and a rationale for cognitive and behavioral therapies. Educational training also attempts to correct misinformation (e.g., not all spiders are poisonous) or deficits in knowledge (e.g., correct animal handling procedures, the mechanics of flying) regarding the feared situation or object.

2. Self-monitoring and fear hierarchy construction allows the client and the therapist to identify key thoughts, feelings, and behaviors about the feared situation which will be addressed in subsequent exercises.

3. Cognitive restructuring is typically taught as an aide to conducting the behavioral exposure exercises. Cognitive methods focus on probability overestimations of their perceived danger in the situation (e.g., "the plane will crash," "the snake will bite," "I'll be stuck in the elevator forever") and perceived dangers or limitations in one's ability to respond to the situation or object (catastrophizing) (e.g., "I cannot cope," "I'll make a fool of myself on the plane," "I will pass out from fear"). Probability overestimations and catastophizing thinking patterns are targeted with cognitive techniques so that clients challenge these maladaptive beliefs and generate alternative beliefs in order to create a more realistic, and presumably more accurate, view of themselves and the world.

4. Breathing retraining and relaxation training are sometimes used for management of physiological arousal during exposures. However, this strategy should not be utilized to "get rid of the sensations" as that may contribute to ones continued misappraisals of the fear situation and an inability to cope unless the sensations are eliminated.

5. Systematic exposure exercises are conducted either in vivo, imaginally, or by virtual reality, although in vivo is recommended when possible. Exposure exercises help patients face their feared situations/objects (through imagery or in their natural environments) and stay psychologically engaged such that their anxiety response may subside through the processes of habituation and extinction.

6. Exposure for blood, injury injection individuals: Öst, Sterner, and Lindahl (1984) developed a treatment procedure for blood phobic individuals called applied tension to specifically target the fainting response common in blood, injection, injury individuals. In contrast to in vivo exposures for other specific phobias where the main goal is anxiety activation, habituation and extinction, the treatment approach for blood-injury phobias basically involves increasing blood pressure to prevent fainting. First, patients are taught to tense their major body muscles in order to increase blood pressure. Next, they are taught to detect early signs of decreasing blood pressure, such as lightheadedness, which eventually prompts body tensing.

7. Combined exposure and cognitive restructuring treatments integrate the utilization of cognitive skills with behavioral exposure to feared situations and/or objects. The focus during exposure is then to provide an opportunity for patients to gather information that may serve to disconfirm misappraisals about themselves in situations they fear.

Several treatment studies of specific phobias over the past 30 years point to the efficacy of the CBT techniques described above. Most research points to the advantage of in-vivo exposure over imaginal exposure (see Barlow, Leitenberg, Agras, & Wincze, 1969; Emmelkamp & Wessels, 1975; Ultee, Griffioen, & Schellekens, 1982). Although Hecker (1990) reported that imaginal exposure was similarly effective to in vivo exposure. More recently, virtual reality exposures have been used to bridge the gap between imaginal and in vivo exposure and offer another treatment option for certain specific phobias (e.g., Emmelkamp et al., 2002). Cognitive strategies alone have demonstrated some utility (Booth & Rachman, 1992), and there is evidence that those strategies may strengthen behavioral approaches to treating specific phobias (Emmelkamp & Felton, 1985). A series of studies by Öst and colleagues provide additional outcome data on the percentage of individuals treated that experienced clinically significant improvement. These studies incorporated exposure, relaxation, modeling, and applied tension techniques and averaged approximately five therapy hours (see Öst, 1989; Öst, Hellstrom, & Kaver, 1992; Öst, Johansson, & Jerremalm, 1982; Öst, Sterner, & Fellenius, 1989). On average, 85% of phobic clients showed clinically significant improvement at the end of treatment and at nearly 2 years follow-up, 76% maintained their treatment gains. Drop-out rates were only 4% and treatments generalized to all phobic situations and not just the specific phobic stimuli that were targeted in treatment.

Thus, research supports the effectiveness of CBT for treating specific phobias, in that it is highly effective within a relatively short period of time and significant treatment gains are maintained over time. Cognitive restructuring and exposure appear to be the most important treatment components.

What are Effective Self-Help Treatments?

The self-help books, listed below, include many elements of effective CBT techniques for specific phobias and anxiety. Of note, however, there is no empirical support for these self-help books when used as the only source of treatment.

- Antony, M. M., Craske, M. G., & Barlow, D. H. (1995). *Mastery of your specific phobias.* San Antonio, TX: Harcourt Brace
- Antony, M. M., & McCabe R. E. (2005). *Overcoming animal and insect phobias: How to conquer fear of dogs, snakes, rodents, bees, spiders, & more.* Oakland, CA: New Harbinger Publications.
- Antony, M., & Watling, M. (2005). *Overcoming medical phobias.* New Harbinger Publications.
- Barlow, D. H., & Craske, M. G. (2000). *Mastery of your anxiety and panic (MAP-3): Client workbook for agoraphobia.* San Antonio, TX: Harcourt Brace.
- Bourne, E. (1995). *Driving far from home (I can do it).* Oakland, CA: New Harbinger Publications.
- Bourne, E. (2001). *Beyond anxiety and phobia: A step-by-step guide to lifetime recovery.* Oakland, CA: New Harbinger Publications.
- Brown, D. (1996). *Flying without fear.* Oakland, CA: New Harbinger Publications
- *http:// www.fearfighter.com/index.htm* (self-guided, web-based specific phobia treatment)
- *http:// www.phobiascured.com/ebook2.htm* (The Phobia Self-help Book)
  Useful informational websites about specific phobia and related resources include:
- *http://www.adaa.org* (Anxiety Disorders Association of America)
- *http://www.adaa. org/ADAA%20web%20fin/Factsheets/phobias.pdf* (ADAA—specific phobia fact sheet)
- *www.aabt.org* (Association for Advancement of Behavior Therapy)
- *http://www. apa.org—http://helping.apa.org/* (American Psychological Association)
- *http://www.psych.org* (American Psychiatric Association)
- *http://www.mentalhealth. ucla.edu/projects/anxiety/behavioralanxietydisorders.htm* (UCLA—Department of Psychology -Anxiety Disorders Behavioral Research Program)
- *http://www.mentalhealth. ucla.edu/projects/anxiety/index.htm* (UCLA Anxiety Disorders Program)
- *http://www. nimh.nih.gov/publicat/adfacts.cfm* (National Institute of Mental Health)
- *http:// www.freedomfromfear.com* (Freedom From Fear)

- *http://www.anxietytreatment.ca/specificP.htm* (Anxiety and Treatment Centre—McMaster University, Hamilton, Ontario)
- *http://www.nmha.org/infoctr/factsheets/template.cfm* (National Mental Health Association)

What is Effective Medical Treatment?

Medications are generally considered to be of limited effectiveness for specific phobias. Specific phobias by definition are fears that are limited to circumscribed situations or objects and therefore medication is typically only needed in those specific instances. The few studies conducted with medication found no additional benefit from adding pharmacological treatments with behavioral treatments. The evidence for efficacy of behavioral treatments is solid even in the absence of pharmacotherapy, and it is widely accepted that medication is not necessary to treat clients with specific phobias.

If a patient is on a stable dose of medication, there is little evidence to suggest that it will interfere with exposure-based treatments. Patients may want to taper off a stable dose with the supervision of the prescribing physician during the latter CBT sessions. For those patients taking medication as needed (e.g., benzodiazepines or beta-adrenergic blockers for fear of flying), the preferred approach is to perform exposure sessions without the medication, as there is some evidence that individuals who associate their treatment gains to medication are less likely to maintain improvement than clients who attribute improvement to exposure-based exercises.

Generally, use of benzodiazepines to treat specific phobias runs contrary to the aim of exposure exercises in that they decrease the fear response. Carrying or taking such medications in anticipation of or during exposure to a feared situation may take the form of a safety behavior (i.e., strategy to limit anxiety). When confronted with a feared situation, individuals engage in these safety behaviors to prevent the feared consequence, which allows them to feel more comfortable in the threatening situation. Safety behaviors diminish the effectiveness of exposure and result in decreased treatment response. Therefore, at posttreatment when patients who have used benzodiazepines confront the feared situation/object there may be a concern of relapse.

Combination Treatments

Some benefits to a combined approach are found with regard to specific phobias. Early on, Marks, Viswanathan, Lipsedge, and Gardner (1972) used a modified crossover design in which eighteen individuals received two hours of in vivo exposure, combined with .1 mg/kg of diazepam (valium) either immediately before exposure (waxing condition), or fours hours before exposure (waning condition), or a waxing or waning placebo. Overall, diazepam potentiated exposure, with the waning condition showing a slight advantage over the waxing condition on some measures. Interestingly, the result was apparently *not* due to lessened unpleasantness of exposure. Next, Whitehead, Blackwell, and Robinson (1978) examined the effect of 10 mg of diazepam on behavioral approach test performance for specific phobias. Compared to the placebo condition, ability to approach phobic objects was increased and self-reported anxiety was decreased in the diazepam condition. In a second study, Whitehead, Robinson, Blackwell, and Stutz (1978) examined flooding therapy with either chronic use of diazepam (15 mg/day) or placebo for the treatment of small animal phobia. Flooding treatment occurred two times a week for three weeks. There was little difference between the two conditions. Taken together, Whitehead, Robinson, et al. (1978) concluded that behavioral treatment may be facilitated by single doses of short acting tranquilizers, but not by chronic dose regimens. Unfortunately, these studies did not assess functioning in the long-term.

A recent development involves the use of D-cycloserine, a cognitive enhancer, which appears to facilitate exposure and the extinction of conditioned fear (Davis, 2003; Walker, Ressler, Lu, & Davis, 2002).

How Does One Select Among Treatments?

There are several areas to consider prior to beginning treatment for specific phobia. As previously noted, CBT is the treatment of choice and while patients are likely to benefit from such treatment the exposure exercises may be quite challenging for some to undergo. Additionally patients may experience and *increase* in anxiety during the beginning phases of treatment and therefore, it may be helpful to assess the acceptability and motivation of the patient to participate in CBT prior to commencing treatment. For those unwilling or unable to partake in a course of CBT, then a medication consultation may be an appropriate alternative option.

REFERENCES (DOES NOT INCLUDE LIST OF SELF-HELP BOOKS UNLESS OTHERWISE CITED)

American Psychiatric Association (1994). *Diagnostic and statistical manual of mental disorders* (4th ed.). Washington, DC: Author.

Antony, M. M., Craske, M. G., & Barlow, D. H. (Eds.) (1995). *Mastery of your specific phobias.* San Antonio, TX: Harcourt Brace.

Barlow, D. H., Leitenberg, H., Agras, W. S., & Wincze J. P. (1969). The transfer gap in systematic desensitization: An analogue study. *Behaviour Research and Therapy, 7,* 191–196.

Barlow, D. H., Vermilyea, J., Blanchard, E. B., Vermilyea, B. B., Di Nardo, P. A., & Cer&ngrave;y, J. A. (1985). The phenomenon of panic. *Journal of Abnormal Psychology, 94,* 320–328.

Booth, R., & Rachman, S. (1992). The reduction of claustrophobia-I. *Behaviour Research and Therapy, 30,* 207–221.

Brown, T. A., & Barlow, D. H. (1992). Comorbidity among anxiety disorders: Implications for treatment and DSM-IV. *Journal of Consulting and Clinical Psychology, 60,* 835–844.

Brown, T. A., Chorpita, B. F., & Barlow, D. H. (1998). Structural relationships among dimensions of the DSM-IV anxiety and mood disorders and dimensions of negative affect, positive affect, and autonomic arousal. *Journal of Abnormal Psychology, 107,* 179–192.

Chambless, D. L., Sanderson, W. C., Shoham, V., Bennett Johnson, S., Pope, K. S., Crits-Christoph, P., et al. (1996). An update on empirically validated therapies. *The Clinical Psychologist, 49,* 5–18.

Chapman, T. F., Fyer, A. J., Mannuzza, S., & Klein, D. F. (1993). A comparison of treated and untreated simple phobia. *American Journal of Psychiatry, 150,* 816–818.

Cohen, D. C. (1977). Comparison of self-report and overt-behavioral procedures for assessing acrophobia, *Behavior Therapy, 8,* 17–23.

Craske, M. G., Antony, M. M., & Barlow, D. H. (1997). *Mastery of your specific phobia: Therapist guide.* USA: Graywind Publications.

Craske, M. G. (2003). *Origins of phobias and anxiety disorders: Why more women than Men?* Oxford, UK: Elsevier.

Craske, M. G., Lang, A. J., Aikins, D., & Mystkowski, J. (2005). Cognitive behavioral therapy for nocturnal panic disorder.

Craske, M. G., Zarate, R., Burton, T., & Barlow, D. H. (1993). Specific fears and panic attacks: A survey of clinical and nonclinical samples. *Journal of Anxiety Disorders, 7,* 1–19.

Curtis, G. C., Hill, E. M., & Lewis, J. A. (1998). Heterogeneity of DSM-III-R simple phobia and the simple phobia/agoraphobia boundary: Evidence from the ECA study. In T. A. Widiger, A. J. Frances, H. A. Pincuss, R. Ross, M. B. First, W. Davis, & M. Kline (Eds.), *DSM-IV source book* (Vol. 4, pp. 245–257). Washington, DC: American Psychiatric Association.

Davis, M. (2003). The role of NMDA receptors in extinction. In Society for Neuroscience 2003 Abstract Viewer/Itinerary Planner (Washington, DC, Society for Neuroscience). Program number 327.322.

DiNardo, P. A., Brown, T. A., & Barlow, d. H. (1994). *Anxiety Disorders Interview Schedule for DSM-IV: Lifetime version (ADIS-IV-L).* San Antonio, TX: The Psychological Corporation.

Ehlers, A. (1993). Somatic symptoms and panic attacks: A retrospective study of learning experiences. *Behaviour Research and Therapy, 31,* 269–278.

Ehlers, A., Hofmann, S. G., Herda, C. A., & Roth, W. T. (1994). Clinical characteristics of driving phobia. *Journal of Anxiety Disorders, 8,* 323–339.

Emmelkamp, P. M. G., & Felten, M. (1985). The process of exposure *in vivo*: Cognitive and physiological changes during treatment of acrophobia. *Behaviour Research and Therapy, 23,* 219–223.

Emmelkamp, P. M. G., Krijn, M., Hulsbosch, A. M., de Vries, S., Schuemie, M. J., & van der Mast, C. A. P. G. (2002). Virtual reality treatment versus exposure in vivo: A comparative evaluation in acrophobia. *Behaviour Research and Therapy, 40,* 509–516.

First, M. B., Spitzer, R. L., Gibbon, M., & Williams, J. (1996). *Structured Clinical Interview for DSM-IV Axis I disorders—Patient Edition* (SCID-I/P, Version 2.0). New York State Psychiatric Institute, New York.

Febbraro, G. A. R., & Clum, G. A. (1995). A dimensional analysis of claustrophobia. *Journal of Psychopathology and Behavioral Assessment, 17,* 335–351.

Fredrikson, M. Annas, P., Fischer, H., & Wik, G. (1966). Gender and age differences in the prevalence of specific fears and phobias. *Behaviour Research and Therapy, 34,* 33–39.

Geer, J. H. (1965). The development of a scale to measure fear. *Behavior Research and Therapy, 3,* 45–53.

Harb, G. C., Eng, W., Zaider, T., & Heimberg, R. G. (2003). Behavioral assessment of public speaking anxiety using a modified version of the Social Performance Rating Scale. *Behaviour Research and Therapy, 41,* 1373–1380.

Haug, T., Brenne, L., Johnsen, B. H., Berntzen, D., et al. (1987). A three-systems analysis of fear of flying: A comparison of a consonant vs a non-consonant treatment method. *Behaviour Research & Therapy, 25,* 187–194

Hecker, J. E. (1990). Emotional processing in the treatment of simple phobia: A comparison of imaginal and in vivo exposure. *Behavioral Psychotherapy, 18,* 21–34.

Himle, J. A., McPhee, K., Cameron, O. G., & Curtis, G. C. (1989). Simple phobia: Evidence for heterogeneity. *Psychiatry Research, 28,* 25–30.

Kendler, K. S., Neale, M. C., Kessler, R. C., Heath, A. C., & Eaves, L. J. (1993). Major depression and phobias: The genetic and environmental sources of comorbidity. *Psychological Medicine, 23,* 361–371.

Kessler, R. C., Berglund, P., Demler, O., Jin, R., Walters, E. E. (2005). Lifetime prevalence and age-of-onset distributions of DSM-IV disorders in the National Comorbidity Survey replication. *Archives of General Psychiatry, 62,* 593–602.

Kessler, R. C., McGonagle, K., Zhao, S., Nelson, C., Hughes, M., Eshelman, S., et al. (1994). Lifetime and 12-month prevalence of DSM-III-R psychiatric disorders in the United States: Results from the National Comorbidity Survey. *Archives of General Psychiatry, 51,* 8–19.

King, N. J., Ollier, K., Iacuone, R., Schuster, S., Bays, K., Gullone, E., et al. (1989). Fears of children and adolescents: A cross-sectional Australian study using the Revised-Fear Survey Schedule for Children. *Journal of Child Psychology and Psychiatry and Allied Disciplines, 30,* 775–784.

Kleinknecht, R. A., Thorndike, R. M., & Walls, M. M. (1996). Factorial dimensions and correlates of blood, injury, injection and related medical fears: Cross validation of the Medical Fear Survey. *Behavior Research and Therapy, 34,* 323–331.

Klorman, R., Hastings, J. E., Weerts, T. C., Melamed, B. G., & Lang, P. J. (1974). Psychometric description of some specific-fear questions. *Behavior Therapy, 5,* 401–409.

Lang, P. J. (1971). The application of psychophysiological methods to the study of psychotherapy and behaviour modification. In A. Bergin & S. Garfield (Eds.), *Handbook of psychotherapy and behaviour change.* New York: Wiley.

Marks, I. M., Lovell, K., Noshirvani, H., Livanou, M., & Thrasher, S. (1998). Treatment of posttraumatic stress disorder by exposure and/or cognitive restructuring: A controlled study. *Archives of General Psychiatry, 55,* 317–325.

Marks, I. M., Viswanathan, R., Lipsedge, M. S., & Gardner, R. (1972). Enhanced relief of phobias by flooding during waning diazepam effect. *British Journal of Psychiatry, 121,* 493–505.

Öst, L. G. (1987). Age of onset in different phobias. *Journal of Abnormal Psychology, 96,* 223–229.

Öst, L. G. (1989). One-session treatment for Specific Phobias. *Behavior Research and Therapy, 27,* 1–7.

Öst, L. G., Hellstrom, K., & Kaver, A. (1992). One versus five sessions of exposure in the treatment of injection phobia. *Behavior Therapy, 23,* 263–282.

Öst, L. G., Johansson, J., & Jerremalm, A. (1982). Individual response patterns and the effects of different behavioral methods in the treatment of claustrophobia. *Behaviour Research and Therapy, 20,* 445–460.

Öst, L. G., Sterner, U., & Fellenius, J. (1989). Applied tension, applied relaxation, and the combination in the treatment of blood phobia. *Behaviour Research and Therapy, 27,* 109–121.

Öst, L. G., Sterner, U., & Lindahl, I. L. (1984). Physiological responses in blood phobics. *Behaviour Research and Therapy, 22,* 109–117.

Öst, L. G., & Treffers, P. D. A. (2001). Onset, course, and outcome for anxiety disorders in children. In W. K. Silverman & P. D. A. Treffers (Eds.), *Anxiety disorders in children and adolescents: Research, assessment and intervention* (pp. 293–312). Cambridge: Cambridge University Press.

Rachman, S., & Hodgson, R. S. (1974). Synchrony and desynchrony in fear and avoidance. *Behaviour Research and Therapy, 12,* 311–318.

Strauss, C. C., & Last, C. G. (1993). Social and simple phobias in children. *Journal of Anxiety Disorders, 7,* 141–152.

Verburg., K., Griez, E., Meijer, J. (1994). A 35% carbon dioxide challenge in simple phobias. *Acta Psychiatrica Scandinavica, 90,* 420–423.

Walker, D. L., Ressler, K. J., Lu, K. T., & Davis, M. (2002). Facilitation of conditioned fear extinction by systemic administration or intra-amygdala infusions of D-cycloserine as assessed with fear-potentiated startle in rats. *Journal of Neuroscience, 22,* 2343–2351.

Whitehead, W. E., Blackwell, B., & Robinson, A. (1978). Effects of diazepam on phobic avoidance behavior and phobic anxiety. *Biological Psychiatry, 13,* 59–64.

Whitehead, W. E., Robinson, A., Blackwell, B., Stutz, R. M. (1978). Flooding treatment of phobias: Does ćhronic diazepam increase effectiveness? *Journal of Behavior Therapy and Experimental Psychiatry, 9,* 219–225.

Williams, S. L., & Falbo, J. (1996). Cognitive and performance-based treatments for panic attacks in people with varying degrees of agoraphobic disability. *Behaviour Research and Therapy, 34,* 253–264.

Wittchen, H. U. (1988). Natural course and spontaneous remissions of untreated anxiety disorder: Results of the Munich Follow-up Study (MFS). In H. Hand & H. Wittchen (Eds.), *Panic and phobias: Treatments and variables affecting course and outcome* (pp. 3–17). Berlin: Springer-Verlag.

Wolpe, J. (1958). *Psychotherapy by reciprocal inhibition.* Oxford, England: Stanford University Press.

Wolpe, J., & Lang, P. J. (1969). A Fear Survey Schedule for use in behaviour therapy. *Behaviour Research and Therapy, 3,* 27–30.

Yonkers, K. A., Dyck, I. R., & Keller, M. B. (2001). An eight-year longitudinal comparison of clinical course and characteristics of social phobia among men and women. *Psychiatric Services, 52,* 637–643.

Zinbarg, R. E., & Barlow, D. H. (1996). Structure of anxiety and the anxiety disorders: A hierarchical model. *Journal of Abnormal Psychology, 105,* 184–193.

Sleep Terrors

V. Mark Durand

SLEEP TERRORS

Sleep disturbances are highly prevalent in our society. Unfortunately, most people do not get enough sleep and one out of every four Americans report that they sleep less than seven hours per night during the work week—which works out to about an hour and a half less than a century ago (National Sleep Foundation, 2002). And, one of the most common reasons for referring children to mental health professionals is a sleep disturbance (Whyte & Schaefer, 1995). Difficulties surrounding sleep can include bedtime tantrums, disruptive night waking, nightmares, sleep terrors, and excessive daytime sleepiness. Over 25% of all children exhibit some form of significant problem involving sleep (Mindell, 1993) and, among these problems, sleep terrors are often the most disturbing.

Sleep terrors are a form of parasomnia (abnormal behavioral or physiological events during sleep) that involve a sudden arousal from slow wave sleep and present as intense emotional upset. These episodes are often mistaken for nightmares, although unlike nightmares sleep terrors are not manifestations of a dream and occur during the deeper stages (Stages 3 and 4) of nonrapid eye movement (NREM) sleep. Called "incubus" in adults, and "pavor nocturnus" in children, these events can be extremely upsetting, especially for an observer (Lask, 1995). Sleep terrors usually commence with a piercing scream, the person appears to be extremely upset, and the episode is often accompanied by sweating and a rapid heartbeat. The person cannot be easily awakened and comforted, as is possible when someone has a nightmare. And, in the case of sleep terror, the individual does not remember the incident, despite its often dramatic presentation (American Sleep Disorders Association, 1990).

Approximately 3% of otherwise healthy young children have sleep terrors at some point, and less than 1% of adults also display this problem. The occurrence in males and females appears equal. Fortunately, most instances of sleep terrors among children decrease in frequency over time, and are usually gone by the time the child is a teenager (Giles & Buysse, 1993). Relatively little is known about this sleep problem, although several theories of the cause of sleep terrors have been proposed (Lask, 1995). Psychological influences were proposed at one time, although research seems to suggest that they may not be an important consideration (Kales et al., 1980). Biological theories have implicated enlarged adenoids as well as an immature central nervous system as the cause of this problem, although there is very little evidence to support or discount these ideas (Karacan, 1988). Members of the same family tend to have this disorder, and there appears to be a strong genetic component but the specific genes or mechanism of action has not yet been found (Abe, Oda, Ikenaga, & Yamada, 1993; Broughton, 2000).

ASSESSMENT

Assessment of sleep terrors usually takes the form of a clinical interview with someone who witnesses the events—typically a bed partner or the parent of a child suspected

Durand, V. M. (2006). Sleep terrors. In J. E. Fisher & W. T. O'Donohue (Eds.), *Practitioner's guide to evidence-based psychotherapy*. New York: Springer.

has having the problem. Along with a descriptive assessment of the reported episodes, the clinician attempts to determine if the episodes occur during the first third of the night and if they are accompanied by full or partial amnesia of the event (Broughton, 2000). The routine use of overnight polysomnography (assessment of physiological measures including sleep stages, breathing, limb activity, etc.) usually is not recommended unless there are concerns about comorbid breathing or limb movement difficulties (Littner et al., 2003). An assessment of the quality and duration of sleep is important, since sleep terrors may be triggered by insufficient sleep.

Differential diagnosis is essential in order to rule out the presence of nightmares or other similar sleep-related interruptions. Information about the timing of the events and the ability to recall the episodes is useful for ruling out the presence of nightmares, which are typically present later in the sleep cycle and can be recalled by the affected person. An additional important piece of information is whether or not the person moves about or speaks during the episode. Nightmares occur during dream sleep (rapid eye movement or REM sleep) when the muscles of the body are relatively immobile-making it impossible for a person to sit up, walk around the room, or speak. In contrast, sleep terrors occur during nonREM (or NREM) sleep, where a person can speak and move. In addition to eliminating the role of nightmares, a medical evaluation is recommended concurrent with the sleep assessment to rule out potential medical causes including seizures. Nocturnal panic attacks can sometimes resemble sleep terrors, although with panic attacks the person awakens, while it is difficult to awaken a person during a sleep terror event.

The DSM-IV-TR criteria for sleep terrors (referred to as Sleep Terror Disorder; American Psychiatric Association, 2000) include:

- Recurrent episodes of abrupt awakening from sleep, usually occurring during the first third of the major sleep episode and beginning with a panicky scream.
- Intense fear and signs of autonomic arousal, such as tachycardia, rapid breathing, and sweating, during each episode.
- Relative unresponsiveness to efforts of others to comfort the person during the episode.
- No detailed dream is recalled and there is amnesia for the episode.
- The episodes cause clinically significant distress or impairment in social, occupational, or other important areas of functioning.
- The disturbance is not due to the direct physiological effects of a substance (e.g., a drug of abuse, a medication) or a general medical condition.
These criteria are generally accepted and are supported by the existing research literature (Neylan, Reynolds, & Kupfer, 2003).

TREATMENT

Treatment for sleep terrors usually begins with the recommendation to wait them out to see if they disappear on their own. When the problem is more frequent or persists over a long period of time, sometimes medications such as antidepressants (e.g., imipramine) or benzodiazepines are recommended for treatment (Neylan, et al., 2003). These medications tend to reduce the amount of time spent in deep (Stages 3 and 4) sleep, which in theory should reduce the number of sleep terror episodes which occur during these stages of sleep. However, the effectiveness of these drugs on chronic sleep terrors has yet to be clearly demonstrated (Lask, 1995; Mindell, 1993). In addition, their side effects-which can include daytime drowsiness—make them a less than ideal solution, especially for children.

Our still limited understanding about the nature of sleep terrors suggests that having the person get more sleep may help to reduce these episodes, a frequently reported clinical finding. Sleep terrors occur during the deepest stages of sleep. There are four stages of NREM sleep, with Stages 1 and 2 being a time of relatively light sleep, and Stages 3 and 4 representing deeper periods of sleep. The sleep terrors a child or adult experience happen while the person is in the deep Stages 3 and 4 sleep. When we are sleep deprived, we tend to have more Stages 3 and 4, or deeper, sleep. This suggests that sleep terrors may be partly the result of the person not getting enough sleep. In contrast, sleeping more hours at night tends to decrease the amount of deep sleep. This is obviously not recommended for children who have night waking problems, since sleeping more hours will tend to produce lighter sleep and therefore can increase wakings. However, if a child has frequent sleep terrors but does not experience other sleep disturbances, it may be helpful to have the child sleep more hours at night, or take a nap during the day.

Unfortunately, sleep in general is typically problematic for many, so that success at increasing the length and quality of sleep may prove elusive. Behavioral interventions for sleep disorders have been used for some time (Durand, Mindell, Mapstone, & Gernert-Dott, 1998) and include, graduated extinction (Ferber, 1985; Mindell, 1997), time-out and social reinforcement (Ronen, 1991), the establishment of stable bedtime and wake-up routines (Christodulu & Durand, in press; Weissbluth, 1982), relaxation training (Anderson, 1979), and sleep restriction (Durand & Christodulu, 2004). One difficulty with using some of these behavioral interventions for sleep terrors is that they assume social attention serves a role in the maintenance of these problems. Unfortunately, unlike many other sleep disturbances, sleep terrors occur while the person is still asleep, and he or she is therefore presumably unaware of the presence or absence of others.

One intervention that does not rely on the withdrawal of attention is scheduled awakening. Scheduled awakening involves waking the person approximately 30 minutes before a spontaneous awakening. As the frequency of spontaneous waking decreases, scheduled awakenings are eliminated. Scheduled awakening has been used in a number of studies to successfully reduce night waking in children (Johnson, Bradley-Johnson, & Stack, 1981; Johnson & Lerner, 1985; Rickert & Johnson, 1988) and for another slow wave sleep disturbance—sleepwalking (Frank, Spirito, Stark, & Owens-Stively, 1997; Tobin, 1993).

Two studies document the potential of scheduled awakening for the treatment of sleep terrors (Durand & Mindell, 1999; Durand, 2002). Durand and Mindell (1999) used this technique to address the chronic sleep terrors of three young children. These sleep disturbances were essentially eliminated with the results maintained over 12 months. A second study replicated these results with children having disabilities (Durand, 2002). These studies represent the first successful demonstration of treatment effectiveness for sleep terrors, although the preliminary nature of these data warrants caution. This initial empirical support scheduled awakening is characterized by one review (Kuhn & Elliott, 2003) as a "promising" intervention for sleep terrors according to criteria outlined by the Society of Pediatric Psychology Task Force.

Scheduled awakening involves waking the individual some time prior to a typical waking. A case of a child who had a many year history of this problem and for whom we were ultimately able to help may prove illustrative (adapted from Durand, 1998).

Case Study

Alfie was 11-years-old and had a 7-year history of sleep terrors. He was born in Jamaica and was living in the United States with an aunt. His aunt told us that he had a learning disability and that his parents sent him to school here because they felt he would receive a better education. Alfie's aunt reported that he would go to bed easily at night and would usually not awaken until the morning. However, about three nights each week, Alfie would cry out loudly. He would appear extremely upset, his heart would race as if he was running and he would sweat profusely. At first his aunt thought he was hurt or that he was getting sick. However, when it became clear that he was fine the next day, she became more concerned. She thought that because he was separated from his parents that he was having horrifying nightmares. After an initial consultation, she was told that these episodes were not nightmares and was asked to contact Alfie's parents to see if this was something new, or if he ever had these episodes before. Alfie's aunt was surprised (and a bit annoyed) to learn that Alfie had these episodes off and on for most of his life.

In order to try to help Alfie avoid these sleep terrors, a plan was designed for his aunt. After several weeks of charting when these sleep terror episodes occurred, it became clear that it usually happened at around 12:30 p.m. Based on this information, his aunt was instructed to wake up at midnight, go into his room, and gently shake him until his eyes opened. Once he briefly opened his eyes, his aunt was to let him go back to sleep. She was to repeat this pattern each night for at least two weeks.

On the first night of the plan, she had a little trouble waking Alfie who appeared to be in a very deep sleep. We told her that this was probably a good sign, and an indication that the midnight waking was a good one. She repeated the waking each night for two weeks and did not observe Alfie having any sleep terror episodes. After the first two weeks, we suggested that she skip one night the next week, two nights the second week, and one more night each subsequent week. With the exception of one instance of a sleep terror incident, Alfie was free from these nighttime problems for the next six months. The intervention plan seemed to help him with sleep terrors and it did not seem to negatively affect him in any way.

Scheduled awakening was successful in helping Alfie's aunt reduce his sleep terrors. One main difficulty with this technique is that it can be difficult for some parents to get up at night to awaken their child. Because the wakings can usually be faded out over several weeks, it does not have to be an overwhelming burden, but depending on the timing of the waking, it still can be challenging. Below is an overview of the steps necessary to implement a scheduled awakening plan.

Scheduled Awakening

- Use a sleep diary to determine the time or times that the person typically experiences a sleep terror during the night. Sleep terrors usually occur at approximately the same time each evening.
- On the night you are to begin the plan, awaken the person approximately 30 minutes prior to the typical sleep terror time. For example, if the person usually has a sleep terror episode at 12:30 a.m., wake him or her at 12:00 a.m. If the person seems to awaken very easily, move back the time 15 minutes the next night and on all subsequent nights (11:45 p.m.).
- If there is a broad range in the times the person has sleep terrors (for example, from 12:00 a.m. to 1:30 a.m.), awaken him or her about 30 minutes prior to the earliest time (in this case, 11:30 p.m.).
- Do not fully awaken the person. Gently touch and/or talk to the person until he or she opens his or her eyes, then let him or her fall back to sleep.
- Repeat this plan each night until the person goes for a full seven nights without a sleep terror. If the program has achieved this level of success, skip one night (that

is, no scheduled waking) for a week. If the person has an episode, go back to every night. Slowly reduce the number of nights with scheduled wakings until the person is no longer having sleep terrors during the night.

Unfortunately, the mechanism of action for the putative success of scheduled awakening in reducing sleep terrors is currently unclear. One theory about the role of scheduled awakening is that awakening during the deep stage of sleep may prevent the person from spending too much time during this part of sleep. The scheduled awakening may help the person sleep a "shallower" but more consistent sleep schedule and that may account for the reduction in sleep terrors. It is hoped that future research will help provide a better understanding of this puzzling sleep problem, and will also lead to more techniques to help people who suffer from sleep terrors.

General Sleep Pages

Sleep medicine home page This home page lists resources regarding all aspects of sleep, including the physiology of sleep, clinical sleep medicine, sleep research, federal and state information, patient information, and business-related groups. (http://www.users.cloud9.net/%7ethorpy/)

The sleep well The Sleep Well was created as a reservoir of information on sleep and sleep disorders. It provides a calendar of important sleep events and meetings, information on sleep disorders, and a way to search Mental HealthNet for more information on sleep disorders (http://www.sleepquest.com).

NIH—National Center on Sleep Disorders Research This is a site hosted by the National Institutes of Health and provides information on research, education and general information related to sleep disorders. (http://www.nhlbi.nih.gov/about/ncsdr/index.htm)

Children's sleep problems The American Academy of Child and Adolescent Psychiatry provides this Facts for Families page as a public service to assist parents and families in their most important roles. It provides a very brief overview of sleep problems in children. (http://www.med.umich.edu/1 libr/child/child42.htm)

KEY READINGS

Durand, V. M. (1998). *Sleep better! A guide to improving sleep for children with special needs.* Baltimore, MD: Paul H. Brookes.

Kryger, M. H., Roth, T., & Dement, W. C. (2000) (Eds). *Principles and practice of sleep medicine* (3rd ed., pp. 693–706). Philadelphia: W. B. Saunders Company.

Mindell, J. A. (1997). *Sleeping through the night: How infants, toddlers, and their parents can get a good night's sleep.* New York: Harper Collins.

REFERENCES

Abe, K., Oda, N., Ikenaga, K., & Yamada, T. (1993). Twin study on night terrors, fears and some physiological and behavioural characteristics in children. *Psychiatric Genetics, 3,* 39–43.

American Psychiatric Association. (2000). *Diagnostic and statistical manual of mental disorders* (4th ed., Text rev.). Washington, DC: Author.

American Sleep Disorders Association. (1990). *The international classification of sleep disorders: Diagnostic and coding manual.* Rochester, MN: Author.

Anderson, D. (1979). Treatment of insomnia in a 13 year old boy by relaxation training and reduction of parental attention. *Journal of Behavior Therapy and Experimental Psychiatry, 10,* 263–265.

Broughton, R. J. (2000). NREM arousal parasomnias. In M. H. Kryger, T. Roth, & W. C. Dement (Eds.). *Principles and practice of sleep medicine* (3rd ed., pp. 693–706). Philadelphia: W. B. Saunders Company.

Christodulu, K. V., & Durand, V. M. (in press). Reducing bedtime disturbance and night waking using positive bedtime routines and sleep restriction. *Focus on Autism and Other Developmental Disabilities.*

Durand, V. M. (1998). *Sleep better! A guide to improving sleep for children with special needs.* Baltimore, MD: Paul H. Brookes.

Durand, V. M. (2002). Treating sleep terrors in children with autism. *Journal of Positive Behavioral Interventions, 4,* 66–72.

Durand, V. M., & Christodulu, K. V. (2004). A description of a sleep restriction program to reduce bedtime disturbances and night waking. *Journal of Positive Behavioral Interventions, 6,* 83–91.

Durand, V. M., & Mindell, J. A. (1999). Behavioral intervention for childhood sleep terrors. *Behavior Therapy, 30,* 705–715.

Durand, V. M., Mindell, J. A., Mapstone, E., & Gernert-Dott, P. (1998). Sleep problems. In T. S. Watson and F. M. Gresham (Eds.), *Handbook of child behavior therapy* (pp. 203–219). New York: Plenum Press.

Ferber, R. (1985). *Solve your child's sleep problems.* New York: Simon and Schuster.

Frank, N. C., Spirito, A., Stark, L., & Owens-Stively, J. (1997). The use of scheduled awakenings to eliminate childhood sleepwalking. *Journal of Pediatric Psychology, 22,* 345–353.

Giles, D. E., & Buysse, D. J. (1993). Parasomnias. In D. L. Dunner (Ed.), *Current psychiatric therapy* (pp. 361–372). Philadelphia: W. B. Saunders Company.

Johnson, C. M., Bradley-Johnson, S., & Stack, J. M. (1981). Decreasing the frequency of infant's nocturnal crying with the use of scheduled awakenings. *Family Practice Research Journal, 1,* 98–104.

Johnson, C. M., & Lerner, M. (1985). Amelioration of infant sleep disturbances: II. Effects of scheduled awakenings by compliant parents. *Infant Mental Health Journal, 6,* 21–30.

Kales, J. D., Kales, A., Soldatos, C. R., Caldwell, A. B., Charney, D. S., & Martin, E. D. (1980). Night terrors: Clinical characteristics and personality patterns. *Archives of General Psychiatry, 37,* 1406–1410.

Karacan, I. (1988). Parasomnias. In R. L. Williams, I. Karacan, & C. A. Moore (Eds.), *Sleep disorders: Diagnosis and treatment* (pp. 131–144). New York: John Wiley & Sons.

Kuhn, B. R., & Elliott, A. J. (2003). Treatment efficacy in behavioral pediatric sleep medicine. *Journal of Psychosomatic Research, 54,* 587–597.

Lask, B. (1995). Night terrors. In C. E. Schaefer (Ed.), *Clinical handbook of sleep disorders in children* (pp. 125–134). Northvale, NJ: Jason Aronson Inc.

Littner, M., Hirshkowitz, M., Kramer, M., Kapen, S., Anderson, W. M., Bailey, D., et al. (2003). Practice parameters for using polysomnography to evaluate insomnia: an update. *Sleep, 26,* 754–60.

Mindell, J. A. (1993). Sleep disorders in children. *Health Psychology, 12,* 151–162.

Mindell, J. A. (1997). *Sleeping through the night: How infants, toddlers, and their parents can get a good night's sleep.* New York: Harper Collins.

National Sleep Foundation (2002). *2002 "Sleep in America Poll."* Washington, DC: Author.

Neylan, T. C., Reynolds, C. F. III, & Kupfer, D. J. (2003). Sleep disorders. In R. E. Hales & S. C. Yudofsky (Eds.), *Textbook of clinical psychiatry* (4th ed.) (pp. 975–1000). Washington, DC: American Psychiatric Publishing.

Rickert, V. I., & Johnson, C. M. (1988). Reducing nocturnal awakenings and crying episodes in infants and children: A comparison between scheduled awakenings and systematic ignoring. *Pediatrics, 81,* 203–212.

Ronen, T. (1991). Intervention package for treating sleep disorders in a four-year-old girl. *Journal of Behavior Therapy and Experimental Psychiatry, 22,* 141–148.

Tobin, J. (1993). Treatment of somnambulism with anticipatory awakening. *Journal of Pediatrics, 122,* 426–427.

Weissbluth, M. (1982). Modification of sleep schedule with reduction of night waking: A case report. *Sleep, 5,* 262–266.

Whyte, J., & Schaefer, C. (1995). Introduction to sleep and its disorders. In C. Schaefer (Ed.), *Clinical handbook of sleep disorders in children* (pp. 1–14). Northvale, NJ: Jason Aronson.

Smoking (Nicotine Dependence)

David O. Antonuccio • Jarrod M. Mosier

WHAT IS NICOTINE DEPENDENCE?

Nicotine dependence is a learned behavior initiated by psychosocial variables and propagated by a physiological dependence on nicotine. This usually takes the form of smoking tobacco or using smokeless tobacco products. This chapter will focus primarily on smoking behavior but the basic principles can be applied to use of nicotine in any form. Environmental stimuli become conditioned to elicit cravings for smoking, making smoking a constantly reinforced and over-learned behavior. The combination of these physical and psychosocial effects of smoking can lead to nicotine dependence. Although the pathophysiological effects are the most physically damaging, the psychological effects can negatively affect a smoker's self-image.

BASIC FACTS ABOUT NICOTINE DEPENDENCE

Smoking is the number one cause of preventable disease in the United States. It has been linked to numerous diseases including 30% of all cancers (Bartechhi, Mackenzie, & Schrier, 1994), increased risk of wound infections (Sorensen, Karlsmark, & Gottrup, 2003), coronary artery disease, peripheral vascular disease, stroke, and lung disease (US Department of Health and Human Services, 1983).

- Nicotine is possibly the most addictive of all drugs (Antonuccio, 2001)
- 1.1 billion people worldwide smoke cigarettes, a number that is expected to rise to 1.6 billion by 2025, with an annual death toll of 10 million by 2030 (WHO, 2003).
- About 1.3 million Americans quit smoking each year, while about 1 million Americans take up smoking each year (Antonuccio, 1993a, b). Those who take up smoking are mostly teenagers, with about 13% of middle school students, and 29% of college students using tobacco (Rigotti, Lee, & Wechsler, 2000).
- 30% of senior high school girls report smoking, a rate that has contributed to the rise of lung cancer in women (Antonuccio, 2004).
- 23% of adult Americans smoke (CDC, 2002), and up to 9% of adult Americans report using smokeless tobacco (CDC, 1993).
- About half of all lifetime smokers die from smoking related disease with half of these deaths occurring between 35 and 69 years of age (Antonuccio, in press).
- Smokers die from Coronary Heart Disease 70% more often than nonsmokers (Antonuccio, 2001).
- Two pack-a-day smokers have lung cancer death rates 12–25 times higher than non-smokers (Antonuccio, 2001).
- Each cigarette reduces lifespan by about 11 minutes (Shaw, Mitchell, & Dorling, 2000).
- Even light smoking (1–4 cigarettes per day) has been shown to significantly increase risk (Willett, Green, Stampfer et al., 1987).

Smoking causes temporary improvements in performance and affect. The mechanism of these improvements is via periodic patterns of arousal and alertness, cycled

Antonuccio, D. O., & Mosier, J. M. (2006). Smoking (nicotine dependence). In J. E. Fisher & W. T. O'Donohue (Eds.), *Practitioner's guide to evidence-based psychotherapy*. New York: Springer.

with calming and a reduction in tension (Pomerleau & Pomerleau, 1985). At low doses, nicotine is a stimulant and not only improves performance, but also enhances every day emotions. At high doses, nicotine acts as a sedative. Thus, the smoker can use nicotine for multiple purposes throughout the day (Antonuccio, 2001).

- The average smoker puffs 160 times a day. At this frequency, a wide variety of environmental factors become "cues" to smoke by means of operant conditioning (Lichtenstein & Antonuccio, 1981).
- Between 70% and 85% of all smokers say they want to quit (Gallup Organization, 1999). Of those who quit, most smokers quit without the help of any treatment program, leaving the medical community with the more challenging task of helping the more severe smokers (Cohen, et al., 1989).
- About half of all patients using the transdermal nicotine patch for 12 weeks still smoke, raising the risk of nicotine toxicities in the body (McClanahan & Antonuccio, 2004).
- Beta-endorphins (natural stimulants) and vasopressin (antidiuretic hormone or ADH) are produced in greater amounts after smoking which tend to decrease pain, increase stress tolerance, improve memory, concentration, and information processing, all leading to positive reinforcement of the behavior (McClanahan & Antonuccio, 2004). The increased production of these hormones also leads to increased blood pressure and vascular resistance, increasing the risk for cardiovascular disease (Joseph, et al., 1996).
- Tobacco smoke contains not only nicotine, but also other toxic substances including but not limited to acetone, ammonia, hexamine (lighter fluid), toluene, urethane, formaldehyde, arsenic, cyanide, etc. Some 43 of these chemicals are known carcinogens (Antonuccio, 2001).
- In addition to the effects of direct smoking, second-hand smoke kills an estimated 53,000 people annually (Glantz & Parmley, 1991).

ASSESSMENT

What Should be Ruled Out?

When evaluating a patient who smokes, it is important to distinguish between the dependent user and the casual user. The best ways to do this are through the patient's history and biometrics (eg., carbon monoxide feedback). Smokers who smoke less than 10 cigarettes per day may be considered light smokers; 11–20 cigarettes per day are considered moderate smokers; and more than 20 cigarettes per day, heavy smokers. Carbon monoxide levels greater than or equal to 10 ppm are considered to be in the unhealthy range.

What is Involved in Effective Assessment?

The US Public Health Service recommends the "5 A's approach" to treatment to smoking (Fiore et al., 2000):

- *Ask* about tobacco use. This also involves addressing myths about quitting. For example, it is a myth that past attempts decrease ability to quit or that older smokers do not benefit from quitting.
- *Advise* users to stop. Provide the patient with information on the medical benefits.
- *Assess* willingness to quit. An important factor is to match the intervention with the stage of quitting (see below).
- *Assist* in quitting.
- *Arrange* for follow-up.

Smoking cessation may be grouped into five stages: precontemplation, contemplation, preparation, action, and maintenance (DiClemente, et al. 1991).

- *Precontemplation stage.* Approximately 15% of all smokers are at this stage. This stage involves no desire or consideration to quit smoking. Smokers in this stage are unwilling to quit smoking and are least likely to benefit from treatment. Helpful feedback from the health care provider to precontemplation smokers is information on the adverse effects of smoking, the benefits of quitting, and tangible information (e.g., CO levels) to allow patients to begin thinking about quitting.
- *Contemplation stage.* Advancement to this stage requires the identification of smoking as a problem. Smokers in this stage are interested in learning more about how to quit, consider the advantages and disadvantages of quitting, and are weighing their options. Helpful intervention from the practitioner includes advice on the medical benefits of quitting, and encouragement to join a smoking cessation class to educate the patient on the process. Intervention techniques that are useful at this stage are "wrap sheets" (Antonuccio, 2004), the Reasons for Quitting Scale (Curry, Wagner, & Grothaus, 1990), the Therapeutic Reactance Scale (Dowd, Milne, & Wise, 1991), the Partner Interaction Questionnaire (Mermelstein, Lichtenstein, & McIntyre, 1983), and the Fagerstrom Nicotine Dependence Scale (Fagerstrom, 1978). "Wrap Sheets" are useful for providing the smoker with a baseline frequency of smoking. They "wrap" around the cigarette box and allow easy tracking. They also reinforce a reduction in smoking frequency. The Reasons for Quitting scale evaluates the nature of motivation for quitting (i.e., intrinsic vs. extrinsic). The Therapeutic Reactance Scale evaluates the smoker's resistance to instruction. The Partner Interaction Questionnaire evaluates the impact of the smoker's partner on smoking behavior. The Fagerstrom Nicotine Dependence Scale evaluates the strength of the smoker's addiction to nicotine.
- *Preparation stage.* A smoker progresses to this stage when he or she sets a target quit date 2–4 weeks into the future. In this stage of quitting, smokers feel ready for change and are setting goals to achieve that change. Useful interventions from the practitioner involve relaxation training to dampen the anxiety that accompanies this process, self-hypnosis training, and encouragement of a spouse or significant other to eliminate negative and punishing behaviors while supporting and reinforcing cessation (Antonuccio, 2004).
- *Action stage.* This stage involves actually changing smoking behavior (McClanahan & Antonuccio, 2004). The process involves strategies designed to reduce smoking behavior, alter environmental reinforcers, and eventually eliminate smoking. Examples of these strategies include leaving the cigarettes in the trunk rather than in the car while driving and overcoming the subsequent urge, nicotine fading (i.e., switching to lower nicotine cigarettes) to reduce dependence, and taste aversion or "smoke holding."
- *Maintenance stage.* This stage involves the continued abstinence from smoking and prevention of relapse. This requires goals that are short term, and achievable with monetary rewards. For example, some smokers like to set an initial goal of quitting for three days. If the three-day goal is achieved, the money is used as a reward. If the goal is not achieved, they have agreed to send the money to their least favorite politician. This stage also requires a gradual decline in nicotine replacement therapy, recognition, and alteration of environmental cues for relapse. Effective interventions from the practitioner include CO monitoring to provide positive feedback, and the administration of the Smoking Self-Efficacy Questionnaire (Baer, Holt, & Lichtenstein, 1986) that predicts situations most likely to elicit relapse (McClanahan & Antonuccio, 2004).

What Assessments are Not Helpful?

Pulmonary function tests are useful for determining lung capacity, but may not be useful for determining the level of dependence on nicotine (Gorecka et al., 2003).

TREATMENT

What Treatments are Effective?

In general, most treatments programs are moderately successful. However, there is a large relapse rate regardless of the type of treatment. For example, behavioral programs show initial cessation rates of 50–100% with relapse rates of 70–80%. Because of such staggering relapse rates, the most effective treatments emphasize relapse prevention. Light smokers generally have higher abstinence rates than heavier smokers, regardless of the treatment program used (McClanahan & Antonuccio, 2004).

What are Effective Self-Help Treatments?

Cost-effective self-help books include (McClanahan & Antonuccio, 2004):

- "Butt out"
- "Quit Smart"
- "Freedom from Smoking"
- "Freshstart"

Carbon monoxide monitoring can provide tangible feedback to the patient about their success and verify abstinence for the provider (Antonuccio, 2004). Although carbon monoxide monitoring requires office visits to the practitioner, it is a quick and easy way of providing feedback about the success of treatment.

Useful Websites:

http://www.cdc.gov/tobacco/
http://cancercontrol.cancer.gov/tcrb.smokersrisk/
http://www.helpself.com/directory/stopsmoking.htm
http://www.smoking-cessation.org/
http://www.surgeongeneral.gov/tobacco/
http://www.nlm.nih.gov/medlineplus/smokingcessation. html
http://www.lungusa.org/tobacco/

What are Effective Therapist Based Treatments?

Typical behavioral programs focus on antecedents and consequences of smoking (Lichtenstein, 2002). Coping skills are taught along with cognitive strategies for addressing smoking triggers. Thus, the aim of these cognitive–behavioral techniques is to confront and overcome these positive and negative reinforcements (McClanahan & Antonuccio, 2004).

Some techniques include:

- smoke holding, rapid smoking, and noxious imagery all designed to be aversive to the experience of smoking
- nicotine fading and controlled smoking
- self control, self monitoring, and substitution strategies designed to identify and modify situations, cognitions, and other cues that elicit the urge or craving
- partner support
- hypnosis
- acceptance based strategies
- relapse prevention

What is Effective Medical Treatment?

Medical treatments for nicotine dependence include nicotine replacement methods and antidepressant medications. However, none of the medical therapies (nicotine gum, transdermal nicotine patches, or bupropion) have been shown to be particularly successful without a behavioral component (McClanahan & Antonuccio, 2004).

- Abstinence rates for behavior therapy and nicotine replacement have typically been about 27% for the combined therapy and 18% for the behavioral methods alone at six months, 23% for the combined therapy and 13% for the behavioral methods alone at 12 months. In studies with minimal behavioral interventions, abstinence rates have been shown to be 11% for both gum and placebo (McClanahan & Antonuccio, 2004).
- Both psychosocial and physiological components of smoking must be addressed to help smokers quit. Thus, the purpose of combining medical treatments with behavioral strategies is to reduce the initial withdrawal symptoms experienced by the smoker.
- The transdermal nicotine patch is an example of a treatment designed as an adjunct to behavioral intervention. Although the optimal duration of use is not defined, studies have shown that use of the transdermal patch combined with behavioral strategies for 12 weeks does not show an advantage to using the patch combined with behavioral strategies for three weeks. Three months after the last patch abstinence rates are 29% and 28%, respectively (Bolin, Antonuccio, Follette, & Krumpe, 1999).
- Antidepressants such as bupropion have also been shown to be successful when combined with behavioral therapy showing abstinence rates as high as 35% at one year when used in conjunction with behavioral therapy (Jorenby, et al., 1999). However, when used alone, success rates have been disappointing, less than 5% in one study (Gifford et al., 2002). Therefore, antidepressants should not be given as the sole treatment option.
- A meta-analysis of the over-the-counter nicotine patch resulted in an average abstinence rate of about 7% (Hughes, Shiffman, Callas, & Zhang, 2003).

Other Issues in Management

The practitioner should consider the following guidelines when treating nicotine dependence and aiding the patient in quitting:

- Require some form of self-help, individual, or group cognitive-behavioral treatment. With the wide availability of over-the-counter nicotine replacement therapies, it is increasingly difficult for the practitioner to regulate access to these therapies. However, health care plans and medical settings can control whether the medication is subsidized.
- Build in maintenance sessions and withdrawal from nicotine replacement.
- Strongly warn patients not to smoke on the patch if for no other reason than it significantly decreases chances of quitting.
- Use CO monitoring to give feedback, reinforce success, and verify abstinence.
- Encourage weaning of the patch if the patient is still smoking after two weeks. Have the patient set a new target date and try again.
- Consider a three-week rapid deployment of nicotine replacement.
- Encourage termination of the patch after six weeks.
- Do not routinely prescribe bupropion unless or until more data become available to support its efficacy when used alone.

The practitioner should be cognizant of the operant conditioning that takes place with smoking. Not only do environmental cues become classically conditioned to elicit urges to smoke, but internal craving become operantly conditioned to elicit the cravings as well. This presents a challenge to the practitioner in that environmental cues can be removed but internal cues cannot. The negative and positive reinforcement of both internal and external cues need to be addressed in a treatment plan for the smoker. These internal and external cues can become so powerful that they cloud out other thoughts, leading to scheduling daily activities around the need and gratification cycles of smokers (Antonuccio, 2001).

The aversiveness of withdrawal must be considered. Withdrawal symptoms typcially reach a peak severity in the first week after cessation and gradually decrease with time to at or near baseline by six weeks of abstinence (Antonuccio, 2004; Lawrence, Amode, & Murray, 1982).

These symptoms include:

- coughing
- craving
- feelings of aggression
- increased appetite
- irritability
- nervousness
- restlessness

Although most symptoms are at or near baseline by six weeks of abstinence, symptoms of constipation and craving for sweets have been seen to persist for longer (Antonuccio, 2004).

Advantageous health effects can be seen with cessation regardless of the age or duration of smoking (Antonuccio, 2004).

Patients should not smoke while on a nicotine replacement therapy, and should discontinue use if smoking has not stopped after two weeks of nicotine replacement. Though the risk is thought to be small, smoking while on nicotine replacement can expose the smoker to toxic levels of nicotine (McClanahan & Antonuccio, 2004).

How Does One Select Among Treatments?

The practitioner should consider that it is impossible to avoid withdrawal symptoms during smoking cessation. Treatments are designed to dampen withdrawal but more importantly, they are tools to help address the behavioral component of smoking. As such, an extended use of the patch can prolong withdrawal or lengthen its duration. Withdrawal is normally overcome in the first week after cessation but can be extended and last from 6 to 16 weeks with extended use of the patch (McClanahan & Antonuccio, 2004).

- When exploring nicotine replacement options, consider that the patch delivers a constant dose of nicotine, while the nicotine gum delivers self-administered doses (McClanahan & Antonuccio, 2004).
- Smokers are more likely to attempt quitting if nicotine replacement techniques are used in conjunction with behavioral strategies (Antonuccio, 2004).

KEY READINGS

Antonuccio, D. O. (1993a). *Butt out, the smoker's book: A compassionate guide to helping yourself quit smoking, with or without a partner.* Saratoga, CA: R and E Publishers.

Antonuccio, D. O. (1993b). *Butt out, the partner's book: A compassionate guide to helping your friend or loved one quit smoking without nagging.* Saratoga, CA: R and E Publishers.

Antonuccio, D. O. (2001) Toward a tobacco free society. In. P. Insel & W. Roth (Eds.), *Core concepts in health.* New Year: The McGraw-Hill Companies, Inc.

Antonuccio, D. O. (2004). Integrating behavioral interventions for smoking into primary care. In N. A. Cummings, M. P. Duckworth, W. T. O'Donohue, & K. E. Ferguson (Eds.), *Detection and treatment of substance abuse in prmary care.* Reno, NV: Context Press.

Baer, J. S., Holt, C. S., & Lichtenstein, E. (1986). Self-efficacy and smoking reexamined: Construct validity and clinical utility, 846–852.

Bartecchi, C. E., Mackenzie, T. D., & Schrier, R. W. (1994). The human costs of tobacco use (first of two parts). *New England Journal of Medicine, 330,* 907–912.

Bolin, L., Antonuccio, D., Follette, W., & Krumpe, P. (1999). Transdermal nicotine: The long and the short of it. *Psychology of Addictive Behaviors, 13,* 152–156.

Centers for Disease Control and Prevention (1993). Use of smokeless tobacco among adults—United States, 1991, *Morbidity and Mortality Weekly Report, 42,* 263–266.

Centers for Disease Control and Prevention (2002). Tobacco information and prevention source: OSH summary for 2002. http://www.cdc.gove/tobacco/overview/oshsummary02.htm.

Cohen, S., Lichtenstein, E., Prochaska, J. O., Rossi, J. S., Gritz, E. R., Carr, K. C. R., et al. (1989). Debunking myths about self-quitting. Evidence from 10 prospective studies of persons who attempt to quit smoking by themselves. *American Psychologist, 44,* 1355–1365.

Curry, S. J., Wagner, E. H., & Grothaus, L. C. (1990). Intrinsic and extrinsic motivation for smoking cessation. *Journal of Consulting and Clinical Psychology, 58(3),* 310–316.

DiClemente, C. C., Prochaska, J. O., Fairhurst, S. K., Velicer, W. F., Velasquez, M. M., & Rossi, J. S. (1991). The process of smoking cessation: An analysis of precontemplation, contemplation, and preparation stages of change. *Journal of Cosulting and Clinical Psychology, 59(2),* 295–304.

Dowd, E. T., Milne, C. R., & Wise, S. L. (1991) The Therapeutic Reactance Scale: A measure of psychological reactance. *Journal of Counseling and Development, 69,* 541–545.

Fagerstrom, K. O. (1978). Measuring degree of physical dependence to tobacco smoking with reference to individualization of treatment. *Addictive Behaviors, 3,* 235–241.

Fiore, M. C. et al. (2000). Treating tobacco use and dependence. *Clinical practice guidelines.* Rockville, MD.: US Department of Health and Human Services.

Gallup Organization, 1999. Majority of smokers want to quit, consider themselves addicted (http://www.gallup.com/poll/releases/pr991118.asp)

Gifford, E. V., Kohlenberg, B. S., Piasecki, M. P., Palm, K. M., Antonuccio, D. O., & Hayes, S. C. (2002). Therapy for smoking cessation: Results from a randomized controlled trial. Paper presented at the annual meeting of the Association for the Advancement of Behavior Therapy, Reno, NV.

Glantz, S. A., & Parmley, W. W. (1991). Passive smoking and heart disease: Epidemiology, physiology, and biochemistry. *Circulation, 83,* 1–12.

Gorecka, D., Bednarek, M., Nowinshi, A., Puscinska, E., Goljan-Geremek, A, & Zielinski, J. (2003). Diagnosis of Airflow Limitation combined with smoking cessation advice increases stop-smoking rate. *Chest, 123,* 1916–1923.

Hughes, J. R., Shiffman, S., Callas, P., & Zhang, J. (2003). A meta-analysis of the efficacy of over-the-counter nicotine replacement. *Tobacco Control, 12,* 21–27.

Jorenby, D. E., Leischow, S. J., Nides, M. A., Rennard, S. I., Johnston, J. A., Hughes, A. R., et al. (1999). A controlled trial of sustained release bupropion, a nicotine patch, or both for smoking cessation. *New England Journal of Medicine, 340,* 685–691.

Joseph, A. M., Norman, S., Ferry, L., Prochazka, A., Westman, E., Steele, B., et al. (1996). The safety of transdermal nicotine therapy as an aid to smoking cessation in patients with cardiac disease. *New England Journal of Medicine, 335(24),* 1792–1798.

Lawrence, P. S., Amodei, N., & Murray, A. L. (1982). *Withdrawal symptoms associated with smoking cessation.* Paper presented at the 21st convention of the Association for Advancement of Behavior Therapy, Los Angeles.

Lichtenstein, E., & Antonuccio, D. O. (1981). Dimensions of smoking. *Addictive Behaviors, 6,* 365–367.

Lichtenstein, E. (2002). From rapid smoking to the Internet: Five decades of cessation research. *Nicotine & Tobacco Research, 4,* 139–145.

McClanahan, T. M., & Antonuccio, D. O. (2004). Behavioral treatment of cigarette smoking. In Hersen (Ed.) *Psychopathology in the workplace: Recognition and adaptation.* New York: Brunner-Routledge

Mermelstein, R., Lichtenstein, E., & McIntyre, K. (1983). Partner support and relapse in smoking—cessation programs. *Journal of Consulting and Clinical Psychology, 51(3),* 465–466.

Pomerleau, O. F., & Pomerleau, C. S. (1985). Neuroregulators and the reinforcement of smoking: Towards a biobehavioral explanation. *Neuroscience and Boibehavioral Reviews, 8,* 503–513.

Rigotti, N. A., Lee, J. E., & Wechsler, H. (2000). U.S. college students' use of tobacco products: Results of a national survey. *Journal of the American Medical Association, 284,* 699–705.

Shaw, M., Mitchell, R., & Dorling, D. (2000). Time for a smoke? One cigarette reduces your life by 11 minutes. *British Medical Journal, 320,* 53.

Sorensen, L. T., Karlsmark, T., & Gottrup, F. (2003). Abstinence from smoking reduces incisional wound infection: a randomized controlled trial. *Annals of Surgery, 238,* 1–5.

US Department of Health and Human Services (1983). *The health consequences of smoking: Cardiovascular disease.* US Department of Health and Human Services, Public Health Service, Office of the Assistant Secretary for Health, Office on Smoking and Health.

US Department of Health and Human Services (1990). *The health benefits of smoking cessation.* US Department of Health and Human Services, Public Health Service, Centers for Disease Control, Center for Chronic Disease Prevention and Health Promotion, Office on Smoking and Health. DHHS Publication No. (CDC) 90-8416.

Willett, W. C., Green, A., Stampfer, M. J., et al. (1987). Relative and absolute risks of coronary heart disease among women who smoke cigarettes. *New England Journal of Medicine, 317,* 1303–1309.

World Health Organization (2003). *Tobacco free initiative: The tobacco atlas.* http://www.who.int/tobacco/statistics/tobacco_atlas/en/

CHAPTER 67

Social Anxiety Disorder

Gerlinde C. Harb • Richard G. Heimberg

WHAT IS SOCIAL ANXIETY DISORDER?

Social anxiety disorder, also known as social phobia, is the persistent fear of negative evaluation in one or more situations that involve social interaction and/or performance in front of others (American Psychiatric Association, 1994). Individuals with social anxiety disorder fear embarrassment or humiliation in these situations although they may recognize that their fears are excessive or unreasonable. When anticipating feared situations, they tend to experience severe discomfort and, when exposed to feared situations, they may attempt to escape the situation or else endure it with great distress. This distress is often accompanied by physical symptoms such as palpitations, sweating, blushing, and trembling, which may take the form of situationally bound panic attacks. As a result, feared situations are often avoided. Fear and avoidance interfere significantly with functioning; affected persons may change their normal routine, decline educational or occupational opportunities, or restrict their social relationships in order to avoid social interactions and/or performance in front of others.

Frequently feared situations include initiating or maintaining conversations, informal interpersonal contact (e.g., small talk at the office), participating in small groups, public speaking, eating in public, dating, dealing with authority figures, attending social gatherings, and assertively saying no to unreasonable requests or asking others to change their behavior.

The one recognized subtype of social anxiety disorder is the generalized subtype, which refers to the experience of fear in most social situations. Other individuals with social anxiety disorder may experience fears in only one or a more narrow range of social interaction or performance situations. The generalized subtype tends to be characterized by greater severity of symptoms, more frequent comorbidity (including avoidant personality disorder), and greater functional impairment.

BASIC FACTS ABOUT SOCIAL ANXIETY DISORDER

Comorbidity. Comorbidity with other disorders is very common; most patients have one or more comorbid diagnoses (Schneier, Johnson, Horing, Lie bowitz, & Weissman, 1992). The most frequent comorbid disorders are depression, panic disorder, generalized anxiety disorder, and substance use disorders. The onset of social anxiety disorder most frequently precedes the onset of these comorbid conditions (Kessler, Stang, Wittchen, Stein, & Walters, 1999). Although some have reported that the existence of any comorbid conditions tends to be associated with a poorer prognosis (Davidson, Hughes, George, & Blazer, 1993), others (Erwin, Heimberg, Juster, & Mindlin, 2002) have noted that comorbid anxiety disorders do not interfere with the outcome of cognitive–behavioral treatment for social anxiety disorder.

Harb, G. C., Heimberg, R. G. (2006). Social anxiety disorder. In J. E. Fisher & W. O'Donohue (Eds.), *Practitioner's Guide to evidence-based psychotherapy.* New York: Springer.

Prevalence. Social anxiety disorder is among the most prevalent psychiatric disorders in the general population. It has been estimated that 13.3% of individuals in the United States will suffer from social anxiety disorder at some point in their lives (Kessler et al., 1994). However, the percentage of persons with truly clinically significant social anxiety disorder may be closer to 4% (Narrow, Rae, Robins, & Regier, 2002).

Age at onset. The majority of individuals with social anxiety disorder report the onset of difficulties by adolescence (the mid-teens), and most clients are symptomatic by their early 20s (Öst, 1987). However, a great number of individuals report a history of either clinical social anxiety disorder or significant symptoms beginning in early childhood.

Gender. Women are more likely than men to receive this diagnosis with a ratio of approximately 1.5:1 (Kessler et al., 1994). However, men appear slightly more likely than women to seek treatment, possibly because social anxiety disorder interferes with instrumental role function that is expected more of men than women in many cultures (Turk et al., 1998).

Course. Children described as behaviorally inhibited are at increased risk for the later development of social anxiety disorder (e.g., Schwartz, Snidman, & Kagan, 1999). Although most patients recall an insidious onset of the disorder, some recall one or more humiliating experiences which directly preceded their symptoms. In adulthood, the course of social anxiety disorder tends to be chronic and unremitting (Reich, Goldenberg, Vasile, Goisman, & Keller, 1994).

Impairment and other demographic characteristics. Social anxiety disorder is associated with significant impairment in daily functioning. Increased incidence of suicidal thoughts, poor social supports, poor work and school performance, and increased utilization of health care services are factors associated with poorer quality of life among individuals with social anxiety disorder. Social anxiety disorder disrupts individuals' social relationships and is associated with a limited social network, less satisfaction with relationships, and difficulty getting along with coworkers and superiors. Social fears often limit patients' achievements in educational and occupational pursuits due to their difficulty with participation in classes or meetings, with assertiveness, and in dealings with authority figures. Individuals with social anxiety disorder are more likely to be single or divorced, less educated and make less money than their nonaffected peers (Schneier et al., 1992; Wittchen et al., 1999).

ASSESSMENT

What Should be Ruled Out?

Social anxiety disorder is only diagnosed when the presenting symptoms are not better accounted for by another mental disorder. Some individuals with social anxiety disorder experience panic attacks in feared situations. For these individuals, a diagnosis of panic disorder should be ruled out, as they may experience nonsituationally bound attacks and apprehension about future attacks. Atypical depression also frequently shares the symptom of interpersonal rejection sensitivity with social anxiety disorder and should be ruled out as a primary diagnosis. Children should be evaluated for symptoms of separation anxiety disorder. The criteria for generalized social anxiety disorder demonstrate some overlap with those of avoidant personality disorder. Although it is useful to assess avoidant personality disorder, some believe that this personality disorder is best conceived as the most severe presentation of generalized social anxiety disorder (Heimberg, 1996).

TABLE 67.1

• DSM-IV criteria for social anxiety disorder	• Range of feared situations (social and/or performance situations)	• Frequency and severity of avoidance behavior	• Severity of anticipatory anxiety
• Severity of social anxiety	• Severity of overall anxiety	• Symptoms of comorbid depression	• Suicidal ideation and past attempts
• Substance use to self-mediate anxiety	• Underemployment, underachievement in school	• Degree of social support/ isolation	• Functional impairment

What is Involved in Effective Assessment?

A thorough psychological assessment of social anxiety disorder should include examination of Table 67.1.

Clinician-administered measures. Structured clinical interviews, such as the Anxiety Disorders Interview Schedule for DSM-IV, Lifetime version (DiNardo, Brown, & Barlow, 1994), provide substantial information about the presence of diagnostic features and fear and avoidance of specific social and performance situations. The Liebowitz Social Anxiety Scale (Heimberg et al., 1999; Liebowitz, 1987) assesses fear and avoidance of 11 social interaction (e.g., "initiating a conversation") and 13 performance (e.g., "working while being observed") situations.

Self-report measures. Two 20-item self-report scales measure a person's anxiety when interacting with others, either in groups of in dyads (Social Interaction Anxiety Scale; Mattick & Clarke, 1998), and anxiety about being observed by others (Social Phobia Scale; Mattick & Clarke, 1998). One of the most widely used self-report scales to assess fears of being judged negatively by others is the 30-item Fear of Negative Evaluation Scale (Watson & Friend, 1969), although the newer 12-item version of the scale (Leary, 1983) may be more sensitive to treatment effects (Weeks et al., 2004). The Social Phobia and Anxiety Inventory (Turner et al., 1989) is a more extensive and lengthy questionnaire assessing somatic, cognitive and behavioral symptoms of social anxiety in a wide range of situations. The 17-item Social Phobia Inventory (Connor et al., 2000) and its 3-item short form (Connor Kobak, Churchill, Katzelnick, & Davidson, 2001) have been widely used in recent years. Self-report screens for depressive symptoms and suicidal ideation (such as the Beck Depression Inventory-II [Beck, Steer, & Brown, 1996] and the Beck Hopelessness Scale [Beck, Weissman, Lester, & Trexler, 1974]) are recommended for individuals with social anxiety and comorbid depression.

Behavioral assessment. Observation of behavior in anxiety-provoking situations may be helpful in understanding the way the individual's anxiety manifests itself in social situations. Behavioral observation may be informal or standardized in the form of behavioral assessment tests (e.g., Harb, Eng, Zaider, & Heimberg, 2003). However, behavioral assessment of some sort is important in the assessment of social anxiety disorder as patients routinely under-report the adequacy of their social behavior (Rapee & Lim, 1992) and overestimate the visibility of their anxiety to others (Alden & Wallace, 1995).

What Assessments are Not Helpful?

Traditional psychological tests such as the MMPI, projective tests and neuropsychological tests are not useful in assessing social anxiety disorder, nor are there medical tests for its diagnosis.

TREATMENT

What Treatments are Effective?

Although many psychosocial therapies have been applied to the treatment of social anxiety, only cognitive–behavioral therapy (CBT) has the empirical support of randomized controlled trials. Cognitive–behavioral interventions share several common characteristics: treatments are time-limited, present-oriented, and aimed at increasing the range of patients' cognitive and behavioral skills in a collaborative working relationship between patient and therapist. Most CBT interventions for socially anxious individuals involve one or more of the following cognitive and behavioral treatment strategies (for a detailed review and description of these strategies, see Heimberg, 2002):

1. Social Skills Training teaches patients the basic skills of competent interpersonal performance in social situations.
2. Relaxation Training helps patients reduce physiologic arousal in anxiety-provoking situations.
3. Cognitive Restructuring instructs patients to challenge their maladaptive beliefs, in order to create a more realistic, and presumably more accurate, view of themselves and the world.
4. Exposure Therapy helps patients face their feared situations (through imagery or in their natural environments) and stay psychologically engaged such that their anxiety reaction may subside through the processes of habituation and extinction.
5. Combined Exposure and Cognitive Restructuring Treatments integrate the teaching of cognitive skills with behavioral exposure to feared situations. The emphasis during exposure is then to provide an opportunity for patients to gather information that may serve to disconfirm maladaptive beliefs about themselves in social and performance situations.

Several meta-analytic reviews of the outcome literature have investigated the efficacy of these treatment methods for social anxiety disorder (e.g., Fedoroff & Taylor, 2001; Feske & Chambless, 1995; Gould, Buckminster, Pollack, Otto, & Yap, 1997; Taylor, 1996). The results of the meta-analyses suggest that patients receiving any of the variety of CBT treatments demonstrate substantial improvements in social anxiety symptoms, functional impairment and other associated symptoms (such as depression). Moreover, in Taylor's (1996) meta-analysis, the overall effect size for these treatments increased significantly after an average follow-up period of three months. Thus, research suggests that these treatments not only allow individuals with social anxiety disorder to make significant and meaningful changes which last beyond their involvement in therapy, but also help them make additional progress after therapy has ended.

Thus, research has clearly established that CBT treatments are able to produce meaningful and significant improvements in patients' lives. However, the question of which treatment components may be important in achieving these outcomes, that is, which types of CBT may be more or less efficacious has not been resolved. All meta-analyses have addressed this question by comparing the average magnitude of the effect obtained by different types of CBT, but there have been few differences between the types of CBT. Treatments using cognitive restructuring alone or social skills training alone appear somewhat less effective, resulting in moderate treatment gains. In addition, relaxation training may only be effective when patients were specifically instructed in its application to feared situations. Evidence to date points to exposure and the combined use of cognitive restructuring techniques and exposure as the most effective strategies. However, in one of the meta-analyses (Taylor, 1996), combined exposure and cognitive restructuring was superior to placebo treatments whereas exposure alone was not. More evidence suggests that the combination treatment may also aid in protecting patients again relapse.

What are Effective Self-Help Treatments?

Several self-help books, listed below, include many elements of effective cognitive-behavioral treatment methods for social anxiety disorder. There has been no empirical evaluation of these self-help books as sole treatment interventions. However, a 16-week therapist-administered treatment utilizing Hope, Heimberg, Juster, & Turk's (2000) client workbook has shown positive outcomes (Zaider, Heimberg, Roth, Hope, & Turk, 2003).

- Antony, M. M., & Swinson, R. P. (2000). *The shyness & and social anxiety workbook: Proven techniques for overcoming your fears.* Oakland, CA: New Harbinger Publications.
- Butler, G. (2001). *Overcoming social anxiety and shyness: A self-help guide using cognitive behavioral techniques.* Washington Square, NY: New York University Press.
- Hope, D. A., Heimberg, R. G., Juster, H. R., & Turk, C. L. (2000). *Managing social anxiety: aA cognitive–behavioral therapy approach.* Therapy Works/ San Antonio, TX: The Psychological Corporation.
- Markway, B. G., Carmin, C. N., Pollard, C. A. & Flynn, T. (1992). *Dying of Embarrassmentembarrassment: Help for social anxiety & and phobia.* Oakland, CA: New Harbinger Publications, Inc.
- Markway, B. G., & Markway, G. P. (2001). *Painfully shy: How to overcome social anxiety and reclaim your life.* New York, NY: Thomas Dunne Books, St. Martins Press.
- Rapee, R. M. (1998). *Overcoming shyness and social phobia: A step-by-step guide.* Northvale, NJ: Jason Aronson.
- Soifer, S., Zgourides, G. D., Himle, J. & Pickering, N. L. (2001). *Shy bladder syndrome: Your step-by-step guide to overcoming paruresis.* Oakland, CA: New Harbinger Publications.
- Stein, M. B., & Walker, J. R. (2001). *Triumph over shyness: Conquering shyness and social anxiety.* New York, NY: McGraw-Hill.

Useful informational websites about social anxiety and related resources include:

- http://www.temple.edu/phobia (Adult Anxiety Clinic of Temple, PA)
- http://www.toastmasters.org (Toastmasters International)
- http://www.adaa.org/AnxietyDisorderInfor/SocialPhobia.cfm (Anxiety Disorders Association of America)
- http://www.nimh.nih.gov/HealthInformation/socialphobiamenu.cfm (National Institute of Mental Health)
- http://www.freedomfromfear.com/aanx_factsheet.asp?id=20 (Freedom From Fear)
- http://www.paruresis.org/ (International Paruresis Association)
- http://www.cognitive-therapy.com/soc-anx.htm (Center for Cognitive Therapy, NC)
- http://www.nmha.org/pbedu/anxiety/social.cfm (National Mental Health Association)
- http://www.anxietynetwork.com/sphome.html#sp1 (Anxiety Network International)

What are Effective Therapist Based Treatments?

Cognitive–behavioral group therapy (CBGT; Heimberg & Becker, 2002) is based on the cognitive–behavioral model of social anxiety advanced by Rapee and Heimberg (1997) and has received the most research attention. CBGT typically involves 12 weekly 2.5-hour group sessions with approximately six members. After a presentation of the rationale for treatment, psychoeducation and instruction on cognitive restructuring, self-monitoring and exposure, the group sessions focus on in-session exposures integrated with cognitive restructuring practice. Individualized homework assignments (including between-session exposures) are also a prominent part of treatment. Hope et al.'s (2000) adaptation of the CBGT protocol for individual therapy is a 16-week treatment based on the same CBT principles of psychoeducation, self-monitoring, cognitive restructuring and exposures. Preliminary data from a recent controlled trial of this treatment manual demonstrated a significant reduction in symptomatology compared to a wait-list control group, with effect sizes roughly equivalent to those produced by group treatment (Zaider et al., 2003).

Another CBT program is based on a slightly different model of social anxiety disorder, which emphasizes cognitive factors in the maintenance of social anxiety (Clark & Wells, 1995). This treatment consists of 16 weekly 75-minute individual sessions and involves developing a personal model of the patient's anxiety-related thoughts and symptoms; experiments addressing the patient's tendency to engage in safety behaviors and self-focused attention; shifting the patient's attention to the external social situation; video feedback to challenge distorted self-images; identification of problems in anticipatory and postevent cognitive processing; and cognitive restructuring of dysfunctional assumptions. A placebocontrolled trial of this treatment showed that it effectively reduced social anxiety symptoms and resulted in outcomes superior to those of two other treatment groups (fluoxetine plus self-exposure and placebo plus self-exposure) after treatment as well as during the 12-month follow-up period (Clark et al., 2003).

What is Effective Medical Treatment?

Selective serotonin reuptake inhibitors (SSRIs) have emerged as a first-line pharmacotherapy for social anxiety disorder based upon results of several large scale placebo-controlled trials (e.g., Stein et al., 1998). Paroxetine, sertraline, and the serotonin–norepenephrine reuptake inhibitor venlafaxine have been approved by the USA Food and Drug Administration for the treatment of social anxiety disorder, although only sertraline has been approved for long-term treatment. Patients treated with these medications show approximately the same amount of reduction in social anxiety symptoms as those treated with CBT immediately after treatment. However, there is significant risk for relapse after discontinuation of medication.

Benzodiazepines have long been used to treat different types of anxiety, including social anxiety. However, there are several limitations of benzodiazepine treatment in social anxiety disorder, including their contraindication in the presence of substance abuse, their lack of efficacy for comorbid depression, and their potential for the development of dependence. Although MAOIs such as phenelzine have established efficacy for social anxiety disorder (e.g., Liebowitz et al., 1992), they have become second line treatments given their risk of hypertensive reactions and the inconvenience of dietary restrictions. For the treatment of performance-related anxiety, beta-adrenergic blockers have been used, however, no controlled trials have supported their efficacy in clinical populations. Tricyclic antidepressants appear ineffective in the treatment of social anxiety disorder (Simpson et al., 1998).

Combination Treatments

With strong empirical support for both SSRIs and CBT, it is intuitively appealing to combine these treatments for maximum efficacy. However, the literature to date does not clearly support the superiority of combined treatments. Davidson et al. (in press) found no difference in efficacy between CBT, fluoxetine and their combination in the treatment of social anxiety disorder, and Heimberg and Liebowitz (unpublished, reported in Heimberg, 2002) reported only a small benefit for the combination of CBGT and phenezine. Others (e.g., Haug et al., 2003) have suggested that medication treatment (e.g., sertraline) may actually detract from the efficacy of CBT. For a more extensive review of this literature see Zaider and Heimberg (2004).

Other Issues in Management

Medical treatment There appears to be a lag between initiation of SSRI medication and treatment response. Treatment with SSRIs appears to become superior to placebo control groups at about 6–8 weeks, with continued improvement on medication for up to 20 weeks (Van Ameringen et al., 2001). With regard to medication discontinuation, all medications should be tapered gradually, under the supervision of a medical doctor. Although the number of controlled studies comparing medication and psychotherapy is limited, the literature to date suggests that medications may offer somewhat greater initial symptom relief, although CBT may provide better protection against relapse (see Heimberg, 2002).

Psychotherapy A typical course of CBT is usually about 12–16 sessions. Although patients with severe generalized social anxiety disorder tend to improve as much as their less impaired peers, they may require more extensive therapy to achieve their treatment goals.

Several factors are important determinants of response to CBT. First, although the research is not wholly consistent, greater homework compliance is associated with greater treatment gains, both after treatment and at follow-up assessments (Edelman & Chambless, 1995; Leung & Heimberg, 1996). Second, patients often engage in a variety of safety behaviors (i.e., anxiety management strategies) during exposures. Individuals engage in these (subtle) avoidance and escape behaviors when confronted with a feared situation because they believe that the behavior "saves" them from feared consequences, allowing them to deflect the full impact of the anxiety associated with the threatening situation. Thus, engaging in safety behaviors diminishes the efficacy of exposure and results in decreased treatment response (Morgan & Raffle, 1999). It is therefore important that clinicians attend to and these behaviors and help patients to abandon them. Third, patients who are encouraged to shift their attention away from the self and toward the external social environment show improved treatment response (Woody, Chambless, & Glass, 1997; Wells & Papageorgiou, 1998). This shift allows patients to attend to positive social feedback, increase their social performance, and attend to information that may disconfirm their negative beliefs about social situations.

How Does One Select Among Treatments?

With regard to medication treatment, possible side effects and should be discussed. In addition, physical health and possible pregnancy should be considered and discussed with the patient before medication treatment is initiated. Finally, prior medication treatment for a psychiatric problem may suggest the patient's likely response and compliance with medication regimens.

Several areas are to be considered when offering a patient the option of CBT. First, although patients are likely to improve after receiving CBT for social anxiety disorder, the exposure to feared situations can be difficult for some to endure. Often an increase in anxiety occurs in the initial stages of treatment despite the typically graduated nature of exposures, and the patient's willingness and/or ability to endure this increase in anxiety should be considered. Patients who are at high risk for suicide due to severe comorbid depression may fall into this category, and comprehensive risk assessment is indicated. Second, patients' expectancy that the treatment will be effective in ameliorating their symptoms may affect treatment outcome (Safren, Heimberg, & Juster, 1997). Third, for patients with previous therapy experience, their level of compliance with therapeutic interventions (e.g., homework assignments) should be assessed. Finally, when choosing a CBT treatment modality, the choice between group and individual therapy, when available, should be made based upon patient preference, cost and severity of social anxiety symptoms/comorbidity.

REFERENCES (DOES NOT INCLUDE LIST OF SELF-HELP BOOKS UNLESS OTHERWISE CITED)

Alden, L. E., & Wallace, S. T. (1995). Social phobia and social appraisal in successful and unsuccessful social interactions. *Behaviour Research and Therapy, 33,* 497–505.

American Psychiatric Association (1994). *Diagnostic and statistical manual of mental disorders* (4th ed.). Washington, DC: Author.

Beck, A. T., Steer, R. A. & Brown, G. K. (1996). *Beck Depression Inventory manual* (2nd ed.). San Antonio: The Psychological Corporation.

Beck, A. T., Weissman, A., Lester, D., & Trexler, L. (1974). The measurement of pessimism: The Hopelessness Scale. *Journal of Consulting and Clinical Psychology, 42,* 861–865.

Clark, D. M., Ehlers, A., McManus, F., Hackmann, A., Fennell, M., Campbell, H., et al. (2003). Cognitive therapy vs fluoxetine in generalized social phobia: A randomized placebo controlled trial. *Journal of Consulting and Clinical Psychology, 71,* 1058–1067.

Clark, D. M., & Wells, A. (1995). A cognitive model of social phobia. In R. G. Heimberg, M. R. Liebowitz, D. A. Hope, & F. R. Schneier (Eds), *Social phobia: Diagnosis, assessment, and treatment* (pp. 69–93). New York, NY: Guilford Press.

Connor, K. M., Davidson, J. R. T., Churchill, L. E., Sherwood, A., Foa, E., & Weisler, R. H. (2000). Psychometric properties of the Social Phobia Inventory (SPIN). *British Journal of Psychiatry, 176,* 379–386.

Connor, K. M., Kobak, K. A., Churchill, L. E., Katzelnick, D., & Davidson, J. R. T. (2001). Mini-SPIN: A brief screening assessment for generalized social anxiety disorder. *Depression and Anxiety, 14,* 137–140.

Davidson, J. R. T., Foa, E., Huppert, J., Keefe, F., Franklin, M., Compton, J., et al. (in press). Fluoxetine, comprehensive cognitive behavioral therapy (CCBT) and placebo in generalized social phobia. *Archives of General Psychiatry.*

Davidson, J. R. T., Hughes, D. L., George, L. K., & Blazer, D. G. (1993). The epidemiology of social phobia: Findings from the Duke Epidemiological Catchment Area study. *Psychological Medicine, 23,* 709–718.

DiNardo, P. A., Brown, T. A., & Barlow, D. H. (1994). *Anxiety Disorders Interview Schedule for DSM-IV: Lifetime version (ADIS-IV-L).* San Antonio, TX: The Psychological Corporation.

Erwin, B. A., Heimberg, R. G., Juster, H. R., & Mindlin, M. (2002). Comorbid anxiety and mood disorders among persons with social anxiety disorder. *Behaviour Research and Therapy, 40,* 19–35.

Edelman, R. E., & Chambless, D. L. (1995). Adherence during session and homework in cognitive–behavioral group treatment of social phobia. *Behaviour Research and Therapy, 33,* 573–577.

Federoff, I. C., & Taylor, S. (2001). Psychological and pharmacological treatments for social phobia: A meta-analysis. *Journal of Clinical Psychopharmacology, 21,* 311–324.

Feske, U., & Chambless, D. L. (1995). Cognitive behavioral versus exposure only treatment for social phobia: A meta-analysis. *Behavior Therapy, 26,* 295–720

Gould, R. A., Buckminster, S., Pollack, M. H., Otto, M. W., & Yap, L. (1997). Cognitive–behavioral and pharmacological treatment for social phobia: A meta-analysis. *Clinical Psychology: Science and Practice, 4,* 291–306.

Harb, G. C., Eng, W., Zaider, T., & Heimberg, R. G. (2003). Behavioral assessment of public speaking anxiety using a modified version of the Social Performance Rating Scale. *Behaviour Research and Therapy, 41,* 1373–1380.

Haug, T. T., Blomhoff, S., Hellström, K., Holme, I., Humble, M., Madsbu, H. P., et al. (2003). Exposure therapy and sertraline in social phobia: 1-year follow-up of a randomised controlled trial. *British Journal of Psychiatry, 182,* 312–318.

Heimberg, R. G. (1996). Social phobia, avoidant personality disorder, and the multiaxial conceptualization of interpersonal anxiety. In P. Salkovskis (Ed.), *Trends in cognitive and behavioural therapies* (pp. 43–62). Sussex, England: John Wiley & Sons Ltd.

Heimberg, R. G. (2002). Cognitive–behavioral therapy for social anxiety disorder: Current status and future directions. *Biological Psychiatry, 51,* 101–108.

Heimberg, R. G., & Becker, R. E. (2002). *Cognitive-behavioral group therapy for social phobia: Basic mechanisms and clinical strategies.* New York, NY: Guilford Press.

Heimberg, R. G., Horner, K. J., Juster, H. R., Safren, S. A., Brown, E. J., Schneier, F. R., et al. (1999). Psychometric properties of the Liebowitz Social Anxiety Scale. *Psychological Medicine, 29,* 199–212.

Hope, D. A., Heimberg, R. G., Juster, H., & Turk, C.L. (2000). *Managing social anxiety: A cognitive–behavioral therapy approach* (Client Workbook). San Antonio, TX: The Psychological Corporation.

Kessler, R. C., McGonagle, K.A., Zhao, S., Nelson, C.B., Hughes, M., Eshleman, S., et al. (1994). Lifetime and 12-month prevalence of DSM-III-R psychiatric disorders in the United States: Results from the National Comorbidity Survey. *Archives of General Psychiatry, 51,* 8–19.

Kessler, R. C., Stang, P., Wittchen, H.-U., Stein, M., & Walters, E. E. (1999). Lifetime comorbidities between social phobia and mood disorders in the U.S. National Comorbidity Survey. *Psychological Medicine, 29,* 555–567.

Leary, M. R. (1983). A brief version of the Fear of Negative Evaluation Scale. *Personality and Social Psychology Bulletin, 9,* 371–375.

Leung, A. W., & Heimberg, R. G. (1996). Homework compliance, perceptions of control, and outcome of cognitive–behavioral treatment of social phobia. *Behaviour Research and Therapy, 34,* 423–432.

Liebowitz, M. R. (1987). Social phobia. *Modern Problems in Pharmacopsychiatry, 22,* 141–173.

Liebowitz, M. R., Schneier, F., Campeas, R., Hollander, E., Hatterer, J., Fyer, A., et al. (1992). Phenelzine vs. atenolol in social phobia: A placebo-controlled comparison. *Archives of General Psychiatry, 49,* 290–300.

Mattick, R. P., & Clarke, J. C. (1998). Development and validation of measures of social phobia scrutiny fear and social interaction anxiety. *Behaviour Research and Therapy, 36,* 455–470.

Morgan, H., & Raffle, C. (1999). Does reducing safety behaviours improve treatment response in patients with social phobia? *Australian and New Zealand Journal of Psychiatry, 33,* 503–510.

Narrow, W. E., Rae, D. S., Robins, L. N., & Regier, D. A. (2002). Revised prevalence estimates of mental disorders in the United States: Using a clinical significance criterion to reconcile 2 surveys' estimates. *Archives of General Psychiatry, 59,* 115–123.

Öst, L. G. (1987). Age of onset in different phobias. *Journal of Abnormal Psychology, 96,* 223–229.

Rapee, R. M., & Heimberg, R. G. (1997). A cognitive–behavioral model of anxiety in social phobia. *Behaviour Research and Therapy, 35,* 741–756.

Rapee, R. M., & Lim, L. (1992). Discrepancy between self- and observer ratings of performance in social phobics. *Journal of Abnormal Psychology, 101,* 728–731.

Reich, J., Goldenberg, I., Vasile, R., Goisman, R., & Keller, M. (1994). A prospective follow-along study of the course of social phobia. *Psychiatry Research, 54,* 249–258

Safren, S. A., Heimberg, R. G., & Juster, H. R. (1997). Client expectancies and their relationship to pretreatment symtomatology and outcome of cognitive–behavioral group treatment for social phobia. *Journal of Consulting and Clinical Psychology, 65,* 694–698.

Schneier, F. R., Johnson, J., Hornig, C. D., Liebowitz, M. R., & Weissman, M. M. (1992). Social phobia: Comorbidity and morbidity in an epidemiologic sample. *Archives of General Psychiatry, 49,* 282–288.

Schwartz, C. E., Snidman, N., & Kagan, J. (1999). Adolescent social anxiety as an outcome of inhibited temperament in childhood. *Journal of the American Academy of Child and Adolescent Psychiatry, 38,* 1008–1015.

Simpson, H. B., Schneier, F. R., Campeas, R.B., Marshall, R.D., Fallon, B.A., Davies, S., et al. (1998). Imipramine in the treatment of social phobia. *Journal of Clinical Psychopharmacology, 18,* 132–135.

Stein, M. B., Liebowitz, M. R., Lydiard, R. B., Pitts, C. D., Bushnell, W., & Gergel, I. (1998). Paroxetine treatment of generalized social phobia (social anxiety disorder): A randomized, double-blind, placebo-controlled study. *Journal of the American Medical Association, 280,* 708–713.

Taylor, (1996). Meta-analysis of cognitive–behavioral treatments for social phobia. *Journal of Behavior Therapy and Experimental Psychiatry, 27,* 1–9.

Turk, C. L., Heimberg, R. G, Orsillo, S. M., Holt, C. S., Gitow, A., Street, L. L., et al. (1998). An investigation of gender differences in social phobia. *Journal of Anxiety Disorders, 12,* 209–223.

Turner, S. M., Beidel, D. C., Dancu, C. V. & Stanley, M. A. (1989). An empirically derived inventory to measure social fears and anxiety: The Social Phobia and Anxiety Inventory. *Psychological Assessment, 1,* 35–40.

Van Ameringen, M., Lane, R. M., Walker, J. R., Bowen, R. C., Chokka, P. R, Goldner, E. M., et al. (2001). Sertraline treatment of generalized social phobia: A 20-week, double-blind, placebo-controlled study. *American Journal of Psychiatry, 158,* 275–281.

Watson, D., & Friend, R. (1969). Measurement of social-evaluative anxiety. *Journal of Consulting and Clinical Psychology, 33,* 448–457.

Weeks, J. W., Heimberg., R. G., Fresco, D. M., Hart, T. A., Turk, C. L., Schneier, F. R., et al. R. (2004). *Empirical validation and psychometric evaluation of the Brief Fear of Negative Evaluation Scale in patients with social anxiety disorder.*

Wells, A., & Papageorgiou, C. (1998). Social phobia: Effects of external attention on anxiety, negative beliefs, and perspective taking. *Behavior Therapy, 29,* 357–370.

Wittchen, H.-U., Stein, M. B., & Kessler, R. C. (1999). Social fears and social phobia in a community sample of adolescents and young adults: Prevalence, risk factors, and co-morbidity. *Psychological Medicine, 29,* 309–323.

Woody, S. R., Chambless, D. L., & Glass, C. R. (1997). Self-focused attention in the treatment of social phobia. *Behaviour Research and Therapy, 35,* 117–129.

Zaider, T. I., & Heimberg, R. G. (2004). The relationship between psychotherapy and pharmacotherapy for social anxiety disorder. In B. Bandelow & D.J. Stein (Eds.), *Social anxiety disorder* (pp. 299–314). New York, NY: Marcel Dekker, Inc.

Zaider, T., Heimberg, R. G., Roth, D. A., Hope, D. A., & Turk, C. L. (2003, November). *Individual CBT for social anxiety disorder: Preliminary findings.* A paper presented at the annual meeting of the Association for Advancement of Behavior Therapy, Boston, MA.

Stress

Lauren Woodward • Lindsay Fletcher • W. O'Donohue

WHAT IS STRESS?

Lazarus (1993) in one of the more influential definitions has defined stress in terms of four components: (1) an external stimuli, often called a stressor, is present, (2) the individual who is encountered with this stimuli must evaluate, or appraise the situation or stimuli as being stress-evoking (e.g, they must determine what is threatening or noxious from what is harmless), (3) the individual attempts to cope with these stressful demands, and (4) a complex set of reactions takes place both in the mind and the body.

One of the earliest contributions to stress research came from Walter Cannon's (1932) description of the fight or flight response. This response was originally thought to be adaptive for humans when faced with the possibility of physical threat (e.g. when cavemen were faced with saber-toothed tigers), however, still occurs today. When faced with a threat (stressor), the body becomes rapidly aroused from activation of the sympathetic nervous system. This physiological response prepares the body to either attack the threat (fight) or to flee (flight). Cannon (1932) reasoned that though common stressors individuals are faced with no longer entail an actual physical threat (e.g., deadlines, traffic, running late, uncertainties, etc.), the response persists, which can lead to various physical and psychological maladies.

Another important stress researcher, Selye (1956), developed the concept of "general adaptation syndrome" in which an individual experiences the same sequence of physiological reactions regardless of the type of stressor. Over time, the repeated or ongoing response to these stressors leads to exhaustion. Selye (1974) outlined two types of stress: distress is harmful and damaging, and eustress involves positive life events that are stressful (e.g. weddings, vacations, a new baby, or dating). Whether a stress is classified as eustress or distress frequently depends on how the stressful event is perceived.

McEwen (1998) has more recently expanded Selye's definition by describing the specific physiologic effects of chronic stress in terms of "allostatic load." According to this model, perception of stress is due to one's experiences, genetics, and behavior, and the body responds to stress with elevations in stress-related hormones, glucocorticoids and catecholamines. Normally once the stressor is gone the physiologic response returns to baseline. However, if inactivation of the stress response is not complete, then increases in allostatic load occur over time. Thus stress has effects on the neural, immune, and endocrine systems, which negatively impact organ systems, causing disease. In fact, a growing body of research has shown that stress is related to many physical problems, such as diabetes, ulcers, irritable bowel syndrome, and cancer (Hafen, Karren, Frandsen, & Smith, 1996).

In addition to physical disease, stress manifests in individuals in a number of different ways, including cognitive, emotional, behavioral, somatic, and social symptoms. Stress has been found to impair cognitive functioning such as attention and can lead to negative rumination about the stressor (Lepore, 1997). Individuals may

Woodward, L., Fletcher, L. & O'Donohue, W. (2006). Stress. In J. E. Fisher & W. T. O'Donohue (Eds.), *Practitioner's Guide to evidence-based psychotherapy*. New York: Springer.

also exhibit emotional symptoms of stress, including feeling overwhelmed, anxious, or depressed (Lazarus, 1999; Sarafino, 2002). If individuals are feeling stressed they may engage in unhealthy behaviors such as overeating, smoking or drinking (Sarafino, 2002), and such behaviors can in turn serve to reduce a person's ability to cope. Also, individuals may experience somatic symptoms in response to stress such as sweaty hands, racing heart, nausea, headaches or muscle tension (Guthrie, Verstraete, Deines, & Stern, 1975). Finally, individuals may exhibit social manifestations of stress where they may be hostile or irritable towards others, or they may try to isolate themselves from others (Sarafino, 2002).

BASIC FACTS ABOUT STRESS

Comorbidity. Stress is not a DSM diagnosis and therefore should only be assessed for after other possible diagnoses are ruled out (see section "Assessment"). Stress is often referred to in the literature as a predisposing factor to the onset of other problems as wide-ranging as depression (Voelkner, 2004), substance abuse (McQuaid et al., 2000), diabetes (Hagglof, Blom, Dahlquist, Lonnberg, & Sahlin, 1991; Thernlund, et al., 1995), asthma (Mrazek & Klinnert, 1996), and gambling addiction (Coman, Burrows, & Evans, 1997). Many adverse health effects have been found to be associated with stress including coronary heart disease, hypertension, high blood pressure, gastrointestinal disorders, low back pain, ulcers, skin disorders, tension headaches, and irritable bowel syndrome (Brand, Hanson & Godaert, 2000; Hafen et al., 1996; Krantz & McCeney, 2002; Robert-McComb, 2001; Taylor, 1999).

Prevalence. Every individual will experience stress more than once in their lifetime. In fact, stress is such a common occurrence that an estimated 75% of all office visits to a primary care physician in the United States are for stress-related complaints (Hughes, Pearson, & Reinhart, 1984).

Age at onset. The age at onset of an elevated stress response depends on the presence of a stressor. Stress may be present at any age.

Gender. Women have been found to report having experienced more major and minor life stressors than men do (Davis, Matthews, & Twamley, 1999). Social support has been found to have a stronger buffering effect for females than males in stress (Sherman & Walls, 1995). Also, males who are highly reactive to stress and exhibit Type A behaviors are more likely to develop coronary heart disease (Carver, Diamond, & Humphreys, 1985).

Course. Stress can present itself in response to acute or chronic stressors. An example of an acute stressor would be the sudden death of a loved one or a natural disaster. Chronic stressors could include a dysfunctional marriage or a demanding job. Also, an acute stressor could lead to chronic stress depending on the coping style of the individual and subsequent related events.

Impairment and other demographic characteristics. Chronic stress can lead to impairment in daily functioning, such as lowered immune functioning which leads to higher susceptibility to infection and illness (Sternberg & Gold, 1997). Younger adults are better equipped with strong immune systems to recover from these illnesses, whereas the elderly, whose immune systems may already be compromised, may not recover as quickly. Individuals with lower socioeconomic status, poor social support systems, negative coping styles, and whose perceived control is low may be more prone to the effects of stress (Brummett, et al. 2004; Klein, Faraday, Quigley & Grunberg, 2004; Sarafino, 2000; Scott, 2004). Finally, research on ethnicity and stress has been inconclusive. Ethnic identity, cultural racism, and race-related stress have all been found to be important predictors of stress levels (Utsey, Chae, Brown, & Kelly, 2002).

ASSESSMENT

What Should be Ruled Out?

Treatment for stress is implemented only after other diagnoses have been ruled out. Symptoms of stress will inevitably overlap with many of the DSM disorders because having a psychological problem is inherently stressful. Clinicians will want to pay special attention to ruling out posttraumatic stress disorder (PTSD), acute stress disorder, depression, and anxiety disorders. Many individuals may find treatment for stress to be more socially and personally more acceptable than diagnosis of a psychiatric disorder. Clinicians should also be careful not to ask such broad questions as to be sure that there is an affirmative response, e.g., "Do you experience any stress?"

What is Involved in Effective Assessment?

A complete assessment of stress should include the analysis of:

- Recent life events
- Frequently occurring stressful situations
- Substance use to self-medicate stress
- Symptoms of comorbid anxiety
- Symptoms of comorbid depression
- Comorbid physical illness
- Functional impairment
- Degree of social support
- Perceived control
- Suicidal ideation and past attempts
- Expression of Type A behaviors
- Appraisal of stressful situations

Clinician-administered measures. The commonly used measures for stress are all self-report. Clinical interviews can be used in conjunction with self-report measures.

Self-report measures. The Derogatis Stress Profile (DSP) is a self-report measure that is used for screening and outcome of stress (Derogatis, 1984). Individuals respond to 77 items on a 5-point Likert scale in the degree to which the given statement is true of them. The measure has 11 subscales which include: Time Pressure, Driven Behavior, Attitude Posture, Relaxation Potential, Role Definition, Vocational Environment, Domestic Environment, Health Environment, Hostility, Anxiety, and Depression. This measure can be useful in identifying individuals' stress levels. The Hassles and Uplifts Scale (Lazarus & Folkman, 1989) consists of three scales (the Daily Hassles Scale, the Daily Uplifts Scale, and the Combined Hassles and Uplifts Scale) designed to measure the appraisal of daily life experiences, either minor annoyances, positive experiences, or a combination of the two. The Daily Hassles scale is a good way to understand the degree to which individuals appraise annoyances as stressful and is widely used. The 15-item Impact of Events Scale (IES) is a widely used measure to assess the psychological impact of traumatic life events and stress reactions (Horowitz, Wilner, & Alvarez, 1979). The measure has often been used with individuals exhibiting symptoms of Posttraumatic Stress Disorder (PTSD) although was originally designed to be used for bereavement. Finally, the Ways of Coping Questionnaire (Folkman & Lazarus, 1988) is a 66-item measure that examines aspects of coping that are relevant to stress such as tension reduction and self-isolation. It also includes assessment of whether an individual uses emotion-focused or problem-focused coping strategies.

Behavioral assessment. Sudden changes in negative health behaviors, such as over- or undereating, sleep problems, smoking, and binge drinking should be carefully assessed as possible symptoms of stress. As previously mentioned, social behavior may be affected such that individuals under severe stress may exhibit moodiness in relationships and they may try to isolate themselves.

What Assessments are Not Helpful?

Traditional psychological measures such as the MMPI, projective tests such as the Rorschach, and neuropsychological tests are not useful in assessing stress.

TREATMENT

What Treatments are Effective?

There are several psychosocial interventions with empirical support that focus on cognitive behavioral techniques. One of these is Stress Inoculation Training (SIT), which has been found to be successful across a broad range of individuals who experience varying degrees of stress and is designed to teach skills to alleviate stress and achieve personal goals. It is composed of three phases: Conceptualization, Skills Acquisition and Rehearsal, and Application and Follow-Through. Conceptualization involves teaching the individual about the nature of stress and how people react to it (Meichenbaum, 2003). In the second phase, Skills Acquisition and Rehearsal, the individual learns cognitive and behavioral skills used in emotion and problem-focused coping. In this phase, other CBT components are added, including relaxation training and cognitive restructuring (Sheehy & Horan, 2004). The third component of SIT, Application and Follow-Through, deals with using the skills taught in the first two phases and applying them when individuals are faced with stressful situations in vivo. Relapse prevention procedures, bolstering self-efficacy, and having clients coach others with similar stress situations are all techniques commonly used with SIT (Meichenbaum, 2003).

Other CBT techniques commonly and effectively used in alleviating the symptoms of stress include social skills training, relaxation training, and cognitive restructuring (Pierce, 1995; Kaplan & Laygo, 2003; Haney, 2004). Social skills training involves educating the individual about how social skills deficits are related to stress and then teaching them basic skills of adaptive social interaction (Kaplan & Laygo, 2003). Relaxation training helps patients to become more aware of how tension is carried in the body when they are feeling stressed and teaches breathing and imaging exercises to help patients release the tension. Finally, cognitive restructuring consists of training the client to identify and become aware of irrational, maladaptive thoughts and statements, and to eventually apply more adaptive thoughts to guide them through stressful situations. CBT treatments implementing all three of these components into an intervention have been found to be efficacious (Tolman & Rose, 1985).

Several group treatments that focus on mind/body awareness have been empirically validated to treat a variety of stress-related symptoms and medical problems. Kabat-Zinn's (1990) mindfulness-based stress reduction (MBSR) is a 6–12 week structured group program that teaches mindfulness meditation. It has been demonstrated by controlled trials to be effective in coping with a wide range of problems, including stress and psychosomatic complaints (for a recent meta-analysis see Grossman et al., 2004). The course was the first of its kind developed in the United States and is offered at numerous locations around the country and the world. Another program with some similar components is The Personal Health Improvement Program™ (PHIP) (formerly Ways to Wellness; WTW). It is 6-week group program that employs readings, meditation, classroom exercises and coaching, and out-of-class discussions with study partners. In a randomized controlled trial, decreases in somatization, anxiety, and depression were found for the treatment group (McLeod, Budd, & McClelland, 1997) and similar effects were found when the program was field tested at seven sites around the country (Locke et al., 1999; contact the author for information).

What are Effective Self-Help Treatments?

Several self-help books use many components of CBTs in conjunction with different healthy lifestyle behaviors, including exercise, enjoying pleasurable activities, and meditation. Listed below are some self-help books that may be helpful in alleviating symptoms of stress, although their effectiveness in treating stress has not been clinically tested.

- Benson, H., & Klipper, M. Z. (1975). *The relaxation response.* New York, NY: Harper Collins Publishers, Inc.
- Carlson, R. (1998). *The don't sweat the small stuff workbook: Exercises, questions, and self-tests to help you keep the little things from taking over your life.* New York: Hyperion.
- Davidson, J. (1999). *The complete idiot's guide to managing stress.* Indianapolis, IN: Alpha Books.
- Davis, M., Eshelman, E. R., & McKay, M. (2000). *The relaxation and stress reduction workbook.* Oakland, CA: New Harbinger Publications Inc.
- Kabat-Zinn, J. (1990). *Full catastrophe living: Using the wisdom of your body and mind to face stress, pain, and illness.* New York, NY: Dell Publishing.
- Kundtz, D. (2000). *Quiet mind one-minute retreats from a busy world.* York Beach, ME: Conari Press.

Useful information websites about stress and related internet links include:

- *www.dontsweat.com* (from the Don't Sweat the Small stuff books)
- *www.mindtools.com*
- *www.nlh.nih.gov/medlineplus/stress.html* (Med Line — national library of medicine's consumer site)
- *www.stress.org* (American Institute of Stress)
- *www.stressrelease.com* (Stress Busters)

What are Effective Therapist Based Treatments?

CBT stress management groups have received empirical support. Usually, the groups use similar techniques to individual therapy including cognitive restructuring, relaxation and assertiveness training (Tallant, Rose & Tolman, 1989). Groups allow individual clients to practice their newly acquired cognitive–behavioral stress management strategies as well as provide encouragement and peer reinforcement to others in the group (Tolman & Rose, 1985). Cognitive Behavioral Group Therapy (CBGT) has also been found to be helpful in reducing the effects of stress in medical populations such as breast cancer, epilepsy and HIV (Au, Chan, Li, Leung, Li, & Chan, 2003; Cruess, et al., 2002; McGregor, et al. 2004).

In addition, MBSR is offered at hospitals and clinics around the United States; in 1997, over 240 sites here and abroad were offering stress reduction programs based on mindfulness training (Salmon, Santorelli & Kabat-Zinn, 1998).

What is Effective Medical Treatment?

To help manage stress, physicians frequently prescribe either benzodiazepines or beta blockers, both of which reduce physiologic arousal and feelings associated with anxiety (Sarafino, 2002). More specifically, Buspar, Buspirone, Paxil, Wellbutrin,

Zoloft, Effexa, and Celexa are commonly prescribed medications to alleviate the symptoms of stress.

REFERENCES

Au, A., Chan, F., Li, K., Leung, P., Li, P., & Chan, J. (2003). Cognitive–behavioral group treatment program for adults with epilepsy in Hong Kong. *Epilepsy & Behavior 4(4)*, 441–446.

Brand, N., Hanson, E., & Godaert, G. (2000). Chronic stress affects blood pressure and speed of short term memory. *Perceptual and Motor Skills 91(1)*, 291–298.

Brummett, B. H., Babyak, M. A., Mark, D. B., Clapp-Channing, N. E., Siegler, I. C., & Barefoot, J. C. (2004). Prospective study of perceived stress in cardiac patients. *Annals of Behavioral Medicine 27(1)*, 22–30.

Cannon, W. B. (1932). *The wisdom of the body*. New York: Norton.

Carver, C. S., Diamond, E. L., & Humphries, C. (1985). Coronary prone behavior. In N. Schneiderman & J. T. Tapp (Eds.), *Behvaioral medicine: The biopsychosocial approach*. Hillsdale, NJ: Erlbaum.

Coman, G. J., Burrows, G. D., & Evans, B. J. (1997) Stress and anxiety as factors in the onset of problem gambling: Implications for treatment. *Stress Medicine 13(4)*, 235–244.

Cruess, S., Antoni, M. H., Hayes, A., Penedo, F., Ironson, G., Fletcher, M. A., et al. (2002). Changes in mood and depressive symptoms and related change processes during cognitive-behavioral stress management in HIV-infected men. *Cognitive Therapy & Research 26(3)*, 373–392.

Davis, M. C., Matthews, K. A., & Twamley, E. W. (1999). Is life more difficult on Mars or Venus? A meta-analytic review of sex differences in major and minor life events. *Annals of Behavioral Medicine, 21*, 83–97.

Derogatis, L. R. (1987). The Derogatis Stress Profile (DSP): Quantification of psychological stress. *Advances in Psychosomatic Medicine 17*, 30–54.

Folkman, S., & Lazarus, R. S. (1988). *Ways of coping questionnaire: Research edition*. Palo Alto, CA: Consulting Psychologists Press.

Grossman, P., Neimann, L., Schmidt, S., & Walach, H. (2004). Mindfulness-based stress reduction and health benefits: A meta-analysis. *Journal of Psychosomatic Research 57*, 35–43.

Guthrie, G. M., Verstraete, A., Deines, M. M., & Stern, R. M. (1975). Symptoms of stress in four societies. *The Journal of Social Psychology 95*, 165–172.

Hafen, B. Q., Karren, K. J., Frandsen, K. J., & Smith N. L. (1996) *Mind/Body health: The effects of attitudes, emotions and relationships*. Needham Heights, MA: Allyn & Bacon.

Hagglof, B., Blom, L., Dahlquist, G., Lonnberg, G., & Sahlin, B. (1991). The Swedish childhood diabetes study: Indications of severe psychological stress as a risk factor for type 1 (insulin-dependent) diabetes mellitus in childhood. *Diabetologia 34(8)*: 579–83.

Haney, C. J. (2004). Stress management interventions for female athletes: Relaxation and cognitive restructuring. *International Journal of Sports Psychology 35*, 109–118.

Horowitz, M. J., Wilner, N. R., & Alvarez, W. (1979). Impact of events scale. A measure of subjective stress. *Psychosomatic Medicine 41*, 209–218.

Hughes, G. H., Pearson, M. A., & Reinhart, G. R. (1984). Stress: Sources, effects and management. *Family & Community Health 7(1)*, 47–58.

Kabat-Zinn, J. (1990). *Full catastrophe living: Using the wisdom of your body and mind to face stress, pain, and illness*. New York, NY: Dell Publishing.

Kaplan, A. & Laygo, R. (2003). Stress management. In W. O'Donohue, J. E. Fisher & S. C. Hayes (Eds.), *Cognitive behavior therapy: Applying empirically supported techniques in your practice*. Hoboken, NJ: John Wiley & Sons, Inc.

Klein, L. C., Faraday, M. M., Quigley, K. S., & Grunberg, N. E. (2004). Gender differences in biobehavioral aftereffects of stress on eating, frustration, and cardiovascular responses. *Journal of Applied Social Psychology 34(3)*, 538–562.

Krantz, D. S., & McCeney, M. K. (2002). Effects of psychological and social factors on organic disease: A critical assessment of research on coronary heart disease. *Annual Review of Psychology 53(1)*, 341–368.

Lazarus, R. S. (1993). From psychological stress to the emotions: A history of changing outlooks. *Annual Review of Psychology 44*, 1–21.

Lazarus, R. S. (1999). *Stress and emotion: A new synthesis*. New York: Springer.

Lazarus, R. S., & Folkman, S. (1984). *Stress, appraisal and coping*. New York: Springer.

Lepore, S. J. (1997). Social–environmental influences on the chronic stress process. In B. H. Gottlieb (Ed.), *Coping with chronic stress*. New York: Plenum.

Locke, S. E., Chan, P.P., Morley, D.S., McLeod, C.C., Budd, M.A., & Orlowski, M. (1999). Behavioral medicine group intervention for high-utilising somatising patients: Evaluation across 7 unrelated healthcare organizations. *Dis Manage Health Outcomes 6(6)*, 387–404.

McEwen, B. S. (1998). Protective and damaging effects of stress mediators. *New England Journal of Medicine, 338*, 171–179.

McGregor, B. A., Antoni, M. H., Boyers, A., Alferi, S. M., Blomberg, B. B., & Carver, C. S. (2004). Cognitive–behavioral stress management increases benefit finding and immune function among women with early-stage breast cancer. *Journal of Psychosomatic Research 56(1)*, 1–8.

McLeod, C. C., Budd, M. A., McClelland, D. C. (1997). Treatment of somatization in primary care. *General Hospital Psychiatry 19*, 251–258.

McQuaid, J. R., Brown, S. A., Aarons, G. A., Smith, T. L., Patterson, T. L., & Schuckit, M. A. (2000). Correlates of life stress in an alcohol treatment sample. *Addictive Behaviors 25(1)*, 131–137.

Meichenbaum, D. (2003). Stress inoculation training. In W. O'Donohue, J. E. Fisher & S. C. Hayes (Eds.), *Cognitive behavior therapy: Applying empirically supported techniques in your practice.*

Mrazek, D. A. & Klinnert, M. (1996). Emotional stressors and the onset of asthma. In: Pfeffer, C. R. (Ed.) *Severe stress and mental disturbance in children.* Washington, DC: American Psychiatric Association.

Pierce, T. W. (1995). Skills training in stress management. In W. O'Donohue & L. Krasner (Eds.) *Handbook of psychological skills training: Clinical techniques and applications.* Needham Heights, MA: Allyn & Bacon.

Robert-McComb, J. J. (2001). *Eating disorders in women and children: Prevention stress management and treatment.* Boca Raton, FL: CRC Press.

Salmon P. G., Santorelli, S. F., & Kabat-Zinn, J. (1998) Intervention elements promoting adherence to mindfulness-based stress reduction programs in the clinical behavioral medicine setting. In S. A. Shumaker, E. B. Schron, J. K. Ockene, & W. L. Bee (Eds.), *Handbook of health behavior change* (2nd ed., pp. 239–268). New York: Springer.

Sarafino, E. P. (2002). *Health psychology: Biopsychosocial interactions.* New York: John Wiley & Sons, Inc.

Scott, L. D. (2004). Correlates of coping with perceived discriminatory experiences among African American adolescents. *Journal of Adolescence 27(2)*, 123–137.

Selye, H. (1956). *The stress of life.* New York: McGraw–Hill.

Selye, H. (1974). *Stress without distress.* Philadelphia: Lippincott.

Sheehy, R., & Horan, J. J. (2004). Effects of stress innoculation training for 1st-year law students. *International Journal of Stress Management 11(1)*, 41–55.

Sternberg, E. M., & Gold, P. W. (1997). The mind–body interaction in disease. *Scientific American 7(1)*, 8–15.

Sherman, A. C., & Walls, J. W. (1995). Gender differences in the relationship of moderator variables to stress and symptoms. *Psychology & Health 10*, 321–331.

Tallant, S., Rose, S. D., & Tolman, R. M. (1989). New evidence for the effectiveness of stress management training in groups. *Behavior Modification 13(4)*, 431–446.

Taylor, S. E. (1999). *Health psychology.* New York: McGraw-Hill.

Thernlund, G. M., Dahlquist, G., Hansson, K., Ivarsson, S. A., Ludvigsson, J., Sjoblad, S., & Hagglof, B. (1995). Psychological stress and the onset of IDDM in children. *Diabetes Care 18 (10):* 1323–1329.

Tolman, R., & Rose, S. D. (1985). Coping with stress: A multimodal approach. *Social Work 30(2)*, 151–158.

Utsey, S. O., Chae, M. H., Brown, C. F., & Kelly, D. (2002). Effects of ethnic group membership on ethnic identity: Race-related stress and quality of life. *Cultural Diversity and Ethnic Minority Psychology 8(4)*, 366–377.

Voelkner, R. (2004). Stress, sleep loss, and substance abuse create potent recipe for college depression. *Journal of the American Medical Association 291(18)*, 2177–2179.

Stuttering

Bruce P. Ryan

WHAT IS STUTTERING?

Stuttering is defined as "Disturbance in the normal fluency and time patterning of speech. Primary characteristics include (a) audible or silent blocking; (b) sound and syllable repetitions; (c) sound prolongations, (d) interjections, (e) broken words (e.g., ca-ar); (f) circumlocutions; or (g) words produced with excess of tension (struggle). Secondary characteristics include the habitual use of speech musculature or other body parts which the stutterer (person who stutters) employs along with the primary characteristics (e.g., head jerk, or stare, or sniff)..." (Nicolosi, Harryman, & Kreschek, 1996). There are many characteristics of social anxiety coexisting in adults who stutter which are probably a result of the stuttering, because many of these disappear after successful instatement of speech fluency. These manifest themselves in avoidance of speaking, especially on the telephone, selection of occupations that require little speaking, limitations in dating, and many more (Krasimaat, Vanryckeghem, & Van Dam-Baggen, 2002).

Most stuttering may be referred to as "developmental stuttering" (due to no known cause except that it develops during childhood) whereas there are also forms of neurological stuttering. These occur commonly after a known trauma such as car accident, CVA, or other brain damage in a person who was known as nonstutterer before the incident. Some authorities believe stuttering should be differentiated from cluttering; the latter is characterized by a high rate of speech, occasional articulation disorders, and minor language problems, and little client concern about the problem (Bloodstein, 1995).

Theories about what causes stuttering abound. These can be sorted into physical (brain variance in anatomy and/or physiology), psychosocial (emotional trauma), and learned. Current interest is high in the physiological basis due to the many new brain measurement instruments such as MRI and PET scans available for such research. A most interesting current, functional thought is that stuttering may come from the use of the right cerebral hemisphere, which is less able to process speech than the left hemisphere (Moore, 1993). This could explain the high incidence of spontaneous recovery as the stuttering child shifts back to the left hemisphere after temporarily using the right. Further, researchers have observed a shift of hemispheric use from the right to the left after successful treatment in adults (Yeudall, 1985). This premise, however, is not supported by extensive, definitive research and other aspects of brain activity are presently being explored as described in Ingham (1998, 2004) and R. Ingham, J. Ingham, Finn, and Fox (2003). There appears to be a hereditary factor, possibly related to physiological and anatomical brain variations (Bloodstein, 1995).

BASIC FACTS ABOUT STUTTERING

Comorbidity. The disorder of stuttering commonly cooccurs with the disorders of misarticulation (Bloodstein, 1995).

Ryan, B. P. (2006). Stuttering. In J.E. Fisher & W. T. O'Donohue (Eds.), *Practitioner's guide for evidence-based psychotherapy.* New York: Springer.

Fluency. The average of stuttering for people who stutter is about 6% words stuttered (Ryan, 2001b) and they can be fluent in one or more of the situations when they: sing, speak in unison with others, speak with delayed auditory feedback, cannot hear their own speech, speak when alone, speak to animals or younger people, speak in time with metronome, and repeat memorized materials such as poems and parts in a play. Exactly why this occurs is not clear. Possibly altered self-hearing or novel production of their own speech may explain these phenomena.

Prevalence. Stuttering is the least frequent of the speech problems of four general categories of speech-language problems (articulation, language, stuttering, and voice). Most authorities suggest both incidence and prevalence to be about 1% whereas 3–4% of the population may be described as having ever stuttered (Bloodstein, 1995).

Age at onset. Stuttering is believed to start around three years of age concurrent with the learning of language at the sentence level. Neurological stuttering may be caused by brain damage at any age.

Gender. Males are more likely to stutter at a ratio of 3 to 1. The ratio is 1:1 in the early phases, but apparently more females naturally or spontaneously recover.

Course. Stuttering begins around three years of age. Most studies have shown that 75–80% of children who ever stuttered spontaneously or naturally recover (Bloodstein, 1995; Yairi & Ambrose, 1999). It is difficult to differentiate between those who will recover and those who will not. Even severity is not predictive of persistence, unless it is very extreme (e.g., 1-minute blocks or extreme struggle).

IMPAIRMENT IN OTHER ACTIVITIES.

Stuttering is associated with significant impairment in daily functioning. People who stutter report being teased as children about their stuttering, avoiding speaking such as public speaking and telephone use, receiving less opportunities to speak, and constant fear about their stuttering in most social situations, especially when introducing themselves or doing public speaking. They often describe themselves as underemployed or taking occupations that require little talking.

ASSESSMENT

What Should be Ruled Out?

For children under eight, spontaneous recovery should be ruled out. Historically, the speech pathology profession has not been able to predict spontaneous recovery (Bloodstein, 1995; Guitar, 1998). Ryan (2001a, 2001b) believes that longitudinal research has suggested that it is possible to predict spontaneous recovery from trend analysis. Spontaneous recovery may continue up to eight years of age (Bloodstein, 1995; Yairi & Ambrose, 1999).

Effort should also be made to differentiate neurological stuttering (late onset, post eight years of age, usually accompanied by subtle or obvious brain insult or processing) from developmental stuttering (early onset with no neurological symptoms). Diagnosis of neurological problems is usually is made because stuttering suddenly occurs after head injury or disease, with no previous history. Those who have been stuttering since childhood are referred to as developmental stutterers. Psychogenic stuttering, also late onset, is very rare.

Preschool children. It is important to take a case history from the parent as to time of onset, child's reaction to onset, the course of stuttering from onset to now, what the parent has done to help the child, and more, contingent on the clinician's training and experience. There are no standard interviews for preschoolers, but

TABLE 69.1 What is Involved in Effective Assessment?

Age	Case history	Standard Attitude Interviews	Speech Sample
Preschool 2–5	Parent	None Self-generated administered to parent asking about improvement posttreatment	Conversation with clinician and with mother or other person in a different setting. Speech sample tool such as Fluency Interview (FI)(Ryan, 2001b). Measure stuttering and speaking rate at least three times for at least 15 months
School age 6–12	Parent and client	A-19 Scale (Guitar, 1998) or Communication Attitude Scale (CAT) (Brutten & Dunham, 1989) Self-generated administered to parent/client asking about improvement posttreatment	Read/conversation, or FI. Measure stuttering and speaking rate
13–18	Parent and client	Same as above, or see adult below, contingent on child's perceived maturity. Self-generated administered to parent/client asking about improvement posttreatment	Read/Conversation, telephone, or FI. Measure stuttering and speaking rate
Adult 19+	Client	Modified Erickson Scale of Communicative Attitudes (S–24) (Andrews & Cutler, 1974), or Stutterer's Self-rating of Reactions to Speech Situations (Johnson, Darley, & Spriestersbach (1952), or Perceptions of Stuttering Inventory (PSI) (Woolf, 1967). (Optional) Social Anxiety Test (Krasimaat, et al. 2002). Self-generated administered to client asking about improvement posttreatment	Read/conversation, telephone, or FI. Measure stuttering and speaking rate

many clinics give posttreatment self-generated interviews about effects of treatment (e.g., has _____[child] improved at home?) It is important to obtain at least three direct measures of stuttering rate (usually percent syllables stuttered, %SS) and speaking rate (usually syllables per minute, SPM) during at least a 15-month period to obtain a trend to detect which children will spontaneously or naturally recover: flat or up = persistence, down = spontaneous recovery (Ryan, 2001a, 2001b). Often younger preschoolers will not talk with the clinician, so having the mother converse while the clinician observes is a method commonly used to obtain a speech sample. The clinician may administer the Fluency Interview (FI) (a set of 10 different speaking items such as singing, reading, talking about a TV show, conversing, etc.) to obtain a speaking sample across different speaking tasks with the reading and telephone tasks omitted and the mother substituted for the stranger item.

School age children. Older children may be able to give case history information along with their parent. Questions concern items like the course of stuttering, previous treatment, and the child's response. Interviews are conducted with older children themselves. The ones suggested here are two of those in use. They both ask questions about speaking (e.g., Is it fun to talk to your dad? Yes or No) and feelings about speaking (e.g., I am not a good talker, T or F). Similar speech samples should be taken. Many clinics give posttreatment self-generated interviews about effects of treatment (e.g., has _____[child] improved at home?). Speech samples including the telephone, extraclinic settings, and other people are helpful.These will be found on the FI.

Adults. The interviews for adults are similar in many ways to those for children. All three ask about feelings about speaking (e.g., I am sometimes embarrassed by the way I talk, Yes__ No__) and/or speaking behavior in real life situations (e.g., I find it easy to talk to anyone. Yes__ No___). The interviews have been tested on both people who stutter and those who do not and do discriminate between the two groups (Bloodstein, 1995). They also show changes posttreatment. Besides in-clinic talking or reading, speech samples including the telephone, and people in extra-clinic settings are helpful. These will be found on the FI.

What Assessments are Not Helpful?

Traditional psychological tests such as the MMPI, projective tests, neuropsycholog-ical tests, and those for assessing general social anxiety are not useful in assessing stuttering, nor are there medical tests for its diagnosis. The interviews or attitude or social anxiety scales discussed above are used mostly to determine the extent of the client's concern about the stuttering and its affect on life activities. They have also been used to measure improvement in those areas posttreatment. Many clients have been helped to speak fluently without the use of any of these assessment pro-cedures (e.g., Ingham, 1984; Ryan, 2001b). The value of these interviews for treat-ment has not been established.

TREATMENT

What Treatments are Effective?

As an introduction into treatment there are several basic considerations. First, most speech therapy is carried out in the public schools by clinicians who often do not feel comfortable treating stuttering, partly because they were not well-trained to do so. Next is that speech–language pathologists are unevenly split on whether speech modification (e.g., Guitar, 1998; Van Riper, 1973) or fluency shaping (Ingham, 1984; Onslow, 1996; Ryan, 2001b) produces better results. Speech modification usually refers to changing stuttering from unacceptable forms (e.g., extreme strug-gle) to more acceptable forms (e.g., whole-word or part-word repetitions) using procedures like cancellations (saying the stuttered word over) and prolongation (saying the expected stuttered word with a prolonged vowel or first consonant), usually resulting in mild, but noticeable stuttering. Such treatment is often accom-panied by cognitive and affect training (Guitar, 1998; Van Riper, 1973) to accept and live with the stuttering remaining posttreatment. A large majority of speech language pathologists practice some form of speech modification along with coun-seling for perceived associated cognitive, affective, stuttering-related social anxiety, or attitude problems.

Fluency shaping includes reinforcement of the client for normally fluent speech (e.g., "Good") and punishment of stuttering (e.g., "Stop, speak fluently") gradual steps from words to conversation or from slow, prolonged speech (PS) to normal fluency and usually result in normally fluent speech. The preponderance of treatment efficacy research including meta analyses support the fluency shaping procedures (Bothe, 2002, 2004; Bothe, et al. Brutten, 1993; Conture, 1996; Cordes, 1998, J. Ingham, 2003). These programs are commonly conducted without attention to affective or cognitive, or social anxiety aspects of stuttering (e.g., R. Ingham, et al. 2001) although changes do occur in these areas after fluency has been gained (Ingham, 1984). Most authorities agree that it is the long-term follow-up data, which are the gold standard of the measure of the efficacy of any fluency training. These are available and they do demonstrate persistent fluency, but they are sparse (Onslow, O'Brien, Packman, & Rousseau, 2004; Ryan, 1981, 2001b). The fluency shaping procedures are also known as operant conditioning procedures, contingency management, behavior management, and programmed instruction. Most of the behavioral treatment is based on learning principles, primarily those of operant conditioning (e.g., Skinner, 1953). These treatment programs include overt behavior, small steps, and contingent stimulation (positive or aversive). Since the 1970's fluency treatment has been described to occur in three phases: establishment (in-clinic fluency with the clinician), transfer (out-of-clinic fluency with and without the clinician present) and maintenance (faded rechecks, commonly over a two-year period). These procedures commonly require between 10 and 30 hours of treatment. Follow-up has been conducted reported from 1 (Ryan, 2001b) to 10 years later (Onslow et al. 2004). Only the most effective behavioral procedures, evaluated as being best practice in meta analyses (see above), will be discussed below. There are essentially three different well-supported procedures: The Lidcombe Program for preschool children, the Gradual Increase in Length and Complexity of Utterance (GILCU) for preschool, school age, and adults and the PS program, also known as continuous phonation for school age and adults.

The Lidcombe Program The Lidcombe Program is administered by the parent in the home after receiving an average of 10 hours of training by the clinician in the clinic to provide consequences (e.g., "Good talking") after fluent utterances, or (e.g., "Say that again") after stuttering (Onslow, 1996; Onslow, Andrews, Lincoln, 1994; Onslow, Packman & Harrison, 2003; see also the Onslow website below for many additional publications). This procedure has built-in transfer as it is conducted in the home by the parent. As discussed above, it is important to apply these procedures only to clients (estimated 20% of those who ever stuttered) who will persist in stuttering using trend analyses to identify them.

Gradual Increase in Length and Complexity of Utterance (GILCU) and Extended Length of Utterance (ELU) These programs both employ starting with a single word or syllable increasing eventually to conversational speech before going to transfer and maintenance (Davidow, Crowe, & Bothe, 2004; J. Ingham, 1999; Ryan, 2001b). These programs are relatively easy to administer and do not alter the naturalness of speech. Although these programs have been applied mostly to children, there is treatment efficacy research, which suggest they are successful with adults, too (Rustin, Ryan, & Ryan, 1987; Ryan, 2001b; Ryan & Ryan, 1995).

PS There are several different programs of PS. Some employ the use of a delayed auditory feedback (DAF) apparatus and teaching the client to use continuous phonation at about 40 words per minute (Ingham, 1984; Onslow & Packman, 1997; Ryan, 1981, 2001b; Ryan & Van Kirk, 1974). Current programs employ only hand shaping the prolonged speech by the clinician (Onslow, 1996). The PS is shaped up to be faster and faster until it approaches normalcy of 200 syllables per minute and sounds natural as graded by the client and clinician. There has been some criticism of this procedure for the clients not sounding normal, but that has been resolved for the most part by adding in a program feature of shaping normal-sounding speech along with fluency (Onslow & Packman, 1997).

Other Procedures

These do not have as much treatment efficacy research to support them, especially, long-term follow-up data, but they are in use at the present time and offer promise in the near future after additional treatment efficacy research has been conducted. *Modifying Phonation Interval (MPI)*. The MPI procedure, employing special feedback equipment, requires the client to gradually decrease the silent or stuttered intervals between syllables (R. Ingham, 1999). Ingham et al. (2001) provided data on five young adult clients who generalized and maintained their normal fluency over a two-year period.

Drugs. The past history of drug treatment for stuttering has not been impressive. Most research was flawed by simple short-term designs employing only reading and no long-term follow-up. Maguire, Yu, Franklin, and Riley (2004) offer a current review of modern drug treatment for children older than eight and adults with reference to a number of treatment efficacy research studies. They conclude, "...novel dopamine antagonists, as well as olanzapine and risperidone are useful, well-tolerated medications for the treatment of stuttering..." (p. 6). These may be used alone or in combination with speech therapy.

Speecheasy®. This device and its ancestors are well-described in Stuart, Kalinowski, Rastetter, Saltuklaroglu, and Dayalu (2003) and some treatment efficacy research data presented and/or referenced. The delayed auditory feedback (DAF) effect on stuttering (produces slow, prolonged fluent speech in an effort to "beat" the device) was first noted by Goldiamond (1965). The present in-the-ear (like a hearing aid), small, expensive, delayed auditory feedback device, the Speecheasy®, on the market for the past two years through distributors in every state, has been well accepted by stuttering clients including the national media and unaccepted by professional speech language pathologists, mostly because of the failure of the progenitors to produce extensive, believable treatment efficacy research similar to that described above for the three "best practices" programs. The procedure is very simple. Find the best DAF setting for the individual client, that is, "fit the client," usually between 50 and 100 ms of delay, put a small device with that setting in his preferred ear and send him home with instructions to wear it all the time when he is talking. Most agree that, historically, DAF procedures along with the PS produced, which is then shaped into normally fluent speech by gradually fading DAF, has been effective in reducing stuttering (e.g., Ingham, 1984; Ryan, 2001b, Ryan & Van Kirk, 1974), but most await appropriate treatment efficacy research on the present device itself, before final judgment. Many distributors of the device report that not all people are helped by the device or will wear it constantly. Further treatment efficacy research is needed.

What are Effective Self-Help Treatments?

There are several self-help groups for people who stutter both nationally and internationally (see websites below). Some of these groups have started their own internal research projects about stuttering experiences and treatment of stuttering efficacy. In the author's opinion, little of useful treatment value has yet come out of the present research except that previous treatments were not successful; most of the members of these groups still noticeably stutter. Many people who stutter do join these groups and report, "receiving support" from them. Books for self-help will be found on the websites listed below especially in the one of the Stuttering Foundation.

Websites

Useful informational websites about stuttering treatment include:

http://www.asha.org/public/speech/disorders/stuttering.htm (American Speech-language Hearing Association)

http://www.WeStutter.org (National Stuttering Association SFA, self-help)

http://www.stutteringsfa.org (Stuttering Foundation, SF, self-help, directory of clinicians, general information)

http://www.nidcd.nih.gov/health/voice/stutter.asp (National Institute of Deafness and Communicative Disorders NIDCD).

http://www.stutterisa.org (International Stuttering association, ISA, self-help).

http://www.asrc@fhs.usyd.edu.au (Australian Stuttering Research Centre, Mark Onslow, world-wide impact).

http://www.mnsu.edu/dept/comdis/kuster/stutter.html (Communicative Disorders, including stuttering, one of the best, with many links to other sites).

http://www.speecheasy.com (Home site of the device).

Combination Treatments

The three most effective treatments described above are seldom conducted with any of the other three procedures, but it is worthwhile to consider the possibility of combining treatments, such as GILCU with PS, or drug treatment with PS or GILCU, although none of this has been done in careful treatment efficacy research designs, only anecdotally reported (Onslow, 1996).

Other Issues in Management

The major issue is that the large majority of the American Speech-language and Hearing Association (ASHA) does not generally accept, practice, and teach in university training programs any of the three preferred programs discussed above. Any person who stutters must look long and hard to find a speech clinician who is skilled in the conduction of one or more of these programs.

How Does One Select Among Treatments?

The three treatments described above are all effective (reduction to less than 1% syllables stuttered) and efficient (average 10–30 hours of treatment) with 1–10 years of published follow-up available for examination. The major criterion of choice is age with Lidcombe and GILCU programs used for children, and PS employed with adults. The second criterion is severity. PS has been demonstrated in several studies to be effective, after GILCU was not, for clients with severe struggle behavior, some of them who have difficulty in speaking even the first word fluently.

Choice among the other treatments should be done very carefully, following the guide of seeking out only those clinicians or researchers with a great deal of experience and expertise, such as the authors of articles, or their students, on these generally minimally or unused treatments.

REFERENCES

Andrews, G. & Cutler, J. (1974). Stuttering therapy: The relation between changes in symptom level and attitudes. *Journal of Speech and Hearing Disorders, 48*, 226–246.

Bloodstein, O. (1995). *A handbook of stuttering* (5th ed.). San Diego, CA: Singular Publishing Company.

Bothe, A (2002). Speech-modification approaches to stuttering treatment in schools. In J. S. Yaruss (Ed.), Facing the challenge of treating stuttering, Part 1: Selecting goals and strategies for success. *Seminars in Speech and Language, 23*, 181–186.

Bothe, A. (Ed.) (2004). *Evidence-based treatment of stuttering: Empirical bases and clinical applications*. Mahwah, NJ: Lawrence Erlbaum Associates, Inc.

Bothe, A., Davidow, J., Ingham, R., Crowe, B, Bramlett, R., Levy, J., et al. (2003, November). *Systematic review of stuttering literature*. Paper presented at the meeting of the American Speech-Language Association meeting, Chicago, IL.

Brutten, G. (Ed.) (1993). Proceedings of the NIDCD Workshop on Treatment Efficacy Research in Stuttering, September 21–22, 1992 [Special Issue]. *Journal of fluency Disorders. 18*, 121–361.

Brutten, E. & Dunham, S. (1989). The communication attitude test: A normative study of grade school children. *Journal of Fluency Disorders, 14*, 371–377.

Conture, E. (1996). Toward efficacy: Stuttering. *Journal of Speech and Hearing Research, 39*, S18–S26.

Cordes, A. (1998). Current status of the stuttering treatment literature. In A Cordes & R. Ingham (Eds.) Treatment efficacy for stuttering: A search for empirical bases (pp. 117–144). San Diego, CA: Singular Publishing Group, Inc.

Cordes, A. & Ingham, R. (Eds.) (1998). *Treatment efficacy for stuttering: A search for Empirical Bases*. San Diego, CA: Singular Publishing Group, Inc.

Davidow, J., Crowe, B, & Bothe, A. (2004). "Gradual Increase in Length and Complexity of Utterance" and "Extended Length of Utterance," treatment programs: Assessing the strong, but limited evidence. In A. Bothe (Ed.), *Evidence-based Treatment of Stuttering: Empirical Bases and Clinical Applications (pp. 201–230)*. Mahwah, NJ: Lawrence Erlbaum Associates, Publishers.

Goldiamond, I. (1965). Stuttering and fluency as manipulable operant response classes. In L. Krasner & L. Ullman (Eds.), *Research in behavior modification: New developments and implications* (pp. 106–156). New York: Holt, Rinehart, & Winston.

Guitar, B. (1998). *Stuttering: An integrated approach to its nature and treatment*. Baltimore, MD: Williams and Wilkins Publishing Group, Inc.

Ingham, J. (1999). Behavior treatment of young children who stutter: An extended length of utterance method. In R. Curlee (Ed.), *Stuttering and related disorders* (pp. 80–109). New York: Thieme.

Ingham, J. (2003), Evidence-based treatment of stuttering: I. Definition and application. *Journal of Fluency Disorders, 28*, 197–207.

Ingham, R. (1984). *Stuttering and behavioral therapy: Current status and experimental foundations*. San Diego, CA: College Hill.

Ingham, R. (1998). On learning from speech-motor control research on stuttering. In A. Cordes & R. Ingham (Eds.), *Treatment efficacy for stuttering: A search for empirical bases* (pp. 67–103). San Diego, CA: Singular Publishing Group, Inc.

Ingham, R. (1999). Performance contingent management in stuttering in adolescents and adults. In R. Curlee (Ed.), *Stuttering and related disorders of fluency* (pp. 200–221). New York: Thieme.

Ingham, R. (2004). Emerging controversies, findings, and directions neuroimaging and developmental stuttering: On avoiding petard hoisting in Athens. In A. Bothe (Ed.), *Evidence-based treatment of stuttering: Empirical bases and clinical* application (pp. 27–64). Mahwah, NJ: Lawrence Erlbaum Associates, Inc.

Ingham, R., Ingham, J., Finn, P., & Fox, P. (2003). Towards a functional neural systems model of developmental stuttering. *Journal of fluency Disorders, 28*, 297–318.

Ingham, R., Kilgo, M., Ingham, J., Moglia, R., Belknap, H., & Sanchez, T. (2001). Evaluation of a stuttering treatment based on reduction of short phonation intervals. *Journal of Speech, Language, and Hearing Research, 44*, 1229–1244.

Johnson, W., Darley, F. & Spriestersbach, D. (1963*). Diagnostic methods in speech pathology*. New York: Harper & Row, Publishers.

Krasimaat, F., Vanryckeghem, M., & Van Dam-Baggen, R. (2002). Stuttering and social anxiety, *Journal of Fluency Disorders, 27*, 319–330.

Maguire, G., Yu, B., Franklyn, D., & Riley, G. (2004). Alleviating stuttering with pharmacological interventions. Expert Opinion. *Ashley Publications.www.ashley -pub.com*.

Moore, W. (1993). Hemispheric processing research: Past, present, and future. In E. Boberg (Ed.), *Neuropsychology of stuttering* (pp. 39–72). Edmonton, Alberta: University of Alberta Press.

Nicolosi, L., Harryman, E., & Kreschek, J. (1996). *Terminology of communication disorders: Speech-language Hearing* (4th ed.). Baltimore: MD: Williams & Williams.

Onslow, M. (1996). Behavioral management of stuttering. San Diego, CA: Singular Publishing Company.

Onslow, M., Andrews, C., & Lincoln, M. (1994). A control/experimental trial of an operant treatment for early stuttering. *Journal of Speech and Hearing Disorders, 37*, 1244–1259.

Onslow, M., O'Brien, S., Packman, A., & Rousseau, I. (2004). Long-term follow up of speech outcomes for prolonged speech treatment for stuttering: The effects of paradox on stuttering treatment research. In A. Bothe (Ed.), *Evidence-based treatment of stuttering: Empirical bases and clinical applications* (pp. 231–244). Mahwah, NJ: Lawrence Erlbaum Associates, Publisher.

Onslow, M., & Packman, A. (1997). Designing and implementing a strategy to control stuttered speech. In R. Curlee & G. Siegel (Eds.), *Nature and treatment of stuttering: New directions* (pp. 356–376). Boston: Allyn and Bacon.

Onslow, M., Packman, A., & Harrison, E. (2003). *The Lidcombe Program for early stuttering intervention: A clinician's guide*. Austin, TX: Pro-Ed.

Rustin, L., Ryan, B., & Ryan, B. (1987). Use of the Monterey programmed stuttering treatment in Great Britain. British Journal of Disorders of Communication, 22, 151–162.

Ryan, B. (1981). Maintenance programs in progress. II. In E. Boberg (Ed.), *Maintenance of fluency: Proceedings of Banff Conference, Banff, Alberta, Canada, June, 1979* (pp. 113–146). New York: Elsevier North-Holland, Inc.

Ryan, B., (2001a) Prediction of spontaneous recovery in preschool children who stutter. In H. Bosshardt, J. Yaruss, & H. Peters (Eds.), *Proceedings of the third world congress of fluency disorders in Nyberg, Denmark: Theory, research, treatment, and self-help* (pp. 206–210). International Fluency Association: Nijemen Press.

(Ryan, 2001b) *Programmed stuttering therapy for children and adults* (2nd ed.). Springfield, IL: CC Thomas Publishers.

Ryan, B. & Ryan, B. (1995). Programmed stuttering treatment for children: Comparison of two establishment programs through transfer, maintenance, and follow-up. *Journal of Speech and Hearing Research, 38,* 61–75.

Ryan, B., & Van Kirk, B. (1974). The establishment, transfer, and maintenance of fluent speech in 50 stutterers using delayed auditory feedback and operant procedures. *Journal of Speech and Hearing Disorders, 39,* 3–10.

Skinner, B. F. (1953). *The science of human behavior.* New York, NY: Macmillan.

Stuart, A., Kalinowski, J., Rastatter, M., Saltuklaroglu, T., & Dayalu, V. (2003). *International Journal of Language and Communication Disorders, 38,* 1–21.

Van Riper, C. (1973). *The treatment of stuttering.* Englewood Cliffs, NJ: Prentice-Hall, Inc.

Woolf, G. (1967). The assessment of stuttering as struggle, avoidance, and expectancy. *British Journal of Disorders of Communication, 2, 158–171.*

Yairi, E. & Ambrose, N. (1999). Early childhood stuttering 1: Persistence and recovery rates. *Journal of Speech, Language, and Hearing Research, 42,* 1097–1112.

Yeudall, L. (1985). A neurophysiological theory of stuttering. *Seminars in Speech and Language, 6,* 197–223.

Substance Use Disorders

G. Alan Marlatt • Katie Witkiewitz

WHAT IS A SUBSTANCE USE DISORDER?

Based on the 2002 National Survey on Drug Use and Health approximately 46% of individuals (aged 12 and older) report lifetime use of illicit drugs, 69% report lifetime use of cigarettes, and 83% report lifetime use of alcohol. Less than 10% of the population, 22 million Americans, meet criteria for a current diagnosis of substance dependence or abuse (SAMSHA, 2002). Of these individuals, 7.7 million may require treatment for a drug use disorder and 17.6 million may require treatment for an alcohol use disorder.

The estimated social costs of substance use disorders are in excess of $300 billion, including costs of treatment, related health problems, absenteeism, productivity loss, crime and incarceration, and education and prevention. Of these costs, treatment and prevention efforts are significantly less costly than the cost of incarceration and crimes (SAMSHA, 1997). A study in California estimated that every dollar spent on substance abuse treatment saves $7 in costs related to health, crime, and work productivity (Delaney, Gable, & Kendell, 2000).

Substance use disorders are classified by the American Psychiatric Association (1994) as two distinct, but often cooccurring, disorders: substance dependence and substance abuse.

DSM-IV CRITERIA FOR SUBSTANCE DEPENDENCE AND ABUSE

Criteria for Substance Dependence

A maladaptive pattern of substance use, leading to clinically significant impairment or distress, as manifested by three (or more) of the following, occurring at any time in the same 12-month period:

1. tolerance, as defined by either of the following:
    a. a need for markedly increased amounts of the substance to achieve intoxication or desired effect
    b. markedly diminished effect with continued use of the same amount of the substance
2. withdrawal, as manifested by either of the following:
    a. the characteristic withdrawal syndrome for the substance . . .
    b. the same (or a closely related) substance is taken to relieve or avoid withdrawal symptoms
3. the substance is often taken in larger amounts or over a longer period than was intended
4. there is a persistent desire or unsuccessful efforts to cut down or control substance use
5. a great deal of time is spent in activities necessary to obtain the substance (e.g., visiting multiple doctors or driving long distances), use the substance (e.g., chain-smoking), or recover from its effects

Marlatt, G. A. & Witkiewitz, K. (2006). Substance use disorder. In J. E. Fisher & W. T. O'Donohue (Eds.), *Practitioner's guide to evidence-based psychotherapy*. New York: Springer.

6. important social, occupational, or recreational activities are given up or reduced because of substance use
7. the substance use is continued despite knowledge of having a persistent or recurrent physical or psychological problem that is likely to have been caused or exacerbated by the substance (e.g., current cocaine use despite recognition of cocaine-induced depression, or continued drinking despite recognition that an ulcer was made worse by alcohol consumption)

Specify whether substance dependence is with physiological dependence (i.e., there is evidence of tolerance or withdrawal) or without physiological dependence (i.e., no evidence of tolerance or withdrawal).

2. Criteria for Substance Abuse

a. A maladaptive pattern of substance use leading to clinically significant impairment or distress, as manifested by one (or more) of the following, occurring within a 12-month period:
   1. recurrent substance use resulting in a failure to fulfill major role obligations at work, school, or home (e.g., repeated absences or poor work performance related to substance use; substance-related absences, suspensions, or expulsions from school; neglect of children or household)
   2. recurrent substance use in situations in which it is physically hazardous (e.g., driving an automobile or operating a machine when impaired by substance use)
   3. recurrent substance-related legal problems (e.g., arrests for substance related disorderly conduct)
   4. continued substance use despite having persistent or recurrent social or interpersonal problems caused or exacerbated by the effects of the substance (e.g., arguments with spouse about consequences of intoxication, physical fights)

b. The symptoms have never met the criteria for substance dependence for this class of substance.

In addition, patients may be variously classified as currently manifesting a pattern of abuse or dependence or as in remission. Those in remission can be divided into four subtypes-full, early partial, sustained, and sustained partial-based on the interval of time that has elapsed since the cessation of Dependence. The remission category can also be used for patients receiving agonist therapy (e.g., methadone maintenance) or for those living in a controlled drug-free environment.

BASIC FACTS ABOUT SUBSTANCE USE DISORDERS

Commonly Abused Substances

Alcohol is the most commonly abused substance. Prevalence rates for alcohol use and abuse/dependence in the United States are approximately 51.0% and 7.5%, respectively. Tobacco is the second most widely used substance, with a prevalence of 30.4% of the population over aged 12 using tobacco products, including cigarettes, cigars (SAMHSA, 2002).

Table 70.1 (taken from the National Institute of Drug Abuse; available online at *http://www.drugabuse.gov/DrugPages/DrugsofAbuse.html*) provides a brief overview of the major substances of abuse and information regarding street names, method of administration, and intoxication effects/health consequences.

TABLE 70.1

Substance: Category and Name	Examples of Commercial and Street Names	DEA Schedule[a]/ Administered[b]	Intoxication Effects and Potential Health Consequences
Cannabinoids			
Hashish	Boom, chronic, gangster, hash, hemp	I/ swallowed, smoked	*Euphoria, slowed thinking and reaction time, confusion, impaired balance and coordination*/cough, frequent respiratory infections; impaired memory and learning; increased heart rate, anxiety; panic attacks; tolerance, addiction
Marijuana	Blunt, dope, ganja, grass, herb, joints, Mary Jane, pot, reefer, skunk, weed	I /swallowed, smoked	
Depressants			
Barbiturates	Amytal, Nembutal, Seconal, Pheobarbital; barbs, reds, red birds, phennies, tooies, yellows yellow jackets	II, III, V/injected, swallowed	*Reduced anxiety; feeling of well-being; lowered inhibitions; slowed pulse and breathing; lowered blood pressure; poor concentration/* fatigue; confusion; impaired
Benzodia-zepines	Ativan, Halcion, Librium, Valium, Xanax; candy, downers, sleeping pills	IV/injected, swallowed	Coordination, memory, judgment; addiction; respiratory depression and arrest, death
flunitrazepam[c]	Rohypnol; forget-me pill, Mexican Valium, R2, Roche, roofies, roofinol, rope, rophies	IV/swallowed, snorted	*Also, for barbiturates—sedation, drowsiness/*depression, unusual excitement, fever, irritability, poor judgment, slurred speech, dizziness, life-threatening withdrawal.
GHB[c]	*gamma-hydroxybutyrate;* G, Georgia home boy, grievous bodily harm, liquid ecstasy	I/swallowed	
Methaqualone	*Quaalude, Sopor, Parest;* ludes, mandrex, quad, quay	I/injected, swallowed	*For benzodiazepines—sedation, drowsiness/*dizziness
			*For flunitrazepam—*visual and gastrointestinal disturbances, urinary retention, memory loss for the time under the drug's effects
			*For GHB—*drowsiness, nausea/ vomiting, headache, loss of consciousness, loss of reflexes, seizures, coma, death
			*For methaqualone—euphoria/*depression, poor reflexes, slurred speech, coma
Dissociative Anesthetics			
ketamine	*Ketalar SV;* cat Valiums, K, Special K, vitamin K	III/injected, snorted, smoked	*Increased heart rate and blood pressure, impaired motor function/*memory loss; numbness; nausea/vomiting
PCP and analogs	*Phencyclidine;* angel dust, boat, hog, love boat, peace pill	I, II/injected, swallowed, smoked	*Also, for ketamine—at high doses, delirium, depression, respiratory depression and arrest For PCP and analogs—possible decrease in blood pressure and heart rate, panic, aggression, violence/*loss of appetite, depression

TABLE 70.1 (Continued)

Substance: Category and Name	Examples of Commercial and Street Names	DEA Schedule[a]/ Administered[b]	Intoxication Effects and Potential Health Consequences
Hallucinogens			
LSD	*Lysergic acid diethylamide;* acid, blotter, boomers, cubes, microdot, yellow sunshines	I/swallowed, absorbed through mouth tissues	*Altered states of perception and feeling; nausea;* persisting perception disorder (flashbacks)
Mescaline	Buttons, cactus, mesc, peyote	I/swallowed, smoked	*Also, for LSD and mescaline—increased body temperature, heart rate, blood pressure; loss of appetite, sleeplessness, numbness, weakness, tremors*
Psilocybin	Magic mushroom, purple passion, shrooms	I/swallowed	*For LSD —persistent mental disorders* *For psilocybin—nervousness, paranoia*
Opioids and Morphine Derivatives			
Codeine	*Empirin with Codeine, Fiorinal with Codeine, Robitussin A-C, Tylenol with Codeine;* Captain Cody, Cody, schoolboy; (with glutethimide) doors & fours, loads, pancakes and syrup	II, III, IV/injected, swallowed	*Pain relief, euphoria, drowsiness/nausea,* constipation, confusion, sedation, respiratory depression and arrest, tolerance, addiction, unconsciousness, coma, death *Also, for codeine—less analgesia, sedation, and respiratory depression than morphine*
Fentanyl and fentanyl analogs	*Actiq, Duragesic, Sublimaze;* Apache, China girl, China white, dance fever, friend, goodfella, jackpot, murder 8, TNT, Tango and Cash	I, II/injected, smoked, snorted	*For heroin—staggering gait*
Heroin	*diacetylmorphine;* brown sugar, dope, H, horse, junk, skag, skunk, smack, white horse	I/injected, smoked, snorted	
Morphine	*Roxanol, Duramorph;* M, Miss Emma, monkey, white stuff	II, III/injected, swallowed, smoked	
Opium	*Laudanum, paregoric;* big O, black stuff, block, gum, hop	II, III, V/swallowed, smoked	
Oxycodone HCL	*Oxycontin;* Oxy, O.C., killer	II/swallowed, snorted, injected	
Hydrocodone bitartrate, acetaminophen	*Vicodin;* vike, Watson-387	II/swallowed	
Stimulants			
Amphetamine	*Biphetamine, Dexedrine;* bennies, black beauties, crosses, hearts, LA turnaround, speed, truck drivers, uppers	II/injected, swallowed, smoked, snorted	*Increased heart rate, blood pressure, metabolism; feelings of exhilaration, energy, increased mental alertness/* rapid or irregular heart beat; reduced appetite, weight loss, heart failure, nervousness, insomnia
Cocaine	*Cocaine hydrochloride;* blow, bump, C, candy, Charlie, coke, crack, flake, rock, snow, toot	II/ injected, smoked, snorted	*Also, for amphetamine—rapid breathing/* tremor, loss of coordination; irritability, anxiousness, restlessness, delirium, panic, paranoia, impulsive behavior, aggressiveness, tolerance, addiction, psychosis
MDMA (methylene-dioxymetham-mphetamine)	Adam, clarity, ecstasy, Eve, lover's speed, peace, STP, X, XTC	I/ swallowed	

TABLE 70.1 (Continued)

Substance: Category and Name	Examples of Commercial and Street Names	DEA Schedule[a] / Administered[b]	Intoxication Effects and Potential Health Consequences
			*for cocaine—increased temperature/*chest pain, respiratory failure, nausea, abdominal pain, strokes, seizures, headaches, malnutrition, panic attacks
Methamphetamine	*Desoxyn;* chalk, crank, crystal, fire, glass, go fast, ice, meth, speed	II/injected, swallowed, smoked, snorted	
Methylphenidate (safe and effective for treatment of ADHD)	*Ritalin;* JIF, MPH, R-ball, Skippy, the smart drug, vitamin R	II/injected, swallowed, snorted	*For MDMA—mild hallucinogenic effects, increased tactile sensitivity, empathic feelings/*impaired memory and learning, hyperthermia, cardiac toxicity, renal failure, liver toxicity
Nicotine	Cigarettes, cigars, smokeless tobacco, snuff, spit tobacco, bidis, chew	Not scheduled/ smoked, snorted, taken in snuff and spit tobacco	*For methamphetamine—aggression, violence, psychotic behavior/*memory loss, cardiac and neurological damage; impaired memory and learning, tolerance, addiction *For nicotine—*additional effects attributable to tobacco exposure,adverse pregnancy outcomes, chronic lung disease, cardiovascular disease, stroke, cancer, tolerance, addiction
Other Compounds			
Anabolic steroids	*Anadrol, oxandrin, durabolin, depo-testosterone, equipoise;* roids, juice	III/injected, swallowed, applied to skin	*No intoxication effects/* hypertension, blood clotting and cholesterol changes, liver cysts and cancer, kidney cancer, hostility and aggression, acne; in adolescents, premature stoppage of growth; in males, prostate cancer, reduced sperm production, shrunken testicles, breast enlargement; in females, menstrual irregularities, development of beard and other masculine characteristics
Inhalants	*Solvents (paint thinners, gasoline, glues), gases (butane, propane, aerosol propellants, nitrous oxide), nitrites (isoamyl, isobutyl, cyclohexyl);* laughing gas, poppers, snappers, whippets	Not scheduled/ inhaled through nose or mouth	*Stimulation, loss of inhibition; headache; nausea or vomiting; slurred speech, loss of motor coordination; wheezing/* unconsciousness, cramps, weight loss, muscle weakness, depression, memory impairment, damage to cardiovascular and nervous systems, sudden death

[a] Schedule I and II drugs have a high potential for abuse. They require greater storage security and have a quota on manufacturing, among other restrictions. Schedule I drugs are available for research only and have no approved medical use; Schedule II drugs are available only by prescription (unrefillable) and require a form for ordering. Schedule III and IV drugs are available by prescription, may have five refills in six months, and may be ordered orally. Most Schedule V drugs are available over the counter.

[b] Taking drugs by injection can increase the risk of infection through needle contamination with staphylococci, HIV, hepatitis, and other organisms.

[c] Associated with sexual assaults.

Course and Chronicity

Lapses, the return to substance use behavior after achievement of a treatment goal, are the most common outcome following treatment for substance use disorders. Such that, repeated treatment attempts are common. In fact, an SAMHSA survey found that approximately 58% of clients admitted to a substance abuse treatment program had at least one prior treatment episode (SAMSHA, 1999).

McLellan, Lewis, O'Brien, & Kleber (2000) described substance abuse/dependence as a chronic illness comparable to other chronic medical conditions, such as diabetes and hypertension. From a behavioral perspective, Witkiewitz and Marlatt (2004) argued that relapse to substance use can be characterized as a continuous process of behavior change. From both perspectives, it is recommended that lapses are not viewed as a treatment failure, but rather as part of the process.

Several risk factors predict the occurrence of lapses. These risk factors have been characterized as both distal (predispositions) and proximal (precipitants) risks. In general, distal risks for lapsing include: family history of substance use disorders, the age of first substance use, and the severity of substance dependence. Proximal risks tend to be highly individual and contextualized, but commonly reported lapse precipitants include: negative affect, urges to use, peer influences, lack of social support, physical withdrawal symptoms, and many others.

Comorbidity

Comorbid psychiatric diagnoses are common among substance users and substance use disorders are the most frequently cooccurring disorders among those with mental disorders. In general, increased severity of other psychiatric symptoms is predictive of poorer treatment outcomes. In the United States, tobacco is the leading preventable cause of death, with one in every five deaths attributed to smoking-related illnesses (Center for Disease Control and Prevention, 2004).

Differential diagnosis is an important part of treatment planning, particularly to determine the chronology of the substance use disorder in relation to comorbid diagnoses. Did the substance abuse/dependence diagnosis predate the other psychiatric symptoms? And, are other psychiatric symptoms present during extensive periods of abstinence (longer than three-months)? When the comorbid psychiatric symptoms begin prior to substance abuse/dependence symptoms, then it is important to consider the possibility of substance use as "self-medication" (Khantzian, 1985). Treatment of comorbid mental disorders may be beneficial for many substance users and individual treatment plans should attempt to integrate substance and nonsubstance use treatment modalities.

Consequences of Sustained Use, Abuse, and Dependence

The long-term consequences of substance abuse and dependence far outweigh the benefits of the immediate "rewards" of using the substance (e.g., the short-term altered state the individual using the substance is trying to achieve), however, many substance users do not recognize the delayed consequences. Overdose, negative physiological reactions (e.g., arrhythmia), nausea, paranoia, poor decision making (e.g., risky sex), risk of injury or death, driving-related accidents, and legal consequences are a few of the immediate consequences of substance use. Some of the long term consequences of substance use include: social, financial, and legal problems, neurological impairments, cancer, cardiovascular disease, liver disease, reproductive disorders.

Demographic Characteristics of Substance Users

Age Rates of illicit drug use are highly variable across different age groups. For most drugs, the average yearly use peaks during the late teens and early to mid-20s, with a steady decline in prevalence as age increases. Younger individuals, aged 12–25 years old, comprised almost half (47%) of the current illicit drug users in 2002 (SAMHSA, 2002). The majority of inhalant users (71%) were in this age group. Individuals older than 25 are more likely to abuse cocaine and nonmedical psychotropic drugs, than individuals who are in the 12–25 year old group. Research has demonstrated that earlier onset of substance abuse is related to greater risk for substance dependence and poorer treatment outcomes.

Gender In 2002, men were more likely to abuse illicit drugs than women, but abuse of nonmedical psychotropic drugs was similar for men (2.7%) and women (2.6%). For individuals over 17 years old, men are more likely to abuse alcohol and tobacco, but for the 12–17 year old age group women and men have comparable rates of alcohol and tobacco abuse.

Ethnicity Ethnic minority groups are underrepresented in the treatment of substance abuse and dependence (SAMHSA, 2001). Prevalence estimates gathered from a variety of sources suggest that non-Hispanic Whites, Blacks, and Hispanic American subgroups have indistinguishable levels of illicit drug use; individuals who are of Puerto Rican heritage, American Indian, and Alaskan Native report higher rates of illicit drug use and Asian Americans are least likely to report illicit drug use (National Institute of Drug Abuse, 2003; SAMHSA, 2003). Substance abuse treatment may need to be adapted for ethnic and cultural minority clients, preferably on a case-by-case basis. A few resources for selecting and implementing evidence-based treatments for specific minority groups include: the *Journal of Ethnicity in Substance Abuse* published by Haworth Press; *Ethnicity and Substance Abuse: Prevention and Intervention* (2002) by Xuegin and Henderson (Eds) published by Charles C Thomas, Ltd; *Ethnocultural Factors in Substance Abuse Treatment* (2001) by Straussner (Ed.) published by Guilford Press.

Socioeconomic status Individuals who abuse illicit drugs, meet criteria for alcohol dependence, and who are in need of drug and/or alcohol treatment are more likely to be unemployed, have lower family incomes, and have fewer years of education. It has been estimated that 38% of homeless individuals are dependent on alcohol and other drugs. Unfortunately fewer than half of these individuals will receive treatment. On the other end of the income spectrum, recent research has shown that children and adolescents from affluent families tend to be at higher risk for substance use than middle class peers (Luthar, 2003).

It is important to consider socioeconomic status when developing treatment plans and gathering information about substance abuse history and comorbid psychiatric diagnoses. Individuals who are struggling to meet basic needs are less likely to seek treatment and adhere to treatment regimens. Furthermore, unemployment, stress, lack of social support, and other life stressors tend to be predictive of both treatment retention and outcomes. Suicidal behavior may also increase among individuals with low socioeconomic status and high substance use, particularly in individuals who are also high on impulsivity.

ASSESSMENT

Assessment of substance use and abuse can be conducted on many levels. Ideally, clinicians would have multiple sources of information prior to developing a treatment plan, but realistically a short interview may be the only resource. In this case, clinicians should be concerned about getting a detailed overview of the individuals current level of use (or previous level of use if the individual has been incarcerated or hospitalized prior to the interview), history and severity of use, consequences related to substance use, social support, barriers to treatment, motivation and readiness to change, life stressors, comorbid mental and/or physical health problems (including chronology), previous treatment attempts, risk factors for relapse, and personal strengths.

Functional analysis of substance use, contextual analysis of high-risk situations, and the role of individual risk factors in predicting substance use are likely to help inform treatment planning. Drug-testing can be used to determine degree of substance use, however, mandatory drug-testing as a part of a treatment program may be contraindicated. For abstinence-based treatments, drug testing to guarantee abstinence during treatment may elicit defensiveness among clients. For treatments with moderation goals, drug testing is unlikely to detect differences between moderation and heavier use, and may also bring out distrust.

Given the constraints often placed on clinicians and care workers it is important to minimize assessments that are unnecessary or not likely to be helpful. Projective and personality testing (MMPI) will provide little information about the function of substance use behavior. Neuropsychological tests may be informative for determining severity of substance-related neurological impairment and prognosis for individuals who are highly cognitive-impaired, but are often expensive and time-consuming.

TREATMENT

National Institute of Drug Abuse—13 Principles of Effective Drug Addiction Treatment
1. No single treatment is appropriate for all individuals
2. Treatment needs to be readily available
3. Effective treatment attends to multiple needs
4. Treatment needs to be flexible
5. Remaining in treatment for an adequate period of time is critical for treatment effectiveness
6. Individual and/or group counseling and other behavioral therapies are critical components of effective treatment for addiction
7. Medications are an important element of treatment for many patients
8. Addicted or drug-abusing individuals with coexisting mental disorders should have both disorders treated in an integrated way
9. Medical detoxification is only the first stage of addiction treatment
10. Treatment does not need to be voluntary to be effective
11. Possible drug use during treatment must be monitored continuously
12. Treatment programs should provide assessment for HIV/AIDS, hepatitis B and C, tuberculosis and other infectious diseases
13. Recovery from drug addiction can be a long-term process

Psychological Treatments
Psychological treatment for substance use disorders can be conducted individually or in groups; in outpatient or inpatient settings; as aftercare following inpatient treatment (e.g., relapse prevention programs) and as brief interventions (Miller & Rollnick, 2002; Moyer, Finney, Swearingen, & Vergun, 2002). Oftentimes the therapist will be responsible for assigning homework, facilitating individual or group

discussion, identifying and addressing high-risk situations for lapses, and educating about physical withdrawal, outcome expectancies, and the abstinence violation effect.

Borrowing from Miller and Rollnick (2002), the term FRAMES can be used as an acronym for six therapists skills that are essential for effective, brief substance abuse interventions:

- **F**eedback is given to the individual about personal risk or impairment
- **R**esponsibility for change is placed on the participant
- **A**dvice to change is given by the clinician
- **M**enu of alternative self-help or treatment options is offered to the participant
- **E**mpathic style is used by the counselor
- **S**elf-efficacy or optimistic empowerment is engendered in the participant

Cognitive–behavioral, interpersonal, and motivational treatments; multidimensional family therapy; the community reinforcement approach; and voucher-based reinforcement treatment are the most widely disseminated and empirically supported psychological treatments for substance use disorders.

Cognitive–behavioral treatments are based on the theory that addictive behaviors are learned behaviors. Cognitive-behavioral treatments often focus on the identification of maladaptive behavioral patterns related to drug and alcohol use and the implementation of cognitive and behavioral strategies (e.g., self-monitoring, psychoeducation, cognitive-restructuring, coping skills training). *http://www.drugabuse.gov/pdf/ CBT.pdf*

1. relapse prevention—*http:// www.bhrm.org/guidelines/RPT%20guideline.pdf*
2. coping skills training—*http:// www.bhrm.org/guidelines/CBT-Kadden.pdf*
3. Matrix model—*http:// www.matrixinstitute.org/Treatment.htm*

Interpersonal treatments are focused on the interpersonal relationships of the substance abuser. In supportive–expressive psychotherapy and individualized drug counseling one focus of the treatment is on the relationship between the client and the treatment provider. Behavioral couples therapy is a specific interpersonal treatment that is designed to increase support for treatment goals and improve interpersonal functioning among married or cohabitating individuals in substance abuse treatment. The treatment focuses on communication, shared activities, positive feelings, and education about substance abuse and dependence.

http://www.nida.nih.gov/BTDP/Effective/ McLellan.html.
http://www.bhrm.org/guidelines/ couples%20therapy.pdf

Motivational enhancement treatments are client-centered treatment approaches that attempt to reduce ambivalence and increase client readiness to change. Motivational statements, supportive feedback, and reducing resistance are key components of the treatment, which are all based on the principles of motivational interviewing (Miller & Rollnick, 2002). *http://www.bhrm.org/guidelines/ motiveint.pdf*

Multidimensional family therapy is a treatment designed for adolescent substance abusers and their families. MDFT treats adolescent substance use by incorporating a systems perspective, including the individual, family, peer, and community relationships. Treatment includes individual, family, and extrafamilial sessions in a variety of contexts.

http://www.nida.nih.gov/BTDP/Effective/ Liddle.html

Community reinforcement approaches are based on the premise that environmental factors and contingencies exert a large influence on drinking and drug use. CRA tends focus on improving interpersonal relationships, increasing recreational and vocational opportunities, minimizing drug use, and learning life skills to sustain abstinence. *http:// www.nida.nih.gov/BTDP/Effective/Higgins.html*

Voucher-based treatments. CRA plus Vouchers is an intensive outpatient therapy that incorporates the use of voucher incentives (which can be exchanged for retail goods) to increase engagement in treatment and sustain longer periods of abstinence. Voucher-based reinforcement therapy is similar to CRA in that the goal is to help patients maintain abstinence by providing vouchers, which are "earned" for drug-free urines and can be exchanged for goods and services that are determined by specific treatment goals.

http://www.bhrm.org/guidelines/ CRAmanual.pdf

http://www.nida.nih.gov/BTDP/Effective/ Silverman.html

Pharmacological Treatments Pharmacotherapy has often been the first line of defense in the treatment of substance use disorders. Disulfiram (antabuse) has been widely used as a behavioral control agent designed to condition an aversive response (sickness) to drinking alcohol. Compliance with disulfiram treatment is extremely low and it has not been shown to be superior to placebo in double-blind studies. More recently, naltrexone and acamprosate have both been shown to be better than placebo at reducing alcohol cravings following treatment. Currently the National Institute of Alcohol Abuse and Alcoholism is launching a multi-site study, called Project COMBINE, investigating the effectiveness of behavioral treatments alone and combined with pharmacotherapy (naltrexone or acamprosate) in the treatment of alcohol use disorders.

Smoking cessation has been successfully treated using nicotine replacement therapy (e.g., nicotine chewing gum, nicotine patch) and more successful outcomes have been found when NRT is combined with a behavioral treatment. Opiate addiction has been primarily treated with a variety of opioid replacement agents, such as methadone, LAAM (l-α-acetylmethadol), buprenorphine, and naltrexone. The efficacy of methadone, an opioid agonist, in reducing relapse to heroin use has been well-demonstrated. LAAM has a longer duration of action than methadone, although higher doses of LAAM may have undesirable and/or unsafe side-effects. Ling, Rawson, & Compton (1994) demonstrated that buprenorphine may result in less physical dependence than methadone. Cocaine has been treated with a variety of acute and maintenance treatments. Both desipiramine and naltrexone have been shown to reduce cocaine use. Other studies have demonstrated that disulfiram is effective in the treatment of polysubstance (cocaine and alcohol) abuse.

Effective Self-Help Treatments

Twelve-step treatments are the most commonly utilized and mandated programs for substance abuse and dependence. Over two million individuals are considered members of Alcoholics Anonymous and 31,000 meetings of Narcotics Anonymous are held daily in over 100 countries. Alternative mutual support groups, which are not based on the 12-step model, include: Secular Organizations for Sobriety, SMART Recovery, Moderation Management, and Rational Recovery. Online mutual support groups are becoming more accessible and popular, including:

http://www.smartrecovery.org/ onlinemeetings.htm and *http://www.egetgoing.com.*

There are several self-help books that incorporate elements of effective treatments these include:

Daley, D. C. *Kicking Addictive Habits Once & for All: A Relapse Prevention Guide.* $23.

Fletcher, A. *Sober for Good.* $14.

Gregson, D., Efran, J., & Marlatt, G. A. *The Tao of Sobriety.* $15.

Other Issues in Management

Response to psychotherapy and medication varies, with some research showing a 10 minute brief intervention can have lasting effects. Simply asking about a person's substance use and providing education about consequences associated with use can lead to reductions in consumption. Although lasting, clinically significant reductions in substance use and substance related consequences will often require more intensive treatment. Maintenance treatments, aftercare, booster sessions, and relapse prevention planning can sustain treatment gains.

Length of treatment stay varies widely, ranging from brief interventions (1 hour or less) to intensive inpatient treatment programs. Estimates from the Treatment Episode Data set suggest shorter stays for detoxification (median = 5 days) and longer time till the completion of outpatient treatment (median = 91 days). According to the Center for Disease Control, methadone maintenance treatments should last a minimum of 12-months.

How Does One Select Among Treatments?

Treatment goal setting is possibly the most important and controversial factor in choosing among different treatments. Most treatment programs require abstinence, whereby any substance use is considered a failure. Alternatively, moderation goals are individually determined goals that do not prohibit abstinence, but also provide increased flexibility and the opportunity to learn from mistakes (lapses), without the guilt associated with failing to meet an abstinence treatment goal. Moderation goals remain a controversial issue in addiction treatment. The recognition that abstinence-based programs can be iatrogenic has led some researchers, clinicians, and treatment agencies to lean toward harm reduction approaches. Harm reduction goals are based on each individual's unique substance-related consequences, severity of substance abuse or dependence, self-efficacy, and beliefs about substance use. For example, an individual who is not physically dependent on alcohol, but who has experienced consequences from drinking under the influence, may work towards the treatment goal of not driving after drinking. If this goal is achieved, then the person may work toward reducing the quantity or frequency of drinking. After reducing quantity and frequency, the same person may work toward the treatment goal of only drinking during special occasions or abstinence.

Patient–treatment matching is a popular approach to treatment selection. Several clinicians have identified client characteristics that moderate the effectiveness of some treatments. For example, it has been shown that cognitive-impairment can limit the effectiveness of interventions that require higher levels of cognitive functioning (e.g., cognitive–behavioral treatment). The National Institute of Alcohol Abuse and Alcoholism funded a multisite, multimillion dollar study (Project MATCH) to test matching hypotheses for three alcohol treatments (cognitive–behavioral, 12-step, and motivation enhancement). The results did not support the matching hypotheses, leading some to doubt the utility of selecting treatments based on client characteristics.

The lack of treatment matching effects in Project MATCH may be partially explained by the complexity of the alcohol relapse process, and it is important to consider the possibility that treatment matching effects were not identified due to the idiosyncratic and dynamic relationship between client characteristics, treatment-type, and treatment outcomes. Many clinicians do treatment matching on a daily/momentary basis when working with patients, yet this level of analysis has never been conducted in a large scale research study.

Costs of treatment can be an important factor in selecting among available treatments. The Alcohol and Drug Services Study–Cost Study (SAMHSA, 2002) estimated the mean cost per admission was greatest for outpatient methadone treatment (average cost per admission = $7,415) and lowest for standard outpatient care (without methadone, $1,433). For those with health insurance, addiction treatment copayments and allowances often do not cover the costs of longer-term treatment programs.

"Addiction parity," which means alcohol and drug treatment be given equal insurance coverage as other chronic disorders could increase treatment options and reduce the cost of substance use treatments to individuals and society, as a whole. Recent studies have shown that providing full and equal coverage for alcohol and drug addiction will only increase insurance premiums by 0.2% (less than $1 per month). The Rand Corporation estimates that this increase in insurance coverage will save taxpayers over $5 billion dollars in costs related to substance abuse and dependence.

REFERENCES

American Psychiatric Association. (1994). Diagnostic and statistical manual of mental disorders (4th ed.). Washington, DC: APA.

Centers for Disease Control and Prevention. (2004). *The burden of chronic diseases and their risk factors: National and state perspectives.* Available: *http://www.cdc.gov/ nccdphp/burdenbook*

Delaney, T., Gable, A., & Kendell, N. (2000). Treatment of alcoholism and drug addiction: What legislators need to know. Washington, DC: National Conference of State Legislatures.

Khantzian, E. J. (1985), The self-medication hypothesis of addictive disorders: Focus on heroin and cocaine dependence. *American Journal of Psychiatry, 142,* 1259–1264.

Ling, W. L., Rawson, R. A., & Compton, M. A. (1994). Substitution pharmacotherapies for opioid addiction: From methadone to LAAM to buprenorphine. *Journal of Psychoactive Drugs, 26,* 119–128.

Luthar, S. (2003). The culture of affluence: Psychological costs of material wealth. *Child Development, 74* (6), 1581–1593.

McLellan, A. T., Lewis, D. C., O'Brien, C. P., & Kleber, H. D. (2000). Drug dependence, a chronic mental illness: Implications for treatment, insurance, and outcomes evaluation. *JAMA, 284,* 1689–1695.

Miller, W. R., & Rollnick, S. (2002). *Motivational interviewing: Preparing people for change.* New York: Guilford Press.

Moyer, A., Finney, J., Swearingen, C., & Vergun, P. (2002). Brief interventions for alcohol problems: A meta-analytic review of controlled investigations in treatment-seeking and non-treatment seeking populations. *Addiction, 97,* 279–292.

National Institute of Drug Abuse (2003). *Drug Use among Racial/Ethnic Minorities.* Bethesda, MD: US Department of Health and Human Services.

Substance Abuse and Mental Health Services Administration (1997). *National Estimates of Expenditures for Substance Abuse Treatments.* Rockville, MD: SAMSHA.

Substance Abuse and Mental Health Services Administration (1999). *Treatment episode data set 1994–1999: National admissions to substance abuse treatment services.* Rockville, MD: SAMSHA.

Substance Abuse and Mental Health Services Administration (2002). *National survey on drug use and health.* Rockville, MD: SAMSHA.

Substance Abuse and Mental Health Services Administration (2003). *Prevalence of substance use among racial and ethnic subgroups in the US* Rockville, MD: SAMSHA.

Substance Abuse and Mental Health Services Administration (2001). *Mental health: Culture, race, and ethnicity, a supplement to mental health: A report of the surgeon general.* Rockville, MD: SAMSHA.

Witkiewitz, K., & Marlatt, G. A. (2004). Relapse prevention for alcohol and drug problems: That was Zen, this is Tao. *American Psychologist, 59(4),* 224–235.

Suicidal and Self-Destructive Behavior

Kirk D. Strosahl • John A. Chiles

WHAT IS SUICIDAL AND SELF-DESTRUCTIVE BEHAVIOR?

Suicidal and self-destructive behavior is one of the most common clinical problems encountered in both out-patient and in-patient behavioral health settings. Studies suggest that as many as 20% of out-patients and 50% of in-patients report suicidal behavior as a significant clinical issue (Crosby, Cheltenham & Sacks, 1999; Chiles & Strosahl 2004). Unlike many of the other mental health conditions described in this text, suicidal behavior is not considered to be a mental disorder; it spans a range of clinical diagnostic groups, including mood disorders, anxiety disorders, addictive disorders, psychotic disorders, and personality disorders. DSM-IV uses suicidal behavior as part of the diagnostic criteria for both Depression and Borderline Personality Disorder. There are several forms of suicidal and self destructive behavior that are encountered in clinical practice. Ranging from the most common to the least frequent they are:

Suicidal ideation/verbalization. The act of thinking about killing oneself or verbalizing thoughts of suicide to other individuals.

Suicide attempt. The act of deliberately inflicting a self injury which at the time of the injury is labeled by the patient or someone else close to the patient as an attempt at suicide.

Suicide. The act of taking one's own life, when the resulting death is determined by a medical examiner to be a self-inflicted death.

Parasuicide. Originally introduced by Kreitman (1977) to describe a pattern of chronic, repetitive suicide attempting that "mimics" suicide attempts in form, but often involves less lethal methods and seems to serve a different function for the patient. This behavior pattern is often observed in patients diagnosed with borderline personality disorder.

Self-mutilation. The act of inflicting self-injury, most commonly lacerating or burning the trunk or a limb, which is not described by the patient as a suicide attempt. Typically, the patient will use self injurious behavior to regulate intolerable mood states by diverting attention from emotional pain to physical pain. This behavior pattern is often observed in patients who exhibit parasuicidal behavior patterns, leading some theorists to claim that they are functionally correlated behaviors (Nock & Prinstein, 2004).

WHAT IS A SUICIDAL CRISIS?

A suicidal crisis is defined in two basic ways. *First, the patient experiences acute emotional pain that is viewed as intolerable, inescapable and interminable. (The Three I's; Chiles and Strosahl, 1995). Associated with this emotional turmoil are strong urges to act in self-destructive ways that may be potentially life threatening.* At this point, the patient will view suicide as a way to stop the problem of feeling bad inside and this may be accompanied by other

Strosahl, K. D., & Chiles, J. A. (2006). Suicidal and self-destructive behavior. In J. E. Fisher & W. T. O'Donohue (Eds.), *Practitioner's guide to evidence-based psychotherapy*. New York: Springer.

perceived benefits of selfdestructive acts (i.e., gain revenge, expressing anger, and escaping intolerable situational stress). Second, a suicidal crisis is always defined as a deviation from a preexisting level of suicidality. In highly functional patients, the preexisting level is no presence of suicidality at all. In chronically suicidal patients, the crisis is an aggravation of what may be daily thoughts of suicide. *It is important to understand that all suicidal crises are time limited.* A crisis will seldom last more than 24–48 hours before it dissipates. This means most crisis intervention measures will only be needed for a relatively short period of time.

BASIC FACTS ABOUT SUICIDAL AND SELF-DESTRUCTIVE BEHAVIOR

Prevalence

Estimates of the population prevalence of the nonfatal forms of suicidal behavior vary greatly because of differing definitions of suicidal behaviors, whether studies measure the point prevalence versus lifetime prevalence of the behaviors in question and methodological inconsistencies. Suicidologists agree that suicide ideation/verbalization is by far the most common form of suicidal behavior; with point prevalence rates ranging from 4% to 17% (Crosby et al., 1999). The lifetime prevalence of significant suicidal ideation in the general population may be as high as 40% (Strosahl, Linehan, & Chiles, 1984). Estimating the rate of suicide attempts in the general population on a point prevalence basis is nearly impossible given the inadequacy of current data sets. Lifetime prevalence rates are more typically the focus of study and a surprisingly high rate has been observed, ranging from 10% to 15% of the general population. For example, the 1997 national youth health risk survey found that one in five of all adolescents reported some serious suicidal ideation, while nearly 7% reported making a suicide attempt. The population rate for suicide is the best kept statistic and typically ranges between 11 and 13 per 100,000 people in the United States. Thus, suicide is an extremely rare phenomenon, even in the highest risk populations where the rate may be as high as 1,200:100,000. Current research on the prevalence of self-mutilative behavior suggests that it is widespread, particularly among adolescents. Studies indicate that from 14% to 39% of adolescents in the community (Lloyd, 1998; Ross & Heath, 2002) and 40–61% of adolescent psychiatric in-patients (Briere & Gill, 2002; Darche, 1990; DiClemente, Ponton, & Hartley, 1991).

Comorbidity of suicidal behaviors and mental disorders/addictions

The social prohibition and stigma associated with suicide has led to the common belief that the presence of suicidality itself is evidence of a mental disorder. Various DSM-IV disorders such as major depressive disorder and borderline personality disorder incorporate suicidality as core diagnostic criteria. However, studies suggest that patients with schizoaffective disorders account for the highest rates of suicide among patients with documented mental disorders followed by patients with drug and alcohol disorders. The rate of suicide appears to be as high in anxiety disorders (particularly Panic Disorder) as it is in depression and roughly the same percentage of suicides occur among personality disorders as among depressive disorders. Studies attempting to assess rates of psychiatric morbidity in completed suicides suffer from major methodological flaws that limit the validity and generalizability of results. With these caveats, the range of comorbidity observed is quite large, from 50% to 90%, in patients that complete suicide (Chiles & Strosahl, 2005). However, the comorbidity Axis I and Axis II disorders may be somewhat lower in suicide attempters and little is known about the comorbidity in the vast population of suicide ideators. The rate of Axis II morbidity is very high in parasuicidal patients. The clinical significance of these results is as follows: *A clinician should not assume that the presence of suicidality is de facto evidence of the presence of a mental or addictive disorder in the absence of a carefully conducted diagnostic evaluation.*

IMPORTANT CLINICAL FEATURES OF SUICIDAL BEHAVIOR

Suicidal Behavior is Not a Monolithic Phenomenon

There are many reasons to believe that the different forms of suicidal behavior, while inter-related to some degree, may not be representative of a single at risk population. An important caveat is that these data are based on western studies, conducted primarily in the US and Great Britain. Crosscultural studies are emerging indicating that suicidal behavior may follow different patterns in other parts of the world. For example, in China women are more likely to commit suicide than men, and the most common method of suicide is poison ingestion (Phillips, Yang, & Li 2004). With this limitation in mind, the following characteristics point to the possibility that there may several different subpopulations within the larger cohort of suicidal patients:

- Men are 2–3 times more likely to commit suicide than women
- Women are 2–3 times more like to make a suicide attempt than men
- The suicide rate increases steadily with age (the rate of suicide in people over 65 is twice as large as in the 15–24 age group), whereas the rate of suicide attempting decreases after 40
- The chief methods used in suicides are guns and hanging, whereas the chief method used in suicide attempting is overdosing
- There are a vast number of patients with suicidal ideation/attempts in relation to a very small percentage of patients that die from suicide
- Less than 10% of suicide attempters die over the course of a lifetime from self-inflicted injuries

The clinical significance of this distinction is as follows: *a clinician should not assume that the presence of suicidal ideation/behavior itself is indicative of an eminent risk of completed suicide. Suicidal behavior may serve a variety of functions apart from the motivation to end life. A careful assessment is required to understand the patient's expectations about suicidal behavior and how such behavior functions in the patient's life space.*

Suicidal Behavior is a Learned Behavior

Suicidal behavior is a learned behavior that is shaped by both external and internal reinforcements. External reinforcements include removal from a stressful environment via hospitalization, a reduction in interpersonal conflicts or changes in the expectations of family, spouse or friends. Internal reinforcements include reductions in negative affect, unpleasant thoughts, memories, or physical sensations. The internal reinforcement for suicidal behavior often occurs after the fact of a suicide attempt, a parasuicidal act or self-mutilation. At this point, there is insufficient evidence to conclude that suicidal behavior is genetically transmitted, although it is well known that suicide risk increases within families with a history of prior suicide (Brent, Bridge, Johnson, & Connoly, 1996). This correlation could be related to genetics, temperament and/or social role modeling, or a combination of the three (Chiles, Strosahl, McMurtrey, & Linehan, 1985).

Suicidal Behavior Contains Both Instrumental and Expressive Functions

Suicidal and self-destructive behavior can serve many functions for the individual, apart from the desire to die. *Instrumental functions* include regulating negative emotional arousal, changing relationship dynamics, escaping from a stress filled living situation, strengthening a disability claim, or escaping from unbearable feelings by ending one's life. *Expressive functions* include help seeking, communicating distress to someone that is seemingly inattentive, or gaining a measure of revenge for a lost relationship. The key point is that both instrumental and expressive functions may be involved in single suicidal event. It appears that self-mutilation functions similarly (Nock & Prinstein, 2004).

Personality and Social/Interpersonal Attributes of Suicidal Patients

A large number of cross sectional studies have examined the unique attributes of suicidal and self-destructive individuals. Typically, such studies suggest that these individuals suffer from an inability to regulate negative emotional states, leading to a state of prolonged emotional and physiological over-arousal. One likely function of suicidal behavior is to regulate such aversive arousal (Brown, Comtois & Linehan, 2002; Chiles & Strosahl, 2005; Linehan, 1997). Aversive emotional states are thought to be related to the cognitive rigidity and lack of effective problem solving that is the sine qua non of suicidal crisis. In numerous studies, suicidal patients have been shown to exhibit ineffective and passive problem solving skills (Linehan Camper, Chiles, Strosahl, & Shearin, 1987; Pollock & Williams, 2001; Rudd, Joiner, & Rajab, 1996; Schotte & Clum, 1987). Because of these deficits, suicidal patients tend to experience heightened interpersonal conflict, socially isolated and unable to marshal competent social support in times of crisis (Darche, 1991; Chiles, Strosahl, Cowden, Grahem, & Linehan, 1986). There is a significant relationship between suicidal/self destructive behavior and substance abuse. Studies consistently reveal that as many as 50% of all completed suicides screen positive for drug or alcohol levels upon autopsy (Chiles & Strosahl, 1995).

ASSESSMENT

Behavioral Assessment

Suicidal and self-destructive behavior, whatever its form, can be described as occurring along three dimensions:

- The *frequency* of suicidal episodes, such as how often a patient thinks about suicide, verbalizes those thoughts to others, the number of suicide attempts, parasuicidal behaviors or self-mutilation episodes within a given time period.
- The *duration* of episodes, such as how long the ideation or verbalizations last or the time frame of a suicide attempts, or the time spent is parasuicidal or self-injurious behaviors within an episode.
- The *intensity* of the episodes, such as how specific and concentrated are the periods of ideation or verbalization, or the degree of cognitive and behavioral preparation prior to an attempt, or the severity of laceration/burning that occurs during an episode of self-mutilation.

It is also important to assess the *situational triggers* for suicidality, using traditional behavioral assessment strategies such as self-monitoring or daily records. Most patients respond to a limited number of specific situations with suicidal and self-destructive behaviors. One example of a behavioral assessment strategy is to have the patient complete a Daily Suicidal Behaviors Diary that elicits trigger events, mood states, and cognitions associated with suicidal behaviors and the impact of suicidal behaviors as a response to the trigger situation (cf. Chiles & Strosahl, 2005 for an example of a daily diary).

There are also some well established self-report and/or interview scales used to directly measure suicidal behavior. One is the Suicidal Thinking and Behaviors Questionnaire (Chiles & Strosahl, 1995, 2005), a 9 item self report measure that measures current suicidal behavior, expectations about the problem solving efficacy of suicide and historical information (i.e., number of prior attempts, suicidal role models, competent social support). The Beck Suicide Intent Scale (SIS; Beck, Scheyler, & Herman, 1974) is designed to measure the intent level associated with an index suicide attempt. It can be administered in either a self report or interview format. The scale focuses on cognitive (i.e., belief that the attempt would be fatal) and behavior (i.e., making a will in anticipation of death) aspects of the suicidal act.

Suicide Risk Indicators

For several decades, research has been conducted to identify the historical, personality, familial, and social risk factors for suicide (Clark & Fawcett, 1992). A variety of research methods, most of them cross sectional, have been used to isolate those factors that are thought to predict suicide risk. Some studies have focused on an intensive review of the psychiatric and social history of completed suicides via medical chart reviews and interviews with significant others. Other studies have employed comprehensive reviews of psychiatric charts, comparing completed suicides with psychiatric patients who did not commit suicide. These studies collectively have produced a large array of risk indicators in two categories. *Background indicators* are either demographic or historical aspects of the patient's life that are static. For example, common background factors are a history of prior suicide attempts, family history of suicide, increasing age, sex, history of psychiatric, or substance abuse disorder. *Foreground indicators* are immediate life events or psychological states that may influence the patient's current suicidal risk such as a recent interpersonal loss, diagnosis of a terminal medical illness, presence of physical pain, intoxication, depression, and/or hopelessness. In most suicide risk prediction systems, the most important foreground indicators are the patient's level of suicidal ideation and suicidal intent (Does the patient have a well detailed plan? Is the plan lethal? Are the means available to execute the plan?)

Predictive Validity of Suicide Risk Indicators

As mentioned previously, almost all of the available suicide risk indicators have been generated in cross sectional research designs. The ultimate test of these indicators is to use them in a prospective research design to examine their specificity and sensitivity. Two large multiyear studies (Pokorney, 1983; Goldstein et al., 1991) have examined the predictive validity of existing suicide risk indicators. *Both studies demonstrated that current risk indicators do not accurately predict risk of suicide and tend to yield an unacceptably high false positive prediction rate (i.e., predicting that a patient is an eminent threat to commit suicide when in fact the patient never dies from suicide). Both studies conclude that at the present time, it is not possible to accurately predict who will and who will not commit suicide.*

Self-report scales

The Beck Hopelessness Scale (BHS; Beck, Weissman, Lester, & Trexler, 1974) is a 20-item instrument that measures the patient's general level of pessimism about the future. Hopelessness has been proposed as the mediating variable between negative mood states such as depression and the risk of suicidal behavior. The Reasons for Living Scale (RFL—Linehan, Goodstein, Nielson, & Chiles, 1983) is a 48 item scale, divided into six subscales. This instrument assesses the importance of reasons an individual has for NOT committing suicide, should the urge arise. The most important subscale for present purposes is the 24-item Survival and Coping Beliefs scale. This subscale assesses the individual's confidence in the future, beliefs about being persistent through hard times and beliefs about the inevitability of change for the better.

Predictive validity of self-report scales

Two small studies of the Beck Hopelessness Scale revealed that it predicts a statistically significant percentage of suicides over a multiple year period in a population of individuals diagnosed with depression (Beck, Steer & Kovacs, 1985; Beck, Brown & Steer, 1989). However, it took several years in each study to accumulate a statistically significant prediction effect, whereas the typical clinical requirement is to predict eminent risk of suicide within the next 24–72 hours. With respect to that requirement, another study of the BHS showed that it misclassified 100% of hospitalized high intent suicide attempters (Strosahl et al., 1984), indicating that it may not predict immediate suicidal risk. Two studies (Strosahl, Chiles and Linehan, 1992; Chiles et. al., 1989) compared the BHS with the Reasons for Living, Survival and Coping Beliefs subscale (RFL—SCB). This scale assesses the reasons an individual has for NOT committing suicide, should the thoughts arise. The results of both studies suggested that the RFL—SCB performed better than the BHS in predicting suicidal intent. Finally, one of these studies (Chiles et al., 1989 also compared a patient generated rating of the efficacy of suicidal behavior as a way of solving one's problems. This rating generally performed as well as either the RFL—SCB or the BHS in the prediction of immediate suicidal intent.

The following conclusions can be drawn from the empirical literature pertaining to the prediction of suicide:

- There is no evidence that any combination of existing suicide risk indicators can accurately predict suicide on a case by case basis in the time frame needed for clinical practice.
- Conventional suicide risk indicators consistently misclassify risk levels in a false positive direction, leading to treatment decisions that may be potentially harmful to the patient.
- The clinical evidence suggests that the best self-report assessment of current suicidality is obtained using the following assessment methods:

1. Beck Hopeless Scale
2. Reasons for Living—Survival and Coping Beliefs Subscale
3. A 1–5 point rating scale measuring the patient's belief in the problem solving efficacy of suicide (i.e., would suicide be an effective way of solving your problems?)

What Assessments Should not be Used?

Many suicide risk prediction instruments are currently marketed and sold to clinicians and agency administrators with the claim that they can identify suicidal patients and estimate suicide risk. There is no evidence that any of these instruments can perform the latter function (predicting suicide). Use of these instruments not only may result in harmful treatment planning decisions, but also may lull clinicians into thinking that a "low risk" patient poses no threat of suicide.

TREATMENT

Given the clinical importance of suicidal and self-destructive behavior, it is surprising to see such limited clinical research on the efficacy of in-patient and outpatient treatments. This is due to a number of factors. One is that there are different forms of suicidal behavior that may share some processes in common, but also may have unique characteristics. In other words, the type of treatment required may vary depending upon the type of suicidal behavior that is being targeted. Two, suicidal outcomes typically have been regarded as "adverse events" in studies investigating treatment of some other condition such as depression, alcohol dependence, or panic disorder. Often, any form of suicidal behavior has been a reason to exclude patients from studies of treatments for these conditions. Third, unified, evidence based clinical models of suicidality did not appear until the early 1990s and this tended to suppress treatment development. Finally there are ethical issues associated with the use of control/placebo comparison group strategies in clinical trials specifically targeting suicidal patients. Until "usual care" treatment control groups were accepted as legitimate research strategy, it was nearly impossible to conduct a well-controlled study of treatment models.

Are There Out-Patient Psychosocial Treatments that Prevent Suicide?

Even though there is a great deal of empirical evidence supporting the effectiveness of psychotherapy for conditions that are known to be associated with suicide, there is no evidence that these treatments prevent suicides. For example, the actual suicide rates observed in pooled data sets from depression clinical trials are very close to the rates predicted for depression in the general population. Given the extremely low prevalence of completed suicide, and the lack of predictive validity of existing suicide risk indicators, this finding is not surprising.

Are There In-Patient Treatments that Prevent Suicide?

Psychiatric in-patient treatment has not been shown to be an effective treatment for the prevention of suicide. Numerous studies of this question have failed to reveal a treatment effect and some studies suggest that the risk of suicide is increased posthospitalization (Chiles & Strosahl, 2005). In addition, 5% of all suicides occur on psychiatric units, dispelling the myth that putting a suicidal patient in the hospital for "safety reasons" is a legitimate clinical response. In a subsequent section, alternatives to hospitalization will be discussed as well as conditions under which a limited in-patient stay may be clinically necessary.

Do Psychopharmacology Treatments Prevent Suicide?

There is scant evidence that psychotropic medications of any sort provide protection from suicidal behavior in any psychiatrically ill population. The most notable exception is the mood stabilizing agent lithium, used primarily in the treatment of bipolar illness. Multiple studies have shown that this agent has consistent positive effects on the rate of death by suicide (Tondo, Hennen, & Baldessarini, 2001). One study has specifically assessed the effect of an antipsychotic medication on suicidal behavior. The InterSePT trial (Metzer et. al., 2003) compared the effects of clozapine versus olanzapine in patients with schizophrenia or schizoaffective disorder who were considered at high risk for suicide, and found clozapine superior in decreasing nonlethal forms of suicidality. A comparison of risperidone and haloperidol for the prevention of relapse in patients with schizophrenia used suicidal behavior as one of several indications for relapse. While respiridone had a lower risk of relapse, the effects of each drug on suicidal behavior were not reported (Csernansky, Mahmoud, & Brenner, 2002). No specific studies on suicidal behavior have been done with either antianxiety or antidepressant medication. Most antidepressant studies have excluded patients deemed to be at risk for suicide.

Many patients with a psychiatric illness are treated with medication. For those patients manifesting suicidal behavior, it is possible that, when the medications are effective, suicidality can be reduced as the problems produced by the mental illness diminish. However, problems of adherence, overdose, and iatrogenesis come with the territory. Iatrogenesis, negative effects on suicidal behavior caused by the medication, is of significant current concern. *A number of serotonin-based antidepressants have now been shown, via a reassessment of pharmaceutical company data bases, to have a suicidogenic effect (Healy, 2003).* For example, in depressed patients treated with serotonin-based antidepressants, the relative risk of suicide increases about 200% compared to the relative risk associated with the use of tricyclic antidepressants. *The clinical features associated with iatrogenic suicidality are intense emotional turmoil, dysphoria and an agitated restlessness reminiscent of akathisia. These symptoms are mostly likely to appear upon initiation of medicine and when dosing titrations occur.*

The data on youth treated with serotonin-based antidepressants are particularly worrisome. A recent FDA review of 22 placebo controlled studies involving 4,250 pediatric patients found that youths taking these drugs were twice as likely to become suicidal as those given placebo. At the time of this writing, the FDA is considering extending its "black box" warning of increased suicidal behavior with certain antidepressants to include all antidepressants. These evaluations are ongoing, and there is increasing pressure on the FDA from the US Congress to make all drug study results available in the public domain. This is a fast moving area, and can best be followed by consulting the FDA website (*www.fda.gov/cder/drug/antidepressants/ default.htm*).

A possible exception to these negative effects may occur with the use of a specific antidepressant, fluoxetine, in combination with cognitive–behavior therapy in adolescents (TADS, 2004). Antipsychotic medications may also have a similar iatrogenic effect, although the evidence for this claim at present remains anecdotal. The neurological side effects of akathisia and akinesia, and the metabolic side-effects of type 2 diabetes and obesity may, separately or combined, be instrumental in producing suicidality. Recently, the makers of several newer antipsychotic medications have conducted studies on bipolar illness. These studies measure suicidal behavior, but, to date, none have reported effects on suicidal behavior. Perhaps, particularly given the FDA's current emphasis on evaluating all study results, more information on antipsychotics and suicidality will be forthcoming.

Are There Treatments that Work with Suicide Attempting?

There is evidence that Dialectical Behavior Therapy (DBT), a contextualistic form of cognitive behavior therapy, reduces both the frequency and lethality of parasuicidal acts (Linehan, Armstrong, Suarez, Allman & Heard 1991, Linehan, 1993; Linehan, 1997). It is important to note that most patients in these studies made subsequent suicide attempts, but generally they were fewer in number and less medically dangerous. Long-term follow up studies indicated that DBT produces modest gains in social functioning. There is also evidence that other more traditional cognitive–behavioral approaches, focusing on personal problem solving skills, also are effective with suicide attempters (Liberman & Eckman, 1981; Salkovskis, Atha, & Storer, 1990).

Several other studies have examined the effectiveness of enhanced treatment follow-up, community-based outreach such as home visits, telephone support, intensive case management services, and methods for improving access to care. For the most part, these studies have been both flawed methodologically and, in most cases, failed to find a significant positive effect. The one exception (Morgan, Jones, & Owen, 1993) found that offering hospitalized suicide attempters improved access to emergency room services (i.e., giving patient a crisis card with key numbers, encouraging help seeking) resulted in a significant reduction in suicide attempts over a one year period. Thus, it appears that successful intervention programs for suicide attempters typically require a longer time period and a more intensive treatment and/or follow up care structure.

Are There Treatments that Work with Suicidal Ideation?

In contrast to the rather mixed picture for suicide attempts, there are several studies showing that time limited in-patient and/or out-patient cognitive–behavioral treatment has a positive impact upon suicidal ideation (Jobes, Jacoby, Cimbolic, & Hustead, 1997; Lerner & Clum, 1990; Liberman & Eckman, 1981; Patsiokas & Clum, 1985; Rudd, Rajab, Stulman, Joiner, & Dixon, 1996; Salkovskis et al. 1990). Most of these treatment models emphasize a personal problem solving focus, which would be predicted given the strong research indications of personal problem solving deficits in suicial patients. Most of these studies provided treatment in the out-patient setting, indicating that most suicidal patients can be safely treated without recourse to in-patient care. The evidence also suggests that such problem solving based behavioral treatments appear to work in relatively brief periods of time.

What are the Alternatives to Hospitalization for Suicidal Patients?

As discussed previously, psychiatric hospitalization has not received empirical support as a treatment for suicidality. The decision to hospitalize should not be made lightly, because it is an invasive treatment that may create more problems than it solves. *Whenever possible, the guiding principle is to find short term alternatives to hospitalization such as crisis respite units or 23 hour hospital beds. If no resource other than an in-patient facility is available, the goal should be to limit the length of stay to 24–48 hours (cf. Chiles and Strosahl, 2005).* The goal of such short stay strategies is to help the patient weather the suicidal crisis (normally 24–48 hours in length) without offering excessive reinforcement for suicidal. From the reinforcement perspective, hospitalization is contra-indicated for patients with chronic, repetitious suicidality. Generally, hospitalization may be indicated in one of the following three circumstances:

- An underlying serious mental disorder (with accompanying suicidality) that can best be managed within the increased structure of a psychiatric unit (i.e., a decompensation patient hearing command hallucinations to commit suicide). Here, the goal is to treat the underlying mental disorder, NOT the suicidal risk.
- When the patients presents with atypical symptoms that need to be ruled out using the types of resources that are only available in the hospital setting (i.e., a patient with an unusual depression with impulsive self destructive acts that might be indicative of organic brain syndrome). Here, the goal is to obtain an accurate differential diagnosis, NOT to treat the impulsive suicidality.
- When hospitalization is used to behaviorally modify a pattern of frequent hospital admissions for parasuicidal behavior (i.e., planning admissions to the hospital on a scheduled basis, regardless of the patient's emotional status). Here, the goal is to change the pattern of reinforcing suicidal behavior by admitting the patient to the hospital.

What Interventions Should not be Used?

The clinical evidence fails to support the use of the "no suicide contract" as a suicide prevention strategy (Chiles & Strosahl, 2005). No suicide contracts are a standard part of many clinic and hospital based risk assessment and management protocols for suicidal patients. Patients who are unwilling to contract for safety are often referred for evaluation for involuntary admission. The danger of relying on a no suicide contract is that it can breed a false sense of security. The clinician assumes that the suicide risk has been managed and therefore may miss the clear signs of a recurrent suicidal crisis.

SELF-HELP AND ON-LINE RESOURCES

There are several associations whose mission it is to better understand, treat and prevent suicidal behavior:

American Association of Suicidology: *www.suicidology.org*
American Foundation for Suicide Prevention: *www.afsp.org*
International Association for Suicide Prevention: *iasp@aol.com*

Self help books for suicidal individuals and/or involved others are very limited in number and may be potentially useful:

Ellis, T., & Newman, C. (1996). *Choosing to live: How to defeat suicide through cognitive therapy.* Oakland, CA: New Harbinger Publications.
Jacobs, D. (1999). *The Harvard Medical School guide to suicide assessment and intervention.* San Francisco: Jossey-Bass.
Survivors of suicide face special challenges in moving on with their lives after such a devastating event as the loss of a loved one to suicide. The following readings may be of help:

Robinson, P. (2005). Understanding and providing care to the survivors of suicide (pp. 273–303). In J. Chiles & K. Strosahl (2005). Clinical manual for the assessment and treatment of suicidal patients. Washington DC: American Psychiatric Publishing.
Alexander, V. (1991). *Words I never thought to speak: Stories of life in the wake of suicide.* New York: Lexington Books.
Carlson, T. (1995). *Suicide survivors handbook: A guide for those bereaved and those who wish to help them.* Duluth, MN: Benline Press.

REFERENCES

Beck, A., Brown, G., & Steer, R. (1989). Prediction of eventual suicide in psychiatric inpatients by clinical ratings of hopelessness. *Journal of Consulting and Clinical Psychology, 57,* 309–310.

Beck, A., Steer, R., & Kovacs, M. (1985). Hopelessness and eventual suicide: A 10 year prospective study of patients hospitalized with suicidal ideation. *American Journal of Psychiatry, 142,* 559–563.

Beck, A., Schuyler, D., & Herman, I. (1974). Development of suicidal intent scales. In A. Beck, H. Resnick, & D. Lettieri (Eds.), *The prediction of suicide (pp. 45–56).* Bowie, MD: Charles Thomas Press.

Beck, A., Weissman, A., Lester, D., & Trexler, L. (1974). The measurement of pessimism: The Hopelessness Scale. *Journal of Consulting and Clinical Psychology, 42,* 861–865.

Brent D., Bridge J., Johnson B., & Connoly J. (1996). Suicidal behavior runs in families: a controlled family study of adolescent suicide victims. *Archives of General Psychiatry, 53,* 1145–1152.

Briere, J., & Gil, E. (2002). Self-mutilation in clinical and general population samples: Prevalence, correlates, and functions. *American Journal of Orthopsychiatry, 68,* 609–620.

Brown, M., Comtois, K., & Linehan, M. (2002). Reasons for suicide attempts and non-suicidal self-injury in women with borderline personality disorder. *Journal of Abnormal Psychology, 111,* 198–202.

Chiles, J. & Strosahl, K. (1995). *The suicidal patient: Principles of assessment, treatment and case management*. Washington DC: American Psychiatric Press.

Chiles, J. & Strosahl, K. (2005). *Clinical manual for the assessment and treatment of suicidal patients*. Washington DC: American Psychiatric Publishing.

Chiles, J., Strosahl, K., Cowden, L., Graham, R., & Linehan, M. (1986). The 24 hours before suicide attempting. *Suicide and Life Threatening Behavior, 16*, 335–342.

Chiles, J., Strosahl, K., McMurtray, L., & Linehan, M. (1985). Social learning effects upon suicidal behavior. *Journal of Nervous and Mental Disease, 173*, 477–481.

Chiles, J., Strosahl, K., Ping, Z. Michael, M., Hall, K., Jemelka, R., et al. (1989). Depression, hopelessness and suicidal behavior in Chinese and American psychiatric patients. *American Journal of Psychiatry, 146*, 339–344.

Clark, D. & Fawcett, J. (1992). Review of empirical risk factors for evaluation of the suicidal patient. In B. Bongar (Ed.), *Suicide: Guidelines for assessment, management and treatment* (pp. 16–48). New York: Oxford Press.

Crosby, A., Cheltenham, M., & Sachs, J. (1999). Incidence of suicidal ideation and behavior in the United States. *Suicide and Life Threatening Behavior, 29*, 131–140.

Csernansky, M., Mahmoud, R., & Brenner, R. for the Risperidone-USA-79 Study Group (2002). A comparison of risperidone and haloperidol for the prevention of relapse in patients with schizophrenia. *New England Journal of Medicine, 346*, 16–22.

Darche, M. (1990). Psychological factors differentiating self-mutilating and non-self-mutilating adolescent in-patient females. *The Psychiatric Hospital, 21*, 31–35.

DiClemente, R., Ponton, L., & Hartley, D. (1991). Prevalence and correlates of cutting behavior: Risk for HIV transmission. *Journal of the American Academy of Child and Adolescent Psychiatry, 30*, 735–739.

Goldstein, R., Black, D., Nasrallah, A., & Winkour, G. (1991). The prediction of suicide: Sensitivity, specificity and predictive value of a multivariate model applied to suicide among 1906 patients with affective disorders. *Archives of General Psychiatry, 48*, 418–422.

Healy, D. (2003). Lines of evidence on the risks of suicide with serotonin reuptake inhibitors. *Psychotherapy and Psychosomatic Medicine, 72*, 71–79.

Jobes, D., Jacoby, A., Cimbolic, P., & Hustead, L. (1997). Assessment and treatment of suicidal clients in a university counseling center. *Journal of Counseling Psychology, 44*, 368–377.

Kreitman, N. (1977). *Parasuicide*. New York: John Wiley.

Lerner, M., & Clum, G. (1990). Treatment of suicide ideators: A problem solving approach. *Behavior Therapy, 21*, 403–411.

Liberman, R., & Eckman, T. (1981). Behavior therapy vs. insight therapy for repeated suicide attempters. *Archives of General Psychiatry, 38*, 1126–1130.

Linehan, M. (1993). *Cognitive behavioral treatment of borderline personality disorder*. New York: Guilford Press.

Linehan, M. (1997). Behavioral treatments of suicidal behaviors. In D. Soff, J. Mann, et al. (Eds.), *Annals of the New York Academy of Sciences: The neurobiology of suicidal behavior* (pp. 302–338). New York: New York Academy of Sciences.

Linehan, M., Armstrong, H., Suarez, A., Allman, D., & Heard, H. (1991). Cognitive–behavioral treatment of chronically parasuicidal borderline patients. *Archives of General Psychiatry, 48*, 1060–1064.

Linehan, M., Camper, P., Chiles, J., Strosahl, K., & Shearin, E. (1987). Interpersonal problem solving and parasuicide. *Cognitive Therapy and Research, 11*, 1–12.

Linehan, M., Goodstein, J., Nielsen, S., & Chiles, J. (1983). Reasons for staying alive when you're thinking of killing yourself: The Reasons for Living Inventory. *Journal of Consulting and Clinical Psychology, 51*, 276–286.

Lloyd, E. (1998). Self-mutilation in a community sample of adolescents (Doctoral dissertation: Louisiana State University, 1998). *Dissertation Abstracts International, 58*, 5127.

Melzer, D., Alphs, L., Green, A., Altamura, A., Anand, R., Bertoldi, A., et al. (2003). Clozapine treatment for suicidality in schizophrenia: International Suicide Prevention Trial. *Archives of General Psychiatry, 60*, 82–91.

Morgan, H., Jones, E., & Owen, J. (1993). Secondary prevention of non-fatal deliberate self-harm: The green card study. *British Journal of Psychiatry, 163*, 111–112.

Nock, M., & Prinstein, M. (2004). A functional approach to the assessment of self-mutilative behavior. *Journal of Consulting and Clinical Psychology, 72*, 885–890.

Patsiokas, A., & Clum, G. (1985). Effects of psychotherapeutic strategies in the treatment of suicide attempters. *Psychotherapy, 22*, 281–290.

Phillips, M., Yang, G., & Li, Y. (2004). Suicide and the unique prevalence pattern of schizophrenia in mainland China: A retrospective observational study, *Lancet, 364*, 1062–1068.

Pollock, L., & Williams, M. (2001). Effective problem solving in suicide attempters depends upon specific autobiographical recall. *Suicide and Life Threatening Behavior, 31*, 386–396.

Porkorney, A. (1983). Prediction of suicide in psychiatric patients: Results of a prospective study. *Archives of General Psychiatry, 40*, 249–257.

Ross, S., & Heath, N. (2002). A study of the frequency of self-mutilation in a community sample of adolescents. *Journal of Youth and Adolescence, 31*, 67–77.

Rudd, M., Rajab, H., Stulman, D., Joiner, T., & Dixon, W. (1996). Effectiveness of an outpatient intervention targeting suicidal young adults: Preliminary results. *Journal of Consulting and Clinical Psychology, 64,* 179–190.

Rudd, M., Joiner, T., & Rajab, H. (1996). Relationship among suicide ideators, attempters and multiple attempters in a young adult sample. *Journal of Abnormal Psychology, 105,* 541–550.

Salkovskis, P., Atha, C., & Storer, D. (1990). Cognitive–behavioral problem-solving in the treatment of patients who repeatedly attempt suicide. *British Journal of Psychiatry, 157,* 871–876.

Schotte, D., & Clum, G. (1987). Problem solving skills of suicidal patients. *Journal of Consulting and Clinical Psychology, 55,* 49–54

Strosahl, K., Chiles, J., & Linehan, M. (1992). Prediction of suicide intent in hospitalized parasuicides: Depression, hopelessness and reasons for living. *Comprehensive Psychiatry, 33,* 366–373.

Strosahl, K., Linehan, M., & Chiles, J. (1984). Will the real social desirability please stand up? Hopelessness, depression, social desirability and the prediction of suicidal behavior. *Journal of Consulting and Clinical Psychology, 52,* 449–457.

Tondo L., Hennen J., & Baldessarini R. (2001). Lower suicidal risk with long term lithium treatment in major affective illness: A meta-analysis. *Acta Psychiatrica Scandanavia, 104,* 163–172.

Treatment for adolescents with depression study [TADS] team. (2004). Fluoxetine, cognitive–behavior therapy, and their combination for adolescents with depression. *Journal of the American Medical Association, 922,* 807–820.

Oral-Digital Habits of Childhood: Thumb Sucking

Michelle R. Byrd • Elizabeth M. Nelson • Lisa M. Manthey

WHAT IS THUMB SUCKING?

Thumb sucking is a common behavior in infancy and early childhood. The skill of sucking is a component of the rooting reflex present at birth, although it does not serve the nutritive function of feeding-related sucking. Most infants will spontaneously begin to suck their fingers and thumbs in their first months of life (the two behaviors will be described interchangeably in this chapter), and many have been observed to do so in utero (Kravitz & Boehm, 1971). In fact, some obstetricians have described infants born with blisters on their thumbs because of having so voraciously sucked them prior to birth.

Historically, there has been some conflict regarding whether thumb sucking should be conceptualized as a simple habit or a symptom of underlying psychopathology (e.g., Davidson, Haryett, Sandilands, & Hansen, 1967). Early psychoanalytic theorists hypothesized that thumb sucking is an autoerotic behavior associated with later masturbatory behavior and underlying psychopathology (e.g., Bakwin, 1948). However, there is little evidence to support this contention. Although a limited number of studies have found increases in psychological/behavior problems in children who suck their thumb (e.g. Mahalski & Stanton, 1992), there is no indication that these elevations are clinically significant. Moreover, the overwhelming majority of studies have not found significant increases in behavioral or psychological problems in thumb sucking children (e.g., Davidson, et al., 1967; Friman, Larzelere, & Finney, 1994; Tyron, 1968).

Therefore, though thumb sucking may be a focus of clinical attention, it may be more appropriate to conceptualize thumb sucking as a simple habit rather than a sign of significant psychopathology. Correspondingly, as with other oral-digital habits such as nail biting, thumb sucking is not a DSM-IV diagnosable disorder (Friman, Byrd, & Oksol, 2001). As such, thumb sucking is commonly viewed as a normal phenomenon in at least the first two years of life (Klein, 1971) and has been hypothesized to serve adaptive functions for infants and toddlers by providing stimulation or self-soothing (Friman, 1987).

However, thumb sucking may become the focus of clinical attention when either the duration or the intensity of the behavior exceeds normative functions. The purpose of this chapter is to describe thumb sucking, how to assess whether or not thumb sucking should be treated, and outline how to treat the behavior when doing so is deemed necessary.

FACTS ABOUT THUMB SUCKING

Comorbidity. Thumb sucking has been indirectly observed to significantly covary with trichotillomania, though epidemiological estimates are not available. Specifically,

Byrd, M. R., Nelson, E. M., & Manthey, L. (2006). Oral-digital habits of childhood: Thumb sucking In J. E. Fisher & W. T. O'Donohue (Eds.), *Practitioner's Guide to evidence based psychotherapy*. New York: Springer Publishing Company.

several studies have successfully reduced hair pulling by targeting thumb sucking (e.g. Friman & Hove, 1987; Watson & Allen, 1993).

Prevalence. The prevalence of thumb sucking in neonates has been estimated to be as high as 95% (Leung, 1991), dropping to approximately 50% in two to four year olds (Infante, 1976, Larsson & Dahlin, 1985; Ozturk & Ozturk, 1977, Popvich & Thompson, 1947) and 25% in five year olds (Mahalski & Stanton, 1992). Prevalence rates for school age children vary widely, ranging from 5.9% to 28% for 11 years olds (Gellin, 1978; Mahalski & Stranton, 1992; Popvich and Thompson, 1947).

Age at onset. The majority of children who suck their thumbs begin doing so in the first months of life. Thumb sucking tends to become the focus of clinical attention when the behavior becomes chronic, operationally defined as occurring in two or more settings (such as home and school) beyond the age of five (Friman & Schmitt, 1989).

Gender. Thumb sucking appears to be more prevalent in girls than boys (Friman, 1987; Infante, 1976; Larsson & Dahlin, 1985; Mahalski & Stanton, 1992).

Course. The majority of young children who suck their thumbs spontaneously discontinue the habit by the age of four (Peterson, 1982) when a more developmentally sophisticated repertoire of self-management skills develops. When the transition to topographically more mature skills fails to occur and thumb sucking persists beyond early childhood and/or becomes problematic for either parent or child as indicated by self-report, the behavior may become the focus of clinical attention.

Impairment and other demographic characteristics. There are several known negative medical/dental outcomes associated with chronic thumb sucking. The most frequent concern related to chronic thumb sucking is the development of dental problems including malocclusion (Brenchley, 1991; Infante, 1976), crossbite, increased overjet, and anterior openbite (Infante, 1976; Peterson, 1982; Rugh & Lemke, 1984). These problems may not self-correct if the thumb sucking persists beyond age four (Peterson, 1982). Though not as common as dental problems, children who engage in thumb sucking have been documented to experience a variety of medical problems such as deformity or impaired growth of the face and/or the digit itself (e.g., Moore, McNeill, & D'Anna, 1972; Rankin, Jabaley, Blair, & Fraser, 1988), skin or cuticle infection (e.g., Vogel, 1998), and speech problems (e.g., Josell, 1995). Moreover, hand-mouth behavior has been cited as the leading cause of lead poisoning (Finney & Friman, 1988).

In addition, there is some evidence that children who engage in thumb sucking may face an increased likelihood of reduced peer acceptance. Friman, McPherson, Warzak, and Evans (1993) found that first grade students found their thumb sucking peers less likable than their nonsucking peers.

ASSESSMENT

What Should be Ruled Out?

Thumb sucking may present as a symptom of several behavior disorders which should be ruled out before thumb sucking can be treated as a simple habit. Thumb or finger sucking may be seen as a symptom of Stereotypic Movement Disorder, an anxiety disorder (such as OCD), and/or a tic disorder. However, when assessed carefully, it is unlikely that thumb sucking will actually meet the functional criterion described in the DSM-IV to be consistent with these diagnoses (Friman, et al., 2001). For example, though it may serve the purpose of self-soothing, thumb sucking is not typically associated with clinical levels of anxiety (e.g., Friman et al., 1994) and appears to be under greater volitional control than other behaviors more commonly seen as symptoms of these disorders. Furthermore, thumb sucking has been noted in individuals who meet criteria for disorders that may include regressive features (i.e., major depressive disorder, dissociative disorders; Friman et al., 2001) but will usually present as one of the many regressive behaviors observed in affected individuals and is not, in and of itself, indicative of caseness. Adequate clinical assessment for each of these disorders should be completed prior to developing a thumb sucking treatment plan.

What is Involved in Effective Assessment?

The primary assessment question with regard to thumb sucking is whether or not treatment is warranted. As described above, thumb sucking which becomes chronic (multiple environments after age 5) may be considered for treatment. When sucking only occurs at night and at home (the most common pattern of behavior), and is, therefore, not chronic, it is less likely to result in physical or psychological problems. In these cases, a "wait and see" approach may be appropriate. In addition, whether or not the habit is chronic, if the behavior begins to jeopardize biopsychosocial functioning, treatment is recommended.

When a child requests help with quitting, whether or not their habit is considered chronic, and especially when this request is attributed to social concerns, this request should be honored. Furthermore, if the child has been evaluated by a medical professional and has been diagnosed with a habit-related medical or dental condition, it would be appropriate to treat the problem. Finally, many parents may request treatment for a variety of social reasons of their own (i.e., embarrassment regarding the sucking behavior). However, parental requests alone are not a good indicator that treatment is necessary. Oftentimes parental education regarding the normative nature and spontaneous remission of thumb sucking is all that is clinically indicated, however, if parental reactions are severe and may negatively impact child–parent relationships, then treatment should be considered.

To best assess how the habit occurs in context, it is recommended that the clinician conduct a thorough functional analysis. Data may be most easily gathered through behavioral interviewing of both parents and child. Clients and their parents should be encouraged to collect data documenting the antecedents, specific behaviors, and consequences observed in relation to thumb sucking. For example, it would be important to note whether the child sucks his or her thumb in multiple environments or only in their bed at night and if they happen to do so only when they are holding their teddy bear, as each of these details may matter in treatment planning. Because the child themselves will likely not be aware of the behavior each time it occurs, especially if they tend to suck their thumb at night or at times when they are otherwise occupied (such as watching television), parents should take primary responsibility for recording data. Many parents find using time sample recording (periodically checking on their child during times when they may be sucking their thumb and recording whether or not the behavior was observed and details about the behavior if it did occur) as a useful strategy to collect data. While it will probably not be necessary to continue recording antecedents, behaviors, and consequences throughout treatment, a frequency count should be sustained throughout treatment and even beyond termination to track outcomes and determine if additional booster sessions may be necessary to prevent relapse.

In addition, if the child has not been recently evaluated by their pediatric primary care provider and a dentist, it should be recommended that they do so to ensure that any medical/dental problems related to the thumb sucking are adequately diagnosed and treated.

What Assessments are Not Helpful?

Traditional inferential assessment tools would not be useful in assessing thumb sucking as the behavior is conceptualized as a simple habit without underlying psychopathology.

TREATMENT

What Treatments are Effective?

Oral-digital habits are among the most treatable behavior problems. Treatment for oral digital habits has been approached using various methods including psychodynamic therapy, mechanical devices, and behavior modification. Of these, the empirical data clearly support the use of behavioral strategies.

Specific behavior modification techniques which have been demonstrated to be effective in treating habit disorders include a comprehensive habit reversal treatment package (e.g., Miltenberger, Fuqua, & Woods, 1998), response prevention (e.g., Watson & Allen, 1993; Van Houten & Rolider, 1984), changing establishing operations (Friman, 2000), differential reinforcement of alternative behavior (DRO/DRA) (e.g., Friman, 1987; Long, Miltenberger, Ellingson & Ott, 1999; Rapp, Miltenberger, Galensky, Roberts & Ellingson, 1999), assigning a response cost (e.g., Long et al., 1999), use of awareness enhancement devices (AEDs) (Ellingson et al., 2000), treatment to eliminate covarying behavior or the use of an attachment object (Friman, 1988; Friman & Hove, 1987), and aversive taste treatment (Friman & Hove, 1987). Of these empirically supported strategies, habit reversal, or components of habit reversal, are the most commonly cited treatment techniques in addressing problematic thumb sucking. As such, we will focus the remainder of this chapter on applying habit reversal strategies to changing thumb sucking behavior.

Habit reversal Habit reversal is considered the first-choice treatment for eliminating oral-digital habits (Woods et al., 1999; Long et al., 1999). Habit reversal is currently typically defined as consisting of several components including procedures designed to improve the motivation of the client to eliminate the habit, awareness training to enhance the child's ability to notice when they are engaging in the undesirable behavior, training a competing response that will effectively block the thumb sucking, and generalization procedures (e.g., Miltenberger et al., 1998; Rapp et al., 1998). Relaxation training is also often added to habit reversal protocols (e.g. Finney, Rapoff, Hall, & Christopherson, 1983). Several comprehensive procedural guides to conducting habit reversal have been recently published which provide detail beyond the scope of this chapter (please consult Adams, Adams, & Miltenberger, 2003, or Christophersen & Mortweet, 2001 for excellent descriptions).

As described above, several of the strategies included in habit reversal protocols have also been demonstrated to be effective independently (e.g. awareness training) and in combination with other methods, such as the application of a response cost (Long et al., 1999). In the treatment of thumb sucking, improving awareness of the habit and training competing responses appear to be the most critical components of habit reversal. Because the focus of treatment is changing the behavior of a child, implementing reinforcement procedures to increase and maintain motivation are also important. Other treatment components may be employed as clinically indicated.

Awareness training Both parents and the child themselves should attempt to notice each time thumb sucking occurs. Parents should be instructed to bring their child's attention to the behavior when they notice it but to do so in a nonpunitive, supportive manner that does not embarrass the child. Because thumb sucking is frequently a private behavior, the child will likely have to take some responsibility for noticing when the behavior occurs such that it can be changed.

Several tools may help children "catch themselves" sucking their thumb. First, temporary modifications to the thumb itself which alter its stimulus properties may improve awareness. For example, a bandage or rubber thimble may be applied to the thumb (or preferred finger) such that when the child inserts the thumb in his or her mouth the previously pleasurable sensation will be absent, drawing their attention to the problem behavior and allowing them to curtail the activity. Mildly unpleasant tasting substances which are safe for consumption may also be applied to the nail or finger such that the child will experience an unusual taste upon insertion of the thumb. Nail polish may be sufficient to serve this purpose and, if not, several products are sold commercially at drug stores for this purpose. When this technique is used to improve awareness, it is recommended that the child actively participate in the application (and reapplication, after a sucking event) of "reminder fluid" such that the function of applying the substance remains raising awareness and does not become punishment (Friman & Hove, 1987). We do not recommend the use of hot sauce or other similar substances to improve awareness as the potential for the procedure to be painful, and, hence, punishing, is too great.

When these more subtle (and virtually invisible) methods fail to improve awareness, more invasive strategies, such as having the child wear mittens (and ensuring that the mittens remain on), may be implemented. This strategy not only raises awareness of when thumb sucking happens, but also serves as a competing response. With older children who are highly motivated to stop sucking their thumbs, negative practice may be employed to raise awareness, such as having the child frequently, repeatedly, and painstakingly suck their thumb in front of a mirror.

Competing response training The principle of training a competing response is to have the child engage in a behavior that is of a mutually exclusive class of behavior than thumb sucking such that it is physically impossible for them to do the competing response and suck their thumb simultaneously. Competing behaviors should be practiced each time the child (or supportive parent) notices that they have begun sucking their thumb and as a preventive measure when the child is in a situation in which it is likely that they will suck their thumb (e.g., lying down to sleep).

Fortunately for our clients, there are a great many behaviors incompatible with thumb sucking, some of which may even serve a similar function. Choosing an appropriate competing response is dependent upon understanding when the thumb sucking behavior occurs and finding a replacement behavior which is more acceptable than the problematic habit. For children who engage in thumb sucking to reduce anxiety in social situations, for example, an effective competing response may be to place their hands in their pockets either when they begin to feel afraid or when they notice themselves bringing their thumb to their mouth. We treated one child who enhanced this strategy by always keeping a "lucky penny" in his pocket which he would then rub whenever he felt nervous. Because many children engage in thumb sucking to help fall asleep, suggestions as simple as going to sleep with their hands clenched or under their pillow may be helpful. For others, holding on to a treasured toy which either requires the use of their thumb to hold (such as a baseball) or blocks access to their thumb (such as a baseball mitt) may be an effective competing response.

Motivation enhancement strategies As with changing any behavior, it is helpful to be mindful of the problematic consequences of the habit prior to beginning treatment. Children who suck their thumbs may want to quit for a variety of reasons including social, behavioral, and physical. To improve their motivation to stop sucking their thumbs, clients should be queried regarding their reasons for wanting to stop to highlight the negative consequences of continuing the behavior. For example, children may be embarrassed to be observed sucking their thumbs by family members or friends. This fear of social ridicule or rejection may be more salient if older siblings become aware of the behavior, if the child naps in a group setting (e.g., all day kindergarten) and/or if they reach an age when they would want to sleep over at another child's house and fear being observed sucking their thumbs. Furthermore, thumb sucking may begin to interfere behaviorally with activities the older child finds desirable to engage in. For example, it is virtually impossible to learn to ride a two-wheel bike without training wheels, a highly desirable skill, while also sucking one's thumb. For truly chronic thumbsuckers, the behavior itself may become physically painful when lesions in the skin cannot heal due to being repeatedly irritated and exposed to moisture while sucking. While these are some commonly reported negative consequences, the clinician should take care to adequately investigate and enhance, when possible, each child's reasons for wanting to stop.

Once treatment has begun, few factors will help to motivate as effectively as the social support of important family members. Though many parents will naturally reinforce their children for their efforts to change their behavior, clinicians may be helpful by reminding parents of their power to influence their child's behavior, providing novel ideas about how to encourage their child that the parents may not have previously utilized, and strongly discouraging the use of punishment to eliminate oral-digital habits. In fact, some findings suggest that parents should increase the amount of time spent in intense positive interactions with their child prior to beginning a thumb sucking protocol (Friman, Barone, & Christophersen, 1986).

First and foremost, parents should be instructed to notice when their child does not engage in the problem behavior, instead of just noticing when thumb sucking does occur. Each of these occasions should prompt praise from the parent. Furthermore, parents should praise their child each time the child complies with any component of the treatment plan, from attending therapy sessions to practicing a competing response when they notice that they have brought their thumb to their mouth. Parents should be coached to praise their child in ways which are specific to the behavior being reinforced (e.g., "I noticed how you caught yourself starting to suck your thumb and put your hand in your pocket. That was awesome!") and to remain positive and encouraging with regard to their child's efforts to change (e.g., "I know how hard you are trying; keep up the good work.").

Parents should also be persuaded to provide other forms of reinforcement in addition to social support whenever possible. Like praise, other reinforcers should be delivered whenever the child engages in behavior consistent with the treatment plan. Clinicians may remind parents that reinforcement may take many forms including, but not limited to, tangible reinforcers such as small gifts or treats, special privileges, access to home resources, and the opportunity to engage in desirable activities. A variety of reinforcers can and should be planned to maximize the probability to treatment efforts being successful.

Generalization When the habit has been eliminated in one situation (such as bedtime), it will be necessary to work toward generalization of skills to all relevant occasions (naptime, while watching TV). For most children, once strategies have been employed successfully in the presence of one set of stimuli, these same strategies may then be applied to other situations, particularly if the two contexts are similar, with excellent results. Parents may facilitate generalization by reminding their child to use their skills in multiple circumstances and of the similarities between different contexts. When appears to have multiple functions, such as when a child sucks her thumb both to help fall asleep and to decrease anxiety when she is in a novel social situation, it may be necessary to employ unique sets of strategies to address the habit in the presence of each set of stimuli.

How Does One Select Among Treatments?

In addition to the treatment outcome data, when deciding on a treatment plan for a specific case, the clinician must remain mindful of three additional variables.

First, the acceptability of various strategies to both parents and the child-client must be considered. For this reason, it is recommended that treatments which inherently require higher levels of commitment on the part of the family because of their intensive and/or aversive nature be avoided unless less invasive methods have been tried and failed. Second, depending on the availability of family resources (such as time and energy to devote to solving the problem of thumb sucking) and the level of motivation/cognitive development of the child, clinicians may choose to employ either a single strategy or several in a comprehensive treatment package. Finally, any relevant assessment data which would suggest including particular treatment components should be carefully considered. For example, if a functional analysis revealed that thumb sucking was being used as an anxiety management strategy, it would be appropriate and necessary to include relaxation training in the treatment package. Or, as another example, if thumb sucking occurred only in the presence of an attachment object, removing the attachment object may well solve the problem of thumb sucking.

REFERENCES

Adams, A. N., Adams, M. A., & Miltenberger, R. G. (2003). Habit reversal. In W. T. O'Donohue, J. E. Fisher & S. C. Hayes (Eds.), Empirically Supported Techniques of Cognitive Behavior Therapy: A Step-By-Step Guide for Clinicians, (pp. 189–195). New York: John Wiley.

Bakwin, H. (1948). Thumb and finger sucking in children. *Journal of Pediatrics, 32,* 99–101.

Brenchley, M. L. (1991). Is digit of signficance? *British Dental Journal, 171,* 357–362.

Christophersen, E. R., & Mortweet, S. L. (2001). *Treatments That Work With Children: Empirically Supported Strategies for Managing Childhood Problems.* Washington, DC: American Psychological Association.

Davidson, P. O., Haryett, R. D., Sandilands, & R. Hansen, F. C. (1967). Thumb sucking: Habit or symptom? *Journal of Dentistry for Children, 34,* 252–259.

Ellingson, S. A., et al. (2000). Analysis and treatment of finger sucking. *Journal of Applied Behavior Analysis, 33,* 41–52.

Finney, J. W., & Friman, P. C. (1988). Behavioral medicine approaches to the prevention of mental retardation. In D. C. Russo & J. H. Kedesdy (Eds.), Behavioral Medicine with the Developmentally Disabled (pp. 173–200). New York: Plenum Press.

Finney, J. W., Rapoff, M. A., Hall, C. L., & Christophersen, E. R. (1983). Replication and social validation of habit reversal treatment for tics. *Behavior Therapy, 14,* 116–126.

Friman, P. C. (2000). "Transitional objects" as establishing operations for thumb sucking: A case study. Journal of Applied Behavior Analysis, 33, 507–509.

Friman, P. C. (1987). Thumb sucking in childhood. Feelings: Their medical significance. *The Ross Laboratories Newsletter, 29,* 11–14.

Friman, P. C., Byrd, M. R., & Oksol, E. M. (2001). Characteristics of oral-digital habits. In D. W. Woods & R. G. Miltenberger (Eds.), *Tic Disorders, Trichotillomania, and Other Repetitive Behavioral Disorders: Behavioral Approaches to Analysis and Treatment* (pp. 197–222). Norwell, MA: Kluwer.

Friman, P. C., Barone, V. J., & Christophersen, E. R. (1986). Aversive taste treatment of finger and thumb sucking. *Pediatrics, 78,* 174–176.

Friman, P. C., & Hove G. (1987). Apparent covariation between child habit disorders: Effects of successful treatment for thumb sucking on untargeted chronic hair pulling. *Journal of Applied Behavior Analysis, 20,* 421–425.

Friman, P. C., Larzelere, R., & Finney, J. W. (1994). *Journal of Pediatric Psychology, 19,* 431–441.

Friman, P. C., McPherson, K. M., Warzak, W. J., & Evans, J. (1993). Influence of thumb sucking on peer social acceptance in first-grade children. *Pediatrics, 91,* 784–786.

Friman, P. C., & Schmitt, B. D. (1989). Thumb sucking: Pediatricians' Guidelines. *Clinical Pediatrics, 28,* 438–440.

Gellin, M. E. (1978). Digital sucking and tongue thrusting in children. *Dental Clinics of North America, 22,* 603–619.

Infante, P. F. (1976). An epidemiologic study of finger habits in preschool children, as related to malocclusion, socioeconomic status, race, sex, and size of community. *Journal of Dentistry for Children, 43,* 33–38.

Josell, S. D. (1995). Habits affecting dental and maxillo facial growth and development. *Dental Clinics of North America, 39,* 851–860.

Klein, E. T. (1971). The thumbsucking habit: Meaningful or empty? *American Journal of Orthodontics, 59* 283–289. has not been included.

Kravitz, H., & Boehm, J. J. (1971). Rhythmic habit patterns in infancy: Their sequence, age of onset, and frequency. *Child Development, 42,* 399–413.

Larsson, E. F., & Dahlin, K. G. (1985). The prevalence and the etiology of the initial dummy- and finger-sucking habit. *American Journal of Orthodontics, 87,* 432–435.

Leung, A. K., & Robson, W. L. (1991). Thumb sucking. *American Family Physician, 44,* 1724–1728.

Long, E. S., Miltenberger, R. G., Ellingson, S. A., & Ott, S. M. (1999). Augmenting simplified habit reversal in the treatment of oral-digital habits exhibited by individuals with mental retardation. *Journal of Applied Behavior Analysis, 32,* 353–365.

Mahalski, P. A., & Stanton, W. R. (1992). The relationship between digit sucking and behaviour problems: a longitudinal study over 10 years. *Journal of Child Psychology and Psychiatry, 33,* 913–923.

Miltenberger, R. G., Fuqua, R. W., & Woods, D. W. (1998). Applying behavior analysis to clinical problems: Review and analysis of habit reversal. *Journal of Applied Behavior Analysis, 31,* 447–469.

Moore, G. J., McNeill, R. W., & D'Anna, J. A. (1972). The effects of digit sucking on facial growth. *Journal of the American Dental Association, 84,* 592–599.

Ozturk, M., & Ozturk, O. M. (1977). Thumb sucking a falling asleep. *British Journal of Medical Psychology, 50,* 95–103.

Peterson, J. E. (1982). Pediatric oral habits. In R. E. Stewart, T. K. Barber, K. C. Troutman, & S. H. I. Wei (Eds.), *Pediatric dentistry: Scientific foundations and clinical practice* (pp. 361–372). St. Louis, MO: The C.V. Mosby Company.

Popovich, F., & Thompson, G. W. (1974). Thumb and finger sucking: Analysis of contributory factors in 1,258 children. *Canadian Journal of Public Health, 65,* 277–280.

Rankin, E. A., Jabaley, M. E., Blair, S. J., & Fraser, K. E. (1988). Acquired rotational digital deformity in children as a result of finger sucking. *The Journal of Hand Surgery, 13,* 535–539.

Rapp, J. T., Miltenberger, R. G., Galensky, T. L., Roberts, J., & Ellington, S. A. (1999). Brief functional analysis and simplified habit reversal treatment of thumb sucking in fraternal twin brothers. *Child & Family Behavior Therapy, 21*(2), 1–17.

Rugh, J. D., & Lemke, R. R. (1984). Significance of oral habits. In J. D. Matarazzo, S. M. Weiss, J. A. Herd, N. E. Miller, & S. M. Weiss (Eds.) *Handbook of health enhancement and disease prevention* (pp. 947–966). New York: John Wiley and Sons.

Tryon, A. F. (1968). Thumb sucking and manifest anxiety: A note. *Child Development, 39,* 1159–1163.

Van Houten, R., & Rolider, A. (1984). The use of response prevention to eliminate nocturnal thumbsucking. *Journal of Applied Behavior Analysis, 17,* 509–520.

Vogel, L. D. (1998). When children put their fingers in their mouths. Should parents and dentists care? *The New York State Dental Journal, 64,* 48–53. has not been included.

Watson, T. S., & Allen, K. D. (1993). Elimination of thumb sucking as a treatment for severe trichotillomania. *Journal of American Academy of Child and Adolescent Psychiatry, 32,* 830–834.

Tic Disorders

Douglas W. Woods • Michael B. Himle • Christopher A. Flessner

WHAT IS A TIC DISORDER?

Tics are "sudden, rapid, recurrent, nonrhythmic, stereotyped motor movements (motor tics), or vocalizations (vocal tics)." (American Psychiatric Association, 2001, p. 108). The Diagnostic and Statistic Manual of Mental Disorders, Fourth Edition—Text Revision (DSM-IVTR; APA), describes four different tic disorders (TDs) (e.g., chronic tic disorder (CTD), Tourette's disorder, transient tic disorder, and tic disorder not otherwise specified). Single or multiple motor or vocal tics, but not both, persisting for at least 1 year characterize CTD, whereas multiple motor tics and one or more vocal tics persisting for at least 1 year characterize TD. Although not studied as frequently, transient tic disorder (TTD) is characterized by single or multiple motor and/or vocal tics occurring for at least 4 weeks but no longer than 12 months. All of the tic disorders described above require onset before age 18.

Basic Facts about Tic Disorders

Comorbidity As many as 95% of individuals diagnosed with a TD meet diagnostic criteria for another psychiatric condition (Coffey et al., 2000ab). One-half to two-thirds of TD patients may also meet diagnostic criteria for attention-deficit hyperactivity disorder (ADHD: Cohen, Friedhoff, Leckman, & Chase, 1992; Comings & Comings, 1985; Gadow, Nolan, Sprafkin, & Schwarz, 2002; Kadesjo & Gillberg, 2000). Similarly high comorbidity rates have been shown with respect to obsessive–compulsive disorder (OCD; Cohen et al., 1992; Comings & Comings, 1985; Hebebrand et al., 1997; Santangelo et al., 1994; Shapiro, Shapiro, Wayne, Clarkin, & Bruun, 1973; Spencer, Biederman, Harding, Wilens, & Farlone, 1995). Individuals diagnosed with TD also frequently suffer from learning disorders and/or learning difficulties (e.g., problems with arithmetic; Caine et al., 1988; Cohen et al., 1992; Comings & Comings, 1985; Dykens et al., 1990; Kadesjo & Gillberg, 2000). Psychiatric conditions such as simple phobia, overanxious disorder, separation anxiety, major depressive disorder, bipolar disorder, conduct disorder, and oppositional defiant disorder have also been found to cooccur with TD more frequently than the general prevalence rates for these disorders would predict (Coffey et al., 2000a, 2000b; Gadow et al., 2002; Kadesjo & Gillberg, 2000; Mason, Banerjee, Eapen, Zeitlin, & Robertson, 1998; Spencer et al., 1995).

Prevalence Reports on to the prevalence of TD suggest the disorder is present in approximately 1% of the population (Robertson, 2003), although estimates vary from 0.04% to 3.0% (Khalifa & Knorring, 2003; Kadesjo & Gillberg, 2000; Mason, Banerjee, Eapen, Zeitlin, & Robertson, 1998). Research suggests that approximately 0.8% of the population suffer from chronic motor tics, 0.5% suffer from chronic vocal tics, and as many as 4.8% suffer from transient tics (Khalifa & Knorring, 2003).

Woods, D. W., Himle, M. B., & Flessner, C. A. (2006). Tic disorders. In J. E. Fisher & W. T. O'Donohue (Eds.), *Practitioner's guide to evidence-based psychotherapy*. New York: Springer.

Age at onset The median age of onset for the development of tics in TD is approximately 7 years of age (APA, 2001; Burd, Kerbeshian, Cook, Bornhoeft, & Fisher, 1988; Caine et al., 1988; Shapiro, et al., 1973). However, tics may first appear at as young an age as 2–4 years (APA, 2001; Caine et al., 1988; Santangelo et al., 1994).

Gender and ethnicity Tourette's disorder has been reported across many races and ethnicity (APA, 2001) and research suggests that tic disorders are more common in males than females (e.g., Caine et al., 1988; Kadesjo & Gillberg, 2000; Gadow et al., 2002; Khalifa & Knorring, 2003; Robertson, 2003), by a ratio of 3–9:1 (Khalifa & Knorring, 2003; Robertson, 2003).

Course. Tics typically wax and wane in both frequency and severity and in many cases decrease significantly or disappear as the person enters adulthood (APA, 2001). Most available epidemiological data suggest the prevalence of tic disorders, particularly the prevalence of TD, is considerably lower among adults than children (APA, 2001; Leckman, King, & Cohen, 1999).

ASSESSMENT

What Should be Ruled Out?

When conducting an assessment for tic disorders, the clinician should conduct a thorough examination of the client's behavior and assess whether it is the direct, physiological effect of a substance or a general medical condition. Certain neuroleptic medications can produce behaviors that may be mistaken for a tic disorder. In addition, the clinician should take care to ensure that the behavior the client displays is not the result of another physical condition (e.g., Sydenham's chorea, Huntington's disease, multiple sclerosis, head injury, stroke, etc.). Finally, the clinician must be ready to distinguish tics from movements commonly associated with other psychiatric conditions, such as OCD, stereotypic movement disorder and stereotypic behaviors associated with pervasive developmental disorders (APA, 2001).

What is Involved in Effective Assessment?

Clinician-administered measures To aid in the assessment of tic severity, several clinician administered tic-rating scales, including the Yale Global Tic Severity Scale (YGTSS), have been developed. The YGTSS (Leckman et al., 1989) has been shown to be a reliable and valid, clinician-rated measure of tic severity providing an evaluation of tic frequency, intensity, complexity, number, and resultant social interference. Examples of other assessment measures include the Tourette's Disorder Scale (TDOS) (Shytle et al., 2003) and the Yale Tourette Syndrome Symptom List (YTSSL), but for a more thorough examination of tic-related measures the reader is urged to read Scahill, King, Schultz, and Leckman (1999).

Diagnostic interview It is also important for the clinician to obtain as accurate and as detailed a family and personal history as possible. In addition to determining age of onset and duration of tic free periods, it is useful to assess for a family history of TD and the possibility of onset of tic symptoms immediately following a streptoccal infection (e.g., Lougee, Perlmutter, Nicolson, Garvey, & Swedo, 2000). The latter issue is important as a positive report of such a history may indicate the presence of a separate condition, (pediatric autoimmune neurpsychiatric disorder associated with streptoccal infection PANDAS), which may require an alternative treatment strategy. It is also important to develop a conceptualization of events, situations, and other environmental factors preceding the tics, as these environmental variables may aid in explaining the common phenomena of symptom waxing and waning. These events, possibly unbeknownst to the client or the client's parent(s), may exacerbate tics.

Current level of functioning In the treatment of TD, it is especially important to evaluate other area of functioning that may be impacted. The clinician should obtain as much information as possible regarding the effects tics have on social, academic, and occupational functioning. Clients with TD may experience problems in peer relationships, social acceptability, and occupational satisfaction (Friedrich, Morgan, & Devine, 1999; Stokes, Bawden, Camfield, Backman, & Dooley, 1991). The clinician must also assess for cooccurring diagnoses, such as depression, ADHD, learning disabilities, and/or anxiety disorders and how these problems interact with the tic disorder (e.g., the presence of tics may lead to the exacerbation or development of major depressive disorder or other psychiatric conditions). An assessment for the presence of these conditions is necessary before a proper case conceptualization can be developed and adequate treatment recommendations made. In addition, this information must be collected to determine if the TD in question should be the primary focus of concern.

What Assessments are Not Helpful?

Traditional psychological tests such as personality tests (e.g., MMPI, MCMI, etc.) and projective tests are not useful in assessing tic disorders.

TREATMENT

What Treatments are Effective?

Behavioral and pharmacological interventions have shown the most empirical support for the treatment of TDs. Habit reversal training (HRT) is the most widely used behavioral intervention for TDs, and a variety of pharmacological interventions have shown varying degrees of success in their effectiveness at reducing both the frequency and severity of tics. What follows is a brief review of research supporting therapist based and medical treatments for tics disorders and some of the limitations associated with these respective intervention strategies.

What are Effective Medical Treatments?

Pharmacological interventions have traditionally been the treatment of choice for TDs. The most commonly prescribed pharmaceuticals are dopamine antagonists (i.e., reuptake inhibitors) such as typical and atypical neuroleptics. A few of the most frequently prescribed typical neuroleptics are haloperidol (Haldol) and pimozide (Orap). Common atypical neuroleptics include olanzapine (Zyprexa) and risperidone (Risperdal). Neuroleptics, although somewhat efficacious, are not well tolerated by many individuals and have side effect profiles ranging from benign, irritating symptoms (e.g., fatigue, weight gain, sedation, akathisia) to longer term effects such as tardive dyskinesia (Carpenter, Leckman, Scahill, & McDougle, 1999; Watson, Howell, & Smith, 2001).

Other pharmaceuticals that are frequently used to treat tics include α-adrenergic receptor agonists, the most common of which include clonidine (Catapres) and guanfacine (Tenex). Although these agents typically have fewer side-effects, efficacy studies have shown that only about one-quarter of individuals benefit significantly from these drugs (Carpenter et al., 1999; Watson et al., 2001). Nevertheless, they are often prescribed due to their mild attention-enhancing effects and relatively benign side effect profile (Carpenter et al., 1999). The existing body of research concerning the efficacy of pharmacological interventions for TS is extensive, complex, and well beyond the scope of this chapter. However, several detailed reviews have been published, and we refer interested readers to these reviews (Peterson & Azrin, 1993; Carpenter et al., 1999). Perhaps it is sufficient to summarize that pharmacological interventions, though effective for some individuals with TS, are not universally efficacious, rarely result in an absolute amelioration of symptoms, and often have side effect profiles sufficient to prevent their use with some patients.

What are Effective Psychosocial Treatments?

Behavioral interventions: Habit reversal Nonpharmacological interventions are becoming increasingly popular as adjuncts or alternatives to pharmacotherapy. The most widely used behavioral intervention for TD is a multicomponent treatment package called habit reversal training (HRT; Azrin & Nunn, 1973). As originally developed, the principle components of HRT were self-monitoring, inconvenience reviews, stimulus control, awareness training, relaxation training, competing response training, social support, and public display. The goal of the procedure is to help an individual become more aware of situations in which they perform a tic and contingently engage in an alternative, incompatible behavior (Azrin & Nunn, 1973).

Between 1973 and 1985, several studies demonstrated the effectiveness of HRT for the treatment of repetitive behaviors (see Carr & Chong, in press; Peterson & Azrin, 1993, for reviews). More recently, analyses of the unique contributions of the various components of HRT have shown that the entire package may not be needed for many individuals. In fact, an abbreviated version of the procedure has been shown to be equally as effective as the original (Miltenberger, Fuqua, & McKinley, 1985). This modified version includes only three components: awareness training, competing response training, and social support (Woods, 2001).

The first component of modified HRT is awareness training. During awareness training, the client is taught to recognize each discrete tic. Through instruction and practice, the client learns to describe and recognize his or her tic(s) and any premonitory sensations or warning signs (e.g., the beginning of the tic movement) that precede the tic(s), both before they occur and when they are exhibited. After the client becomes aware of his/her tics, he/she is taught to engage in a behavior that is incompatible with the tic (called the "competing response") contingent on each incidence of the tic or pre-tic warning signs. Social support provides motivation and reminders for using the competing response. Friends or family members are taught to praise the client intermittently for therapy progress and each time he or she uses the competing response. The social support person also reminds the client to use the competing response whenever a tic is observed and the competing response is not used.

Several empirical studies demonstrate HRT to be efficacious in the treatment of TS (for a review see Carr & Chong, in press) and in a recent study HRT was shown to be significantly more efficacious than supportive psychotherapy for individuals with TS (Wilhelm et al., 2003). Although the literature showing HRT to be effective for TS supports its use as a primary treatment for tics, not all individuals with TS benefit from self-management strategies. In fact, there is growing evidence that some individuals may not respond to HRT or may require ancillary treatments. For example, research has shown that individuals with developmental disabilities may not benefit from traditional HRT unless the procedures are supplemented with awareness enhancement procedures or contrived reinforcement for using the procedures (e.g., Rapp, Miltenberger, Long, Elliot, & Lumley, 1998; Woods, Fuqua, & Waltz, 1997). The same has been shown for children below six years of age (Long, Miltenberger, & Rapp, 1999; Woods et al., 1999).

Alternative behavioral interventions Other behavioral interventions have also been used to treat TS, with varying degrees of success. Varni, Boyd, and Cataldo (1978) successfully treated a seven-year-old boy with multiple motor and vocal tics (who was also hyperactive) using self-monitoring, operant reinforcement, and time-out procedures. Other studies have also shown reinforcement and punishment may be an effective treatment for some individuals with TS (e.g., Lahey, McNees, & McNees, 1973; Doleys & Kurtz, 1974). Unfortunately, more rigorous, controlled studies have not been conducted, thus limiting conclusions about the efficacy and effectiveness of such procedures for TS.

Massed negative practice (MNP) has also been used to treat tics. When using MNP, a therapist instructs a patient to "practice" his/her tic movements continuously for some period of time, several times each day. For example, Nicassio, Liberman, Patterson, Ramirez, & Sanders (1972) instructed two individuals with motor tics to practice their tics continuously for 10 minutes each day and to self-monitor their rate of tics throughout the day. The efficacy of MNP reported in the literature is mixed (Azrin, Nunn, & Frantz, 1980; Kaliappan & Murthy, 1982). Nicassio et al. (1972) demonstrated MNP to be successful for one participant but not another. Other studies have shown MNP to have paradoxical effects in which tics worsened enough that treatment was discontinued.

Like many neurobiological conditions, the symptoms of TS are influenced by environmental events. Emotional and physical states such as fatigue, boredom, anxiety, excitement, and fear have all been associated with exacerbation or amelioration of tics (Silva, Munoz, Barickman, & Friedhoff, 1995). Social events such as public gatherings, talking to friends, and doctor visits have also been shown to influence tics (Silva et al., 1995). Woods, Watson, Wolfe, Twohig, & Firman (2001) demonstrated that talking about tics can increase vocal tics in some individuals with TS, and Woods and Himle (in press) demonstrated that when environmental conditions reinforce tic suppression, tics decreased substantially in some children with multiple motor and vocal tics. Given the reactive nature of tics, a thorough, idiopathic functional assessment of contextual events is warranted when assessing or treating individuals with TS. In addition, environmental restructuring to minimize events that exacerbate tics and strategically establishing contexts that minimizes tics may be warranted.

What are Effective Self-Help Treatments?

A small, yet growing, collection of books exists which include many elements of HRT and other effective treatment strategies for the treatment of TDs. In addition, several Internet sites exist providing a variety of resources for information about TD and other tic disorders. Nevertheless, research has not established the efficacy of these modes of intervention in ameliorating tic symptoms. What follows is a short list of self-help materials, books, and internet sources which may prove beneficial for individuals looking to obtain more information regarding tic disorders.

- Kurlan, R. (Ed.). (1993). *Handbook of Tourette's syndrome and related tic and behavioral disorders.* New York, NY: Marcel Dekker Publishing
- Leckman, J. F., & Cohen, D. J. (1999). *Tourette syndrome: Tics, obsessions, and compulsions.* New, York, NY: Harper Collins
- Shimberg, E. F. (1995). *Living with Tourette syndrome.* New York: Simon & Schuster.

- Woods, D. W., & Miltenberger, R. G. (Eds.). (2001). *Tic disorders, Trichotillomania, and other repetitive behavior disorders: Behavioral approaches to analysis and treatment.* Boston, MA: Kluwer Academic Publishers.

Useful informational websites about TS and other TDs and related resources include:

- *http://www.tsa-usa.org* (Tourette Syndrome Association, official website)
- *http:// www.tourettesyndrome.net/* (Tourette Syndrome Plus, home page)
- *http://info. med.yale.edu/chldstdy/tsocd* (Yale Child Study Center and TS/OCS Clinic)
- *http://www.nlm.nih.gov/medlineplus/tourettesyndrome.html* (National Institute of Mental Health)
- *http://www.tourette-syndrome.com/* (Tourette Syndrome online)
- *http://www.tourette.net/* (source for additional links with information regarding TS)

How Does One Select Among Treatments?

A decision upon which form of treatment (pharmacological, nonpharmacological, or combination) should be implemented for a given client should be based upon a clear and coherent conceptualization of the client's case. Given the relatively high prevalence of psychiatric comorbidity in the tic disordered population, it is often the case the comorbid conditions require more urgent clinical attention. Nevertheless, should tic symptoms require intervention, the decision must be made to use medication, psychosocial interventions, or a combination. Ultimately, the client's care provider should be knowledgeable of the options and present them to the client in a clear fashion. Typically, medications are not prescribed for mild tics, and indeed, psychosocial monotherapy may be an desirable treatment strategy. Medication is often considered with more moderate to severe tics. With regard to medication, side effects should be discussed with the client, and physical complaints which may restrict the use of this medication should be examined. Past history obtained from previous psychiatrists and/or psychologists with regard to the client's compliance with treatment procedures (e.g., did he/she take his/her medication regularly, did he/she attend sessions on a regular basis, etc.) should also play a major role in the clinician's decision as to which intervention he/she decides upon. Psychosocial intervention can also be effective for moderately severe tics, but its efficacy with the most severe cases remains unclear. Although it is becoming a relatively common clinical practice, the efficacy of combined therapies has not been empirically established.

REFERENCES

American Psychiatric Association (2001). *Diagnostic and statistical manual of mental disorders (4th ed., text revision).* Washington, DC Author.

Azrin, N. H., & Nunn, R. G. (1973). Habit Reversal: a method of eliminating nervous habits and tics. *Behaviour Research and Therapy, 11*, 619–628.

Azrin, N. H., Nunn, R. G., & Frantz, S. E. (1980). Habit reversal vs. negative practice treatment of nervous tics. *Behavior Therapy, 11*, 169–178.

Caine, E. D., McBride, M. C., Chiverton, P., Bamford, K. A., Rediess, S., & Shiao, J. (1988). Tourette syndrome in Monroe county school children. *Neurology, 38*, 472–475.

Carpenter, L. L., Leckman, J. F., Scahill, L., & McDougle, C. J. (1999). Pharmocological and other somatic approaches to treatment. In J. F. Leckman, & D. J. Cohen (Eds.), *Tourette syndrome—tics, obsessions, and compulsions: Developmental psychopathology and clinical care* (pp. 370–398). New York: John Wiley, & Sons, Inc.

Carr, J. E., & Chong, I. M. (in press). Habit reversal treatment of tic disorders: A methodological critique of the literature. *Behavior Modification.*

Coffey, B. A., Biederman, J., Geller, D. A., Spe, T. J., Kim, G. S., Bellordre, C. A., et al. (2000a). Distinguishing illness severity from tic severity in children and adolescents with Tourette's disorder. *Journal of the American Academy of Child and Adolescent Psychiatry, 39(5)*, 556–561.

Coffey, B. A., Biederman, J., Smoller, J. W., Geller, D. A., Sarin, P., Schwartz, S., et al. (2000b). Anxiety disorders and tic severity in juveniles with Tourette's disorder. *Journal of the American Academy of Child and Adolescent Psychiatry, 39(5)*, 562–568.

Cohen, D. J., Friedhoff, A. J., Leckman, J. F., & Chase, T. N. (1992). Tourette syndrome: Extending basic research to clinical care. In T. N. Chase, A. J. Friedhoff, & D. J. Cohen (Eds.). *Advances in neurology*, New York; Raven Press, Ltd.

Comings, D. E., & Comings, B. G. (1985). Tourette syndrome: Clinical and psychological aspects of 250 cases. *American Journal of Human Genetics, 37*, 435–450.

Doleys, D. M., & Kurtz, P.S. (1974). A behavioral treatment program for the Gilles de la Tourette Syndrome. *Psychological Reports, 35*, 43–48.

Dykens, E., Leckman, J., Riddle, M., Hardin, M., Schwartz, S., & Cohen, D. (1990). Intellectual, academic, and adaptive functioning of Tourette syndrome children with and without attention deficit disorder. *Journal of Abnormal Child Psychology, 18(6)*, 607–615.

Friedrich, S., Morgan, S. B., & Devine, C. (1996). Children's attitudes and behavioral intentions toward a peer with Tourette's syndrome, *Journal of Pediatric Psychology, 21(3)*, 307–319.

Gadow, K. D., Nolan, E. E., Sprafkin, J., & Schwarz, J. (2002). Tics and comorbidity in children and adolescents. *Developmental Medicine & Child Neurology, 44*, 330–338.

Kadesjo, B., & Gillberg, C. (2000). Tourette disorder: Epedemiology and comorbidity in primary school children. *Journal of the American Academy of Child and Adolescent Psychiatry, 39(5)*, 545–555.

Kaliappan, K. V., & Murthy, H. N. (1982). Negative practice and tics—a case analysis. *Journal of Psychological Researchers, 26(2)*, 61–62.

Khalifa, N., & von Knorring, A. (2003). Prevalence of tic disorders and Tourette syndrome in a Swedish school population. *Developmental Medicine & Child Neurology, 45*, 315–319.

Lahey, B. B., McNees, M. P., & McNees, M. C. (1973). Control of an obscene "verbal tic" through time out in an elementary classroom. *Journal of Applied Behavior Analysis, 6*, 101–104.

Leckman, J. F., Riddle, M. A., Hardin, M. T., Ort, S. I., Swartz, K. L., Stevenson, J., et al. (1989). The Yale global tic severity scale: Initial testing of a clinician-rated scale of tic severity. *Journal of the American Academy of Child and Adolescent Psychiatry, 28(4)*, 566–573.

Leckman, J. F., King, R. A., & Cohen, D. J. (1999). Tics and tic disorders. In J. F. Leckman, & D. J. Cohen (Eds.). *Tourette's syndrome—tics, obsessions, compulsions: Developmental psychopathology and clinical care* (pp. 23–42). New York: John Wiley & Sons Inc.

Long, E. S., Miltenberger, R. G., & Rapp, J. T. (1999). Simplified habit reversal plus Adjunct contingencies in the treatment of thumb sucking and hair pulling in a young child. *Child and Family Behavior Therapy, 21*, 45–58.

Lougee, L., Perlmutter, S. J., Nicolson, R., Garvey, M. A., & Swedo, S. E. (2000). Psychiatric disorders in first-degree relatives of children with pediatric autoimmune neuropsychiatric disorders associated with streptococcal infections (PANDAS). *Journal of the American Academy of Child and Adolescent Psychiatry, 39(9)*, 1120–1126.

Mason, A., Banerjee, S., Eapen, V., Zeitlin, H., Robertson, M. M. (1998). The prevalence of Tourette syndrome in a mainstream school population. *Developmental Medicine & Child Neurology, 40*, 292–296.

Miltenberger, R. G., Fuqua, R. W., & McKinley, T. (1985). Habit reversal with muscle tics: Replication and component analysis. *Behavior Therapy, 16*, 39–50.

Nicassio, F. J., Liberman, R. P., Patterson, R. L., Ramirez, E., & Sanders, N. (1972). The treatment of tics by negative practice. *Journal of Behavior Therapy & Experimental Psychiatry, 3*, 281–287.

Peterson, A. L., & Azrin, N. H. (1993). Behavioral and pharmacological treatments for Tourette syndrome: A review. *Applied & Preventative Psychology, 2*, 231–242.

Rapp, J. T., Miltenberger, R. G., Long, E. S., Elliot, A. J., & Lumley, V. A. (1998). Simplified habit reversal treatment for chronic hair pulling in three adolescents: A clinical replication with direct observation. *Journal of Applied Behavior Analysis, 31*, 299–302.

Robertson, M. M. (2003). Diagnosing Tourette syndrome: Is it a common disorder? *Journal of Psychosomatic Research, 55*, 3–6.

Santangelo, S. L., Pauls, L., Goldstein, J. M., Faraone, S. V., Tsuan, M. T., & Leckman, F. (1994). Tourette's syndrome: What are the influences of gender and comorbid obsessive–compulsive disorder. *Journal of the American Academy of Child and Adolescent Psychiatry, 33(6)*, 795–804.

Scahill, L. S., King, R. A., Schultz, R. T., & Leckman, J. F. (1999). Selection and use of diagnostic and clinical rating instruments. In J. F. Leckman & D. J. Cohen (Eds.). *Tourette's Syndrome—tics, obsessions, compulsions: Developmental psychopathology and clinical care*. New York: John Wiley & Sons, Inc.

Shapiro, A. K., Shapiro, E., Wayne, H., Clarkin, J., & Bruun, R. D. (1973). Tourette's syndrome: Summary of data on 34 patients. *Psychosomatic Medicine, 35(5)*, 419–435.

Shytle, R. D., Silver, A. A., Sheehan, K. H., Wilkinson, B. J., Newman, M., Sanberg, P. R., et al. (2003). The Tourette's disorder scale (TODS): Development, reliability, and validity. *Assessment, 10(3)*, 273–287.

Silva, R. R., Munoz, D. M., Barickman, J., & Friedhoff, A. J. (1995). Environmental factors and related fluctuations of symptoms in children and adolescents with Tourette's disorder. *Journal of Child Psychology and Psychiatry, 36*, 305–312.

Spencer, T., Biederman, J., Harding, M., Wilens, T., & Faraone, S. (1995). The relationship between tic disorders and Tourette's syndrome revisited. *Journal of the American Academy of Child and Adolescent Psychiatry, 34(9)*, 1133–1139.

Stokes, A., Bawden, H. N., Camfield, P. R., Backman, J. E., & Dooley, J. M. (1991). Peer problems in Tourette's disorder, *Pediatrics, 87(6)*, 936–942.

Varni, J. W., Boyd, E. F., & Cataldo, M. F. (1978). Self-monitoring, external reinforcement, and timeout procedures in the control of high rate tic behaviors in a hyperactive child. *Journal of Behavior Therapy and Experimental Psychiatry, 9*, 353–358.

Watson, T. S., Howell, L. A., & Smith, S. L. (2001). Behavioral interventions for tic disorders. In D. W. Woods, & R. G. Miltenberger (Eds.), Tic Disorders, trichotillomania, and other repetitive behavior disorders: Behavioral approaches to analysis and treatment (pp. 73–96). Boston, MA: Kluwer Academic Publishers.

Wilhelm, S., Deckersbach, T., Coffey, B. J., Bohne, A., Peterson, A. L., & Baer, L. (2003). Habit reversal versus supportive psychotherapy for Tourette's disorder: A randomized controlled trial. *American Journal of Psychiatry, 160*, 1175–1176.

Woods, D. W. (2001). Habit reversal treatment manual for tic disorders. In D. W. Woods, & R. G. Miltenberger (Eds). *Tic disorders, trichotillomania, and other repetitive behavior disorders: Behavior approaches to analysis and treatment* (pp. 73–96). Boston: Kluwer Academic Publishers

Woods, D. W., Fuqua, R. W., & Waltz, T. J. (1997). Evaluation and elimination of an avoidance response in a child who stutters: A case study. *Journal of Fluency Disorders, 22*, 287–297.

Woods, D. W., & Himle, M. (in press). Understanding tic "suppression": Differential effects of two environmental variables on the rate of tic expression. *Journal of Applied Behavior Analysis.*

Woods, D. W., Murray, L. K., Fuqua, R. W., Seif, T. A., Boyer, L. J., & Siah, A. (1999). Comparing the effectiveness of similar and dissimilar competing responses in evaluating the habit reversal treatment for oral-digital habits in children. *Journal of Behavior Therapy an Experimental Psychiatry, 30*, 289–300.

Woods, D. W., Watson, T. S., Wolfe, E., Twohig, M. P., & Friman, P. C. (2001). Analyzing the influence of tic-related talk on vocal and motor tics in children with Tourette's syndrome. *Journal of Applied Behavior Analysis, 34*, 353–356.

Weight Loss

Brie A. Moore • Adrian Bowers

WHAT IS WEIGHT LOSS?

Weight loss is a decrease in body weight that occurs when energy expenditure exceeds energy input over time. For each individual, body weight is determined by genetic, metabolic, behavioral, environmental, cultural, and socioeconomic factors. The rapid increase in the prevalence of overweight and obesity strongly indicate that behavioral and environmental factors have played a significant role in contributing to the current epidemic. Many underscore a "toxic environment" (Horgen & Brownell, 1998), characterized by the promotion and accessibility of energy dense foods and increasingly sedentary lifestyles, as the primary contributing factor. This chapter will focus primarily on the behavioral treatment of overweight and obesity, including implementing and maintaining increases in energy expenditure (i.e., physical activity) and decreases in energy intake (i.e., food consumption).

Basic Facts about Overweight and Obesity

Overweight refers to an increased body weight in relation to height as compared to some standard of acceptable or desirable weight (CDC, 2004). Individuals with a Body Bass Index (BMI), or ratio of weight-to-height, of 25–25.9 are considered overweight.

Obesity is defined as an excessively high amount of body fat or adipose tissue in relation to lean body mass (CDC, 2004). Individuals with a BMI of 30 or greater are considered obese.

- Obesity is the number two cause of *preventable* death in the United States (Mokdad, Marks, Stroup, & Gerberding, 2004). It is a chronic disease that has reached global epidemic proportions (WHO, 2003).
- An estimated 64 % of adults in the United States are overweight or obese (NHANES, 1999–2000). The prevalence of obesity in adults has doubled from 15 to an estimated 31 percent in the last 25 years (NHANES, 1976–1980; 1999–2000).
  - According to the CDC's Behavioral Risk Factor Surveillance System, in 2002:
    18 states reported obesity prevalence rates of 15–19%
    29 states reported obesity prevalence rates of 20–24%
    3 states reported obesity prevalence rates greater than 25%
- In children and adolescents, approximately 1 in 5 children meet criteria for overweight or obesity (Dietz, 1998). Prevalence rates have nearly doubled in the last 25 years.
  - According to National Health and Nutrition Examination Survey data (NHANES II and III), prevalence rates increased from an estimated:
    7–11% in 6–11-year old children;
    5–11% in 12–19-year old children.
- In children, overweight is associated with increased risk for adult morbidity and mortality. Moreover, overweight children are at a heightened risk of becoming overweight adults.

Moore, B. A., & Bowers, A. (2006). Weight loss. In J. E. Fisher & W. T. O'Donohue (Eds.), *Practitioner's guide to evidence-based psychotherapy*. New York: Springer.

Mokdad et al. (1999, 2000, 2001, 2003) have examined prevalence data on the obesity epidemic since 1991. Their data show:

- These trends apply across all ages, educational levels, racial and ethnic groups and both genders.
- For all racial and ethnic groups combined, women of lower socioeconomic status (income less than 130% of the poverty threshold) are approximately 50% more likely to be obese than those of higher socioeconomic status.
- The prevalence of overweight and obesity increases until about age 60, after which it begins to decline.
- Overweight adolescents have a 70% chance of becoming overweight or obese adults. If one parent is overweight or obese, this risk increases to 80%.

- According to the National Institutes of Health Clinical Guidelines on the Identification, Evaluation and Treatment of Overweight and Obesity in Adults (1998), overweight and obese individuals are considered at-risk for premature death and disability.
- As BMI increases, risk for some diseases increases. Overweight and obese individuals are at increased risk for physical ailments such as (NIH, 1998; CDC, 2004):
  - high blood pressure, hypertension
  - high blood cholesterol, dyslipidemia
  - type 2 (noninsulin dependent) diabetes mellitus
  - resistance, glucose intolerance
  - hyperinsulinemia
  - heart disease
  - pectoris
  - congestive heart failure
  - stroke
  - gallstones
  - cholescystitis and cholelithiasis
  - gout
  - osteoarthritis
  - obstructive sleep apnea syndrome and respiratory problems
  - endometirial, breast, prostrate, and colon cancer
  - pregnancy complications (e.g., gestational diabetes, gestational hypertension, preeclampsia, fetal neural tube defects, and delivery complications)
  - Poor female reproductive health (e.g., menstrual irregularities, infertility, irregular ovulation)
  - uric acid nephrolithiasis
  - psychological disorders (e.g., depression, eating disorders, distorted body image, low self-esteem)
  - Individuals who gain 11–18-pounds have an increased risk of developing type 2 diabetes mellitus twice that of those who have not gained weight (Surgeon General's Call to Action, 2004).
  - Females who gain more than 20-pounds from 18-years-old to midlife double their risk of postmenopausal breast cancer, compared to those whose weight remains stable.
  - Obesity during pregnancy is associated with increased risk of death in both the mother and newborn and a tenfold increased risk in maternal high blood pressure.
- In 2000, poor diet and physical inactivity accounted for 400,000 deaths in the United States (Mokdad, 2004).

- Even moderate excess weight (10—20-pounds) increases the risk of death, particularly among adults age 30–64-years-old.
- Compared to individuals with a health weight, persons with a BMI greater than or equal to 30 have a 50–100% increased risk of premature death from all causes.

The economic cost of obesity in the United States in 2000 approached $117 billion (CDC, 2004).

- According to the Behavioral Risk Factor Surveillance System in 2000, physical activity is important in preventing and treating overweight and obesity.
  - Two-thirds of adults do not engage in the recommended amount of physical activity.
  - More than 26% of adults in the United States do not participate in any leisure time physical activity.
  - 43% of adolescents watch more than two hours of television each day.

ASSESSMENT

What Should be Ruled Out?

Because obesity is a complex and multidetermined problem, a through assessment involves both medical and behavioral components. Medical etiologies may contribute to weight gain. Due to discrimination of the overweight or obese individual (Atkinson, 2002), physicians may ignore complaints that could indicate an underlying medical problem (e.g., hypoglycemia, bone fractures or cold intolerance). A thorough medical assessment should rule-out:

- Endocrine dysfunction
  - thyroid disease (hypothyroidism or hyperthyroidism)
  - insulinoma (excess insulin), nesidioblastosis
  - cushing's syndrome (adrenocorticoid excess)
  - polycystic ovary syndrome
  - hypogonadism
  - hypothalamic damage or disease
  - growth hormone deficiency
  - leptin deficiency or receptor defect
  - pseudohypoparathyroidism
- Endocrine dysfunctions are among the rarest causes of obesity. However, identifying and treating an underlying disorder may resolve or improve the condition considerably.
  - Genetic or dysmorphic syndromes
  - Prader-Willi
  - Bardet-Biedl
  - Ahlstrom
  - Coehn
  - Carpenter
- Some medications, such as steroids and some antidepressants may also cause weight gain. A thorough assessment of current prescribed and over the counter medications should be completed.

A thorough behavioral assessment should consider the role of psychological etiologies or sequelae of weight gain. Overweight or obesity presenting with depression, a history of child physical or sexual abuse or problems in interpersonal relationships should be addressed with adjunct psychotherapy.

What is Involved in Effective Assessment?

Wadden and Phelan (2002) recommend the "**BEST T**reatment" approach to behavioral assessment of overweight and obesity.

- *Biological Factors.* Collecting a thorough history can provide information about degree of overweight, the patient's risk of weight-related health complications, and provide motivation for treatment. Asking about *age of onset* and progression of obesity and *family history* of obesity can set the stage for a discussion of the role of both genetic and environmental contributions to obesity. For example, learning that genetic factors could contribute to a slower metabolic rate and a potential to gain weight can help assuage persons that their weight status is not all their fault. However, noting the behavioral factors that allowed a genetic potential to be realized highlights the individual's responsibility to change key health behaviors and provides hope for future weight loss.

- *Anthropometric measures.* The NIH clinical guidelines for the identification, evaluation and treatment of overweight and obesity in adults (1998) recommended use of *Body Mass Index* (BMI) to classify overweight and obesity. BMI is the most global, widely accepted and practical means of calculating body fat for the majority of people. However, BMI can overestimate body fat in persons who are very muscular and underestimate body fat in individuals who have lost muscle mass, such as the elderly. BMI is a mathematical formula expressing the ratio of weight to height. The formula for BMI is:

$$\text{Weight (kg)}/\text{Height (m)}^2$$
$$\text{or}$$
$$(\text{Weight (lbs)}/\text{Height (in.)}^2) \text{ times } 703.,$$

Or, refer to the National Institutes of Health Body Mass Index table at *http://www.nhlbi.nih.gov/guidelines/obesity/bmi_tbl.htm*

For adults:

Healthy Weight:	18.5–24.9
Overweight:	25.0–29.9
Obesity:	
Class I:	30.0–34.9
Class II:	35.0–39.9
Class III:	> 40.0

Assessment of overweight in children and adolescent requires consideration of child's age, height, weight, and growth patterns. To calculate BMI for children ages 2- to 20-years-old go to the sex appropriate (Boys: BMI-by-age or Girls: BMI-by-age) growth charts at:

http://www.cdc.gov/nchs/about/major/nhanes/ growthcharts/clinical_charts.htm
For children ages 2- to 20-years-old, BMI-by-age and sex:

At-risk for Overweight:	85th < 95th percentile
Overweight:	≥ 95th percentile

A BMI-by-age at the 85th percentile means that compared to children of the same sex and age, 85% have a lower BMI.

- *Environmental influences.* Treatment can be best informed by determining the environmental and behavioral contributions to overweight and obesity. Assessment should include current *daily food intake* for three weekdays and one weekend day. Food diaries should include amount of caloric intake, diet composition (e.g., fruit and vegetable consumption, fat intake), and an assessment of the environmental cues associated with food consumption (e.g., time, people, place, emotion, appetite). MEASURE

The degree to which an individual engages in *physical activity* must also be assessed. Physical activity not only includes programmed or structured exercise (e.g., basketball, aerobics, etc.), but also activities like walking to the store, taking the stairs at work, gardening or cleaning the house. The amount of time spent in sedentary activities, such as watching television, reading, or using the computer, should also be examined.

With an eye toward treatment, diet and activity *strengths* should also be assessed. Treatment can be appropriately tailored by learning whether an individual prefers, for example, walking or riding a bicycle or exercising alone or with a companion. Identifying specific *barriers* to engaging in healthy diet and physical activity behaviors is also an essential component in designing an individualized treatment approach.

- *Social/psychological status.* In assessing the social and psychological context in which the obese individual lives, it is first important to learn more about the weights, eating habits and attitudes of friends, *family* members and significant others. With this information, a family-based treatment may be selected if both the identified client and his or her significant others are also struggling with overweight.

Obesity is also associated with a number of *social and psychological sequelae*, including depression, low self-esteem, impaired social relationships, distorted body image, and overall reductions in perceived quality of life. Investigation of these factors allows us to learn more about the individual's motivation and *expectations* for weight loss. For example, the obese individual may hope for weight loss to save a failing marriage or facilitate a job promotion. Some studies have indicated that at least 20% of obese individuals report significant symptoms of depression (Wadden & Phelan, 2002). In children and adolescents, overweight children report significant difficulties in peer relationships (Ebbeling, Pawlak, Ludwig, 2002). Assessment of sleep patterns, energy levels, and overall life satisfaction can provide valuable information about the individual's current mood. Well-validated clinical instruments, such as the Beck Depression Inventory (BDI; Beck, Steer, & Brown, 1996) can also be integrated into the assessment process.

Assessment of social and historical contributors to obesity can also inform treatment. As previously mentioned, a *history* of physical or sexual abuse may have played an important role in the development of obesity. An individual's current struggle with *substance abuse* or addiction also must be identified to prevent compromising the efficacy of weight loss treatment. In such instances, ensuring access to supportive, adjunctive treatment should be the provider's main goal.

- *Timing of the weight loss effort.* Participation in weight loss treatment requires motivation, concentration, and time. The probability of treatment success increases when 2- to 3-months of *uninterrupted time*, relatively free of *life stressors*, is dedicated to treatment. For example, attending vacation 3-weeks into treatment, or moving into a new home, may sabotage otherwise successful treatment efforts. With this information, providers and patients together can determine if engaging in treatment at a later date could be beneficial. Asking *why now* allows the provider to access information regarding the individual's current motivation for engaging in weight loss treatment. Motivational interviewing can be a skillfully integrated into assessment to evaluate the nature of the patient's motivation to lose weight (i.e., intrinsic or extrinsic) and his or her level of resistance to recommendations for health promotion (Smith, Heckemeyer, Kratt & Mason, 1997; DiLillo, Siegfried, & West, 2003). For example, an individual may report that he is adamantly opposed to exercising at a health club, due to embarrassment, but would enjoy taking the dog on long walks in the afternoon. This information is valuable to the provider in designing an effective, individualized treatment plan.

- *Treatment option.* After a through assessment is completed, both provider and patient together can decide upon specific treatment goals and the most appropriate treatment option. Discussing goals allows providers to educate patients about the gradual nature of weight loss and realistic weight loss goals (e.g., losing 10% of total body weight is usually considered a treatment success; Wadden & Osei, 2002). Although a target weight may be agreed upon, focusing on nonweight-related goals is advised. Goals may emphasize improvements in health, health complications, mood and overall lifestyle changes. For example, an individual's goal may be to have enough energy to play with her children. Adjunctive treatments, such as Cognitive Behavior Therapy (see effective therapist-based treatments below) may be indicated if one's goals are to improve relationships, self-esteem and overall life satisfaction. Once goals are agreed upon, an individualized treatment plan can be developed. To maximize outcomes, before commencing treatment providers should assess the individual's confidence in his or her ability to attain the decided upon goals. This provides an opportunity to inquire which skills the patient needs to embark on treatment feeling confident and efficacious.

At the conclusion of the assessment process, the individual should leave with new knowledge about the nature and cause of overweight or obesity, a clear understanding of the course of the proposed treatment, the behavioral repertoire necessary for obtaining desired outcomes, and with a sense of hope for treatment success.

What Assessments are Not Helpful?

Anthropometric assessments such as waist-to-hip (WHR) circumference ratio, skinfold calipers, ultrasound, Computed Tomography (CT), Magnetic Resonance Imaging (MRI), underwater weighing, dual-energy X-ray absorptiometry may not be warranted. WHR and calipers are limited in their accuracy and no longer recognized as a tool for evaluating morbidity risk (Atkinson, 2002). More technologically advanced assessments are costly and may not have direct treatment implications in many cases.

TREATMENT

What Treatments are Effective?

In general, most treatments programs are moderately successful. For example, both behavioral programs and pharmacotherapy induce average weight reductions of approximately 8–10% of initial body weight during the first 4- to 6-months of treatment (Wing, 2002). Moreover, approximately 80–85% of participants complete behavioral treatments (Wadden & Osei, 2002). However, there is a large relapse rate regardless of the type of treatment. Without ongoing contact, most patients experience either partial or full relapse within 3–5 years after treatment (NHLBI, NIDDK, 1998). Some hold that the maintenance of treatment effects represents the single greatest challenge in the long-term management of obesity (Perri, 1998). However, there is a large relapse rate regardless of the type of treatment. Without ongoing contact, patients typically regain 30–35% of the weight lost by 1-year post-treatment (Wadden, Sarwer, & Berkowitz, 1999) and nearly, if not all of the weight lost within 3- to 5-years after treatment (National Heart, Lung, and Blood Institute, 1998). Some hold that the maintenance of treatment effects represents the single greatest challenge in the long-term management of obesity (Perri, 1998). Because of the magnitude of the problem of relapse, the most effective treatments emphasize continuous care, lifestyle behavior modification and relapse prevention.

What are Effective Self-Help Treatments?

Cost-effective self-help books include:

- *"Weight Watchers Stop Stuffing Yourself : 7 Steps To Conquering Overeating"* by Weight Watchers. Wiley: 1998. ($14.95).
- *"Exercising Your Way to Better Mental Health : Combat Stress, Fight Depression, and Improve Your Overall Mood and Self-Concept With These Simple Exercises"* by Larry M. Leith. Fitness Information Technology, Incorporated: 1998. ($14.95).
- *"The Pocket Food and Exercise Diary"* by Allan Borushek. Allan Borushek & Associates: 1996. ($3.95). with *"The Doctor's Pocket Calorie, Fat, & Carbohydrate Counter 2004"* by Allan Borushek. Family Health Publications: 2003. ($6.99).
- *"Helping Your Overweight Child"* by Caroline J. Cederquist. Advance Medical Press: 2002 ($14.95).
- *"Dieting for Dummies"* by Jane Kirby. For Dummies: 1998. ($21.99).

Useful Websites

http://www.cdc.gov/nccdphp/dnpa/obesity/index.htm
http://www.eatright.org/Public/
http://www.surgeongeneral.gov/publichealthpriorities.html#overweight
http://www.nhlbi.nih.gov/health/public/heart/obesity/lose_wt/
http://www.niddk.nih.gov/health/nutrit/nutrit.htm
http://www.bodyforlife.com/
http://www.gymamerica.com

What are Effective Therapist Based Treatments?

Cognitive Behavioral Treatment of Obesity.
Typical behavioral programs are goal-oriented and involve identifying and modifying antecedents and consequences. Treatment sessions focus on homework assignments and developing interventions to address barriers to adherence. For example, *The LEARN Program for Weight Management 2000, first developed by Kelly Brownell in 1976* (Brownell, 2000; Womble et al., 2004), is a manualized treatment approach focusing on lifestyle, exercise, attitude, relationships and nutrition that has been well-validated in over 25 empirical studies.
Some techniques include:

- *Motivational Interviewing* at treatment onset and as a relapse prevention strategy by identifying personal goals, examining discrepancies between goals and current behavior, and acknowledging ambivalence about behavior change (e.g., DiLillo et al., 2003; Smith et al., 1997).
- *Self-monitoring* of food and fluid intake, including time, place, and comments, total daily calorie consumption, portion sizes, emotions, negative cognitions, exercise behaviors, and weight. Self-monitoring is important for calculating energy intake as well as identifying triggers for overeating and barriers to treatment adherence (e.g, Tate, Wing, & Winett, 2001).
- *Stimulus control* including structured diets and grocery lists, meal replacements, and/or limiting access to energy dense foods and sedentary activities (e.g., television) while increasing access to healthy food options and stimuli likely to elicit physical activity (e.g., exercise equipment; e.g., Faith et al., 2001).

- *Problem solving* including adopting a future-oriented perspective to promote identification to barriers to program adherence such as frequent snacking, motivational issues, binge eating, consumption of restricted or energy dense (e.g., high fat) foods, or eating in response to negative emotional arousal (e.g., Perri et al., 2001; Epstein et al., 2000; Leermakers, Perri, Shigaki, & Fuller, 1999).
- *Cognitive restructuring* focusing on cognitive obstacles to the acceptance of weight maintenance (Cooper, Fairburn, Hawker, 2003), body image concerns, determining realistic and attainable expectations and motivations for weight loss.
- *Social support* to create a supportive environment for weight loss including adherent dietary and lifestyle behaviors in the home and supportive attitudes about weight management for treatment adherence and long-term maintenance of behavior change (e.g., Wing & Jeffery, 1999).
- *Nutrition education* including composition of health diets (based on US Department of Agriculture, 1995 nutritional guidelines) and the nature of energy balance (calorie consumption vs. expenditure). Participants may be limited to between 1,200 and 1,500 kcal daily (Cooper et al., 2003). Programs may also construct individualized diets based on personal food preferences.
- *Increasing physical activity* by setting specific behavioral goals (short or more extended bouts), self-monitoring, and encouraging lifestyle physical activity for long-term weight maintenance strategy, as well as programmed exercise (e.g., Jeffery, Wing, Sherwood & Tate, 2003).
- *Relapse prevention* including addressing cognitive and environmental barriers to weight maintenance, motivational factors, goals, and expectations (e.g., Perri, 1998). Relapse prevention may focus on discouraging additional weight loss, as the weight loss "plateau" may discourage long-term adherence. Some models advocate a minimum of 14 weeks for the acquisition and practice of long-term weight maintenance skills (Cooper et al., 2003).

Others promote the inclusion of stress management techniques to address the tension and stress in overeating and relapse (Poston & Foreyt, 2000). Strategies proven effective for numerous health-related problems, including diaphragmatic breathing, progressive muscle relaxation, and meditation may reduce tension, serve as a distraction and reduce sympathetic nervous system arousal for obese patients.

What is Effective Medical Treatment?

Pharmacotherapy for obesity include appetite suppressants (e.g., noradrenergic drugs), antidepressants, metabolic altering drugs (e.g. Orlistat), drugs that increase energy expenditure (e.g., thyroid hormones, ephedrine, and caffeine). Long-term drug therapy is typically considered for individuals who are considered for surgical treatment of obesity and for those with a BMI above 35 (Bray, 1998). However, low-calorie, very low calorie diets (VLCD), structured meal plans and liquid diets are also treatment options for individuals with a BMI greater than 30 (Wadden & Osei, 2002). As well as a myriad of other side effects, pharmacotherapy can be associated with adverse effects such as depression, neurotoxicity, valvular heart disease, primary pulmonary hypertension, and the potential for abuse or the development of tolerance to a specific agent (Poston & Foreyt, 2000). Interested readers are directed to existing reviews of drug treatment for weight management (National Task Force on the Prevention and Treatment of Obesity, 1996; Bray, 1998).

Bariatric surgery is the last step in stepped care model of obesity treatment and is presented as a viable option for persons with a BMI greater than or equal to 40 and those experiencing serious weight-related health complications (Latifi, Kellum, De Maria, & Sugerman, 2002). These procedures may include vertical banded gastroplasty, gastric bypass, and gastric banding procedures. Gastric bypass procedures, although not without risk, induces average weight loss of 25–30% and is associated with long-term maintenance of results and improvement of comorbid conditions (Wadden & Osei, 2002).

Other Issues in Management

The practitioner should consider the following guidelines when treating overweight and obesity:

- Gradual, lifestyle changes are more likely to persist in the individual's repertoire over the long-term.
- Encourage expression of positive behaviors that already existing in the individual's diet and activity repertoire.
- Self-help, individual, or group cognitive–behavioral treatment addresses the cognitive barriers to effective short- and long-term weight management.
- Obesity is best thought of and treated as a chronic disease requiring ongoing care.
- Use self-monitoring to give feedback, reinforce success, and address barriers to adherence.
- Encourage specific diet and activity goals and gradual increase in exercise duration and intensity.
- Discourage use of over-the-counter weight-loss drugs and "fad diets." Educate patients about lifestyle health promotion.

Discussing and validating difficulties associated with making changes may facilitate treatment motivation and program adherence. Losing even a modest amount of body weight (5–15%) can improve health.

How Does One Select Among Treatments?

The practitioner and patient should together consider the individual's BMI, health risks and complications, the history of weight loss efforts, as well as the safety, efficacy and cost of the selected treatment.

- Studies involving pharmacotherapy with dietary modifications shows modest benefits when compared to behavior modification plus placebo (National Heart, Lung and Blood Institute, 1998).
- Behavioral interventions are less expensive and associated with fewer risks of health complications.
- When exploring pharmacotherapy options, consider that behavioral interventions and behavioral interventions plus pharmacotherapy typically produce greater outcomes than pharmacotherapy alone (Poston & Foreyt, 2000).

KEY READINGS

Atkinson, R. L. (2002). Medical evaluation of the obese patient. In T.A. Wadden & A. J. Stunkard (Eds.), *Handbook of obesity treatment* (2nd ed., pp. 173–185).

Beck, A., Steer, R., & Brown, G. (1996). *Beck Depression Inventory–II (BDI-II) manual.* San Antonio, TX: Harcourt Brace.

Brownell, K. (2000). *The LEARN program for weight management 2000.* Dallas, TX: American Health.

Centers for Disease Control and Prevention (2004). Overweight and obesity: Defining overweight and obesity. Nutrition and physical activity. Available: http://www.cdc.gov/nccdphp/dnpa/obesity/defining.htm

Dietz, W. H. (1998). Health consequences of obesity in youth: childhood predictors of adult disease. *Pediatrics, 101(3)*, 554–570.

DiLillo, V., Siegfried, N., & West, D. (2003). Incorporating motivational interviewing into behavioral obesity treatment. *Cognitive & Behavioral Practice, 10(2)*, 120–130.

Ebbeling, C. B., Pawlak, D., Ludwig, D. (2002). Childhood obesity: Public-health crisis, common sense cure. *Lancet, 10(360)*, 473–483.

Faith, M., Berman, N., Moonsoeong, H., Pietrobelli, A. Gallagher, D., Epstein, L., et al. (2001). Effects of contingent television on physical activity and television viewing in obse children. *Pediatrics, 107(5)*, 1043–1048.

Jeffery, R. W., Wing, R. R., Sherwood, N. E., & Tate, D. F. (2003). Physical activity and weight loss: does prescribing higher physical activity goals improve outcome? *American Journal of Clinical Nutrition, 78(4)*, 684–489.

Horgan, K., & Brownell, K. (1998). Policy change as a means for reducing the prevalence and impact of alcoholism, smoking, and obesity. In W.R. Miller & N. Heather (Eds.), *Treating addictive behaviors* (2nd ed., pp. 105–118).

Latifi, R., Kellum, J., De Maria, E., & Sugerman, H. (2002). Surgical treatment of obesity. In T.A.Wadden & A.J Stunkard (Eds.), *Handbook of obesity treatment* (2nd ed., pp. 339–356).

Leermakers, E., Perri, M., Shigaki, C., & Fuller, P. (1999). Effects of exercise-focused versus weight-focused maintenance programs on the management of obesity. *Addictive Behaviors, 24(2)*, 219–227.

Mokdad, A., Serdula, M., Dietz, W., et al. (1999). The spread of the obesity epidemic in the United States, 1991–1998. *Journal of the American Medical Association, 282*, 1519–1522.

Mokdad, A., Serdula, M., Dietz, W., et al. (2000). The continuing obesity epidemic in the United States. *Journal of the American Medical Association, 284*, 1650–1651.

Mokdad, A., Bowman, B., Ford, E., et al. (2001). The continuing epidemics of obesity and diabetes in the United States. *Journal of the American Medical Association, 286(10)*, 1195–1200.

Mokdad, A., Ford, E., Bowman, B., Dietz, W., Vinicor, F., Bales, V., & Marks, J. (2003). Prevalence of obesity, diabetes, and obesity-related health risk factors, 2001. *Journal of the American Medical Association, 289*, 76–79.

Mokdad, A., Marks, J., Stroup, D., & Gerberding, J. (2004). Actual causes of death in the United States, 2000. *Journal of the American Medical Association, 291*, 1238–1245.

National Institutes of Health (1998). *Clinical guidelines on the identification, evaluation, and treatment of overweight and obesity in adults.* Bethesda, MD: Department of Health and Human Services, National Institutes of Health, National Heart, Lung, and Blood Institute, 1998.

Perri, M. G. (1998). The maintenance of treatment effects in the long-term management of obesity. *Clinical Psychology: Science and Practice, 5*, 526–543.

Perri, M. G., Nezu, A. M., McKelvey, W. F., Shermer, R., Renjilian, D., & Viegener, B. (2001). Relapse prevention training and problem-solving therapy in the long-term management of obesity. *Journal of Consulting and Clinical Psychology, 69(4)*, 722–726.

Poston, W., & Foreyt, J. (2000). Successful management of the obese patient. *American Family Physician, 61*, 3615–3622.

Surgeon General's Call to Action to Prevent and Decrease Overweight and Obesity. Available: www.surgeongeneral.gov/topics/obesity/

Tate, D., Wing, R., & Winett, R. (2001). Using Internet technology to deliver a behavioral weight loss program. *Journal of the American Medical Association, 285(9)*, 1172–1177.

Wadden, T., & Osei, S. (2002). The treatment of obesity: an overview. In T.A.Wadden & A.J Stunkard (Eds.), *Handbook of obesity treatment* (2nd ed., pp.229–248).

Wadden, T., & Phelan, S. (2002). Behavioral assessment of the obese patient. In T. A.Wadden & A. J Stunkard (Eds.), *Handbook of obesity treatment* (2nd ed., pp. 186–226).

Wadden, T., Sarwer, D., & Berkowitz, R. (1999). Behavioral treatment of the overweight patient *Balliere's Clinical Endocrinology and Metabolism, 13*, 93–107.

Wing, R. (2002). Behavioral Weight Control. In T. A. Wadden & A. J. Stunkard (Eds.), *Handbook of obesity treatment* (2nd ed., pp. 301–316).

Wing, R. R. & Jeffery, R. W. (1999). Benefits of recruiting participants with friends and increasing social support for weight loss and maintenance. *Journal of Consulting and Clinical Psychology, 67(1)*, 132–138.

Womble, L., Wadden, T., McGuckin, B., Sargent, S., Rothman, R., & Krauthamer-Ewing, E. (2004). A randomized controlled trial of a commercial weight loss program. *Obesity Research, 12*, 1011–1018.

World Health Organization (2003). Controlling the global obesity epidemic. *Nutrition.* Available: http://www.who.int/nut/obs.htm

INDEX

Page numbers followed by f and t indicates figures and tables, respectively.